ABOUT THE EDITORS

Mark S. Blumberg

Mark S. Blumberg is the F. Wendell Miller Professor of Psychology at the University of Iowa. He is the author of three books and more than eighty journal articles and book chapters on a wide variety of subjects. He currently serves as Editor-in-Chief of the journal *Behavioral Neuroscience*.

John H. Freeman

John H. Freeman is Professor of Psychology at the University of Iowa. He is the author of more than sixty journal articles and currently serves as Associate Editor of the journal *Behavioral Neuroscience*.

Scott R. Robinson

Scott R. Robinson is Associate Professor of Psychology and head of the Laboratory for Comparative Ethogenesis at the University of Iowa. He has authored more than 100 journal articles and chapters on various subjects in ethology and developmental psychobiology. He has also edited one book on fetal behavioral development.

CONTRIBUTORS

Elizabeth Adkins-Regan
Department of Psychology
Department of Neurobiology and Behavior
Cornell University
Ithaca, NY

Jeffrey R. Alberts
Department of Psychological and
  Brain Sciences
Indiana University
Bloomington, IN

Maria C. Alvarado
Yerkes National Primate Research Center
Emory University
Atlanta, GA

Evan L. Ardiel
Brain Research Centre
Department of Psychology
University of British Columbia
Vancouver, Canada

Anthony P. Auger
Neuroscience Training Program
Department of Psychology
University of Wisconsin
Madison, WI

Jocelyne Bachevalier
Yerkes National Primate Research Center
Emory University
Atlanta, GA

Patrick Bateson
Sub-Department of Animal Behaviour
University of Cambridge
Cambridge, UK

Peter Blaesse
Department of Biological and
  Environmental Sciences
University of Helsinki
Helsinki, Finland

Mark S. Blumberg
Department of Psychology and Delta
  Center
University of Iowa
Iowa City, IA

Michele R. Brumley
Department of Psychology
Idaho State University
Pocatello, ID

Gyorgy Buzsáki
Center for Molecular & Behavioral
  Neuroscience
Rutgers University
Newark, NJ

Michèle Carlier
Cognitive Psychology
Aix-Marseille Université
Marseille, France

Frances A. Champagne
Department of Psychology
Columbia University
New York, NY

Dragana Ivkovich Claflin
Department of Psychology
Wright State University
Dayton, OH

François Clarac
Laboratoire Plasticité et Physio-Pathologie
  de la Motricité
Centre National de la Recherche
  Scientifique
Aix-Marseille Université
Marseille, France

Michael Colombo
Department of Psychology
University of Otago
Dunedin, New Zealand

James P. Curley
Sub-Department of Animal Behavior
University of Cambridge
Cambridge, UK

Terrence W. Deacon
Department of Anthropology
University of California, Berkeley
Berkeley, CA

Tony del Rio
Division of Biological Sciences
University of California, San Diego
La Jolla, CA

Theodore C. Dumas
Department of Molecular Neuroscience
Krasnow Institute for Advanced Study
George Mason University
Fairfax, VA

Reha S. Erzurumlu
Department of Anatomy and Neurobiology
University of Maryland School
  of Medicine
Baltimore, MD

Marla B. Feller
Division of Biological Sciences
University of California, San Diego
La Jolla, CA

John H. Freeman
Department of Psychology, Delta Center,
  and Interdisciplinary Neuroscience
  Program
University of Iowa
Iowa City, IA

Robbin Gibb
Canadian Centre for Behavioural
  Neuroscience
University of Lethbridge
Lethbridge, Canada

Michael H. Goldstein
Department of Psychology
Cornell University
Ithaca, NY

Julie Gros-Louis
Department of Psychology
  and Delta Center
University of Iowa
Iowa City, IA

Celeste Halliwell
Canadian Centre for Behavioural
  Neuroscience
University of Lethbridge
Lethbridge, Canada

Harlene Hayne
Department of Psychology
University of Otago
Dunedin, New Zealand

Jane Herbert
Department of Psychology
University of Sheffield
Sheffield, UK

Hunter Honeycutt
Department of Psychology
Bridgewater College
Bridgewater, VA

Deborah L. Hunt
Center for Neuroscience
Department of Psychology
University of California, Davis
Davis, CA

Pamela S. Hunt
Department of Psychology
College of William & Mary
Williamsburg, VA

Marc Jamon
Génomique Médicale et Génomique
  Fonctionnelle
Aix-Marseille Université
Marseille, France

Timothy D. Johnston
College of Arts and Sciences
University of North Carolina at
  Greensboro
Greensboro, NC

Kai Kaila
Department of Biological and
  Environmental Sciences
Neuroscience Center
University of Helsinki
Helsinki, Finland

Sarah J. Karlen
Center for Neuroscience
University of California, Davis
Davis, CA

Rustem Khazipov
INMED, INSERM U29
Marseille, France

Andrew P. King
Department of Psychological
and Brain Sciences
Indiana University
Bloomington, IN

Thomas J. Koehnle
Department of Neuroscience
University of Pittsburgh
Pittsburgh, PA

Bryan Kolb
Canadian Centre for Behavioural
Neuroscience
University of Lethbridge
Lethbridge, Canada

Leah Krubitzer
Center for Neuroscience
Department of Psychology
University of California, Davis
Davis, CA

Robert Lickliter
Department of Psychology
Florida International University
Miami, FL

Joseph S. Lonstein
Neuroscience Program
Department of Psychology
Michigan State University
East Lansing, MI

Jill M. Mateo
Department of Comparative Human
Development
Committee on Evolutionary
Biology, and the Institute for
Mind and Biology
University of Chicago
Chicago, IL

Carol Milligan
Department of Neurobiology and Anatomy
The Neuroscience Program
Wake Forest University School
of Medicine
Winston-Salem, NC

Stephanie Moriceau
Emotional Brain Institute
Nathan S. Kline Institute for Psychiatric
Research
New York University Langone Medical
Center
New York, NY

Ronald W. Oppenheim
Department of Neurobiology and Anatomy
The Neuroscience Program
Wake Forest University School of Medicine
Winston-Salem, NC

Edouard Pearlstein
Laboratoire Plasticité et
Physio-Pathologie de la Motricité
Centre National de la Recherche
Scientifique
Aix-Marseille Université
Marseille, France

Susan Rai
Brain Research Centre
Department of Psychology
University of British Columbia
Vancouver, Canada

Catharine H. Rankin
Brain Research Centre
Department of Psychology
University of British Columbia
Vancouver, Canada

Rick Richardson
School of Psychology
University of New South Wales
Sydney, Australia

Linda Rinaman
Department of Neuroscience
University of Pittsburgh
Pittsburgh, PA

Scott R. Robinson
Laboratory of Comparative
Ethogenesis
Department of Psychology
and Delta Center
University of Iowa
Iowa City, IA

Tania Roth
Emotional Brain Institute
Nathan S. Kline Institute for Psychiatric
 Research
New York University Langone Medical
 Center
New York, NY

Pierre L. Roubertoux
Génomique Médicale et Génomique
 Fonctionnelle
Aix Marseille University
Marseille, France

Jerry W. Rudy
Department of Psychology
University of Colorado
Boulder, CO

Jeffrey C. Schank
Department of Psychology
University of California, Davis
Davis, CA

Jens Schouenborg
Group of Neurophysiology
Neuronanoscience Research
 Center
Department of Experimental
 Medical Research
Lund University
Lund, Sweden

Jennifer A. Schwade
Department of Psychology
Cornell University
Ithaca, NY

Adele M. H. Seelke
Center for Neuroscience
University of California, Davis
Davis, CA

Kiseko Shionoya
Department of Zoology
University of Oklahoma
Norman, OK

Keith Sillar
School of Biology
University of St. Andrews
Fife, UK

Sampsa T. Sipilä
Department of Biological and
 Environmental Sciences
University of Helsinki
Helsinki, Finland

Mark E. Stanton
Department of Psychology
University of Delaware
Newark, DE

Regina M. Sullivan
Emotional Brain Institute
Nathan S. Kline Institute for Psychiatric
 Research
New York University Langone Medical
 Center
New York, NY

Woong Sun
Department of Anatomy
Korea University College of Medicine
Seoul, South Korea

Susan E. Swithers
Department of Psychological Sciences
Ingestive Behavior Research Center
Purdue University
West Lafayette, IN

Daniel J. Tollin
Department of Physiology
 and Biophysics
University of Colorado at Denver
Denver, CO

Laurent Vinay
Laboratoire Plasticité et Physio-Pathologie
 de la Motricité
Centre National de la Recherche
 Scientifique
Aix-Marseille Université
Marseille, France

Meredith J. West
Department of Psychological and Brain
 Sciences
Indiana University
Bloomington, IN

Alyson Zeamer
Department of Psychology
Emory University
Atlanta, GA

Introduction: A New Frontier for Developmental Behavioral Neuroscience

Mark S. Blumberg, John H. Freeman, *and* Scott R. Robinson

As editors of this volume, we wrestled with alternative titles to capture what we felt was a theoretically connected but highly interdisciplinary field of science. Previous edited volumes that have addressed related content areas were published over a 15-year span beginning in the mid-1980s under the label of "developmental psychobiology" (e.g., Blass, 1986, 1988, 2001; Krasnegor, Blass, Hofer, & Smotherman, 1987; Shair, Hofer, & Barr, 1991). Although all three of the editors of the present volume have longstanding ties to the field of developmental psychobiology (DP) and its parent society (the International Society for Developmental Psychobiology), we also view our work as part of a larger community of researchers in behavioral neuroscience, comparative psychology, developmental science, and evolutionary biology. This volume is aimed at this larger research community concerned with empirical and theoretical issues about behavioral and neural development.

DP has traditionally concerned itself with investigations of the biological bases of behavior and how they change during development. The rich tradition of DP is seen in the many advances it has provided to our understanding of behavior and behavioral development. Moreover, DP has been distinguished by its adherence to an epigenetic perspective, that is, a perspective that embraces all contributions to individual development, from the molecular to the social. DP remains a productive and innovative discipline, but it now faces new challenges posed by rapid advances and the advent of powerful technologies in molecular biology, neuroscience, and evolutionary biology. These challenges, however, are also opportunities. Thus, our goal for this volume is twofold: (1) to communicate the central research perspectives of DP to a wider community interested in behavioral and neural development and (2) to highlight current opportunities to advance our understanding of behavioral and neural development through enhanced interactions between DP and its sister disciplines.

In 1975, in his influential book *Sociobiology: The New Synthesis,* E. O. Wilson famously looked forward to the year 2000 when, he predicted, the various subdisciplines of behavioral biology could be represented by a figure in the shape of a barbell—the narrow shaft representing the dwindling domain of the whole organism (i.e., ethology and comparative psychology) and the two bulging orbs at each end comprising the burgeoning fields of sociobiology and neurophysiology. Wilson's prediction that the study of the whole organism would be "cannibalized" by population and reductionistic approaches seemed, to many behavioral researchers over the last quarter century, to be relentlessly fulfilled. But ultimately, the "death of the organism" has proven greatly exaggerated. On the contrary, we are witnessing a resurgence of interest in a diversity of mechanisms—especially developmental mechanisms—that contribute to the form and function of the organism. Most importantly (for this volume), the behavior of whole organisms has emerged as a central product and causal influence of developmental change.

Wilson's view of the future from his 1975 perch reflected two biological themes–cell theory and evolutionary theory–that were central to the rise of modern biology in the nineteenth century and which were greatly refined and expanded in their influence in the twentieth century. By the mid-twentieth century, these two perspectives culminated in the rise of the Modern Synthesis, the discovery of DNA, and the success of the molecular revolution. The new emphasis on parts and populations anchored Wilson's barbell and relegated the organism to a transient vessel, a mere conveyance for selfish genes (Dawkins, 1977). On the one hand, the Modern Synthesis succeeded in reconciling Darwinian evolution with population genetics (Provine, 1971); on the other, the successes of molecular biology convinced many that whole organisms could be reduced to individual traits and crucial biochemicals produced through the actions of single genes (Keller, 2000; Moore, 2001). Although many prominent scientists tried very hard to offer plausible alternatives and amendments to these two dominant perspectives (Alberch, 1982; Gottlieb, 1992; Gould & Lewontin, 1979; Lehrman, 1953; Stent, 1977), they were unable to stem the tide.

Proximate causes are the immediate conditions that give rise to behavior. Such causes include activity in particular neural circuits, the actions of neurotransmitters at specific receptors, the modulating influence of hormone molecules, and the transduction of sensory stimuli into neural responses. In contrast, *ultimate* causes refer to the function or purpose of behavior, which in evolutionary terms is the result of natural selection acting on populations. Although the distinction between proximate and ultimate causation is evident in the early writings of both biologists (Baker, 1938; Huxley, 1916; Lack, 1954) and comparative psychologists (Craig, 1918; Dewsbury, 1999), this dichotomy of causes was promoted most effectively by Ernst Mayr (Beatty, 1994; Mayr, 1961), a central figure in the rise of the Modern Synthesis. Interestingly, Mayr used proximate and ultimate causation as independent explanations to defend evolutionary interpretations from criticisms coming from mechanistic physiologists and molecular biologists (Amundson, 2005; Dewsbury, 1999; Mayr, 1974). In effect, Mayr appealed to the explanatory categories of proximate and ultimate causation to delineate the fields of molecular–cellular and population biology, thereby creating the very barbell that Wilson conveniently "predicted" in 1975.

Of course, what was missing from both the Modern Synthesis and the reductionism of molecular biology was an adequate appreciation for the role of development as a mediating cause of organic change. As long as genes were viewed as root causes of individual characteristics (necessary for a modern synthetic interpretation of evolution), and gene frequencies in populations were viewed as sufficient metrics of evolution, it was possible to skip over the messy details of how a fertilized egg is transformed into an organism that can, in turn, be a target of natural selection. Tinbergen (1963) and Hailman

(1967) at least called attention to the value of developmental analyses of behavior and expanded the traditional dichotomy of causes into four "causes and origins" of behavior: (1) causation or control (immediate physiological mechanisms), (2) development (history of change in the individual), (3) adaptive significance (mechanisms acting on past populations, such as natural selection), and (4) evolution (history of change in the population). But whether viewed as two, four, or even more classes of cause, such classification schemes have reified the notion that biological causes can be treated as distinct and independent entities.

Tinbergen's four-question scheme has been widely adopted in textbooks and behavioral training programs and has contributed a great deal to the clearer formulation of research questions in ethology and comparative psychology (Dewsbury, 1994; Hailman, 1982; Hogan, 1994; Sherman, 1988). But it also has obscured deep underlying connections between these areas of inquiry. For instance, we are coming to appreciate that—in contrast to the comparative anatomy of behavior espoused by Lorenz (1937, 1981)—behavior is not an entity such as a bone or internal organ that has a continuous existence. Rather, each behavioral performance is unique and ephemeral, although it may be recognizably similar to other performances by the same individual in the past or other individuals of the same species. Behavior is elaborated in time despite the common research practice of treating individual behavioral acts as instantaneous for purposes of analysis. From these perspectives, the causation of behavior, which encompasses the "proximate" physiological mechanisms that generate behavior, also should be seen as a question of historical origins, albeit on a much briefer time scale and therefore within the same continuum of phenomena as development.

Theorists since Darwin also have recognized parallels in patterns of change on developmental and evolutionary time scales. Early attempts to explain the phylogenetic information evident in embryological development were founded on notions such as Haeckel's biogenetic law, which stated that embryos pass through the same sequence of stages during development as the adult forms of ancestral species during evolution (Haeckel, 1866). Although strong forms of recapitulation have long since been discredited (Gould, 1977), developmental issues have risen in prominence again over the last several decades within both the evolutionary (Kirschner & Gerhart, 2005; West-Eberhard, 2003) and molecular (Carroll,

INTRODUCTION: A NEW FRONTIER FOR DEVELOPMENTAL BEHAVIORAL NEUROSCIENCE

2005) domains. Moreover, the success of unsupervised processes such as natural selection in explaining evolutionary change has led to similar shifts of emphasis on emergent process and multicausal interactions in changes occurring within the lifetime of an individual. For example, the twin processes of variation and selection have been proposed as general principles leading to greater organization without preexisting instructions in various domains of development, including antibody production in the immune system (Burnet, 1957; Jerne, 1955), operant learning (Hull, Langman, & Glenn, 2001; Skinner, 1981), motor development (Sporns & Edelman, 1993), neural development (Changeaux, 1985; Sporns, 1994), and moment-to-moment functioning of the nervous system (Edelman, 1987).

Despite a plethora of metaphors about developmental programs encoded in genetic blueprints, and the repeated appeals of nativists to genetically determined modules governing specific aspects of behavior and cognition, the study of behavioral development has never been more vibrant. A clear example is the "new" concept of epigenetics and its role in development. In modern genetics, epigenetics refers to changes in developmental outcomes, including regulation of gene expression, that are based on mechanisms other than DNA itself. At a molecular level, gene expression can be affected by experience and sensory-dependent activation of immediate early genes (e.g., c-fos), alternative and contingent editing and translation of mRNA transcripts, methylation and chromatin remodeling in the regulation of gene expression, and chaperoned folding and other posttranslational modifications of newly synthesized proteins. Thus, the discovery that gene function is modulated by epigenetic factors has recapitulated, at a molecular level, what developmental psychobiologists working at a behavioral level have known for decades: that development is multicausal, multilevel, embodied, contextual, conditional, and most importantly, not preformed in a genetic blueprint or program (Kuo, 1967; Lehrman, 1953).

Moreover, a renewed appreciation for the formative role of experience—not just in the sense of explicit learning but in the broader sense that Lehrman (1953) emphasized—in the self-organization of complex nervous systems is dramatically altering the developmental and neurophysiological landscape. What is emerging is a science of developmental systems and epigenesis that places all of the factors that guide development and evolution—from genes to social systems—in proper balance (Blumberg,

2005, 2009; Gottlieb, 1997; Oyama, Griffiths, & Gray, 2001; West, King, & Arberg, 1988). Although Wilson's barbell may have seemed inevitable 30 years ago, it now appears that researchers working at both molecular and population levels of analysis are returning to the whole organism in general and development in particular. Perhaps we are beginning to see glimpses of a new kind of synthesis—elaborated from conceptual foundations in developmental psychobiology and developmental systems theory—which will unify time scales from the neurophysiological to the developmental to the evolutionary.

The foregoing are just a few of the recent trends in developmental behavioral neuroscience that originally spurred us to assemble the present volume. In seeking contributions for this volume, we have attempted to bring together a diverse group of individuals who have been investigating the development of behavior from a variety of perspectives using a variety of techniques. Our criteria for inclusion were nonstandard: we invited contributions from individuals based less on their academic affiliations and more on their topics of research and conceptual perspectives. We believe that this approach to assembling these contributions will help to reveal common themes that have otherwise been hidden within the subdisciplines that most of us inhabit. As a consequence, we hope that this volume will encourage future cross-disciplinary work and spur new insights and, perhaps, even new collaborations.

References

Alberch, P. (1982). The generative and regulatory roles of development in evolution. In D. Mossakowski & G. Roth (Eds.), *Environmental adaptation and evolution* (pp. 19–36). Stuttgart, Germany: Gustav Fischer.

Amundson, R. (2005). *The changing role of the embryo in evolutionary thought.* New York: Cambridge University Press.

Baker, J. R. (1938). The evolution of breeding seasons. In: G. R. de Beer (Ed.), *Essays on aspects of functional biology* (pp. 161–177). Oxford: Clarendon Press.

Beatty, J. (1994). The proximate/ultimate distinction in the multiple careers of Ernst Mayr. *Biological Philosophy, 9,* 333–356.

Blass, E. M. (1986). *Handbook of behavioral neurobiology: Developmental psychobiology and developmental neurobiology* (Vol. 8). New York: Plenum Press.

Blass, E. M. (1988). *Handbook of behavioral neurobiology: Developmental psychobiology and behavioral ecology* (Vol. 9). New York: Plenum Press.

Blass, E. M. (2001). *Handbook of behavioral neurobiology: Developmental psychobiology* (Vol. 13). New York: Plenum Press.

Blumberg, M. S. (2005). *Basic instinct: The genesis of behavior.* New York: Thunder's Mouth Press.

Blumberg, M. S. (2009). *Freaks of nature: What anomalies tell us about development and evolution.* New York: Oxford University Press.

Burnet, F. M. (1957), A modification of Jerne's theory of antibody production using the concept of clonal selection, *The Australian Journal of Science, 20*, 67–69.

Carroll, S. B. (2005). *Endless forms most beautiful: The new science of Evo Devo.* New York: W. W. Norton.

Changeaux, J. -P. (1985). *Neuronal man.* Princeton, NJ: Princeton University Press.

Craig, W. (1918). Appetites and aversions as constituents of instincts. *Biological Bulletin, 34*, 91–107.

Dawkins, R. (1977). *The selfish gene.* New York: Oxford University Press.

Dewsbury, D. A. (1994). On the utility of the proximate–ultimate distinction in the study of animal behavior. *Ethology, 96*, 63–68.

Dewsbury, D. A. (1999). The proximate and the ultimate: past, present, and future. *Behavioural Processes, 46*, 189–199.

Edelman, G. (1987). *Neural Darwinism: The theory of neuronal group selection.* New York: Basic Books.

Gottlieb, G. (1992). *Individual development and evolution.* New York: Oxford University Press.

Gottlieb, G. (1997). *Synthesizing nature–nurture: Prenatal roots of instinctive behavior.* Mahway: Lawrence Erlbaum Associates.

Gould, S. J. (1977). *Ontogeny and phylogeny.* Cambridge: The Belknap Press of Harvard University Press.

Gould, S. J., & Lewontin, R. C. (1979). The spandrels of San Marco and the Panglossian paradigm: A critique of the adaptationist programme. *Proceedings of the Royal Society of London, B205*, 581–598.

Haeckel, E. (1866). *Generelle Morphologie der Organismen: Allgemeine Grundzüge der organischen Formen-Wissenschaft, mechanisch begründet durch die von Charles Darwin reformirte Descendenz-Theorie* (2 vols.), Berlin: Georg Reimer.

Hailman, J. P. (1967). Ontogeny of an instinct. *Behaviour Supplement, 15*, 1–159.

Hailman, J. P. (1982). Ontogeny: toward a general theoretical framework for ethology. In: Bateson, P. P. G., & Klopfer, P. H. (Eds.), *Perspectives in ethology* (Vol. 5, pp. 133–189). New York: Plenum Press.

Hogan, J. A. (1994). The concept of cause in the study of behavior. In: Hogan, J. A., & Bolhuis, J. J. (Eds.), *Causal mechanisms of behavioural development* (pp. 3–15). Cambridge: Cambridge University Press.

Hull, D. L., Langman, R. E., & Glenn, S. S. (2001). A general account of selection: Biology, immunology, and behavior. *Behavioral and Brain Sciences, 24*, 511–573.

Huxley, J. (1916). Bird-watching and biological science. *Auk, 33*, 142–161, 256–270.

Jerne. N. K. (1955). The natural-selection theory of antibody formation, *Proceedings of the National Academy of Sciences, 41*, 849–857.

Keller, E. F. (2000). *The century of the gene.* Cambridge, MA: Harvard University Press.

Kirschner, M. W., & Gerhart, J. C. (2005). *The plausibility of life: Resolving Darwin's dilemma.* New Haven, CT: Yale University Press.

Krasnegor, N. A., Blass, E. M., Hofer, M. A., & Smotherman, W. P. (Eds.) (1987). *Perinatal development: A psychobiological perspective.* Orlando, FL: Academic Press.

Kuo, Z.-Y. (1967). *The dynamics of behavior development: An epigenetic view.* New York: Random House.

Lack, D. (1954). *The natural regulation of population numbers.* Oxford: Clarendon Press.

Lehrman, D. S. (1953). A critique of Konrad Lorenz's theory of instinctive behavior. *The Quarterly Review of Biology, 4*, 337–363.

Lorenz, K. (1937). The companion in the bird's world. *Auk, 54*, 245–273.

Lorenz, K. (1981). *The foundations of ethology.* New York: Springer-Verlag.

Mayr, E. (1961). Cause and effect in biology. *Science, 134*, 1501–1506.

Mayr, E. (1974). Teleological and teleonomic, a new analysis. *Boston Studies in the Philosophy of Science, 14*, 91–117.

Moore, D. S. (2001). *The dependent gene: The fallacy of "nature vs. nurture".* New York: W. H. Freeman & Company.

Oyama, S., Griffiths, P. E., & Gray, R. D. (Eds.). (2001). *Cycles of contingency: Developmental systems and evolution.* Cambridge, MA: MIT Press.

Provine, W. B. (1971). *The origins of theoretical population genetics.* Chicago: University of Chicago Press.

Shair, H. N., Hofer, M. A., & Barr, G. (Eds.) (1991). *Developmental psychobiology: New methods and changing concepts.* New York: Oxford University Press.

Sherman, P. W. (1988). The levels of analysis. *Animal Behaviour, 36*, 616–619.

Skinner, B. F. (1981). Selection by consequences. *Science, 213*, 501–504.

Sporns, O. (1994). *Selectionism and the brain.* New York: Elsevier.

Sporns, O., & Edelman, G. M. (1993). Solving Bernstein's problem: a proposal for the development of coordinated movement by selection. *Child Development, 64*, 960–981.

Stent, G. S. (1977). Explicit and implicit semantic content of the genetic information. In Butts, R.E., & Hintikka, J. (Eds.), *Foundational problems in the special sciences* (pp. 131–149). Dordrecht: D. Reidel Publishing Company.

Tinbergen, N. (1963). On aims and methods of ethology. *Zeitschrift fur Tierpsychologie, 20*, 410–433.

West, M. J., King, A. P., & Arberg, A. A. (1988). The inheritance of niches: The role of ecological legacies in ontogeny. In E. M. Blass (Ed.), *Handbook of Behavioral Neurobiology* (Vol. 9, pp. 41–62). New York: Plenum Press.

West-Eberhard, M. J. (2003). *Developmental plasticity and evolution.* Oxford: Oxford University Press.

Wilson, E. O. (1975). *Sociobiology: The new synthesis.* Cambridge: Harvard University Press.

PART 1

Comparative and Epigenetic Perspectives

to a mathematician to help formalize the problem of how a neural system operates. I appreciate that this is not a message that everyone will want to hear. For some, their research is driven by clear and explicit theories. Other people suppose that when enough information has been collected, the explanations for behavior will stare them in the face. Some push a theory for all it is worth until it overwhelms the opposition or collapses from weakness. Others, revelling in curiosity, simply enjoy the diversity of individuals and species. The opposition between these contrasting styles is easily overstated for they complement each other and, when those who work in different ways find a way of coming together, my optimistic hope is that they will find such a union highly productive in answering all of Tinbergen's four questions.

References

Bateson, P. (1991). Are there principles of behavioural development? In P. Bateson (Ed.), *The development and integration of behaviour* (pp. 19–39). Cambridge: Cambridge University Press.

Bateson, P. (2006). The nest's tale: a reply to Richard Dawkins. *Biology and Philosophy, 21*, 553–558.

Dawkins, R. (1976). *The selfish gene.* Oxford: Oxford University Press.

Dawkins, R. (1982). *The extended phenotype.* Oxford: Freeman.

Jablonka, E., & Lamb, M. J. (2005). *Evolution in four dimensions.* Cambridge, MA: MIT Press.

Krebs, H. A. (1975). The August Krogh principle: 'For many problems there is an animal on which it can be most conveniently studied.' *Journal of Experimental Zoology, 194*, 221–226.

Lorenz, K. (1941). Vergleichende Bewegungstudien an Anatinen. *Journal of Ornithology Supplement, 89*, 194–294.

Noble, D. (2006). *The music of life: Biology beyond the genome.* Oxford: Oxford University Press.

Pagel, M. (1999). Inferring the historical patterns of biological evolution. *Nature, 40*, 877–884.

Reader, S. A., & Laland, K. N. (2002). Social intelligence, innovation and enhanced brain size in primates. *Proceedings of the National Academy of Sciences USA, 99*, 4436–4441.

Real, L. A. (1994). *Behavioural mechanisms in evolutionary ecology.* Chicago: University of Chicago Press.

Schwarts, J., Brumbaugh, R. C., & Chiu, M. (1987). Short stature, growth hormone, insulin-like growth factors and serum protein in Mountain Ok people of Papua New Guinea. *Journal of Clinical Endocrinology and Metabolism, 65*, 901–905.

Tinbergen, N. (1963). On aims and methods of ethology. *Zeitschrift für Tierpsychologie, 20*, 410–433.

Developmental Systems Theory

Timothy D. Johnston

Abstract

Developmental systems theory (DST) provides a framework for understanding behavioral development that transcends the misleading dichotomies that have characterized the field. Drawing on Kuo's criticisms of the concept of instinct in the 1920s, T. C. Schneirla and Daniel S. Lehrman laid the conceptual groundwork for contemporary DST during the middle of the twentieth century, work that was later built on by Gilbert Gottlieb, who developed his theory of probabilistic epigenesis. DST incorporates a concept of experience that goes beyond the traditional equation of experience with learning, which has helped to sustain dichotomies such as that between learning and instinct, and replaces unhelpful genetic metaphors with a molecular understanding of gene action during the course of development.

Keywords: DST, Kuo, T. C. Schneirla, Daniel S. Lehrman, Gilbert Gottlieb, probabilistic epigenesis

Developmental systems theory (DST) is a theoretical framework that provides an alternative to the very pervasive tendency to think about behavior in dichotomous terms, to attribute patterns or aspects of behavior either to genetic influences (nature) or to experience (nurture) separately. Proponents of DST have argued that the attempt to partition behavior in this way is based on a fundamental misconception about the way in which living systems develop and articulated an alternative theoretical approach with a number of distinctive themes. The following list of themes is a modification of the list presented by Oyama, Griffiths, and Gray (2001a):

1. *Behavior is jointly determined by multiple causes:* Behavior cannot be attributed separately to individual developmental causes (such as genes or experience). Every pattern of behavior has multiple determinants (also called developmental resources; Griffiths & Gray, 1994) and the task of developmental analysis is to specify the ways in which the determinants act together in particular cases.

2. *Genetic influences are not privileged in development:* Although this theme can logically be subsumed under the first theme, it is worth identifying separately because a great deal of work in DST has been devoted to finding alternatives to the view that genes can be said to determine, control, or specify certain patterns or features of behavior. For a variety of reasons (discussed later in this chapter), the idea of genetic specification has been especially hard to eliminate from the analysis of behavior.

3. *Development is context sensitive:* The way in which one developmental factor (such as a particular

experience or the activation of a particular gene) affects development depends on the current state of the developing system and on the presence of other developmental factors.

4. *Organisms inherit resources for development, not traits or specifications of traits:* Inheritance involves not just a set of genes but a variety of other developmental resources that are reliably transmitted between generations. In particular, organisms inherit typical environments within which development takes place. These resources support the construction of the behavioral phenotype, which is neither inherited itself nor specified by inherited programs or instructions. This concept has also been referred to as "extended inheritance" (Jablonka, 2001; Sterelny, 2001; Sterelny, Smith, & Dickison, 1996).

5. *The developing system extends beyond the skin of the organism:* All behaviors involve interactions between the organism and its environment, including (in many cases) a social environment made up of conspecifics. These interactions are themselves part of the developing system and also serve as resources supporting developmental change.

6. *Evolution involves change over time in entire developmental systems, not just in the genetic makeup of populations:* Because DST rejects the idea that genes alone specify any aspects of behavior, it also has been critical of the idea that behavioral evolution can be explained in genetic terms alone. While DST does not deny that change in the genetics of populations is one important source of behavioral evolution, it also postulates additional, nongenetic sources of evolutionary change (Gottlieb, 1987; Johnston & Gottlieb, 1990; see Lickliter & Honeycutt, 2003, and Chapter 3, for a thorough discussion).

Many people have contributed to DST and not all of them agree on every theoretical point (see Oyama, Griffiths, & Gray, 2001b), but all, I believe, accept the main ideas embodied in these themes. Although DST itself is of relatively recent origin (Gray, 1992; Oyama, 1985, 2000; Schaffner, 1998), the ideas it embodies grew out of attempts to understand behavioral development that date at least to the early part of the twentieth century and, indeed, long before.

Historical Background

The theoretical issues and puzzles that led to the articulation of DST have a long history in both biology and psychology. It is self-evident that organisms grow not only in size but also in complexity; the question of where the increase in complexity comes from has a long history stretching back into antiquity, but was focused especially by anatomical investigations beginning in the seventeenth century. Two broad positions emerged from the debates engendered by these investigations (see Chapter 3; Oppenheim, 1982, 1992). On one side were the preformationists, who argued that the complex structures we see arising in development are present even in the fertilized egg and that development is simply an unfolding of this preexisting structure. On the other side were the epigeneticists, who contended that organisms really do become more complex during development and that anatomical structures emerge from an unformed germinal material.

Both positions were problematic. If the preformationists were correct, then the origin of complexity in development simply seemed to be replaced by the even deeper puzzle of how that complexity got into the fertilized egg. But the epigenetic position seemed to require the existence of some mysterious force to account for the appearance of complex structure out of nothing, an unattractive feature in an age seeking scientific explanations of the natural world, with the mechanical explanations of classical physics serving as a model. In many respects, preformationism seemed the more scientifically tenable position. Accepting, as most people did, the initial creation of all living things *ex nihilo*, the origin of organismic complexity could be attributed to God's design, leaving its unfolding in successive individual organisms merely a mechanical problem, well-suited to scientific investigation. The debate between these two positions continued well into the nineteenth century, although the terms of the debate changed as scientific understanding advanced. The idea that perfectly formed anatomical structures exist in miniature from the very beginning of development was soon called in question by improved microscopes but the same technology also revealed that the cytoplasm of the egg is not entirely homogeneous and undifferentiated. Thus, by the nineteenth century, neopreformationists were arguing that an initial heterogeneity in the egg cytoplasm gives rise to anatomical structure as a result of a mechanical process of maturation.

Nature versus Nurture: Instinct versus Learning

The epigenesis–preformation debate was conducted almost entirely in relation to anatomical structure and hardly communicated at all with the inquiries, mostly within philosophy, that would eventually lead to the emergence of psychology. However, its major theme, pitting preexisting complexity against the gradual emergence of order, finds an echo in philosophical debates between nativists and empiricists about the origins of knowledge. Nativists (such as Plato, Descartes, and Kant) have maintained in general that knowledge is preexisting in the mind, or the soul, and is awakened or unearthed by experience, which plays no role in shaping or structuring what we know. Empiricists (such as Aristotle, Bacon, and Hume) argue that the mind is empty prior to experience (the *tabula rasa* of the seventeenth-century British philosopher John Locke) and that experience constructs and shapes knowledge as we interact with the world through our senses.

Although this very brief description caricatures two complex and highly differentiated epistemologies, it identifies an underlying theme that is common to the two great currents of inquiry that most influenced theories of behavioral development as they emerged in the late nineteenth and early twentieth centuries—a biological current that runs through evolutionary biology, anatomy, and genetics, and a philosophical current that emerges in psychology. These currents met and mingled in complex ways to shape thinking about behavioral development but they both helped to legitimize the view that one can reasonably ask whether a particular feature (a behavior, an idea, a psychological ability) is part of an organism's preexisting structure or, alternatively, emerges de novo in the course of its lifetime.

By the beginning of the twentieth century, scientists studying behavior, whether human or nonhuman, had mostly accepted Darwinian evolution as the foundation of their analyses (Richards, 1987). It was becoming widely understood that principles drawn from the study of nonhuman animals could be applied to humans and, in particular, that at least a portion of human behavior could be attributed to instinct. Instincts had been prominent in writings on the behavior of nonhuman animals since well before Darwin, but it was the widespread acceptance of evolutionary thinking that extended their application to humans as well. People had long marveled at the precision with which the instinctive behavior of animals fit the most exacting demands of the environment, a characteristic attributed to the careful design of a benevolent Creator. This is the position of natural theology, associated especially with the eighteenth-century naturalist and theologian William Paley (e.g., Paley, 1848; see Richards, 1981). With Darwin's theory at hand, natural selection gradually came to replace divine creation as the explanation for the fit between instinct and environment.

Evolutionary theory had several important influences on the landscape of American psychology at the end of the nineteenth century (see Cravens & Burnham, 1971; Richards, 1987, especially Chapters 9 and 10). The comparative psychology of learning grew out of the application of experimental methods imported from German psychological laboratories to problems of animal behavior articulated by British evolutionary naturalists, such as George Romanes (1884) and Conwy Lloyd Morgan (1895; see Dewsbury, 1984). The early work of Edward Thorndike (1898) and others on animal learning included the careful design of experiments that would separate learning from instinct so that the former could be studied in isolation (see pp. 15–16). The existence of instinct, far from being denied, was viewed as a powerful influence on behavior that could easily obscure the effects of learning, which was the primary focus of interest for these researchers.

In a rather different vein, the convergence of Darwinian evolutionary theory and philosophical pragmatism gave rise to the functionalist school of psychology in which instinct played a prominent role. In his *Principles of Psychology* (1890), William James listed more than 20 human instincts and, in the following decades, that list was expanded by other writers until it seemed that virtually every identifiable form of behavior was to be explained by a specific instinct. Bernard (1924) cataloged over 850 proposed instincts from the psychological literature up to 1920. Perhaps the most influential instinct theorist during this period was William McDougall (1908), whose "hormic psychology" (from *horme* [Greek], impulse or urge) sought to explain all behavior in terms of underlying instinctive mechanisms. In McDougall's tripartite theory, each instinct has an affective core responsible for the impulse associated with the instinct, a cognitive component that provides knowledge of objects relevant to the instinct, and a conative (or motor) component that generates action with respect to these objects. The core is innate and unmodifiable and is responsible for the goal-directedness of the instinctive behavior. The cognitive and conative components are much more variable and can be modified by experience. Thus the instinct of fear, for example, ensures that the organism will always experience fear and attempt to flee from the presence of danger (the affective core), but the particular objects that evoke fear and the particular actions taken to avoid the danger it connotes may vary from one individual to another. McDougall argued that in nonhuman animals, instincts are not much subject to modification by experience, but in humans, the role of learning has become much more important. As a result, it is harder to discern the innate affective core of human behavior, a problem made more acute because human instincts are also more numerous than are those of nonhuman animals.

The Anti-Instinct Movement

Starting around 1920, the concept of instinct was subjected to a series of highly critical analyses, beginning with a paper by Dunlap (1919). Dunlap distinguished between the *teleological* and the *physiological* uses of the concept, the former corresponding to McDougall's theory of instinct, with its inherently goal-directed affective core, the latter to the more mechanistic theories proposed by Lloyd Morgan and others working from a naturalistic perspective. Dunlap acknowledged the value of the physiological concept of instinct for understanding behavior but criticized the teleological concept as vague and nonspecific. The criticism initiated by Dunlap was echoed and further developed by a number of other authors, most especially Zing-Yang Kuo, who published a series of papers highly critical of the concept of instinct during the 1920s (Kuo, 1921, 1922, 1924, 1928, 1929). The details of Kuo's arguments changed over the course of the decade, becoming more radical in its rejection of any instinctive or innate components of behavior, but his fundamental point remained unchanged. Calling patterns of behavior instinctive provides only a label, not an explanation, because it gives no account of how those patterns come into being over the course of an individual's life. Instinct, Kuo said, provides a "finished psychology"—finished in the sense that it assumes an explanation of the developmental origins of a behavior simply by giving it a label. Kuo (1921, 1922) initially accepted that some simple elements of behavior, which he called "unlearned reaction units," were inherited, but later (Kuo, 1924) he rejected even this limited concession, asserting that "*in a strictly behavioristic psychology...there is practically no room for the concept of heredity*" (p. 428; italics in original).

Although Kuo's was the most radical position, several writers took issue with the vagueness and circularity in the way that the concepts of instinct and heredity were used to explain behavior, resulting in wide-ranging debate over the utility of the concept of instinct in psychology during the 1920s and 1930s (e.g., Bernard, 1921; Chein, 1936; Dunlap, 1922; Marquis, 1930; Tolman, 1922). There were many reasons to criticize the instinct concept as it had been articulated by James, McDougall, and other writers around the turn of the twentieth century. Kuo's main criticism was aimed at the nondevelopmental (even antidevelopmental) claim that instincts were determined by heredity, whereas other behaviors result from learning. When instinct theorists considered development at all, they maintained that instincts were the result of maturation, the passive unfolding of behavior from an inherited germ that was passed from parent to offspring (Gesell, 1929, 1933; Witty & Lehman, 1933; see Oyama, 1982). Kuo's dissatisfaction with that preformationist (or nativist) position was echoed by Leonard Carmichael (1925), an embryologist who pointed out that even the development of anatomical structure could not be explained simply by assuming a passive maturational unfolding. Carmichael described experimental results from embryology showing that many supposedly inherited anatomical features, such as the number and position of eyes in fish, depend on the environment for their normal development. Based on such findings, Carmichael argued that attributing some features of the organism to heredity alone, or attempting to separate the effects of environment and heredity in development, were quite futile. "Heredity and environment are not antithetical, nor can they expediently be separated," he wrote; "for in all maturation there is learning: in all learning there is hereditary maturation" (Carmichael, 1925, p. 260).

During the 1930s and 1940s, behaviorism became the dominant influence in American psychology, bringing with it an almost exclusive emphasis on the role of learning in shaping behavior. Although most behaviorists rejected the utility of the concept of instinct, and de-emphasized the role of heredity, they nonetheless adopted a position that was sympathetic to a sharp distinction between experience and heredity as determinants of behavior. At the turn of the century, Thorndike (1898, 1911) had devised techniques for studying animal learning that were intended to "get the association process free from the helping hand of instinct" (Thorndike, 1911, p. 30). The puzzle boxes and mazes that he used in his experiments were intended to pose challenges that, while within the general scope of the animal's behavioral repertoire, were sufficiently unlike its natural environment that they could only be solved by learning. Thorndike, and those like John B. Watson who followed him in building the behaviorist tradition, accepted the distinction between learning and instinct (or experience and heredity) as a basis for their work. Watson certainly accepted the utility of instinct in his early work; only after 1920, when he had left academia and was writing primarily for a nonscientific audience (e.g., Watson, 1924), did he adopt the radical environmentalist position that has become so strongly associated with his name. Behaviorists in general argued that experience was far more important than heredity in shaping behavior but they did not, for the most part, question that some behavior is due to heredity and some to experience (Herrnstein, 1972; Skinner, 1966). Even more than that, within the behaviorist tradition, "experience" was narrowly interpreted to mean learning as defined by the prevailing theoretical paradigms.

The distinction between heredity and experience, and the equating of experience with laboratory paradigms of learning, gave behaviorism a very nondevelopmental perspective. And because behaviorism was so dominant in American experimental psychology, much of the discipline tended to ignore important developmental questions. A major exception to this generalization was the "child study movement" and the study of child development to which it gave rise. Initiated by G. Stanley Hall at Clark University around the turn of the twentieth century, child study sought to apply observational and experimental methods to the understanding of children's behavior so as to benefit both child rearing and educational practice. Even within this developmental approach, however, the idea of instinctive behavior played an important role. The pages of the *Pedagogical Seminary*, the journal that Hall founded at Clark, are filled with articles identifying one or another instinct in children and proposing ways to use the child's instinctive impulses to guide educational or parenting practice. Hall had little influence on mainstream experimental psychology, partly because of his unsystematic and uncontrolled methods of data collection, primarily involving questionnaires (Brooks-Gunn & Johnson, 2006; Davidson & Benjamin, 1987). As the study of child development grew during the middle part of the century, it drew on the work of experimental embryologists such as Carmichael and Coghill and acquired both a biological and a maturational perspective, as represented especially in the work of Arnold Gesell (1929, 1933). Although strongly influenced by Gesell, Myrtle McGraw (1946) offered a different view of development in which genetic and environmental influences were much more closely integrated (see Dalton & Bergenn, 1995). However, this branch of the discipline of psychology had only a limited impact on DST, which grew from a different set of roots in the second half of the twentieth century.

Ethological Instinct Theory

During the same period in which behaviorism and the experimental study of animal learning began to dominate American psychology, a very different approach to the study of animal behavior was emerging in Europe. Led by Konrad Lorenz and Nikolaas Tinbergen, ethology involved the naturalistic study of behavior, based primarily on observation of animals under natural conditions (see Tinbergen, 1951). The concept of instinct was as central to ethological theory as learning was to behaviorist psychology. Although ethologists readily accepted that animals learn (just as behaviorists acknowledged that they have instincts), learning was not their primary interest and they looked for ways to minimize its effects so as to gain an unimpeded view of instinct (just as behaviorists devised experiments to minimize the contributions of instinct to the process of learning). An important part of the rationale for this separation between learning and instinct was the focus of ethological theory on the evolution and adaptedness of behavior, and it was instinctive, not learned behavior, that was to be explained in evolutionary terms. The importance of separating learned and instinctive behavior is especially evident in the writings of Lorenz.

Lorenz's training in anatomy encouraged him to apply the methods of comparative anatomists to the analysis of behavioral evolution. By treating patterns of behavior as analogous to anatomical structures, Lorenz was able to work out phylogenetic relationships among species based on their behavior. For a behavior to be useful in phylogeny, however, it cannot be greatly affected by learning (which he presumed would result in unpredictable variation having nothing to do with evolutionary relatedness) and so Lorenz restricted his attention to behavior patterns that he could classify as strictly instinctive, such as courtship rituals in waterfowl. Lorenz conducted numerous studies of waterfowl behavior, including the following response of young ducklings, which led to his influential theory of imprinting as an explanation for species recognition (Lorenz, 1935). Imprinting provided Lorenz with an especially clear example of the relationship between learning and instinct in behavior. Since the propensity to follow a moving object can be seen even in newly hatched ducklings, he classified that tendency as an innate or instinctive reaction, not dependent on experience. However, although the first moving object that a duckling typically sees is its mother, Lorenz demonstrated that it would follow any of a wide variety of objects and would come to treat as its mother the first one it encountered. The initial following response is innate, but the specific characteristics of the object followed are learned.

This sharp and essential distinction between patterns of behavior that are innate or instinctive and patterns that are learned is a central theme in all of Lorenz's writing on behavior. It is crystallized in his account of the experimental procedure that he proposed for differentiating between learning and innate behavior—the deprivation experiment. If an animal is raised under conditions that deprive it of any opportunity to learn a particular behavior—in particular, no contact with conspecifics and no opportunity for practice—and the behavior nonetheless appears in its usual form at the usual time, then it must be innate. Innate behavior depends on maturational processes that are intrinsic to the developing animal and arises independently of its experience. The behavior is inherited and is subject to evolutionary modification via the natural selection of variant forms in the same way as anatomical structures, permitting the construction of behavioral phylogenies. Instinct also has primacy over learned behavior, because in order for learning to occur at all (say, by the selective reinforcement of a particular response) something must be present in advance of the opportunity to learn and that something must, by definition, be an innate reaction.

Daniel Lehrman's Critique of Lorenz's Instinct Theory

Lorenz's theory of instinct provided a far more detailed account than had been available in the earlier writings of psychologists such as James and McDougall and so it provided the opportunity for an equally detailed critique. The critique was provided by Daniel Lehrman (1953) in a paper that, although now more than half a century old, still merits careful study for the clarity with which it articulates many of the essential features of a systems approach to developmental theory (see Johnston, 2001). Lehrman's developmental critique of Lorenz followed directly in the tradition of Kuo's criticisms of the concept of instinct and drew also on the work of his mentor T. C. Schneirla (1949, 1956). At the root of Lehrman's argument was a rejection of the longstanding idea that behavior can be neatly divided into two categories: learning or acquired behavior, resulting from experience, and innate or instinctive behavior, resulting from inherited genetic influences. Following Kuo and Schneirla, Lehrman argued that the development of all behavior is a result of interactions between the developing organism and its environment and that these interactions involve both experiential and hereditary influences.

Lehrman took special aim at the deprivation experiment that Lorenz proposed as a clear and conceptually unproblematic way to distinguish learned from innate behavior. Lorenz (1937) had argued that if a behavior develops normally in animals reared in isolation and deprived of all experience, then the behavior is shown to be innate. If the behavior fails to develop at all, or develops only in an imperfect form, then it (or some component) can be diagnosed as learned. Lehrman pointed out that there is in fact no way to entirely deprive an animal of experience. No matter how impoverished the circumstances under which development takes place, some environmental influences are present whereas others are excluded. By treating the experiment as if it completely eliminates experience, and arguing that the behavior that emerges can thus be diagnosed as innate, Lorenz provided spurious support for a dichotomy that does not exist. Lerhman reviewed experimental evidence showing that at least some patterns of supposedly instinctive behavior can be modified by altering the conditions under which animals are reared. He pointed out that even isolated animals gain experience from self-stimulation, which may play a role in development, an insight that was subsequently elaborated especially by Gottlieb (1976b; see pp. 18–19). He also emphasized the importance of analyzing behavioral development in the context of the entire developing organism, noting that the development of pecking in chicks, for example, involves changes in muscular strength and balance and cannot simply be due to maturation of particular neural circuits controlling pecking (Lerhman, 1953, p. 344).

Genes and Experience in Developmental Systems Theory

Lehrman's work can justifiably be seen as the first articulation of what later came to be known as developmental systems theory (Johnston, 2001). The ideas that he introduced have been extended, developed, and supplemented in various ways to establish a distinctive theoretical approach characterized by the six themes identified at the beginning of this chapter. The most important contribution of DST to our understanding of behavioral development is that it allows us to transcend the ancient dichotomies between nature and nurture, learning and instinct, and genes and experience to provide a unified account of development as the outcome of interactions among a variety of factors. It does so primarily by adopting accounts of both experience and genes that are different from those historically used in the explanations of development that have given rise to these dichotomies.

Contributions of Experience to Behavior

Traditionally, the way in which experience affects the development of behavior is through the mechanisms of learning, as described in the work of experimental psychologists (see Pearce & Boulton, 2001; Rescorla & Holland, 1982). Learning is undeniably important in the development of behavior but, from the standpoint of DST, a number of caveats are in order. First, because of the historical opposition of learning and instinct, the study of learning adopted from early in its history a set of methodologies that bear little resemblance to the natural circumstances under which animals normally learn. As noted earlier, this was done deliberately, because the idea was to separate the animal's instinctive repertoire of behavior from whatever it might learn in the laboratory, ensuring that whatever change in behavior was seen would represent only the contribution of learning (Johnston, 1981). Since DST rejects the dichotomy on which this methodological strategy is based, its advocates have not generally been satisfied with traditional learning theory as an account of experiential contributions to development.

Lehrman (1953) pointed out that "experience" encompasses a much broader range of phenomena than those addressed by theories of learning and noted that one consequence of treating learning and instinct as the only possible sources of behavior is to ignore a wide range of possible inputs to development. It is ironic that many European ethologists (e.g., Eibl-Eibesfeldt, 1961; Eibl-Eibesfeldt & Kramer, 1958; Hess, 1962; Lorenz, 1956) read Lehrman's rejection of the dichotomy between learning and instinct as a claim that all behavior depends on learning, missing entirely his point that *both* terms in the dichotomy are inadequate to the analysis of behavioral development (Johnston, 2001).[1]

Responding to the inadequacy of traditional conceptions of learning, Gottlieb (1976a, 1976b, 1981) proposed three roles that experience may play in the development of a behavior: *induction*, in which the behavior does not appear at all in the absence of the experience; *facilitation*, in which the experience is required for the behavior to develop at the normal time; and *maintenance*, in which the experience is required to ensure the continued persistence of a behavior that has already developed. Aslin (1981) suggested a fourth role, *attunement*, in which experience is required to bring the behavior to the typical level of performance.[2]

Gottlieb's classification of roles readily incorporates results from the study of learning (mostly as examples of induction or attunement) but provides a considerably expanded vocabulary for thinking about experiential contributions to development. Certainly it encourages us to go beyond the question of *whether* experience influences development and gives us analytical tools to ask the broader and more helpful question of *how* experience influences development.

One important feature of Gottlieb's roles of experience is that they accommodate relationships between experience and development that are nonobvious. Gottlieb's own research on the development of ducklings' responses to their mother's call illustrates this nonobvious relationship. If eggs of the mallard duck (*Anas platyrhynchos*) are incubated and allowed to hatch in isolation in a soundproof incubator, the ducklings nonetheless show the normal selective approach response to a recording of the mallard maternal assembly call, which the mother uses under natural conditions to lead her brood off the nest after hatching and keep the ducklings together. Such isolated ducklings will approach the mallard call in preference to the calls of other species or to recordings of the mallard call that have been experimentally altered in various ways (Gottlieb, 1971, 1997). Thus the approach response would appear to be a classic example of instinctive behavior, as defined by Lorenz. However, an isolated duckling provides its own auditory stimulation by producing calls while still in the egg, just before hatching. If it is prevented from making these calls, by being surgically devocalized just before the calls start to be produced, it no longer shows the same response to the maternal call after hatching. Unlike the case in which an animal comes to approach an object as a result of previous exposure to that object (as in the case of imprinting), in this example, the crucial experience (exposure to self-produced embryonic calls) and the resultant behavior (a response to the maternal call) are not obviously related to one another. This is not an example of learning, in any sense of that term, and it poses problems for theoretical accounts of development that group all experiential contributions into the category of learning.

In learning as traditionally defined, the crucial experience and the behavior that is learned stand in what I have called a "rational relationship" to one another (Johnston, 1997). That is, one can quite readily imagine that the experience could, in principle, contribute to the development of the behavior, as when the repeated pairing of shock with a stimulus leads to avoidance of that stimulus in an avoidance learning paradigm. It is reasonable a priori that such a relationship might hold and the experimental data provide confirmation of that expectation and lead to more detailed analyses of the exact conditions under which learning does and does not occur. In nonobvious relationships, such that identified by Gottlieb's data, no such a priori reasonableness exists.

Although experience typically is thought of as being provided for the developing animal by the environment, organisms also actively seek out and structure their perceptual experience (E. J. Gibson, 1969; J. J. Gibson, 1966, 1979; Reed, 1996) and much of that experience is created by the animal's own activity. Gottlieb's research on mallard ducklings, summarized above, provides one clear example of the importance of self-stimulation (Michel, 2007) and similar findings have been reported by Miller (1997) for the development of responsiveness to the alarm call in the same species. In other cases, the necessary physical stimulation comes from the animal's environment, rather than from the animal itself, but it must be self-generated if it is to be effective for normal development. Held and Hein (1963) showed that kittens reared in darkness do not develop the ability to control their movements using visual information. A few minutes per day of exposure to light permits normal development, but only if the exposure involves self-produced movement through a lighted environment. Control kittens given exactly the same type and amount of exposure, but with their experience passively imposed rather than actively produced, show the same deficits as dark-reared animals. Similar results were obtained by Held and Bauer (1974; Bauer & Held, 1975) for the development of visually guided reaching in monkeys. As a further example, the self-produced stimulation provided by play and exercise in young mammals are important contributors to the development of both muscular strength and motor coordination (Bekoff, 1988; Byers & Walker, 1995).

Contributions of Genes to Behavior

The idea that genes can be said to specify, code for, or otherwise determine behavior directly has perhaps elicited more sustained attention from developmental systems theorists than any other issue. From Kuo's early anti-instinct writings to the present day, developmentalists have attempted to counter the claim that the genes (or, in earlier formulations, instinct or inheritance) directly specify or cause behavior. Lehrman's criticism of ethological instinct theory was partly aimed at the dichotomy between learned and innate behavior, but it also focused on Lorenz's claim that innate behavior is causally distinct from learned behavior, being part of the organism's evolutionary inheritance and unfolding in development through strictly determined maturation. In his lengthy reply to Lehrman, Lorenz (1965) wrote of innate behavior being determined by "phylogenetic information," encoded in the genes and constituting a genetic blueprint analogous to the blueprint used in building a house. In this metaphor, the genes completely define the organization of innate behavior, including the ways in which experience may supplement it, as in the case of imprinting discussed earlier. The environment plays only a supportive role, allowing the information in the genes to unfold, but making no contribution to the behavioral organization that they specify. On careful analysis, Lorenz's information metaphor cannot sustain the work that he intended it to do (see Griffiths & Gray, 1994; Johnston, 1987) although it has remained a popular way of talking about genetic influences on development (see Griffiths, 2001; Lewontin, 2000; Moss, 2003; Newson, 2004).

Since DST categorically rejects the claim that an organism's genes directly specify any of its behavior, we can ask what alternative account it provides of genetic contributions to development. It is first worth reiterating that modern versions of DST do not attempt to minimize the importance of the genes (see Griffiths & Gray, 2005). It is true that Kuo (at least in his later writings) wanted to eliminate heredity entirely from his developmental approach, but from Lehrman on, the architects of DST have understood very clearly that any account of development must recognize and incorporate genetic influences. Lehrman had little to say about how genes affect the development of behavior, a feature of his article that may have encouraged the view that his was an anti-hereditarian position in which genetic influences are simply not very important. This was a common misreading of Lehrman's position at the time, especially by ethologists responding to his criticisms (Johnston, 2001), and it has continued to be a misreading of later theoretical positions based on Lehrman's insights (Griffiths & Gray, 2005). The history of genetic knowledge makes it unsurprising that theorists writing in the middle of the twentieth century could offer few details, even hypothetically, about the role of the genes in the development of behavior. At the time Lehrman was writing, little was known about the molecular structure of the genes. Indeed, it had not even been established that DNA was the molecule responsible for inheritance, with many geneticists arguing that the protein component of chromosomes was a more likely candidate because of its greater molecular complexity.

Just a few months before Lerhman's critique appeared, James Watson and Francis Crick had published their seminal paper in which they elucidated the molecular structure of DNA (Watson & Crick, 1953) and noted (in the last sentence) its implications for understanding the mechanisms of heredity. With a persuasive account based on the molecular structure of DNA now available to explain how information might be stored and transmitted between generations, it was a straightforward step simply to attribute complex organization in the phenotype (e.g., patterns of instinctive behavior) to complex genetic information stored as base sequences in DNA molecules. Exactly how this was supposed to work was unclear, but the idea gave rise to the metaphor of a blueprint for behavior, in which the DNA base sequences stand in the same relation to behavior as the lines and architectural symbols on a blueprint do to the finished structure of the building it represents.

In the late 1960s, evidence began to emerge that gene transcription could be affected by experience, something that was completely inconsistent with the idea of the genetic blueprint. In that view, the relationship between genes and experience is seen to be entirely one way: genes determine the possible contributions of experience and specify when and how experience has its effects (Lorenz, 1965; Mayr, 1974), but experience has no comparable effect on the genes. Rose (1967) showed that exposure to light increases protein synthesis in the visual cortex of rats, implying that this experience somehow stimulates the gene transcription responsible for protein synthesis. Subsequently, other investigators provided more direct evidence of experimental effects on the genes by demonstrating an increase in RNA diversity as a function of complexity of rearing experience (Grouse, Schrier, Bennett, Rosenzweig, & Nelson, 1978; Grouse, Schrier, & Nelson, 1979; Uphouse & Bonner, 1975). This apparent sensitivity of genes to experience was quite compatible with DST and could be incorporated into its emerging theoretical structure. In 1970, Gottlieb had proposed the term "probabilistic epigenesis" for a view of development that he contrasted with "predetermined epigenesis" (Gottlieb, 1970). In the latter view, the genes directly and inexorably specify a particular neural structure, which in turn determines the animal's functional activity and its behavior (Genes → Structural maturation → Function → Behavior). In his probabilistic alternative, behavior can have reciprocal influences on physiological function, which in turn can alter structure (Genes → Structural maturation ↔ Function ↔ Behavior). Later, Gottlieb (1976a, 1983), drawing on the results of Rose, Grouse and others, extended the bidirectional arrows to include the relationship between genes and structure, allowing the "downward" influence of behavior and experience to extend into the formerly autonomous realm of genetic activity.

Recent advances in genetics have made it possible to specify the ways in which genes contribute to the development of behavior in far greater detail than ever before. In particular, we can now replace the largely metaphorical language of earlier writing with a different and more concrete account. The most important shift of perspective is to abandon the seductive language in which genes are cast as sources of information, plans, or blueprints and replace it with the language of molecular interactions that describe the realm in which genes operate during development. Psychologists tend to resist using such molecular language, in part because it seems so remote from the main theoretical concerns of the discipline. The language of information, by contrast, resonates favorably with psychological theory, providing (false) assurance that genetic and psychological explanations will turn out to connect smoothly through the information metaphor. A major challenge for DST has been to provide an account of genetic contributions to development that treats the genes as molecular structures rather than information carriers without losing sight of the organismal end points (outcomes that are psychological and behavioral, rather than molecular) at which our explanations aim.

Johnston and Edwards (2002) tackled this problem by conceiving of three major contributions to development, each of which can be thought of as a class of developmental resources, to use the language of Griffiths and Gray (1994), as shown in Figure 2.1. "Sensory stimulation" comprises influences on development that are transduced through the organism's sensory/perceptual systems. They include the familiar resources of visual, auditory, gustatory, and olfactory stimuli whose developmental effects have been thoroughly investigated in a wide variety of species by developmental psychologists and psychobiologists (e.g., Michel & Moore, 1995). Although we might have used the term "experience" rather than "sensory stimulation," we chose the latter to emphasize that experience, no matter abstractly defined (parental care, practice in reading, exposure to conspecific song or to the French language) can only affect the developing organism through its sensory systems. Most of the sensory resources that have been studied developmentally come from the external environment, but the developing organism itself is also an important source of sensory stimulation, as shown

by Gottlieb's studies of the development of auditory responsiveness in ducklings and the work of Held and his colleagues on sensory-motor development described earlier.

"Physical influences" are influences on development that are not transduced by the sensory systems. Of course, all sensory influences are also physical or chemical. Visual stimuli only affect development because of the physical effects of reflected or transmitted light on photosensitive cells. However, recognizing physical influences as a separate class of developmental resources points out the importance of acknowledging that the physical environment is important for development even when its effects are not mediated by sensory receptors. For example, the development of locomotor behavior depends to a great extent on the growth of bones and muscle and these structures are themselves heavily influenced by physical forces (such as gravity and self-produced muscular force) acting on the developing organism. Thelen's elegant studies of locomotor development in human infants demonstrate clearly that "learning to walk" is a developmental process both constrained and facilitated by considerations of force and mass (Thelen, 1995; Thelen, Kelso, & Fogel, 1987). "Genetic activity," of course, begins with the organism's DNA, although, as we shall see, it is more than a simple matter of genes producing proteins. This figure shows all of these resources acting from outside the developing system, although a central tenet of DST is that genes are part of the system, not separate from it. The separation, however, is only temporary and will disappear as the figure is elaborated.

The preliminary outline represented by Figure 2.1 can be elaborated by identifying the next step in the cascade of developmental interactions that follows from the action of each of the three classes of developmental resources (Figure 2.2). Thus, the immediate effect of sensory stimulation is on the activity of some ensemble of nerve cells—depending on the situation, the effect may be to sustain an existing pattern or to produce a new pattern. Similarly, the immediate effect of gene activity (transcription) is the production of a messenger RNA molecule (mRNA) that will result in protein synthesis. The relationship between transcription and protein synthesis is considerably more complex than suggested by the conventional dictum of "one gene, one protein." If we define the gene as a transcribable segment of DNA (a definition that is by no means universally accepted), then a single gene may in fact specify the amino acid sequence of many

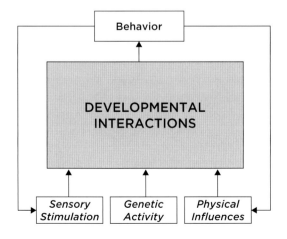

Figure 2.1 Three basic classes of developmental resources. (From Johnston and Edwards (2002). Copyright American Psychological Association. Reproduced by permission.)

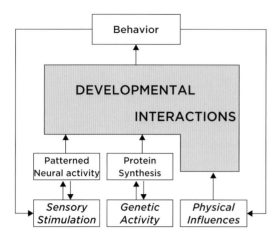

Figure 2.2 The first stage in unpacking the developmental interactions. (From Johnston and Edwards (2002). Copyright American Psychological Association. Reproduced by permission.)

proteins, a finding that accounts for the fact that the number of genes in the human genome (about 25,000) is several times smaller than the number of proteins they produce (in excess of 85,000). This is accomplished in a variety of ways: alternative transcription, in which different mRNAs are produced from a single stretch of DNA depending on the precise starting point; alternative splicing of the initial product of transcription (an mRNA precursor) to produce different mRNA molecules, each of which will be translated to produce a different protein (Ast, 2005); and posttranslational modification, or protein splicing, in which protein molecules are modified to produce alternative molecular structures (Wallace, 1993). For present purposes, we can treat protein synthesis as the immediate consequence of gene activity (that is, of DNA transcription), recognizing that the single arrow in the diagram conceals considerable complexity. It may be that to achieve a satisfactory explanation of the ways in which gene activity contributes to some aspects of behavioral development, it will be necessary to unpack some of this complexity.

In Figure 2.3, the various interactions involved in the development of behavior have been fully unpacked. That is not to say that the various elements of the system (boxes) and the possible interactions between them (arrows) could not be explicated in further detail. However, the diagram represents a systems model of developmental interactions that achieves several things. First, it incorporates all of the resources that decades of research have shown to contribute in one way or another to the development of behavior. Not all of them are identified explicitly in the model, but all are in principle capable of being described in terms of its elements. For example, Shanahan and Hofer (2005, p. 71) pointed out that the diagram seems to say nothing about a set of developmental resources that are particularly important to human development, namely contextual (i.e., social and cultural) influences. Although such influences are not explicitly represented here, the model certainly provides a place for them, as the social and cultural environment can only affect development by providing sensory or physicochemical resources for development. Sometimes, we know at least roughly what sensory input corresponds to a particular sociocultural influence. Language, for example, affects development through particular auditory stimuli, modulated most likely by visual and tactile stimuli provided by caretakers. The study of language development has as one of its goals the detailed specification of the sensory stimuli involved in the process (e.g., Werker & Tees, 1999). If this approach seems to account less well for other cases where the sociocultural environment affects development (peer-group influences on academic performance, for example), this may be because we are much further from being able to identify the specific developmental resources involved. However, such resources must exist, and it must, in principle, be possible to specify the ways in which they act through the nervous system and other organ systems of the developing child.

Second, the model forcefully rejects any metaphorical components, in particular those relating to the contributions of genetic resources. In constructing the model, and identifying its various elements and interactions, we repeatedly asked "What *actually* takes place at the genetic, cellular, or organismic level when one element affects another in the course of development?" We sought a balance between adding so much detail and specificity that the model would offer no general conceptual guidance, and leaving so much out that it would provide nothing more than an unhelpfully superficial gloss on the process of development. The model has no room for blueprints, plans, or instructions—it presents the genes as molecular structures, located within cell nuclei, from where they affect behavior development through molecular and cellular pathways. This view places the genes squarely within the system whose development they affect, rather than outside it, operating in some strange metaphorical realm where causal relationships are obscured.

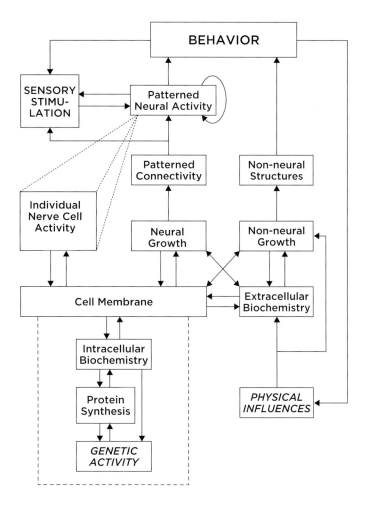

Experience has its effects on behavior by changing the underlying neural circuitry—creating new synaptic connections, strengthening some existing ones, and weakening or eliminating others. The model makes clear that these effects are implemented through changes in the activity of genes, as shown by the fact that there is no direct route (arrow) connecting sensory stimulation and neural connectivity. Experience directly affects the electrochemical activity of nerve cells and thus indirectly produces changes in the activity of genes within their nuclei. These changes in genetic activity, in turn, are responsible for the changes in neural growth and hence connectivity that produce experience-dependent changes in behavior. This feature of the model represents a critical feature of DST, namely the intimate connection between experiential and genetic influences on behavioral development.

Of particular importance in the response of the organism's genome to experiential effects is a class of genes known as immediate-early genes (IEGs). A number of such genes have been identified (such as *c-fos*, *c-jun*, *ZENK*, and *CREB*), all of which have the common characteristic that their transcription responds quickly to changes in experience (Morgan & Curran, 1989, 1991). Changes in IEG transcription have been found in virtually every system studied in which experience produces a change in behavior, whether in adult or immature animals. IEG involvement has been extensively studied in relation to birdsong,[3] which is well understood at both the behavioral and neurobiological levels (Clayton, 2000), making it an excellent system for elucidating genetic mechanisms in development (Clayton, 2004). For example, transcription of the IEGs *ZENK*, *c-fos*, and *c-jun* occurs in auditory areas of the brain involved in song recognition when songbirds hear conspecific song (e.g., Mello & Clayton, 1994) and occurs in motor areas during singing (Jarvis & Nottebohm, 1997; Jarvis et al., 2000; Kimpo & Doupe, 1997). Only a very brief exposure to song (as little as 2 s) is necessary to induce the expression of ZENK (Kruse, Stripling, & Clayton, 2000). The IEG response to song is greater for conspecific than for heterospecific song (Mello, Vicario, & Clayton, 1992), and for the song of birds reared with a song tutor than for that of birds reared without tutoring, which sing an abnormal, impoverished song as a result (Tomaszycki, Sluzas, Sundberg, Newman, & DeVoogd, 2006).

A variety of evidence shows that stimulus-driven gene expression is regulated by experience. Transcription in areas of the brain known to be involved in song is enhanced when birds are exposed to songs that they learned as juveniles (Marler & Doupe, 2000) and the response to the familiar song of tutors is correlated with the number of elements that have been copied from the tutor song (Bolhuis, Hetebrij, den Boer-Visser, De Groot, & Zijistra, 2001; Bolhuis, Zijlstra, den Boer-Visser, & Van Der Zee, 2000). Birds that have been reared in the presence of song tutors show a greater overall response to conspecific song than birds reared without tutors and tutored birds show a stronger response to the songs of tutored than of untutored males, whereas birds reared without tutors do not show any difference (Tomaszycki et al., 2006). Interestingly, similar results are found in both male and female subjects, suggesting that the genetic response is important for the development of song perception as well as song production, since females do not sing (Tomaszycki et al., 2006; Bailey & Wade, 2005).

The proteins produced as a result of IEG expression are transcription factors that regulate the expression of other genes by binding to promoter regions of DNA, initiating a complex cascade of molecular events that produce the structural changes in the nervous system that underlie developmental change in behavior (Pfenning, Schwartz, & Barth, 2007; Rose, 1991; Shaw, Lanius, & van den Doel, 1994). For example, the proteins produced by the IEGs c-fos and c-jun (Fos and Jun, respectively) combine to form a protein complex called a dimer that regulates subsequent gene activity by binding to specific regions of DNA (Morgan & Curran, 1989, 1991). The ZENK protein binds to the promoter region of many genes, including those for synapsin I and synapsin II (Petersohn, Schoch, Brinkmann, & Thiel, 1995; Thiel, Schoch, & Petersohn, 1994), suggesting ways in which ZENK induction may affect neuronal growth and synaptic modification (see Ribeiro & Mello, 2000). Other studies have also begun to explore

the downstream consequences of stimulus-induced IEG induction (e.g., Chew, Mello, Nottebohm, Jarvis, & Vicario, 1995; Hong, Li, Becker, Dawson, & Dawson, 2004).

Exposure to song induces the expression of at least one gene that directly influences neuronal physiology, rather than regulating the expression of other genes. Velho, Pinaud, Rodrigues, and Mello (2005) examined the expression of two IEGs (ZENK and c-fos) and the activity-regulated cytoskeletal-associated gene (Arc), expression of which is required for synaptic changes in the hippocampus underlying memory and learning in certain tasks (Guzowski, Setlow, Wagner, & McGaugh, 2001). They found that expression of ZENK and c-fos in the zebra finch auditory system following exposure to song is soon followed by expression of Arc and that all three genes are expressed in the same cells. Because Arc expression occurs before Fos and ZENK proteins have accumulated significantly, Velho et al. infer that song affects Arc expression directly, rather than indirectly through the DNA-binding activity of Fos and ZENK.

Velho et al.'s (2005) results show that Arc mRNA migrates from the nucleus to the dendrites and that Arc protein appears at postsynaptic sites soon after sensory stimulation. Several studies have shown that translation of protein from mRNA, previously thought to occur only in the nucleus, also occurs in the cytoplasm, specifically at the synapse (Steward & Schuman, 2001; Sutton & Schuman, 2006; Wang & Tiedge, 2004) and that posttranslational modification of proteins also occurs at the synapse (Routtenberg & Rekart, 2005).

All of these results are beginning to paint a picture of a relationship between gene expression and experience and of genetic contributions to development in general, that is far more subtle and complex than anything implied by the seductive genetic metaphors against which DST has been struggling for over 50 years. On the other hand, none of these recent molecular and genetic discoveries are at all incompatible with the view of development presented by DST (Figure 2.3; see Johnston & Edwards, 2002). While most of the results could not have been predicted by the early theorists who laid the foundations for DST, they would almost certainly have been embraced as entirely consistent with the view those founders were setting forth.[4]

Conclusions

The systems view of development that is explicated by DST transcends the obsolete and misleading dichotomies of nature and nurture, genes and environment, instinct and learning that have pervaded (and obstructed) thinking about development for centuries. In recent years, the technical accounts that are the foundation of this chapter have been supplemented by a number of thoughtful and engaging books on development that may help to spread the systems viewpoint to a larger audience of general scientists and lay readers (e.g., Coen, 1999; Lewontin, 2000; Moore, 2002; Morange, 2001; Noble, 2006; Ridley, 2003).

The great strengths of DST are that it offers a more complete account of development than anything provided by the alternative, dichotomous views and that it receives increasing support as we learn more about the ways in which the molecular genetic machinery actually functions. Those who would view the genes as determining or specifying patterns or aspects of behavior increasingly find themselves having to adopt some version of DST in order to be consistent with what the data show. Even though the primary architects of DST, such as Lehrman and Gottlieb, had access to only very limited information about the mechanisms of gene action at the time they developed their ideas in the middle of the last century, their intuitions about development, and their sense of how genes and experience most likely worked together to bring about behavior, have turned out to be remarkably prescient.

Difficult as it may be, we should now permanently set aside the idea that it is useful to search for genes that code for or specify behavior. Of course, it remains important to identify candidate genes that may have especially strong effects on the way in which particular behavior develops (e.g., Moffitt, Caspi, & Rutter, 2005, 2006). Identifying such genes is the first step toward explicating how they act in the course of development, but it does not imply that they specify or determine the behavior. New technologies will undoubtedly provide important insights into the developmental roles of genes that influence behavior, and psychologists must become conversant with those technologies and the results they produce, even if they cannot implement them themselves. The study of behavioral development increasingly depends on interdisciplinary collaborations between behavioral and molecular scientists; DST provides a conceptual framework within which these collaborating disciplines can speak to each other to achieve a deeper understanding of the complex and difficult problems they face.

References

Aslin, R. (1981). Experiential influences and sensitive periods in perceptual development: A unified model. In R. N. Aslin, J. R. Alberts, & M. R. Petersen (Eds.), *Development of perception* (Vol. 1, pp. 5–44). New York: Academic Press.

Ast, G. (2005). The alternative genome. *Scientific American, 292(4),* 58–65.

Bailey, D. J., & Wade, J . (2005). *FOS* and *ZENK* responses in 45-day-old zebra finches vary with auditory stimulus and brain region, but not sex. *Behavioral Brain Research, 162,* 108–115.

Bauer, J., & Held, R . (1975). Comparison of visual guided reaching in normal and deprived infant monkeys. *Journal of Experimental Psychology: Animal Behavior Processes, 1,* 298–308.

Bekoff, M. (1988). Motor training and physical fitness: Possible short- and long-term influences on the development of individual differences in behavior. *Developmental Psychobiology, 21,* 601–612.

Bernard, L. L. (1921). The misuse of instinct in the social sciences. *Psychological Review, 28,* 96–119.

Bernard, L. L. (1924). *Instinct: A study in social psychology.* New York: Henry Holt.

Bolhuis, J. J, Hetebrij, E., den Boer-Visser, A. M., De Groot, J. H., & Zijistra, G. G. O . (2001). Localized immediate early gene expression related to the strength of song learning in socially reared zebra finches. *European Journal of Neuroscience, 13,* 2165–2170.

Bolhuis, J. J., Zijlstra, G. G., den Boer-Visser, A. M., & Van Der Zee, E. A. (2000). Localized neuronal activation in the zebra finch brain is related to the strength of song learning. *Proceedings of the National Academy of Sciences, 97,* 2282–2285.

Brooks-Gunn, J., & Johnson, A. D. (2006). G. Stanley Hall's contribution to science, practice, and policy: The child study, parent education, and child welfare movements. *History of Psychology, 9,* 247–258.

Byers, J. A., & Walker, C. (1995). Refining the motor training hypothesis for the evolution of play. *American Naturalist, 146,* 25–40.

Carmichael, L . (1925). Heredity and environment: are they antithetical? *Journal of Abnormal and Social Psychology, 20,* 245–260.

Chein, I. (1936). The problems of heredity and environment. *Journal of Psychology, 2,* 229–244.

Chew, S. J., Mello, C., Nottebohm, F., Jarvis, E., & Vicario D. S. (1995). Decrements in auditory responses to a repeated conspecific song are long-lasting and require two periods of protein synthesis in the songbird forebrain. *Proceedings of the National Academy of Sciences, 92,* 3406–3410.

Clayton, D. F. (2000). The neural basis of avian song learning and perception. In J. J. Bolhuis (Ed.), *Brain, perception, memory* (pp. 113–125). New York: Oxford University Press.

Clayton, D. F. (2004). Songbird genomics: Methods, mechanisms, opportunities, and pitfalls. *Annals of the New York Academy of Sciences, 1016,* 45–60.

Coen, E. (1999). *The art of genes: How organisms make themselves.* Oxford, Oxford University Press.

Cravens, H., & Burnham, J. C. (1971). Psychology and evolutionary naturalism in American thought, 1890–1940. *American Quarterly, 23,* 635–657.

Dalton, T. C., & Bergenn, V. W. (1995). *Beyond heredity and environment: Myrtle McGraw and the maturation controversy.* Boulder, CO: Westview Press.

Davidson, E. S., & Benjamin, L. T. (1987). A history of the child study movement in America. In J. A. Glover & R. R. Ronning (Eds.), *Historical foundations of educational psychology* (pp. 41–60). New York: Plenum Press.

Dewsbury, D. A. (1984). *Comparative psychology in the twentieth century.* Stroudsburg, PA: Hutchinson Ross Co.

Dunlap, K. (1919). Are there any instincts? *Journal of Abnormal Psychology, 14,* 307–311.

Dunlap, K. (1922). The identity of instinct and habit. *Journal of Philosophy, 19,* 85–94.

Eibl-Eibesfeldt, I . (1961). The interactions of unlearned behaviour patterns and learning in mammals. In J. M. Delafresnaye (Ed.), *Brain mechanisms and learning* (pp. 53–73). Oxford: Blackwell.

Eibl-Eibesfeldt, I., & Kramer, S. (1958). Ethology, the comparative study of animal behavior. *Quarterly Review of Biology, 33,* 181–211.

Gesell, A. (1929). Maturation and infant behavior pattern. *Psychological Review, 36,* 307–319.

Gesell, A. (1933). Maturation and the patterning of behavior. In C. Murchison (Ed.), *Handbook of child psychology* (2nd ed., pp. 209–235). New York: Russell & Russell.

Gibson, E. J. (1969). *Principles of perceptual learning and development.* New York: Appleton-Century-Crofts.

Gibson, J. J. (1966). *The senses considered as perceptual systems.* Boston: Houghton-Mifflin.

Gibson, J. J. (1979). *The ecological approach to visual perception.* Boston: Houghton Mifflin.

Gottlieb, G . (1970). Conceptions of prenatal behavior. In L. R. Aronson, E. Tobach, D. S. Lehrman, & J. S. Rosenblatt (Eds.), *Development and evolution of behavior: Essays in memory of T. C. Schneirla* (pp. 111–137). San Francisco: W. H. Freeman.

Gottlieb, G. (1971). *Development of species identification in birds: An inquiry into the prenatal determinants of perception.* Chicago: University of Chicago Press.

Gottlieb, G. (1976a). Conceptions of prenatal development: Behavioral embryology. *Psychological Review, 83,* 215–234.

Gottlieb, G. (1976b). The roles of experience in the development of behavior and the nervous system. In G. Gottlieb (Ed.), *Studies on the development of behavior and the nervous system, Vol. 3: Neural and behavioral specificity* (pp. 25–54). New York: Academic Press.

Gottlieb, G. (1981). Roles of early experience in species-specific perceptual development. In R. N. Aslin, J. R. Alberts, & M. R. Petersen (Eds.), *Development of perception* (Vol. 1, pp. 5–44). New York: Academic Press.

Gottlieb, G. (1983). The psychobiological approach to developmental issues. In P. H. Mussen (Ed.), *Handbook of child psychology. Vol. II: Infancy and developmental psychobiology* (pp. 1–26). New York, Wiley.

Gottlieb, G. (1987). The developmental basis of evolutionary change. *Journal of Comparative Psychology, 101,* 262–271.

Gottlieb, G. (1997). *Synthesizing nature–nurture: Prenatal roots of instinctive behavior.* Mahwah, NJ: Erlbaum Associates.

Gottlieb, G. (2001). A developmental psychobiological systems view: Early formulation and current status. In S. Oyama, P. E. Griffiths, & R. D. Gray (Eds.), *Cycles of contingency: Developmental systems and evolution* (pp. 41–54). Cambridge, MA: MIT Press.

Gray, R. (1992). Death of the gene: Developmental systems strike back. In P. Griffiths (Ed.), *Trees of life: Essays in philosophy of biology* (pp. 165–209). Dordrecht, The Netherlands: Kluwer.

Griffiths, P. E . (2001). Genetic information: A metaphor in search of a theory. *Philosophy of Science, 68,* 394–412.

Griffiths, P. E., & Gray, R. D. (1994). Developmental systems and evolutionary explanation. *Journal of Philosophy, 91,* 277–305.

Griffiths, P. E., & Gray, R. D. (2005). Discussion: Three ways to misunderstand developmental systems theory. *Biology and Philosophy, 20,* 417–425.

Grouse, L. D., Schrier, B. K., Bennett, E. L., Rosenzweig, M. R., & Nelson, P. G. (1978). Sequence diversity studies of rat brain RNA: effects of environmental complexity in rat brain RNA diversity. *Journal of Neurochemistry, 30,* 191–203.

Grouse, L. D., Schrier, B. K., & Nelson, P. G. (1979). Effect of visual experience on gene expression during the development of stimulus specificity in cat brain. *Experimental Neurology, 64,* 354–364.

Guzowski, J. F., Setlow, B., Wagner, E. K., & McGaugh, J. L. (2001). Experience-dependent gene expression in the rat hippocampus after spatial learning: A comparison of the immediate-early genes *Arc, c-fos,* and *zif268. Journal of Neuroscience 21,* 5089–5098.

Held, R., & Bauer, J. A. (1974). Development of sensorially-guided reaching in infant monkeys. *Brain Research 71,* 265–271.

Held, R., & Hein, A. (1963). Movement-produced stimulation in development of visually guided behavior. *Journal of Comparative and Physiological Psychology, 56,* 872–876.

Herrnstein, R. J. (1972). Nature as nurture: Behaviorism and the instinct doctrine. *Behaviorism, 1,* 23–52.

Hess, E. H. (1962). Ethology: An approach toward the complete analysis of behavior. *New Directions in Psychology, 1,* 157–266.

Hong, S. J., Li, H., Becker, K. G., Dawson, V. L., & Dawson, T. M. (2004). Identification and analysis of plasticity-induced late-response genes. *Proceedings of the National Academy of Sciences, 101,* 2145–2150.

Jablonka, E. (2001). The systems of inheritance. In S. Oyama, P. E. Griffiths, & R. D. Gray (Eds.), *Cycles of contingency: Developmental systems and evolution* (pp. 99–116). Cambridge, MA: MIT Press.

James, W. (1890). *Principles of psychology.* New York: Henry Holt.

Jarvis, E. D., & Nottebohm, F. (1997). Motor-driven gene expression. *Proceedings of the National Academy of Sciences, 94,* 4097–4102.

Jarvis, E. D., Ribeiro, S., da Silva, M. L., Ventura, D., Vielliard, J., & Mello, C. V. (2000). Behaviourally driven gene expression reveals song nuclei in hummingbird brain. *Nature, 406,* 628–632.

Johnston, T. D. (1981). Contrasting approaches to a theory of learning. *Behavioral and Brain Sciences, 4,* 125–173.

Johnston, T. D. (1987). The persistence of dichotomies in the study of behavioral development. *Developmental Review, 7,* 149–182.

Johnston, T. D. (1997). Comment on Miller. In C. Dent-Read & P. Zukow-Goldring (Eds.), *Evolving explanations of development: Ecological approaches to organism–environment systems* (pp. 509–513). Washington, D.C.: American Psychological Association.

Johnston, T. D. (2001). Towards a systems view of development: An appraisal of Lehrman's critique of Lorenz. In S. Oyama, P. E. Griffiths, & R. D. Gray (Eds.), *Cycles of contingency: Developmental systems and evolution* (pp.15–23). Cambridge, MA: MIT Press.

Johnston, T. D., & Edwards, L. (2002). Genes, interactions, and the development of behavior. *Psychological Review, 109,* 26–34.

Johnston, T. D., & Gottlieb, G. (1990). Neophenogenesis: A developmental theory of phenotypic evolution. *Journal of Theoretical Biology, 147,* 471–495.

Kimpo, R. R., & Doupe, A. J. (1997). FOS is induced by singing in distinct neuronal populations in a motor network. *Neuron, 18,* 315–325.

Kruse, A. A., Stripling, R., & Clayton, D. F. (2000). Minimal experience required for immediate-early gene induction in zebra finch neostriatum. *Neurobiology of Learning & Memory, 76,* 179–184.

Kuo, Z.-Y. (1921). Giving up instincts in psychology. *Journal of Philosophy, 18,* 645–664.

Kuo, Z.-Y. (1922). How are our instincts acquired? *Psychological Review, 29,* 344–365.

Kuo, Z.-Y. (1924). A psychology without heredity. *Psychological Review 31,* 427–448.

Kuo, Z.-Y. (1928). The fundamental error of the concept of purpose and the trial and error fallacy. *Psychological Review, 35,* 414–433.

Kuo, Z.-Y. (1929). The net result of the anti-heredity movement in psychology. *Psychological Review, 36,* 181–199.

Lehrman, D. S. (1953). A critique of Konrad Lorenz's theory of instinctive behavior. *Quarterly Review of Biology, 28,* 337–363.

Lewontin, R. C. (2000). *The triple helix: Gene, organism, and environment.* Cambridge, MA: Harvard University Press.

Lickliter, R., & Honeycutt, H. (2003). Developmental dynamics: Towards a biologically plausible evolutionary psychology. *Psychological Bulletin, 129,* 819–835.

Lorenz, K. Z. (1935). Der Kumpan in der Umwelt des Vogels. *Journal für Ornithologie, 83,* 137–213, 289–413.

Lorenz, K. Z. (1937). Uber die Bildung des Instinktbegriffes. *Naturwissenschaften, 25,* 289–300, 307–318, 324–331.

Lorenz, K. Z. (1956). The objectivistic theory of instinct. In P. P. Grassé (Ed.), *L'Instinct dans le comportement des animaux et de l'homme* (pp. 51–76). Paris: Masson.

Lorenz, K. Z. (1965). *Evolution and modification of behavior.* Chicago: University of Chicago Press.

Marler, P., & Doupe, A. J. (2000). Singing in the brain. *Proceedings of the National Academy of Sciences, 97,* 2965–2967.

Marquis, D. G. (1930). The criterion of innate behavior. *Psychological Review, 37,* 334–349.

Mayr, E. (1974). Behavior programs and evolutionary strategies. *American Scientist, 62,* 650–659.

McDougall, W. (1908). *Introduction to social psychology.* London: Methuen & Co.

McGraw, M. (1946). Maturation of behavior. In L. Carmichael (Ed.), *Manual of child psychology* (pp. 332–369). New York: Wiley.

Mello, C. V., & Clayton, D. S. (1994). Song-induced *ZENK* gene expression in auditory pathways of songbird brain and its relation to the song control system. *Journal of Neuroscience, 14,* 6652–6666.

Mello, C. V., Vicario, D. S., & Clayton, D. F. (1992). Song presentation induces gene expression in the songbird forebrain. *Proceedings of the National Academy of Sciences, 89,* 6818–6822.

Michel, G. F. (2007). Doing what comes naturally: The role of self-generated experience in behavioral development. *European Journal of Developmental Science, 2,* 155–164.

Michel, G. F., & Moore, C. L. (1995). *Developmental psychobiology: An interdisciplinary science.* Cambridge, MA: MIT Press.

Miller, D. B. (1997). The effects of nonobvious forms of experience on the development of instinctive behavior. In C. Dent-Read & P. Zukow-Goldring (Eds.), *Evolving explanations of development: Ecological approaches to organism–environment systems* (pp. 457–507). Washington, D.C.: American Psychological Association.

Moffitt, T. E., Caspi, A., & Rutter, M. (2005). Strategy for investigating interactions between measured genes and measured environments. *Archives of General Psychiatry, 62,* 473–481.

Moffitt, T. E., Caspi, A., & Rutter, M. (2006). Measured gene–environment interactions in psychopathology: Concepts, research strategies, and implications for research, intervention, and public understanding of genetics. *Perspectives on Psychological Science, 1,* 5–27.

Moore, D. S. (2002). *The dependent gene: The fallacy of "nature" vs. "nurture."* New York: W. H. Freeman.

Morange, M. (2001). *The misunderstood gene.* Cambridge, MA: Harvard University Press.

Morgan, C. L. (1895). *An introduction to comparative psychology.* London: Walter Scott.

Morgan, J. I., & Curran, T. (1989). Stimulus–transcription coupling in neurons: Role of cellular immediate-early genes. *Trends in Neurosciences, 12,* 459–462.

Morgan, J. I., & Curran, T. (1991). Stimulus-transcription coupling in the nervous system: Involvement of the inducible proto-oncogenes *fos* and *jun. Annual Review of Neuroscience, 14,* 421–451.

Moss, L. (2003). *What genes can't do.* Cambridge, MA: MIT Press.

Nelson, D.A., Marler, P., & Palleroni, A. (1995). A comparative approach to vocal learning: Intraspecific variation in the learning process. *Animal Behaviour, 50,* 83–97.

Newson, A . (2004). The nature and significance of behavioural genetic information. *Theoretical Medicine, 25,* 89–111.

Noble, D. (2006). *The music of life: Biology beyond the genome.* Oxford: Oxford University Press.

Oppenheim, R. W. (1982). Preformation and epigenesis in the origins of the nervous system and behavior: Issues, concepts, and their history. In P. P. G. Bateson & P. H. Klopfer (Eds.), *Perspectives in ethology* (Vol. 5, pp. 1–100). New York: Plenum Press.

Oppenheim, R. W. (1992). Pathways in the emergence of developmental neuroethology: Antecedents to current views of neurobehavioral ontogeny. *Journal of Neurobiology, 23,* 1370–1403.

Oyama, S. (1982). A reformulation of the idea of maturation. In P. P. G. Bateson & P. H. Klopfer (Eds.), *Perspectives in ethology* (Vol. 5, pp. 101–131). New York, Plenum Press.

Oyama, S. (1985). *The ontogeny of information: Developmental systems and evolution.* Cambridge: Cambridge University Press.

Oyama, S. (2000). *The ontogeny of information: Developmental systems and evolution,* 2nd edition. Durham, NC: Duke University Press.

Oyama, S., Griffiths, P. E., & Gray, R. D. (2001a). Introduction: What is developmental systems theory? In S. Oyama, P. E. Griffiths, & R. D. Gray (Eds.), *Cycles of contingency: Developmental systems and evolution* (pp. 1–23). Cambridge, MA: MIT Press.

Oyama, S., Griffiths, P. E., & Gray, R. D. (2001b). *Cycles of contingency: Developmental systems and evolution.* Cambridge, MA: MIT Press.

Paley, W. (1848). *Natural theology.* New York: American Tract Society.

Pearce, J. M., & Boulton, M. E. (2001). Theories of associative learning in animals. *Annual Review of Psychology, 41,* 169–211.

Petersohn, D., Schoch, S., Brinkmann, D. R., & Thiel, G. (1995). The human synapsin II gene promotor: Possible role for the transcription factors zif268/egr-1, polyoma enhancer activator 3, and AP2. *Journal of Biological Chemistry, 270,* 24361–24369.

Pfenning, A. R., Schwartz, R., & Barth, A. L. (2007). A comparative genomics approach to identifying the plasticity transcriptome. *BMC Neuroscience* 8(20). Retrieved August 7, 2007, from http://www.biomedicalcentral.com/1471–2202/8/20

Reed, E. S. (1996). *Encountering the world: Towards an ecological psychology.* New York: Oxford University Press.

Rescorla, R. A., & Holland, P. C. (1982). Behavioral studies of associative learning in animals. *Annual Review of Psychology, 33,* 265–308.

Ribeiro, S., & Mello, C. V. (2000). Gene expression and synaptic plasticity in the auditory forebrain of songbirds. *Learning and Memory, 7,* 235–243.

Richards, R. J. (1981). Instinct and intelligence in British natural theology: some contributions to Darwin's theory of the evolution of behavior. *Journal of the History of Biology, 14,* 193–230.

Richards, R. J. (1987). *Darwin and the emergence of evolutionary theories of mind and behavior.* Chicago: University of Chicago Press.

Ridley, M. (2003). *Nature via nurture: Genes, experience, and what makes us human.* New York: Harper Collins.

Romanes, G. J. (1884). *Mental evolution in animals. With a posthumous essay on instinct, by Charles Darwin.* New York: Appleton.

Rose, S. P. R. (1967). Changes in visual cortex on first exposure of rats to light: Effect on incorporation of tritiated lysine into protein. *Nature, 215,* 253–255.

Rose, S. P. R. (1991). How chicks make memories: the cellular cascade from c-fos to dendritic remodeling. *Trends in Neurosciences, 14,* 390–397.

Routtenberg, A., & Rekart, J. L. (2005). Post-translational protein modification as the substrate for long-lasting memory. *Trends in Neurosciences, 28,* 12–19.

Schaffner, K. F. (1998). Genes, behavior, and developmental emergentism: One process, indivisible? *Philosophy of Science, 65,* 209–252.

Schneirla, T. C. (1949). Levels in the psychological capacities of animals. In R. W. Sellars, V. J. McGill, & M. Farber (Eds.), *Philosophy for the future* (pp. 243–286). New York: Macmillan.

Schneirla, T. C. (1956). Interrelationships of the "innate" and the "acquired" in instinctive behavior. In P. P. Grassé (Ed.), *L'Instinct dans le comportement des animaux et de l'homme* (pp. 387–452). Paris: Masson.

Seligman, M. E. P. (1970). On the generality of the laws of learning. *Psychological Review, 77,* 406–418.

Shanahan, M. J., & Hofer, S. M. (2005). Social context in gene-environment interactions: Retrospect and prospect. *Journal of Gerontology, 60B,* 65–76.

Shaw, C.A., Lanius, R. A., & van den Doel, K. (1994). The origin of synaptic neuroplasticity: Crucial molecules or a dynamical cascade? *Brain Research Reviews, 19,* 241–263.

Shettleworth, S. J. (1972). Constraints on learning. *Advances in the Study of Behavior, 4,* 1–68.

Skinner, B. F. (1966). Phylogeny and ontogeny of behavior. *Science, 153,* 1205–1213.

Sterelny, K. (2001). Niche construction and the extended replicator. In S. Oyama, P. E. Griffiths, & R. D. Gray (Eds.), *Cycles of contingency: Developmental systems and evolution* (pp. 333–349). Cambridge, MA: MIT Press.

Sterelny, K., Smith, K., & Dickison. M. (1996). The extended replicator. *Biology and Philosophy, 11,* 377–403.

Steward, O., & Schuman, E. M. (2001). Protein synthesis at synaptic sites on dendrites. *Annual Review of Neuroscience, 24,* 299–325.

Sutton, M. A., & Schuman, E. M. (2006). Dendritic protein synthesis, synaptic plasticity, and memory. *Cell, 127,* 49–58.

Thelen, E. (1995). Motor development: A new synthesis. *American Psychologist, 50,* 79–95.

Thelen, E., Kelso, J. A. S., & Fogel, A. (1987). Self-organizing systems and infant motor development. *Developmental Review, 7,* 39–65.

Thiel, G., Schoch, S., & Petersohn, D. (1994). Regulation of *synapsin 1* gene expression by the zinc finger transcription factor zif268/egr-1. *Journal of Biological Chemistry, 269,* 15294–15301.

Thorndike, E. L. (1898). Animal intelligence: An experimental study of the associative process in animals. *Psychological Review (Monograph Supplement), 2(4),* 1–109.

Thorndike, E. L. (1911). *Animal intelligence.* New York: MacMillan.

Tinbergen, N. (1951). *The study of instinct.* Oxford: Oxford University Press.

Tolman, E. C. (1922). Can instincts be given up in psychology? *Journal of Abnormal and Social Psychology, 17,* 139–152.

Tomaszycki, M. L., Sluzas, E. .M, Sundberg, K. A., Newman, S. W., & DeVoogd, T. J. (2006). Immediate early gene (*ZENK*) responses to song in juvenile female and male zebra finches: Effects of rearing environment. *Journal of Neurobiology, 66,* 1175–1182.

Uphouse, L. L., & Bonner, J. (1975). Preliminary evidence for effects of environmental complexity on hybridization of rat-brain RNA to rat unique DNA. *Developmental Psychobiology, 8,* 171–178.

Velho, T. A. F., Pinaud, R., Rodrigues, P. V., & Mello, C. V. (2005). Co-induction of activity-dependent genes in songbirds. *European Journal of Neuroscience, 22,* 1667–1678.

Wallace, C. J. A. (1993). The curious case of protein splicing: Mechanistic insights suggested by protein semisynthesis. *Protein Science, 2,* 697–705.

Wang, H. D., & Tiedge, H. (2004). Translational control at the synapse. *Neuroscientist, 10,* 456–466.

Watson, J. B. (1924). *Behaviorism.* New York: W. W. Norton & Co.

Watson, J. D., & Crick, F. H. C. (1953). A structure for deoxyribose nucleic acid. *Nature, 171,* 737–738.

Werker, J. F., & Tees, R. C. (1999). Influences on infant speech processing: Toward a new synthesis. *Annual Review of Psychology*, *50*, 509–535.

Witty, P. A., & Lehman, H. C. (1933). The instinct hypothesis versus the maturation hypothesis. *Psychological Review*, *40*, 33–59.

Notes

1   The limitations of analyses of learning that rely on artificial laboratory paradigms were also identified in the so-called "biological boundaries" approach to learning that advocated more naturalistic experimental designs (e.g., Seligman, 1970; Shettleworth, 1972).

2   Aslin (1981, Figure 2.2) also identified maturation as a sixth role of experience, but since he defined maturation as the case in which experience has no influence, there is no justification for also describing it as a role of experience. An experiment showing that a particular experience has no influence on the development of some behavior is simply a null result, with all of the interpretative difficulties posed by such results.

3   The results summarized in this section are drawn primarily from research on the zebra finch (*Taeniopygia guttata*).

There are interesting and important species differences in the way in which song develops (e.g., Nelson, Marler, & Palleroni, 1995), and genetic correlates of song development have also been studied in song sparrows, hummingbirds, starlings, and a few other species (Clayton, 2004). However, insufficient data are available to draw many useful inferences about species differences at present.

4   In a semiautobiographical essay written just a few years before his death, Gottlieb (2001, pp. 45–46) described how he tried, in about 1965, to get a neurobiologist colleague to compare RNA and protein levels in the brains of normally reared ducklings with those in ducklings that had been devocalized and raised in auditory isolation. That he made this attempt even before the earliest publications on experiential effects on RNA and protein production by Grouse and his colleagues (Grouse et al., 1978; Grouse, Schrier, & Nelson, 1979) suggests the extent to which his probabilistic epigenesis, one of the precursors of DST, allowed him to encompass the kinds of reciprocal gene–experience interactions that have only recently been clearly and conclusively demonstrated.

Rethinking Epigenesis and Evolution in Light of Developmental Science

Robert Lickliter *and* Hunter Honeycutt

Abstract

The dynamic and contingent nature of development revealed by work in developmental biology, neuroscience, and developmental psychology has challenged the notion of genes as the primary cause of development and renewed interest in the nature of the relations between developmental and evolutionary processes. To situate this shift in thinking currently underway across the life sciences, this chapter provides an overview of the ideas used to explain the connection between development and evolution over the last several centuries. It critiques several of these enduring ideas in light of recent findings from developmental and evolutionary science, particularly the notions that instructions for building organisms reside in their genes, that genes are the exclusive vehicles by which these instructions are transmitted from one generation to the next, and that there is no meaningful feedback from the environment to the genes.

Keywords: genes, development, developmental processes, evolutionary processes, environment

How individual organisms develop and how lineages of organisms evolve remain among the most interesting and challenging topics of investigation in contemporary biology. To anyone unfamiliar with the history of theorizing on these topics, it might seem natural to presume that knowledge of developmental processes would be necessary to understand evolutionary processes. Indeed, this supposition was widely held by biologists for much of the nineteenth century (including Charles Darwin), only to be abandoned by the dominant school of evolutionary theory (the "modern" or "neo-Darwinian" synthesis) in the twentieth century. Attempts to integrate Darwin's theory of evolution by natural selection with Mendel's theory of genetics during the first half of the twentieth century gave rise to the science of population genetics, whose proponents assumed that knowledge of developmental processes was superfluous to understanding the ways and means of evolution.

The split between development and evolution evident in the writings of the architects of the so-called Modern Synthesis of evolutionary biology (e.g., Dobzhansky, 1937; Mayr, 1942; Simpson, 1944) was achieved by stripping developmental processes of any meaningful role in bringing about evolutionary change. Development was described as being "programmed" in the genes (Mayr, 1988) and any evolutionarily significant changes in this program for development were thought to be complete at fertilization, prior to the onset of individual development (Simpson, 1967). Viewing development as the result of preformed programs encoded in the organism's genes permitted evolutionary biologists to effectively sidestep developmental questions and instead focus their conceptual and empirical efforts on a population-level perspective of evolutionary change. This population-level focus advanced our understanding of speciation, selection, and the spread of traits in populations (e.g., Mayr, 1982). Moreover, the priority assigned to genes in development and evolution unified much of biology around the goal of understanding gene structure, function, and transmission.

Despite the significant advances in genetics, molecular biology, and cellular biology achieved in the last half of the twentieth century, it has become clear to a growing number of life scientists that understanding development or evolution simply in terms of genes is implausible. An increased appreciation of the dynamic, contingent, and complex nature of development revealed by work in developmental biology and developmental psychology has led a number of investigators to challenge the established notion of genes as the primary cause of development and to reexamine the nature of the relations between developmental and evolutionary processes. To situate this shift in thinking currently underway across the life sciences, in this chapter, we provide an overview of the ideas and principles that have been applied to explain the connection between development and evolution over the course of the last several centuries. We then critique several of these enduring principles in light of recent findings from developmental and evolutionary science. We conclude with a discussion of the dividends of reintegrating developmental and evolutionary inquiry.

Accounting for the Phenomenon of Development

The process of development involves progression from simpler to a more complex organization, repeatedly bringing into being structures and responses of the organism that were not there before. As the developmental psychologists Linda Smith and Esther Thelen put it, "development is about creating something more from something less" (2003, p. 343). This pattern of increasing complexity across individual development has been appreciated since at least the time of the ancients Greeks, particularly in the work of Aristotle (388–322 B.C.), and came to be referred to as *epigenesis*. To the Greeks, the term *epi* (upon, on top of) *genesis* (origin) referred to that idea that embryos gradually develop by the successive formation of new parts. Development was viewed as the emergence of new

characters and traits in an organized embryo from a relatively unstructured egg.

This view of development was in sharp contrast to an opposing framework of development also evident among the ancients, *preformationism*. One proponent of preformationistic thinking was Hippocrates (460–370 B.C.), who like many of his contemporaries proposed that all structures of the adult organism were present in the fertilized egg. In this view, development was seen as merely the growth of a preformed miniature and did not require significant qualitative change or an increase in overall complexity during the course of the individual's lifetime. For example, Anaxagoras (499–428 B.C.) proposed that all parts of the child were preformed in the paternal semen. Various versions of this "morphological" preformationism persisted across the centuries (see Richards, 1992; Roe, 1981) but are now removed from scientific thinking about development and evolution.

Morphological preformationism was largely abandoned due to evidence provided by the experimental efforts of a small group of nineteenth century embryologists. Building on the earlier work of the epigenesist Casper Wolff (1722–1794), who challenged the validity of morphological preformationism by careful descriptions of chick embryo development, experiments and observations of nineteenth century embryologists combined to make it clear that the progression from relatively simple egg to fully formed adult occurs in a temporal and spatial coordination of processes and events, with one stage of complexity leading to the next (see Gottlieb, 1992, Moore, 1993 for overviews). For example, a butterfly begins life as an egg, emerges as a caterpillar, and then undergoes a complete change in body form during pupal development, emerging as an adult butterfly. A monkey begins life as an egg, then reorganizes into a zygote, embryo, fetus, infant, juvenile, and eventually adult monkey. Karl Ernst von Baer's discovery of the mammalian egg in 1827 allowed him to experimentally confirm an idea proposed by Aristotle, some 2,100 years earlier, that the animal embryo develops from a relatively undifferentiated state to a highly differentiated one. His detailed descriptions of embryological sequences provided an initial map of the process of differentiation and set the stage for the growth of experimental embryology in the second half of the nineteenth century.

These advances in embryology (inspired in part by the availability of better microscopes) effectively dismissed the plausibility of morphological preformationism. They did not, however, eliminate preformationistic thinking from the life sciences. Since its inception, the notion of epigenesis had struggled with a daunting and enduring problem: If the egg is relatively unstructured, what could account for the continuity and species-specificity of development within any given species? For example, we all know and expect that the fertilized eggs of a chicken will produce more chickens (and not turkeys) and those of a mouse will produce other mice (and not hamsters). Further, assuming the absence of preformed structures, where does the increasing complexity and differentiation of form and function observed as the egg divides and grows come from? Efforts at answering these difficult questions by the epigenesists of the eighteenth and nineteenth centuries typically led to appeals to an *élan vital*, some ethereal vital force that was thought to animate and direct the transformation of the embryo into an adult (also called *vis essentialis* or *essential nature*, see Gould, 1977; Mayr, 1982 for overviews). However, epigenesists could not explain what this mysterious force was or why it was so specific for each different species. As a result, the notion of epigenesis was again challenged by a new form of preformationism, one that had its roots in the eighteenth century and gained considerable strength by the turn of the twentieth century.

Material Predispositions for Developmental Outcomes

Morphological preformationism was only one of several variants of preformationistic thought entertained during the Enlightenment. The preformationist Charles Bonnet (1720–1793), for instance, did not believe a miniature adult existed in the germ cells. Instead, he proposed the idea (which we will henceforth call "potential" preformationism) that all the adult parts of an organism are represented in the germ as elementary particles, which corresponded to the parts of the adult and directed their development and growth (also referred to as "predelineation," see Russell, 1930). From this view, what were preformed were not the actual parts of the organism in miniature, but rather organic particles that corresponded to and determined the growth of the parts. Even though Bonnet's notion of potential preformationism fell out of favor during his lifetime (due in part to the arguments of the epigenesist Caspar Wolff), his ideas anticipated a view of development and heredity that was to become widely embraced in the nineteenth and twentieth centuries.

As a case in point, Charles Darwin struggled for much of his career with how to account for the fact that "like begets like" and eventually settled on the notion of *pangenesis* to explain the inheritance of traits and the guidance of development across generations. Darwin's theory of pangenesis held that as the cells of the body grow and divide during the various stages of development, they release very small invisible particles, called gemmules, which disperse throughout the developing organism's body. As the individual matures, these very small particles, contributed by different cells from all parts of the body, were thought to flow throughout the body in the bloodstream and become concentrated in the sex cells (egg and sperm). At reproduction, the gemmules that had collected in the germ cells were passed on to the offspring, thereby allowing for the fertilized embryo to contain the basic cellular ingredients for the specific features of all its organs and body parts. Darwin assumed that there was a gemmule corresponding to every trait and that was specific to only one trait. These and other details and mechanisms of Darwin's theory of pangenesis were widely debated following the publication of his *Variation of Animals and Plants Under Domestication* in 1868, but received little support from experimental embryology. For example, Francis Galton (Darwin's cousin) injected the blood of white-furred rabbits (which presumably contained gemmules for white fur) into gray-furred rabbits (and vice versa) and found that these injections had no influence on the fur color of their offspring. The lack of experimental support for gemmules, as well as the challenges presented by advances in cell theory during the latter half of the nineteenth century, led to the eventual demise of Darwin's pangenesis theory. However, the basic idea underlying Darwin's notion of pangenesis that heredity involved germinal substance transmission from generation to generation continued to grow in popularity across the next several decades.

Indeed, by the end of the nineteenth century, many prominent biologists argued that heredity must involve the transmission of germinal substances. These substances were referred to as "determinants" by August Weismann, "pangenes" by Hugo DeVries, "plastidules" by Ernst Haeckel, "physiological units" by Herbert Spencer, and "stirps" by Francis Galton. The influential writings of these and other popular biologists of the day fueled an almost obsessive search to locate the elusive substance of heredity (see Churchill, 1987). This search for the material basis of heredity gained additional momentum upon the rediscovery of the experimental work of Gregor Mendel at the turn of the twentieth century.

Mendel's research on the laws of inheritance in garden peas (resurrected some four decades after its initial publication in 1865) suggested to him that heredity came packaged in discrete units that were combinable in predictable ways. Mendel proposed that each of these discrete units or factors was associated with a particular phenotypic trait or character. Further, he proposed that each character was represented in the fertilized egg by two factors, one derived from the father and the other from the mother. Mendel's research thus provided a basis for a conceptual dichotomy between the characters and qualities of individual organisms and the factors or "units" of heredity that passed from parent to offspring in the process of reproduction. This dichotomy was eventually formalized into the terms "genotype" (the total repertoire of hereditary units acquired at conception) and "phenotype" (the appearance and function of the individual organism).

During the early years of the twentieth century, a growing cadre of prominent biologists (including Hugo de Vries, William Bateson, and Thomas Hunt Morgan) were busy using Mendel's proposed principles to solidify the view that heredity (and the resulting stability and variability of traits and qualities observed across generations) involved the passing on of discrete internal factors situated somewhere in the structure of fertilized cells. These internal factors were termed "genes" by the Danish botanist Wilhelm Johannsen in 1909 and soon came to be seen by most biologists as the (still unknown) physical units that determined the development of the physical appearance and behavioral characteristics of all organisms.

This gene-based version of potential preformationism came to dominate thinking about development in the life sciences during the twentieth century, contributing to the formulation of the Modern Synthesis of evolutionary biology (the attempt to integrate Darwin's theory of evolution with Mendel's theory of genetics) during the first half of the century and facilitating significant advances in genetics and molecular and cellular biology in the second half of the century. Many of these advances, however, challenged the viability of strict versions of potential preformationism. For example, close correspondences between particular genes and particular phenotypes were found to be exceptional rather than typical. Moreover, new types of genes were identified that made up a large portion of the genome and did not seem to code for any products or traits, but instead regulated the activity of other genes.

Such findings from molecular and cellular biology gradually ushered in a more epigenetic (but still decidedly preformationistic) metaphor in biology's vernacular, the "genetic program." As the philosopher Jason Robert pointed out: "in modern incarnations of preformationism, miniature encapsulated adults or their parts have been replaced by coded information or instructions contained within a genetic program, executed epigenetically" (2004, p. 40). This view of the epigenetic execution of preformed programs was termed *predetermined epigenesis* by Gottlieb (1970). The basic assumptions of this framework are captured in a quote from the prominent evolutionary biologist Ernst Mayr: "The process of development, the unfolding phenotype, is epigenetic. However, development is also preformationist because the zygote contains an inherited genetic program that largely determines the phenotype" (1997, p.158).

On this view, genes acquired at conception both orchestrate an organism's growth and development and provide for the intergenerational stability and variability of traits and qualities observed within species (see Keller, 2000; Sapp, 2003 for overviews). Nongenetic factors such as hormones, diet, or social interactions simply support or activate the developmental programs prespecified in the individual's genome. This dualistic causal framework was the established view for many decades in evolutionary biology (Dobzhansky, 1937; Fisher, 1930; Mayr, 1942; Simpson, 1944; Williams, 1966), molecular and cellular biology (Bonner, 1965; Gehring, 1998; Jacob, 1977), and ethology and animal behavior (Hamilton, 1964; Lorenz, 1965; Wilson, 1975), to highlight but a few prominent examples.

Rendering Development Superfluous to Evolutionary Theory

The successful split between developmental and evolutionary inquiry achieved by the Modern Synthesis involved linking the notion of predetermined epigenesis with two other related presumptions: (1) genes are the exclusive source of biological heredity and (2) genes are buffered from any effects of the individual's experience during its development. The notion of a barrier between the genes and an individual's activities or experiences during development (*genetic encapsulation*) is usually credited to the influential nineteenth century German biologist August Weismann. Like Darwin, Weismann wrote widely on heredity, development, and evolution (see Johnston, 1995). Also like Darwin (and other influential biologists of the time), Weismann thought that heredity involved particles transmitted from parent to offspring, which he termed "determinants." Unlike Darwin, however, Weismann came to believe that the germ plasm containing these particles (which were passed on to the next generation) was largely sequestered from any influences arising during an individual's development.

Ideologically, Weismann was reacting to the notion of the inheritance of acquired characteristics, an idea that dated back to Aristotle's time and was a popular view of development in the early nineteenth century. The idea of the inheritance of acquired characteristics held that structural and functional changes that stem from direct environmental factors or the use or disuse of organs during one generation could be inherited to some (usually small) extent by offspring. As is well known to many, the inheritance of acquired characteristics was incorporated in Jean Baptiste de Lamark's (1744–1829) theory of evolutionary transformations, which stands as the first major attempt to explain evolution at the level of species. Lamark's writings on the mechanisms of heredity during the early years of the eighteenth century influenced several generations of scientists concerned with evolution, including Darwin. According to Lamark, the activities of individuals in response to the specific demands of their environment often resulted in adaptive changes in anatomy, physiology, or behavior that could be passed on to their offspring.

Darwin and many of his colleagues accepted this view of development and evolution. In his theory of pangenesis, for example, Darwin argued that the type and number of gemmules released by parts of the body reflected the use and disuse of those parts. In other words, body parts that were underutilized would not throw off as many gemmules as other parts of the body, and as a result, offspring would have a relatively underdeveloped corresponding part of the body that had been underutilized in the parent. For Darwin, a full understanding of heredity thus required knowledge of development. If body parts were modified by use or disuse, they produced modified gemmules, which were then passed on to the next generation.

Darwin also grappled with how the timing of environmental effects during individual ontogeny was reflected in the development of descendents (Winther, 2000). He observed "at whatever period of life a peculiarity first appears, it tends to appear in the offspring at a corresponding age, though sometimes earlier" (Darwin, 1859, p. 13). For Darwin, predicting the development of offspring thus required some understanding of the development of the previous generation. In this sense, Darwin can be characterized as a developmentalist, who viewed characters or traits as resulting from changes in the process of individual growth and reproduction (Bowler, 1989). He insisted that all inheritance must be epigenetic, a product of both the transmission and the development of traits (see West-Eberhard, 2003 for further discussion).

Weismann opposed this view of inheritance and set out to disprove it. Unlike Darwin's gemmules (which flowed freely throughout the body), Weismann's "determinants" were strictly contained inside each cell. Further, the type and number of determinants present at conception were thought to remain unchanged throughout the organism's lifetime. Moreover, Weismann argued that there was a complete separation of the germ plasm from its expression in the phenotype. As a result, only changes in the determinants in the "germ line" (contained in the sperm and egg) could contribute to heredity and ultimately to evolution (Weismann, 1889). From this view, the fertilized egg contained all the necessary information for the development of the organism and this preformed information was insulated from any environmental influences occurring during the individual's lifetime. Like most other preformationists, he was convinced that "epigenetic development is an impossibility" (Weismann, 1893, p. xiv). Weismann argued that this was necessarily the case because the separation of the germ cells from all other cells of the body (what he called the "somatic line") occurred so early in the course of the individual's development that what happened to somatic cells over the individual's ontogeny had no opportunity to affect the makeup or activity of the germ cells. This separation between the germ plasm and the somatic cells thus prevented the effects of individual experience from being inherited. Changes in determinants (which came to be termed "genes" following the turn of the century) and any resulting evolutionary change would have to come from somewhere other than an organism's life experience.

The rediscovery of Mendel's work completed this conceptual split between development and heredity that Weismann had put into play (see Amundson, 2005; Winther, 2001 for alternative views of Weismann's perspective on development and heredity). The geneticist Richard Lewontin has highlighted the nature of this split: "the essential feature of Mendelism is the rupture between the processes of inheritance and the processes of development. What is inherited…is the set of internal factors, the genes, and the internal genetic state of any organism is a consequence of the dynamic laws of those entities as they pass from parent to offspring." (1992, p. 137). Widespread acceptance of this view of Mendelism and Weismannism by mainstream biology in the early decades of the twentieth century resulted in developmental issues becoming more and more divorced from evolutionary issues. If genes contained all the necessary information for phenotypic traits and if events during individual development could not directly influence the traits or characteristics of offspring, then any role or influence of development in evolution had to be minimal (but see Baldwin, 1896; Lloyd Morgan, 1896; Osborn, 1896 for early arguments that learned behaviors could affect the direction and rate of evolutionary change).

Over the next several decades, evolutionary biology came to distance itself from its earlier concerns with embryology and embrace the new science of population genetics (see Gilbert, 1994; Gottlieb, 1992 for overviews). Population genetics focused on how genetic mutation, recombination, and selection could lead to changes in gene frequencies found within a population of breeding organisms over generations. It assumed that modification and transmission of genes, directed by mechanisms summarized quantitatively by basic principles of probability at the population level, were the sole source of evolutionary change. Adherents of the population genetics approach virtually ignored the possibility that developmental processes could also be involved in evolutionary change.

This shift in focus away from development, solidified by the Modern Synthesis of evolutionary biology in the 1930s and 1940s, ultimately resulted in a very narrow definition of evolution as "a change in gene frequencies in populations" (e.g., Ayala & Valentine, 1979; Dobzhansky, 1951). This narrow definition of evolution was widely embraced by several generations of scientists and continues to be the dominant metric in the biological sciences for what qualifies as evolution. This established definition of evolution was made possible by accepting three related assumptions about development and heredity highlighted above:

1. Instructions for building organisms reside in their genes (*predetermined epigenesis*).

2. Genes are the exclusive vehicles by which these instructions are faithfully transmitted from one generation to the next (*heredity as gene transmission*).

3. There is no meaningful feedback from the environment or the experience of the organism to the genes (*genetic encapsulation*).

These three assumptions fit squarely within the conceptual framework of population genetics. The architects of the "Modern Synthesis" of evolutionary biology saw no need to integrate disciplines primarily concerned with development (for example, embryology and developmental biology) into their collective attempts to forge a synthesis of the tenets of Darwinism and Mendelism. As a result, discussion of the possible importance of development to evolutionary issues was relatively absent from biological discourse for more than four decades (but see Gottlieb, 1987, 1992; Gould, 1977; Matsuda, 1987; van Valen, 1973; West-Eberhard, 1989 for notable exceptions). This is no longer the case.

Taking Development Seriously

By the last decades of the twentieth century, each of the three assumptions of the Modern Synthesis regarding the role of genes in development, heredity, and evolution (predetermined epigenesis, heredity as gene transmission, genetic encapsulation) was being called into question. Evidence drawn from research in genetics, molecular and cellular biology, developmental biology, comparative and developmental psychology, psychobiology, and the neurosciences began to converge to suggest a view of epigenesis radically different from the gene-centered perspective that had dominated views of development and evolution for most of the century. For example, studies of experience-dependent synaptic pruning and cell death, brain reorganization following insult, and other illustrations of brain plasticity demanded a more dynamic and context-contingent view of epigenesis. As we briefly review below, this alternative view of epigenesis, termed *probabilistic epigenesis* by Gottlieb (1970, 1997), challenged several of the established assumptions of the Modern Synthesis of evolutionary biology (for additional perspectives, see Bjorklund, 2006; Jablonka & Lamb, 2005; Müller & Newman, 2003; Neumann-Held & Rehmann-Sutter, 2006; Overton, 2006; Oyama, 2000; Oyama, Griffiths, & Gray, 2001). In addition, this new view of epigenesis contributed to the coalescence of one of the most rapidly growing fields within contemporary biology, evolutionary developmental biology. Evolutionary developmental biology (often referred to as *evo-devo*) involves a partnership among evolutionary, developmental, and molecular biologists and attempts to integrate our understanding of developmental processes operating during ontogeny with those operating across generations (e.g., Arthur, 1997; Gilbert, 2001; Hall, 1999, 2003; Kirschner & Gerhart, 2005; Raff, 2000).

It is beyond the scope of this chapter to review the emerging themes and tenets of evolutionary developmental biology (see Hall & Olson, 2003). However, given that many psychologists and neuroscientists are likely unfamiliar with how several of the key assumptions of the Modern Synthesis of evolutionary biology are being called into question by recent findings from developmental and evolutionary science, we briefly review current challenges to three of these assumptions. It should be noted that the challenges and questions that arise in our discussion are often similar or overlapping, a result of the recurrent genocentric theme of what still stands as the established explanatory framework for understanding the relations between development, heredity, and evolution (e.g., Alberts et al., 1994; Futuyma, 1998, Stearns & Hoekstra, 2000).

Assumption # 1: Predetermined Epigenesis

The assumption of prespecification, which holds that the bodily forms, physiological processes, and behavioral dispositions of organisms can be specified in advance of the organism's development, lies at the heart of the idea of predetermined epigenesis. As we have seen, this view dominated biological thought over the twentieth century and still remains prominent in some quarters of biology and psychology. This view of epigenesis assumes that phenotypic features preexist in the form of latent information or instructions before they become "realized" during development (Mahner & Bunge, 1997).

The notion that a program or recipe for an organism's traits, characters, and dispositions can somehow be present prior to development is a key metatheoretical assumption of several disciplines within biology and psychology, including evolutionary psychology and sociobiology. Although enormously influential, this established framework has recently been questioned in terms of its adequacy for explaining the dynamics of the developmental process and its varied outcomes (e.g., Johnston & Gottlieb, 1990; Lickliter & Honeycutt,

2003; Michel & Moore, 1995; Moore, 2002, 2003). A growing number of scientists working in genetics, developmental biology, comparative psychology, and the neurosciences are coming to realize that development is not the expression of a preexistent form. Rather, *development is the very process by which form and function is generated and maintained within and across generations* (Ingold, 2000; Oyama, 2000; Robert, 2004). As the astute biologist E.S. Russell (1930) noted more than 75 years ago, the fault of all preformationistic or predetermined theories of development is that they translate the future possibilities of development into "material" predispositions. However, these potentialities are purely virtual and conceptual, not material. They do not exist in gemmules, determinants, or genes. Their actual appearance or realization is entirely dependent on the resources, relations, and interactions that make up the process of development. Simply put, *all* phenotypes are the result of developmental processes.

If instructions for development actually resided somewhere within the fertilized egg, then one should be able to accurately predict specific aspects of the organism's phenotype simply based on the genetic strain from which its egg is derived. In 1958, McLaren and Michie provided a striking challenge to this supposition by demonstrating the context-contingency involved in mammalian skeletal morphology. They transferred fertilized mouse eggs from a strain that had five lumbar vertebrae into the uteri of a strain of mouse that had six lumbar vertebrae. Those embryos that implanted and successfully gestated following transfer developed six lumbar vertebrae rather than five! In this case, knowledge of the genetic (and phenotypic) makeup of the strain was simply insufficient to predict the actual number of vertebrae present in the transplanted embryo. Some years later, the developmental biologist Lewis Wolpert posed the question if "given a total description of the fertilized egg—the total DNA sequence and the location of all proteins and RNA—could one predict how the embryo will develop?" (1994, p. 572). Although still not widely appreciated by many (particularly in the popular media), we now know the answer to this question is *no*, as all development depends on interactions between genes, cells, and the physical, biological, and social environments in which the organism develops.

To illustrate this key point, let us consider the role of embryonic activity on avian skeletal morphology. The fibular crest is a leg bone that connects the tibia to the fibula in most bird species. It allows the force of the iliofibularis muscle to pull directly from the femur bone to the tibia bone. This direct connection between the femur and tibia is important, as it allows the reduction in size of the femur bone seen in birds when compared to mammals. When developmental biologists prevented chicken embryos from moving within the egg during periods of their prenatal development, they found that the fibular crest bone fails to develop (Müller & Steicher, 1989). In other words, embryonic movements appear necessary to induce the development of the fibular crest bone in the chick embryo. No prenatal movement, no leg bone.

Under the normal conditions of prenatal development, the bird embryo is subjected to stimulation from a host of factors, including gravity, amnion contraction, maternal stimulation, and also from self-stimulation of its own muscles, joints, and sensory systems as it moves and positions itself in the egg (or in the case of the mammalian embryo, the uterus). The prenatal environment (and later the more complex postnatal environment) thus provides a range of stimulation and activity that turns out to be essential for normal anatomical, physiological, and behavioral development (see Gottlieb, 1997; Lickliter, 2005 for other examples). In the case of avian skeletal development, the use and exercise of the chick embryo's leg turns out to influence gene expression, the activity of nerve cells and their processes, as well as the release of various neurochemical and endocrine secretions during prenatal development. All of these factors turn out to be necessary resources for the normal development of the skeleton of the young bird.

Moreover, in the case of avian brain development, the coaction of organismic and environmental factors has been shown to induce the patterns of lateralization and forebrain function commonly observed in several precocial bird species. During the later stages of prenatal development, the precocial avian embryo is oriented in the egg such that its left eye (and ear) is occluded by the body and yolk sac, whereas the right eye is exposed to diffuse light passing through the egg shell when the hen is off the nest during the incubation period. The differential prenatal visual experience resulting from this postural orientation prior to hatching facilitates the development of the left hemisphere of the brain in advance of the right and influences the direction of hemispheric specialization for a variety of postnatal behaviors, including visual discrimination, spatial orientation, feeding behavior, and various visual and motor asymmetries (Rogers, 1995). Altering the conditions of prenatal development alters this typical pattern of brain and behavioral development. For example, a left visual bias can be established by experimentally occluding the right eye and stimulating the left eye with light. Likewise, lateralization can be prevented by rearing eggs in darkness or providing light to both eyes in the period prior to hatching (Casey & Lickliter, 1998; Rogers, 1995).

Proponents of the prespecification view of phenotypic traits typically explain such instances of context-contingency in developmental outcomes by claims that environmental factors encountered during individual development simply trigger or activate latent developmental programs. In our view, this line of reasoning does more to obscure rather than advance our understanding of the realization of phenotypes. At the very least, relying on explanations of the phenotype that refer to latent or hidden programs inside the organism sidesteps the issue of development and minimizes the role of the environment, much like the morphological preformationists who argued preexisting adult form in the fertilized egg.

The complex interactions between genes, gene products, and external influences involved in phenotypic development underscores a basic tenet of the probabilistic epigenesis framework—what a gene (or any other developmental resource) does in terms of what it provides the developmental process depends on the organization and relations of genetic and nongenetic factors internal and external to the organism (see Chapter 2; Johnston & Edwards, 2002 for overviews). This complex self-regulating network is comprised of at least three interacting components: genetic material, other components of the cell and cell aggregates, and various environmental and experiential factors.[1] Because of the interdependency and causal contingency within and between these components (and contrary to the established tenets of the Modern Synthesis) *genetic and nongenetic factors cannot be meaningfully partitioned when accounting for developmental outcomes.*

Assumption #2: Heredity as Gene Transmission

The study of heredity is typically synonymous with the study of genetics in contemporary biology, reflecting the longstanding belief that genes are the exclusive vehicles of biological inheritance (Figure 3.1). As discussed earlier, this key

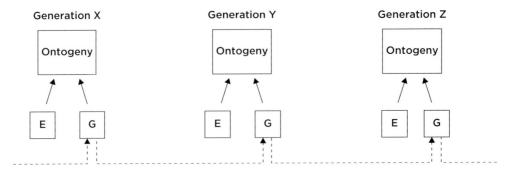

Figure 3.1 Predetermined epigenetic model of development and heredity. Genetic (G) and environmental (E) factors are treated as separate sources of developmental information that combine additively during development. The dashed arrows depict how heredity is characterized as only gene transmission across generations.

assumption of the Modern Synthesis can be traced back to the influential writings of August Weismann in the late nineteenth century and received an additional boost from the experimental work of the geneticist Thomas Hunt Morgan and his colleagues following the rediscovery of Mendel's work in the early years of the twentieth century. Recall that Weismann assumed that if a trait or feature could not be passed on at conception in the germ line, then it could not be passed on at all. This narrow view of heredity became solidified in the writings of the architects of the Modern Synthesis and turned into dogma with the discovery of the double-helical structure of DNA by Watson and Crick in 1953. DNA, transferred from parents to offspring at conception, was the ideal vehicle for reaffirming the strict Weismannian view of heredity (see Mameli, 2005; Sapp, 2003 for further discussion). A new form of potential preformationism thus took center stage in biology and psychology—this time proposing that only one kind of heredity information existed, which is contained in DNA (see Maynard-Smith, 2000 for a recent example).

Thinking on the scope and nature of inheritance has been undergoing a considerable shift in recent years, due in large part to converging discoveries showing that a variety of developmental resources beyond the genes reliably reoccur across generations. Consistent with the probabilistic epigenesis view of development (e.g., Gottlieb, 2003; Gottlieb, Wahlsten, & Lickliter, 2006), there is now considerable evidence that parents transfer to offspring a variety of nongenetic factors in reproduction that can directly influence phenotypic outcomes, including DNA methylation patterns, other chromatin marking systems, RNA interference, cytoplasmic chemical gradients, and a range

of sensory stimulation necessary for normal development (reviewed in Harper, 2005; Jablonka & Lamb, 1995, 2005; Lickliter, 2005; Mameli, 2004). In mammals, where the embryo develops within the body of the female, these factors can include noncytoplasmic maternal effects, including uterine effects (vom Saal & Dhar, 1992).

The McLaren and Michie (1958) study discussed above showing how the number of verterate in mice depends on the uterine environment in which the mice gestate represents a striking example of uterine effects on morphological development. Clark and Galef (1995) have provided evidence that uterine experiences can also have *transgenerational* effects. For example, when a female gerbil embryo develops in a uterine environment in which most adjoining embryos are male, its prenatal exposure to the relatively high level of testosterone produced by its male siblings results in later physical maturation and the display of more aggressive and territorial behavior than that displayed by other females. These testosterone-exposed females go on to produce litters in which the proportion of male offspring is greater than the normal 1:1 sex ratio, and as a result their daughters also develop in a testosterone-rich uterine environment. This results in maternal lineages differing over generations in the sex ratio and behavioral tendencies of the offspring they produce without initial changes in gene frequencies between the lineages. Based on these and similar results documenting how early subtle environmental factors can establish morphological, physiological, neural, perceptual, and behavioral variation between and within sexes, Crews and Groothuis (2005) have argued that patterns of mate choice and sexual and aggressive behavior observed across reptiles, birds, and mammals are best understood in the context of an individual's entire life history, including maternal and other environmental effects at play during the embryonic period, and not simply in terms of the passing on of genes.

A persistent change in any of the networks of coactions involved in the reproduction and maturation of an organism can lead to anatomical, physiological, or behavioral modifications in that individual and in many cases in their offspring as well (see Harper, 2005; Honeycutt, 2006; Jablonka & Lamb, 1995; Moore, 2003; West-Eberhard, 2003 for reviews). As a result, definitions of inheritance that do not include all components of the developmental system that are replicated in each generation and which play a role in the production or maintenance of the life cycle of the organism cannot be complete (Gray, 1992; Lickliter & Ness, 1990; Oyama et al., 2001). In keeping with this insight, Matteo Mameli has recently defined inheritance as "the intergenerational process or processes that explain the reliable reoccurrence of features within lineages" (2005, p. 368). This expanded definition of heredity transmission recognizes that genes *and* recurring nongenetic resources for development routinely pass between one generation and the next (Figure 3.2). Moreover, this definition implies that the scope of what constitutes inheritance cannot complete at the moment of fertilization (see Griffiths & Gray, 1994; Honeycutt, 2007; West, King, & Arburg, 1988 for further discussion).

The developmentalist Susan Oyama (1989) captured this important idea in a discussion of the transmission of developmental means between generations—she includes the genes, the cellular machinery necessary for their functioning, the extracellular environment, and the larger developmental context, which may include maternal reproductive system, parental care or interactions with conspecifics, as well as relations with other aspects of the animate and inanimate world. In some species, these developmental means can be regulated by interaction with other species (see Gilbert, 2002 for examples). For example, several hundred species of symbiotic microbes reside in the gut of mammalian species. Colonization of the digestive system by these microbes begins during or immediately after birth for many species. Many of these microbial colonies aid in important digestive and metabolic functions and some are known to be required for normal gut differentiation and morphology (see Gilbert, 2005 for a review). Further, the inheritance of these microbial symbionts is evolutionarily stable and reliable (Sterelny, 2004) but is not prescribed by the genes of the host species.

It is important to emphasize that such an expanded view of heredity does not imply that genes do not play a necessary and significant role in development, nor does it argue against heritable changes in the phenotype originating in the genotype. The passing on of genes from one generation to the next is not, however, a sufficient explanation for the achievement of any phenotypic outcome (although it is certainly a necessary one). What is passed on from one generation to the next are genes and a host of other necessary internal and external factors that contribute to the development of

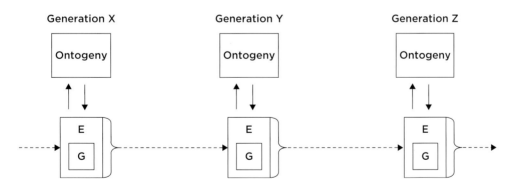

Figure 3.2 Probabilistic epigenetic model of development and heredity. The box containing genetic factors (G) is embedded within environmental factors (E) to represent the developmental system and illustrates that the effects of G and E are interdependent and causally contingent. The dashed arrows running between generations indicate that it is the developmental system that is "transmitted" across generations. The double arrows running between the ontogeny boxes and the developmental system boxes indicate that (1) the information going into ontogeny is itself a product of ontogenetic processes, which makes prespecification impossible and (2) events that occur during one generation can effect the hereditary endowment (i.e., the developmental system) made available to subsequent generations.

an organism's traits and qualities. Contrary to the genocentric assumptions of the Modern Synthesis, the complex and contingent interrelations between these developmental resources are the source of both the *stability* and the *variability* of development, eliminating the need for notions of preformed genetic programs or blueprints.

Assumption #3: Genetic Encapsulation

If one accepts that (1) development is fully contextualized, emergent, and epigenetic and (2) inheritance involves the recurrence of numerous developmental resources across various timescales (and not just genes at conception), then the debate over whether genes are sequestered or buffered during development carries far less significance than in years past. That being said, genes are an enormously important developmental resource, so understanding how, when, and under what circumstances they can be modified during individual development remains an important developmental and evolutionary topic.

Recall that Weismann's "barrier" held that other cells of the body could in no way influence determinants in the germ cells. This barrier was restated and expanded in the so-called central dogma of molecular biology in the mid-twentieth century. The central dogma (proposed by Francis Crick in 1958) held that in all cells (not just germ cells) information always flows outward from DNA to RNA to proteins and never in the reverse order. That is, there is no backtranslation of information from proteins to RNA or back transcription from RNA to DNA. As Gottlieb (1998) has pointed out, the view of genes that emerges from the central dogma is one of genetic encapsulation, in which genes are set off from all nongenetic influences, and a feed-forward information process, implying that genes contain a blueprint that is read out to determine the phenotype of the organism. In other words, genetic causes are different in kind than all other developmental causes (Maynard-Smith, 2000).

The central dogma has been challenged on a number of fronts in recent years. For example, inspired in large part by the pioneering work of the geneticist Barbara McClintock, a great deal of research has been devoted to understanding the extent and effects of transposable gene elements (called "transposons" or "jumping" genes). Transposons have been found in every species of plant and animal studied and they are estimated to make up 40% to 50% of the human genome. These genetic elements can jump from one part of a chromosome and insert itself (or a copy of itself) into the same or other chromosomes, often in response to extreme or unusual environmental conditions. In most cases, transposons are silenced by the process of DNA methylation, in which a quartet of atoms called a methyl group attaches to a gene at a specific point and induces changes in the way the gene is expressed. Different patterns of methylation determine which genes are silent and which can be transcribed. In some cases, jumping genes can influence transcription patterns of neighboring genes. Typically these alterations in genetic activity are detrimental to the organism and transposons have been linked to numerous disorders (Bernstein & Bernstein, 1991; Kidwell & Lisch, 2001). Recently, however, Shapiro (1999) argued that transposon activity can have beneficial effects of potential evolutionary significance.

In any case, the discovery of transposons and other avenues of DNA rearrangement have raised important questions regarding whether the genome is a static and immutable entity during development. The developmental biologist Mae-Wan Ho captured this shift in thinking over two decades ago: "The classical view of an ultraconservative genome—the unmoved mover of development—is completely turned around. Not only is there no master tape to be read out automatically, but the 'tape' itself can get variously chopped, rearranged, transposed, and amplified in different cells at different times" (1984, p. 285).

Advances in molecular, cellular, and developmental biology over the last several decades have also shown that the expression of genes is routinely affected or modified not only by other genes, but also by the local cellular as well as the extracellular environment of the developing organism (reviewed in Davidson, 2001; Jablonka & Lamb, 2005; Gerhart & Kirschner, 1997; Gottlieb, 1998). The inherited microbial symbionts discussed earlier, for example, influence gut differentiation by turning on specific genes that otherwise would not be activated (Gilbert, 2005). Other environmental regulators of gene activity include cell cytoplasmic factors, hormones, and even sensory stimulation provided or denied to the developing organism (Clayton, 2000; Hughes & Dragunow, 1995; Tischmeyer & Grimm, 1999). For example, external environmental factors such as social interactions can cause hormones to be secreted and these hormones result in the activation of DNA transcription inside the nucleus of the cell. Recently, Meaney and his colleagues (Champagne, Francis,

Mar, & Meaney, 2003; Meaney, 2001) have provided examples of how variations in maternal care in rodents can influence gene expression and the transmission of individual differences in stress reactivity across generations. These types of findings have led some to question if genes can really be characterized as occupying a privileged position in the development of an organism, as they are themselves participants in the developmental process, which includes influences and interactions taking place at many hierarchically arranged levels, including nucleus–cytoplasm, cell–cell, cell–tissue, and organism–organism interactions (Gottlieb, 1992; Noble, 2006; Oyama, 2000; Rose, 1997; Solé & Goodwin, 2000).

Recent studies with monozygotic human twins provide dramatic demonstration of how an individual's activity and experience can influence gene expression and activity. Cancer researchers working in Spain found that 35% of 80 sets of identical twins (who share the same genotype) had significant differences in their DNA methylation and histone modification profiles, which are useful markers of patterns of gene activity and expression (Fraga et al., 2005). Twins who spent less time together during their lives or who had different medical histories had the greatest differences. Further, the older the twin pair, the more different they were when compared to younger twins. For example, a 50-year-old pair of twins had four times as many differently expressed genes as did a 3-year-old pair. These findings indicate a significant influence of environmental and experiential factors on gene activity and help explain how genetically identical individuals can nonetheless differ in their phenotypic traits and qualities, a common observation of the parents and friends of twins.

A similar example of this insight comes from medical researchers, who regularly report that only one twin of an identical twin pair will develop a health problem, even when traditional genetics would predict that both of them should. For example, in some pairs of identical twins, only one of the pair develops rheumatoid arthritis. Several genes are known to be overexpressed in individuals with rheumatoid arthritis and a recent study indicates that as yet unknown nongenetic factors influence the expression of these genes. Further, expression patterns can differ significantly between identical twins (Haas et al., 2006). Differences in the expression of these genes can modify DNA activity and in turn modify the severity and symptoms of the disease and the response of the individual patient to various treatment regimes.

It is important to note that the examples we have reviewed above may not occur in DNA in the germ cells (and thus would not violate Weismann's barrier). However, given that inheritance is not complete at conception and that higher-order levels of the organism–environment system are known to control gene activity and expression, it seems to us that this distinction has less import than the Modern Synthesis supposed. For example, evidence is available from both vertebrate and invertebrate species that some environmental events in one generation can have lasting influences on subsequent generations, even in the absence of these environmental events for offspring and later descendents (see Campbell & Perkins, 1988; Harper, 2005; Honeycutt, 2006; Rossiter, 1996). As a case in point, there is an autosomal recessive mutation associated with the development of short antennae present in the Mediterranean flour moth. Pavelka and Koudelova (2001) manipulated the incubation temperature of these flour moth mutants during the early stages of their development. Some were incubated in their typical 20°C incubation range, while others were incubated in a warmer 25°C environment. Although all of the moths in these two incubation conditions carried the short-antennae mutation, those reared in the warmer environment nonetheless developed normal-size antennae. What is most striking about this research is that offspring from these normal-size antennae mutants continued to show normal-sized antennae across the next five generations *even when they were incubated in the original 20°C incubation environment*. A change in the developmental context of one generation was thus able to influence gene expression and phenotypic development across multiple generations of offspring.

These types of findings clearly argue against the view that genes are strictly encapsulated, somehow buffered or protected from any influences occurring during an individual's lifetime. As the philosopher Richard Burian (2005) recently noted, "the context-dependence of the effects of nucleotide sequences entails that what a sequence-defined gene does cannot be understood except by placing it in the context of the higher-order organizations of the particular organisms in which it is located and in the particular environments in which those organisms live" (p. 177). It is now clear that a wide range of nongenetic and environmental factors are key participants in gene activity and gene expression, in some cases well beyond the timescale of individual development.

Reintegrating Developmental and Evolutionary Inquiry

We are a long way from fully understanding development, even in the simplest organisms. Integrating our understanding of development with evolution is an even more daunting task. As Griesemer (2000) has pointed out, existing accounts of evolution and development each tend to "black box" the other: development is typically ignored in transmission-based population genetics and transmission genetics is often ignored in concerns with the developmental dynamics of an individual's phenotype. In our view, any successful integration of development and evolution must ultimately bring these phenomena together to account for (1) the emergence and growth of complexity of organization by differentiation, (2) the stability of structure and function across generations, and (3) the origin and range of variability across individuals of a species. Attempts at this intellectual synthesis have engaged (and frustrated) scientists for centuries. As we have seen, in the twentieth century life, scientists converged on a bottom-up approach to the challenge of accounting for the similarities and differences observed across individuals and lineages, holding that genes were the key to understanding the fundamental characteristics of both development and evolution. We and a growing number of biologists and psychologists believe that this genocentric view is in need of significant revision. At the very least, it is time to take seriously the dynamics of development in discussions of evolution (e.g., Bjorklund, 2006; Johnston & Gottlieb, 1990; Gottlieb, 2002; Ho, 1998; Lickliter & Schneider, 2006; Mahner & Bunge, 1997; Moore, 2003;Overton, 2006; Oyama, 2000; Robert, 2004). West-Eberhard promotes this point throughout her encyclopedic text, *Developmental Plasticity and Evolution*, arguing that: "Any comprehensive theory of adaptive evolution has to feature development. Development produces the phenotypic variation that is screened by selection…In order to understand phenotypic change during evolution, one has to understand phenotypic change during development" (2003, p. 89).

This insight was put forward in the 1980s by the morphologist Pere Alberch (1980, 1982), who realized that development both (a) generates the reliable reproduction of phenotypes across generations and (b) introduces phenotypic variations and novelties of potential evolutionary significance. In the first case, the process of development constrains phenotypic variation such that the traits and characters presented to the filter of natural selection are not random or arbitrary. This is can be viewed as the *regulatory* function of development in evolution. It results from the physical properties of biological materials and the temporal and spatial limitations on the coactions of the internal, external, and ecological factors involved in the developmental process. These constraints collectively serve to restrict the "range of the possible" in terms of phenotypic form and function. The limited number of body plans observed across animal taxa serves to highlight this regulatory role of development. On the other hand, the availability, coordination, and persistence of formative functional and structural influences involved in the process of development can vary across individuals and the dynamics of these developmental interactions can result in modified phenotypic outcomes. This production of phenotypic novelties can be viewed as the *generative* function of development and has significant implications for the sources of evolutionary change (Gottlieb, 2002; Johnston & Gottlieb, 1990; Lickliter & Schneider, 2006).

Contrary to the assumptive base of the Modern Synthesis, a number of evolutionary theorists are now proposing that both intergenenerational stability and the introduction of phenotypic variation upon which natural selection acts are the result of a wide range of epigenetic processes, involving internal *and* external factors contributing to individual ontogeny (e.g., Arthur, 2004; Pigliucci, 2001; Rossiter, 1996: West-Eberhard, 2003). Although phenotypic plasticity has long been considered to be genetically determined (e.g., Mayr, 1942; Via & Lande, 1985), in recent years, developmental and evolutionary biologists have emphasized the necessity of considering the complex interactions between genetics, development, and ecology in order to understand the range of morphological structures, shifts in behavioral repertoires, and other instances of phenotypic plasticity observed across plant and animal species (e.g., Gilbert, 2001; Nijhout, 2003; Schlichting & Pigliucci, 1998; West-Eberhard, 2003). This contingent and probabilistic view of epigenesis sees the novelty-generating aspects of evolution as the result of the developmental dynamics of living organisms, situated and competing in specific ecological contexts, and not simply the result of random genetic mutations, genetic drift, or recombination.

The "genes-eye-view" of life that defined notions of epigenesis and evolution in the twentieth century overlooked the fact that evolutionary theory is ultimately about explaining phenotypes, about explaining how organisms come to be similar or differ anatomically, physiologically, and behaviorally from their ancestors. It is the phenotypic continuity across generations and the plasticity of the development of the phenotype that provides the material for natural selection to act (Alberch, 1982; Jablonka, 2006). Reintegrating developmental and evolutionary inquiry can refocus our collective attention back to the phenotype and provide a new general approach to evolution built around explaining the ways and means of the transgenerational stability *and* variability of phenotypic form and function.

In this light, it is interesting to note that some emerging theories of phenotypic evolution have proposed that changes in the frequency and distribution of genes may often be an effect of evolution (here defined as *enduring transgenerational phenotypic change*) rather than its cause (Gottlieb, 1992; Johnston & Gottlieb, 1990). For example, Gottlieb (1992) argues that changes in development that result in novel behavioral shifts that recur across generations can facilitate new organism–environment relationships and these new relationships can bring out latent possibilities for gene activity and expression, as well as morphological, physiological, or further behavioral change (see also Gottlieb, 2002). Eventually, a change in gene frequencies may also occur as a result of geographically or behaviorally isolated breeding populations. As a case in point, the apple maggot fly has historically laid its eggs on haws (the fruit of hawthorn trees). When domestic apple trees were introduced into their home ranges, maggot fly females began to also lay their eggs on apples. After several centuries, there are now two variants of the maggot fly, one that lays its eggs only on haws and one that lays its eggs only on apples. Because apples mature earlier in the fall than haws, the two fly variants have different mating seasons and thus no longer mate with one another. Further, evidence indicates that this change in developmental and reproductive timing has resulted in observed differences in gene frequencies between the two populations (Feder, Roethele, Wlazlo, & Berlocher, 1997). Thus, changes in behavior can be the first step in creating new phenotypic variants on which natural selection can act. In this view of evolutionary change, genetic change is often a secondary or tertiary consequence of enduring transgenerational behavioral changes brought about by alterations of normal or species-typical development. This epigenetic scenario introduces a plurality of possible pathways to evolutionary change, complementing genetic factors such as mutation, recombination, and drift (see Avital & Jablonka, 2000; Jablonka & Lamb, 2005).

This developmental–relational network of causation is central to the probabilistic epigenetic approach we have outlined in this chapter. It directly challenges the longstanding notion that one can meaningfully separate genetic and environmental influences on development or evolution. Whereas most accounts of development and evolution have traditionally focused on partitioning the organism's phenotypic characters among those genetically determined and those produced by the environment, we argue that no such partitioning is possible, even in principle. All phenotypes have a specific developmental history that explains their emergence, and a developmental mode of analysis is the only method that has the potential to fully explicate the structures and functions of maturing and mature organisms. One important consequence of the developmental point of view is that by placing changes in behavior, context, and development at the forefront of evolutionary inquiry, systematic investigations of the various mechanisms involved in evolutionary change can be pursued at several different levels of analysis (and not simply in terms of population genetics).

Identifying the varied resources, processes, and relations involved in constructing phenotypic traits during ontogenesis and maintaining traits in a lineage over generations will necessarily involve investigators from multiple disciplines. A deeper understanding of the interdependence of development and evolution will require both description and experimentation, with the goal of explaining how one generation and its environments sets up or provides the necessary developmental conditions and resources for the next. In other words, understanding the persistence and change of phenotypic forms over time will require an empirical focus on the activities and resources that generate them. For instance, behavioral scientists can focus on determining how and when organisms change their activity patterns, enter new habitats or inhabit new ecological niches, and how these new activities can be perpetuated across generations (e.g., Yeh & Price, 2004). Physiologists, endocrinologists, developmental biologists, and developmental psychologists can focus on how changes in the activities and ecologies of organisms alter physiological and morphological development in members of a population, and how these changes can be transmitted and maintained transgenerationally (e.g., Crews, 2003).

These types of investigations can include a focus on environmental regulation of gene expression and cellular function and the effects of sensory stimulation and social interaction on neural and hormonal responsiveness, to name but a few examples. These individual-level transformational approaches can be integrated with the group-level, variational approach of population genetics, which has traditionally emphasized the dynamics of selection pressures and the modes of speciation. We are confident that this pluralism of methods, timescales, and levels of analyses will ultimately provide a richer and more complete account of how individuals develop and how lineages of organisms evolve.

Acknowledgments

The writing of this chapter was supported in part by NICHD grant RO1 HD048423 and NSF grant SBE-0350201 awarded to R.L. We thank Bill Overton and Susan Schneider for constructive comments.

References

Alberch, P. (1980). Ontogenesis and morphological diversification. *American Zoologist, 20*, 653–667.

Alberch, P. (1982). The generative and regulatory roles of development in evolution. In D. Mosakowski & G. Roth (Eds.), *Environmental adaptation and evolution* (pp. 19–36). Stuttgart, Germany: Fischer-Verlag.

Alberts, B., Bray, D., Lewis, J., Raff, M., Roberts, K., & Watson, J. D. (1994). *Molecular biology of the cell*. New York: Garland.

Amundson, R. (2005). *The changing role of the embryo in evolutionary thought: Roots of evo-devo*. Cambridge: Cambridge University Press.

Arthur, W. (1997). *The origin of animal body plans: A study in evolutionary developmental biology*. Cambridge: Cambridge University Press.

Arthur, W. (2004). *Biased embryos and evolution*. Cambridge: Cambridge University Press.

Avital, E., & Jablonka, E. (2000). *Animal traditions: Behavioural inheritance in evolution*. Cambridge: Cambridge University Press.

Ayala, F. J., & Valentine, J. W. (1979). *Evolving: The theory and processes of organic evolution*. Menlo Park, CA: Benjamin/ Cummings.

Baldwin, J. M. (1896). A new factor in evolution. *American Naturalist, 30*, 441–451, 536–553.

Bernstein, C., & Bernstein, H. (1991). *Aging, sex, and DNA repair*. San Diego, CA: Academic Press.

Bjorklund, D. F. (2006). Mother knows best: Epigenetic inheritance, maternal effects, and the evolution of human intelligence. *Developmental Review, 26*, 213–242.

Bonner, J. T. (1965). *Size and cycle*. Princeton, NJ: Princeton University Press.

Bowler, P. J. (1989). *The Mendelian revolution: The emergence of hereditarian concepts in modern science and society*. New York: Blackwell.

Burian, R. M. (2005). *The epistemology of development, evolution, and genetics*. New York: Cambridge University Press.

Campbell, J. H., & Perkins, P. (1988). Transgenerational effects of drug and hormonal treatments in mammals: a review of observations and ideas. In G. J. Boer, M. G. P. Feenstra, M. Mimiran, D. F. Swaab, & F. Van Haaren (Eds.), *Progress in brain research* (Vol. 73, pp. 535–552). Amsterdam: Elsevier.

Casey, M. B., & Lickliter, R. (1998). Prenatal visual experience influences the development of turning bias in bobwhite quail. *Developmental Psychobiology, 32*, 327–338.

Champagne, F. A., Francis, D. D., Mar, A., & Meaney, M. J. (2003). Variations in maternal care in the rat as a mediating influence for the effects of the environment on development. *Physiology and Behavior, 79*, 359–371.

Churchill, F. B. (1987). From heredity theory to *Vererbung*: The transmission problem, 1850–1915. *ISIS, 78*, 337–364.

Clark, M. M., & Galef Jr., B. G. (1995). Parental influence on reproductive life history strategies. *Trends in Ecology and Evolution, 10*, 151–153.

Clayton, D. (2000). The genomic action potential. *Neurobiology of Learning and Memory, 74*, 185–216.

Crews, D. (2003). The development of phenotypic plasticity: Where biology and psychology meet. *Developmental Psychobiology, 43*, 1–10.

Crews, D., & Groothuis, T. (2005). Tinbergen's fourth questions, ontogeny: Sexual and individual differentiation. *Animal Biology, 55*, 343–370.

Curtis, W. J., & Cicchetti, D. (2003). Moving research on resilience into the 21st century: Theoretical and methodological considerations. *Development and Psychopathology, 15*, 773–810.

Darwin, C. (1964). *On the origin of species: A facsimile of the first edition*. Cambridge, MA: Harvard University Press. (Original work published in 1859.)

Davidson, E. H. (2001). *Genomic regulatory systems: Evolution and development*. San Diego, CA: Academic Press.

Dobzhansky, T. (1937). *Genetics and the origin of species* (1st ed). New York: Columbia University Press.

Dobzhansky, T. (1951). *Genetics and the origin of species* (3rd ed.). New York: Columbia University Press.

Feder, J. L., Roethele, J. B., Wlazlo, B., & Berlocher, S. H. (1997). Selective maintenance of allozyme differences among sympatric host races of the apple maggot fly. *Proceedings of the National Academy of Sciences, USA, 94*, 11417–11421.

Fisher, R. A. (1930). *The genetical theory of natural selection*. Oxford: Clarendon Press.

Fraga, M. F., Ballestar, E., Paz, M. F., Ropero, S., Setien, F., Ballestar, M. L., et al. (2005). Epigenetic differences arise during the lifetime of monozygotic twins. *Proceedings of the National Academy of Sciences USA, 102*, 10604–10609.

Futuyma, D. J. (1998). *Evolutionary biology* (3rd ed.). Sunderland, MA, Sinauer.

Gehring, W. J. (1998). *Master control genes in development and evolution: The homeobox story*. New Haven, CT: Yale University Press.

Gerhart, J., & Kirschner, M. (1997). *Cells, embryos, and evolution: Toward a cellular and developmental understanding of phenotypic variation and evolutionary adaptability*. Boston: Blackwell Science.

Gilbert, S. F. (1994). Dobzhansky, Waddington, and Schmalhaussen: Embryology and the modern synthesis. In M. B. Adams (Ed.), *The evolution of Theodosius Dobzhansky* (pp. 143–154). Princeton, NJ: Princeton University Press.

Gilbert, S. F. (2001). Ecological developmental biology: Developmental biology meets the real world. *Developmental Biology, 233,* 1–12.

Gilbert, S. F. (2002). The genome in its ecological context: Philosophical perspectives on interspecies epigenesis. *Annals of the New York Academy of Science, 981,* 202–218.

Gilbert, S. F. (2005). Mechanisms for the regulation of gene expression: Ecological aspects of animal development. *Journal of Bioscience, 30,* 101–110.

Gottlieb, G. (1970). Conceptions of prenatal behavior. In L. R. Aronson, E. Tobach., D. S. Lehrman, & J. S. Rosenblatt (Eds.), *Development and evolution of behavior* (pp. 111–137). San Francisco: W. H. Freeman and Company.

Gottlieb, G. (1987). The developmental basis of evolutionary change. *Journal of Comparative Psychology, 101,* 262–271.

Gottlieb, G. (1992). *Individual development and evolution: The genesis of novel behavior.* New York: Oxford University Press.

Gottlieb, G. (1997). *Synthesizing nature–nurture: Prenatal roots of instinctive behavior.* Mahwah, NJ: Erlbaum.

Gottlieb, G. (1998). Normally occurring environmental and behavioral influences on gene activity: From central dogma to probabilistic epigenesis. *Psychological Review, 105,* 792–802.

Gottlieb, G. (2002). Developmental–behavioral initiation of evolutionary change. *Psychological Review, 109,* 211–218.

Gottlieb, G. (2003). Probabilistic epigenesis of development. In: J. Valsiner & K. J. Connolly (Eds.), *Handbook of developmental psychology* (pp. 3–17). London: Sage.

Gottlieb, G., Wahlsten, D., & Lickliter, R. (2006). The significance of biology for human development: A developmental psychobiological systems view. In R. Lerner (Ed.), *Handbook of child psychology, Vol. 1: Theoretical models of human development* (6th ed., pp. 210–257). New York: Wiley.

Gould, S. J. (1977). *Ontogeny and phylogeny.* Cambridge, MA: Harvard University Press.

Gray, R. (1992). Death of the gene: Developmental systems strike back. In P. E. Griffiths (Ed.), *Trees of Life: Essays in the philosophy of biology* (pp. 163–209). Boston: Kluwer.

Griesemer, (2000). Reproduction and the reduction of genetics. In P. Beurton, R. Falk, & H. J. Rheinberger (Eds.), *The concept of the gene in development and evolution: Historical and epistemological perspectives* (pp. 240–285). New York: Cambridge University Press.

Griffiths, P. E., & Gray, R. D. (1994). Developmental systems and evolutionary explanation. *Journal of Philosophy, 91,* 277–304.

Haas, C. S., Creighton, C. J., Pi, X., Maine, I., Koch, A. E., Haines, G. K. III, et al. (2006). Identification of genes modulated in rheumatoid arthritis using complementary DNA analysis of lymphoblastoid B cell lines from disease-discordant monozygotic twins. *Arthritis and Rheumatism, 54,* 2047–2060.

Hall, B. K. (1999). *Evolutionary developmental biology* (2nd Ed.). Dordrecht: Kluwer.

Hall, B. K. (2003). Unlocking the black box between genotype and phenotype: Cells and cell condensations as morphogenetic (modular) units. *Biology and Philosophy, 18,* 219–247.

Hall, B. K., & Olson, W. (2003). *Keywords and concepts in evolutionary developmental biology.* Cambridge, MA: Harvard University Press.

Hamilton, W. D. (1964). The genetical evolution of social behaviour. I. *Journal of Theoretical Biology, 7,* 1–16.

Harper, L. V. (2005). Epigenetic inheritance and the intergenerational transfer of experience. *Psychological Bulletin, 131,* 340–360.

Ho, M.-W. (1984). Environment and heredity in development and evolution. In M.-W. Ho & P. T. Saunders (Eds.), *Beyond neo-Darwinism: An introduction to the new evolutionary paradigm* (pp. 267–289). London: Academic Press.

Ho, M.-W. (1998). Evolution. In G. Greenberg and M. M. Haraway (Eds.), *Comparative psychology: A handbook* (pp. 107–119). New York: Garland Publishing.

Honeycutt, H. (2006). Studying evolution in action: Foundations for a transgenerational comparative psychology. *International Journal of Comparative Psychology, 19,* 170–184.

Hughes, P., & Dragunow, M. (1995). Induction of immediate-early genes and the control of neurotransmitter-regulated gene expression within the nervous system. *Pharmacological Review, 47,* 133–178

Ingold, T. (2000). Evolving skills. In H. Rose & S. Rose (Eds.), *Alas, poor Darwin: Arguments against evolutionary psychology* (pp. 225–246). New York: Harmony Books.

Jablonka, E. (2006). Genes as followers in evolution: A post-synthesis synthesis? *Biology and Philosophy, 21,* 143–154.

Jablonka, E., & Lamb, M. J. (1995). *Epigenetic inheritance and evolution.* New York: Oxford University Press.

Jablonka, E., & Lamb, M. J. (2005). *Evolution in four dimensions: Genetic, epigenetic, behavioral, and symbolic variation in the history of life.* Cambridge, MA: MIT Press.

Jacob, F. (1977). Evolution and tinkering. *Science, 196,* 1161–1166.

Johnston, T. D. (1995). The influence of Weismann's germ-plasm theory on the distinction between learned and innate behavior. *Journal of the History of the Behavioral Sciences, 31,* 115–128.

Johnston, T. D., & Edwards, L. (2002). Genes, interactions, and development. *Psychological Review, 109,* 26–34.

Johnston, T. D., & Gottlieb, G. (1990). Neophenogenesis: A developmental theory of phenotypic evolution. *Journal of Theoretical Biology, 147,* 471–495.

Keller, E. F. (2000). *The century of the gene.* Cambridge, MA: Harvard University Press.

Kidwell, M. G., & Lisch, D. R. (2001). Perspective: transposable elements, parasitic DNA, and genome evolution. *Evolution, 55,* 1–24.

Kirschner, M., & Gerhart, J. (2005). *The plausibility of life: Resolving Darwin's dilemma.* New Haven, CT: Yale University Press.

Lewontin, R. C. (1992). Genotype and phenotype. In E. F. Keller & E. A. Lloyd (Eds.). *Keywords in evolutionary biology* (pp. 137–144). Cambridge, MA: Harvard University Press.

Lickliter, R. (2005). Prenatal sensory ecology and experience: Implications for perceptual and behavioral development in precocial birds. *Advances in the Study of Behavior, 35,* 235–274.

Lickliter, R. L., & Honeycutt, H. G. (2003). Developmental dynamics: Toward a biologically plausible evolutionary psychology. *Psychological Bulletin, 129,* 819–835.

Lickliter, R. L., & Ness, J. W. (1990). Domestication and comparative psychology: Status and strategy. *Journal of Comparative Psychology, 104,* 211–218.

Lickliter, R., & Schneider, S. M. (2006). The role of development in evolution: A view from comparative psychology. *International Journal of Comparative Psychology, 19,* 150–167.

Lloyd Morgan, C. (1896). Of modification and variation. *Science, 4,* 733–739.

Lorenz, K. (1965). *Evolution and the modification of behavior.* Chicago: Chicago University Press.

Mahner, M., & Bunge, M. (1997). *Foundations of biophilosophy.* New York: Springer.

Mameli, M. (2004). Nongenetic selection and nongenetic inheritance. *British Journal of the Philosophy of Science, 55,* 35–71.

Mameli, M. (2005). The inheritance of features. *Biology and Philosophy, 20,* 365–399.

Matsuda, R. (1987). *Animal evolution in changing environments with special reference to abnormal metamorphosis.* New York: Wiley.

Maynard-Smith, J. (2000). The concept of information in biology. *Philosophy of Science, 67,* 177–194.

Mayr, E. (1942). *Systematics and the origins of species.* New York: Columbia University Press.

Mayr, E. (1982). *The growth of biological thought.* Cambridge, MA: Harvard University Press.

Mayr, E. (1988). *Toward a new philosophy of biology: Observations of an evolutionist.* Cambridge, MA: Harvard University Press.

Mayr, E. (1997). *This is biology: The science of the living world.* Cambridge, MA: Belknap Press.

McLaren, A. & Michie, D. (1958, April 19). An effect of uterine environment upon skeletal morphology in the mouse. *Nature, 181,* 1147–1148.

Meaney, M. J. (2001). Maternal care, gene expression, and the transmission of individual differences in the stress reactivity across generations. *Annual Review of Neuroscience, 24,* 1161–1192.

Michel, G., & Moore, C. (1995). *Developmental psychobiology: An integrative science.* Cambridge, MA: MIT Press.

Moore, C. L. (2003). Evolution, development, and the individual acquisition of traits: What we have learned since Baldwin. In B. H. Weber & D. J. Depew (Eds.), *Evolution and learning: The Baldwin effect reconsidered* (pp. 115–139). Cambridge, MA: MIT Press.

Moore, D. S. (2002). *The dependent gene: The fallacy of nature vs. nurture.* New York: Freeman.

Moore, J. A. (1993). *Science as a way of knowing: Foundations of modern biology.* Cambridge, MA: Harvard University Press.

Müller, G. B., & Newman, S. A. (Eds.). (2003). *Origination of organismal form: Beyond the gene in developmental and evolutionary biology.* Cambridge, MA: MIT Press.

Müller, G. B., & Steicher, J. (1989). Ontogeny of the syndesmosis tibiofibularis and the evolution of the bird hindlimb: A caenogenetic feature triggers phenotypic novelty. *Anatomical Embryology, 179,* 327–339.

Neumann-Held, E. M., & Rehmann-Sutter, C. (Eds.). (2006). *Genes in development and evolution: Re-reading the molecular paradigm.* Durham, NC: Duke University Press.

Nijhout, H. F. (2003). Development and evolution of adaptive polyphenisms. *Evolution and Development, 5,* 9–18.

Noble, D. (2006). *The music of life: Biology beyond the genome.* New York: Oxford University Press.

Osborn, H. F. (1896). A mode of evolution requiring neither natural selection nor the inheritance of acquired characteristics. *Transactions of the New York Academy of Science, 15,* 141–148.

Overton, W. F. (2006). Developmental psychology: Philosophy, concepts, methodology. In R. Lerner (Ed.), *Handbook of child psychology, Vol. 1: Theoretical models of human development* (6th ed., pp. 18–88). New York: Wiley.

Oyama, S. (1989). Ontogeny and the central dogma: Do we need the concept of genetic programming in order to have an evolutionary perspective? In M. R. Gunnar & E. Thelen (Eds.), *Systems and development. The Minnesota symposia on child psychology* (Vol. 22, pp. 1–34.). Hillsdale, NJ: Erlbaum.

Oyama, S. (2000). *The ontogeny of information: Developmental systems and evolution* (2nd Ed.). Durham, NC: Duke University Press.

Oyama, S., Griffith, P. E., & Gray, R. D. (Eds.). (2001). *Cycles of contingency: Developmental systems and evolution.* Cambridge, MA: MIT Press.

Pavelka, J., & Koudelova, J. (2001). Inheritance of a temperature-modified phenotype of the short antennae (*sa*) mutation in a moth, *Ephestia kuehniella* (Lepidoptera Pyralidae). *Journal of Heredity, 92,* 234–242.

Pigliucci, M. (2001). *Phenotypic plasticity: Beyond nature and nurture.* Baltimore, MD: Johns Hopkins University Press.

Raff, R. A. (2000). Evo-devo: The evolution of a new discipline. *Nature Review: Genetics, 1,* 74–79.

Richards, R. J. (1992). *The meaning of evolution.* Chicago: University of Chicago Press.

Robert, J. S. (2004). *Embryology, epigenesis, and evolution: Taking development seriously.* New York: Cambridge University Press.

Roe, S. (1981). *Matter, life, and generation.* Cambridge: Cambridge University Press.

Rogers, L. J. (1995). *The development of brain and behavior in the chicken.* Wallingford, UK: CAB International.

Rose, S. (1997). *Lifelines: Biology beyond determinism.* New York: Oxford University Press.

Rossiter, M. C. (1996). Incidence and consequence of inherited environmental effects. *Annual Review of Ecology and Systematics, 27,* 451–476.

Russell, E. S. (1930). *The interpretation of development and heredity.* Freeport, NY: Books for Libraries Press.

Sapp, J. (2003). *Genesis: The evolution of biology.* Oxford, UK: Oxford University Press.

Schlichting, C., & Pigliucci, M. (1998). *Phenotypic evolution: A reaction norm perspective.* Sunderland, MA: Sinauer.

Shapiro, J. A. (1999). Transposable elements as the key to a 21st century view of evolution. *Genetica, 107,* 171–179.

Simpson, G. G. (1944). *Tempo and mode in evolution.* New York: Columbia University Press.

Simpson, G. G. (1967). The study of evolution: methods and present status of theory. In A. Roe and G. G. Simpson (Eds.), *Behavior and evolution* (pp. 7–26). New Haven, CT: Yale University Press.

Smith, L. B., & Thelen, E. (2003). Development as a dynamic system. *Trends in Cognitive Sciences, 7,* 343–348.

Solé, R., & Goodwin, B. (2000). *Signs of life: How complexity pervades biology.* New York: Basic Books.

Stearns, S. C., & Hoekstra, R. F. (2000). *Evolution: An introduction.* New York: Oxford University Press.

Sterelny, K. (2004). Symbiosis, evolvability and modularity. In G. Schlosser & G. Wagner (Eds.), *Modularity in development and evolution* (pp. 490–516). Chicago: University of Chicago Press.

Stiles, J. (2000). Neural plasticity and cognitive development. *Developmental Neuropsychology, 18*, 237–272.

Tischmeyer, W., & Grimm, R. (1999). Activation of immediate early genes and memory formation. *Cellular and Molecular Life Sciences, 55*, 564–574.

Van Valen, L. (1973). A new evolutionary law. *Evolutionary Theory, 1*, 1–30.

Via, S., & Lande, R. (1985). Genotype-environment interaction and the evolution of phenotypic plasticity. *Evolution, 39*, 505–522.

vom Saal, F. S., & Dhar, M. G. (1992). Blood flow in the uterine loop artery and loop vein is bidirectional in the mouse: Implications for transport of steroids between fetuses. *Physiology and Behavior, 52*, 163–171.

Weismann, A. (1889). *Essays upon heredity*. Oxford, England: Clarendon Press.

Weismann, A. (1893). *The germ-plasm: A theory of heredity*. London: Walter Scott.

West, M., King, A., & Arburg, (1988). The inheritance of niches: The role of ecological legacies in ontogeny. In: E.M. Blass (Ed.), *Handbook of behavioral neurobiology, Vol. 9: Developmental psychobiology and behavioral ecology* (pp. 41–62). New York: Academic Press.

West-Eberhard, M. J. (1989). Phenotypic plasticity and the origins of diversity. *Annual Review of Ecology and Systematics, 20*, 249–278.

West-Eberhard, M. J. (2003). *Developmental plasticity and evolution*. New York: Oxford University Press.

Westermann, G., Mareschal, D., Johnson, M. H., Sirois, S., Spratling, M., & Thomas, M. S. (2007). Neuroconstructivism. *Developmental Science, 10*, 75–83.

Williams, G. C. (1966). *Adaptation and natural selection*. Princeton, NJ: Princeton University Press.

Wilson, E. O. (1975). *Sociobiology: The new synthesis*. Cambridge, MA: Belknap Press.

Winther, R. G. (2000). Darwin on variation and heredity. *Journal of the History of Biology, 33*, 425–455.

Winther, R. G. (2001). August Weismann on germ-plasm variation. *Journal of the History of Biology, 34*, 517–555.

Wolpert, L. (1994). Do we understand development? *Science, 266*, 571–572.

Yeh, P. J., & Price, T. D. (2004). Adaptive phenotypic plasticity and the successful colonization of a novel environment. *American Naturalist, 164*, 531–542.

Note

1 In her review of the literature on brain plasticity, Stiles (2000) presents of view of development consistent with the one we present here. In particular, she argues that neural development is "not a passive unfolding of predetermined systems, or even as well defined systems awaiting an external trigger" (p. 266). Instead, "the developing brain is a dynamic, responsive, and to some extent self-organizing system" (p. 266). She also notes that "in the normal course of neural development, specification and stabilization of neural systems relies on dynamic processes that are the product of multidirectional interaction of genetic processes, neural systems, and input" (p. 252). See also Curtis and Cicchetti (2003) and Westermann et al. (2007) for additional examples.

PART 2

Foundations of Neural Development

Brain Development: Genes, Epigenetic Events, and Maternal Environments

Pierre L. Roubertoux, Marc Jamon, *and* Michèle Carlier

Abstract

The major question "What does the genome do in the development of the brain?" includes three subquestions. Firstly, are there genes specifically involved in brain development? The part played by growth factor genes and homeogenes in brain development is reviewed in this chapter. Secondly, given that all the cells of an organism share the same genome, how can differentiated cells emerge from the same genome? The mechanism by which the genes contribute to brain differentiation is examined. Thirdly, individuals have the same genes within the same species. Although their development follows the general pattern of the species, large individual differences can be seen in the rate of development. So which are the genes that contribute to individual differences in the rate of development? Do we know some environmental factors also contributing to these individual differences? A brief survey of existing knowledge is given with the focus on the mouse.

Keywords: genome, brain development, homeogenes, brain differentiation, rate of development, environmental factors, mouse

Development is defined by biological changes that correlate with chronological age. Changes in the morphology, chemistry, and functioning of cells (or part of a cell), of organs, or of the entire organism are indicators of development. Development is measured by comparing the present state to an earlier state. In longitudinal studies, individuals are compared to their own status at different ages, whereas cross-sectional studies compare groups of individuals in different age groups. The measurements are a single index, or a pattern of measurements, that show developmental change, and in all studies, the rate of development is infered.

What does the genome do in the development of the brain? This chapter is not intended to be a state-of-the-art report on genes and brain development. One book alone would not suffice to analyze the 20,000 publications on the topic indexed in PubMed and to discuss the techniques used; that challenge is not taken up here. This chapter is a compromise, presenting the general genetic framework in which brain development occurs described for neurobiologists, psychologists, and psychiatrists who may not be familiar with genetics, embryology, and proteomics.

The study of the genetic bases of brain development addresses questions in three major domains:

1. The brain differs from other organs, such as the liver, which have quite homogeneous cells with similar structure and function; the brain is a collection of structures that differ in their anatomy, morphology, neurochemistry, and in the functioning of the cells that compose the structures. The human

brain has approximately 50 cytoarchitecturally different regions (Broadman, 1909). The amygdala and hippocampus, for example, do not have many cytological, neurochemical, or functional similarities, but operate jointly for learning tasks and exploration. The brain functions in an integrated way. The brain's ability to integrate the activities of different structures is dependent upon the development of structures, and even of substructures, with cytological and functional specificity. This requires a stringent timing in the development process that is the price to pay for the harmonious functioning of the brain. "Which genes control development?" or rather "How do genes control the development of brain structures and how is their development coordinated?" Is the development of a structure controlled solely by endogenous factors, that is genes, or is it jointly determined by exogenous elements such as the neighboring tissue? The general process of development, the succession of steps in development, is invariant within a species, but several characteristics of development are common to all species, suggesting that species-specific genetic programs share common genetic elements. What are the common elements in the genetic bases of the program of development? What do these common bases mean in the context of evolution?

2. Cells go through an undifferentiated stage of development, being first pluripotent and then, after a transitional stage, multipotent. All the cells of an organism share the same genes, and all the cells of a given individual bear the same allelic forms. It is amazing to see that the same undifferentiated stem cells sharing identical genes with identical alleles can become either a neuron or a liver cell. It is even more amazing that the same stem cell can become either a serotonin neuron or a dopamine neuron depending on the cellular context. The challenge of developmental genetics is to uncover the rules of cell differentiation and cell specification. "Is it an intrinsic (i.e., genetic) process or is it an extrinsic (i.e., environmental) mechanism?" In either case, the molecular mechanism of cell differentiation needs to be deciphered. What are the genetic mechanisms that determine the specification of a cell?

3. Individual differences in the rate of development have been reported for a wide range of species. Differences do not occur between the succession of developmental events, with certain exceptions resulting in abnormal and often unviable phenotypes, but individual differences are observed in the rate of development. There is a considerable difference between individuals in the age when an organ reaches maturity, when a milestone of development is reached, when a function becomes operational, and when a childhood pattern disappears and an adult pattern appears. Purebred Basenji dogs display adult behavior patterns at much the same age, whereas cocker spaniels and beagles display the same characteristic at a different age (Scott & Fuller, 1965). Developmental differences in both brain and behavioral characteristics have been observed in strains of laboratory mice. In pediatrics, any departure from development chart averages is a quantitative assessment of an individual difference. Are genes involved in these differences? Are the differences caused by allelic variants of genes regulating development sequences? Which are these genes? Are development factors related to genes? Do epigenetic factors, that is, factors occurring between the DNA template and the protein, contribute to individual differences? What are these epigenetic factors? Do pre- and postnatal environmental events modulate the differences?

The three sections that follow will address each of these major issues concerning the roles of genes in brain development: (1) growth factors and homeogenes, (2) specification of nerve cells, and (3) the origin of individual differences in rates of development.

Growth Factor Genes and Homeogenes

Genes contributing to the development of the brain belong to two main categories: (i) growth factor genes and (ii) genes encoding for transcription factors. The first set of genes could be seen as providing the cellular energy needed for development, while the second set of genes provide the spatial and temporal expression of growth factor genes.

Growth Factors

Growth factors are polypeptides that stimulate cell proliferation and differentiation, and many polypeptides play a crucial role in the development of neurons and glial cells. Transforming growth factor β (TGF-β) is found in cells where it inhibits growth and proliferation. The granulocyte-colony-stimulating factor stimulates granulocytes, bone marrow, and the production of stem cells. The nerve growth factor (NGF) plays a crucial role in the maintenance of sympathetic and sensory neurons. Neurotrophic factors (1) differentiate the progenitor cells that are then transformed into neurons and (2) protect neurons from cell death. Different subcategories of neurotrophic factors have been characterized: brain-derived neurotrophic factor (BDNF) is present in the peripheral and central nervous systems; neurotrophin-3 plays a role in synaptic differentiation and contributes to the development and maintenance of the synapses; neurotrophin-1 (NT-1) interacts with different neurotransmitters; and neurotrophin-4 interacts with tyrosine kinase, initiating cascades in the nerve cell.

The contribution of neurotrophic factors is not limited to neurons but extends to all cells in the nervous system. A glial-derived neurotrophic factor, and its receptor that leads to modifications of ion channel functioning and dopaminergic activity, has been reported. The platelet-derived growth factor and basic fibroblast growth factor contribute to angiogenesis. The epidermal growth factor contributes to cell proliferation by modifying tyrosine kinase activity, resulting in changes in cell calcium levels, glycolysis, and protein synthesis. Hepatocyte growth factor/scatter factor is a morphogenic factor that acts on epithelial and endothelial cells and has an important part to play in organ development. Other growth factors, such as myostatin, erythroprotein, growth differentiation factor-9, and thromboprotein, do not have any direct action on the development of the nervous system. Growth factors, also referred to as "growth hormones," act in a similar manner as hormones with respect to growth factor production, receptor, and binding protein.

Most genes involved in growth factor activities have been characterized; 160 genes have been identified so far. Figure 4.1 shows the chromosomal location of the genes encoding for growth factors in the mouse (*Mus musculus*). The list is temporarily limited to the 69 genes currently known to contribute to brain and peripheral nervous system development. The figure gives the name of the gene and its target nerve tissue. The effects of the genes were identified by using transgenic and gene targeting technologies and by observing mutations in the mouse and fruit fly. Target organs for the growth factors were deduced from the analysis of papers published and referenced on the Mouse Genome Informatics Web site as of March 2007 (Gene Expression Database [GXD], 2007). Each paper cited on the Web site was analyzed and recorded when the results showed direct or indirect involvement in the development of the nervous system.

The number of genes identified as coding for growth factors is surprisingly small (160), too small to be compatible with the hypothesis that one gene could be found to correspond to the development of one given category of nerve cells. The analysis of Figure 4.1 shows that several genes can contribute to the growth of one single type of nerve cell. The growth of each type of cell is thus "overdetermined." This is clearly illustrated by the genes coding for factors that contribute to the development of the hippocampus (*Egr4, Igf1, Egr4, Igf1r, Igf2, Ing1, Sf3b1*) and factors contributing to retinal development (*Fgfrl1, Fgf8, Fgfbp1, Efemp1 Crebzf, Apaf1, Fgfr3-ps*). One gene may have several different target cells; for example, the fibroblast growth factor 17 (*Fgf17*) gene is found in both the inferior colliculus and anterior vermis of the brain.

The relationships between growth factor genes and phenotype is not linear. The first consequence is that the products of growth factor genes affecting development are not specific to a category of tissue. The second consequence is that there is a gap between the huge number of brain and neural functions and the relatively small number of growth factor genes involved in the development of nerve tissue. This is particularly relevant for the discrepancy between the small number of genes carried by the genome and the enormous number of gene-dependent phenotypes. Several nonexclusive hypotheses have been suggested as explanations for this apparent paradox, one being interactions with transcription factors that are also involved in development (Roubertoux & Carlier, 2007).

Transcription Factor Genes

Transcription factors are "interactive factors," which control the expression of other genes and the expression of growth factor genes. Transcription factor genes are a heterogeneous category of genes sharing a common sequence called the "homeobox." Homeobox was first described by a Swiss group (Garber, Kuroiwa, & Gehring, 1983) and an American group from Bloomington (Scott et al., 1983). Three researchers were awarded the Nobel Prize in Medicine in 1995 for their work on the genetics of development (Edward Lewis, California Institute of Technology; Christiane Nuesslein-Volhard, Max-Planck Institute; and Eric Wieschaus, Princeton University).

Transcription is a process by which the DNA sequence is copied into an RNA sequence. The transcription factor either allows or blocks transcription. All homeogenes share a common sequence of 180 bp DNA called the homeobox, coding for the homeodomain. The homeodomain is a protein made up of 60 amino acids in a three-dimensional configuration. The protein

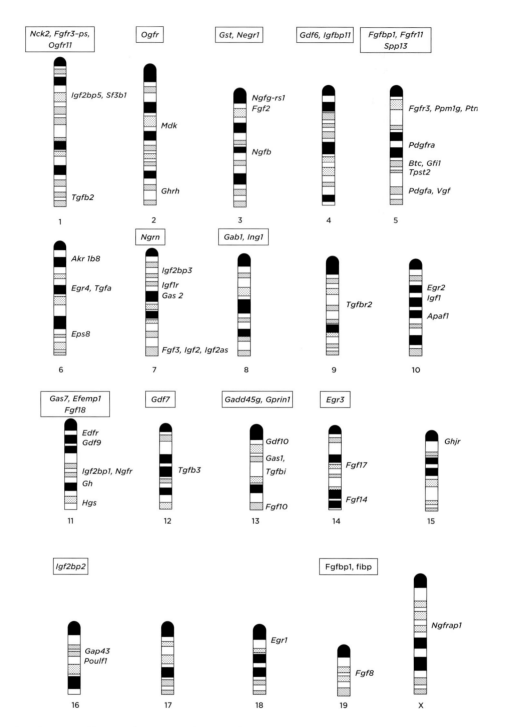

Figure 4.1 Chromosomal location of genes coding for growth factors and contributing to the nerve tissues in mammals. The symbol of the gene is in italics. Symbols, followed by the full names of the genes, and the targets on which the growth factors act, are listed below. Akr1b8: aldo-keto reductase family 1, member B8, aldolase reductase; Apaf1: apoptotic peptidase activating factor 1, retina; Btc: betacellulin, epidermal growth factor family member, gray matter; Crebzf: CREB/ATF bZIP transcription factor, retina; Efemp1:epidermal growth factor-containing fibulin-like extracellular matrix protein 1, retina; Egfr: epidermal growth factor receptor, eye, whisker; Egr1: early growth response 1, luteinizing hormone-beta expression, Memory defects; Egr2: early growth response 2, rhombomeres 3 and 5, myelination of Schwann cells; Egr3:early growth response 3, cell bodies of proprioceptive neurons within dorsal root ganglia; Egr4: early growth response 4, dentate gyrus of the hippocampus; Eps8: epidermal growth factor receptor pathway substrate 8, resistant intoxicating effects of ethanol, Eps8 part of NMDA receptor complex; Egf10: fibroblast growth factor 10, eye; Fgf14, fibroblast growth factor 14, balance and grip strength, Fgf17, fibroblast growth factor 17, inferior colliculus and the anterior vermis of the brain, Fgf17, transforming growth factor, beta receptor II, neural crest, Fgf18, fibroblast growth

includes a coil peptide chain and three α-helices. The three helices are positioned at right angles in space, forming a helix-loop-helix motif. Helix 1 helps stabilize the homeodomain protein during interactions with DNA and binds the sugar–phosphate backbone by entering into the minor groove of the DNA. The homeodomain protein usually recognizes the DNA sequence located within the promoter region; this is done by the third helix, sometimes referred to as the recognition helix, which binds with the TAAT or ATTA patterns of DNA bases of the regulatory sequences of the gene (Wolberger, Vershon, Liu, Johnson, & Pabo 1991; Billeter,1996) by coming within the major groove of DNA (Kissinger, Liu, Martin-Blanco, Kornberg, & Pabo, 1990; see Ades & Sauer, 1995 for the specificity of the grooves).

The gene to be transcribed carries a sequence that must be recognized by the transcription factor. Transcription is initiated by opening of the double helix and separation of the two DNA strands. For transcription to be initiated, the promoter region needs to be recognized by the gene to be transcribed. The recognized region is always inside the promoter region (Gehring, Affolter, & Bürglin, 1994a; Gehring et al., 1994b). The regulating sequences of the promoter are common to several promoters and the specificity of the sequence of recognition is therefore small. Sequences carried in addition to the homeobox improve the transcription factor's recognition capacity (Laughon, 1991). The homeobox is common to all genes encoding transcription factors, while the three-dimensional structure of the protein and its recognition capacities are preserved.

Several families of transcription factors contribute to the development of the brain. The canonical homeobox described above alone defines the Hox domain family. In addition to the canonical homeobox, the Cut, Dlsx, Dlx, Emx, En, LIM, Msx, Nk, Pax, POU, six, and TALE families specify the transcription of genes that contribute to brain development (Dekker et al., 1993; Patarnello et al., 1997; Banerjee-Basu, Landsman, & Baxevanis, 1999;

factor 18, Patterning of frontal cortex subdivisions, Fgf2,, fibroblast growth factor 2, cortical neuronal density, Fgf3, fibroblast growth factor 3, inner ear, Fgf8, fibroblast growth factor 8, thymus, Fgfbp1, fibroblast growth factor binding protein 1, retina, Fgfbp3, fibroblast growth factor binding protein 3, neuronal differentiation in the developing midbrain-hindbrain, Fgfr3, fibroblast growth factor receptor 3, cochlea; Fgfr3-ps: fibroblast growth factor receptor 3, pseudogene, tyrosine kinase; Fgfrl1: fibroblast growth factor receptor-like 1, retina, Fibp: fibroblast growth factor (acidic) intracellular binding protein, intracellular binding protein; Gab1:growth factor receptor bound protein 2-associated protein, eye; Gadd45g: growth arrest and DNA-damage-inducible 45 gamma, cortical patterning; Gadd45g: growth arrest and DNA-damage-inducible 45 gamma, eye; Gap43: growth associated protein 43, olfactory neurogenesis; Gas1:growth arrest specific 1,eye cerebellum; Gas2: growth arrest specific 2, modifier for holoprosencephalon; Gas7: growth arrest specific, PC12 cells; Gdf10: growth differentiation factor 10, neural precursors in cerebellar vermis formatio; Gdf6: growth differentiation factor 6, inner ear; Gdf7: growth differentiation factor 7, spinal cord neurons; Gdf9: growth differentiation factor 9, granulosa cell proliferation; Gfi1: growth factor independent 1, ear, neuroendorine cell; Gh: growth hormone, pituitary gland; Ghr: growth hormone receptor, pituitary gland; Ghrh: growth hormone releasing hormone, pituitary gland; Ghsr: growth hormone secretagogue receptor, growth hormone release; Gprin1: G protein-regulated inducer of neurite outgrowth 1, control growth of neuritis; Hgs: HGF-regulated tyrosine kinase substrate, tyrosine phosphorylation; Igf1: insulin-like growth factor 1, brain size, hypomyelination, hippocampal granule, striatal parvalbumin-containing neurons; Igf1r: insulin-like growth factor I receptor, neuronal proliferation, phosphorylation of tau in the hippocampus; Igf2, insulin-like growth factor 2, interactions with kainic acid; Igf2bp1 I: insulin-like growth factor 2 mRNA binding protein 1, anxiety, exploratory behavior; Igf2bp2: insulin-like growth factor 2 mRNA binding protein 2, neuron; Igf2bp3: insulin-like growth factor 2 mRNA binding protein 3, neuron; Igfbp5: insulin-like growth factor binding protein 5, midbrain, hindbrain; Igfbpl1: insulin-like growth factor binding protein-like 1, neopallium, dorsal thalamus, hippocampus; Ing1: inhibitor of growth family, member 1, apoptosis; Mdk: midkine, glucocorticoid receptor; Nck2, non-catalytic region of tyrosine kinase adaptor protein 2, ephrinB reverse signals modulating spine morphogenesis and synapse formation; Negr1:neuronal growth regulator 1, neurotractin →neurite outgrowth of telencephalic neurons, neurotractin →regulation of neurite outgrowth in developing brain; Ngfb, nerve growth factor, beta, neuron; Ngfg-rs1: nerve growth factor gamma, related sequence 1, sympathetic neurons; Ngfr: nerve growth factor receptor (TNFR superfamily, member 16), sensory innervation, pain; Ngfrap1: nerve growth factor receptor (TNFRSF16) associated protein 1, apoptosis; Ngrn: neugrin, neurite outgrowth associated, neurons; Ogfr: opioid growth factor receptor, opioid growth factor receptor; Ogfrl1: opioid growth factor receptor-like 1; opioid growth factor receptor; Pdgfa: platelet derived growth factor, alpha, numbers of oligodendrocytes; Pdgfra: platelet derived growth factor receptor, alpha polypeptide, neural crest cells; Ppm1g: protein phosphatase 1G (formerly 2C), magnesium-dependent, gamma isoform, prepulse inhibition; Ptn: pleiotrophin, subcortical projection neurons in cerebral cortex; Sf3b1: splicing factor 3b, subunit, hippocampus, cerebellum; Sppl3: signal peptide peptidase 3, hippocampus, cerebellum; Tgfa: transforming growth factor alpha, eye; Tgfb2: transforming growth factor, beta 2, spinal column, eye, inner ear; Tgfb3: transforming growth factor, beta 3, central mechanism of respiration; Tgfbi: transforming growth factor, beta induced, extracellular matrix proteins; Tpst2: protein-tyrosine sulfotransferase 2, tyrosylprotein sulfotransferase; Vgf: VGF nerve growth factor inducible, leptin, proopiomelanocortin, neuropeptide Y, hypothalamus.

Kim, Choi, Lee, Conti, & Kim, 1998). Transcription factors in the Cut domain add three repeated Cut domains to the Hox domain, each of these being defined by 80 amino acids. Cut binds to DNA. The homeobox is longer in the Dlsx and Dlx domain families than in the canonical homeobox. The LIM domain consists of two repeated zinc fingers motifs, resulting in 60 amino acids (Konrat, Weiskirchen, Krautler, & Bister, 1997). The LIM domain appears to initiate protein–protein interactions. The paired box or Pax families are characterized by two extra paired sequences. The paired domain is a 128-amino-acid DNA-binding domain. The POU domain (POU is derived from the names of three mammalian transcription factors: pituitary-specific Pit-1, octamer-binding proteins Oct-1 and Oct-2, and neural Unc-86 from *Caenorhabditis elegans*) is characterized by a 75-amino-acid domain and seems to recognize transcription cofactors (Chu-Lagraff, Wright, McNeil, & Doe, 1991; Andersen & Rosenfeld, 2001).

Most investigations into genetic mechanisms of development have been performed on mice and flies. Most genes coding for growth factors or transcription factor genes are present in all species, including humans. Genes have strong homology, that is, the same DNA sequences are present across species, and genetic homology results in similar phenotypes with similar development mechanisms. A good illustration of this characteristic is found with a mutation affecting the size of the eye in different species

(Cheyette et al., 1994; Chauhan, Zhang, Cveklova, Kantorow, & Cvekl, 2002), including the "eyeless" mutation for drosophila, "small eye" for the mouse, and "aniridia" for humans (Hanson et al., 1993, 1994). Sequencing of the gene showed that they (1) share common sequences, proving that they are homologous and (2) carry a homeotic sequence plus a paired box sequence that are the signature of *Pax* genes (Ton et al., 1991). The gene is called *Pax6* and the phenotypes are similar in different species. Drosophila with the mutation have no eyes or tiny eyes, mice with the mutation have small eyes, and in humans, homozygous cases present aniridia (no iris) and heterozygous cases have small eyes.

Figure 4.2 shows the chromosomal location of transcription factor genes contributing to the development of the brain in the mouse. Table 4.1 lists the nerve tissue where each of the genes is expressed and the nerve tissue where development is modified by the gene. We analyzed the papers referenced by Vollmer and Clerc (1998) and the papers referenced for the period 1997 to March 2007 on the Mouse Genome Informatics Web site (Mouse Genome Database [MGD], 2007) The number of transcription factors producing a modification in brain development is relatively small (80) compared to the total number of transcription factor genes (255). As is the case for growth factor genes, the same tissue is usually targeted by several transcription factor genes and one transcription factor gene targets several different tissues.

---

cluster including Hoxb1-9, homeo box B1-B9. Hoxb13: homeo box B1; Hoxc: homeo box C cluster including Hoxc 4-6, homeo box C 4 - 6, Hoxc 8-13 Homeo box C 8-13; Hoxd: homeo box D cluster including Hoxd1, homeo box D1, homeo box D3-4, homeo box D8-D13; Irx1: Iroquois related homeobox 1; Irx2: Iroquois related homeobox 2; Irx3: Iroquois related homeobox 3; Irx4: Iroquois related homeobox 4; Irx5: Iroquois related homeobox 5; Irx6: Iroquois related homeobox 6; Isl1: ISL1 transcription factor, LIM/homeodomain; Lbx1: ladybird homeobox homolog 1; Lbx2: ladybird homeobox homolog 2; Lhx2, LIM homeobox protein 2; Lhx3, LIM homeobox protein 3; Lhx4, LIM homeobox protein 4; Lhx5, LIM homeobox protein 5; Lhx6, LIM homeobox protein 6; Lhx8, LIM homeobox protein 8; Lmx1a, LIM homeobox transcription factor 1 alpha; Lmx1b, LIM homeobox transcription factor 1 beta; Meis1: myeloid ecotropic viral integration site 1; Meox1, mesenchyme homeobox 1; Mixl1, Mix1 homeobox-like 1, Xenopus laevis; Msx2: homeo box, msh-like 2; Msx3: homeo box, msh-like 3; Nkx1-2: NK1 transcription factor related, locus 2, Drosophila; Noto: notochord homolog, Xenopus laevis; Otp, orthopedia homolog, Drosophila; Otx1: orthodenticle homolog 1, Drosophila; Otx2: orthodenticle homolog 2, Drosophila; Pax1: paired box gene 1; Pax2: paired box gene 2; Pax3: paired box gene 3; Pax4: paired box gene 4; Pax5: paired box gene 5; Pax6: paired box gene 6; Pax7: paired box gene 7; Pax8: paired box gene 8; Pbx3: pre B-cell leukemia transcription factor 3; Phox2a: paired-like homeobox 2a; Phtf1: putative homeodomain transcription factor 1; Phtf1: putative homeodomain transcription factor 1; Phtf2: putative homeodomain transcription factor 2;; Pit1-rs1: pituitary specific transcription factor 1, related sequence 1; Pitx1: paired-like homeodomain transcription factor 1; Pitx2: paired-like homeodomain transcription factor 2; Pitx3: paired-like homeodomain transcription factor 3; Pou3f1: POU domain, class 3, transcription factor 1; Pou3f2: POU domain, class 3, transcription factor 2; Pou3f3: POU domain, class 3, transcription factor 3; Pou3f4: POU domain, class 3, transcription factor 4; Pou4f1: POU domain, class 4, transcription factor 1; Prop1: paired like homeodomain factor 1; Prrxl1: paired related homeobox protein-like 1 (chord); Rax: retina and anterior neural fold homeobox; Six2: sine oculis-related homeobox 2 homolog (Drosophila); Six6: sine oculis-related homeobox 6 homolog, Drosophila; Tgif1: TG interacting factor 1; Tgifx1: TGIF homeobox 1; Tlx3: T-cell leukemia, homeobox 3; Vax: ventral anterior homeobox containing gene 1; Vax2: ventral anterior homeobox containing gene 2; Vsx1: visual system homeobox 1 homolog, zebrafish; Zfhx2: zinc finger homeobox 2; Zfhx2as: zinc finger homeobox 2, antisense; Zhx2: zinc fingers and homeoboxes protein 2.

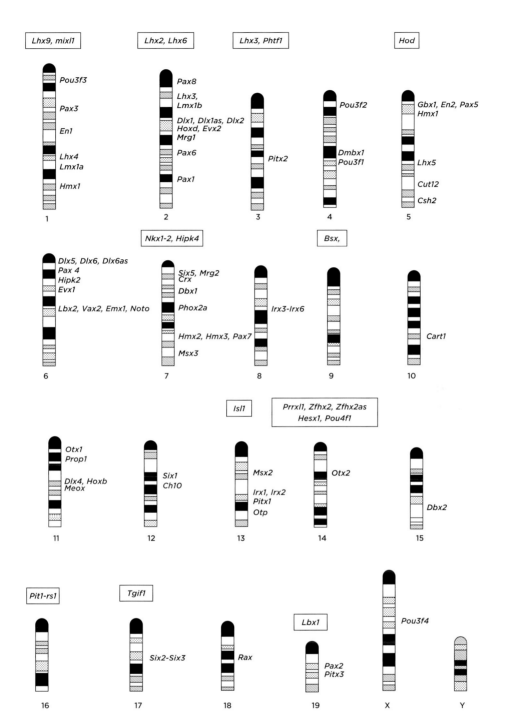

Figure 4.2 Transcription factor genes that contribute to the development of nerve tissue. The symbols for the genes are in italics. Symbols, followed by the full names of the genes, are listed below. Arx: aristaless related homeobox gene; Bsx: brain specific homeobox; Cart1: cartilage homeo protein 1; Ch10: C. elegans ceh-10 homeo domain containing homolog; Crx: cone-rod homeobox containing gene; Cutl2: cut-like 2 (Drosophila); Dbx1: developing brain homeobox; Dlx1: distal-less homeobox 1; Dlx1as: distal-less homeobox 1, antisense.; Dlx2: distal-less homeobox 2; Dlx4: distal-less homeobox 4.; Dlx5:distal-less homeobox 5; Dlx5as : distal-less homeobox 6 antisense; Dmbx1: diencephalon/mesencephalon homeobox 1; Emx1: empty spiracles homolog 1, Drosophila; Emx2: empty spiracles homolog 2, Drosophila; En1: engrailed 1; En2: engrailed 2; Evx1: even skipped homeotic gene 1 homolog; Gbx1: gastrulation brain homeobox 1; Gbx2: gastrulation brain homeobox 2; Gsh2: genomic screened homeo box 2; Hesx1: homeo box gene expressed in ES cells (skeleton, CNS); Hhex-rs3: hematopoietically expressed homeobox, related sequence 3. (blood); Hipk2: homeodomain interacting protein kinase 2; Hlxb9: homeobox gene HB9; Hmx1: H6 homeo box 1; Hmx2: H6 homeo box 2; Hmx3: H6 homeo box 3 (nteraction with Pax2); Hod: homeobox only domain; Hoxb: homeo box B

Table 4.1 Transcription Factor Genes Implicated in Brain Development in Mice

Homeobox Family	Gene	Brain Region of Expression	CNS Target
Cut			
	Cut12	Telencephalon, pons	PNS in Drosophila
Dlx			
	Dlx1	Diencephalon, optic chiasma	Forebrain, striatum (with *Dlx2*)
	Dlx2	Ventral thalamus, undifferentiated neurons	Olfactory central neurons
	Dlx5, Dlx6	Basal ganglia, diencephalon	
Emx			
	Emx1	Cerebral cortex, hippocampus	Forebrain
	Emx2	Cerebral cortex, hippocampus, thalamus, hypothalamus, mesencephalon	Dentate gyrus, limbic cortex,
En			
	En1	Mesencephalon, colliculus, periaqueductal gray matter, cerebellum	Mesencephalon, telencephalon, cerebellum, colliculus
	En2	Mesencephalon, colliculus, periaqueductal gray matter, cerebellum	Mesencephalon-metencephalon differentiation
Hox			
	Hoxa1	Rhombomere 4	Rhombomere defects, respiratory impairment
	Hoxa2	Myelencephalon, rhombomere 3	
	Hoxa4	PNS-medula limit	
	Hoxa5	Myelencephalon	
	Hoxa6	Myelencephalon	
	Hoxb1	Rhombomere 4 & 2	Motor neuron axon guidance in hindbrain
	Hoxb2	Rhombomere 3	
	Hoxb3	Rhombomere 5	
	Hoxb4	Rhombomere 7	
	Hoxb13		Notchord and spinal ganglia
	Hoxc4	Rostral region of rhombomere 7	
	Hoxd1		Patterning mouse hindbrain
	Hoxd3	Myelencephalon	
	Hoxd4	Myelencephalon	
	Irx1	Diencephalon	Sodium channel function
	Irx2	Hindbrain, midbrain	Hindbrain–midbrain boundaries
	Irx3	Hindbrain	Midbrain dorsoventral patterning
	Irx6	Optic cup	Retina
Homeo domain related			
	Gbx1	Ventral telencephalon	Neuronal migration, neuronal differentiation, brain
	Gbx2	Hindbrain	Thalamocortical axon guidance
	Pitx1	Hindbrain	Pro-opiomelanocortin, pituitary gland
	Pitx2	Chord	Eye, dopaminergic neurons of the substantia nigra
LIM			
	Lhx1	Lateral diencephalons, midbrain, hindbrain, then telencephalon	Differentiation of sensorial receptors
	Lhx2	Roof of the developing mouth, front of buccopharyngal membrane	Eye, cerebral cortex
	Lhx3	Pons, medulla, raphe	Pituitary gland
	Lhx4	4th ventricle	Central control of respiration
	Lhx5	Fore and mid brain, thalamus, hypothalamus, then pons and medulla	Forebrain patterning

(Continued)

Table 4.1 Continued

Homeobox Family	Gene	Brain Region of Expression	CNS Target
	Lhx6	Medial forebrain	Expansion of neuronal progenitors
	Lhx8:	Forebrain	Cholinergic neurons
	Lhx9	Medulla, forebrain	Interneurons in the mouse spinal cord Progenitors of cortical neuton
	Lmx1a	Medulla	Specification of spinal cord neurons
	Lmx1b	Developing interneurons	Central serotonergic neurons
Msx			
	Msx1:	Roof of the developing mouth, front of buccopharyngal membrane, thalamus, ventricles then in retina	Craniofacial, diencephalic epithelium
	Msx2	Optic cup	Eye
	Msx3	Dorsal part of the neurotube, rhombomeres 1, 2 and 6	
Nk			
	Nkx1–1	Ventral telencephalic vesicle, striatum, hypothalamus, thalamus	
	Nkx1–2	Hypothalamus, thalamus	Anterior hypothalamus
	Nkx2–5	Hipothalamus, thalamus, tegmentum	Specification of neuronal progenitors
Otx			
	Otx1	Ubiquitous in brain structures	Forebrain and cerebral cortex
	Otx2	Ubiquitous in brain structures	Forebrain and cerebral cortex, neural tube
Pax			
	Pax1	Mesoderm	
	Pax2	Eye, myelencephalon, cerebellum	Eye, including retina and chiasma Chochlea and its spinal projections
	Pax3	Myelencephalon, hindbrain	Patterning of neural tube
	Pax4		
	Pax5	Myelencephalon, cerebellum, pons	Colliculus, patterns of cerebellar foliation
	Pax6	Ubiquitous in the telencephalon	Eye, hypothalamus, cerebral regionalisation
	Pax7	Myelencephalon, cerebellum, pons	Neural tube
	Pax8	Myelencephalon, cerebellum	Thyroid
Pax related			
	Arx	Dorsal telencephalon, diencephalon	Neuronal migration and differentiation in ventral telencephalon
	Ch10	Rhombencepalon	Retinal inter cellular channels, size of the eye, optic nerve
	Phox2a	Rhombencepalon, mesencephalon, metencephalon, locus coeruleus	Autonomic ganglia, locus coeruleus; dorsoventral patterning of the mouse hindbrain
	Prop1	Telencephalon	Anterior pituitary gland
	Prrx1	Telencephalic vesicles, ventral hypothalamus	Vascular system
	Prrxl1:	Telencephalon	Tactile projections in the chord
	Rax,	Basal forebrain, optic nerve	Retina, forebrain/midbrain structures, hypothalamus.
	Uncx4.1	Mesencephalon, tegmentum, hypothalamus then cerebellum	Central mechanisms of respiration
Pou domain			
	Pou3f3	Hypothalamus	Organization of the cells in the hippocampus and adjacent transitional cortex

(Continued)

Table 4.1 Continued

Homeobox Family	Gene	Brain Region of Expression	CNS Target
	Pou3f2	Hypothalamus	Hypothalamic pituitary axis, hypothalamic neuron
	Pou4f1	Mesencephalon, chord, pons	Brain cranial nerves
	Pou3f4	Hypothalamus	Hearing
	Pou3f1	Fore and midbrain	Schwann cell maturation
	Pit1-rs1		Pituitary gland
Six			
	Six3	Midbrain tegmentum, eye	Eye
TALE			
	Meis1	Ubiquitous	
	TGIF1	Ventricles, cerebellar plate	Cerebellar external granular layer? cell proliferation
Homeo domain-interacting protein kinases			
	Hipk2	Midbrain	Apoptosis, neuron numbers in trigeminal ganglion, dopamine neuron
	Cart1	Neural tube	Neural tube, forebrain
	Phtf1	Forebrain	Retina

The homeodomain class is indicated in column 1, the symbol of the gene is reported in column 2; see the legend of Figure 4.2 for the full names. The regions of expression are reported in column 3. Column 4 indicate the target of the gene in the nervous tissues as they result from spontaneous variants, gene targeting or transgenesis.

The structure or nerve tissue where the gene is expressed, and the structure or tissue where the gene acts, are two different things and were considered independently. The measurement of expression raises numerous questions. The quantity of RNA is assayed in most cases, but not the quantity of the protein, and many processes take place between RNA formation and protein production. The transcription factor gene is sometimes expressed in a brain structure that will not appear as the target organ of the product of the gene. The expression of a gene is the prerequisite for its action, but expression alone is not enough for it to act. However, it was possible to draw conclusions from expression studies of development provided comparable techniques and probes or primers were used.

Expression follows a spatial rule. Transcription factors are not expressed ubiquitously in the brain; expression can occur in certain structures and not in others, and it is not territory-dependent. A gene can be expressed in the thalamus and not in the cerebral cortex, as can be seen from the patterns of expression of the gene *Emx1* in the brain (Table 4.2). The presence of RNA in two structures is not determined by anatomical proximity. The *Emx1* gene is expressed, or not expressed, in neighboring regions of the brain. The expression of a transcription factor may also differ within the same structure. In the mouse, at postconception day 13.5, the organs are well shaped and it is possible to isolate brain structures to study the expression of genes in the substructures. *Pax6* is expressed in the cortex, but not in the striatum, yet both are in the telencephalon. *Pax6* is not expressed in the spinal cord, but is expressed in neighboring territories such as the cranial ganglia and root ganglia, all of which are in the myelencephalon. What are the determinants of gene expression? The crucial role played by the Hox system and Pax system in the specification of nerve cells is discussed in the next section.

Expression also follows temporal rules. Genes encoding transcription factors are expressed later than genes coding for growth factors. The age when the first signal is detected varies from one brain structure to another and within each brain structure. In the mouse, a number of transcription factors are not detected on the same day in the gyrus dentatus and CA3. Figure 4.3 illustrates the clear lack of synchrony of transcription factor genes in different structures of the brain. The *Pax6* gene is expressed earlier in the olfactory bulbs than in the cortex. The expression of transcription factor genes is not constant and may fluctuate with time. For some genes, it disappears at around postnatal day 29. Two structures in Figure 4.3

Table 4.2 Expression of the Transcription Factor Gene. *Emx1* at 13.5 Days Post Conception in the Mouse

Emx1

13.5 days PC
Telencephalon present
Cerebral cortex present
Striatum absent
Thalamus absent
Hypothalamus absent
Ventricular layer absent
Olfactory bulb present
Ear present
Retina absent
Spinal chord absent
Cranial ganglion present
Root ganglions present

Source: From a Review of Published Papers or Unpublished Data Referenced by http://www.informatics.jax.org/mgihome/other/citation.shtml

show an occasional interruption of expression for one day during embryonic life.

The foregoing two sections emphasize the fact that the number of growth factor genes and transcription factor genes is too small to provide an explanation of the development of the brain by direct gene–phenotype correspondence. This is part of the general paradox of the finite number of genes (around 24,000) and the infinite number of phenotypes that are all gene-dependent. Interactions between the two categories of genes provide a plausible hypothesis for how this paradox may be partially resolved. The question is "How are the interactions between these genes carried out?," which leads to another question: "How do genes manage the specification of nerve cells?" Because of the time-based organization of development, interactions between genes need to be closely timed, and it appears that this timing is accomplished by transcription factor genes.

Processes of Nerve Cell Specification

There is incredible variety in the cells of an organism. Red and white blood cells, bipolar cells in the retina, neurons, and astrocytes are just a few examples of the diverse range of cells. Cell morphology, physiology, and function are determined by genes, with morphological, physiological, and functional variations depending on the allelic forms they carry. And it is in this diversity of cell types

and functions that the difficulty arises, as all the cells in an organism carry the same genes and the same alleles. All cells descend from a single cell by mitotic division and are copies of the original single cell of the zygote. As cells have the same genes, they should have the same shape and function, but this obviously is not the case. Why? Not all genes are activated/repressed at the same time in the same cell. Each cell possesses the same potentialities but not all cells use all those potentialities.

Role of Transcription Factors

Transcription factors interact with other genes that contribute to development via the mechanism of transcription. The *Hox* gene, via the recognition helix, initiates or blocks transcription. Other motifs, such as POU, CUT, or Pax, improve the specificity of the recognition. Only a small number of the 24,000 genes in a mammalian embryonic stem cell are expressed at any one time and other genes are repressed. Neurons and epidermal cells, or dopamine neurons and serotonin neurons, do not require the same gene products for development. The development of a stem cell into Cell A rather Cell B is the result of a different pattern of genetic expression. Experimental studies have investigated the molecular and phenotypic effects of transcription factors, taking them one by one. Gene targeting technology has provided a powerful tool for investigating the role of transcription factors in development. The technique consists of replacing a functional gene with a neutral gene. A gene of resistance to neomycin has been used in most studies of development. Other techniques, such as lox-cre, are now available, and several "double transgenic" and "double targeted genes" have been derived. The effects are not simply additive; the effects of a double genetic modification cannot be deduced from the effect of each modification. *Dlx2* knockout mice have abnormal development of the olfactory bulb, while mice with this deletion plus the deletion of the *Dlx1* gene have abnormal development of the striatum.

The observation that the specific development of a cell requires a selected number of proteins, or that a small number of genes are expressed in a cell, is a first step toward understanding the mechanisms of cell specification. What is the process involved in selecting genes to be expressed? Not all genes are expressed all the time, as is evident in patterns of gene expression summarized in Figure 4.3 and Table 4.2. How is the timing of this expression

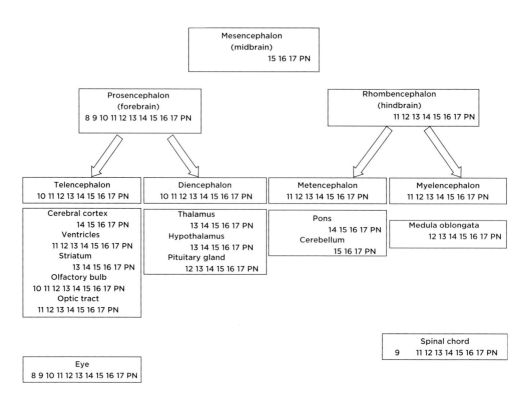

Figure 4.3 Expression of the transcription factor gene Pax 6 in different regions of the brain. The day (post-conception age) when the expression was detected is given. Postnatal period = PN.

controlled? The expression of genes involved in the cell specification is tissue-dependent, as can be seen in Table 4.1. Which regulation process causes a gene to be expressed in one tissue and not another, or, more surprisingly, causes a gene to be expressed in one tissue at one point in time and in another at another point in time (see Figure 4.3 and Table 4.2)?

Hox and Pax Genes and Cell Specification

Cell specification is crucial in brain development. Certain cases of cognitive impairment, pervasive development disorders, and psychiatric disorders have been associated with incomplete neuronal specification that may cause abnormal neuronal migration. The position of a neuron in a structure during embryonic development and its final location are required for normal brain development. More generally, the position of a cell in a given organ is a prerequisite for normal development and viability. The position of a cell in the embryo is determined by a system operating along two axes (as illustrated in Figure 4.4).

The first axis of development sets the rostra-caudal specification (also known as anterocaudal patterning) of the cells. The first axis gives information to the cell about its position in the embryo and determines the region where an organ will develop. *Hox* genes determine the specification of the cells in anterocaudal direction. The second axis is dorsoventral and *Pax* genes determine dorsoventral cell specification. The cell is thus specified by two coordinates.

In mammals, the *Hox* system is located on four chromosomes (see Table 4.3) and encompasses the homeobox A cluster (*Hoxa*) with 11 genes, the homeobox B cluster (*Hoxb*) with 10 genes, the homeobox C cluster (*Hoxa*) with 13 genes, and the homeobox D cluster (*Hoxd*) with 8 genes. The patterning of the digestive tract, notochord, and later differentiated motoneurons, skeleton and limb positions, and hindbrain is determined by *Hoxa*, *Hoxb*, *Hoxc*, and *Hoxd*. The *Hox* complex of different species comes from a common ancestor, as shown in Figure 4.5. One copy of the *Hox* is believed to be present in the initial genome of the ancestor of mammals. The four *Hox* copies should have arisen from two chromosomal duplications occurring in the course of evolution. Table 4.3 shows the similarity of the four complexes. Some genes do not

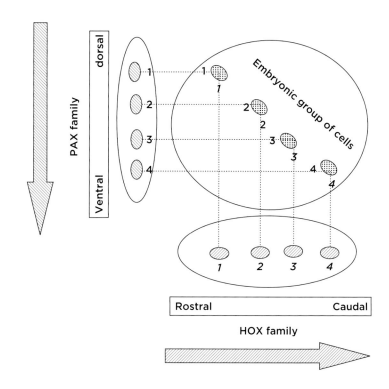

Figure 4.4 Specification of the cells during the development by the Hox and the Pax system. The cells (numbered 1–4) are specified in the rostracaudal dimension by the Hox system and in the dorsoventral dimension by the Pax system. The system with two coordinates specifies the position of the cells in the developing organ.

Table 4.3 The Hox System in Insects and Mammals Derives from a Common Hypothetical Ancestor. The Arrows Indicate the Correspondences Between the Hypothetical Ancestral Genes and Those of the Hox System in Insects and Mammals

	Drosophila		Common ancestor (hypothetical)		Mouse			
					Chromosome 11	Chromosome 6	Chromosome 15	Chromosome 2
5′	*lab*	←	lab	→	*Hoxb1*	*Hoxa1*		*Hox1d*
	Pb	←	Pb	→	*Hoxb2*	*Hoxa2*		*Hoxb3*
					Hoxb3	*Hoxa3*		
	zen							
	Dfd	←	Dfd	→	*Hoxb4*	*Hoxa4*	*Hoxc4*	*Hoxd4*
	Ser				*Hoxb5*	*Hoxa5*	*Hoxc5*	
	Antp	←	Antp	→	*Hoxb6*	*Hoxa6*	*Hoxc6*	
	Ubx				*Hoxb7*	*Hoxa7*		
	abd-A				*Hoxb8*		*Hoxc8*	*Hoxd8*
	abd-B	←	abd-B	→	*Hoxb9*	*Hoxa9*	*Hoxc9*	*Hoxd9*
						Hoxa10	*Hoxc10*	*Hoxd10*
						Hoxa11	*Hoxc11*	*Hoxd11*
							Hoxc12	*Hoxd12*
3′					*Hoxb13*	*Hoxa13*	*Hoxc13*	*Hoxd13*

Source: Adapted from Ruddle et al., 1994.

tally in all the complexes, but the same order and functions of the genes that are present are found in all the four complexes.

The *Hox* complexes control the development of different systems such as the skeleton, brain, and digestive tract, but genes located towards the 5′ extremity are expressed in the rostral regions and expressed first, whereas genes located at extremity 3′ are expressed in the caudal regions and expressed later. For this reason, the genes of the four *Hox*

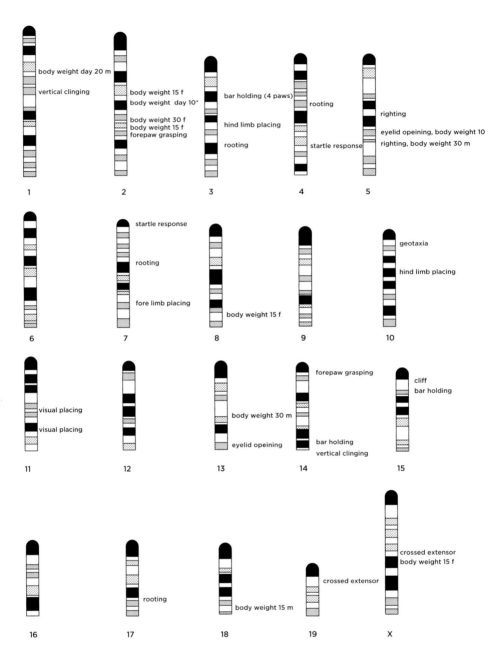

Figure 4.5 Chromosomal regions associated with sensory and motor development in mice; data from Roubertoux et al., 1987; Le Roy, Perez-Diaz, Cherfouh, & Roubertoux, 1999). The battery is from Fox (1965) adapted by Carlier, Roubertoux, and Cohen-Salmon (1983). Righting: The pup was placed on its back and immediately tried to right itself. The day when the pup turned over within 10 s was recorded. Cliff Drop Aversion (abbreviated "cliff"): The pup was placed on the edge of a cliff, the forepaws and head over the edge. It turned and crawled away from the cliff. Forepaw Grasping: When the inside of one paw was gently stroked with an object, the paw flexed to grasp the object. Forelimb Placing and Hindlimb Placing: When the dorsum of the paw came into contact with the edge of an object, the pup raised its paw and placed it on the object. Age of Disappearance of Rooting (rooting): Bilateral stimulation of the face stimulated the pups to crawl forwards, pushing the head in a rooting fashion. Age of Disappearance of Crossed Extensor (crossed extensor): When pinched, the stimulated limb flexed while the opposite hindlimb extended. Geotaxia: The pup turned upwards when placed on a 45° angle with its head pointing down the incline. Vibrissae Placing: The pup was suspended by the tail and lowered towards the tip of a pencil. When the vibrissae touched the pencil the pup raised its head and performed a placing response with the extended forelimb. Bar Holding (bar holding): The forepaws were placed on a round wooden bar. Bar Holding (bar holding four paws): The pup also put the hindpaw on the bar, a movement that insures a longer period of stability. Vertical Clinging and Vertical Climbing: The pup was held against a vertical metal grid. Two behavioral responses were scored: clinging for 10 s and climbing after clinging. Startle response: A composite sound was delivered above the head of the pup and the startle response observed visually. Age at Eyelid Opening (eyelid opening): The score is the age in days when the pup opened its eyes. Visual Placing: The day after eye-opening, the pup was suspended by the tail and lowered towards the tip of the pencil without the vibrissae touching it. It extended the paw to grasp the pencil. Body Weight was measured at day 10, 15, 20, and 30 (m for males, f for females, * for m and f).

complexes are said to be paralogous. These properties explain why development sequences are non-transitional within a species and are subjected to minor variations between species.

The effect of the *Hox* genes is lasting. If we consider an organ divided into four segments A, B, C, and D, going from rostral to caudal, *Hoxa1* is expressed first and helps specify the cells in the rostral segment (segment A); later, *Hoxa2* specifies the B segment, then *Hoxa3* specifies C segment, and finally *Hoxa4* specifies the D fragment. In this way, segments A, B, C, and D are specified by genes 1, 2, 3, and 4 respectively.

The nine genes in the *Pax* system determining the dorsoventral specification of the cells are not grouped together in a complex, as shown in Figure 4.2. One hypothesis is that they are derived from homeogenes with the adjunction of the paired domain. The dorsoventral direction of the *Pax* genes contributes to the specification of the cells. Some *Pax* genes are expressed in the dorsal part only and not in the ventral part of an organ; this is the case of *Pax3* and *Pax7* genes in the neural tube. The mode of action of the *Pax* system is not the same as the *Hox* system, with *Pax* genes acting by successive cascades of expression (van Heyningen & Williamson, 2002). The number of genes successively expressed by a *Pax* trigger is high. The most famous example is the "master gene," *Pax6*. The name "master" is given to genes that trigger dozens of cascades of expression. The hunt for "mastermind" is in progress (Wu, Sun, Kobayash, Gao, & Griffin, 2002) but the idea of a master gene for brain development is compatible neither with the modular characteristic of brain function nor with the experimental data.

The conjunction of the *Hox* and *Pax* system increases the specification of cells in the embryo. Figure 4.4 shows how a group of embryonic cells can be specified by both the rostrocaudal and the dorsoventral positions. We have already noted the spatial and temporal characteristics and patterns in gene expression in the course of development, and space and time appear to be inextricably linked in genetics.

Plasticity of Hox genes

In this chapter, which endeavors to shed light on genetic factors contributing to brain development, readers may be struck by the strictness of the genetic rules applying to development. There is, however, a longstanding debate on the relative impact of intrinsic/genetic and extrinsic/environmental factors in the specification of brain structures, but it seems more rational to investigate the plasticity of the *Hox*, *Pax*, *Lim*, and *Pou* systems, rather than repeat the errors of the nature–nurture debate in a bid to estimate the respective impact of the environment and genes.

Transcription factors do not operate in a binary mode; their effects are subtle (Holland & Takahashi, 2005). Normal brain development requires a delicate balance between the products and the different genes. The role of *Otx1* and *Otx2* genes in brain patterning provides an illustration of this requirement, and their role in brain morphogenesis is shown in Figure 4.2 and Table 4.1. *Otx1* and *Otx2* interact during the process of brain specification; a minimum level of OTX1 and/or OTX2 is required for the specification of brain cells, and this can be achieved by either one dose of both OTX1 and OTX2, or two doses of OTX2. Does this leave any scope for vicarious processes in the specification of brain cells? Experiments have shown that cellular specification requires more than just one protein and that a threshold protein level must be reached for neuronal specification.

The effect of the transcription factor gene is not the same for all the cells of the brain; it is associated with the expression of a gene in a group of embryonic cells and the inhibition of the same gene in the neighboring population of embryonic cells. This can be interpreted as intrinsic control by genetic mechanisms or as extrinsic factors that may be distinct signals emitted by different brain territories (Trainor & Krumlauf, 2000). The fact that the expression of *Hox* genes in rhombomeres varies when the embryonic tissue is grafted in different locations casts doubt on the autonomy of the *Hox* system (Grapin-Botton, Bonnin, McNaughton, Krumlauf, & Le Douarin, 1995; Couly, Grapin-Botton, Coltey, & Le Douarin, 1996). The expression of a sample of *Hox* genes (*Hoxb-4*, *Hoxb-1*, *Hoxa-3*, *Hoxb-3*, *Hoxa-4*, and *Hoxd-4*) was analyzed before and after caudal-to-rostral transplantation and after rostral-to-caudal transplantation. The patterns of expression do not change in the caudal-to-rostral situation, but do change in the reverse situation. In the rostral-to-caudal transplantation, the rostral tissues express the genes usually expressed in the caudal region. Several experiments suggest that *Hox* expression is modulated by the integration of signals coming from the cells (Trainor & Krumlauf, 2000). Modulation of *Hox* expression could be greater in certain tissues (Job & Tan, 2003). The complexity of the tissues, the multiplicity of interactions, and the correlative entropy of the signals increase as development progresses. Complexity reaches its apex with the neocortex. It could be speculated that the neocortex is the most recent structure in brain evolution and that it has been subjected to less genetic constraint.

Individual Differences in Brain and Behavioral Development

Genes that specify the course of development are defined by the genome of the species. There is no genomic difference between individuals of the same species, even when they are different breeds or are from domesticated breeds (e.g., horses, cows, and dogs), or inbred strains (mouse, rat, and drosophila). Exceptions may occur when individuals lack a gene or set of genes or carry an extra copy of a chromosomal segment. While all individuals of one species have the same genome, they do not have the same genotype; in other words, individuals of the same species differ in the alleles that the genes carry. The question therefore is to establish whether the allelic forms contribute to individual differences observed in the rate of development. Do allelic forms belong to the genes that determine the program of development? Here again, it would be better to investigate the plasticity of the processes triggered by the alleles rather than embark upon the nature–nurture conflict.

Impaired Development in Genetic Disorders

The genetic approach to the rate of development is a long story. Our field of research started with the comparison of intrapair similarities in monozygotic (MZ) and dizygotic twins (DZ). Papousek and Papousek (1983)) compared babies from MZ and DZ twin pairs for social development. They concluded that the steps of socialization were more similar for MZ twins than for DZ twins (which differed genetically as siblings). Wilson (1972) reported that MZ twins developed quite similarly from 3 to 72 months compared to DZ for the onset of cognitive performances. Since these publications, a number of twin pairs have been observed from birth to senescence, confirming the greater similarity in MZ than in DZ twin pairs for psychological development. Recent studies use twins rather than siblings to detect genes associated with complex traits using wide genome scan (Oliver & Plomin, 2007).

However, brain correlates of behavioral development in these studies are not provided. Brain characteristics could be obtained with brain imaging techniques. Developmental disorders have been reported in relation to chromosomal anomalies, either an extra copy or a deletion. Therefore, by establishing which genes are carried by the extra or deleted chromosomal region, it should be possible to link the developmental disorder to one of the aberrant genes. The strategy is controversial because of the nonspecificity of some developmental disorders in the genetic diseases characterized by cognitive impairment. It sometimes has been assumed that developmental and cognitive disorders were the result of some general brain dysfunction, but this has been challenged by comparing neuropsychological profiles. Hemizygous deletions of large chromosomal fragments, 7q11.23 in Williams–Beuren (Mervis & Klein-Tasman, 2000) and 22q11 deletion syndromes (Swillen et al., 1997; De Smedt et al., 2007) are associated with distinct profiles of cognitive dysfunction typical of each syndrome (Carlier & Ayoun, 2007). The mean cognitive level is higher in patients with 22q11 deletion than in Williams–Beuren syndrome and the psychotic disorders that are frequent in 22q.11 syndrome are rarely seen in Williams–Beuren syndrome. Trisomy 21 (TRS21), caused by an extra copy of all or part of chromosome 21, presents a neuropsychological profile that is different from the Williams–Beuren profile (see Vicari, 2006 for a general review). The development of laterality differs in patients with Williams–Beuren syndrome and TRS21 (Carlier et al., 2006, Gérard-Desplanches et al., 2006). Several phenotypes are known to be the result of trisomies affecting only one gene. Recent investigations of gene–brain–behavior relationships have led to considerable advances in the understanding of TRS21 and could be used as a model for other chromosomal anomalies. Genetic analysis of abnormal behavioral development appears to be useful for characterizing the functions of allelic forms. More than 1,400 genes have been identified as playing a role in brain impairment. By drawing up a developmental profile of a given gene, we should produce a more accurate description of the function of the gene in question.

Animal models of development, and mouse models in particular, operate with two technologies: (1) the gene-to-phenotype approach (transgenics, gene targeting, spontaneous mutants) and (2) the trait-to-genes approach (wide genome scan). In experiments on mice, several mutants have been tested (Anagnostopoulos, Mobraaten, Sharp, & Davisson, 2000) and they have shown overlapping characteristics but also specificities (Noël, 1989; Marzetta & Nash, 1979, Cripps & Nash, 1983; Mikuni & Nash, 1979) for a battery of sensorial and motor tests (adapted from Fox, 1965). Mice carrying extra copies of HAS21 contiguous fragments, encompassing the genes of the D21S17–ETS2 region (previously referred to as "Down syndrome critical region 1"), display specific profiles of sensory and motor development. The extra copies of the three regions do not alter development, whereas three copies of a region encompassing *Dyrk1A* gene delay sensorial and motor development (Roubertoux et al., 2006). The cross-transfer of mitochondrial DNA in congenic strains of mice also had an impact on the sensory and motor development that interacted with the nuclear genes (Roubertoux et al., 2003).

Two exhaustive genome scans were performed to measure sensory and motor development in the mouse. The first used the recombinant inbred strain strategy (Roubertoux, Semal, & Ragueneau, 1985) and the second a screening of an intercrossed generation of two strains of mice with a significant difference in the rate of preweaning development (from birth to 20 days). A number of observations can be made on the basis of the findings (Figure 4.5).

1. A factor analysis showed no general development factor and the wide genome scan showed no general genetic development factor.

2. No link could be detected between one chromosomal region and most of the sensory and motor development indices common to the loci mapped. Some regions showed links to several indices: eyelid opening, body weight at day 10 and at day 30 in males, and the age of appearance of the righting response were all on the same region of chromosome 5; body weight at days 15 and day 30 in females and forepaw grasping were on the same chromosomal fragment on chromosome 2. The confidence interval of each potential locus is large and it is impossible to conclude that two loci with overlapping confidence intervals are the same.

3. The same observation applies to the candidate genes of these putative genes. Some genes involved in the program of development of the species are close to the loci linked to sensory and motor development. Are they the same genes? The confidence interval is too large to confirm or refute the hypothesis. The use of mutants in drosophila has shown that some transcription factor such as *Prospero* may modify adult behavior (Grosjean, Guenin, Bardet, & Ferveur, 2007). The bsx homeobox factor contributes to motor behavior and food consumption after complex metabolic pathways (Sakkou et al., 2007).

4. Most development indices are linked to several regions.

5. Most of the linkages here contributed to a small percentage of the variance, which was never greater than 15% of total variance. As genetic variance was higher, the undetected loci account for a very small percentage of the variance. This suggests that the number of loci involved was high.

6. In several cases, the allelic forms at two loci interact.

7. The linkage changes when the polymorphism changes; the alleles linked with the traits are not necessarily the same in different populations. The locus contributing to age at disappearance of rooting response that was the first identified gene for a behavioral trait (Roubertoux, Bauman, Ragueneau, & Semal, 1987) has a major effect on a C57Bl/6by × Balbc/by background and a minor effect in epistasis with other locus on a NZB/BlNJ × C57Bl/6by background.

The main difficulty with the wide genome scan is the size of the confidence interval, which limits possibilities for performing fine linkage mapping. Several solutions have been proposed to reduce the confidence interval (Darvasi & Soller, 1995).

Plasticity of the Effects of Genes Involved in Development: Epigenetic Factors

In all cases, the role of genes must be argued in a deterministic framework (Roubertoux & Carlier, 2007). Many molecular events can occur in the course of epigenesis, which is defined as the gap between the DNA template and the functional protein. One class of events is how RNA is spliced to generate mature transcripts. Introns but not exons can be spliced, which is called constitutive splicing. Or one to several exons can be eliminated as the flanking introns are spliced, which is called alternative splicing. Alternative splicing factors recently studied in the mouse, the fruit fly, and the nematode shed light on the way alternative splicing contributes to the plasticity of the transcription factor genes.

Several studies of brain development, pervasive developmental disorders, and cognitive impairment have shown that alternative splicing plays a crucial role in the molecular regulation of the brain (see, among others, Hyman, 2000 for autism or Yu et al., 2000 for Alzheimer disease). In simple terms, an alternative splicing protein binds to either an exonic cluster, blocking exon inclusion, or an intronic cluster, enhancing exon inclusion (Ule et al., 2006). Alternative splicing thus appears to breach the "one gene–one protein" law. Each gene contains several exons. The loss of one exon creates a new form of RNA and the combination of several lost exons can generate a large set of spliced RNA for a single gene. The drosophila *Dscam* gene (Down syndrome cell adhesion molecule) encodes an axon guidance receptor that can express 38,016 splicing RNAs and 38,016 functions (Schmucker et al., 2000). This is three times the size of the drosophila genome that encompasses some 13,000 genes.

The characteristics of alternative splicing alone can explain its potentially substantial contribution to the plasticity of genes: (1) Individual differences in splicing frequency in organ territories may be the result of allelic forms of the gene encoding the splicing factor. (2) The splicing effect is amplified by the high number of receptors, e.g., postsynaptic tissue encompasses 6,000 acetylcholine receptors per μm^2. The splicing effects may be diverse, as splicing events do not occur the same way in the different receptors.

Plasticity of the Effects of Genes Involved in Development: Maternal Factors

Maternal factor means the phenotype of the progeny derives more from the mother's characteristics than from the father's. Several components contribute to maternal effects; two are related to genetic mechanisms (nuclear genomic imprinting and mitochondrial DNA transmission) and three are environmental (cytoplasmic, uterine and postnatal). The uterine source of variation covers the effects mediated by the genotype of the mother and all environmental events affecting the embryo. The postnatal maternal source of variation includes pup care and the biochemical characteristics of the milk. It is difficult to distinguish the contribution of each source of variation and the respective effects on the genes.

All sources of variation coming from the mother interact with the genotypes and modulate the effect of the allelic forms. We have known for a long time (Mistretta & Bradley, 1975) that the human fetus presents elaborated forms of sensitivity and behavior and that he/she can react to external events. Behavior, sensitivity, and reactions to events may depend on the genotype of the fetus. The treatments to which the fetus is subjected may also vary according to his/her genotype. We demonstrated that cryo preservation in mice may modify the rate of sensorial and motor development. The size and the direction of the effect depend on the genotype of the embryos that were cryopreserved (Dulioust et al., 1995). Wahlsten (1982) observed that the size of corpus callosum was reduced when the pups were carried by a lactating mother. The reduction of the corpus callosum was observed in Balb-c mice.

Several experimental designs have been used to test the impact of the components of the maternal environment, either in addition to or in interaction with the genotype (Carlier, Nosten-Bertrand, & Michard-Vahnée, 1992). The use of adoption and ovary transplantation or embryo transfer in experiments can help identify the effect of one component and its interaction with others or with the genotype. This strategy has been used to study anxiety, maternal behavior, and attack behavior, but has only been used once to investigate the origin of individual differences in sensory and motor development. The following conclusions were obtained from a study designed with ovary transplantation and adoption. The findings from the first study were similar to the first conclusion drawn from wide genome scan, i.e., that there is no general environmental factor. The uterine and postnatal environments can have effects, but these effects can be in opposing directions (Carlier, Roubertoux, & Cohen-Salmon, 1983; Nosten & Roubertoux, 1988; Nosten, 1989; see Roubertoux, Nosten-Bertrand, & Carlier, 1990; Carlier, Roubertoux, & Wahlsten, 1999, for reviews). The effect of an environmental component is neither good nor bad as there is no good or bad genotype. A source of variation will accelerate development for one genotype and slow down the rate of development for another or vice versa. A source of uterine variation will accelerate or slow down sensory and motor development for one postnatal environment, but not for another. Things appear more complex. When components in the postnatal maternal environment are taken into consideration. Maternal care and the biochemical constituents of milk affect the rate of development in an interactive manner (as shown by multiple regression analysis).

Uterine Component in Humans: The Chorion Effect

Experimental designs available for rodents, and mice in particular, cannot be applied to the human species. The adoption method alone cannot disentangle the genetic and the prenatal environmental contributions. Characteristics at birth are the result of both genotype and maternal factors (genetic and uterine). Any investigation of sources of variation should focus on naturally occurring situations.

Twin pregnancies offer possibilities for testing prenatal effects on the development of biological and behavioral traits. For almost 100 years, twin studies have been used to assess the contribution of the additive genetic effect (heritability), shared or common family environmental effects, and unique, individual-specific within-family environmental effects (Neale & Cardon, 1992). To interpret such quantitative estimates of variance components, a number of postulates have to be accepted or rejected. The most popular hypothesis is the so-called "equal environment assumption," i.e., "that monozygotic (MZ) and dizygotic (DZ) twins experience equally correlated environments" (Eaves, Foley, & Silberg, 2003). Most authors testing this postulate have focused on postnatal environmental variables, but some teams have conducted research on prenatal effects on the development of biological and behavioral traits.

Twins occupy the same uterus, but do not always experience the same prenatal environmental events. Placentation (or chorionicity) is related to zygosity and four rules apply (Machin, 2001).

1. Unlike-sexed twins are DZ (with some exceptions, i.e., in a pair of MZ twins, one twin is a male 46,XY and the other is a female 45,X with Turner syndrome). Monochorionic (MC) twins are MZ with very rare exceptions. Souter et al. (2003) reported the case of MC DZ twins and speculated on the embryological events producing this MC placentation. The twins were conceived by in vitro fertilization without intracytoplasmic sperm injection, and the trophoblasts from the two embryos might have fused before implantation. After this paper was published, other investigators reported cases of MC DZ twins (see Chan, Mannino, & Benirschke, 2007 for a review) conceived by in vitro fertilization.

2. Same-sexed dichorionic (DC) twins may be MZ or DZ.

3. DZ twins are DC in almost all cases.

4. MZ twins are MC or DC but approximately two-thirds of MZ placentas are MC.

The type of placentation is determined by the timing of the zygotic division: if the split occurs within the first 3 days of development, MZ twins are DC diamniotic; if the split occurs between days 4 and 7, the two embryos share the same chorion but have two separate amnions (monochorionic diamniotic twins); when the split occurs even later, the two embryos share both membranes (monochorionic monoamniotic twins).

Special complications have been reported to affect MC twins more than DC twins: preterm birth, lower birth weight, fetal entanglement of umbilical cords, fetal thrombosis, neurological impairment, and twin–twin transfusion syndrome. Prenatal and perinatal mortality is higher for MC twins than for DC twins. For example, a population-based, retrospective cohort study was conducted of all twin deliveries in Nova Scotia, Canada, from 1988 to 1997 (Dubé, Dodds, & Armson, 2002). Perinatal death was defined as the death of a fetus with a weight ≥ 500 g or death of a live-born infant before 28 days of age. Of the 1,008 twin pregnancies analyzed, the rate of perinatal mortality of one or both twins, adjusted for maternal age, small size for gestational age, and major anomalies, was significantly higher for MC MZ twins compared to DC DZ twins (relative risk, 2.5; 95% CI, 1.1–2.5).

Placental differences in twins are well known to researchers studying twins, but unfortunately the information on the number of chorions is not always available or is incorrectly diagnosed at birth. Derom, Derom, Loos, Jacobs, and Vlietinck (2003) reported that retrospective determination of chorion type with a simple questionnaire filled out by parents was unreliable. We confirmed their conclusion (Carlier & Spitz, 2004), finding it was impossible to obtain valid retrospective information from parents. Reed and coauthors attempted to find other criteria for a posteriori classification of MZ twins as MC or DC. Reed, Uchida, Norton, and Christian (1978) reported that, in MZ twins, within-pair differences for a number of dermatoglyphic traits correlated to the placental type and used the data to calculate an index score discriminating between the two groups of MZ according to the chorion type. Unfortunately a cross-validation study with new twin samples of known chorionicity concluded that the mean score of the index differed between MC MZ and DC MZ, but that the size of the difference was too small to make any accurate classification of the type of chorion (Reed, Spitz, Vacher-Lavenu, & Carlier, 1997). It is therefore essential to have accurate information from birth records. Methods used for analysis included ultrasound examinations (although no definite diagnosis can be based on ultrasound examination), macroscopic description of the placenta by the obstetrician and/or midwife at the time of delivery, and, in cases of uncertainty, the pathologist's examination of the placenta (see Derom, Bryan, Derom, Keith, & Vlietinck, 2001 for details).

Tables 4.4 and 4.5 present a summary of data on twins of known chorionicity. Repeated observations showed greater within-pair variability in the birth weight of MC twins compared to DC twins. A similar trend was found for tooth size. The picture is more complicated for psychological traits. The chorion effect was significant for certain variables but in the opposite direction: within-pair variance was greater in DC twins than in MC twins in all cases but one. How can these differences be explained? For birth weight, the interpretation is obvious: MC twins often have common blood circulation and a twin–twin transfusion imbalance often occurs, producing a substantial difference in weight. The embryological development of permanent dentition begins at week 20 in utero and may

be disturbed by certain postnatal environmental factors. The same explanation can be put forward for the chorion-related effect on dermatoglyphics, which are formed at approximately Week 20 in utero. Race, Townsend, and Hughes (2006) have suggested that the sharing of the chorion by MC twins increases environmental stress and discordance within pairs of MC twins.

Findings on behavioral traits showing within-pair differences, which are greater in DC twins compared to MC twins, are more puzzling. Some hypotheses have been put forward (Jacobs et al., 2001). As MC twins have shared blood circulation, fetal programming could be more similar in MC twins than in DC twins. In females, another source of variation could be linked to the X-inactivation patterns that often differ in DC twins but not in MC twins (Monteiro et al., 1998). It could be

Table 4.4 Chorion Effect on Biological Variables and/or Anthropometry (Papers Arranged from the Younger Twins to the Older)

Authors, year of publication	Number of twin pairs	Variable	Main Results[a]
Corey et al., 1979	118 MC 54 DC	Birth weight	MC > DC
Vlietinck et al., 1989	246 MC[b] 133 DC	Birth weight	MC > DC The chorion effect accounts for 12% of the variance
Loos et al., 2001	138 MC[b] 103 DC	Birth weight Adults: body mass and height	MC > DC No effect
Race et al., 2006	14 MC 13 DC	Birth weight Permanent tooth-size variability	MC > DC MC > DC
Corey et al., 1976	30 MC 22 DC	Cord blood cholesterol level	DC > MC
Melnick et al., 1980	117 MC 56 DC	Anterior fontanelle development	No chorion effect
Spitz et al., 1996	20 MC 24 DC	Birth weight 10 years: Weight height Body mass	MC > DC MC > DC No effect MC > DC
Gutknecht et al., 1999	16 MC[c] 22 DC	13 years: Weight height Body mass	MC > DC No effect MC > DC
Reed et al., 1997	136 MC 92 DC	8 dermatoglyphic variables used in the calculation of an index score (in children or adults)	MC pairs have a more positive scores in the index
Fagard et al., 2003	128 MC[b] 96 DC	Blood pressure Young adults	No effect

[a] MC > DC means that the within pair difference is larger in MC than DC.
[b] Sample was drawn from the East Flanders Prospective Twin Survey.
[c] Longitudinal study.

Table 4.5   Chorion Effects on Behavioral Traits (Papers Arranged from the Younger Twins to the Older)

Authors, year of publication	Variables and test used	Number of MZ twin pairs	Mean age	Main results
Riese, 1999	Temperament	48 MC 29 DC	neonates	Not significant
Welch et al., 1978	Cognition Bayley scales	20 MC 12 DC	18 months	Not significant
Sokol et al., 1995	Cognition McCarthy scales Personality Inventory	23 MC 21 DC	6 years	Difference in 3/19 subtests DC > MC in two cases, DC < MC in one case. For the global scales: no difference Difference in three scales and in 8/12 clinical scales: DC > MC
Melnick et al., 1978	WISC	23 MC 9 DC	7 years	DC > MC on IQ
Spitz et al., 1996; Carlier et al., 1996	WISC: vocabulary and Block design K-ABC Laterality WISC	20 MC 24 DC	10 years	DC > MC only on Bloc design
Gutknecht et al., 1999	Test of figurative reasoning	16 MC 22 DC	13 years	DC >MC only on Perceptive Organisation Index DC > MC in visualisation score (1/4 scores)
Blekher et al., 1998	Eye saccadic movements	17 MC 16 DC	13 years	DC > MC for latency of saccades
Jacobs et al., 2001	WISC	175 MC 95 DC	Between 8 and 14 years	DC > MC on Vocabulary and Arithmetic. The chorion effect explains respectively 14% and 10% of the variance of these subtests.
Wichers et al., 2002	CBCL	202 MC 125 DC	Children	Not significant
Rose et al., 1981	WAIS: vocabulary and block design	17 MC 15 DC	Adults	DC > MC on Block design

ᵃSample was drawn from the East Flanders Prospective Twin Survey.
WISC and WAIS: Wechsler intelligence scales for children and adults; K-ABC: Kaufman Intelligence Scale; CBCL: Child Behavior Check List (measures behavioral and emotional problems).

also argued that some differences observed across studies may be due to artifacts (e.g., small samples, random statistical effects, or low power of the statistical test) and that further studies are needed to gain a clearer picture.

Conclusions

Genetic techniques now offer opportunities to identify genes and their functions. A survey of the published literature shows a huge number of genes reported as contributing to a great variety of phenotypes. Four thousand genes are involved in mouse behavior and the same number was found for brain functions. These figures are obtained from available knockout, transgenic, and spontaneous mutants (to date, less than 3,000). The number of gene–phenotype links is greater than the 24,000 genes carried by the genome. If we factor in the number of gene–phenotype links that will be discovered when knockout and transgenic mice are available for the 21,000 genes remaining, the number of genes needed will be more than 100,000. A solution to this paradox has been suggested (Roubertoux & Carlier, 2007): the hypothesis of strict correspondence between each gene and each phenotype, which was supported at the time the genome was sequenced, should be abandoned. This means that one gene can have multiple functions. Several processes are needed to achieve such a versatile, polyvalent state as alternative splicing, epistasis, cascades, and, for the brain, neuronal integration. The genetic "basis" of a phenotype is no longer the gene, but a network of genetic events, a concept that means less causality, with all the scientific, medical, and ethical consequences that it may entail.

References

Ades, S. E., & Sauer, R. T. (1995). Specificity of minor-groove and major-groove interactions in a homeodomain–DNA complex. *Biochemistry 34*, 14601–14608.

Anagnostopoulos, A. V., Mobraaten, L. E., Sharp, J. J., & Davisson, M. T. (2000). Transgenic and knockout databases: Behavioral profiles of mouse mutants. *Physiology and Behavior, 73*, 675–689.

Andersen, B., & Rosenfeld, M. G. (2001). POU domain factors in the neuroendocrine system: Lessons from developmental biology provide insights into human disease. *Endocrinology Review, 22*, 2–35.

Banerjee-Basu, S., Landsman, D., & Baxevanis, A. D. (1999). Threading analysis of prospero-type homeodomains. In *Silico Biology, 3*, 163–173.

Billeter, M. (1996). Homeodomain-type DNA recognition. *Progress in Biophysics and Molecular Biology, 66*, 211–225.

Blekher, T., Christian, J. C., Abel, L. A., & Yee R. D. (1998). Influence of chorion type on saccadic eye movements in twins. *Investigate Ophthalmology & Visual Science, 39*, 2186–2190.

Broadman, K. (1909). *Vergleichende Lokalisationslehre der Grosshirnrinde*. Leipzig, Germany: Barth.

Carlier, M., & Ayoun, C. (2007). *Déficiences intellectuelles et intégration*. Wavre, Belgium: Mardaga.

Carlier, M., Nosten-Bertrand, M., & Michard-Vahnée, C. (1992). Separating genetic effect from maternal environmental effect. In D. Goldowitz, D. Wahsten, & R. E. Wimer (Eds.), *Techniques for the genetic analysis of brain and behavior* (pp. 111–126). Amsterdam: Elsevier.

Carlier, M., Roubertoux, P. L., & Cohen-Salmon, Ch. (1983). Early development in mice: I genotype and post-natal maternal effects. *Physiology and Behavior; 80*, 837–844.

Carlier, M., Roubertoux, P. L., & Wahlsten, D. (1999). Maternal effect in behavior genetic analysis. In B. C. Jones, & P. Mormède (Eds.), *Neurobehavioral genetics, methods and applications* (pp. 187– 200). Boca Raton, FL: CRC Press.

Carlier, M., & Spitz, E. (2004). Failure to obtain reliable determination of chorion type using parent information: Confirmation with French data. *Twin Research, 7*, 13–15.

Carlier, M., Spitz, E., Vacher-Lavenu, M. C., Villéger, P., Martin, B., & Michel, F. (1996). Manual performance and laterality in twins of know chorion type. *Behavior Genetics, 26*, 409–407.

Carlier M., Stefanini S., Deruelle C., Volterra V., Doyen A.-L., Lamard C., et al. (2006). Laterality in persons with intellectual disability. Do patients with Trisomy 21 and Williams–Beuren syndrome differ from typically developing persons? *Behavior Genetics, 36*, 365–376.

Chan, O. T. M., Mannino, F. L., & Benirschke, K. (2007). A retrospective analysis of placentas from twin pregnancies derived from assisted reproductive technology. *Twin Research and Human Genetics, 10*, 385–393.

Chauhan, B. K., Zhang, W., Cveklova, K., Kantorow, M., & Cvekl, A. (2002). Identification of differentially expressed genes in mouse Pax6 heterozygous lenses. *Investigative Ophthalmology & Visual Science, 43*, 1884–1890.

Cheyette, B. N., Green, P. J., Martin, K., Garren, H., Hartenstein, V., & Zipursky, S. L. (1994). The *Drosophila* sine oculis locus encodes homeodomain-containing protein required for the development of the entire visual system. *Neuron, 12*, 977–996.

Chu-Lagraff, Q., Wright, D. M., McNeil, L. K., & Doe, C. Q. (1991). The prospero gene encodes a divergent homeodomain protein that controls neuronal identity in *Drosophila*. *Development, Suppl. 2*, 79–85.

Corey, L. A., Kang, K. W, Christian, J. C., Norton, J. A., Harris, R. E., & Nance, W. E. (1976). Effects of chorion type on variation in cord blood cholesterol of monozygotic twins. *American Journal of Human Genetics, 28*, 433–441.

Corey, L. A., Nance, W. E., Kang, K. W., & Christian, J. C. (1979). Effects of type of placentation on birthweight and its variability in monozygotic and dizygotic twins. *Acta Geneticae Medicae et Gemellologiae, 28*, 41–50.

Couly, G., Grapin-Botton, A., Coltey, P., & Le Douarin, N. M. (1996). The regeneration of the cephalic neural crest, a problem revisited: The regenerating cells originate from the contralateral or from the anterior and posterior neural fold. *Development, 22*, 3393–3407.

Cripps, M. M., & Nash, D. J. (1983). Ontogeny and adult behavior of mice with congenital adult tube defects. *Behavioral and Neural Biology, 38*, 127–132.

Darvasi, A., & Soller, M. (1995) Advanced intercross lines, an experimental design for fine genetic mapping. *Genetics, 141*, 1199–1207.

De Smedt, B., Devriendt, K., Fryns, J.-P., Vogels, A., Gewillig, M., & Swillen, A. (2007). Intellectual abilities in a large sample of children with velo-cardio-facial syndrome: An update. *Journal of Intellectual Disability Research, 51*(9), 666–670.

Dekker, N., Cox, M., Boelens, R., Verrijzer, C. P., van der Vliet, P. C., & Kaptein, R. (1993). Solution structure of the POU-specific DNA-binding domain of *Oct-1*. *Nature 362*, 852–855.

Derom, C., Derom, R., Loos, R. J. B., Jacobs, N., & Vlietinck, R. (2003) Retrospective determination of chorion type in twins using a simple questionnaire. *Twin Research, 26*, 407–408.

Derom, R., Bryan, E., Derom, C., Keith, L., & Vlietinck, R. (2001). Twins, chorionicity and zygosity. *Twin Research, 4*, 134–136.

Dubé, J., Dodds, L., & Armson, B. A. (2002). Does chorionicity or zygosity predict adverse perinatal outcomes in twins? *American Journal of Obstetrics and Gynecology, 186*, 579–583.

Dulioust, E., Toyama, K., Busnel, M.-C., Moutier, R., Carlier, M., Marchaland, C., et al. (1995). Long-term effects of embryo freezing in mice. *Proceedings of the National Academy of Sciences of USA, 92*, 589–593.

Eaves, L., Foley, D., & Silberg, J. (2003). Has the "equal environments" assumption been tested in twin studies? *Twin Research, 6*, 486–489.

Fagard, R. H., Loos, R. J. F., Beunen, G., Derom, C., & Vlietinck, R. (2003). Influence of chorionicity on the heritability estimates of blood pressure:

Fox, M. W. (1965). Neuro-ontogeny of neuromuscular mutant mice. *Journal of Heredity*, 56, 55–60.

Garber, R. L., Kuroiwa, A., & Gehring, W. J. (1983). Genomic and cDNA clones of the homeotic locus Antennapedia in drosophila. *EMBO Journal*, 11, 2027–2036.

Gehring, W. J., Affolter, M., & Bürglin, T. (1994a). Homeodomain proteins. *Annual Review of Biochemistry*, 63, 487–526.

Gehring, W. J., Qian, Y. Q., Billeter, M., Furukubo-Tokunaga, K., Schier, A. F., Resendez-Perez, D., et al. (1994b). Homeodomain–DNA recognition. *Cell*, 78, 211–223.

Gene Expression Database (GXD), Mouse Genome Informatics Web Site, The Jackson Laboratory, Bar Harbor, Maine. Retrieved July, 21, 2007 from http://www.informatics.jax.org.

Gérard-Desplanches, A., Deruelle, C., Stefanini, S., Ayoun, C., Volterra, V., Vicari, S., et al. (2006). Laterality in persons with intellectual disability. II. Hand, foot, ear and eye lateralities in children or adolescent and adults persons with Trisomy 21 and Williams Beuren syndrome. *Developmental Psychobiology*, 48, 482–491.

Grapin-Botton, A., Bonnin, M. A., McNaughton, L. A., Krumlauf, R., & Le Douarin, N. M. (1995). Plasticity of transposed rhombomeres: *Hox* gene induction is correlated with phenotypic modifications. *Development*, 121, 2707–2721.

Grosjean, Y., Guenin, L., Bardet, H. M., & Ferveur, J. P. (2007). Prospero mutants induce precocious sexual behavior in drosophila males. *Behavior Genetics*, 37, 575–584.

Gutknecht, L., Spitz, E., & Carlier, M. (1999). Long term effect of placental type on anthropometrical and psychological traits among monozygotic twins: A follow up study. *Twin Research*, 2, 212–217.

Hanson, I. M., Fletcher, J. M., Jordan, T., Brown, A., Taylor, D., Adams, R. J., et al. (1994). Mutations at the PAX6 locus are found in heterogeneous anterior segment malformations including Peters' anomaly. *Nature Genetics*, 6, 168–173

Hanson, I. M., Seawright, A., Hardman, K., Hodgson, S., Zaletayev, D., Fekete, G., et al. (1993). PAX6 mutations in aniridia. *Human Molecular Genetics* 7, 915–920.

Holland, P. W., & Takahashi, T. (2005). The evolution of homeobox genes: Implications for the study of brain development. *Brain Research Bulletin*, 66, 484–490.

Hyman, S. (2000). Mental illness: Genetically complex disorders of neural circuitry and neural communication. *Neuron*, 28, 321–323.

Jacobs, N., Van Gestel, S., Derom, C., Thierry, E., Vernon, P., Derom, R., et al. (2001). Heritability estimates of intelligence in twins: Effect on chorion type. *Behavior Genetics*, 31, 209–217.

Job, C., & Tan, S. S. (2003). Constructing the mammalian neocortex: The role of intrinsic factors. *Developmental Biology*, 257, 221–232.

Kim, Y. H., Choi, C. Y., Lee, S. J., Conti, M. A., & Kim, Y. (1998). Homeodomain-interacting protein kinases, a novel family of co-repressors for homeodomain transcription factors. *Journal of Biological Chemistry*, 40, 25875–25879.

Kissinger, C. R., Liu, B. S., Martin-Blanco, E., Kornberg, T. B., & Pabo, C. O. (1990). Crystal structure of an engrailed homeodomain–DNA complex at 2.8 Å resolution: A framework for understanding homeodomain–DNA interactions. *Cell*, 63, 579–590.

Konrat, R., Weiskirchen, R., Krautler, B., & Bister, K. (1997). Solution structure of the carboxyl-terminal LIM domain from quail cysteine-rich protein CRP2. *The Journal of Biological Chemistry*, 272, 12001–12007.

Laughon, A. (1991). DNA binding specificity of homeodomains. *Biochemistry*, 30, 11357–11367.

Le Roy, I., Perez-Diaz, F., Cherfouh, A., & Roubertoux, P. L. (1999). Preweanling sensorial and motor development in laboratory mice: Quantitative trait loci mapping. *Developmental Psychobiology*, 34, 139–158.

Loos, R. F., Beunen, G., Fagard, R., Derom, C., & Vlietinck, R. (2001). The influence of zygosity and chorion type on fat distribution in young adult twins: Consequences for twin studies. *Twin Research*, 4, 356–364.

Machin, G. (2001). Placentation in multiple births. *Twin Research*, 4, 150–155.

Marzetta, C. A., & Nash, D. J. (1979) Ontogenetic study of the Miwh gene in mice. *Developmental Psychobiology*, 12, 527–532.

Melnick, M., Myrianthopoulos, N. C., & Christian J. C. (1978). The effects of chorion type on variation in IQ in the NCPP twin population. *American Journal of Human Genetics*, 30, 425–433.

Melnick, M., Myrianthopoulos, N. C., & Christian J. C. (1980). Estimates of genetic variance for anterior fontanelle development in the NCPP twin population. *Acta Geneticae Medicae et Gemellologia*, 29, 151–155.

Mervis, C. B., & Klein-Tasman, B. P. (2000). Williams syndrome: Cognition, personality and adaptive behaviour. *Mental Retardation and Developmental Disabilities Research Reviews*, 6, 148–158.

Mikuni, P. A., & Nash, D. J. (1979). Ontogeny of behavior in mice selected for large size. *Behavior Genetics*, 22, 227–232.

Mistretta, C. M., & Bradley, R. M. (1975). Taste and swallowing in utero. A discussion of fetal sensory function. *British Medical Bulletin*, 31, 80–83.

Monteiro, J., Derom, C., Vlietinck, R., Kohn, N., Lesser, M., & Gregersen, P. (1998). Commitment to X-inactivation precedes the twinning event in monochorionic-monozygotic (MC-MZ) twins. *American Journal of Human Genetics*, 63, 339–346.

Mouse Genome Database (MGD), Mouse Genome Informatics Web Site, The Jackson Laboratory, Bar Harbor, Maine. Retrieved July 14, 2007 from http://www.informatics.jax.org.

Neale, M. C., & Cardon, L. R. (1992). *Methodology for genetic studies of twins and families*. Dordrecht: Kluwer Academic.

Noël, M. (1989). Early development in mice: V. Sensorimotor development of four coisogenic mutant strains. *Physiology and Behavior*, 45, 21–26.

Nosten, M. (1989). Early development in mice. VI. Additive and interactive effects of offspring genotype and maternal environment, *Physiology and Behavior*, 45, 955–961.

Nosten, M., & Roubertoux, P. L. (1988). Uterine and cytoplasmic effects on pup eyelid opening in two inbred strains of mice. *Physiology and Behavior*, 43, 167–71.

Oliver, B. R., & Plomin, R. (2007). Twins' Early Development Study (TEDS): A multivariate, longitudinal genetic investigation of language, cognition and behaviour problems from childhood through adolescence. *Twin Research and Human Genetics*, *10*, 96–105.

Papousek, H., & Papousek, M. (1983). Biological basis of social interactions. *Journal of Child Psychologyand Psychiatry*, *24*, 177–219.

Pardon, M.-C., Gérardin, P., Joubert, C., Pérez-Diaz, F., & Cohen-Salmon, Ch. (2000). Influence on prepartum chronic ultramild stress on maternal pup care behavior in mice. *Biology of Psychiatry*, *47*, 858–863.

Patarnello, T., Bargelloni, L., Boncinelli, E., Spada, F., Pannese, M., & Broccoli V. (1997). Evolution of *Emx* genes and brain development in vertebrates. *Proceedings of the Royal Society, Biological Sciences, 1389*, 1763–1766.

Race, J. P., Townsend, G. C., & Hughes, T. E. (2006). Chorion type, birthweight discordance and tooth-size variability in Australian monozygotic twins. *Twins Research and Human Genetics*, *9*, 285–291.

Reed, T., Spitz, E., Vacher-Lavenu, M. C., & Carlier M. (1997). Evaluation of a dermatoplyphic index to detect placental type variation in MZ twins. *American Journal of Human Biology*, *9*, 609–615.

Reed, T., Uchida, I. A., Norton, J. A., & Christian, J. C. (1978). Comparison of dermatoglyphic patterns in monochorionic and dichorionic monozygotic twins. *American Journal of Human Genetics*, *31*, 315–323.

Riese, M. L. (1999). Effects of chorion type on neonatal temperament differences in monozygotic twin pairs. *Behavior Genetics*, *29*, 87–94.

Rose, R. J, Uchida, I. A, & Christian, J. C. (1981). Placentation effects on cognitive resemblance of adult monozygotes. In *Twin research 3: Intelligence, personality, and development* (pp. 35–41). New York: Alan Liss.

Roubertoux, P. L., Baumann, L, Ragueneau, S., & Semal, C. (1987). Early development in mice: IV. Age at disappearance of the rooting response; Genetic analysis in newborn mice. *Behavior Genetics*, *7*, 453–464.

Roubertoux, P. L., Bichler, Z., Pinoteau, W., Jamon, M., Sérégaza, Z., Smith, D. J., et al. (2006). Pre-weaning sensorial and motor development in mice transpolygenic for the critical region of trisomy 21. *Behavior Genetics*, *36*, 377–386.

Roubertoux, P. L., & Carlier, M. (2007). From DNA to the mind. *EMBO Reports*, *8* [Science & Society Special Issue], S7–S11.

Roubertoux , P. L., Nosten-Bertrand, M., & Carlier, M. (1990). Additive and interactive effects between genotype and maternal environments, concepts and facts. *Advances in the Study of Behavior*, *19*, 205–247.

Roubertoux, P. L., Semal, C., & Raguenau S. (1985). Early development in mice. II—Sensory motor behavior and genetic analysis. *Physiology and Behavior, 35*, 659–666.

Roubertoux, P. L., Sluyter, F., Carlier, M., Marcet, B., Maarouf-Veray, F., Cherif, C., et al. (2003). Mitochondrial DNA modifies cognition in interaction with the nuclear genome and age in mice. *Nature Genetics*, *35*, 65–69.

Ruddle, F. H., Bartels, J. L., Bentley, K. L., Kappen, C., Murtha, M. T. & Pendleton, J. W. (1994). Evolution of Hox genes. *Annual Review of Genetics*, *28*, 423–442.

Sakkou, M., Wiedmer, P., Anlag, K., Hamm, A., Seuntjens, E., Ettwiller, L., et al. (2007). A role for brain-specific homeobox factor *bsx* in the control of hyperphagia and locomotory behavior. *Cell Metabolism*, *6*, 450–463.

Schmucker, D., Clemens, J. C., Shu, H., Worby, C. A., Xiao J., Muda, M., et al. (2000). Drosophila Dscam is an axon guidance receptor exhibiting extraordinary moleculardiversity. *Cell 101*, 671–684.

Scott, J. P., & Fuller, J. L. (1965) *Genetics and the social behavior of the dog.* Chicago: University of Chicago Press.

Scott, M. P., Weiner, A. J., Hazelrigg, T. I., Polisky, B. A., Pirrotta, V., Scalenghe, F., et al. (1983). The molecular organization of the Antennapedia locus of drosophila. *Cell, 35*, 763–776.

Sokol, D. K., Moore, C. A., Rose, R. J., Williams, C. J, Reed, T., & Christian, J. C. (1995). Intra-pair differences in personality and cognitive ability among young monozygotic twins distinguished by chorion type. *Behavior Genetics*, *25*, 457–466.

Souter, V. L., Kapur, R. P., Nyholt, D. R., Skogerboe, K., Myerson, D., Ton, C. C., et al. (2003). A report of dizygous monochorionic twins. *The New England Journal of Medicine. 349*, 154–158.

Spitz, E., Carlier, M., Vacher-Lavenu, M.-C., Reed, T., Moutier, R., Busnel, M.-C., et al. (1996). Long term effect of prenatal heterogeneity among monozygotes. *CPC Cahiers de Psychology Cognitive Current Psychology of Cognition*, *15*, 283–308.

Swillen, A., Devriendt, K., Legius, E., Eyskens, B., Dumoulin, M., Gewillig, M., et al. (1997). Intelligence and psychological adjustment in velocardiofacial syndrome: A study of 37 children and adolescents with VCFS. *Journal of Medical Genetics*, *34*, 453–458.

Ton, C. C., Hiroven, H., Miwa, H., Weil, M. M., Monaghan, P., Jordan, T., et al. (1991). Positional cloning and characterization of a paired box- and homeobox-containing gene from the aniridia region. *Cell*, *67*, 1059–1054.

Trainor, P. A., & Krumlauf, R. (2000). Patterning the cranial neural crest: Hindbrain segmentation and Hox gene plasticity. *Nature Review Neuroscience*, *2*, 116–124.

Ule, J., Stefani, G., Mele, A., Ruggiu, M., Wang, X., Taneri, B., et al. (2006). An RNA map predicting Nova-dependent splicing regulation. *Nature. 444*, 580–586.

van Heyningen, V., & Williamson, K. A. (2002). PAX6 in sensory development. *Human Molecular Genetics, 11*, 1161–1167.

Vicari, S. (2006). Motor development and neuropsychological patterns in persons with Down syndrome. *Behavior Genetics*, *36*, 355–364.

Vlietinck, R., Derom, R., Neale, M. C., Maes H., Van Loon, H., Derom, C., et al. (1989). Genetic and environmental variation in the birth weight of twins. *Behavior Genetics*, *19*, 51–61.

Vollmer, J. Y., & Clerc, R. G. (1998). Homeobox genes in the developing mouse brain, *Journal of Neurochemistry*, *71*, 1–19.

Wahlsten, D. (1982). Mice in utero while their mother is lactating suffer higher frequency of deficient corpus callosum. *Brain Research. 281*, 354–357.

Welch, P., Black, K. N., & Christian, J. C. (1978). Placental type and Bayley mental development scores in 18-month-old twins. In *Twin research: Psychology and methodology* (pp. 145–149). New York: Alan Liss.

Wichers, M. C., Danckaerts, M., Van Gestel, S., Derom, C., Vlietinck, R., & van Os, J. (2002). Chorion type and twin similarity for child psychiatric symptoms. *Archives of General Psychiatry*, *59*, 562–564.

Wilson, R. S. (1972). Twins: Early mental development. *Science, 175*, 914–917.

Wolberger, C., Vershon, A. K., Liu, B., Johnson, A. D., & Pabo, C. O. (1991). Crystal structure of a MAT alpha 2 homeodomain–operator complex suggests a general model for homeodomain–DNA interactions. *Cell, 67*, 517–528.

Wu, L., Sun, T., Kobayashi, K., Gao, P., & Griffin, J. D. (2002). Identification of a family of mastermind-like transcriptional coactivators for mammalian notch receptors, *Molecular and Cellular Biology, 21*, 7688–7700.

Yu, G., Nishimura, M., Arawaka, S., Levitan, D., Zhang, L., Tandon, A., et al. (2000). Nicastrin modulates presenilin-mediated notch/glp-1 signal transduction and β-APP processing. *Nature, 407*, 48–54.

Programmed Cell Death During Nervous System Development: Mechanisms, Regulation, Functions, and Implications for Neurobehavioral Ontogeny

Ronald W. Oppenheim, Carol Milligan, *and* Woong Sun

Abstract

During normal development of the nervous system of most species of vertebrate and invertebrate animals, large numbers of immature neuronal and glial cells are lost by a process of programmed cell death (PCD). PCD occurs by evolutionarily conserved molecular and biochemical pathways that are regulated by the relative activity of pro- and antiapoptotic genes. The decision to live or die is often determined by the availability of survival-promoting neurotrophic factors that act via receptor-mediated signaling pathways. Neuronal activity also plays a role in modulating neuronal survival. The PCD of neurons serves a variety of adaptive functions that are involved in the nervous system development and organization. Finally, pathological cell death may be involved in the dysfunction resulting from injury and in neurodegenerative diseases.

Keywords: PCD, cell death, nervous system, neuronal cells, glial cells, proapoptotic genes, antiapoptotic genes, receptor-mediated signaling, dysfunction

Introduction

During embryonic, fetal, larval, and early postnatal development of many invertebrate and vertebrate species, there is a loss of many mitotic and postmitotic undifferentiated and differentiating cells (precursors, immature neurons and glia) in the central nervous system (CNS) and peripheral nervous system (PNS). This cell loss is a normal part of development and it occurs by a metabolically active, biochemically regulated process known as programmed cell death (PCD). Developmental PCD is defined as the spatially and temporally reproducible, tissue- and species-specific loss of cells. PCD in the nervous system serves diverse functions, is required for normal development, and its perturbation can result in pathology. Although developmental PCD in the nervous system is primarily restricted to prenatal

and early postnatal stages, a major exception involves the CNS regions in which adult neurogenesis occurs. Newly generated adult cells are subject to many of the same major steps of differentiation as embryonically generated cells, including the PCD of a significant proportion of the originally generated cells. For this reason, we also include here a discussion of the PCD of adult-generated neurons.

In view of the diverse functions subserved by PCD in the nervous system (section on "Adaptive Functions of PCD in the Nervous System"), it is not surprising that perturbations of normally occurring PCD can result in a variety of abnormal conditions that directly or indirectly affect nervous system organization and function (neurobehavioral ontogeny). Because the survival of developing and adult-generated neurons can often be regulated by synaptic activity arising from endogenous sources as well as from environmental stimuli via sensory receptors, there are reciprocal influences by which PCD can affect function and in which function can influence PCD. It is this interaction that is the basis for the important role of PCD in neurobehavioral ontogeny.

History

The occurrence of developmental PCD in nonnervous tissues was first reported in the mid-nineteenth century (Clarke & Clarke, 1996) and neuronal PCD was discovered in the 1890s (Clarke, 1990). However, it was not until the middle of the twentieth century that the occurrence and significance of PCD in the nervous system was first appreciated by embryologists (Hamburger, 1992; Oppenheim, 1981a). In a series of seminal papers by Viktor Hamburger and Rita Levi-Montalcini in the 1930s, 1940s, and 1950s (Cowan, 2001; Oppenheim, 1981a, 2001) it was shown that sensory and motor neurons in the spinal cord of the chick embryo are generated in excess during neurogenesis followed by the PCD of approximately one-half of the original population. This period of cell loss was found to occur as sensory and motor neurons were establishing synaptic connections with their peripheral synaptic targets (Figure 5.1). In a conceptual tour de force, Hamburger and Levi-Montalcini proposed that developing neurons compete for limiting amounts of target-derived, survival-promoting signals (the winners survive and losers are eliminated by PCD). In this way, neurons are thought to optimize their innervation of targets (e.g., motoneuron–muscle synapses) by a process known as systems-matching. It was this conceptual framework that led to the discovery of the first target-derived survival factor, the neurotrophic molecule nerve growth factor (NGF), and to the formulation of the neurotrophic theory or hypothesis, which has fostered progress in this field for over 60 years. According to the neurotrophic theory, neurons that compete successfully for neurotrophic factors (NTFs) avoid PCD by receptor-mediated activation of survival-promoting intracellular molecular-genetic programs. The discovery of molecular-genetic programs in the 1980s and 1990s that regulate both the survival and death of developing cells (first observed in the nematode worm, *Caenorhabditis elegans*, and subsequently in vertebrates and mammals [Horvitz, 2003]) revolutionized the study of developmental PCD, resulting in the publication of thousands of papers in the last 15 years, which has led to enormous progress in our understanding of the biochemical, molecular, and genetic regulation of PCD.

Evolution

The occurrence of massive PCD during normal development is, on the face of it, counterintuitive in that embryogenesis is generally considered to be a progressive growth process. However, it is now appreciated that regressive events are also normally required for many aspects of early development (Oppenheim, 1981a, 1981b). The death of occasional cells during development is to be expected in biological systems in which accidental or genetically mediated deleterious events may be lethal to individual cells. However, the stereotypical death of large numbers of developing cells in all members of a species, as occurs in many cases of PCD in the nervous system, cannot be easily explained in this way. Accordingly, this raises two fundamental questions regarding the evolution of this type of PCD: (1) Because PCD occurs by a metabolically active, genetically regulated process, how and why did the molecular mechanisms involved arise during evolution? (2) What are the adaptive reasons for massive developmental PCD in the nervous system? An attempt to answer the second question will be addressed in the section on "Adaptive Functions of PCD in the Nervous System."

With regard to the first question, the loss of cells by PCD was until relatively recently believed to have arisen concomitant with multicellularity in plants and animals as a defense mechanism for eliminating damaged or abnormal cells that threatened the survival of the whole organism (Brodersen et al., 2002; Umansky, 1982; Vaux, Haecker, & Strasser, 1994). According to this scenario, death-promoting mechanisms arose in host cells to defend against viral infection and, at the same time, viruses evolved survival-promoting mechanisms to block the host defenses (Ameisen, 2004). This is not only a reasonable explanation for why PCD evolved but may also explain the origin of the specific genetic mechanisms mediating cellular death and survival (such as pro- and antiapoptotic pathways).

However, PCD has now been identified in several species of unicellular eukaryotes including yeast as well as in prokaryotes, including several species of bacteria that emerged several billion years ago and are one of the oldest forms of life

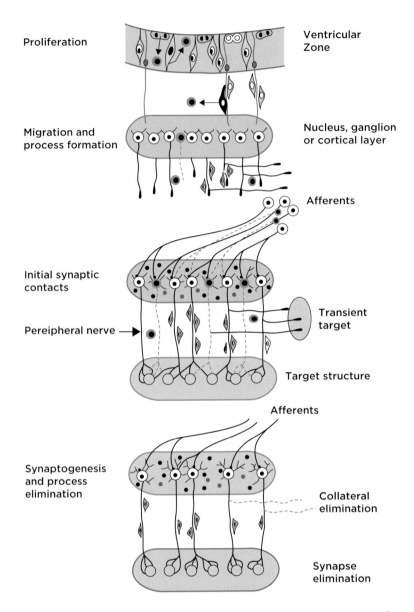

Figure 5.1 Schematic illustration of some key steps in neuronal development. Neurons undergoing PCD (●) are observed during neurogenesis in the ventricular zone, during migration, and while establishing synaptic contacts.

Schwann cells in developing nerves also undergo PCD. (•) represents peripheral glial (Schwann) cells; (◉) represents surviving, differentiating neurons (motoneurons) whose targets are skeletal muscles.

on earth (Ameisen, 2004). When considered in the context of PCD in metazoans, in which the loss of individual cells is a plausible adaptive strategy for the survival of the whole organism, PCD in unicellular protozoa and prokaryotes seems evolutionarily counterintuitive in that it appears analogous to the maladaptive death of individual multicellular animals. One solution to this apparent dilemma that has been suggested is that PCD in these organisms is altruistic (Ameisen, 2004; Frohlich & Madeo, 2000; Lewis, 2000). Unicellular organisms often live in colonies or communities composed of genetic clones in which the death of some individuals and the survival of others may, in fact, be adaptive. For example, in the face of limited resources (e.g., nutrients), the

PCD of some members of the colony may enhance the survival of others.

Mechanisms and Regulation
Programmed Cell Death by Autonomous Versus Conditional Specification

The type of PCD of neurons studied by Hamburger and Levi-Montalcini in which cell death occurs as neurons establish synaptic connections is a classic example of the conditional specification of cell fate during development (Figure 5.2). Developmental biologists have identified two primary kinds of pathways that cells use for specifying their differentiated fate or phenotype (Gilbert, 2003). One, *autonomous specification*, involves the differential segregation of cytoplasmic signals into daughter cells following mitosis (Table 5.1). In this way, the cells become different from one another by the presence or absence of these cytoplasmic signals with little, if any, contribution of signals from neighboring cells. The other pathway, *conditional specification*, requires signals from other cells (cell–cell interactions) to progressively restrict differentiation and determine whether a cell lives or dies (Figure 5.2). These cell–cell interactions can be of four types: (1) *juxtacrine* (direct cell–cell or cell–matrix contact); (2) *autocrine* (a secreted signal acts back on the same cell from which the

signal arose); (3) *paracrine* (a secreted diffusible signal from one cell that acts locally on a different cell type; and (4) *endocrine* (signaling via the bloodstream). In the developing vertebrate nervous system, neuronal and glial survival is largely dependent on conditional specification involving paracrine interactions that utilize NTFs. A third type of specification, *syncytial specification* is most characteristic of insects and combines aspects of autonomous and conditional specification (Table 5.1; Gilbert, 2003).

For neurons, the most commonly used NTFs are members of three major gene families: (1) neurotrophins (NGF, BDNF, NT-3, NT-4); (2) glial cell line–derived NTFs (GDNF, neurturin, persephin, artemin); and (3) ciliary-derived NTFs (CNTF, CT-1, CLC-CLF). The individual members of each family act preferentially on specific types of neurons via distinct membrane-bound receptors (Oppenheim & Johnson, 2003). By contrast, the survival of glial cells depends on different families of trophic factors such as neuregulins and insulin-like growth factors (Jessen & Mirsky, 2005; Winseck, Caldero, Ciutat, Prevette, & Scott, 2002; Winseck & Oppenheim, 2006). Neurons and glial cells utilize paracrine signaling to promote survival by ligand–receptor interactions. However, as discussed below, there are some situations in which paracrine signals can activate receptors that induce the PCD of neurons and glia (i.e., death receptor PCD).

Molecular Regulation of Programmed Cell Death and Survival by Neurotrophic Factors

Neuronal survival and death during development is regulated by extracellular signals that include trophic factors and extracellular matrix proteins (Davies, 2003). The dependence of neurons on NTFs for survival intuitively leads to the conclusion that inactivation of NTF receptors, and the signal transduction pathways associated with them, leads to activation of cell death events (Figure 5.3; Biswas & Greene, 2002; Brunet, Datta, & Greenberg, 2001; Fukunaga & Miyamoto 1998; Grewal, York, & Stork, 1999; Hetman & Zia, 2000). Many trophic factors interact with receptors that have intrinsic tyrosine kinase activity. This has been best studied with neurotrophins and their receptors, notably the Trk receptors and p75 (see Sofroneiw, Howe, & Mobley, 2001). Tyrosine kinase activation of the Trk receptors and other trophic factor receptors

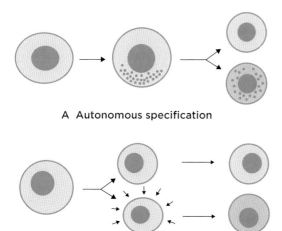

A Autonomous specification

B Conditional specification

Figure 5.2 Two major ways by which developing cells diversify to attain distinct phenotypes. The dots in A represent cytoplasmic determinants (e.g., mRNAs) that are differentially allotted to daughter cells during mitosis (see text and Table 5.1). Copyright 2002, Garland Science.

Table 5.1 Modes of Cell Type Specification and Their Characteristics

I. *Autonomous specification*
- Characteristic of most invertebrates
- Specification by differential acquisition of certain cytoplasmic molecules present in the egg
- Invariant cleavages produce the same lineages in each embryo of the species. Blastomere fates are generally invariant
- Cell type specification precedes any large-scale embryonic cell migration
- Produces "mosaic" development: cells cannot change fate if a blastomere is lost

II. *Conditional specification*
- Characteristic of all vertebrates and some invertebrates
- Specification by interactions between cells. Relative positions are important
- Variable cleavages produce no invariant fate assignments to cells
- Massive cell rearrangements and migrations precede or accompany specification
- Capacity for "regulative" development: allows cells to acquire different functions

III. *Syncytial specification*
- Characteristic of most insect classes
- Specification of body regions by interactions between cytoplasmic regions prior to cellularization of the blastoderm
- Variable cleavage produces no rigid cell fates for particular nuclei
- After cellularization, conditional specification is most often seen

results in activation of associated signal transduction pathways such as PLCγ, PI3K, PKA, PKB/Akt, PKC, and MAPK. Activation of these pathways has been associated with neuronal growth, differentiation, and migration events. Additionally, many of these pathways are also associated with changes in expression, location, or activation of cellular components associated with cell death. For example, Akt, a substrate of PI3-K has been reported to phosphorylate Bad, promoting its association with 14–3-3 and preventing inactivation of Bcl-2 and Bcl-x (Datta et al., 2000). Gsk-3b phosphorylates and inactivates Bax, whereas serine phosphorylation of Bad and Bcl-2 has been associated with activation of PI3K/Akt, ERK1/2, PKC, or PKA (Biswas & Greene 2002; Datta et al., 1997; del Peso, Gonzalez-Garcia, Page, Herrera, & Nunez, 1997; Harada et al., 1999; Jin, Mao, Zhu, & Greenberg, 2002). The survival-promoting activity of phosphorylated Bcl-2, however, is controversial, on the one hand being associated with motoneuron survival, whereas on the other hand, in neurons treated with microtubule destabilizing agents, it appears to promote death (Figueroa-Masot, Hetman, Higgins, Kokot, & Xia, 2001; Hadler et al., 1995 ; Newbern, Taylor, Robinson, & Milligan, 2005). The c-jun N-terminal kinase (JNK) pathway is reported to exhibit increased activity in neurons triggered to die. The activation of one of its substrates, c-jun, is also thought

to play a role in mediating neuronal death (Sun et al., 2005). For example, JNK activation of BH-3 proteins, Bim, and DP5, regulation of the release of Smac from mitochondria, and a JNK-p53-Bax pathway appear to be critical for death in specific cell types (Becker, Howell, Kodama, Barker, & Bonni, 2004; Chauhan et al., 2003; Deng et al., 2001; Donovan, Becker, Konishi, & Bonni, 2002; Gupta, Campbell, Derijard, & Davis, 1995; Harris & Johnson, 2001; Lei & Davis, 2003; Maundrell et al., 1997; Putcha et al., 2003; Sunayama, Tsuruta, Masuyama, & Gotoh, 2005; Tournier et al., 2000; Yamamoto, Ichijo, & Korsmeyer, 1999). Nonetheless, the JNK pathway has also been reported to be a critical mediator of survival-promoting events such as neurite outgrowth (Kuan et al., 1999; Sabapathy et al., 1999). These findings suggest that the JNK pathways may have a dual role in promoting both survival and death depending on changes in intracellular localization and specific activation or inactivation of individual isoforms and/or specific substrates (Waetzig & Herdegen, 2005).

The role of the p75 NGF receptor in promoting neuronal survival or death is also controversial. For example, complexes of p75 and sortilin appear to promote the binding of the proneurotrophins, resulting in the survival of neurons (Bronfman & Fainzilber, 2004; Hempstead, 2006). Activation of p75 in the absence of Trk activation has most

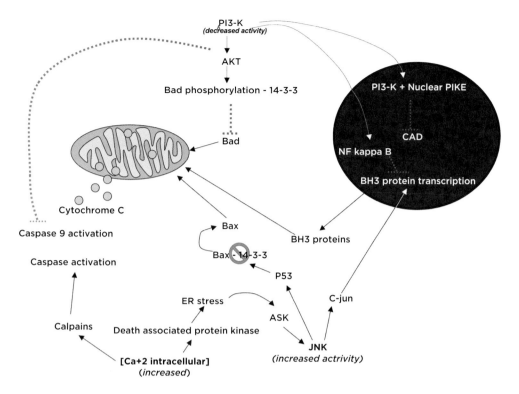

Figure 5.3 Signals to die. Changes in signal transduction pathways, activation of receptors containing a DD, or changes in intracellular calcium concentrations have been identified as events that can lead to activation of cell death–specific events. Loss of trophic support results in decreased activation of the phosphatidylinositol-3 kinase (PI3-K) thereby releasing inhibitory factors linked to this pathway. Alternatively, increases in intracellular calcium concentrations, activation of the Fas receptor, and/or increased c-jun terminal kinase activation are associated with the mitochondrial changes and caspase activation that occurs in cell death.

notably been associated with the death of neurons, but this appears to be developmentally regulated. The precise mechanism by which p75 promotes death is unclear. However, p75 is a member of the tumor necrosis factor receptor family, and another member of this family better known for its death-promoting activity is Fas/CD95 (see Wallach et al., 1999 for review). Engagement of Fas by Fas ligand leads to the activation of caspase 8. This event is dependent on the formation of a death-inducing signaling complex (DISC) (Peter & Krammer, 2003). Homotrimerization is the first step in this process. Engagement of Fas by its ligand can only occur when it is homotrimerized. This family of receptors is characterized by the presence of a death domain (DD) on the cytoplasmic region of the receptors. The Fas-associated death domain–containing protein (FADD) can then bind to Fas. In addition to the DD, FADD also contains a death effector domain (DED). Procaspase 8 binds to the DED. The autolytic nature of caspases leads to active capsase 8 that can then go on to directly

activate caspase 3 (in type 1 cells, e.g., thymocytes) or cleave Bid, leading to changes at the mitochondria (in type 2 cells, e.g., hepatocytes and neurons) and cell death.

Intracellular Regulation of Cell Death

Many of the intracellular mechanisms mediating neuronal cell death were investigated following initial work that suggested that new gene expression was required for the process. Horvitz and coworkers provided some of the first evidence that there was indeed a genetic component of PCD from their work in the 1980s with the free living nematode *C. elegans*, although it was two decades later that the significance of this work was fully appreciated (Figure 5.4; Horvitz, 2003; Lettre & Hengartner, 2006). As these genes were identified, the sequence of events leading to the death of cells was pieced together.

The presence of Bcl-2 family proteins appears critical for mediating survival or death of nervous system cells (Akhtar, Ness, & Roth, 2004; Soane

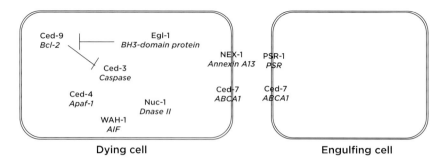

Figure 5.4 Many of the key regulators of cell death are evolutionarily conserved. Many of the genes for these proteins were initially identified through genetic mutations in the free living nematode (bold type), with homologs later being identified in Drosophila and mammals (italics). Genes that mediate interactions between dying and engulfing cells are depicted as extending across the cell membrane.

& Fiskum, 2005). During development, Bcl-2 expression is correlated with neuronal survival. With continued maturation and development, this expression declines, whereas Bcl-x expression increases. The specific mechanisms responsible for this change in expression are currently not known. On the other hand, the expression of pro-death Bcl-2 family proteins such as Bid or Bax appears to be consistent throughout development, whereas the intracellular localization of these proteins appears to change in cells undergoing death. In healthy cells, Bax is localized more in the cytoplasm whereas in dying cells, the majority of Bax localizes to organelle membranes, including the mitochondria. The localization of Bax to the mitochondria corresponds to the release of cytochrome c into the cytoplasm. Once in the cytoplasm, cytochrome c binds Apaf-1, causing a conformational change in Apaf-1 to reveal a caspase recruitment domain (CARD) (Adams & Cory, 2002). In the presence of adenosine triphosphate (ATP), a heptamer of the cytochrome c/Apaf-1 complex is formed. Procaspase 9 has a high affinity for the CARD and localizes to the heptamer. This complex is referred to as the apoptosome. With the increased local concentration of procaspase 9, the autolytic property of caspases leads to the generation of active caspase 9. As an initiator caspase, active caspase 9 can cleave procaspase 3, resulting in the active form of this protease (reviewed in Danial & Korsmeyer, 2004; Yuan, Lipinski, & Degterev, 2003; Figure 5.5). The activation, inactivation, or destruction of specific cytoplasmic and nuclear substrates significantly contributes to the rapid degeneration of the cell (Fischer, Janicke, & Schulze-Osthoff, 2003). Caspase activity leads to activation of endonucleases that may play a role in the changes in nuclear morphologies that are observed in may cell types.

The caspase-dependent cell death pathway outlined above is often referred to as "apoptotic" death and occurs in neurons in response to numerous stimuli, including loss of trophic support. Nonetheless, inhibition or elimination of caspases often results in only a delay in neuronal death followed by death by a caspase-independent pathway (Milligan et al., 1995a; Oppenheim et al., 2001a, 2001b, 2008). This alternative death pathway may also rely on mitochondrial changes and appears to be dependent on BH3 proteins and/or Bax. These changes at the mitochondria can cause energy depletion or generation of free radicals, both leading to cellular dysfunction and death (Gorman, Ceccatelli, & Orrenius, 2000). It is not clear if this pathway occurs only when caspases are inhibited or occurs in parallel but is overshadowed by caspase activation (reviewed in Stefanis, 2005). Another factor thought to play a role in caspase-independent pathways is the apoptosis-inducing factor (AIF; Cregan et al., 2002). AIF is normally present within the mitochondria, but upon appropriate stimulation is released and translocates to the nucleus where it appears to be involved in chromatin condensation. Nonetheless, AIF also appears to have a physiological role in the mitochondria. It may serve as a scavenger of oxidative radicals and may play a role in oxidative phosphorylation and maintenance of the electron transport chain and mitochondrial structure (Cheung et al., 2006; Lipton & Bossy-Wetzel, 2002; Vahsen et al., 2004). Other molecules have also been shown to be involved in regulating neuronal death, and cell cycle molecules are most notable

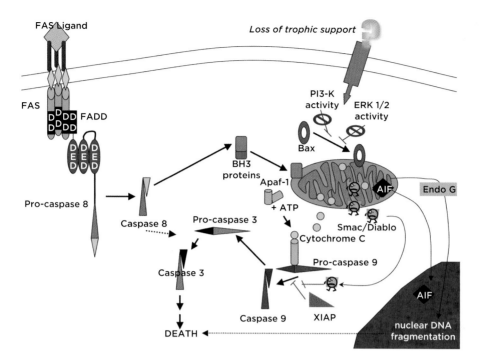

Figure 5.5 Many of the critical components of neuronal death and their apparent sequence of activation during development are illustrated. The mitochondria release many regulators that can lead to death with or without caspase activation. Neurons are considered "type 2" cells where Fas engagement results in minimal caspase 8 activation resulting in cleavage of Bid and its subsequent movement to the mitochondria. The localization of Bax to the mitochondria appears to be a critical event in the death of neurons.

(Freeman, Estus, & Johnson, 1994; Greene, Biswas, & Liu, 2004). Nonetheless, as with many events in cell death, their use appears to be cell-specific, whereas cell cycle events mediate sensory neuron death, but not motoneuron death (Taylor, Prevette, Urioste, Oppenheim, & Milligan, 2003).

The removal of the dying cell is most likely just as critical an event in the cell death process as any of those discussed above (Figure 5.4). This event can be accomplished by nonprofessional phagocytes (e.g., Schwann cells), but more often involves dedicated phagocytes such as tissue macrophages (microglia) or circulating monocytes (Mallat, Marin-Teva, & Cheret, 2005). During early CNS development, resident microglia are often not present in large numbers among dying cell populations. Intuitively, some signal must be sent by the dying cells to recruit the phagocytes into the area (Milligan et al., 1995b). One such chemotactic factor has been identified in nonneuronal cells, and interestingly, this factor is the phospholipid, lysophosphatidylcholine (Lauber et al., 2003). Caspase 3 activation appears to be necessary for release of this factor. Once the phagocytic cells are in the region, they must be able to distinguish dying cells

from healthy cells (Savill, 1997; Savill & Fadok, 2000; Savill, Gregory, & Haslett, 2003). Changes on the dying cell's surface include revealing of thrombospondin 1–binding sites and exposure of phosphatidylserine, ATP-binding cassette (ABC-1) molecules, and carbohydrate changes. The phagocyte in turn expresses the phosphatidylserine receptor, as well as thrombospondin receptors that recognize the thrombospondin bound to the binding site on the dying cell, lectins that bind to the carbohydrate changes, and ABC-1 molecules that bind to like molecules. Phagocytosis occurs only when multiple changes are recognized, and this phagocytosis is limited and does not result in macrophage secretion of cytokines that would normally induce an inflammatory or immune response if foreign antigens were phagocytosed.

Different Types of Neuronal Programmed Cell Death

Many investigators studying cell death often rely on the critical papers of Currie, Kerr, and Wyllie (1980) to define and characterize the different types of cell death. These investigators described in detail two distinct morphological changes associated with cell death. An active process, apoptosis, was characterized by specific morphological changes that included condensation of nuclear chromatin, shrinking of the cytoplasm, and a breaking up of the cell into membrane bound particles (apoptotic bodies) that were phagocytosed. Necrosis, on the other hand, was characterized by a swelling of the cytoplasm with eventual bursting of the cell. In this case, intracellular components are spilled into the extracellular space where they could initiate inflammatory and immune responses. However, electron microscopic studies of the developing nervous system indicated that often neuronal death cannot be so easily defined by only these two modes of death (Figure 5.6; Chu-Wang & Oppenheim, 1978; Clarke, 1990; Pilar & Landmesser, 1976). During the naturally occurring death of some neurons, initial changes in dying cells are observed in the cytoplasm where there is an increase in the diameter of the cisternae of the rough endoplasmic reticulum (RER). Mitochondrial swelling was also observed although it was not clear if these changes occur in the same cell. Nonetheless, during normal development, initial changes are observed in the cytoplasm with little nuclear alterations in dying cells. The cell then appears to round up and break into fragments that are phagocytosed. Although cytoplasmic cell death appears to be more prominent during development, nuclear or apoptotic death also occurs.

A third type of death is autophagy, characterized by the formation of numerous, membrane-bound autophagic vacuoles. Nuclear changes may also occur in this type of death.

It is important to note that all three types of neuronal death appear to reflect a metabolically active process. Accordingly, it would appear that a homogeneous mode of suicide does not occur, but rather processes leading to death appear to be dependent on context, cell type, and development. One example would be a neuronal population undergoing apoptosis where nuclear condensation is a prominent feature but in which following caspase inhibition or genetic deletion, the same neuronal population undergoes a delayed, caspase-independent death with major changes occurring in the cytoplasm (Oppenheim et al., 2008).

Adaptive Functions of Programmed Cell Death in the Nervous System
Background

PCD in the nervous system involves both neurons and glia and occurs in the CNS and PNS of diverse species (Buss, Sun, & Oppenheim, 2006). Accordingly, it is not surprising that the diversity of adaptive roles for PCD differ according to the animal species, cell type, nervous system region, and stage of development. A list of some of the common reasons for PCD in the nervous system

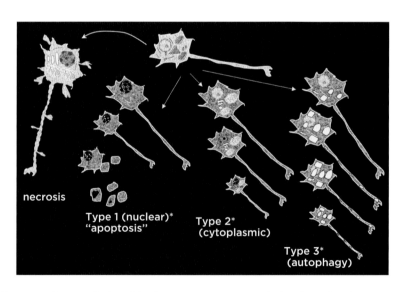

Figure 5.6 An illustration of necrotic death and the three most common types of PCD observed in the nervous system (see Koliatsos & Ratan, 1999). One type (type 1) meets the criteria for apoptosis. Cells undergoing type 2 death show predominant changes in the cytoplasm, with a swelling of the mitochondria and disruption of RNA and protein synthesis machinery. In type 3 death, the appearance of lysosomes is most prominent. Types 1–3 are observed in PCD, and the corpses are removed by phagocytes. Necrosis often occurs as a result of direct injury and can result in inflammation.

is provided in Table 5.2. There is a growing consensus that once the genetic mechanisms evolved for regulating cell death and survival, they could then be co-opted to subserve many different events during development. According to this view, it is not necessary to postulate that each instance of developmental PCD was independently selected. Rather, it seems much more likely that once the pro- and anti-PCD genetic machinery was in place, then excess cells could be deleted or retained using so-called "social" controls (Raff, 1992) involving evolutionarily conserved cell–cell interactions (e.g., trophic factor signaling) that may have been selected for reasons other than the control of cell death (Amiesen, 2004; Jaaro, Beck, Conticello, & Fainzilber, 2001), but that were co-opted in the service of PCD.

In considering the possible adaptive functions of PCD in this chapter, we define the term "adaptive" as a specific event or a process that increases fitness by enhancing the survival of individuals who exhibit the adaptation. Adaptations in this Darwinian sense arise from selection upon genetic variation (mutations). However, we also include in our definition adaptation as an intuitive functional statement about an efficient way of doing something independent of any inferences about its specific origin during evolution. Admittedly, there is a danger in assuming that all developmental events are adaptive and the result of gene mutations and natural selection versus being epiphenomenal or due to allometry, genetic drift, pleiotropy, or developmental plasticity (Gould & Lewontin, 1979; Mayr, 1983; West-Eberhard, 2003). Given the timescale over which evolution by natural selection works, however, even miniscule positive selection pressures resulting in small changes in anatomy or physiology can be adaptive (Haldane, 1932).

One of the first attempts to address the issue of the biological functions of massive developmental PCD was that of Ernst (1926) and Glücksmann (1930, 1951). According to Glücksmann, there are three major categories of PCD that subserve distinct functions: morphogenetic (e.g., creation of digits by interdigital PCD); histogenetic (e.g., PCD during histogenesis, including most neuronal PCD); and phylogenetic (e.g., the loss of vestigial structures such as the tail, the pronephros, and mesonephros, or the loss of larval structures). Historically, this represents an important and thoughtful attempt to understand the biological utility of developmental PCD. Glücksmann, for instance, provided a comprehensive list of examples of PCD in many tissues and organs at all stages of development in diverse species and he attempted to define their adaptive purpose within the three

Table 5.2 Some Possible Functions of Developmental PCD in the Nervous System

1. Differential removal of cells in males and females (sexual dimorphisms)
2. Deletion of some of the progeny of a specific sublineage that are not needed
3. Negative selection of cells of an inappropriate phenotype
4. Pattern formation and morphogenesis
5. Deletion of cells that act as transient targets or that provide transient guidance cues for axon projections
6. Removal of cells and tissues that serve a transient physiological or behavioral function
7. "Systems-matching" by creating optimal quantitative innervation between interconnected groups of developing neurons and between neurons and their targets (e.g., muscles, sensory receptors); may involve synaptic activity–modulated signals (see Figure 5.6).
8. Systems-matching between neurons and their glial partners by regulated glial PCD (e.g., Schwann cells and axons) (see Figure 5.3)
9. Error correction by the removal of ectopically positioned neurons or of neurons with misguided axons or inappropriate synaptic connections
10. Removal of damaged or harmful cells
11. Regulation of the size of mitotically active progenitor populations
12. The production of excess neurons may serve as an ontogenetic buffer for accommodating mutations that require changes in neuronal numbers in order to be evolutionary adaptive (e.g., increases or decreases in limb size may require less or more motoneuron death for optimal innervation)
13. Activity-regulated survival of subpopulations of adult-generated neurons as a means of experience-dependent plasticity

Evidence is support of one or more of the reasons for PCD can be found in the following sources: Buss, Sun, and Oppenheim (2006); Ellis, Yuan, & Horvitz (1991); Forger (2006); Kempermann (2006); Nottebohm (2002a, 2002b); Oppenheim (1991); Oppenheim et al. (2001a, 2001b); Silver (1978); Truman (1984). Copyright 2006, *Annual Reviews*. Reprinted with permission.

major categories described. Over the past 50 years, a number of reviews have appeared that expand on Glücksmann's pioneering efforts by the addition of new examples of developmental PCD and, more importantly, by providing experimental evidence for the adaptive roles of, and the mechanisms that regulate, PCD (Ellis, Yuan, & Horvitz, 1991; Källen, 1965; Moon, 1981; Sanders & Wride, 1995; Saunders, 1966; Silver, 1978; Wyllie et al., 1980). One inference that emerges from these reviews is that it is often far easier to provide convincing evidence for the adaptive roles of PCD in the development of nonnervous tissues than it is for nervous tissues, especially within the morphogenetic and histogenetic categories of Glücksmann. For example, interdigital cell death, the deletion of self-reactive immune cells; the loss of Müllerian ducts in male embryos; the formation of ducts, canals, and openings in many organs; and the loss of larval structures in insects and amphibians are all widely accepted as necessary adaptations mediated by PCD. By contrast, it is less obvious why, for example, thousands of mitotically active precursor cells and immature postmitotic cells in the early embryonic brain undergo PCD (de la Rosa & de Pablo, 2000; Kuan, Roth, Flavell, & Rakic, 2000; Putz, Harwell, & Nedivi, 2005) or why 75% of differentiating neurons in the mesencephalic trigeminal nucleus of the chick embryo degenerate (Rogers & Cowan, 1973; von Bartheld & Bothwell, 1993).

In attempting to understand the biological utility of PCD in the developing nervous system, a reasonable first step is to determine where and when cell death appears evolutionarily as well as in what regions and cell types in the nervous system it is present or absent. Are there common features in where and when PCD occurs and can this information provide clues to putative adaptive roles? If PCD is, in fact, essential for nervous system development, one might expect it to be present in virtually all animals with a nervous system. Alternatively, if PCD serves only a few specific functions required for nervous system development (e.g., optimizing neuronal connectivity), then there may be some species or regions of the nervous system in which this function is either absent or is attained by other developmental mechanisms not requiring PCD.

PCD appears to be dispensable for nervous system development as it is only used to varying degrees, or not at all, in some animals with a nervous system (Buss et al., 2006). Furthermore, genetic prevention of PCD in nematodes has no outwardly noticeable effect on development and in flies, development in the absence of PCD progresses until metamorphosis when morphogenetic PCD is absolutely required. In mammals, the prevention of neuronal PCD during early stages of neurogenesis can result in massive brain pathology (see below), whereas the prevention of the death of postmitotic neurons that are establishing synaptic connections results in only subtle changes in neuronal function and behavior (Buss et al., 2006, 2007). Finally, the consequences of preventing the PCD of adult-generated neurons are currently being investigated (see section on "Functional Significance of Adult-Generated Neurons and the Role of PCD").

The occurrence of developmental PCD in the vertebrate nervous system has been most extensively documented in birds and mammals, whereas less information exists for fishes, reptiles, and amphibians. However, despite over 100 years of investigation, there are still several regions and cell populations even in birds and mammals that have not yet been examined, and, of course, much of what is known is based on observations in only a few popular animal models (e.g., frog, chick, mouse, rat). Nonetheless, by extrapolation from the available information, it appears that PCD occurs in both neurons and glia in many, if not most, regions of the CNS and PNS and involves virtually all major subtypes of cells (motor, sensory, autonomic, enteric, sensory receptors, interneurons as well as Schwann cells, astrocytes, and oligodendrocytes). For neurons in the CNS and PNS, the timing of PCD occurs both prior to the onset of connectivity and involves progenitor or undifferentiated cells, as well as during synaptogenesis when neurons are differentiating (Figure 5.1). Surprisingly, however, there are a few apparent cell types in which PCD is either absent or not detectable by currently available methods (Oppenheim, 1991; Oppenheim et al., 2001a, 2001b). Although there have been attempts to discern common features shared by these populations that might explain the apparent absence of PCD—for example, extensive axon collateral arborization or an abundance of potential targets (Cowan, Fawcett, O'Leary, & Stanfield, 1984; Oppenheim, 1991)—these have never been tested experimentally. Moreover, some populations of neurons may undergo PCD in one class of animals but not in another. For example, spinal interneurons and photoreceptors in the retina exhibit PCD in mammals but not in birds (Cook, Portera-Cailliau, & Adler, 1998; Lowrie & Lawson, 2000), whereas sympathetic preganglionic neurons exhibit PCD in birds but not in mammals (Wetts & Vaughn, 1998).

We provide a detailed discussion of the following adaptive roles of PCD that we consider to represent current key issues in the field: (1) the regulation of PCD in progenitor populations, (2) error correction by PCD, and (3) the regulation of optimal quantitative connectivity between neurons and their afferents and targets ("systems-matching") by PCD.

Programmed Cell Death as a Means of Regulating the Size of Progenitor Populations

One of the most surprising "discoveries" in the last decade regarding developmental PCD in the nervous system is the observation of a significant death of mitotically active cells in germinal zones of the CNS and PNS (Kuan et al., 2000). We use the term "discover" advisedly since if one digs deep enough into the literature, it is clear that this phenomenon was noticed previously (for reviews see Boya & de la Rosa 2005; Homma, Yaginuma, & Oppenheim, 1994; Sanders & Wride, 1995; Yeo & Gautier, 2004), often decades ago (Glücksmann, 1951), although its significance was not well understood. As indicated in the heading for this subsection, however, the significance of this phase of PCD is now being revealed. Whereas reviews published prior to the mid-1990s were silent on this issue (e.g., Hamburger & Oppenheim, 1982; Jacobson, 1991; Oppenheim, 1981a, 1991), all of the more recent reviews acknowledge this early phase of PCD and recognize its apparent biological utility (e.g., Kuan et al., 2000; Mehlen, Mille, & Thibert, 2005; Voyvodic, 1996).

The PCD of significant numbers of proliferative cells has been observed in germinal regions of the vertebrate spinal cord, sensory ganglia, autonomic ganglia, retina, brainstem, thalamus, cerebellum, and cortex (Argenti et al., 2005; Blaschke, Staley, & Chun, 1996; Blaschke, Weiner, & Chun,1998; Frade & Barde, 1999; Haydar, Kuan, Flavell, & Rakic, 1999; Homma et al., 1994; Kuan et al., 2000; Lee et al., 2001) as well as during insect neurogenesis (Bello, Hirth, & Gould, 2003). Although several of the categories listed in Table 5.2 provide plausible explanations for why cells might die during proliferation (deletion of progeny in sublineage, negative selection, morphogenesis, removal of harmful cells, evolutionary change), we favor the idea that the primary role is to regulate the size (number) of the precursor population, which will,

in turn, secondarily affect the size and morphology of the resulting neuronal structures. Strong evidence consistent with this idea comes from gene-targeting studies in mice in which the disruption of genes regulating the PCD of progenitor cells result in the perturbation of brain size and morphology (Depaepe, Suarez-Gonzalez, Dufour, Passante, & Gorski, 2005; Frade & Barde, 1999; Haydar et al., 1999; Kuan et al., 2000; Putz et al., 2005). However, there is some evidence that PCD of proliferating cells may also regulate the phenotypic fate of vertebrate neurons (Yeo & Gautier, 2003) as has been observed in Drosophila. Additionally, some PCDs of proliferating precursors may also be necessary to delete cells with genomic instability as reflected in chromosomal variations (aneuploidy) (Rehen et al., 2001; Yang et al., 2003). Although not the focus of our chapter, it is nonetheless of interest that the proapoptotic *Bcl-2* genes that regulate the PCD of precursor cells versus genes that regulate the PCD of postmitotic differentiating neurons are distinct (Kuan et al., 2000; Sun & Oppenheim 2003; White, Tahaoglu, & Steller, 1996). By contrast, soluble, secreted factors (neurotrophic molecules) appear to regulate the survival of precursor cells as well as postmitotic differentiating neurons in a manner consistent with the NTF hypothesis (Depaepe et al., 2005; Elshamy & Ernfors, 1996; Elshamy, Linnarsson, Lee, Jaenisch, & Ernfors, 1996; Frade & Barde, 1999; Lu, Pang, & Woo, 2005; Ockel, Lewin, & Barde, 1996; Putz et al., 2005). In addition, survival or death may also be promoted by patterning molecules (e.g., Mehlen et al., 2005) involved in early neurogenesis and cell fate decisions.

Error Correction as a Reason for Developmental Programmed Cell Death

Although it is possible to include several of the categories listed in Table 5.2 as performing an error correction function (e.g., deletion of harmful cells, negative selection), we prefer to limit our attention here to category number 9 that is restricted to the selective removal of neurons that have (a) migrated to an ectopic position, (b) axons that go astray during pathfinding, or (c) innervated inappropriate targets relative to their afferent inputs or vice versa.

Because the operation of the nervous system is unique in being dependent on the formation of extensive and specific synaptic circuits, error correction is an intuitively attractive hypothesis that provides a plausible adaptive rationale for neuronal

PCD. In fact, it has been argued that error correction for the establishment and refinement of functional circuitry may be the major role for the PCD of differentiating neurons as they form connections (Clarke et al., 1998; Finlay & Pallas, 1989; Lamb et al., 1988). Although there are several examples, especially in the visual system, of the removal of cells by PCD that have made one or more of the three errors described earlier (Clarke 1998; Oppenheim, 1981a, 1991; Thanos, 1999), these appear to be the exception and not the rule. Many of the populations of neurons in which developmental PCD occurs during the formation of synaptic circuits appear to make few, if any, such errors and in some cases even grossly aberrant errors created experimentally are maintained (Oppenheim, 1991). Similarly, there are many examples of persistent ectopic, malpositioned cells that also are not eliminated by PCD (Jacobson, 1991). It has been suggested that the refinement of synaptic connections by PCD may occur mainly in neuronal systems (e.g., the visual system) whose function is highly dependent on spatially precise topographic mapping (Clarke, 1998). However, throughout the developing nervous system refinements of this kind mainly occur, not by PCD, but rather by another evolutionarily conserved regressive phenomenon, the elimination of neuronal processes and synapses (Jacobson, 1991; Luo & O'Leary, 2005; Wong & Lichtman, 2003; Yakura, Fukuda, & Sawai, 2002). We conclude that although error correction by PCD occurs, it is not likely to be the primary reason for the normal massive loss of postmitotic, differentiating neurons.

Programmed Cell Death as a Means of Quantitatively Optimizing the Connectivity between Neurons and Their Efferent Targets and Afferent Inputs (Systems-Matching)

There must be hundreds of papers in this field in which some variation of the following statement regarding the PCD of postmitotic vertebrate neurons is repeated: "The most generally accepted idea is that neurons are produced in excess in order that they may compete for contacts with their cellular partners and thus adjust their numbers so as to provide sufficient innervation of their targets" (Pettmann & Henderson, 1998). The historical origins of this idea have been well documented (Cowan, 2001; Jacobson, 1991; Oppenheim, 1981a, 2001; Purves & Sanes, 1987) and the considerable evidence supporting it (as well as negative evidence)

has also been extensively reviewed (Burek & Oppenheim, 1999; Cunningham, 1982; Jacobson, 1991; Kuno, 1990; Lamb et al., 1988; Linden, 1994; McLennan, 1988; Oppenheim, 1981a, 1991; Tanaka & Landmesser, 1986; Williams & Herrup, 1988). More recently, this idea has even been extended to include glial PCD involved in "systems-matching" of myelinating cells with their axons (Figure 5.7; Burne, Staple, & Raff, 1996; Winseck et al., 2002). Historically, the context in which the massive PCD of postmitotic neurons was first appreciated

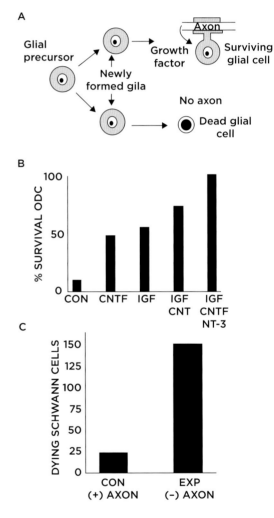

Figure 5.7 PCD of glial cells. (A) Immature glial cells undergo PCD if they fail to obtain sufficient trophic support provided by axon-glial contacts. (B) Developing oligodentrocytes (ODC) in the optic nerve require specific NTFs for their survival (see Barres & Raff, 1994). (C) Developing Schwann cells in peripheral nerves require axon-derived trophic support for their survival. (See Winseck, Caldero, Ciutat, Prevette, & Scott, 2002; Winseck & Oppenheim, 2006.)

involved the issue of developing interactions between neurons and their targets (Oppenheim, 1981a). This line of investigation led to the discovery of the first neurotrophic factor (NGF) and to the formulation of the neurotrophic hypothesis (Cowan, 2001; Oppenheim, 2001). In its original form, this hypothesis stated that neurons compete for limiting amounts of survival-promoting factors provided by targets (the winners survive and the losers die by PCD) as a means of attaining optimal, numerical/quantitative innervation of their targets. More recently, the hypothesis has been expanded to include competition for trophic support from afferent inputs and other cellular partners such as glia (Oppenheim, 1996; Oppenheim et al., 2001a, 2001b). If systems-matching is the major reason for the PCD of postmitotic neurons, then a major challenge is to understand the relative contribution of these different sources of trophic support (e.g., targets, afferents, glia) to the quantitative regulation of cell numbers (Figure 5.8; Bunker & Nishi, 2002; Cunningham, 1982; Galli-Resta & Resta, 1992; Korsching, 1993).

It has sometimes been argued that the PCD of postmitotic neurons in the CNS (vs. the PNS) must serve a function distinct from systems-matching (Bähr, 2000; Lowrie & Lawson, 2000). However, experimental evidence in support of this claim is lacking. Rather, PCD in many CNS populations occurs during synaptogenesis and in some cases has been shown to be regulated by target-derived trophic factors (Burke, 2004; Chu, Hullinger, Schilling, & Oberdick, 2000; Cusato, Stagg, & Reese, 2001; Lotto, Asavaritikrai, Vali, & Price, 2001; Morcuende, Benitez-Temino, Pecero, Pastor, & de la Cruz, 2005; Oliveira et al., 2002; Verney, Takahashi, Bhide, Nowakowski, & Caviness, 2000; Vogel, Sunter, & Herrup, 1989; von Bartheld & Johnson, 2001). Admittedly, however, the most compelling evidence for quantitative systems-matching comes from populations of PNS neurons such as motoneurons and neurons in sensory and autonomic ganglia. With only a few exceptions, the evidence from these populations support the argument that the numbers of interconnected cells are regulated rather precisely by PCD (Jacobson, 1991; Oppenheim, 1991; Tanka & Landmesser, 1985; Williams & Herrup, 1988). One apparent exception that has been widely cited and discussed involves the studies of Lamb and his colleagues (1988). By experimentally forcing lumbar motoneurons in *Xenopus* frog tadpoles from both sides of the spinal cord to innervate a single leg, they reported that, contrary to the systems-matching hypothesis, the single limb

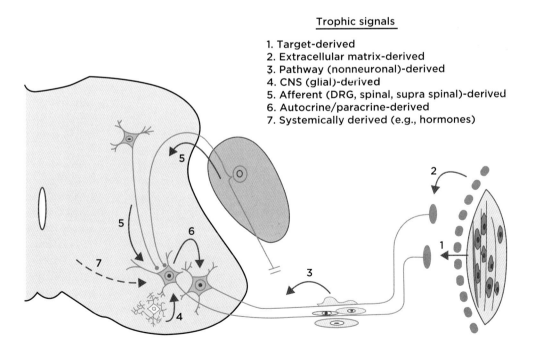

Trophic signals

1. Target-derived
2. Extracellular matrix-derived
3. Pathway (nonneuronal)-derived
4. CNS (glial)-derived
5. Afferent (DRG, spinal, supra spinal)-derived
6. Autocrine/paracrine-derived
7. Systemically derived (e.g., hormones)

Figure 5.8 Spinal motoneurons exemplify the diverse sources of trophic signals that can promote the survival of developing neurons. Copyright 2006, Cell Press.

was able to sustain innervation by significantly more motoneurons than in controls (i.e., fewer cells died and thus motoneuron numbers did not appear to match the target size). Several criticisms of this study have been raised (e.g., Oppenheim, 1991) and although some of these have been addressed, others have not been. Interestingly, in these same animals, the total number of surviving sensory neurons in the dorsal root ganglion (DRG) on the two sides that also innervate a single limb are similar to controls, consistent with a systems-matching function of PCD (Lamb et al., 1988).

As summarized in Table 5.2, the PCD of developing neurons can serve a variety of different roles depending on the stage of development, neuronal subtypes, and species. The evidence is rather compelling for postmitotic vertebrate neurons (especially in birds and mammals) that quantitative systems-matching is likely the primary reason for PCD. This adaptive function of PCD appears to have arisen only in recent vertebrate evolution and does not appear to play a major role in nervous system development of primitive fishes or invertebrates.

Programmed Cell Death, Synaptic Function, and Neurobehavioral Ontogeny

In principle, perturbations of any of the putative biological roles of neuronal PCD delineated in Table 5.2 have the potential to affect the neurobiological mechanisms that mediate behavior. Although studies of the consequences of altered PCD are just beginning (see Alberi, Raggenbass, DeBilbao, & Dubois-Dauphin, 1996; Avery & Horvitz, 1987; Buss et al., 2006; Ellis et al., 1991; Rondi-Reig & Mariani, 2002; Truman, 1984; White, Southgate, & Thomson, 1991), there appear to be powerful intrinsic regulatory mechanisms, which in some situations, may be able to compensate for changes in neuronal numbers (Buss et al., 2006, 2007). However, until further studies are available, the extent to which these regulatory mechanisms are successful in generating normal functional phenotypes in the face of altered cell numbers remains an open question (Rondi-Reig & Mariani, 2002).

The lion's share of normal PCD in the nervous system occurs either during neurogenesis (section on "PCD as a Means of Regulating the Size of Progenitor Populations") or during the formation of neuronal connectivity at later prenatal and early postnatal stages (section on "Error Correction as a Reason for Developmental Programmed Cell Death and Section on PCD as Means of Quantitatively Optimizing the Connectivity between Neurons and Their Efferent Targets and Afferent Inputs Systems-Matching"). However, substantial PCD also occurs among neurons generated during adulthood. Accordingly, in the following section, we discuss prenatal/postnatal PCD and the PCD of adult-generated neurons separately.

Prenatal and Postnatal Development

As neurons begin to differentiate, they establish interactions with neuronal and nonneuronal cellular partners that are the source of signals, which regulate survival as well as other aspects of their differentiation (Figure 5.8). In the context of our focus here on synaptic function and neurobehavioral ontogeny, the role of neurophysiological interactions between neurons and their efferent targets and afferent inputs are especially noteworthy.

Neurons in the CNS and PNS become capable of generating axon potentials, neurotransmitter release, and synaptic transmission prior to their complete differentiation and in some cases this functional activity begins at remarkably early stages of embryogenesis (Milner & Landmesser, 1999; O'Donovan, 1999; Provine, 1973). Overtly, this neuronal function is manifested as embryonic and fetal movements and reflexes that have been the focus of considerable research (Gottlieb, 1973; Hamburger, 1963; Michel & Moore, 1995; Oppenheim, 1982). The developmentally early appearance of neuronal activity and behavior raises the obvious question of what adaptive role, if any, is served by prenatal neurobehavioral functions. Early neural activity may be an epiphenomenon, in that it merely indicates that neuronal differentiation is proceeding normally. Alternatively, this early function may be a necessary feature of early nervous system organization acting to prepare the nervous system for its later role in mediating complex behavioral patterns (Crair, 1999). Finally, early neurobehavioral function may serve some immediate developmental function, a role I have previously called *ontogenetic adaptations* (Hall & Oppenheim, 1986; Oppenheim, 1981, 1984).

Motoneurons (and some other neuronal populations as well, including retinal ganglion cells, neurons in the chick isthmo-optic nucleus (ION), and ciliary neurons) have another interesting property; their target dependency appears to be regulated by physiological synaptic interactions with their targets (Burek & Oppenheim, 1999). Following the formation of synaptic contacts between motoneurons and target muscles, the initiation of synaptic transmission activates the muscle and results in embryo movements. Chronic blockade of this activity during the cell death period with specific drugs or toxins that cause paralysis prevents the death of all motoneurons (Figure 5.9). Although the cellular and molecular mechanisms that mediate this effect are unknown, two major hypotheses have been proposed: the production hypothesis, which predicts that the production of trophic factor by the target is regulated inversely by target muscle activity, and the access hypothesis, which argues that sufficient trophic factor is initially produced by targets to maintain all motoneurons, but that activity regulates access to this factor by modulating axonal branching and the formation of neuromuscular synapses, thus restricting the uptake of the trophic factor to axons and synaptic terminals (Figure 5.6). At present, evidence favors the access hypothesis (Terrado et al., 2001). Regardless of which of these two hypotheses is proven correct, however, it is clear that neuronal activity at both early and later stages of embryogenesis can make fundamental contributions to nervous system development. A recent striking example of this is the observation that in mutant embryonic and neonatal mice lacking all afferent and efferent synaptic transmission, there is a massive PCD of virtually all CNS neurons (Verhage et al., 2002).

PCD is also modulated by specific perturbations of afferent inputs (Harris & Rubel, 2006; Linden, 1994; Oppenheim et al., 2001a, 2001b). Five such cases that have been examined in considerable detail are spinal motoneurons, neurons in the ION, the avian ciliary ganglion (CG), visual receptive neurons in the optic tectum, and neurons in the avian brainstem auditory nuclei. In all these five cases, surgical removal of afferent inputs prior to or during the period of PCD results in significant increases in cell death (Figure 5.10). Because similar changes in PCD also occur after the blockade of afferent synaptic activity, the functional input provided by afferents appears to be of fundamental importance in this situation (Oppenheim et al., 2001a, 2001b). Other examples of the regulation of developmental PCD by afferent synaptic input include: the loss of olfactory input increases PCD in the rat olfactory bulb (OB) (Brunjes & Shurling, 2003; Frazier & Brunjes, 1988; Najbauer & Leon, 1995; Zou et al., 2004); activity blockade in zebrafish larvae reduces the PCD of Rohon-Beard

sensory neurons (Svoboda, Linares, & Ribera, 2001); the loss of vestibular input to the vestibular ganglion increases ganglion cell PCD (Smith, Wang, Wolgemuth, & Murashov, 2003); and reductions of somatosensory input (maternal licking) to neonatal rats results in increased PCD in a sexually dimorphic spinal cord nucleus (Moore, Don, & Juraska, 1992). Finally, a recent study has suggested an interesting link between early neonatal experience and the later vulnerability of adult-generated neurons in the hippocampus of rats to undergo PCD (Weaver, Grant, & Meaney, 2002). Adult offspring of mothers who engage in low levels of licking and grooming of their pups (vs. the offspring of mothers that exhibit high levels of licking and grooming) have increased expression of the proapoptotic gene *Bax* and increased PCD of hippocampal neurons. In other studies, it has been reported that the offspring of mothers who exhibit low levels of licking and grooming perform below normal in tests of hippocampal-dependent learning and memory (Liu et al., 2000) suggesting a possible link between early experience, the survival of adult-generated neurons, and behavioral performance (see section on "Functional Significance of Adult-Generated Neurons and the Role of PCD").

Functional afferent input may act to regulate the survival of postsynaptic neurons by several different mechanisms: (1) depolarization by afferents can alter intracellular calcium levels in postsynaptic cells, which in turn can independently modulate survival; (2) afferent activity can regulate the expression of trophic factors and their receptors in postsynaptic cells; and (3) the release of trophic factors from terminals of afferent axons or adjacent glial cells may be regulated by activity and provide a survival signal to postsynaptic cells. At present, it is not clear which, if any, of these mechanisms mediate the effects of afferent input on PCD. Because the PCD of many developing neurons may be coordinately regulated by signals derived from targets, afferents, and nonneuronal cells, an important unresolved issue is how these different sources interact to control survival. One possibility is that the targets regulate the response of neurons to afferent input and that afferents regulate the response to target-derived signals. In this scheme, the relative influence of targets and afferents would have to be balanced or coordinated in some way for optimal survival (Cunningham, 1982).

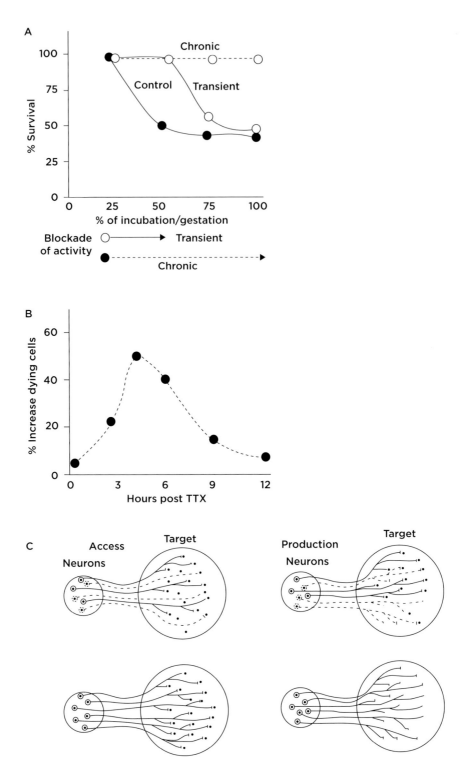

Figure 5.9 Synaptic transmission between neurons and their targets (A and C) or between neurons and their afferents (B) can modulate PCD. (A) Spinal motoneurons in the chick embryo are rescued from normal PCD (control) by blocking neuromuscular transmission. Following a transient blockade of activity (0--0), rescued motoneurons undergo a delayed cell death as activity levels return to normal. Chronic activity blockade maintains rescued neurons. (B) There is a significant increase in the number of dying neurons in the superior colliculus of neonatal rats when afferent electrical activity of retinal ganglion cells is blocked by tetrodotoxin (TTX). (C) The two hypotheses for explaining the role of neuromuscular activity in regulating motoneuron survival are illustrated. Dying cells are indicated by dashed lines. On the left, activity blockade (bottom) is postulated to increase axonal

Functional Significance of Adult-Generated Neurons and the Role of Programmed Cell Death

New neurons are continuously generated in some regions of the adult mammalian brain including the dentate gyrus (DG) of the hippocampal formation and the subventricular zone (SVZ) of the lateral ventricle. It is believed that adult neurogenesis recapitulates events occurring during embryonic development (Esposito et al., 2005; Kintner, 2002), although the precise program for the differentiation of adult-generated neurons appears to be slightly different from that of developmentally produced neurons (Belluzzi, Benedusi, Ackman, & LoTurco, 2003; Overstreet-Wadiche, Bensen, & Westbrook, 2006; Zhao, Teng, Summers, Ming, & Gage, 2006). Similar to the PCD of developing neurons, PCD in the adult brain also occurs during specific periods of neuronal differentiation. For this reason, and because the potential role of adult neurogenesis and PCD in neurobehavioral plasticity has received considerable attention (Kempermann, 2006), we have included this topic in our review of PCD and nervous system development. Birth date– or lineage-tracing methods (e.g., BrdU pulse-labeling or proliferating-cell specific retroviral infection) have been widely used to identify and analyze PCD in the adult brain (Biebl, Cooper, Winkler, & Kuhn, 2000; Dayer, Ford, Cleaver, Yassaee, & Cameron, 2003; Kempermann, Gast, Kronenberg, Yamaguchi, & Gage, 2003; van Praag et al., 2002). These studies demonstrate that, in rodents, 50%–70% of newly produced DG cells undergo PCD between 1 week and 1 month after their birth, and that the extent of PCD is influenced by housing conditions and genetic background (Biebl et al., 2000; Kempermann, Kuhn, & Gage, 1997).

The PCD of adult-produced OB neurons exhibits two distinct waves, one of which eliminates about 50% of the new cells between 1 week and 1 month after their birth followed by a second wave that occurs over an extended period (>6 months) during which time an additional 30% of cells are eliminated (Petreanu & Alvarez-Buylla, 2002; Winner, Cooper-Kuhn, Aigner, Winkler, & Kuhn, 2002). Neurons that survive beyond these periods appear to be maintained for long periods and become integrated into functional neural circuits. One week after their genesis when PCD begins, DG neurons actively extend mossy fiber axons toward the CA3 field and make provisional synaptic connections (Zhao et al., 2006). Similarly, the first wave of PCD of OB neurons occurs during the establishment of dendro-dendritic connections (Petreanu & Alvarez-Buylla, 2002). Adult-generated DG neurons progressively receive GABAergic and glutamatergic inputs, and specialized glutamatergic contacts on dendritic spines appear by 3 weeks in both the DG and OB (Esposito et al., 2005). Electrophysiological studies have identified small sodium currents in 1-week-old adult-generated neurons (Belluzzi et al., 2003; van Praag et al., 2002), suggesting that neuronal death begins after the onset of excitable neuronal properties. Collectively, these data indicated that PCD begins after the initiation of morphological and functional differentiation of newly produced cells (Figure 5.11).

Although the specific role of targets (i.e., CA3 neurons in the DG and preexisting interneurons or mitral/tufted cells in the OB) in the control of PCD has received little attention, neural activity has been shown to play a critical role in the survival of adult-generated neurons. For example, increased neural activity during learning (Gould, Beylin, Tanapat, Reeves, & Shors, 1999), environmental enrichment (Olson, Eadie, Ernst, & Christie, 2006; Rochefort, Gheusi, Vincent, & Lledo, 2002; Young, Lawlor, Leone, Dragunow, & During, 1999), and during in vivo long-term potentiation (LTP) (Bruel-Jungerman, Davis, Rampon, & Laroche, 2006; Chun, Sun, Park, & Jung, 2006; Derrick, York, & Martinez, 2000) all result in the increased survival of newly produced DG cells. Similarly, odor enrichment also enhances the survival of adult-generated OB neurons (Gheusi et al., 2000). Conversely, reduced activity by sensory deprivation or denervation increases PCD (Corotto, Henegar, & Maruniak, 1994; Mandairon, Jourdan, & Didier, 2003). These results suggest that a "use it or lose it" rule may govern PCD in the adult brain. Several factors such as hormones, neurotransmitters, and NTFs are also known to regulate the

branching and synapse formation over control levels (top) and thereby increasing the access to target-derived trophic factors (small black dots in target). By contrast, on the right, activity blockade (bottom) is thought to increase the production of trophic factors (i.e., more dots in target) over control values (top) (A and C are modified from Oppenheim, 1989 and B is modified from Galli-Resta, Ensini, Fusco, Gravina, & Margheritti, 1993).

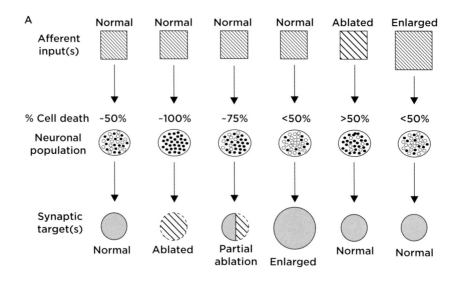

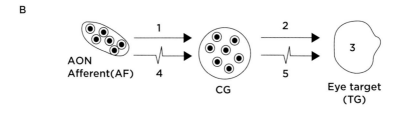

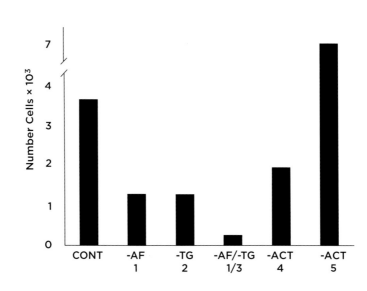

Figure 5.10 The role of targets (TG) and afferents (AF) in regulating survival and PCD of neurons. (A) The predicted outcome of modifying afferent inputs and efferent (synaptic) targets on a neuronal population is shown. The black dots in the neuronal population represent dying cells. (B) Afferent neurons in the accessory oculomotor nucleus (AON) innervate the CG and neurons in the CG innervate muscle targets in the eye. The numbers 1 and 2 indicate anatomical innervation, numbers 2 and 5 indicate synaptic transmission, and number 3 represents the eye muscle targets. (C) The number of surviving CG neurons following removal of afferents (1, -AF), removal of target activity (5, -ACT), and removal of both (1, 3, -AF, -TG). The survival of CG neurons depends on both functional afferent and target connections. (See Furber, Oppenheim, & Prevette, 1987.)

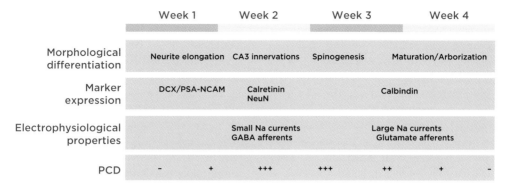

Figure 5.11 The differentiation and PCD of adult-generated DG neurons. Morphological and electrophysiological differentiation of adult-generated neurons is evident before the onset of PCD. Note that the differentiation/maturation of adult-generated neurons continues beyond 4 weeks, and that a subset of newly produced neurons may undergo PCD after this initial maturation period.

survival of adult-generated neurons (Kempermann, 2006), and these may act on neuronal survival by activity-mediated mechanisms (Abrous, Koehl, & Le Moal, 2005; Lehmann, Butz, & Teuchert-Noodt, 2005).

One of the principle roles of competition among developing neurons for limiting amounts of target-derived survival-promoting molecules (the neurotrophic hypothesis) is to regulate optimal target innervation by efferent neurons, a process known as systems-matching (Buss et al., 2006). Recent evidence suggests that a similar competition process among adult-produced neurons is also important for survival. Following infection with a replication-defective virus coding for Cre DNA recombinase, a subpopulation of adult-generated neurons become deficient in *N*-methyl-ᴅ-aspartate (NMDA) receptors and only these cells exhibit increased PCD (Tashiro, Sandler, Toni, Zhao, & Gage, 2006). However, when a glutamate receptor antagonist is administered to suppress overall excitatory input, many receptor-defective neurons were rescued from PCD, suggesting that competition among adult-generated neurons for excitatory NMDA afferent input is related to the survival of new neurons.

In addition to the PCD of immature, adult-generated neurons, other neural populations in the adult hippocampus (e.g., preexisting neurons and neuronal progenitor/stem cells) also undergo PCD as a means of maintaining the net number of adult neurons (Dayer et al., 2003; Sun et al., 2004). Because the continuous addition of new neurons in neurogenic regions does not result in a progressive increase in the number of neurons in the DG and OB, it seems plausible that a homeostasis

exists between the generation of new neurons and the PCD of preexisting neurons. Because some research groups have failed to identify mature (vs. more recently produced) adult-generated neurons that exhibit signs of PCD (e.g., apoptosis), this idea has received little attention. Recently, however, Dayer et al. (2003) demonstrated that the number of DG neurons generated at early postnatal stages is progressively decreased (by 50%) at 6 months. Similarly, adult-generated OB neurons exhibit a second delayed wave of PCD, which progressively eliminates an additional 30% of previously generated mature OB neurons (Petreanu & Alvarez-Buylla, 2002). It has also been recently shown that some subpopulations of postnatally generated OB neurons do not undergo PCD later, suggesting that cell renewal may be limited to only specific populations of OB neurons (Lemasson, Saghatelyan, Olivo-Marin, & Lledo, 2005). The existence and extent of cell renewal are especially important issues regarding the significance of adult neurogenesis and PCD. Some hypotheses regarding the functional significance of adult neurogenesis are based upon the assumption of a homeostatic balance between cell renewal and PCD. For example, it has been postulated that cell replacement optimizes the homeostatic stabilization of neuronal circuits involved in learning, memory, and other hippocampal and olfactory functions (Cecchi, Petreanu, Alvarez-Buylla, & Magnasco, 2001; Chambers, Potenza, Hoffman, & Miranker, 2004; Meltzer, Yabaluri, & Deisseroth, 2005).

The PCD of undifferentiated, mitotically active stem/precursor cell populations can markedly affect the final number of adult-generated neurons.

As discussed earlier (section on "PCD as a Means of Regulating the Size of Progenitor Populations"), prevention of stem cell death during embryonic development results in exencephaly owing to the marked expansion of proliferating precursor cells. There is a progressive reduction in the number of adult neuronal stem/progenitor cells during the aging process, and accordingly the number of new cells produced is reduced in older adult animals (Cameron & McKay, 1999; Enwere et al., 2004; Rao, Hattiangady, Abdel-Rahman, Stanley, & Shetty, 2005). Although cells undergoing PCD are infrequently observed in the SVZ where adult stem cells/progenitor cells are found, the inhibition of PCD in Bax/Bak double knockout (KO) mice results in the survival and expansion of the stem cell population (Lindsten et al., 2003), indicating that PCD of progenitor cells may, in fact, control the size of stem cell populations in the adult brain.

Because a significant population of adult-generated neurons undergo PCD, the functional significance of adult neurogenesis is inextricably linked to the role of PCD in this situation. One strategy for understanding the role of adult neurogenesis and PCD is by comparative and ethological analyses (Clayton, 1998; Gerlai & Clayton, 1999; Nottebohm, 2002a, 2002b). Neurogenesis persists throughout life in many species (Table 5.3) and the major neurogenic regions and their functions are surprisingly well evolutionarily conserved. Brain regions related to learning and memory (e.g., the mushroom body in insects and the hippocampus in mammals), and olfaction are most commonly retained as neurogenic regions. In several vertebrate species, spontaneous neurogenesis is also observed in the retina or optic tectum. Although there is no evidence for spontaneous neurogenesis in the mammalian retina, injury can induce neurogenesis by endogenous retinal progenitor cells (Das et al., 2006).

The correlation of neurogenesis and function in the high vocal center (HVC) neurons of songbirds has received considerable attention (Nottebohm, 2002a, 2002b). Male song birds such as canaries learn new song syllables each year together with the seasonal replacement of old HVC neurons by new neurons (Nottebohm, O'Loughlin, Gould, Yohay, & Alvarez-Buylla, 1994). Marsh tits and black-capped chickadees, in their natural habitat, have increased hippocampal neurogenesis compared to captive wild-caught birds, suggesting that the more complex natural environment, which requires increased spatial learning for locating food sources,

regulates hippocampal neurogenesis (Barnea & Nottebohm et al., 1994; Clayton, 1998; Lipkind, Nottebohm, Rado, & Barnea, 2002). Similar correlations have also been observed in mammals. In the rat, associative learning (Shors et al., 2001) or an enriched environment (Kempermann et al., 1997; Young et al., 1999) enhances the survival of adult-generated neurons. However, some conditions such as physical exercise, which does not specifically involve the hippocampus, also enhance adult neurogenesis (van Praag, Kempermann, & Gage, 1999). Additionally, some types of hippocampal-dependent learning fail to promote adult neurogenesis (Shors, Townsend, Zhao, Kozorovitskiy, & Gould, 2002).

The generation of new neurons in the adult brain may serve either (or both) immediate or future needs. For example, memory storage following learning could be an example of an immediate need, whereas the construction of new, more complex neuronal circuits via environmental inputs at one point in time may adaptively prepare the brain for future contingencies (Kempermann, 2006). Adult neurogenesis is also influenced by many factors, such as spatial memory acquisition and retention (Kempermann & Gage, 2002; Leuner et al., 2004), circadian rhythm (Goergen, Bagay, Rehm, Benton, & Beltz, 2002; Holmes, Galea, Mistlberger, & Kempermann, 2004), pregnancy (Shingo et al., 2003), prenatal stress (Lemaire, Koehl, Le Moal, & Abrous, 2000), maternal deprivation (Mirescu, Peters, & Gould, 2004), and social interactions (Gould, McEwen, Tanapat, Galea, & Fuchs, 1997; Kozorovitskiy & Gould, 2004), some of which may be best understood as serving future needs and others as having an immediate functional role.

Reductions of adult neurogenesis by antimitotic reagents result in hippocampal learning deficits in the rat (Shors et al., 2001), and in insects, gamma irradiation, which selectively eliminates proliferating stem cells, significantly impairs olfactory learning (Scotto-Lomassese et al., 2003). These data support the hypothesis that neurogenesis may be required for cellular neuronal plasticity and enhanced learning ability, although the results remain controversial. For example, reduced neurogenesis following irradiation in rats fails to modify enrichment-dependent enhancement of learning ability (Meshi et al., 2006). Similarly, enrichment-induced neurogenesis in presenilin 1 (PS1)-KO mice is selectively impaired whereas the basal level of neurogenesis is not affected (Feng et al., 2001). Interestingly, PS1-KO mice fail to reduce old

Table 5.3 Adult Neurogenesis in Diverse Species

Species	Neurogenic Regions	Proposed Function	Reference
Insects/Crustacean[a]			
Cricket	Mushroom body (Kenyon cells)	Learning and memory	Scotto Lamassese et al. (2000)
Moth	Mushroom body	Learning and memory	Dufour and Gadenne (2006)
Crab	Hemiellipdoid body	Learning and memory	Schmidt (1997)
	Olfactory	Olfaction	Schmidt (1997)
Mollusca (snails)			
	Procerebrum	Olfaction	Zakharov, Hayes, Ierusalimsky, Nowakowski, and Balaban (1998)
Fishes (zebrafish, goldfish)			
	Olfactory bulb	Olfaction	Byrd and Brunjes (1998)
	Retina, tectum	Visual process	Hitchcock, Lindsey Myhr, Easter, Mangione-Smith, and Jones (1992)
Reptiles (turtles, lizards)			
	Olfactory system	Olfaction	Perez-Canellas and Garacia-Verdugo (1996)
	Medial cerebral cortex	Learning and memory	Perez-Canellas and Garacia-Verdugo (1996)
Birds (zebra finch, chickaree, marsh tits, chicken)			
	HVC (high vocal center)	Vocal (motor) control	Nottebohm, O'Loughlin, Gould, Yohay, and Alvarez-Buylla (1994)
	Hippocampus	Learning and memory	Barnea and Nottebohm (1994); Clayton (1994)
	Nidopallium	Auditory process	Lipkind, Nottebohm, Rado, and Barnea (2002)
	Retina	Visual process	Fischer and Reh (2001)
Rodents (rat, mouse, hamster, rabbit, vole)			
	Hippocampus	Learning and memory	Altman and Das (1965)
	Olfactory bulb	Olfaction	Lois and Alvarez-Buylla (1994)
	Substantial nigra	Motor control	Zhao et al. (2003)
	Hypothalamus	Hormone control	Kokoeva, Yin, and Flier (2005)
Primates (new world monkey, etc.)			
	Hippocampus	Learning and memory	Gould, McEwen, Tanapat, Galea, and Fuchs (1997)
	Olfactory bulb	Olfaction	Kornack and Raki (2001)[b]
Human			
	Hippocampus	Learning and memory	Eriksson et al. (1998)
	Olfactory bulb	Olfaction	Sanai et al. (2004)

[a]In some insects such as Drosophila and honeybees, adult neurogenesis is not evident (Fahrbach, Strande, & Robinson, 1995; Ito & Hotta, 1992).

[b]In this paper, the authors indicate that there is an absence of cortical neurogenesis in the adult primate brain. Recently the absence of cortical neurogenesis was demonstrated in humans using elegant 14C age-tracing methods (Bhardwaj et al., 2006).

memory traces and new learning ability is unaffected, suggesting that neurogenesis and PCD (cell replacement) may be required for the loss of previous memory traces.

Investigations of the significance of neurogenesis and PCD in the adult brain for regulating behavioral plasticity are still in their infancy. Because PCD in the adult brain is apoptotic, perturbation of apoptotic processes by inhibition of caspase 3, deletion of the proapoptotic gene *Bax*, and/or overexpression of the antiapoptotic gene *Bcl-2* inhibits the PCD of adult-generated DG and OB neurons (Biebl, Winner, & Winkler, 2005; Ekdahl, Mohapel, Elmer, & Lindvall, 2001; Kuhn et al., 2005; Sun et al., 2004) and thus provides possible models for examining the role of PCD. The proapoptotic gene *Bax* appears to be essential for the PCD of adult-produced neurons (Sun et al., 2004) (Figure 5.12). Accordingly, the behavior of Bax-KO mice may provide valuable clues

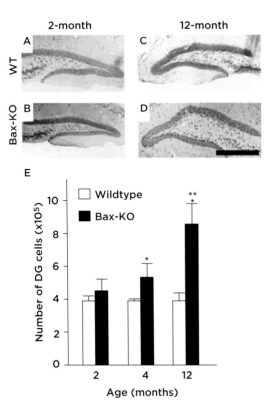

Figure 5.12 The absence of PCD and the age-dependent increase in the total number of DG neurons in Bax-KO mice (A–D). (A) Two-month-old wild type (WT); (B) 2-month-old Bax-KO; (C) 12-month-old wild type; (D) 12-month-old Bax-KO. Representative Nissl-stained sections at a similar anatomical level are presented. (E) The number of DG neurons in WT and Bax-KO mice. The total number of DG neurons was estimated by measuring volume and cell density of DG neurons. (Data from Sun et al., 2004. Copyright Society for Neuroscience, 2004.)

regarding the role of PCD of adult-generated neurons for systems-matching in the adult brain. In adult Bax-KO mice, mossy fiber connections are selectively impaired due to the imbalance in the ratio of mossy fiber afferents versus CA3 synaptic space. Following the prevention of PCD in the DG and the impairment of mossy fiber connections in adult Bax-KO mice, we observed a perturbation of a subset of hippocampal-dependent behaviors related to associative learning (Kim et al., 2009). However, this phenotype is only seen in adult mice, whereas young Bax-KO mice appear normal, despite the accumulation of excess immature neurons; the failure of reduced PCD to affect behavior in younger mice may reflect compensatory mechanisms that prevent the excess neurons from being incorporated into behaviorally relevant neuronal circuits

(Buss et al., 2006; Sun, Gould, Vinsant, Prevette, & Oppenheim, 2003).

Finally, we wish to underscore the admonition that in the future, studies of adult neurogenesis and PCD need to utilize a greater diversity of animal models that are examined in natural or seminatural conditions, with a focus on ethologically relevant behaviors, as a more biologically meaningful approach for elucidating the functional significance of neuron replacement in the adult brain (Clayton, 1998; Gerlai & Clayton, 1999; Nottebohm, 2002a, 2002b).

Developmental Abnormalities Resulting from Inappropriate Cell Death in the Central Nervous System

Mice lacking critical components of the cell death pathway (e.g., Apaf-1, caspase 9, or caspase 3) have gross malformations of the developing brain (Cecconi, Alvarez-Bolado, Meyer, Roth, & Gruss, 1998; Kuida et al., 1996, 1998; Naruse & Keino, 1995; Oppenheim et al., 2001a, 2001b). Likewise, when neuronal death is exacerbated, microencephaly results (McFarland, Wilkes, Koss, Ravichandran, & Mandell, 2006). When Bcl-2 is overexpressed, naturally occurring neuronal death is reduced and these animals have deficits in motor learning, fear-related behavior, and allocentric navigation. These results suggest that neuronal death during CNS development may be necessary for multisensory learning and emotional development (Rondi-Reig et al., 2001). During development, deprivation of active sleep (or rapid eye movement [REM] sleep) results in enhanced cell death resulting in behavior abnormalities (Biswas et al., 2006; Morrissey, Duntley, Anch, & Nonneman, 2004). The deletion of *frizzled 9*, a gene in the Williams Syndrome deletion expanse, results in increases in cell death in the developing DG and the mutant mice have diminished seizure threshold and defects in visuospatial learning and memory (Zhao et al., 2005). Although no definitive genetic linkage with cell death–specific molecules has been identified in individuals with autism spectrum disorders, a reduced occurrence of PCD has been suggested to play a role (reviewed in Persico & Bourgeron, 2006). On the other hand, a significant decrease in the number of neurons in the amygdala and its lateral nucleus has been reported in individuals with autism, although whether this is characteristic of autism remains to be determined (Schumann & Amaral, 2006).

Many of the mechanisms that have been identified to play a role in neuronal death during development are reported to be reactivated in the mature pathological nervous system (Krantic, Mechawar, Reix, & Quirion, 2005). Alterations in expression of Bcl-2 proteins, caspase activation, and other apoptotic events are observed in animal models and postmortem human tissue in Alzheimer's disease (AD), Parkinson's disease (PD), Huntington's chorea (HC), amyotrophic lateral sclerosis (ALS), schizophrenia, and stroke (see Catts et al., 2006; Jarskog, 2006; Kermer, Liman, Weishaupt, & Bahr, 2004; Lopez-Neblina, Toledo, & Toledo-Pereyra, 2005 for reviews). Interestingly, while reports of apoptotic-like cells are present in these conditions, the majority of degenerating cells exhibit morphological changes reminiscent of cytoplasmic or autophagic death. This is most notable in the mutant SOD1 mouse model of ALS. During development, dying motoneurons exhibit many features of apoptosis, including possible Fas activation, Bax translocation, mitochondrial dysfunction, caspase activation, and condensation of nuclear chromatin. By contrast, in the adult spinal cord of SOD1 mice, degenerating motoneurons exhibit cytoplasmic vacuolization, mitochondrial dilation, and protein aggregation. Nonetheless, some of the cell death–associated events that occur during development are also observed. It is becoming increasingly recognized that neuronal dysfunction (and not neuronal death) is most likely the event responsible for clinical symptoms in ALS and other neurodegenerative diseases (Gould & Oppenheim, 2007; Sathasivam & Shaw, 2005). In experiments where motoneuron death is inhibited in the SOD1 mouse, disease progression and survival of the animal are only very modestly affected and muscle denervation still occurs and the animals die prematurely (Gould et al., 2006). Results such as this call into question the practical application of inhibiting cell death as a therapeutic approach for these disorders.

References

Abrous, D. N., Koehl, M., & Le Moal, M. (2005). Adult neurogenesis: From precursors to network and physiology. *Physiological Reviews, 85*(2), 523–569.

Adams, J. M., & Cory, S. (2002). Apoptosomes: Engines for caspase activation. *Current Opinion in Cell Biology, 14*(6), 715–720.

Akhtar, R. S., Ness, J. M., & Roth, K. A. (2004). Bcl-2 family regulation of neuronal development and neurodegeneration. *Biochimica Biophysica Acta, 1644*(2–3), 189–203.

Alberi, S., Raggenbass, M., DeBilbao, F., & Dubois-Dauphin, M. (1996). Axotomized neonatal motoneurons overexpressing the Bcl-2 proto-oncogene retain functional electrophysiological properties. *Proceedings of the National Academy of Science, USA, 39*, 3978–3983.

Altman, J., & Das, G. D. (1965). Autoradiographic and histological evidence of postnatal hippocampal neurogenesis in rats. *Journal of Comparative Neurology, 124*(3), 319–335.

Ameisen, J. C. (2004). Looking for death at the core of life in the light of evolution. *Cell Death and Differentiation, 11*, 4–10.

Argenti, B., Gallo, R., Di Marcotullio, L., Ferretti, E., Napolitano M., Canterini S., et al. (2005). Hedgehog antagonist REN(KCTD11) regulates proliferation and apoptosis of developing granule cell progenitors. *Journal of Neuroscience, 25*, 8338–8346.

Avery, L., & Horvitz, H. R. (1987). A cell that dies during wild-type *C. elegans* development can function as a neuron in a ced-3 mutant. *Cell, 51*, 1071–1078.

Bahr, M. (2000). Live or let die—Retinal ganglion cell death and survival during development and in the lesioned adult CNS. *Trends in Neuroscience, 23*, 483–490.

Barnea, A., & Nottebohm, F. (1994). Seasonal recruitment of hippocampal neurons in adult free-ranging black-capped chickadees. *Proceedings of National Academy of Sciences, USA, 91*(23), 11217–11221.

Barres, B. A., & Raff, M. C. (1994). Control of oligodendrocyte number in the developing rat optic nerve. *Neuron, 12*, 935–942.

Becker, E. B., Howell, J., Kodama, Y., Barker, P. A., & Bonni, A. (2004). Characterization of the c-Jun N-terminal kinase-BimEL signaling pathway in neuronal apoptosis. *Journal of Neuroscience, 24*, 8762–8770.

Bello, B. C., Hirth, F., & Gould, A. P. (2003). A pulse of the Drosophila *Hox* protein abdominal-A schedules the end of neural proliferation via neuroblast apoptosis. *Neuron, 37*, 209–219.

Belluzzi, O., Benedusi, M., Ackman, J., & LoTurco, J. J. (2003). Electrophysiological differentiation of new neurons in the olfactory bulb. *Journal of Neuroscience, 23*(32), 10411–10418.

Bhardwaj, R. D., Curtis, M. A., Spalding, K. L., Buchholz, B. A., Fink, D., Bjork-Eriksson, T., et al. (2006). Neocortical neurogenesis in humans is restricted to development. *Proceedings of National Academy of Sciences, USA, 103*(33), 12564–12568.

Biebl, M., Cooper, C. M., Winkler, J., & Kuhn, H. G. (2000). Analysis of neurogenesis and programmed cell death reveals a self-renewing capacity in the adult rat brain. *Neuroscience Letters, 291*(1), 17–20.

Biebl, M., Winner, B., & Winkler, J. (2005). Caspase inhibition decreases cell death in regions of adult neurogenesis. *Neuroreport, 16*(11), 1147–1150.

Biswas, S., Mishra, P., & Mallick, B. N. (2006). Increased apoptosis in rat brain after rapid eye movement sleep loss. *Neuroscience, 142*(2), 315–313.

Biswas, S. C., & Greene, L. A. (2002). Nerve growth factor (NGF) down-regulates the Bcl-2 homology 3 (BH3) domain-only protein Bim and suppresses its proapoptotic activity by phosphorylation. *Journal of Biological Chemistry, 277*, 49511–49516.

Blaschke, A. J., Staley, K., & Chun, J. (1996). Widespread programmed cell death in proliferative and postmitotic regions of the fetal cerebral cortex. *Development, 122*, 1165–1174.

Blaschke, A. J., Weiner, J. A., & Chun, J. (1998). Programmed cell death is a universal feature of embryonic and postnatal neuroproliferative regions throughout the central nervous system. *Journal of Comparative Neurology, 396*, 39–50.

Boya, P., & de la Rosa, E. J. (2005). Cell death in early neural life. *Birth Defects Research, 75*, 281–293.

Brodersen, P., Petersen, M., Pike, H. M., Olszak, B., Skov, S., Odum, N., et al. (2002). Knockout of Arabidopsis accelerated-cell-death11 encoding a sphingosine transfer protein causes activation of programmed cell death and defense. *Genes and Development, 16*, 490–502.

Bronfman, F. C., & Fainzilber, M. (2004). Multi-tasking by the p75 neurotrophin receptor: Sortilin things out? *European Molecular Biology Organization Report, 5*(9), 867–871.

Bruel-Jungerman, E., Davis, S., Rampon, C., & Laroche, S. (2006). Long-term potentiation enhances neurogenesis in the adult dentate gyrus. *Journal of Neuroscience, 26*(22), 5888–5893.

Brunet, A., Datta, S. R., & Greenberg, M. E. (2001). Transcription-dependent and -independent control of neuronal survival by the PI3K-Akt signaling pathway. *Current Opinion in Neurobiology, 11*(3), 297–305.

Brunjes, C., & Shurling, D. C. (2003). Cell death in the nasal septum of normal and naris-occulded rats. *Developmental Brain Research, 146*, 25–28.

Bunker, G. L., & Nishi, R. (2002). Developmental cell death in vivo: Rescue of neurons independently of changes at target tissues. *Journal of Comparative Neurology, 452*, 80–92.

Burek, M. J., & Oppenheim, R. W. (1999). Cellular interactions that regulate programmed cell death in the developing vertebrate nervous system. In V. E. Koliatsos & R. R. Ratan (Eds.), *Cell death and diseases of the nervous system* (pp. 145–179). Totowa, NJ: Humana Press.

Burke, R. E. (2004). Ontogenic cell death in the nigrostriatal system. *Cell Tissue Research, 318*, 63–72.

Burne, J. F., Staple, J. K., & Raff, M. C. (1996). Glial cells are increased proportionally in transgenic optic nerves with increased numbers of axons. *Journal of Neuroscience, 16*, 2064–2073.

Buss, R. R., Gould, T. W., Ma, J., Vinsant, S., Prevette, D., Winseck, A., et al. (2006). Neuromuscular development in the absence of programmed cell death: Phenotypic alteration of motoneurons and muscle. *Journal of Neuroscience, 26*, 13413–13427.

Buss, R., Sun W., & Oppenheim, R. W. (2006). Adaptive roles of programmed cell death during nervous system development. *Annual Review Neuroscience, 29*, 1–35.

Byrd, C. A., & Brunjes, P. C. (1998). Addition of new cells to the olfactory bulb of adult zebrafish. *Annals of the New York Academy of Sciences, 855*, 274–276.

Cameron, H. A., & McKay, R. D. (1999). Restoring production of hippocampal neurons in old age. *Nature Neuroscience, 2*(10), 894–897.

Catts, V. S., Catts, S. V., McGrath, J. J., Feron, F., McLean, D., Coulson, E. J., et al.(2006). Apoptosis and schizophrenia: A pilot study based on dermal fibroblast cell lines. *Schizophrenia Research, 84*(1), 20–28.

Cecchi, G. A., Petreanu, L. T., Alvarez-Buylla, A., & Magnasco, M. O. (2001). Unsupervised learning and adaptation in a model of adult neurogenesis. *Journal of Computational Neuroscience, 11*(2), 175–182.

Cecconi, F., Alvarez-Bolado, G., Meyer, B. I., Roth, K. A., Gruss, P. (1998). Apaf1 (CED-4 homolog) regulates programmed cell death in mammalian development. *Cell, 94*(6),727–737.

Chambers, R. A., Potenza, M. N., Hoffman, R. E., & Miranker, W. (2004). Simulated apoptosis/neurogenesis regulates learning and memory capabilities of adaptive neural networks. *Neuropsychopharmacology, 29*(4), 747–758.

Chauhan, D., Li, G., Hideshima, T., Podar, K., Mitsiades, C., Mitsiades, N., et al. (2003). JNK-dependent release of mitochondrial protein, Smac, during apoptosis in multiple myeloma (MM) cells. *Journal of Biological Chemistry, 278*, 17593–17596.

Cheung, E. C., Joza, N., Steenaart, N. A., McClellan, K. A., Neuspiel, M., McNamara, S., et al. (2006). Dissociating the dual roles of apoptosis-inducing factor in maintaining mitochondrial structure and apoptosis. *European Molecular Biology Organization Report, 25*(17), 4061–4073.

Chu, T., Hullinger, H., Schilling, K., & Oberdick, J. (2000). Spatial and temporal changes in natural and target deprivation-induced cell death in the mouse inferior olive. *Journal of Neurobiology, 43*, 18–30.

Chun, S. K., Sun, W., Park, J. J., & Jung, M. W. (2006). Enhanced proliferation of progenitor cells following long-term potentiation induction in the rat dentate gyrus. *Neurobiology of Learning and Memory, 86*(3), 322–329.

Chu-Wang, I. W., & Oppenheim, R. W. (1978). Cell death of motoneurons in the chick embryo spinal cord. I. A light and electron microscopic study of naturally occurring and induced cell loss during development. *Journal of Comparative Neurology, 177*(1), 33–57.

Clarke, P. G. (1990). Developmental cell death: Morphological diversity and multiple mechanisms. *Anatomy and Embryology (Berlin), 181*(3), 195–213.

Clarke, P. G., Posada, A., Primi, M. P., & Castagne, V. (1998). Neuronal death in the central nervous system during development. *Biomedical Pharmacotherapeutics, 52*, 356–362.

Clarke, P. G. H., & Clarke, S. (1996). Nineteenth century research on naturally occurring cell death and related phenomena. *Anatomy and Embryology, 193*, 81–99.

Clayton, N. S. (1998). Memory and the hippocampus in food-storing birds: A comparative approach. *Neuropharmacology, 37*(4–5), 441–452.

Cook, B., Portera-Cailliau, C., & Adler, R. (1998). Developmental neuronal death is not a universal phenomenon among cell types in the chick embryo retina. *Journal of Comparative Neurology, 396*, 12–19.

Corotto, F. S., Henegar, J. R., & Maruniak, J. A. (1994). Odor deprivation leads to reduced neurogenesis and reduced neuronal survival in the olfactory bulb of the adult mouse. *Neuroscience, 61*(4), 739–744.

Cowan, W. M. (2001). Viktor Hamburger and Rita Levi-Montalcini: The path to the discovery of nerve growth factor. *Annual Review of Neuroscience, 24*, 551–600.

Cowan, W. M., Fawcett, J. W., O'Leary, D. D., & Stanfield B. B. (1984). Regressive events in neurogenesis. *Science, 225*, 1258–1265.

Cregan, S. P., Fortin, A., MacLaurin, J. G., Callaghan, S. M., Cecconi, F., Yu, S. W., et al. (2006). Apoptosis-inducing factor is involved in the regulation of caspase-independent neuronal cell death. *Journal of Cell Biology, 158*(3), 507–517.

Cunningham, T. J. (1982). Naturally occurring neuron death and its regulation by developing neural pathways. *International Review of Cytology, 74*, 163–186.

Cusato, K., Stagg, S. B., & Reese, B. E. (2001). Two phases of increased cell death in the inner retina following early elimination of the ganglion cell population. *Journal of Comparative Neurology, 439*, 440–449.

Das, A. V., Mallya, K. B., Zhao, X., Ahmad, F., Bhattacharya, S., Thoreson, W. B., et al. (2006). Neural stem cell properties of Muller glia in the mammalian retina: Regulation by Notch and Wnt signaling. *Developmental Biology, 299*(1), 283–302.

Datta, S. R., Dudek, H., Tao, X., Masters, S., Fu, H., Gotoh, Y., et al. (1997). Akt phosphorylation of BAD couples survival signals to the cell-intrinsic death machinery. *Cell, 91*, 231–241.

Datta, S. R., Katsov, A., Hu, L., Petros, A., Fesik, S. W., Yaffe, M. B., et al. (2000). 14-3-3 proteins and survival kinases cooperate to inactivate BAD by BH3 domain phosphorylation. *Molecular Cell, 6*(1), 41–45.

Davies, A. M. (2003). Regulation of neuronal survival and death by extracellular signals during development. *Embryology Journal, 22*(11), 2537–2545.

Dawkins, R. (1971). Selective neurone death as a possible memory mechanism. *Nature, 229*, 118–119.

Dayer, A. G., Ford, A. A., Cleaver, K. M., Yassaee, M., & Cameron, H. A. (2003). Short-term and long-term survival of new neurons in the rat dentate gyrus. *Journal of Comparative Neurology, 460*(4), 563–572.

del Peso, L., Gonzalez-Garcia, M., Page, C., Herrera, R., & Nunez, G. (1997). Interleukin-3-induced phosphorylation of BAD through the protein kinase Akt. *Science, 278*, 687–689.

Deng, X., Xiao, L., Lang, W., Gao, F., Ruvolo, P., & May, W. S., Jr. (2001). Novel role for JNK as a stress-activated Bcl2 kinase. *Journal of Biological Chemistry, 276*, 23681–23688.

Depaepe, V., Suarez-Gonzalez, N., Dufour, A., Passante, L, Gorski, J. A., Jones, K. R., et al. (2005). Ephrin signalling controls brain size by regulating apoptosis of neural progenitors. *Nature, 435*, 1244–1250.

Derrick, B. E., York, A. D., & Martinez, J. L., Jr. (2000). Increased granule cell neurogenesis in the adult dentate gyrus following mossy fiber stimulation sufficient to induce long-term potentiation. *Brain Research, 857*(1–2), 300–307.

Donovan, N., Becker, E. B., Konishi, Y., & Bonni, A. (2002). JNK phosphorylation and activation of BAD couples the stress-activated signaling pathway to the cell death machinery. *Journal of Biological Chemistry, 277*, 40944–40949. [Epub 42002 Aug 40919].

Dufour, M. C., & Gadenne, C. (2006). Adult neurogenesis in a moth brain. *Journal of Comparative Neurology, 495*(5), 635–643.

Ekdahl, C. T., Mohapel, P., Elmer, E., & Lindvall, O. (2001). Caspase inhibitors increase short-term survival of progenitor-cell progeny in the adult rat dentate gyrus following status epilepticus. *European Journal of Neuroscience, 14*(6), 937–945.

Ellis, R. E., Yuan, J. Y., & Horvitz, H. R. (1991). Mechanisms and functions of cell death. *Annual Review of Cell Biology, 7*, 663–698.

Elshamy, W. M., & Ernfors, P. (1996). Requirement of neurotrophin-3 for the survival of proliferating trigeminal ganglion progenitor cells. *Development, 122*, 2405–2414.

Elshamy, W. M., Linnarsson, S., Lee, K. F., Jaenisch, R., & Ernfors, P. (1996). Prenatal and postnatal requirements of NT-3 for sympathetic neuroblast survival and innervation of specific targets. *Development, 122*, 491–500.

Enwere, E., Shingo, T., Gregg, C., Fujikawa, H., Ohta, S., & Weiss, S. (2004). Aging results in reduced epidermal growth factor receptor signaling, diminished olfactory neurogenesis, and deficits in fine olfactory discrimination. *Journal of Neuroscience, 24*(38), 8354–8365.

Eriksson, P. S., Perfilieva, E., Bjork-Eriksson, T., Alborn, A. M., Nordborg, C., Peterson, D. A., et al. (1998). Neurogenesis in the adult human hippocampus. *Nature Medicine, 4*(11), 1313–1317.

Ernst, M. (1926). Untergang von Zellen wahrend der normalen entwickuung bei wirbeltieren. *Zeitschrift Anatomie Entwicklungsgeshichte, 79*, 228–262.

Esposito, M. S., Piatti, V. C., Laplagne, D. A., Morgenstern, N. A., Ferrari, C. C., Pitossi, F. J., et al. (2005). Neuronal differentiation in the adult hippocampus recapitulates embryonic development. *Journal of Neuroscience, 25*(44), 10074–10086.

Fahrbach, S. E., Strande, J. L., & Robinson, G. E. (1995). Neurogenesis is absent in the brains of adult honey bees and does not explain behavioral neuroplasticity. *Neuroscience Letters, 197*(2), 145–148.

Feng, R., Rampon, C., Tang, Y. P., Shrom, D., Jin, J., Kyin, M., et al. (2001). Deficient neurogenesis in forebrain-specific presenilin-1 knockout mice is associated with reduced clearance of hippocampal memory traces. *Neuron, 32*(5), 911–926.

Figueroa-Masot, X. A., Hetman, M., Higgins, M. J., Kokot, N., & Xia, Z. (2001). Taxol induces apoptosis in cortical neurons by a mechanism independent of Bcl-2 phosphorylation. *Journal of Neuroscience, 21*, 4657–4667.

Finlay, B. L., & Pallas, S. L. (1989). Control of cell number in the developing mammalian visual system. *Progress in Neurobiology, 32*, 207–234.

Fischer, A. J., & Reh, T. A. (2001). Muller glia are a potential source of neural regeneration in the postnatal chicken retina. *Nature Neuroscience, 4*(3), 247–252.

Fischer, U., Janicke, R. U., & Schulze-Osthoff, K. (2003). Many cuts to ruin: A comprehensive update of caspase substrates. *Cell Death and Differentiation, 10*(1), 76–100.

Forger, N. G. (2006). Cell death and sexual differentiation of the nervous system. *Neuroscience, 738*, 929–938.

Frade, J. M., & Barde, Y. A. (1999). Genetic evidence for cell death mediated by nerve growth factor and the neurotrophin receptor p75 in the developing mouse retina and spinal cord. *Development, 126*, 683–90.

Frazier, L. L., & Brunjes, P. C. (1988). Unilateral odor deprivation: Early postnatal changes in olfactory bulb cell density and number. *Journal of Comparative Neurology, 269*, 355–370.

Freeman, R. S., Estus, S., & Johnson, E. M., Jr. (1994). Analysis of cell cycle-related gene expression in postmitotic neurons: Selective induction of Cyclin D1 during programmed cell death. *Neuron, 12*(2), 343–355.

Frohlich, K. U., & Madeo, F. (2000). Apoptosis in yeast—A monocellular organism exhibits altruistic behaviour. *FEBS Letters, 473*, 6–9.

Fukunaga, K., & Miyamoto, E. (1998). Role of MAP kinase in neurons. *Molecular Neurobiology, 16*(1), 79–95.

Furber, S., Oppenheim, R. W., & Prevette, D. (1987). Naturally-occurring neuron death in the ciliary ganglion of the chick embryo following removal of preganglionic input: Evidence for the role of afferents in ganglion cell survival. *Journal of Neuroscience, 7*, 1816–1832.

Galli-Resta, L., Ensini, M., Fusco, E., Gravina, A., & Margheritti, B. (1993). Afferent spontaneous electrical activity promotes the survival of target cells in the developing retinotectal system of the rat. *Journal of Neuroscience, 13*, 243–250.

Galli-Resta, L., & Resta, G. (1992). A quantitative model for the regulation of naturally occurring cell death in the developing vertebrate nervous system. *Journal of Neuroscience, 12*, 4586–4594.

Gerlai, R., & Clayton, N. S. (1999). Analysing hippocampal function in transgenic mice: An ethological perspective. *Trends in Neuroscience, 22*(2), 47–51.

Gheusi, G., Cremer, H., McLean, H., Chazal, G., Vincent, J. D., & Lledo, P. M. (2000). Importance of newly generated neurons in the adult olfactory bulb for odor discrimination. *Proceedings of National Academy of Sciences, USA, 97*(4), 1823–1828.

Gilbert, S. F. (2003). *Developmental biology.* Sunderland, MA: Sinauer.

Gluksmann, A. (1930). Ueber die bedeutung von zellvorgangen fur die formbildung epithelialer organe. *Zeitschrift Anatomie Entwicklungsgeshichte, 93*, 35–92.

Gluksmann, A. (1951). Cell deaths in normal vertebrate ontogeny. *Biological Review, 26*, 59–86.

Goergen, E. M., Bagay, L. A., Rehm, K., Benton, J. L., & Beltz, B. S. (2002). Circadian control of neurogenesis. *Journal of Neurobiology, 53*(1), 90–95.

Gorman, A. M., Ceccatelli, S, & Orrenius, S.(2000). Role of mitochondria in neuronal apoptosis. *Developmental Neuroscience, 22*(5–6), 348–358.

Gottlieb, G. (Ed.). (1973). *Studies in the development of behavior and the nervous system: Behavioral embryology.* New York: Academic Press.

Gould, E., Beylin, A., Tanapat, P., Reeves, A., & Shors, T. J. (1999). Learning enhances adult neurogenesis in the hippocampal formation. *Nature Neuroscience, 2*(3), 260–265.

Gould, E., McEwen, B. S., Tanapat, P., Galea, L. A., & Fuchs, E. (1997). Neurogenesis in the dentate gyrus of the adult tree shrew is regulated by psychosocial stress and NMDA receptor activation. *Journal of Neuroscience, 17*(7), 2492–2498.

Gould, S. J., & Lewontin, R. C. (1979). The spandrels of San Marco and the Panglossian paradigm: A critique of the adaptationist programme. *Proceedings of the Royal Society, London B, Biological Sciences, 205*, 581–598.

Gould, T., & Oppenheim, R. W. (2007). Axonal pathology and denervation vs cell death in the pathogenesis of neurological disease and following injury. *Neuroscience and Biobehavioral Reviews, 31,* 1073–1087.

Gould, T. W., Buss, R. R., Vinsant, S., Prevette, D., Sun, W., Knudson, M., et al. (2006 . Complete dissociation of motor neuron death from motor dysfunction by Bax deletion in a mouse model of ALS. *Journal of Neuroscience, 26*(34), 8774–8786.

Greene, L. A., Biswas, S. C., & Liu, D. X. (2004). Cell cycle molecules and vertebrate neuron death: E2F at the hub. *Cell Death and Differentiation, 11*(1), 49–60.

Grewal, S. S., York, R. D., & Stork, P. J. (1999). Extracellular-signal-regulated kinase signalling in neurons. *Current Opinion in Neurobiology, 9*(5), 544–553.

Gupta, S., Campbell, D., Derijard, B., & Davis, R. J. (1995). Transcription factor ATF2 regulation by the JNK signal transduction pathway. *Science, 267*, 389–393.

Haldane, J. B. S. (1932). *The causes of evolution.* New York: Longmans Green.

Haldar, S., Jena, N., & Croce, C. M. (1995). Inactivation of Bcl-2 by phosphorylation. *Proceedings of the National Academy of Science, USA, 92*, 4507–4511.

Hall, W. G., & Oppenheim, R. W. (1986). Developmental psychobiology: Prenatal, perinatal and early postnatal aspects of behavioral development. *Annual Review of Psychology, 38*, 91–128.

Hamburger, V. (1963). Some aspects of the embryology of behavior. *Quarterly Review Biology, 38*, 342–365.

Hamburger, V. (1975). Cell death in the development of the lateral motor column of the chick embryo. *Journal of Comparative Neurology, 160*, 535–546.

Hamburger, V. (1992). History of the discovery of neuronal death in embryos. *Journal of Neurobiology, 23*, 1116–1123.

Hamburger, V., & Oppenheim R. W. (1982). Naturally occurring neuronal death in vertebrates. *Neuroscience Commentaries, 1*, 39–55.

Harada, H., Becknell, B., Wilm, M., Mann, M., Huang, L. J., Taylor, S. S., et al. (1999). Phosphorylation and inactivation of BAD by mitochondria-anchored protein kinase A. *Molecular Cell, 3*, 413–422.

Harris, C. A., & Johnson, E. M., Jr. (2001). BH3-only Bcl-2 family members are coordinately regulated by the JNK pathway and require Bax to induce apoptosis in neurons. *Journal of Biological Chemistry, 276*, 37754–37760.

Harris, J. A., & Rubel, E. W. (2006). Afferent regulation of neuron number in the cochlear nucleus: Cellular and molecular analyses of a critical period. *Hearing Research, 216–217*, 127–137.

Haydar, T. F., Kuan, C. Y., Flavell, R. A., & Rakic, P. (1999). The role of cell death in regulating the size and shape of the mammalian forebrain. *Cerebral Cortex, 9*, 621–626.

Hempstead, B. L. (2006). Dissecting the diverse actions of pro- and mature neurotrophins. *Current Alzheimer Research, 3*(1), 19–24.

Hetman, M., & Xia, Z. (2000). Signaling pathways mediating anti-apoptotic action of neurotrophins. *Acta Neurobiologiae Experimentalis, 60*(4), 531–545.

Hitchcock, P. F., Lindsey Myhr, K. J., Easter, S. S., Jr., Mangione-Smith, R., & Jones, D. D. (1992). Local regeneration in the retina of the goldfish. Journal of Neurobiology, 23(2), 187–203.

Holmes, M. M., Galea, L. A., Mistlberger, R. E., & Kempermann, G. (2004). Adult hippocampal neurogenesis and voluntary running activity: Circadian and dose-dependent effects. *Journal of Neuroscience Research, 76*(2), 216–222.

Homma, S., Yaginuma, H., & Oppenheim, R. W. (1994). Programmed cell death during the earliest stages of spinal cord development in the chick embryo: A possible means of early phenotypic selection. *Journal of Comparative Neurology, 345*, 377–395.

Horvitz, H. R. (2003). Worms, life and death: Nobel lecture. *Chembiochem, 4*, 697–711.

Ito, K., & Hotta, Y. (1992). Proliferation pattern of postembryonic neuroblasts in the brain of Drosophila melanogaster. *Developmental Biology, 149*(1), 134–148.

Jaaro, H., Beck, G., Conticello, & S. G., Fainzilber, M. (2001). Evolving better brains: A need for neurotrophins? *Trends in Neuroscience, 24*, 79–85.

Jacobson, M. (1991). *Developmental neurobiology.* New York: Plenum.

Jarskog, L. F. (2006). Apoptosis in schizophrenia: Pathophysiologic and therapeutic considerations. *Current Opinion in Psychiatry, 19*(3), 307–312.

Jessen, K. R., & Mirsky, R. (2005). The origin and development of glial cells in peripheral nerves. *Nature Neuroscience, 6,* 671–682.

Jin, K., Mao, X. O., Zhu, Y., & Greenberg, D. A. (2002). MEK and ERK protect hypoxic cortical neurons via phosphorylation of Bad. *Journal of Neurochemistry, 80,* 119–125.

Kallen, B. (1965). Degeneration and regeneration in the vertebrate central nervous system during embryogenesis. *Progress in Brain Research,* 14, 77–96.

Kempermann, G. (2006). *Adult neurogenesis: Stem cells and neuronal development in adult brain.* New York: Oxford University Press.

Kempermann, G., & Gage, F. H. (2002). Genetic determinants of adult hippocampal neurogenesis correlate with acquisition, but not probe trial performance, in the water maze task. *European Journal of Neuroscience, 16*(1), 129–136.

Kempermann, G., Gast, D., Kronenberg, G., Yamaguchi, M., & Gage, F. H. (2003). Early determination and long-term persistence of adult-generated new neurons in the hippocampus of mice. *Development, 130*(2), 391–399.

Kempermann, G., Kuhn, H. G., & Gage, F. H. (1997). More hippocampal neurons in adult mice living in an enriched environment. *Nature, 386(6624),* 493–495.

Kermer, P, Liman, J, Weishaupt, JH, & Bahr, M. (2004). Neuronal apoptosis in neurodegenerative diseases: From basic research to clinical application. *Neurodegenerative Disorder, 1*(1), 9–19.

Kim, W., Park, O., Choi, S. C., Choi, S. Y., Park, S., Lee, K., et al. (2009). Th maintance of specific aspects of neuronal function and behavior is dependent on programmed cell death of adult-generated neuorns in the dentate gyrus. *European Journal of Neuroscience* (In Press).

Kintner, C. (2002). Neurogenesis in embryos and in adult neural stem cells. *Journal of Neuroscience, 22*(3), 639–643.

Kokoeva, M. V., Yin, H., & Flier, J. S. (2005). Neurogenesis in the hypothalamus of adult mice: Potential role in energy balance. *Science, 310*(5748), 679–683.

Koliatsos, V., & Ratan, R. (1998). *Cell death in diseases of the nervous system.* Totowa, NJ: Humana Press..

Kornack, D. R., & Rakic, P. (2001). Cell proliferation without neurogenesis in adult primate neocortex. *Science, 294*(5549), 2127–2130.

Korsching, S. (1993). The neurotrophic factor concept: A reexamination. *Journal of Neuroscience, 13,* 2739–2748.

Kozorovitskiy, Y., & Gould, E. (2004). Dominance hierarchy influences adult neurogenesis in the dentate gyrus. *Journal of Neuroscience, 24*(30), 6755–6759.

Krantic, S, Mechawar, N, Reix, S, & Quirion, R. (2005). Molecular basis of programmed cell death involved in neurodegeneration. *Trends in Neuroscience, 28*(12), 670–676.

Kuan, C. Y., Roth, K. A., Flavell, R. A., & Rakic, P. (2000). Mechanisms of programmed cell death in the developing brain. *Trends in Neuroscience,* 23, 291–297.

Kuan, C. Y., Yang, D. D., Samanta Roy, D. R., Davis, R. J., Rakic, P., & Flavell, R. A. (1999). The Jnk1 and Jnk2 protein kinases are required for regional specific apoptosis during early brain development. *Neuron, 22,* 667–676.

Kuhn, H. G., Biebl, M., Wilhelm, D., Li, M., Friedlander, R. M., & Winkler, J. (2005). Increased generation of granule cells in adult Bcl-2-overexpressing mice: A role for

cell death during continued hippocampal neurogenesis. *European Journal of Neuroscience, 22*(8), 1907–1915.

Kuida, K., Haydar, T. F., Kuan, C. Y., Gu, Y., Taya, C., Karasuyama, H., et al. (1998). Reduced apoptosis and cytochrome c-mediated caspase activation in mice lacking caspase 9. *Cell, 94*(3), 325–337.

Kuida, K., Zheng, T. S., Na, S., Kuan, C., Yang, D., Karasuyama, H., et al. (1996). Decreased apoptosis in the brain and premature lethality in CPP32-deficient mice. *Nature, 384*(6607), 368–372.

Kuno, M. (1990). Target dependence of motoneuronal survival: The current status. *Neuroscience Research, 9,* 155–172.

Lauber, K., Bohn, E., Krober, S. M., Xiao, Y. J., Blumenthal, S. G., Lindemann, et al. (2003). Apoptotic cells induce migration of phagocytes via caspase-3-mediated release of a lipid attraction signal. *Cell, 113*(6), 717–730.

Lehmann, K., Butz, M., & Teuchert-Noodt, G. (2005). Offer and demand: Proliferation and survival of neurons in the dentate gyrus. *European Journal of Neuroscience, 21*(12), 3205–3216.

Lei, K., & Davis, R. J., (2003). JNK phosphorylation of Bim-related members of the Bcl2 family induces Bax-dependent apoptosis. *Proceedings of the National Academy of Science, USA,* 100, 2432–2437.

Lemaire, V., Koehl, M., Le Moal, M., & Abrous, D. N. (2000). Prenatal stress produces learning deficits associated with an inhibition of neurogenesis in the hippocampus. *Proceedings of National Academy of Sciences, USA, 97*(20), 11032–11037.

Lemasson, M., Saghatelyan, A., Olivo-Marin, J. C., & Lledo, P. M. (2005). Neonatal and adult neurogenesis provide two distinct populations of newborn neurons to the mouse olfactory bulb. *Journal of Neuroscience, 25*(29), 6816–6825.

Lettre, G., & Hengartner, M. O. (2006). Developmental apoptosis in *C. elegans*: A complex CEDnario. *Nature Reviews Molecular Cell Biology, 7*(2), 97–108.

Leuner, B., Mendolia-Loffredo, S., Kozorovitskiy, Y., Samburg, D., Gould, E., & Shors, T. J. (2004). Learning enhances the survival of new neurons beyond the time when the hippocampus is required for memory. *Journal of Neuroscience, 24*(34), 7477–7481.

Lewis, K. (2000). Programmed death in bacteria. *Microbiology Molecular Biology Review, 64,* 503–514.

Linden, R. (1994). The survival of developing neurons: A review of afferent control. *Neuroscience, 58,* 671–682.

Lindholm, D., & Arumae, U.(2004). Cell differentiation: Reciprocal regulation of Apaf-1 and the inhibitor of apoptosis proteins. *Journal Cell Biology, 167*(2), 193–195.

Lindsten, T., Golden, J. A., Zong, W. X., Minarcik, J., Harris, M. H., & Thompson, C. B. (2003). The proapoptotic activities of Bax and Bak limit the size of the neural stem cell pool. *Journal of Neuroscience, 23*(35), 11112–11119.

Lipkind, D., Nottebohm, F., Rado, R., & Barnea, A. (2002). Social change affects the survival of new neurons in the forebrain of adult songbirds. *Behavioral Brain Research, 133*(1), 31–43.

Lipton, S. A., & Bossy-Wetzel, E. (2002). Dueling activities of AIF in cell death versus survival: DNA binding and redox activity. *Cell, 111*(2), 147–150.

Lois, C., & Alvarez-Buylla, A. (1994). Long-distance neuronal migration in the adult mammalian brain. *Science, 264*(5162), 1145–1148.

Lopez-Neblina, F., Toledo, A. H., & Toledo-Pereyra, L. H. (2005). Molecular biology of apoptosis in ischemia and reperfusion. *Journal Investigative Surgery, 18*(6), 335–350.

Lotto, R. B., Asavaritikrai, P., Vali, L., & Price, D. J. (2001). Target-derived neurotrophic factors regulate the death of developing forebrain neurons after a change in their trophic requirements. *Journal of Neuroscience, 21*, 3904–3910.

Lowrie, M. B., & Lawson, S. J. (2000). Cell death of spinal interneurones. *Progress Neurobiology, 61,* 543–555.

Lu, B., Pang, P. T., & Woo, N. H. (2005). The yin and yang of neurotrophin action. *Nature Reviews Neuroscience, 6,* 603–614.

Lui, D., Diorio, J., Day, J., Francis, D., & Meaney, M. J. (2002). Maternal care, hippocampal synaptogenesis and cognitive development in rats. *Nature Neuroscience, 3,* 799–806.

Luo, L., & O'Leary, D. D. (2005). Axon retraction and degeneration in development and disease. *Annual Review of Neuroscience, 28,* 127–156.

Mallat, M., Marin-Teva, J. L., & Cheret, C. (2005). Phagocytosis in the developing CNS: More than clearing the corpses. *Current Opinion in Neurobiology, 15*(1), 101–107.

Mandairon, N., Jourdan, F., & Didier, A. (2003). Deprivation of sensory inputs to the olfactory bulb up-regulates cell death and proliferation in the subventricular zone of adult mice. *Neuroscience, 119*(2), 507–516.

Maundrell, K., Antonsson, B., Magnenat, E., Camps, M., Muda, M., Chabert, C., et al. (1997). Bcl-2 undergoes phosphorylation by c-Jun N-terminal kinase/stress-activated protein kinases in the presence of the constitutively active GTP-binding protein Rac1. *Journal of Biological Chemistry, 272*, 25238–25242.

Mayr, E. (1983). How to carry out the adaptationist program? *American Naturalist, 121*, 324–334.

McFarland, K. N., Wilkes, S. R., Koss, S. E., Ravichandran, & K. S., Mandell, J. W. (2006). Neural-specific inactivation of ShcA results in increased embryonic neural progenitor apoptosis and microencephaly. *Journal of Neuroscience, 26*(30), 7885–7897.

McLennan, I. S. (1988). Quantitative relationships between motoneuron and muscle development in Xenopus laevis: Implications for motoneuron cell death and motor unit formation. *Journal of Comparative Neurology, 271*, 19–29.

Mehlen, P., Mille, F., & Thibert, C. (2005). Morphogens and cell survival during development. *Journal of Neurobiology, 64*, 357–366.

Meltzer, L. A., Yabaluri, R., & Deisseroth, K. (2005). A role for circuit homeostasis in adult neurogenesis. *Trends in Neuroscience, 28*(12), 653–660.

Meshi, D., Drew, M. R., Saxe, M., Ansorge, M. S., David, D., Santarelli, L., et al. (2006). Hippocampal neurogenesis is not required for behavioral effects of environmental enrichment. *Nature Neuroscience, 9*(6), 729–731.

Michel, G. E., & Moore, C. L. (1995). *Developmental psychobiology.* Cambridge, MA: MIT Press.

Milligan, C. E., Prevette, D., Yaginuma, H., Homma, S., Cardwell, C., Fritz, L. C., et al. (1995a). Peptide inhibitors of the ICE protease family arrest programmed cell death of motoneurons in vivo and in vitro. *Neuron, 15*, 385–393.

Milligan, C. E., Webster, L., Piros, E. T., Evans, C. J., Cunningham, T. J., Levitt, P. (1995b). Induction of opioid receptor-mediated macrophage chemotactic activity after neonatal brain injury. *Journal of Immunology, 154*(12), 6571–6581.

Milner, L. D., & Landmesser, L. T. (1999). Cholinergic and GABAergic inputs drive patterned spontaneous motoneuron activity before target contact. *Journal of Neuroscience, 19*, 3007–3022.

Mirescu, C., Peters, J. D., & Gould, E. (2004). Early life experience alters response of adult neurogenesis to stress. *Nature Neuroscience, 7*(8), 841–846.

Moon, R. T. (1981). Cell death: An integral aspect of development. *The Biologist, 63*, 5–26.

Moore, C. L., Don, H., & Juraska, J. M. (1992). Maternal stimulation affects the number of motor neurons in a sexually dimorphic nucleus of the lumbar spinal cord. *Brain Research, 572*, 52–56.

Morcuende, S., Benitez-Temino, B., Pecero, M. L., Pastor, A. M., & de la Cruz, R. R. (2005). Abducens internuclear neurons depend on their target motoneurons for survival during early postnatal development. *Experimental Neurology, 195*, 244–256.

Morrison, R. S., Kinoshita, Y., Johnson. M. D., Ghatan, S., Ho, J. T., & Garden, G. (2002). Neuronal survival and cell death signaling pathways. *Advances in Experimental Medicine and Biology, 513*, 41–86.

Morrissey, M. J., Duntley, S. P., Anch, A. M., & Nonneman. R. (2004). Active sleep and its role in the prevention of apoptosis in the developing brain. *Medical Hypotheses, 62*(6), 876–879.

Najbauer, J., & Leon, M. (1995). Olfactory experience modulated apoptosis in the developing olfactory bulb. *Brain Research, 674*, 245–251.

Naruse, I., & Keino, H. (1995). Apoptosis in the developing CNS. *Progress in Neurobiology, 47*(2), 135–155.

Newbern, J., Taylor, A., Robinson, M., Li, L., & Milligan, C. E. (2005). Decreases in phosphoinositide-3-kinase/Akt and extracellular signal-regulated kinase 1/2 signaling activate components of spinal motoneuron death. *Journal Neurochemistry, 94*, 1652–1665.

Nicholson, D. W. (1999). Caspase structure, proteolytic substrates, and function during apoptotic cell death. *Cell Death Differ, 6*(11), 1028–1042.

Nottebohm, F. (2002a). Neuronal replacement in adult brain. *Brain Research Bulletin, 57*(6), 737–749.

Nottebohm, F. (2002b). Why are some neurons replaced in adult brain? *Journal of Neuroscience, 22*, 624–628.

Nottebohm, F., O'Loughlin, B., Gould, K., Yohay, K., & Alvarez-Buylla, A. (1994). The life span of new neurons in a song control nucleus of the adult canary brain depends on time of year when these cells are born. *Proceedings of National Academy of Sciences USA, 91*(17), 7849–7853.

Ockel, M., Lewin, G. R., & Barde, Y. A. (1996). In vivo effects of neurotrophin-3 during sensory neurogenesis. *Development, 122*, 301–307.

O'Donovan, M. J. (1999). The origin of spontaneous activity in developing networks of the vertebrate nervous system. *Current Opinion in Neurobiology, 9*, 94–104.

Oliveira, A. L., Risling, M., Negro, A., Langone, F., & Cullheim, S. (2002). Apoptosis of spinal interneurons induced by sciatic nerve axotomy in the neonatal rat is counteracted by nerve growth factor and ciliary neurotrophic factor. *Journal of Comparative Neurology, 447*, 381–393.

Olson, A. K., Eadie, B. D., Ernst, C., & Christie, B. R. (2006). Environmental enrichment and voluntary exercise massively increase neurogenesis in the adult hippocampus via dissociable pathways. *Hippocampus, 16*(3), 250–260.

Oppenheim, R. W. (1981a). Neuronal cell death and some related regressive phenomena during neurogenesis: A selective historical review and progress report. In: W. M. Cowan (Ed.), *Studies in developmental neurobiology essays in honor of Viktor Hamburger* (pp. 74–133). New York: Oxford University Press.

Oppenheim, R. W. (1981b). Ontogenetic adaptations and retrogressive processes in the development of the nervous system and behavior. In K. Connolly & H. F. Prechtl (Eds.). *Maturation and development: Biological and psychological perspectives* (pp. 198–215). Philadelphia, PA: Lippincott.

Oppenheim, R. W. (1982). The neuroembryological study of behavior: Progress, problems, perspectives. *Current Topics in Developmental Biology, 17,* 257–309.

Oppenheim, R. W. (1984). Ontogenetic adaptations in neural and behavioral development: Towards a more ecological developmental psychobiology. In H. F. Prechtl (Ed.). *Continuity of neural functions from prenatal to postnatal life* (pp. 16–30). Philadelphia, PA: Lippincott.

Oppenheim, R. W. (1989). The neurotrophic theory and naturally occurring motoneuron death. *Trends in Neuroscience, 12,* 252–255.

Oppenheim, R. W. (1991). Cell death during development of the nervous system. *Annual Review of Neuroscience, 14,* 453–501.

Oppenheim, R. W. (1996). Neurotrophic survival molecules for motoneurons: An embarrassment of riches. *Neuron, 17,* 195–197.

Oppenheim, R. W. (2001). Viktor Hamburger (1900–2001). Journey of a neuroembryologist to the end of the millennium and beyond. *Neuron, 31,* 179–190.

Oppenheim, R. W., Caldero, J., Esquerda, J., & Gould, T. W. (2001a). Target-independent programmed cell death in the developing nervous system. In: A. F. Kalverboer & A. Gramsbergen (Eds.). *Handbook of brain behaviour in human development* (pp. 343–408). Great Britain: Kluwer

Oppenheim, R. W., Flavell, R. A., Vinsant, S., Prevette, D., Kuan, C. Y., & Rakic, P. (2001b). Programmed cell death of developing mammalian neurons after genetic deletion of caspases. *Journal of Neuroscience, 21*(13), 4752–4760.

Oppenheim, R. W., & Johnson, J. (2003). Programmed cell death and neurotrophic factors. In L. R. Squire, F. E. Bloom, S. K. McConnell, J. L. Roberts, N. C. Spitzer, N. J., & Zigmond, M. J. (Eds.), *Fundamental neuroscience* (pp. 499–532). New York: Elsevier.

Oppenheim, R. W., Blomgrem, K., Ethell, D. W., Koika, K., Komatsu, M., Prevette, D., et al. (2008). Developing postmitotic mammalian neurons in vivo lacking Apaf-1 undego programmed cell death by a caspase-independent, non-apoptotic pathway involving autophagy. *Jounal of Neuroscience, 28,* 1490–1497.

Overstreet-Wadiche, L. S., Bensen, A. L., & Westbrook, G. L. (2006). Delayed development of adult-generated granule cells in dentate gyrus. *Journal of Neuroscience, 26*(8), 2326–2334.

Perez-Canellas, M. M., & Garcia-Verdugo, J. M. (1996). Adult neurogenesis in the telencephalon of a lizard: A [3H]thymidine autoradiographic and bromodeoxyuridine immunocytochemical study. *Brain Research. Developmental Brain Research, 93*(1–2), 49–61.

Persico. A. M., & Bourgeron, T. (2006). Searching for ways out of the autism maze: Genetic, epigenetic and environmental clues. *Trends in Neuroscience, 29*(7), 349–358.

Peter, M. E., & Krammer, P. H. (2003). The CD95(APO-1/Fas) DISC and beyond. *Cell Death and Differentiation, 10*(1), 26–35.

Petreanu, L., & Alvarez-Buylla, A. (2002). Maturation and death of adult-born olfactory bulb granule neurons: Role of olfaction. *Journal of Neuroscience, 22*(14), 6106–6113.

Pilar, G., & Landmesser, L.(1976). Ultrastructural differences during embryonic cell death in normal and peripherally deprived ciliary ganglia. *Journal Cell Biology, 68*(2), 339–356.

Polster, B. M., & Fiskum, G.(2004). Mitochondrial mechanisms of neural cell apoptosis. *Journal of Neurochemistry, 90*(6), 1281–1289.

Provine, R. R. (1973). Neurophysiological aspects of behavior development in the chick embryo. In G. Gottlieb (Ed.), *Studies on the development of behavior and the nervous system: Behavioral embryology* (pp. 77–102). New York: Academic Press.

Purves, D., & Sanes, J. R. (1987). The 1986 Nobel prize in physiology or medicine. *Trends in Neuroscience, 10,* 231–235.

Putcha, G. V., Le, S., Frank, S., Besirli, C. G., Clark, K., Chu, B, et al. (2003). JNK-mediated BIM phosphorylation potentiates BAX-dependent apoptosis. *Neuron, 38,* 899–914.

Putz, U., Harwell, C., & Nedivi, E. (2005). Soluble CPG15 expressed during early development rescues cortical progenitors from apoptosis. *Nature Neuroscience, 8,* 322–331.

Rao, M. S., Hattiangady, B., Abdel-Rahman, A., Stanley, D. P., & Shetty, A. K. (2005). Newly born cells in the ageing dentate gyrus display normal migration, survival and neuronal fate choice but endure retarded early maturation. *European Journal of Neuroscience, 21*(2), 464–476.

Rehen, S. K., McConnell, M. J., Kaushal, D., Kingsbury, M. A., Yang, A. H., & Chun, J. (2001). Chromosomal variation in neurons of the developing and adult mammalian nervous system. *Proceeding of the National Academy of Science USA, 98,* 13361–13366.

Rochefort, C., Gheusi, G., Vincent, J. D., & Lledo, P. M. (2002). Enriched odor exposure increases the number of newborn neurons in the adult olfactory bulb and improves odor memory. *Journal of Neuroscience, 22*(7), 2679–2689.

Rogers, L. A., & Cowan, W. M. (1973). The development of the mesencephalic nucleus of the trigeminal nerve in the chick. *Journal of Comparative Neurology, 147,* 291–320.

Rondi-Reig, L., Lemaigre-Dubreuil, Y., Montecot, C., Muller, D., Martinou, J. C., Caston, J., et al. (2001). Transgenic mice with neuronal overexpression of bcl-2 gene present navigation disabilities in a water task. *Neuroscience, 104*(1), 207–215.

Rondi-Reig, L., & Mariani, J. (2002). To die or not to die, does it change the function? Behavior of transgenic mice reveals a role for developmental cell death. *Brain Research Bulletin, 57,* 85–91.

Ryan, C. A., & Salvesen,G. S. (2003). Caspases and neuronal development. *Biological Chemistry, 384*(6), 855–861.

Sabapathy, K., Jochum, W., Hochedlinger, K., Chang, L., Karin, M., & Wagner, E. F. (1999). Defective neural tube morphogenesis and altered apoptosis in the absence of both JNK1 and JNK2. *Mechanisms of Development, 89,* 115–124.

Sanai, N., Tramontin, A. D., Quinones-Hinojosa, A., Barbaro, N. M., Gupta, N., Kunwar, S., et al. (2004). Unique astrocyte ribbon in adult human brain contains neural stem cells but lacks chain migration. *Nature, 427*(6976), 740–744.

Sanders, E. J., & Wride, M. A. (1995). Programmed cell death in development. *International Review of Cytology, 163*, 105–173.

Sathasivam, S., & Shaw, P. J. (2005). Apoptosis in amyotrophic lateral sclerosis—What is the evidence? *Lancet Neurology, 4*(8), 500–509.

Saunders, J. W., Jr. (1966). Death in embryonic systems. *Science, 154*, 604–612.

Savill, J.(1997). Recognition and phagocytosis of cells undergoing apoptosis. *British Medical Bulletin, 53*(3), 491–508.

Savill, J., & Fadok, V.(2000). Corpse clearance defines the meaning of cell death. *Nature, 407*(6805), 784–788.

Savill, J., Gregory, C., & Haslett, C. (2003). Cell biology. Eat me or die. *Science, 302*(5650), 1516–1517.

Schmidt, M. (1997). Continuous neurogenesis in the olfactory brain of adult shore crabs, Carcinus maenas. *Brain Research, 762*(1–2), 131–143.

Schumann, C. M., & Amaral, D. G. (2006). Stereological analysis of amygdala neuron number in autism. *Journal of Neuroscience, 26*(29), 7674–7649.

Scotto-Lomassese, S., Strambi, C., Strambi, A., Aouane, A., Augier, R., Rougon, G., et al. (2003). Suppression of adult neurogenesis impairs olfactory learning and memory in an adult insect. *Journal of Neuroscience, 23*(28), 9289–9296.

Scotto-Lomassese, S., Strambi, C., Strambi, A., Charpin, P., Augier, R., Aouane, A., et al. (2000). Influence of environmental stimulation on neurogenesis in the adult insect brain. *Journal of Neurobiology, 45*(3), 162–171.

Shingo, T., Gregg, C., Enwere, E., Fujikawa, H., Hassam, R., Geary, C., et al. (2003). Pregnancy-stimulated neurogenesis in the adult female forebrain mediated by prolactin. *Science, 299*(5603), 117–120.

Shors, T. J., Miesegaes, G., Beylin, A., Zhao, M., Rydel, T., & Gould, E. (2001). Neurogenesis in the adult is involved in the formation of trace memories. *Nature, 410*(6826), 372–376.

Shors, T. J., Townsend, D. A., Zhao, M., Kozorovitskiy, Y., & Gould, E. (2002). Neurogenesis may relate to some but not all types of hippocampal-dependent learning. *Hippocampus, 12*(5), 578–584.

Silver, J. (1978). Cell death during development of the nervous system. In: M. Jacobson (Ed.), *Handbook of sensory physiology*, (Vol. IX, pp. 419–436). Berlin: Springer Verlag.

Smith, M., Wang, X. Y., Wolgemuth, D. J., & Murashov, A. K. (2003). Development of the mouse vestibular system in the absence of gravity perception. *Developmental Brain Research, 140*, 133–135.

Soane, L., & Fiskum, G. (2005). Inhibition of mitochondrial neural cell death pathways by protein transduction of Bcl-2 family proteins. *Journal of Bioengineering and Biomembranes, 37*(3), 179–190.

Sofroniew, M. V., Howe, C. L., & Mobley, W. C. (2001). Nerve growth factor signaling, neuroprotection, and neural repair. *Annual Review of Neuroscience, 24*, 1217–1281.

Stefanis, L. (2005). Caspase-dependent and -independent neuronal death: Two distinct pathways to neuronal injury. *Neuroscientist, 11*(1), 50–62.

Sun, W., Gould, T. W., Newbern, J., Milligan, C., Chio, S. Y., Kim, H., et al. (2005). Phosphorylation of c-jun in avian and mammalian motoneurons in vivo during programmed cell death: An early reversible event in the apoptotic cascade. *Journal of Neuroscience, 25*, 5595–5603.

Sun, W., Gould, T. W., Vinsant, S., Prevette, D., & Oppenheim, R. W. (2003). Neuromuscular development after the prevention of naturally occurring neuronal death by Bax deletion. *Journal of Neuroscience, 23*, 7298–7310.

Sun, W., & Oppenheim, R. W. (2003). Response of motoneurons to neonatal sciatic nerve axotomy in Bax-knockout mice. *Molecular Cellular Neuroscience, 24*, 875–886.

Sun, W., Winseck, A., Vinsant, S., Park, O. H., Kim, H., & Oppenheim, R. W. (2004). Programmed cell death of adult-generated hippocampal neurons is mediated by the proapoptotic gene Bax. *Journal of Neuroscience, 24*(49), 11205–11213.

Sunayama, J., Tsuruta, F., Masuyama, N., & Gotoh, Y. (2005). JNK antagonizes Akt-mediated survival signals by phosphorylating 14-3-3. *Journal Cell Biology, 170*, 295–304.

Svoboda, K. R., Linares, A. E., & Ribera, A. B. (2001). Activity regulates programmed cell death of zebrafish. Rohon-Beard neurons. *Development, 128*, 3511–3520.

Tanaka, H., & Landmesser, L. T. (1986). Cell death of lumbosacral motoneurons in chick, quail, and chick-quail chimera embryos: A test of the quantitative matching hypothesis of neuronal cell death. *Journal of Neuroscience, 6*, 2889–2899.

Tashiro, A., Sandler, V. M., Toni, N., Zhao, C., & Gage, F. H. (2006). NMDA-receptor-mediated, cell-specific integration of new neurons in adult dentate gyrus. *Nature, 442*(7105), 929–933.

Taylor, A. R., Prevette, D., Urioste, A. S., Oppenheim, R. W., & Milligan, C. E.(2003). Cell cycle events distinguish sensory neuronal death from motoneuron death as a result of trophic factor deprivation. *Molecular Cellular Neuroscience, 24*(2), 323–339.

Terrado, J., Burgess, R. W., DeChiara, T., Yancopoulos, G., Sanes, J. R., & Kato, A. C. (2001). Motoneuron survival is enhanced in the absence of neuromuscular junction formation in embryos. *Journal of Neuroscience, 21*, 3144–3150.

Thanos, S. (1999). Genesis, neurotrophin responsiveness, and apoptosis of a pronounced direct connection between the two eyes of the chick embryo: A natural error or a meaningful developmental event? *Journal of Neuroscience, 19*, 3900–3917.

Tournier, C., Hess, P., Yang, D. D., Xu, J., Turner, T. K., Nimnual, A., et al. (2000). Requirement of JNK for stress-induced activation of the cytochrome c-mediated death pathway. *Science, 288*, 870–874.

Truman, J. W. (1984). Cell death in invertebrate nervous systems. *Annual Review of Neuroscience, 7*, 171–188.

Umansky, S. R. (1982). The genetic program of cell death. Hypothesis and some applications: Transformation, carcinogenesis, ageing. *Journal of Theoretical Biology, 97*, 591–602.

Vahsen, N., Cande, C., Briere, J. J., Benit, P., Joza, N., Larochette, N., et al. (2004). AIF deficiency compromises oxidative Phosphorylation. *Embryology, 23*(23), 4679–4689.

van Praag, H., Kempermann, G., & Gage, F. H. (1999). Running increases cell proliferation and neurogenesis in the adult mouse dentate gyrus. *Nature Neuroscience, 2*(3), 266–270.

van Praag, H., Schinder, A. F., Christie, B. R., Toni, N., Palmer, T. D., & Gage, F. H. (2002). Functional neurogenesis in the adult hippocampus. *Nature*, *415*(6875), 1030–1034.

Vaux, D. L., Haecker, G., & Strasser, A. (1994). An evolutionary perspective on apoptosis. *Cell*, *76*, 777–779.

Verhage, M., Maia, A. S., Plomp, J. J., Brussard, A. B., Heeroma, J. H., Vermeer, H., et al. (2000). Synaptic assembly of the brain in the absence of neurotransmitter secretion. *Science*, *287*, 864–869.

Verney, C., Takahashi, T., Bhide, P. G., Nowakowski, R. S., & Caviness, V. S., Jr. (2000). Independent controls for neocortical neuron production and histogenetic cell death. *Developmental Neuroscience*, *22*, 125–138.

Vogel, M. W., Sunter, K., & Herrup, K. (1989). Numerical matching between granule and Purkinje cells in lurcher chimeric mice: A hypothesis for the trophic rescue of granule cells from target-related cell death. *Journal of Neuroscience*, *9*, 3454–3462.

von Bartheld, C. S., & Bothwell, M. (1993). Development of the mesencephalic nucleus of the trigeminal nerve in chick embryos: Target innervation, neurotrophin receptors, and cell death. *Journal of Comparative Neurology*, *328*, 185–202.

von Bartheld, C. S., & Johnson, J. E. (2001). Target-derived BDNF (brain-derived neurotrophic factor) is essential for the survival of developing neurons in the isthmo-optic nucleus. *Journal of Comparative Neurology*, *433*, 550–564.

Voyvodic, J. T. (1996). Cell death in cortical development: How much? Why? So what? Neuron, 16, 693–696.

Waetzig, V., & Herdegen, T. (2005). Context-specific inhibition of JNKs: Overcoming the dilemma of protection and damage. *Trends in Pharmacological Sciences*, *26*, 455–461.

Wallach, D., Varfolomeev, E. E., Malinin, N. L., Goltsev, Y. V., Kovalenko, A. V., & Boldin, M. P. (1999). Tumor necrosis factor receptor and Fas signaling mechanisms. *Annual Review of Immunology*, *17*, 331–367.

Weaver, I. C. G., Grant, R. J., & Meaney, M. J. (2002). Maternal abehavior regulates long-term hippocmpal expression of Bax and apoptosis in the offspring. *Journal of Neurochemistry*, *82*, 998–1002.

West-Eberhard, M. J. (2003). *Developmental plasticity and evolution*. Oxford: Oxford University Press.

Wetts, R., & Vaughn, J. E. (1998). Differences in developmental cell death between somatic and autonomic motor neurons of rat spinal cord. *Journal of Comparative Neurology*, *396*, 483–492.

White, J. G., Southgate, E., & Thomson, J. N. (1991). On the nature of undead cells in the nematode *Caenorhabditis elegans*. *Philosophical Transactions of the Royal Society of London (B)*, *331*, 263–271.

White, K., Tahaoglu, E., & Steller, H. (1996). Cell killing by the Drosophila gene reaper. *Science*, *271*, 805–807.

Williams, R. W., & Herrup, K. (1988). The control of neuron number. *Annual Review of Neuroscience*, *11*, 423–453.

Winner, B., Cooper-Kuhn, C. M., Aigner, R., Winkler, J., & Kuhn, H. G. (2002). Long-term survival and cell death of newly generated neurons in the adult rat olfactory bulb. *European Journal of Neuroscience*, *16*(9), 1681–1689.

Winseck, A. K., Caldero, J., Ciutat, D., Prevette, D., Scott, S. A., Wang, G., et al. (2002). In vivo analysis of Schwann cell programmed cell death in the embryonic chick: Regulation by axons and glial growth factor. *Journal of Neuroscience*, *22*, 4509–4521.

Winseck, A. K., & Oppenheim, R. W. (2006). An in vivo analysis of Schwann cell programmed cell death in embryonic mice: The role of axons, glial growth factor and the pro-apoptotic gene *Bax*. *European Journal of Neuroscience*, *24*, 2105–2177.

Wong, R. O. L., & Lichtman, J. W. (2003). Synapse elimination. In L. R. Squire, F. E. Bloom, S. K. McConnell, J. L. Roberts, N. C. Spitzer, & N. J. Zigmond (Eds.), *Fundamental Neuroscience* (pp. 533–554). New York: Academic Press.

Wyllie, A. H., Kerr, J. F., & Currie, A. R. (1980). Cell death: The significance of apoptosis. *International Review of Cytology*, *68*, 251–306.

Yakura, T., Fukuda, Y., & Sawai, H. (2002). Effect of Bcl-2 overexpression on establishment of ipsilateral retinocollicular projection in mice. *Neuroscience*, *110*, 667–673.

Yamamoto, K., Ichijo, H., & Korsmeyer, S. J. (1999). BCL-2 is phosphorylated and inactivated by an ASK1/Jun N-terminal protein kinase pathway normally activated at G(2)/M. *Molecular Cell Biology*, *19*, 8469–8478.

Yang, A. H., Kaushal, D., Rehen, S. K., Kriedt, K., Kingsbury, M. A., McConnell, M. J., et al. (2003). Chromosome segregation defects contribute to aneuploidy in normal neural progenitor cells. *Journal of Neuroscience*, *23*, 10454–10462.

Yeo, W., & Gautier, J. (2004). Early neural cell death: Dying to become neurons. *Developmental Biology*, *274*, 233–244.

Young, D., Lawlor, P. A., Leone, P., Dragunow, M., & During, M. J. (1999). Environmental enrichment inhibits spontaneous apoptosis, prevents seizures and is neuroprotective. *Nature Medicine*, *5*(4), 448–453.

Yuan, J., Lipinski, M., & Degterev, A.(2003). Diversity in the mechanisms of neuronal cell death. *Neuron*, *40*(2), 401–413.

Zakharov, I. S., Hayes, N. L., Ierusalimsky, V. N., Nowakowski, R. S., & Balaban, P. M. (1998). Postembryonic neurogenesis in the procerebrum of the terrestrial snail, *Helix lucorum* L. *Journal of Neurobiology*, *35*(3), 271–276.

Zhao, C., Aviles, C., Abel, R. A., Almli C. R., McQuillen, P., & Pleasure, S. J. (2005). Hippocampal and visuospatial learning defects in mice with a deletion of frizzled 9, a gene in the Williams syndrome deletion interval. *Development*, *132*(12), 2917–2927.

Zhao, C., Teng, E. M., Summers, R. G., Jr., Ming, G. L., & Gage, F. H. (2006). Distinct morphological stages of dentate granule neuron maturation in the adult mouse hippocampus. *Journal of Neuroscience*, *26*(1), 3–11.

Zhao, M., Momma, S., Delfani, K., Carlen, M., Cassidy, R. M., Johansson, C. B., et al. (2003). Evidence for neurogenesis in the adult mammalian substantia nigra. *Proceedings of National Academy of Sciences, USA*, *100*(13), 7925–7930.

Zou, D. J., Feinstein, P., Rivers, A. L., Mathews, G. A., Kim, A., Greer, C. A., et al. (2004). Postnatal refinement of peripheral olfactory projections. *Science*, *304*, 1976–1979.

Development of GABAergic Signaling: From Molecules to Emerging Networks

Sampsa T. Sipilä, Peter Blaesse, *and* **Kai Kaila**

Abstract

GABAergic transmission mediated by anion-permeable $GABA_A$ receptor-channels is one of the most fundamental mechanisms of neuronal communication in the brain at the cellular and systems level. During development, there is a qualitative change in $GABA_A$ signaling from depolarizing and often even excitatory responses, displayed by immature neurons, to the "conventional" inhibitory actions observed in the adult. An increasing amount of evidence points to bidirectional interactions, where GABAergic signaling shapes the functional as well as structural properties of neurons and neuronal networks. This chapter reviews the molecular basis of the ontogeny of GABA actions with an emphasis on $GABA_A$ receptors and ion-transport mechanisms. With a focus on the hippocampus, the chapter shows how this kind of information can be used in understanding the development of endogenous and evoked network events.

Keywords: GABA, neuronal communication, bidirectional interactions, $GABA_A$ receptors, ion-transport mechanisms, hippocampus

Introduction

The history of γ-aminobutyric acid (GABA) as a neurotransmitter dates back to the 1950s when Roberts and Frankel (1950) and others (Awapara, Landua, Fuerst, & Seale, 1950) found that GABA is abundant in extracts of mammalian brain tissue. The canonical signaling function of GABA, postsynaptic inhibition, was first established in electrophysiological experiments on crayfish neurons and muscle fibers (Boistel & Fatt, 1958; Kuffler & Edwards, 1958), and somewhat later in the mammalian central nervous system (CNS) (Krnjevic & Schwartz, 1967; for review, see Krnjevic 2004).

The word "information" is used in a rather loose manner in biological literature. From an engineering point of view, the information content of a message or signal is inversely related to its probability (Shannon & Weaver, 1949). However, the original Shannon–Weaver theory that quantifies information as binary digits or bits is not easy to apply when dealing with communication in the nervous system. Without elaborating further on this topic, it suffices to note that the transfer of information between nerve cells is achieved by allosteric interactions between a ligand (usually released from a presynaptic terminal) and its receptors (located in the target cell). Thus, neuronal communication is "pragmatic" in the sense that the code of the message is defined by the effect of the signaling molecule at its target. This pragmatic nature of communication is also true for electrical signals in the nervous system and, in fact, for molecular and cellular communication in general.

GABA as a Signaling Molecule

GABA is a very simple signaling molecule: a small amino acid with a molecular weight of about 100 Da that is not incorporated into any protein. However, a complex structure is not required for a ligand to produce a change in the stereochemical (quaternary, or 3-D) structure of its receptor. What counts is an exact fit of a conformationally specific part of the GABA molecule into the binding site of the receptor. In the case of the ionotropic GABA$_A$ receptors (GABA$_A$Rs), which are receptor-channels, the change in the 3-D structure is obviously an essential step in the "gating" (i.e., opening and closing) of the GABA$_A$ receptor-channel. As will be evident below, a cooperative action of two GABA molecules is needed for receptor-channel activation. GABA has other physiologically important effects mediated by binding sites in various kinds of molecules (e.g., metabotropic GABA$_B$ receptors [GABA$_B$Rs]) and membrane-located GABA transporters, and in all these distinct cases, the binding site recognizes some specific property in the 3-D structure of the GABA molecule. By constructing molecules that mimic a specific stereochemical property of GABA, it has been possible to produce artificial receptor agonists and other molecules that mimic (or block) a given action of GABA. Here, it is also noteworthy that GABA is conformationally very flexible and its ability to adopt different shapes is a major factor that governs its interactions with distinct binding sites.

The general principles of GABA-mediated signaling discussed above are, of course, true for all neurotransmitters, hormones, and intracellular messengers. A point to emphasize is that (without additional knowledge) it is not possible to deduce the action of a signaling molecule on the basis of its structure. In fact, the action of a signaling molecule can change radically during both evolution and ontogeny—and the latter aspect is one of the main themes of the present chapter. Specifically, we focus here on the actions mediated by the GABA$_A$Rs during development.

Basic Concepts and Terminology

GABA and glycine are widely known as the main inhibitory transmitters in the mammalian CNS. However, the terms "inhibition" and "excitation" should be used with caution. *Postsynaptic inhibition* is a transient decrease in the probability of firing of action potentials by the target cell, while postsynaptic *excitation* has the opposite effect. It is worth emphasizing that *hyperpolarization* and *depolarization* are *not* synonyms with inhibition and excitation. Unfortunately, the literature is fraught with confusions with regard to the usage of the these terminologies. This is reflected in the widely held belief that GABA transmission shifts from excitatory to inhibitory at a fixed time point during development, when the postsynaptic GABA$_A$ response changes from depolarizing to hyperpolarizing. As will be explained below, a depolarizing GABA response can be functionally inhibitory.

GABA$_A$Rs are receptor-channels that are selectively permeable to Cl$^-$ and to a lesser extent to HCO$_3^-$ (bicarbonate). Whether GABA$_A$R-mediated currents are hyperpolarizing or depolarizing depends on the reversal potential (E_{GABA}), which is set by the distribution of Cl$^-$ and HCO$_3^-$ across the plasma membrane of the target neuron (Kaila, 1994). E_{GABA} defines the value of the membrane potential (V_m) where the opening of GABA$_A$R channels does not lead to any net current. In a neuron that actively accumulates Cl$^-$ to produce a high intracellular concentration (a typical property of immature neurons), the HCO$_3^-$ component of the total current is small and can be ignored. In such a cell, GABA$_A$R activation leads to a passive efflux of Cl$^-$ driven by the Cl$^-$ ions' electrochemical gradient, resulting in depolarization. If the cell is experimentally depolarized in a step-wise manner from its physiological resting V_m level (e.g., –70 mV) by current injection, the additional depolarization will lead to a diminishing depolarizing GABA response, and at a sufficiently positive value of V_m (e.g., –30 mV), the GABA responses change their polarity. The point of this reversal defines E_{GABA}. In an analogous manner, it is easy to see that a neuron with an E_{GABA} that is more negative than the resting V_m must be equipped with a transport mechanism that extrudes Cl$^-$ and creates an electrochemical gradient that drives a hyperpolarizing influx of Cl$^-$ when GABA$_A$Rs are activated.

In a Cl$^-$-extruding neuron, bicarbonate (HCO$_3^-$) makes a significant contribution to the GABAergic current (section on "Ionic Selectivity") and, therefore, E_{GABA} is always more positive than the equilibrium potential of Cl$^-$ (E_{Cl}). The relative contribution of HCO$_3^-$ to E_{GABA} and to the electrochemical force that drives GABA$_A$R-mediated currents is strictly dependent on the intraneuronal Cl$^-$ concentration and on the resting V_m (for a quantitative treatment, see Farrant & Kaila, 2007; Kaila, 1994; Kaila et al., 1993). This driving force of the GABAergic current is the voltage difference between E_{GABA} and V_m (defined in this paper as $E_{GABA} - V_m$), and a key topic addressed in the present chapter is the change in the driving force from a positive, depolarizing value characteristic of immature neurons to more negative (and sometimes even hyperpolarizing) levels during neuronal maturation. The early developmental shift in E_{GABA} (section on "GABAergic Depolarization and Excitation in Immature Neurons") can be largely explained by focusing on neuronal Cl^- regulation and $GABA_A$R-mediated Cl^- currents.

For those who are not closely involved in cellular electrophysiology, it may seem surprising that a property of neurons as fundamental as the resting V_m is extremely difficult to measure reliably and there is an ongoing debate on whether direct techniques are valid at all (Kyrozis & Reichling, 1995; Tyzio et al., 2003, 2006; Verheugen, Fricker, & Miles, 1999), especially in immature neurons that have an enormously high input resistance (e.g., Serafini, Valeyev, Barker, & Poulter, 1995; Tyzio et al., 1999). In the present context, it is important to note that the values of the driving force are, by definition, based on the more-or-less controversial values of resting V_m.

GABA released in a vesicular manner from the presynaptic terminals of GABAergic neurons evokes postsynaptic potentials (PSPs) or currents (PSCs) in the target neuron. These responses are not always called inhibitory PSPs or PSCs (IPSP or IPSCs), because GABA can act in an excitatory manner. Thus, the term GABA-PSP/C is used if there is any reason to believe that the PSP/C under consideration might be functionally excitatory. The term excitatory postsynaptic potential (EPSP) is traditionally related to glutamatergic transmission.

$GABA_A$Rs are located throughout the neuronal plasma membrane, and they can be roughly divided into postsynaptic and "extrasynaptic" receptors. As will be described below, the latter do not directly respond to the release of GABA from the presynaptic terminal, but they have a very high agonist affinity and thereby they "sense" the low level of interstitial GABA that is ultimately set by the cellular GABA uptake mechanisms, mainly by the GABA transporter GAT-1 (Chiu et al., 2005; Richerson & Wu, 2003). Hence, in addition to the above postsynaptic or "phasic" action of GABA, a persistent or "tonic" activation of postsynaptic $GABA_A$Rs has been observed in various kinds of neurons (Farrant & Nusser, 2005; Kullmann et al., 2005; Mody, 2001; Semyanov, Walter, Kullmann, & Silver, 2004). Notably, tonic signaling is the only mode of $GABA_A$R-mediated transmission at the early stages of neuronal development, prior to synapse formation (section on "$GABA_A$ Signaling in Immature Neurons Devoid of Synapses").

From a systems-level point of view, the traditional view of GABA as the "main inhibitory transmitter in the mature brain" can easily lead to a bias in the thinking and intuitions of neurobiologists. GABAergic transmission does not simply lead to a suppression of ongoing neuronal activity. Extensive work on cortical structures has shown that GABAergic neurons are crucially involved in the assembly of neurons into functional networks and in shaping transient population events and network oscillations (Buzsaki, 2002, 2006; Buzsaki & Draguhn, 2004; Freund, 2003; Jonas et al., 2004; McBain & Fisahn, 2001; Vida, Bartos, & Jonas, 2006; Whittington & Traub, 2003). Many aspects of these network-level phenomena are attributable to $GABA_A$R-mediated changes in the integrative properties of principal neurons that depend critically on their time constant (e.g., Pouille & Scanziani 2001) as well as on synapse location and on the precise timing of presynaptic activity (Klausberger et al., 2003; Tukker, Fuentealba, Hartwich, Somogyi, & Klausberger, 2007). This complexity is not easily conceptualized on the basis of the term "inhibition." In a nutshell, GABAergic signaling in the living brain and in slice preparations is heavily context-dependent.

The Problem of Cross-Species Calibration of Developmental Stage and Time

Much of the literature reviewed here is based on experiments on rats and mice. These species are "altricial," i.e., the pups are born at a very immature stage of development. Cross-species calibration of developmental time is a major challenge in developmental neurobiology where an extrapolation to the human condition is one of the major goals, both in basic and applied research. Nevertheless, there seems to be a wide consensus that the structural and functional properties of the cortex of a newborn rat correspond to those of the human fetus around the end of the second trimester of pregnancy (Avishai-Eliner, Brunson, Sandman, & Baram, 2002; Clancy, Darlington, & Finlay, 2001). This means that laboratory rodents (see also Danglot, Triller, & Marty, 2006) provide excellent research models for studying processes that are relevant for both pre- and postnatal cortical development in humans.

The time point of birth versus brain developmental stage must be carefully considered in extrapolations from rodent to human data. Talking about "postnatal" or "a newborn" in rodent–human comparisons can lead (and has led) to serious flaws in the literature. In brief, identifying a novel neurobiological mechanism in newborn rats does not imply that a similar mechanism has any significance for newborn full-term human infants. A more rational view is that such findings might be more relevant to human preterm babies. In light of an extremely wide spectrum of functional, structural, and pathophysiological data, the cortex (neocortex and hippocampus) of the rat and mouse around postnatal day 12 (P12) seems to undergo something that is close to a metamorphosis as seen from the molecular, cellular, and network level to behavior (e.g., Capsoni, Tongiorgi, Cattaneo, & Domenici, 1999; Colonnese, Phillips, Constantine-Paton, Kaila, & Jasanoff, 2008; Erecinska, Cherian, & Silver, 2004; Geal-Dor, Freeman, Li, & Sohmer, 1993; Welker, 1964). This is, as could be expected, accompanied by major qualitative changes in the modes of action of GABAergic transmission (section on "Developmental Electrophysiology of GABAergic Transmission") and in the intracellular signaling mechanisms that target the ion transporters and channels involved therein (section on "Role of Ion Transporters in the Maturation of GABA$_A$ Signaling").

Aims of This Chapter

The upper jaw must fit into the lower one during the development of an individual. This basic principle of biological design is also evident in the concerted development of the various functional and structural properties of neurons and neuronal networks. At the level of cellular electrophysiology, immature neurons have a very high input resistance (small currents lead to large voltage changes), and the immature PSPs/PSCs and action potentials are slower than in the adult. In contrast to the strikingly fast changes seen at the structural level, it is as if the whole immature nervous system functions—in electrophysiological terms—at a much lower speed than the mature one. Also, ongoing oscillations are absent and instead the primitive emerging neuronal networks generate intermittent bursts of activity (section on "Intermittent Network Events in the Immature Central Nervous System") which may, among other things, serve as a mechanism whereby individual neurons produce a spatiotemporal signature that is exploited during network formation. "Hebbian" mechanisms supporting long-term plasticity have been implicated in activity-dependent

wiring, and in these phenomena, GABAergic transmission plays an important role (Hensch, 2005; Kanold & Shatz, 2006; Katz & Crowley, 2002; Zhou & Poo, 2004). Notably, cross-talk between GABAergic transmission and activity-dependent release of trophic factors (e.g., Lessmann, Gottmann, & Malcangio, 2003) appears to exist in evolving neuronal circuits, and the early network events to be described at the end of this paper are most likely of fundamental importance in this context (Mohajerani, & Cherubini, 2006; Mohajerani et al., 2007; Rivera, Voipio, & Kaila, 2005). In summary, the molecular, cellular, and network mechanisms underlying brain development are both paralleled by and controlled by changes in the basic properties of GABAergic transmission.

GABA$_A$ Receptors

Membrane receptors activated by GABA are classified into GABA$_A$ and GABA$_B$ receptors. The former are macromolecular structures, where the GABA binding site (the receptor in the strict sense) and the effector (the channel) are incorporated into a single molecule. Hence, GABA$_A$Rs are "receptor-channels" or "ionotropic receptors." In many respects, they are very closely related to ionotropic glycine receptors, and much of what is said below about the biophysical, ion-regulatory, and developmental mechanisms in connection with GABA$_A$R function applies also to ionotropic glycine receptors. In contrast, GABA$_B$Rs are metabotropic receptors (Marshall, Jones, Kaupmann & Bettler, 1999; Misgeld, Bijak, & Jarolimek, 1995) where the interaction of GABA with its binding site triggers the activation of an intracellular messenger cascade that leads to an increase in the K$^+$ conductance of the target cell or inhibits activation of voltage-gated Ca^{2+} channel in presynaptic terminals, whereby GABA release is controlled by negative feedback. In terms of evolution, GABA$_A$Rs and GABA$_B$Rs have little in common. The latter are not dealt with presently, and the term "GABAergic" will imply GABA$_A$R-mediated actions.

Structure of GABA$_A$ Receptors

GABA$_A$ receptors belong to the large family of ligand-gated ion channels, which also includes the nicotinic acetylcholine receptors, glycine receptors, and 5-HT$_3$ receptors. The structure of these receptors is based on the assembly of five subunits, which together form the pentameric receptor-channel. So far, 19 GABA$_A$R subunits have been identified in mammals. They are grouped into eight gene families according to structural similarity: $\alpha 1–6$, $\beta 1–3$, $\gamma 1–3$, δ, ϵ, θ, π, and $\rho 1–3$ (Barnard et al., 1998; Korpi, Grunder, & Luddens, 2002; Rudolph & Mohler, 2004; Sieghart & Ernst, 2005). This diversity is further enhanced at the mRNA level by alternative splicing of pre-mRNAs (Barnard et al., 1998; Simon, Wakimoto, Fujita, Lalande, & Barnard, 2004). It is obvious that the number of theoretically possible combinations at the protein level is astronomically high but, not unexpectedly, there seem to be "rules" whereby only a limited subset of subunit combinations exists in the brain as a whole (Kittler, McAinsh, & Moss, 2002; Luscher & Keller, 2004) from which the expression patterns typical to the various types of neurons are derived (Fritschy & Mohler, 1995; Pirker et al., 2000; Wisden, Laurie, Monyer, & Seeburg, 1992).

Each of the five subunits of ligand-gated channels has four transmembrane domains (M1–4), forming a central ion channel, which is gated by the binding of the transmitter molecule (Lester, Dibas, Dahan, Leite, & Dougherty, 2004; Sine & Engel, 2006; Unwin, 2005). Two GABA molecules bind in a cooperative manner at the extracellular interfaces between α and β subunits to open the GABA$_A$R channel. The subunit composition of a given receptor has a major influence on the kinetics of its gating (for a recent review, see Farrant & Kaila, 2007). In general, the rate of channel activation (opening) and deactivation (closure that is associated with the unbinding of GABA) increases during neuronal maturation. A constant exposure to GABA leads to desensitization, i.e., closure of the channel during a prolonged exposure to its agonist. Typically, GABA$_A$Rs expressed in immature neurons show less desensitization than at later ages, and a particularly slow desensitization (or virtual absence thereof) seems to be characteristic for those GABA$_A$Rs that mediate tonic or extrasynaptic actions. The affinity of a GABA$_A$R to GABA is also dictated by its subunit composition and, obviously, those receptors that mediate the tonic actions of GABA show a particularly high ligand affinity. GABA$_A$R subunit composition is also a major determinant of the profile of actions of numerous exogenous and endogenous molecules, such as ethanol, benzodiazepines, and (neuro)hormones (Maguire & Mody, 2007; Mody, 2008; Rudolph & Mohler, 2004; Sieghart & Ernst, 2005; Stell et al., 2003). Recently, the actions of oxytocin on GABAergic functions in the immature brain have received much attention (Tyzio et al., 2006; section

on "Role of NKCC1 in the Developmental Shift in E_{GABA} in Cortical Neurons").

Subunit Composition and Molecular Diversity of GABA$_A$Rs during Development

In mature neurons, the most abundant GABA$_A$R subtype is formed from α_1, β_2, and γ_2 subunits with a stoichiometry of two α, two β, and one γ subunits (Benke et al., 2004; McKernan & Whiting, 1996; Tretter, Ehya, Fuchs, & Sieghart, 1997). In some neurons, receptors exist where the γ subunit is replaced by a δ subunit (e.g. $\alpha_4\beta_3\delta$ or $\alpha_6\beta_3\delta$) and, as will be described below, these GABA$_A$Rs show an exclusive extrasynaptic localization. The $\rho_{1–3}$ subunits form functional homo- or hetero-oligomeric receptors. This suggests that they present an evolutionarily ancient class of ionotropic GABA receptors (Cutting et al., 1992). They have sometimes been called "GABA$_C$" receptors (Bormann, 2000; Chebib & Johnston, 2000) on the basis of their insensitivity to the GABA$_A$R antagonist bicuculline. Nevertheless, in the light of evolutionary as well as functional and structural data, they should rather be considered a subclass of GABA$_A$Rs (Barnard et al., 1998; Kaila, 1994; Pan & Qian, 2005; Qian & Ripps, 1999).

During the development and maintenance of GABAergic synapses (Huang, Di Cristo, & Ango, 2007), a γ-subunit (most commonly the γ_2) is indispensable for postsynaptic clustering of GABA$_A$ receptors (Baer et al., 1999; Essrich, Lorez, Benson, Fritschy, & Luscher, 1998; Fritschy & Brunig, 2003). In contrast, the δ subunit is present exclusively in extrasynaptic and perisynaptic locations (Nusser, Sieghart, & Somogyi, 1998; Wei, Zhang, Peng, Houser, & Mody, 2003). The δ subunit coassembles with the α_4 subunit in the dentate gyrus and thalamic nuclei and with the α_6 subunit in cerebellar granule cells (Brickley, Cull-Candy, & Farrant, 1996; Bright, Aller, & Brickley, 2007; Chandra et al., 2006; Nusser et al., 1998; Wall & Usowicz, 1997). α_6 is not present in cortical structures. The high-affinity, slowly desensitizing δ subunits work in combination with α_4 or α_6 subunits to generate tonic GABAergic transmission. Other subunit combinations (Glykys et al., 2006) may also produce a tonic current (section on "Structure of GABA$_A$ Receptors").

The molecular diversity of GABA$_A$Rs, seen at distinct points in time, undergoes profound changes during brain development. During the early developmental time window when GABA$_A$R signaling operates in the absence of synapses, expression of

α_1 is low. In proliferating neuronal precursors, the GABA$_A$Rs are mainly composed of $\alpha_4\beta_1\gamma_2$ subunits (Laurie, Wisden, & Seeburg, 1992; Ma & Barker, 1995), which is followed by expression of $\alpha_3\beta_3\gamma_2$ during differentiation. As explained in the section "GABA$_A$ Signaling in Immature Neurons Devoid of Synapses", GABA$_A$R signaling works in a non-synaptic manner at this stage. At the level of synaptic transmission, the developmental changes in GABA$_A$R subunits are associated with faster kinetics of GABA-gated currents and increased desensitization (Dunning, Hoover, Soltesz, Smith, & O'Dowd, 1999; Hollrigel & Soltesz, 1997; Kapur & Macdonald, 1999). It seems that developmental expression of the α_1 subunit is a hallmark of the maturation of GABA$_A$Rs in the brain (see Fritschy, Paysan, Enna, & Mohler, 1994).

Ionic Selectivity

Ion channels show large variations in their selectivity, and none of them are perfectly selective for one ion only. The study of the anion selectivity of GABA$_A$Rs was begun half a century ago, and the first reliable data were obtained using crayfish preparations by Boistel and Fatt (1958), Kuffler and Edwards (1958), as well as Takeuchi and Takeuchi (1971) (for a review of the early work, see Kaila, 1994). Ion selectivity is not simply set by the geometrical properties of the transmembrane channel (the width of its narrowest region) but also by a competitive type of action of water and fixed charges within the channel for binding of the permeant ions. These structural and electrostatic properties define the selectivity of a channel's "ionic filter" (Bormann, Hamill, & Sakmann, 1987; Kaila, 1994; Takeuchi & Takeuchi, 1971).

Cl$^-$ and HCO$_3^-$ are the only anions that have a significant permeability in GABA$_A$Rs under physiological conditions. The first demonstration that HCO$_3^-$ is able to act as a significant carrier of current was, again, based on work using crayfish muscle fibers (that have an inhibitory GABAergic innervation as well as extrasynaptic GABA$_A$Rs) and neurons (Kaila & Voipio, 1987; Voipio, Pasternack, Rydqvist, & Kaila, 1991). The relative permeability of HCO$_3^-$ vs. Cl$^-$ is around 0.2–0.4 (Bormann et al., 1987; Kaila, 1994; Kaila & Voipio, 1987). Hence, it is clear that the standard textbook view that E_{GABA} equals E_{Cl} is not correct. HCO$_3^-$ can act as the major carrier of synaptically evoked GABAergic current under steady-state conditions in mature neurons that have a low intracellular Cl$^-$ concentration (Gulledge & Stuart, 2003; Kaila et al., 1993).

In view of the evolutionarily conserved properties of the ionic filter of GABA$_A$Rs (Kaila, 1994; Wooltorton, Whiting, & Smart, 1995; Wotring, Chang, & Weiss, 1999), there is no reason to believe that the developmental shift in E_{GABA} from depolarizing to more negative values would be attributable to the expression of channels with distinct anion permeability ratios. The contribution of HCO$_3^-$ to depolarizing GABA$_A$ currents is very small in immature neurons because of their high intracellular Cl$^-$ concentration (for a quantitative treatment, see Farrant & Kaila, 2007).

Developmental Electrophysiology of GABAergic Transmission
Postsynaptic Voltage Inhibition and Shunting Inhibition

The input from a GABAergic neuron can evoke various kinds of GABA$_A$R-mediated responses in a target neuron. The best known—and the only one described in many textbooks—is the hyperpolarizing IPSP. As schematically shown in Figure 6.1A, the voltage inhibition brought about by an IPSP acts to counteract the positive voltage deflections caused by simultaneous EPSPs, thereby decreasing the probability of action potential generation. As will be evident, an obligatory requirement for the generation of a genuinely hyperpolarizing IPSP (where E_{GABA} is more negative than the resting V_m) is active Cl$^-$ extrusion by ion transporters located in the target neuron.

The opening of GABA$_A$Rs leads also to another type of effect, known as shunting inhibition. This term refers to the fact that the enhanced Cl$^-$ conductance caused by the activation of a set of GABA$_A$R channels leads, by necessity, to a decrease in the input resistance (R_{in}) of the target neuron with a consequent attenuation of simultaneous EPSPs, and in the summation of temporally successive EPSPs (Figure 6.1B). In other words, shunting inhibition simply means short-circuiting of excitatory inputs. The effect of the fall in R_{in} can be expressed in terms of (i) a decrease in the "time constant" τ of the postsynaptic neuron, where a high τ (defined as $\tau = R_m C_m$, where R_m and C_m are respectively the specific resistance and capacitance of the cell membrane) implies effective temporal summation of successive voltage changes. In addition to this, there is (ii) a decrease in the "space constant" λ (defined as $\lambda = \sqrt{r_m/r_a}$, where r_m and r_a are the membrane and intracellular axial resistance per unit length of cable) where a high λ implies effective spatial summation of voltage changes that take place at various sites on the neuron.

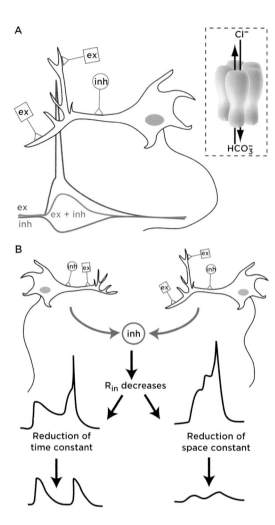

A

B

R$_{in}$ decreases

Reduction of time constant

Reduction of space constant

Figure 6.1 Basic mechanisms of GABA$_A$ receptor-mediated postsynaptic responses: voltage inhibition and shunting inhibition. (A) Voltage inhibition produces a hyperpolarizing shift in the target neuron's membrane potential (blue trace, "*inh*"), thereby attenuating the depolarizing actions (red trace, "*ex*") of simultaneous excitatory synaptic inputs (as schematically depicted by the green trace, "*ex + inh*"). An obligatory requirement for hyperpolarizing postsynaptic GABA$_A$ responses in a resting neuron is a Cl$^-$ electrochemical gradient maintained by active chloride extrusion, which leads to a channel-mediated influx of Cl$^-$ ions during the activation of GABA$_A$Rs (see inset). (B) Shunting inhibition is based on the decrease in the input resistance (R$_{in}$) of the target neuron, which is a direct consequence of the conductance increase caused by GABA$_A$R activation. This leads to a reduction in the efficacy of summation of excitatory synaptic inputs, which occur within a brief time window (reduction of time constant) and/or in spatially distinct sites of the target neuron (reduction of space constant). For further details, see text.

An important point is that postsynaptic voltage inhibition is always accompanied by shunting inhibition, but the opposite is not true. There are various types of neurons with effective

postsynaptic shunting inhibition that is not associated with hyperpolarizing IPSPs. Moreover, it should be emphasized that shunting inhibition associated with a moderate depolarization is often a more efficient type of inhibition than shunting with hyperpolarization (Farrant & Kaila, 2007; Kaila, 1994). A modest depolarization can inactivate fast voltage-gated Na$^+$ channels and activate K$^+$ channels, thereby leading to a decrease in the overall excitability of the neuron. Furthermore, for biophysical reasons discussed elsewhere (Farrant & Kaila, 2007; Kaila, 1994), the GABA-gated conductance associated with an IPSP, and hence the efficacy of shunting inhibition, is higher at slightly depolarized than hyperpolarized values of V_m. In the context of brain development, it is intriguing that the depolarizing GABA action in the neonatal rat neocortex (Yamada et al., 2004) has been shown to be functionally inhibitory (Minlebaev, Ben-Ari, & Khazipov, 2007).

Recent work has shown that Cl$^-$ regulation in neurons can be compartmentalized to the extent that GABA-PSPs have a distinct polarity in distinct subcellular compartments. A striking example here is provided by the axon initial segment (AIS) of cortical and hippocampal pyramidal neurons, where GABAergic inputs evoke depolarizing PSPs, while the somatodendritic compartment generates conventional hyperpolarizing IPSPs (Szabadics et al., 2006; Khirug et al., 2008). This difference reflects a sustained gradient of Cl$^-$ along the axo-somato-dendritic axis, where the highest Cl$^-$ levels are seen in the AIS and the lowest in the dendrites. At an anatomical level, this also means that various kinds of interneurons targeting specific subcellular sites can evoke quantitatively and also qualitatively distinct responses.

GABAergic Depolarization and Excitation in Immature Neurons

Practically all animal cells maintain a high intracellular Cl$^-$ concentration (Pedersen, O'Donnell, Anderson, & Cala, 2006; Russell, 2000). An important exception is provided by most types of adult vertebrate central neurons, which actively extrude Cl$^-$. A corollary of this basic biological fact is that GABAergic responses in immature neurons are depolarizing, because GABA$_A$R activation will lead to an efflux of the negatively charged chloride ions.

In immature brain tissue, GABAergic signaling starts in the absence of synapses in a "paracrine" or "autocrine" manner (section on "GABA$_A$ Signaling in Immature Neurons Devoid of Synapses"), and the depolarizing effects activate voltage-gated Ca^{2+} channels (Ben-Ari, 2002; Owens & Kriegstein, 2002). After the maturation of GABAergic synapses, the responses evoked by synaptically released (and in some cases by ambient) GABA are depolarizing.

Very often, an a priori criterion for a genuinely excitatory, action potential-triggering nature of GABAergic transmission is based on the level of the reversal potential of the GABA$_A$R-gated current. This means that GABA is considered to have an excitatory action if E_{GABA} > action potential threshold. This kind of reasoning has major flaws:

1. Even with a strongly depolarizing GABA response, the conductance increase linked to GABA$_A$R activation will lead to a shunting action that will manifest itself as a positive shift in the action potential threshold to more positive potentials.

2. Already in the classical electrophysiological literature dating back more than half a century (for an excellent review, see Katz, 1966), it was a well-recognized fact that the action potential threshold for an incoming signal is not constant. In particular, while a fast depolarization may readily trigger a spike, a slower change in V_m of identical magnitude may be completely inefficient. This is because the intrinsic properties of the target neuron (including the availability of fast sodium channels and activation of potassium channels) are affected by both the rate and magnitude of the change in V_m.

In neurons with intrinsic bursting characteristics, the relationship between depolarizing inputs and triggering of spikes is even more complicated than in a classical Hodgkin–Huxley-type neuron (see point 2 above). All these facts underscore the context-dependence of GABAergic signaling, and it is therefore not surprising that GABA$_A$R-mediated transmission has frequently been reported to exert "dual" (i.e., both excitatory and inhibitory) actions in neurons and neuronal circuits (Jean-Xavier, Mentis, O'Donovan, Cattaert, & Vinay, 2007; Khalilov, Dzhala, Ben-Ari, & Khazipov, 1999; Lamsa, Palva, Ruusuvuori, Kaila, & Taira, 2000). This context-dependence gains even more weight when considering GABAergic actions in a living brain, where the value of V_m in neurons is continuously fluctuating, and action potential generation is influenced by a multitude of intrinsic and extrinsic factors.

In addition to providing insights into the basic aspects of GABAergic inhibition, the two sections above make it clear that the currently widespread idea of a singular "developmental switch from depolarizing to hyperpolarizing GABA action," which, astonishingly, is often thought to reflect a "developmental switch from GABAergic excitation to inhibition during neuronal maturation," implies a fundamental misconception of how synaptic transmission works. The developmental change in E_{GABA} to more negative values is rather a *shift* than a switch, especially because a change from depolarization to hyperpolarization is not a necessary condition for the emergence of inhibitory transmission, as explained above.

GABA$_A$ Signaling in Immature Neurons Devoid of Synapses

During early development, a tonic GABA$_A$R-mediated conductance is present in cortical neurons prior to formation of functional synapses (Demarque et al., 2002; LoTurco, Owens, Heath, Davis, & Kriegstein, 1995; Owens, Liu, & Kriegstein, 1999; Serafini et al., 1995). There are various sources of GABA that might account for the tonic conductance in early development. For instance, axonal growth cones release GABA in a vesicular manner (Gao & van den Pol, 2000). Moreover, GABA released by astrocytes has been shown to activate GABA$_A$ receptors in cultured embryonic rat hippocampal neurons (Liu, Schaffner, Chang, Maric, & Barker, 2000). Another potential source for interstitial GABA is nonvesicular release via reversal of the GABA transporters (Richerson & Wu, 2003). The main neuronal GABA transporter, GAT-1, has a stoichiometry of 1 GABA:2 Na$^+$:1 Cl$^-$ (Cammack, Rakhilin, & Schwartz, 1994; Richerson & Wu, 2003). Hence, possible developmental changes in the intra- and extracellular ionic concentrations, in addition to the membrane potential, can affect the operation of the transporter. It has been suggested that paracrine GABA signaling is attributable to a lack of GABA uptake during the perinatal period in rats (Demarque et al., 2002; but see Sipilä, Voipio, & Kaila, 2007). Others have shown that GABA can be released via the reversal of transport from axonal growth cones in response to elevated extracellular K$^+$ (Taylor & Gordon-Weeks, 1991).

Although there are various possible sources for interstitial GABA during early development, it should be noted that a pronounced tonic GABA$_A$ current persists in immature cortical pyramidal neurons even under conditions where neuronal vesicular release is strongly suppressed (Demarque et al., 2002; Sipilä et al., 2007; Valeyev, Cruciani, Lange, Smallwood, & Barker, 1993). Blocking the main neuronal GABA transporter GAT-1 (in the absence of added GABA) leads to an increase in the magnitude of the tonic $GABA_A$ conductance. It also prolongs the decay of the slow GABAergic current component seen during spontaneous network events (known as giant depolarizing potentials; section on "Giant Depolarizing Potentials") in rat hippocampal neurons already at birth. These findings indicate that GABA transport is functional and operates in net uptake mode during the perinatal period (Sipilä, Huttu, Voipio, & Kaila, 2004; Sipilä et al., 2007).

In contrast to cortical pyramidal cells where a tonic $GABA_A$ conductance appears to be present throughout development, in cerebellar granule cells, a tonic $GABA_A$ conductance is seen only in neurons with functional GABAergic synapses and its magnitude increases during maturation (Brickley et al., 1996). The tonic $GABA_A$ current appears to result from an "spill-over" of synaptically released GABA in these neurons. Synaptic vesicular release has been ascribed a major role also in mature thalamic relay cells of the dorsal lateral geniculate nucleus and hippocampal neurons (Bright et al., 2007; Glykys & Mody, 2007).

$GABA_A$Rs can be in an open state, albeit with a low probability, even in the absence of agonist binding, which could account for the generation of tonic $GABA_A$ currents (see, e.g., Birnir, Everitt, Lim, & Gage, 2000; Campo-Soria, Chang, & Weiss, 2006; Chang & Weiss, 1999; Jones, Whiting, & Henderson, 2006; McCartney, Deeb, Henderson, & Hales, 2007). However, manipulation of the extracellular GABA concentration alters the magnitude of the tonic current, which is blocked by competitive $GABA_A$R antagonists (Farrant & Nusser, 2005). Hence, an increase in the open probability of extrasynaptic $GABA_A$Rs resulting in a tonic $GABA_A$ conductance is brought about by agonist binding.

In principle, any $GABA_A$R can mediate a tonic conductance. However, extracellular GABA, estimated to have a concentration of 0.2–1.5 µM in mature native tissue (Ding, Asada, & Obata, 1998; Kuntz et al., 2004; Lerma et al., 1986; Tossman & Ungerstedt, 1986), preferentially activates those receptors that have a high affinity for GABA and exhibit little or slow desensitization (Farrant & Nusser, 2005). A key role has been ascribed to the δ subunit of the $GABA_A$R in

the mediation of the tonic $GABA_A$ conductance in mature cerebellar and dentate gyrus granule cells (Brickley et al., 1996; Brickley, Revilla, Cull-Candy, Wisden, & Farrant, 2001; Hamann, Rossi, & Attwell, 2002; Nusser et al., 1998; Stell et al., 2003) as well as in thalamocortical neurons of the dorsal lateral geniculate and ventral basal thalamus (Belelli, Peden, Rosahl, Wafford, & Lambert, 2005; Cope, Hughes, & Crunelli, 2005; Jia et al., 2005). Under standard in vitro conditions, the δ subunit-containing $GABA_A$Rs are activated also in pyramidal neurons of the hippocampus (Scimemi, Semyanov, Sperk, Kullmann, & Walker, 2005), where an increase in the extracellular GABA concentration has been used in order to detect tonic activation of α_5-subunit containing receptors (Caraiscos et al., 2004; Scimemi et al., 2005; but see Prenosil et al., 2005). Hence, the presence and characteristics of a tonic $GABA_A$R-mediated conductance depend on the source and regulation of extracellular GABA and on the GABA subunit composition of the target cell. That a tonic $GABA_A$ current is present in vivo has been shown by Chadderton, Margrie, and Hausser (2004) in mature cerebellar granule cells. It is unlikely that the δ-subunit has a key role in the mediation of the tonic $GABA_A$ conductance in immature hippocampal pyramidal neurons since the neurosteroid tetrahydrodeoxycorticosterone (which enhances the current mediated by δ-subunit containing GABA receptors; see Stell et al., 2003) has little effect on the tonic current in these cells (Marchionni, Omrani, & Cherubini, 2007). The α_5 subunit has been proposed to be involved in the mediation of the tonic GABA current in the immature pyramidal cells (Marchionni et al., 2007).

Depolarizing and Excitatory Effects of GABA in Mature Neurons

A very robust, HCO_3^--dependent depolarization evoked by GABA is seen in adult hippocampal and cortical neurons under a number of conditions where massive activation of $GABA_A$Rs takes place. For instance, in the mature rat hippocampus, exogenous application of $GABA_A$ agonists (Alger & Nicoll, 1979) or high-frequency stimulation (Fujiwara-Tsukamoto, Isomura, Imanishi, Fukai, & Takada, 2007; Grover, Lambert, Schwartzkroin, & Teyler, 1993; Kaila, Lamsa, Smirnov, Taira, & Voipio, 1997) of GABAergic axons evokes a biphasic response in CA 1 pyramidal neurons. This response consists of a fast initial hyperpolarization, followed by a depolarization with a duration of up to several seconds that is strong enough to trigger spike bursts in the pyramids. Thus, during intense interneuronal activity, GABA's signaling role can change qualitatively from inhibitory to excitatory.

A detailed analysis (Kaila et al., 1997; Smirnov, Paalasmaa, Uusisaari, Voipio, & Kaila, 1999) of the ionic bases of the biphasic response has shown that (1) the early hyperpolarization evoked by high-frequency stimulation represents a summation of individual hyperpolarizing IPSPs. (2) The initial phase of the depolarization is caused by anionic redistribution, where the inwardly directed HCO_3^- current drives a depolarization that promotes the uptake of Cl^- and hence leads to a fast positive shift in E_{GABA} (see Figure 7 in Kaila et al., 1997). (3) The prolonged late depolarization that is seen afterwards is caused by an increase in extracellular K^+. This is attributable to the recovery of the neuronal $[Cl^-]_i$ levels which requires a net coefflux of Cl^- and K^+ in a 1:1 stoichiometry. Notably, during the prolonged depolarization, the V_m of the pyramidal neurons achieves a level that is much more depolarized than the simultaneous value of E_{GABA}. The biphasic response cannot be generated by rat CA1 pyramidal neurons before P10–12 because of the lack of intraneuronal carbonic anhydrase activity (section on "Development of HCO_3^--dependent Excitatory GABAergic Signaling".).

Role of Ion Transporters in the Maturation of GABA_A Signaling

In a study that has by now become a classical paper in its field, Obata and coworkers examined chick spinal motor neurons cocultured with muscle fibers, and they used the muscle end-plate potential as a reliable indicator of action potentials generated in the motor neurons (Obata, Oide, & Tanaka, 1978). What they observed was a clear excitatory action of GABA (and glycine) in cultures taken from 6–8-day-old embryos, while an inhibitory effect was seen in more mature cultures, starting at embryonic day 10. Immature neurons have a very high input impedance, and obtaining direct estimates of the resting membrane potential is difficult (section on "Basic Concepts and Terminology"). Nevertheless, the microelectrode recordings made from the motor neurons by Obata and coworkers indicated a shift in GABA_AR action from depolarizing to more negative (and hyperpolarizing) values. As already pointed out, this kind of a developmental shift in

GABA_AR action has now been described throughout the CNS. The underlying mechanisms operate at the level of functional expression of ion transporters that control the plasmalemmal Cl^- gradient and thereby set the value of E_{GABA}. These mechanisms are described below.

Most of the observations on the ontogeny of neuronal chloride regulation are based on work on mammalian cortical neurons, and it is worth noting that such data have often and erroneously been generalized to other types of neurons. It has become increasingly evident that there are major region- and cell-specific differences in the developmental and functional expression patterns of Cl^- transporters (Blaesse et al., 2006). There are also species differences. During avian brain development, nicotinic cholinergic activity plays a crucial role in the maturation of GABAergic transmission (Liu, Neff, & Berg, 2006), and in the avian auditory brain stem, GABA is rendered inhibitory during development because of an increase in low-voltage activated outward currents mediated by Kv1-type K^+ channels (Howard, Burger, & Rubel, 2007).

Ion Transporters: Basic Properties

There are two main types of molecules that provide the basis for electrophysiological activity in excitable cells: (i) ion transporters that actively generate and maintain transmembrane electrochemical ion gradients and (ii) ion channels that (when activated) permit a conductive flux (a current) of one or more ion species driven by these gradients. Active ion transport against the prevailing electrochemical gradient consumes energy, whereas ion flux across channels is a thermodynamically passive ("downhill") process.

With respect to their energy input, ion transporters can be classified into (1) primary active transporters (transport ATPases) that are fueled by ATP and (2) secondary active transporters where the energy for the transport of the driven ion is derived from the electrochemical gradient of some other ion species. The best known example of a primary active transporter is the ubiquitous Na-K ATPase, which maintains a high concentration of intracellular K^+ and a low concentration of intracellular Na^+. The secondary active transporters include cotransporters such as the cation chloride cotransporters (CCCs) that play a key role in neuronal Cl^- regulation. Uptake of Cl^- in many (but perhaps not all) neurons is driven by the Na^+ gradient that acts as the energy source for Na-K-2Cl cotransport (NKCC), while extrusion of Cl^- is based on K-Cl cotransport (KCC) driven by the K⁺ gradient. Ion transporters involved in neuronal HCO_3^-/pH regulation are also of the secondary active type (Chesler, 2003; Romero, Fulton, & Boron 2004) and they include the Na⁺-coupled bicarbonate transporters (NCBTs), the sodium-independent Cl/HCO_3 exchanger, and the Na/H exchangers. Apart from Na/H exchange, all the ion transporters above are schematically depicted in Figure 6.2. The ultimate source of energy for *all* these secondary active transporters is derived from the Na–K ATPase. The neuronal isoform of the Na–K pump shows a steep upregulation in expression during development (Erecinska, Cherian, & Silver, 2004).

Maturation of Neuronal Chloride Regulation

CHLORIDE EXTRUSION

As is the case for most of the fundamental mechanisms underlying GABAergic inhibition, the first observations on K–Cl cotransport were done in crayfish preparations (Aickin, Deisz, & Lux, 1982; Deisz & Lux, 1982) and later in mammalian cortical neurons (Misgeld, Deisz, Dodt, & Lux, 1986; Thompson, Deisz, & Prince, 1988a, 1988b; Thompson & Gähwiler, 1989).

Based on its 1:1 stoichiometry, K–Cl cotransport is at equilibrium when the equilibrium potentials of K⁺ (E_K) and Cl⁻ (E_{Cl}) are equal (Kaila, 1994; Williams & Payne, 2004). This equilibrium is rarely

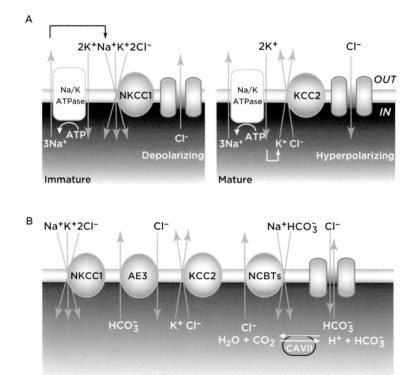

Figure 6.2 Ionic mechanisms underlying GABA$_A$ receptor mediated transmission in immature and mature cortical neurons. (A) NKCC1 mediates Cl⁻ uptake and KCC2 Cl⁻ extrusion in immature and mature cortical neurons, respectively. These secondary active transporters are fuelled by the Na⁺ and K⁺ gradients generated by the Na-K ATPase. Because the intracellular concentration of Cl⁻ is high and controlled mainly by NKCC1 in the immature neurons, the rather positive value of E_{GABA} is not affected by transporters that affect intracellular HCO_3^-. (B) In mature neurons, the Cl⁻ fluxes mediated by the HCO_3^--dependent exchangers (AE3 and the Na⁺-dependent Cl/HCO_3 exchanger, a member of the NCBTs) cannot be ignored. Note, however, that Cl⁻ is not a substrate of all NCBTs (Parker & Boron, 2008). These anion exchangers as well as Na/H exchangers (not illustrated) have a direct influence on the intraneuronal HCO_3^- concentration which, in turn, has a significant effect on E_{GABA} in mature neurons. During intense GABAergic activity, carbonic anhydrase isoform VII (CAVII; expressed around P10–P12) plays a key role in the replenishment of intraneuronal HCO_3^-, which makes it a key molecule in the generation of depolarizing and even excitatory GABAergic responses in mature neurons (cf. Figure 6.3).

achieved, but a most important point here is that in neurons, E_K is more negative than the resting V_m and this is exactly the reason why K–Cl cotransport is able to support hyperpolarizing IPSPs. In most central neurons studied so far, the molecule that acts as the main chloride extruder is the neuron-specific KCC isoform KCC2 (Balakrishnan et al., 2003; DeFazio, Keros, Quick, & Hablitz, 2000; Hubner et al., 2001; Payne, Stevenson, & Donaldson, 1996; Rivera et al., 1999; Williams et al., 1999), but recent data indicate that KCC3 may also have a significant role in certain neurons (Boettger et al., 2003). Some immature neurons express KCC4, at least at the mRNA level (Li, Tornberg, Kaila, Airaksinen, & Rivera, 2002).

The gramicidin-perforated patch clamp technique, where a flux of Cl^- does not occur between the recording pipette and the intracellular compartment (Kyrozis & Reichling, 1995), is thought to be an ideal technique to study the presence and efficacy of Cl^- extrusion in the context of developmental E_{GABA} shift and other phenomena that are accompanied by changes in Cl^- regulation (e.g., neuronal trauma; Payne, Rivera, Voipio, & Kaila, 2003; Rivera et al., 2005). Measuring E_{GABA} in a resting neuron can, however, at best verify the presence of Cl^- extrusion, because without extrusion of Cl^-, E_{GABA} can never attain a steady-state level that is more negative than the resting V_m. If the influx via most or all pathways that mediate Cl^- influx into a neuron (the cellular chloride load) is very small, a very inefficient Cl^- extrusion mechanism would be able to maintain a rather negative or even hyperpolarizing E_{GABA}. Thus, it is much more important to measure the efficacy of Cl^- extrusion (Jarolimek, Lewen, & Misgeld, 1999; Khirug et al., 2005). In order to characterize the physiological importance of a Cl^- extrusion mechanism, experiments should be based on a procedure where a defined Cl^- load is imposed on a cell, and the cell's capability to maintain the level of Cl^-_i provides a valid estimate of the efficacy of extrusion (Khirug et al., 2005). At steady state, the Cl^- influx mediated by the loading procedure gives an estimate of the amount of net Cl^- extrusion. This approach has been used in the study of cellular pH regulation for several decades (Roos & Boron, 1981).

CHLORIDE UPTAKE

Neuronal Cl^- uptake mediated by the Na-K-2Cl cotransporter isoform 1 (NKCC1) is generally thought to underlie the well-known depolarizing action of GABAergic transmission in dorsal root ganglion neurons (Alvarez-Leefmans & Russell,

1990). Recent data also point to NKCC1 as the main Cl^- uptake mechanism in developing hippocampal and neocortical neurons (Achilles et al., 2007; Sipilä, Schuchmann, Voipio, Yamada, & Kaila, 2006b; Yamada et al., 2004). In contrast, the identity of the transporters that account for depolarizing GABA actions in the immature auditory brain stem and retina are not known (Balakrishnan et al., 2003; Vardi, Zhang, Payne, & Sterling, 2000).

Cation-Chloride Transporters in Neuronal Development

STRUCTURE AND MOLECULAR DIVERSITY OF CATION-CHLORIDE COTRANSPORTERS

The CCC family is also known as solute carrier family 12 (*Slc12*) and belongs, according to the transporter classification database, to the amino acid–polyamine–organocation superfamily (Saier, Tran, & Barabote, 2006). Out of the nine CCC family members (*Slc12A1–9*) described so far, seven CCCs have been identified as transporters and the function of two of them remains unknown (Blaesse, Airaksinen, Rivera, & Kaila, 2009; Mercado, Mount, & Gamba, 2004; Payne, Rivera, Voipio, & Kaila, 2003). Three types of CCCs have been described: (i) two members are Na–K–2Cl cotransporters (NKCC1 and NKCC2), (ii) one is a Na–Cl cotransporter (NCC), and (iii) four are K–Cl cotransporters (KCC1–4). The predicted secondary structures for all CCCs contain 12 transmembrane domains flanked by a relatively small intracellular N terminus and a large intracellular C terminus that constitutes about half the protein. Except for NKCC2 and NCC, which are kidney-specific, all other CCCs seem to be expressed in the CNS. The molecular diversity of the CCCs is further increased by alternative splicing. Splice variants are known for NKCC1, NKCC2, KCC1, KCC2, and KCC3 (Adragna, Fulvio, & Lauf, 2004; Gamba, 2005; Mercado et al., 2004; Uvarov et al., 2007).

REGULATION OF TRANSPORT PROTEIN EXPRESSION AND FUNCTIONALITY: AN OVERVIEW

The regulation of the functionality of proteins has to match the physiological "needs" of a neuron and, in addition, there must be a fine balance (or a compromise) between cost effects, resources, and safety factors (see Diamond, 1993). The anion-regulatory transmembrane proteins are rather large (and hence costly), with more than 1000 amino acid residues. On the other hand, a reserve pool of a protein is needed for a cell to react in an adaptive manner within a short timescale. This means that for long-term changes, such as developmental processes, changes in gene expression leading to net changes in protein synthesis are necessary. In contrast, for short-term changes, a cell has to rely on a reserve pool of proteins that can be activated or inactivated within minutes. A classical example here is the trafficking of the Na–K ATPase to the membrane of muscle cells during increased motor activity (Clausen, 1986). Similar situations must be numerous in neurons, but this perspective has not attracted much attention among neurobiologists studying chloride transport functions (but see Senatorov, Stys, & Hu, 2000).

During the development of cortical neurons, there is a close correlation between the mRNA expression levels of NKCC1 and KCC2 and the "functional expression" of these two transporters (i.e., the number of active transporters; Farrant & Kaila, 2007; Payne, Rivera, Voipio, & Kaila, 2003). However, such a clear link from gene expression to protein function is by no means a default situation. NKCC1 expression is not detectable in immature brain stem neurons that, nevertheless, have depolarizing $GABA_A$ responses based on a relatively positive E_{Cl} and, at the same time, KCC2 is already expressed at a high level (Balakrishnan et al., 2003; Blaesse et al., 2006). These findings show that the immature neurons in the brain stem express an as yet unidentified transporter that accumulates Cl^-. In addition, they have two general implications: (i) the available data and conclusions that point to a key role of NKCC1 in Cl^- uptake in immature neocortical and hippocampal neurons cannot be directly extrapolated to other brain regions; (ii) the mere presence of KCC2 protein in a neuron does not necessarily imply the presence of functionally active KCC2. KCC2 protein that is functionally inactive has also been observed in primary cortical cultures during the first few days in vitro (Khirug et al., 2005).

A high level of KCC2 has been detected in the spines of cortical neurons (Gulyas, Sik, Payne, Kaila, & Freund, 2001). This was a surprising observation, because in cortical neurons, the vast majority of glutamatergic synapses are formed on dendritic spines (Hering & Sheng, 2001), while GABAergic synapses are mainly located on the somata and on dendritic shafts devoid of spines (Freund & Buzsaki, 1996). A recent study sheds light on this paradox by showing that, independent of its Cl^- transport function, KCC2 has a structural role in spine formation (Li et al., 2007).

This observation suggests that KCC2 expression in spines acts as a synchronizing factor in the development of inhibitory and excitatory transmission. Moreover, KCC2 appears to have a role in the genesis of GABAergic synapses (Chudotvorova et al., 2005). Thus, these findings demonstrate that the CCCs are not only working as Cl^- pumps, but also show that plasmalemmal proteins are often multifunctional (Denker & Barber, 2002). The multifunctionality of proteins in general and of ion transporters in particular (Bennett & Baines, 2001; Hilgenberg, Su, Gu, O'Dowd, & Smith, 2006; Li et al., 2007; Liang et al., 2007) is, in fact, not unexpected in view of the rather small number of genes (around 20,000) in the mammals.

It is obvious that mechanisms operating at the transcriptional level are not sufficiently fast to account for short-term changes that have been observed in neuronal Cl^- regulation (Fiumelli, Cancedda, & Poo, 2005). Posttranslational modifications, such as phosphorylation, comprise an important set of mechanisms to regulate CCC activity in a fast manner. It has been known for many years that phosphorylation and dephosphorylation play a pivotal role in the regulation of CCC transport activity (Gamba, 2005; Russell, 2000). The effects of pharmacological manipulations of phosphorylation mechanisms on NKCC1 and KCC2 are qualitatively dissimilar because, in general, NKCCs are activated by phosphorylation and KCCs by dephosphorylation (Payne et al., 2003). In addition, a functional interaction of several kinases (e.g., WNK3, WNK4, SPAK, and creatine kinase) with NKCC1 or KCC2 (or both of them) has been demonstrated (Delpire & Gagnon, 2006; Inoue, Ueno, & Fukuda, 2004; Kahle et al., 2006). Evidence for a change of the phosphorylation state of the transporter proteins during development or after manipulations of phosphorylation is rather weak or controversial (Stein, Hermans-Borgmeyer, Jentsch, & Hubner, 2004; Vale, Caminos, Martinez-Galan, & Juiz; 2005; Wake et al., 2007). Recently, however, it has been shown that a direct phosphorylation of KCC2 by protein kinase C (PKC) is involved in KCC2 trafficking (Lee et al., 2007).

The quaternary structure is a crucial determinant of the functions of all proteins, but there is little data on the quaternary structure of functional, plasmalemmal CCCs. Hetero- and homooligomers of the different CCCs have been described for nearly all CCCs (Blaesse et al., 2006; Casula et al., 2001; de Jong et al., 2003; Moore-Hoon and

Turner, 2000; Simard et al., 2007; Starremans, Kersten, van den Heuvel, Knoers, & Bindels, 2003). A dominant-negative effect of a transport-inactive KCC1 mutant and a very strict correlation of the age-dependent oligomerization and the age-dependent activation of KCC2 suggest that oligomerization is essential for KCC activation (Blaesse et al., 2006; Casula et al., 2001). Nevertheless, an important point to make here is that the available data are not conclusive regarding the mechanism whereby oligomerization affects CCC transport functions.

Unsurprisingly, when considering neuronal anion homeostasis as a whole, the regulation of NKCC1 and KCC2 and the regulation of $GABA_A$Rs share some basic mechanisms. As mentioned above, PKC regulates KCC2 trafficking (Lee et al., 2007), and this kinase is also involved in the regulation of $GABA_A$R trafficking (Kittler & Moss, 2003; Michels & Moss, 2007). This kind of synergy becomes even more evident when intrinsic factors that regulate CCCs and $GABA_A$Rs are considered. One of these intrinsic factors is the brain-derived neurotrophic factor (BDNF), which increases KCC2 expression in immature neurons (section on "Changes in KCC2 Expression: Overlapping Mechanisms in Neuronal Differentiation and Damage"; Aguado et al., 2003; Rivera et al., 2004). The transcription factor "early growth response 4" (Egr4), which seems to be under the control of BDNF (O'Donovan, Tourtellotte, Millbrandt, & Baraban, 1999), induces KCC2 expression (Uvarov, Ludwig, Markkanen, Rivera, & Airaksinen, 2006). In more mature neurons, BDNF has the opposite effect and downregulates KCC2 expression (Rivera et al., 2002, 2004; see also Wardle & Poo, 2003). Such an age-dependent BDNF function has also been described for $GABA_A$Rs (Mizoguchi, Ishibashi, & Nabekura, 2003). In immature hippocampal neurons, BDNF potentiates $GABA_A$R-mediated currents, whereas it suppresses them later on.

THE DEVELOPMENTAL SHIFT FROM DEPOLARIZING TO MORE NEGATIVE (AND HYPERPOLARIZING) $GABA_A$ SIGNALING

The subheading of this section looks clumsy, but there is a good reason for this: there is no universal developmental shift from depolarizing to hyperpolarizing. As explained above, virtually all central neurons undergo a developmental change where E_{GABA} is initially at a very positive level, and GABAergic transmission produces depolarizing and often also excitatory responses. To reiterate, the negative shift does not have to achieve a hyperpolarizing value (i.e., a change in polarity, often called the "developmental switch") to render $GABA_A$ signaling inhibitory. Even a depolarizing GABAergic input can be strongly inhibitory.

The negative shift in E_{GABA} appears to be a ubiquitous feature of central neurons, with some notable exceptions described above. In hippocampal and neocortical neurons, the shift is attributable to the developmental upregulation of KCC2 that is thought to be paralleled by a downregulation of NKCC1 (Blaesse, Airaksinen, Rivera, & Kaila, 2009; Lu, Karadsheh, & Delpire, 1999; Plotkin et al., 1997; Rivera et al., 1999, 2005; Yamada et al., 2004).

The first observations related to the molecular mechanisms of the E_{GABA} shift were made by Rivera et al. (1999), who showed that upregulation of KCC2 renders GABA hyperpolarizing in rat CA1 hippocampal neurons. The key to this finding were experiments that showed an increase in KCC2 expression during the first two postnatal weeks, a time window which was known to be associated with a negative shift in E_{GABA}. Because there are no selective drugs to block CCCs in an isoform-specific manner (see Payne, 1997; Payne, Rivera, Voipio, & Kaila, 2003; Russell, 2000), gene knock-down experiments had to be performed to confirm the role of KCC2 in the generation of hyperpolarizing $GABA_A$ responses. We know now that effects at the level of gene expression are not the only mechanisms that influence the functional expression of KCC2 (see section "Regulation of transport protein expression and functionality: an overview"). Indeed, a comparison of the levels of KCC2 expression and functionality in cultured neurons and neurons in slice preparations showed that the delay from the increase in gene and protein expression to functional activation is very brief in native cortical neurons, but a much longer delay is seen in cultured neurons (Khirug et al., 2005). Hence, activation patterns in hippocampal primary cultures appear to mimic the delayed activation of KCC2 that is seen in the brain stem. Recently, it has been observed that the developmental expression of KCC2 shows gender-specific differences in various brain areas (Galanopoulou, 2005; Perrot-Sinal, Sinal, Reader, Speert, & McCarthy, 2007), which may contribute to gender differences in susceptibility to epilepsy.

Some central neurons do not express KCC2. These include the dopaminergic neurons in the substantia nigra (Gulacsi et al., 2003) as well as a population of neurons in the nucleus reticularis thalami (Bartho, Payne, Freund, & Acsady, 2004). Perhaps the weak GABAergic inhibition the KCC2-devoid neurons experience (e.g., Gulacsi et al., 2003) is important for tonic spiking and the consequent secretion of dopamine. One might speculate that a lack of KCC2 (and/or other Cl⁻ extruders, e.g., KCC3) is a general feature of neurons that secrete neuromodulatory amines.

CHANGES IN KCC2 EXPRESSION: OVERLAPPING MECHANISMS IN NEURONAL DIFFERENTIATION AND DAMAGE

With notable exceptions discussed above, the level of expression of KCC2 has turned out to be a useful indicator of the state of neuronal differentiation. The increase in KCC2 mRNA expression levels not only faithfully follows well-established patterns of neuronal maturation (see Rivera et al., 1999, 2005), but there is also a prompt downregulation of KCC2 expression during neuronal damage such as seen in epilepsy and axotomy (Nabekura et al., 2002; Payne et al., 2003; Rivera et al., 2002, 2004; Toyoda et al., 2003). Damage to adult neurons often leads to the expression of genes that are expressed at an embryonic or fetal stage, and this kind of dedifferentiation, is accompanied by downregulation of genes that are characteristically active in mature neurons. These events, a "recapitulation of ontogeny" may reflect a strategy to enable rewiring and repairing of damaged neuronal circuitry (Cohen, Navarro, Le Duigou, & Miles, 2003; Payne et al., 2003).

Based on studies on the consequences of epileptic activity in vivo and in vitro, the molecular mechanisms underlying the down- and upregulation of KCC2 have been at least partly identified. Epileptic activity leads to an increase in the expression of BDNF and its plasmalemmal receptor TrkB (Binder, Croll, Gall, & Scharfman, 2001; Huang & Reichardt, 2001, 2003). Following in vivo kindling, the expression of KCC2 showed a rapid, pronounced fall in those regions of the epileptic hippocampus where BNDF–TrkB upregulation is known to be most salient (Rivera et al., 2002), and parallel in vitro experiments established a direct causal link from TrkB activation to KCC2 downregulation (Rivera et al., 2002, 2004). In experiments on tissue from transgenic mice with point mutations in their TrkB receptors (cf. Minichiello et al., 1998), the downregulation of KCC2 requires the activation of the two major TrkB-mediated signaling cascades, the PLCγ and Shc activated

pathways. Interestingly, activation of the Shc cascade in isolation leads to an increase in KCC2 expression (Rivera et al., 2004), which suggests a role for this pathway in the developmental upregulation of KCC2.

INSIGHTS BASED ON TRANSGENIC KCC2 MICE

Transgenic animals (e.g., knock-out mice) are valuable tools for analyzing the functions of a defined protein. Regarding KCC2, four transgenic mouse strains have been generated: (i) knock-out strains in which the KCC2 expression is completely absent (KCC2⁻/⁻; Hubner et al., 2001; Vilen, Eerikäinen, Tornberg, Airaksinen, & Savilahti, 2001); (ii) a knock-down strain with 5%–8% (Woo et al., 2002); (iii) a hypomorph strain with about 30% (Vilen et al., 2001); and (iv) an intercrossed knock-out/hypomorph strain with 15%–20% of the wild-type KCC2 expression level (Tornberg, Voikar, Savilahti, Rauvala, & Airaksinen, 2005). They provide an exceptional possibility to compare different strains with graded variations in KCC2 expression levels.

Disruption of the *Slc12A5* gene, which inhibits KCC2 expression completely, results in mice that die immediately after birth due to severe motor defects, including respiratory failure (Hubner et al., 2001). In the transgenic knock-down mouse strain, exon 1 of the known *Slc12A5* sequence was targeted (Woo et al., 2002). For an initially unknown reason, 5%–8% of the KCC2 expression was retained. In contrast to the KCC2⁻/⁻ mice, the knock-down mice are viable after birth but die after around two postnatal weeks due to spontaneous generalized seizures (Woo et al., 2002). Meanwhile it has turned out that the residual KCC2 expression in the knock-down animals represents the expression of a new KCC2 splice variant, KCC2a, which contains, compared to the previously described KCC2b, an alternative exon 1 (Uvarov et al., 2007). Both isoforms show a similar transport efficacy, at least in assays based on overexpression in human embryonic kidney cells (Uvarov et al., 2007).

Despite the similar transport function, comparison of the knock-out and the knock-down strains indicates that KCC2a and KCC2b have distinct functions in the brain. The expression of KCC2a in the knock-down strain is sufficient to promote survival for up to three postnatal weeks, but the absence of KCC2b leads to seizures during this period. It seems that KCC2a, which is expressed in the neonatal brain stem and spinal cord at a level similar to KCC2b, is important for some basic functions of these structures. It is worth noting that KCC2b is essential for hyperpolarizing glycinergic responses in auditory brain stem neurons (Balakrishnan et al., 2003). In the mature cortex, KCC2b is the dominant isoform (Blaesse et al., 2009; Uvarov et al., 2007). When looking at the published information on the expression patterns of KCC2, one should bear in mind that the in situ hybridization and immunohistochemical data reflect the expression of both KCC2a and KCC2b, because the mRNA probes as well as antibodies used in these studies detect both isoforms.

The hypomorph mice with about 30% of the wild-type KCC2 expression level are viable (Vilen et al., 2001). The intercrossing of the KCC2$^{-/-}$ and the hypomorph mice resulted in a reduction of the KCC2 expression to 15%–20% of the wild-type level (Tornberg et al., 2005). These compound heterozygous mice display normal locomotor activity and motor coordination. A significant increase compared to the wild-type was found when anxiety, seizure susceptibility, and spatial learning and memory were analyzed. In contrast, the sensitivity to thermal and mechanical stimuli was reduced.

ROLE OF NKCCI IN THE DEVELOPMENTAL SHIFT IN E$_{GABA}$ IN CORTICAL NEURONS

In cortical neurons, active Cl$^-$ uptake is mediated by NKCC1, and this transporter accounts for the depolarizing actions of GABA in immature neurons (Achilles et al., 2007; Sipilä et al., 2006b). Pharmacological blockade of NKCC1 by a specific NKCC inhibitor, bumetanide, resulted in a ~10 mV shift in E$_{GABA}$ in hippocampal pyramidal neurons, resulting in a loss of the depolarizing GABA$_A$ current driving force (Sipilä et al., 2006b). A similar observation (Sipilä et al., 2009) was made in mice with a disruption of the *Slc12A2* gene coding for NKCC1 (Flagella et al., 1999). Hence, the developmental shift in E$_{GABA}$ is a result of the concerted downregulation of NKCC1 and upregulation of KCC2.

Both functional and structural data indicate that NKCC1 and KCCs are coexpressed in certain types of mature neurons (Duebel et al., 2006; Martina, Royer, & Pare, 2001; Marty & Llano, 2005; Vardi, Zhang, Payne, & Sterling, 2000; Khirug et al., 2008). As noted above (Farrant & Kaila, 2007), this seemingly paradoxical push–pull design permits precise of the set-point of the intracellular ion concentration under various physiological conditions (Roos & Boron, 1981).

Various subcellular expression patterns of NKCC1 and KCC2–3 may produce intraneuronal Cl$^-$ gradients (even under "resting" conditions) that shape GABA-PSPs/PSCs in subcellular domains (Duebel et al., 2006; Szabadics et al., 2006; Khirug et al., 2008). The significance of E$_{GABA}$ compartmentalization should be a major focus of future studies on the ontogeny of E$_{GABA}$. It is evident that assigning a singular E$_{GABA}$ value to a given neuron is not correct—a more appropriate approach is to specify the E$_{GABA}$ level of a given GABAergic input in the postsynaptic neuron, because distinct GABAergic interneurons in various brain structures target anatomically distinct subcellular sites in postsynaptic neurons (Freund & Buzsaki, 1996).

In a recent study, Tyzio et al. (2006) reported that maternal oxytocin induces a transient hyperpolarizing shift in E$_{GABA}$ to strikingly negative values (up to –100 mV) in pyramidal neurons in the rat pup hippocampus. The evidence presented points to an oxytocin-induced block of NKCC1. The authors suggest that such an effect protects the newborn brain from anoxic–ischemic damage, a condition that is a major cause of neurological dysfunctions in humans (e.g., see Jacobs, Hunt, Tarnow-Mordi, Inder, & Davis, 2007). Although the observation of Tyzio and coworkers is exciting, it is unclear whether such a mechanism would be important in rats that do not appear to be prone to birth-related anoxia. In addition, an extrapolation based on data on the fetal primate (macaque) hippocampus suggested that depolarizing GABA responses and associated network events are not present in the principal neurons of full-term human babies (Khazipov et al., 2001). Oxytocin is also known to block GABA$_A$Rs (Brussaard, Kits, & de Vlieger 1996), which would be expected to suppress GABAergic depolarizations and consequent intracellular Ca^{2+} transients in the immature rat neurons (cf. Tyzio et al., 2006). Thus, the effects of oxytocin on GABA$_A$Rs add another facet to the spectrum of its actions on the perinatal rodent hippocampus.

Development of HCO$_3^-$-dependent Excitatory GABAergic Signaling

As noted above, E$_{GABA}$ is always more positive than E$_{Cl}$, and this is because all nucleated cells, including neurons, maintain their intracellular pH (pH$_i$) at a level that is higher than what is predicted on the basis of a passive distribution of H$^+$ ions. Under physiological conditions, the equilibrium potentials of H$^+$ and HCO$_3^-$ are equal and, most importantly, they have rather positive values (because of the active regulation of pH_i) of around -10 to -15 mV. This means that the current carried by HCO_3^- is depolarizing (Kaila & Voipio, 1987). The intracellular concentration of HCO_3^- in a mammalian neuron is on the order of 15–20 mM.

In light of quantitative considerations based on the Goldman–Hodgkin–Katz equation (see Figure 2 in Farrant & Kaila, 2007), it is clear that the effect of the HCO_3^- permeability on E_{GABA} is very small in neurons with a high $[Cl^-]_i$ (such as immature neurons and adult dorsal root ganglion neurons), but in neurons with a low $[Cl^-]_i$, HCO_3^- can act as the main carrier of $GABA_A$R-mediated current. This is often the case with, for example, adult cortical neurons, which have a very negative resting membrane potential that is depolarized by fast actions of GABA (Gulledge & Stuart, 2003; Kaila et al., 1993). Thus, KCC2 function (or K–Cl cotransport in general, whichever isoform is involved), is a necessary but not sufficient condition for hyperpolarizing IPSPs, as was clearly stated in the original study on the role of KCC2 in setting E_{GABA} (Rivera et al., 1999). It is also obvious from considerations based on the Hodgkin–Huxley voltage equation that in an intact neuron, E_{GABA} can never attain values as low as -90 mV (Farrant & Kaila, 2007). It is not possible to challenge basic thermodynamic quantifications using electrophysiological data, and hence published estimates of E_{GABA} as low as -100 mV or even more negative must reflect small but significant errors in measurements of V_m.

Neuronal acid extrusion that maintains the HCO_3^- reversal potential at its rather depolarized level is carried out by Na^+-coupled bicarbonate transporters (NCBTs) and the Na^+/H^+ exchangers (Chesler, 2003; Jacobs et al., 2007; Parker & Boron, 2008; Payne et al., 2003; Romero, Fulton, & Boron, 2004). The Na^+-independent anion exchanger (AE3) that extrudes base equivalents in the form of HCO_3^- in exchange for Cl^- is an "acid loader" that takes up Cl^- and thereby can also induce a positive shift of E_{Cl} (Figure 6.2) (Romero et al., 2004). In addition to these plasmalemmal transporters, pH in neuronal tissue is modulated by both extracellular and intracellular carbonic anhydrases (CAs). The isomer that is first expressed in cortical principal neurons is CAVII.

CAs are enzymes that catalyze the reversible hydration of CO_2 into HCO_3^- and hydrogen ions. So far, 12 catalytically active CA isozymes are known, and five of these show a cytosolic localization (Pastorekova, Parkkila, Pastorek, & Supuran, 2004). During a large channel-mediated net efflux of HCO_3^-, the intracellular HCO_3^- is quickly replenished by the activity of a cytosolic CA isoform (Kaila, Saarikoski, & Voipio, 1990; Pasternack, Voipio, & Kaila, 1993). In neonatal pyramidal neurons, CA activity is absent until around P10, and thereafter a steep increase in the expression of the CAVII isoform takes place (Ruusuvuori et al., 2004). The expression of CAVII modulates postsynaptic GABAergic responses in a qualitative manner: the biphasic GABA response, described earlier on, and the associated epileptiform afterdischarges are dependent on intraneuronal CA activity (see also Taira, Lamsa, & Kaila, 1997).

The CA-dependent excitatory GABAergic signaling that is seen after P10 in the rat hippocampus is largely caused by a rise in the extracellular potassium concentration ($[K^+]_o$) that is caused by the HCO_3^-/Cl^- anion shift in pyramidal neurons (Kaila et al., 1997). The GABAergic $[K^+]_o$ transients are obviously nonsynaptic signals that do not affect only those neurons that are postsynaptic with regard to the stimulated ones, but the transient increase in $[K^+]_o$ has a strong depolarizing effect on all nearby neurons, glial cells as well as on presynaptic terminals (Kaila et al., 1997; reviewed by Voipio & Kaila, 2000). This implies that intense GABAergic transmission, such as seen during high-frequency stimulation, may play a role in the induction of long-term potentiation (Collingridge, 1992). Interestingly, high-frequency stimulation does not induce LTP before P12 (Harris & Teyler, 1984; Jackson, Suppes, & Harris, 1993; Muller, Oliver, & Lynch, 1989; see also Chabot et al., 1996). After P12, intense GABAergic activity and the associated CA-dependent $[K^+]_o$ transients are also likely to be involved in the generation of epileptiform activity (cf. Avoli, Louvel, Pumain, & Kohling, 2005; Kaila et al., 1997; Stasheff, Mott, & Wilson, 1993). Hence, the expression of intraneuronal CA is likely to contribute to the high propensity for epileptogenesis that is characteristic of the immature rat hippocampus, and CAVII may prove to be an important target of antiepileptic drugs (Vullo et al., 2005).

GABAergic Mechanisms in Emerging Networks

As is amply evident from what has been described so far, the role of GABAergic signaling in brain development encompasses an extremely wide spectrum of phenomena, and these will of course manifest themselves at the systems level, that is, in the functions of neuronal networks and in an organism's behavior. In fact, GABA's role in the formation of neuronal connectivity starts already during the early stages of neurogenesis (Owens & Kriegstein, 2002). Moreover, GABAergic transmission plays a key role during "critical periods" (see Chapter 7 by del Rio and Feller in this volume), when the nervous system is particularly prone to both normal and aberrant types of input (Hensch, 2005; Kanold & Shatz, 2006; Katagiri, Fagiolini, & Hensch, 2007; Katz & Crowley, 2002).

Depolarization-Mediated Trophic Actions of GABA

In immature neurons, depolarizing GABAergic signaling promotes action potential firing, opening of voltage-gated Ca^{2+} channels, and activation of NMDA receptors (Ben-Ari, 2002; Fukuda et al., 1998; Gao & van den Pol, 2001; Yuste & Katz, 1991). These responses lead to transient elevations of intracellular Ca^{2+} levels and activation of downstream intracellular signaling cascades, which are central in mediating the trophic effects of GABA during development (Owens & Kriegstein, 2002; Represa & Ben Ari, 2005). Trophic effects of GABA have been observed in vitro at various levels of neuronal and network development including DNA synthesis, migration, morphological maturation of individual neurons, and synaptogenesis (Akerman & Cline, 2007; Behar et al., 1996; Haydar, Wang, Schwartz, & Rakic, 2000; Liu, Wang, Haydar, & Bordey, 2005; LoTurco et al., 1995; Marty, Berninger, Carroll, & Thoenen, 1996; Marty, Wehrle, & Sotelo, 2000; Owens & Kriegstein, 2002; Represa & Ben-Ari, 2005; Wolff, Joo, & Dames, 1978). BDNF has been ascribed a key role in the trophic actions of GABA (Berninger et al., 1995; Marty et al., 2000). While it is clear that neuronal activity is needed for the development, fine-tuning, and maintenance of neuronal network connectivity (Katz & Crowley, 2002; Penn & Shatz, 1999), the significance of the specific findings on depolarizing actions in normal neuronal development in vivo is, however, unclear. Somewhat surprisingly, synaptogenesis and early brain development is hardly affected in knock-out mice where GABA synthesis, vesicular transport, or vesicular release are eliminated (Ji, Kanbara, & Obata 1999; Verhage et al., 2000; Varoqueaux et al., 2002; Wojcik et al., 2006). On the other hand, Cancedda, Fiumelli, Chen, and Poo (2007) found that while neuronal migration was not affected (but see Heck et al., 2007), morphological maturation was markedly impaired in immature neurons in vivo that were devoid of depolarizing GABAergic responses. The developmental patterns of GABAergic signaling, including trophic actions on synapse formation and dendritic development are repeated during adult neurogenesis in the dentate gyrus in vivo (Esposito et al., 2005; Ge et al., 2006; Tozuka, Fukuda, Namba, Seki, & Hisatsune, 2005; van Praag et al., 2002). In light of the preponderance of cell culture experiments on the trophic mechanisms of GABA action, it is clear that more in vivo work is needed.

Intermittent Network Events in the Immature Central Nervous System

Spontaneous network events, that is, events that are generated independently of sensory input, are a salient feature of structures in the immature CNS, for example, hippocampus, neocortex, spinal cord, retina, brain stem, and thalamus (Adelsberger, Garaschuk, & Konnerth, 2005; Ben-Ari, 2001; Dupont, Hanganu, Kilb, Hirsch, & Luhmann, 2006; Feller, 1999; Fitzgerald, 1987; Garaschuk, Linn, Eilers, & Konnerth, 2000; Gummer & Mark, 1994; Ho & Waite, 1999; Kandler, 2004; Khazipov et al., 2004b; Kilb & Luhmann, 2003; Maffei & Galli-Resta, 1990; Meister, Wong, Baylor, & Shatz, 1991; Moody & Bosma 2005; O'Donovan, 1999; Pangratz-Fuehrer, Rudolph, & Huguenard, 2007; Wang et al., 2007; Yuste, Peinado, & Katz, 1992). Recently, spontaneous events similar to those observed in animal experiments were detected in the preterm human cortex (Vanhatalo & Kaila, 2006; Vanhatalo et al., 2002, 2005). We prefer not to call these events network oscillations, because in both noninvasive and invasive electroencephalograms (EEGs), they are seen as discrete events rather than ongoing oscillations that evolve later during development (Vanhatalo & Kaila, 2006).

A major issue for debate during the past decades regarding spontaneous network events in immature neural structures is to what degree these early patterns merely reflect the functional maturation of the underlying neuronal network, or whether they are intimately involved in sculpting and maintenance of network connectivity and function (e.g., Dasen, Tice, Brenner-Morton, & Jessell, 2005; Hamburger, 1963; Hinde, 1970). While there is overwhelming evidence that network activity contributes to network formation (see above), it is imperative to identify the mechanisms of early spontaneous activity in order to understand their specific consequences. Importantly, intermittent events also exist in the adult brain; for example, in rodents, sharp positive waves (SPWs) are produced in the hippocampus during consummatory activity and rest (Buzsaki, 1986).

Giant Depolarizing Potentials

Hippocampal spontaneous events in vitro were originally recorded with intracellular electrodes in slice preparations taken from neonatal rats. These events were termed "giant depolarizing potentials" (GDPs). After their initial discovery, GDPs have been investigated extensively (reviewed in Ben-Ari, 2001; Sipilä & Kaila, 2008). Examining the role of GABAergic transmission in their generation may shed light on phenomenologically similar (not necessarily homologous) activity patterns elsewhere in the brain.

CHARACTERISTICS OF GIANT DEPOLARIZING POTENTIALS

Despite their name, GDPs are genuine network phenomena. The acronym stands for the large intracellular response seen in individual neurons (Ben-Ari, Cherubini, Corradetti, & Gaiarsa, 1989), and even the current that is recorded under voltage clamp is also often called a "GDP," again referring to the network nature of these events (Ben-Ari, 2001). A major component of intracellular GDPs in current- or voltage-clamp experiments is blocked by $GABA_A$ receptor-antagonists and has a rather positive reversal potential, which is at a similar level to the E_{GABA} in immature neurons exposed to exogenous $GABA_A$ receptor agonists (Ben-Ari et al., 1989). Moreover, the disappearance of GDPs occurs in parallel with the developmental shift to hyperpolarizing $GABA_A$ receptor-mediated transmission in vitro (Ben-Ari et al., 1989; Khazipov et al., 2004a). Hence, GABAergic transmission and the interneuronal network have been proposed to play a crucial role in GDP generation.

GDPs have been detected in hippocampal slices from rats, mice, monkeys, and rabbits (Aguado et al., 2003; Ben-Ari et al., 1989; Khazipov et al., 2001; Menendez de la Prida, Bolea, & Sanchez-Andres, 1996). They occur at various irregular intervals ranging from seconds to minutes (Sipilä, Huttu, Soltesz, Voipio, & Kaila, 2005) and are also seen in whole hippocampal preparations (Leinekugel, Khalilov, Ben-Ari, & Khazipov, 1998). Both pyramidal cells and interneurons fire during the network events (Ben-Ari et al., 1989;

Khazipov, Leinekugel, Khalilov, Gaiarsa, & Ben-Ari, 1997; Lamsa et al., 2000). Whereas pyramidal cell firing is restricted to a time window of ~0.5 s, the associated GABAergic current component follows a somewhat longer time course (Sipilä et al., 2005). Various hippocampal subregions (i.e., CA1, CA3, and dentate gyrus) can generate GDPs even in isolation (Garaschuk, Hanse, & Konnerth, 1998; Khazipov et al., 1997; Menendez de la Prida, Bolea, & Sanchez-Andres, 1998), but the CA3 area has the highest propensity for GDP generation (Ben-Ari, 2001). In the whole hippocampus preparation, there is apparently a gradient within the CA3 such that the septal pole seems to act as the pacemaker of GDPs (Leinekugel et al., 1998).

GIANT DEPOLARIZING POTENTIALS: THE IN VITRO COUNTERPARTS OF EARLY SHARP WAVES

In the adult hippocampus in vivo, various network rhythms (e.g., SPWs with ripples, theta, gamma) are exhibited depending on the behavioural state of the animal (Buzsaki & Draguhn, 2004; Buzsaki, Leung, & Vanderwolf, 1983). They all have their own specific developmental profiles (Buhl & Buzsaki, 2005; Karlsson & Blumberg, 2003; Lahtinen et al., 2002; Leblanc & Bland, 1979; Leinekugel et al., 2002; Mohns, Karlsson, & Blumberg, 2007), but the SPW is the earliest pattern that has been characterized in vivo (Leinekugel et al., 2002). In the rat, SPWs occur already during the early postnatal period, when they are not associated with ripples (Buhl & Buzsaki, 2005; Mohns et al., 2007) but are sometimes followed by a "tail" event consisting of multiunit bursts (Leinekugel et al., 2002).

GABAergic depolarization has been proposed to be crucial for GDP generation (see previous section) while SPWs in adults are generated by the network of glutamatergic CA3 pyramidal neurons interconnected by recurrent collaterals (Buzsaki, 1986). Hence, a crucial question is whether there is a major reorganization in the hippocampal neuronal network during development in such a way that GDP/SPWs are generated by interneurons in the neonatal rat and by pyramidal cells in the adult. In contrast to this view, we present evidence that GDPs are, in fact, paced by intrinsically bursting pyramidal neurons and, hence, are likely to be in vitro counterparts of neonatal in vivo SPWs.

As described above, GABA has a context- and also dose-dependent "dual" effect in immature neurons: its action can be excitatory or inhibitory.

For instance, while a bath application of GABA$_A$R agonists initially leads to an increase in GDP frequency, a high concentration of these drugs eventually blocks the network events (Khalilov et al., 1999; Lamsa et al., 2000; see also Wells, Porter, & Agmon, 2000). On the other hand, GABA$_A$R antagonists typically reduce the frequency of spontaneous network events but cause an increase in their amplitude (Lamsa et al., 2000; Sipilä et al., unpublished observations). That depolarizing GABAergic signaling has a facilitatory action on GDPs is supported by the finding that the NKCC1 inhibitor, bumetanide, blocks GDPs and abolishes the depolarizing driving force for GABA in immature CA3 pyramidal neurons (Sipilä et al., 2006b).

A clear-cut approach to examine the role of GABA in GDP generation is to block GABA$_A$Rs, which, of course, abolishes the GABAergic current associated with GDPs. Under these conditions, spontaneous network events are typically observed at a lower frequency than the ones seen in control. This effect of GABA$_A$R antagonists has often been interpreted to block the "GABAergic" GDPs and subsequently induce "interictal" events driven by pyramidal neurons (Ben-Ari et al., 1989; Khazipov et al., 1997, 2001; Safiulina, Kasyanov, Giniatullin, & Cherubini, 2005). Nevertheless, there is no evidence that the original pacemaker mechanism is fundamentally different in the presence of GABA$_A$R antagonists. In fact, several lines of evidence, described below and elsewhere (Sipilä & Kaila, 2008), support the opposite conclusion: that the pacemaking mechanism itself remains largely unchanged in the presence or absence of GABAergic transmission.

A strong argument against the view that an interneuronal, GABAergic network generates GDPs is that these events are completely blocked by antagonists of ionotropic glutamate receptors. Notably, this block is achieved by specific AMPA receptor antagonists (Bolea, Avignone, Berretta, Sanchez-Andres, & Cherubini, 1999), and a combined application of AMPA and NMDA antagonists gives the same result (Ben-Ari et al., 1989; Gaiarsa, Corradetti, Cherubini, & Ben-Ari, 1991; Hollrigel, Ross, & Soltesz, 1998; Khazipov et al., 2001; Lamsa et al., 2000; Sipilä et al., 2005; see also Safiulina et al., 2005). Thus, the generation of GDPs is strictly dependent on glutamatergic but not on GABAergic transmission.

The effects of depolarizing GABA on neuronal spiking are strongly influenced by the intrinsic properties of target neurons. In the presence of the glutamatergic blockers, immature CA3 neurons are spontaneously active and fire in bursts, which occur with a temporal pattern similar to GDPs (Sipilä et al., 2005). However, the spontaneous activity of the individual pyramidal neurons is suppressed by GABA$_A$R antagonists, a fact that can be readily explained by the tonic and synaptic GABAergic inputs that depolarize these cells (Sipilä et al., 2005). These data provide a parsimonious explanation for the role of GABAergic signaling in GDP generation: voltage-dependent intrinsic bursting of immature CA3 pyramidal neurons (Menendez de la Prida & Sanchez-Andres, 2000) is facilitated by tonic and synaptic GABAergic depolarizing inputs that, therefore, play a "permissive" role in GDP generation (Sipilä et al., 2005). While these results show that GABAergic transmission is, by definition, clearly excitatory since it increases the probability of firing, the temporal pattern of pyramidal cell bursts is primarily dictated by intrinsic conductances such as a persistent Na$^+$ current and a slow Ca^{2+}-activated K$^+$ current (Sipilä, Huttu, Voipio, & Kaila, 2006a). Whether intrinsically bursting principal neurons generate GDPs also in the isolated CA1 area and the dentate gyrus (see Menendez de la Prida et al., 1998) remains to be studied in future work. That the "GDP pacemaker" is functionally downstream of GABAergic signaling is further supported by the finding that a tonic activation of GABA$_A$Rs promotes the occurrence of GDPs even in the absence of synaptic GABAergic transmission (Sipilä et al., 2005). In line with this, the blocking effect of GABA$_A$R antagonists on GDPs can be consistently unblocked by membrane depolarization imposed by elevation of extracellular K$^+$ concentration (Sipilä et al., 2005)—a maneuver that conveys no temporally structured input whatsoever.

In summary, GABAergic signaling increases the probability of burst initiation in CA3 pyramidal neurons via temporally nonpatterned (non-pacemaking) depolarization and thereby promotes the occurrence of GDPs. The conclusion that GDPs are driven by the network of intrinsically busting pyramidal neurons is fully consistent with the idea that these events are the in vitro counterparts of neonatal SPWs. This is further supported by the finding that both the in vitro and in vivo events are blocked by the NKCC1 inhibitor, bumetanide (Sipilä et al., 2006b). The mechanisms underlying the generation of GDPs and SPWs are summarized in Figure 6.3. From a more general point of view, the bursting activity

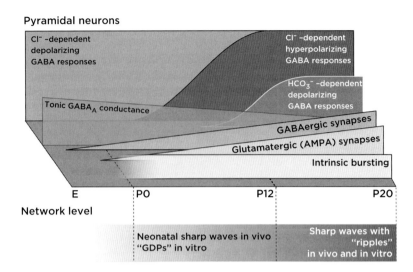

Pyramidal neurons

Cl⁻-dependent depolarizing GABA responses — Cl⁻-dependent hyperpolarizing GABA responses

HCO₃⁻-dependent depolarizing GABA responses

Tonic GABA_A conductance

GABAergic synapses

Glutamatergic (AMPA) synapses

Intrinsic bursting

E · P0 · P12 · P20

Network level

Neonatal sharp waves in vivo "GDPs" in vitro · Sharp waves with "ripples" in vivo and in vitro

Figure 6.3 Developmental profiles of GABAergic signaling and of the generation of intermittent network events (in vitro GDPs and in vivo SPWs) in the rat hippocampus. Developmental milestones of pyramidal neurons: The tonic mode of GABA_A receptor signaling emerges in the absence of synapses, and functional glutamatergic synapses appear after GABAergic ones. GABA_ARs mediate depolarizing Cl⁻ currents in immature pyramidal neurons, and a shift to hyperpolarizing currents is seen during the second postnatal week. The current component that is carried by HCO₃⁻ is depolarizing, irrespective of developmental stage, but it has a significant action on GABAergic responses only at around P12 and later. Developmental milestones at the network level: The occurrence of GDPs decreases as the GABA_A-receptor mediated action shifts from depolarizing to hyperpolarizing. The ability of mature CA3 pyramidal neurons to generate GDPs is enhanced under conditions where the strength of functional recurrent connections is increased or the efficacy of GABAergic inhibition is decreased. In vivo, SPWs are the first endogenous pattern of activity seen during ontogeny. The development of SPWs is further characterized by the emergence of high-frequency "ripple" oscillations. The approximate developmental time scale includes the late embryonic period (E) and the postnatal period from P0 (postnatal day 0; time of birth) to P20.

of pyramidal neurons appears to pace spontaneous physiological as well as pathological network events throughout hippocampal development.

COMPARISON OF NEONATAL NEOCORTICAL AND HIPPOCAMPAL NETWORK EVENTS

Recent data indicate that the role of GABAergic transmission is somewhat different in the generation of the early network events in the neocortex compared to the hippocampus. Neocortical network events with a relatively long duration have been called "slow activity transients" (SATs) in the human (Vanhatalo et al., 2005) and these events include "spindle bursts" in the rodent neocortex (Hanganu, Staiger, Ben-Ari, & Khazipov, 2007; Khazipov et al., 2004b). In electrophysiological recordings in the rat barrel cortex, the probability of spindle-burst initiation is not reduced by GABA_AR antagonists or the NKCC1 blocker, bumetanide (Minlebaev, Ben-Ari, & Khazipov, 2007). On the other hand, the duration and amplitude of the network events is increased by GABA_AR antagonists in the hippocampus (Lamsa et al., 2000), which

is similar to observations in the barrel cortex (Minlebaev et al., 2007). Another notable similarity between neocortical and hippocampal population events is that they are both strongly inhibited by AMPA/kainate antagonists (Minlebaev et al., 2007), which points to a key role for principal neurons in the generation of the intermittent network patterns.

From Intermittent Events to Ongoing Oscillations

Oscillatory network patterns occurring within theta, gamma, and ripple frequency ranges appear after the emergence of intermittent SPWs during hippocampal development (Buhl & Buzsaki, 2005; Karlsson & Blumberg, 2003; Karlsson, Mohns, di Prisco, & Blumberg, 2006; Lahtinen et al., 2002; Leblanc & Bland, 1979; Leinekugel et al., 2002; Mohns et al., 2007). GABAergic mechanisms and the interneuronal network are heavily implicated in the patterning of hippocampal theta and gamma rhythms as well as sharp-wave associated ripple events (Bartos, Vida, & Jonas, 2007; Bragin et al.,

1995; Klausberger et al., 2003; Somogyi & Klausberger, 2005; Tukker, Fuentealba, Hartwich, Somogyi, & Klausberger, 2007; Vida et al., 2006; Ylinen et al., 1995a, 1995b). However, more studies are needed to elucidate the specific roles for different aspects of GABAergic signaling ranging from various interneuron subtypes to ionic regulation in the ontogenesis of oscillatory network patterns.

The molecular and cellular mechanisms that are required for the emergence of ongoing oscillatory activity in cortical structures most likely reflect changes in the various modes of GABAergic transmission reviewed here, and also in the protracted development of the interneuronal network (Danglot et al., 2006). It is likely that an efficient strategy to examine this transitory developmental period is to transfer ideas from the vast literature that is available on oscillatory activity in the mature brain and, in particular, on the roles of GABA in the generation of neuronal network oscillations.

Acknowledgments

We thank Matti Airaksinen, Mark Blumberg, Mark Farrant, Jean-Marc Fritschy, Pepin Marshall, and Liset Menendez de la Prida for constructive comments. The original research work of the authors was supported by the Academy of Finland and the Sigrid Jusélius Foundation (K.K. and S.T.S.), the Jane and Aatos Erkko Foundation (K.K.), the Paulo Foundation (S.T.S.), and the German Academic Exchange Service DAAD (P.B.).

References

Achilles, K., Okabe, A., Ikeda, M., Shimizu-Okabe, C., Yamada, J., Fukuda, A., et al. (2007). Kinetic properties of Cl uptake mediated by Na$^+$-dependent K$^+$-2Cl$^-$ cotransport in immature rat neocortical neurons. *Journal of Neuroscience, 27*(32), 8616–8627.

Adelsberger, H., Garaschuk, O., & Konnerth, A. (2005). Cortical calcium waves in resting newborn mice. *Nature Neuroscience, 8*, 988–990.

Adragna, N. C., Fulvio, M. D., & Lauf, P. K. (2004). Regulation of K–Cl cotransport: From function to genes. *Journal of Membrane Biology, 201*(3), 109–137.

Aguado, F., Carmona, M. A., Pozas, E., Aguilo, A., Martinez-Guijarro, F.J., Alcantara, S., et al. (2003). BDNF regulates spontaneous correlated activity at early developmental stages by increasing synaptogenesis and expression of K+/Cl- co-transport. *Development, 130*, 1287–1280.

Aickin, C. C., Deisz, R. A., & Lux, H. D. (1982). Ammonium action on post-synaptic inhibition in crayfish neurones: Implications for the mechanism of chloride extrusion. *Journal of Physiology, 329*, 319–339.

Akerman, C. J., & Cline, H. T. (2007). Refining the roles of GABAergic signaling during neural circuit formation. *Trends in Neurosciences, 30*, 382–389.

Alger, B. E., & Nicoll, R. A. (1979). GABA-mediated biphasic inhibitory responses in hippocampus. *Nature, 281*(5729), 315–317.

Alvarez-Leefmans, F. J., & Russell, J. M. (Eds.), (1990). *Chloride channels and carriers in nerve, muscle and glial cells.* New York: Plenum Press.

Avishai-Eliner, S., Brunson, K. L., Sandman, C. A., & Baram. T. Z. (2002). Stressed-out, or in (utero)? *Trends in Neurosciences, 25*(10), 518–524.

Avoli, M., Louvel, J., Pumain, R., & Kohling, R. (2005). Cellular and molecular mechanisms of epilepsy in the human brain. *Progress in Neurobiology, 77*(3), 166–200.

Awapara, J., Landua, A.J., Fuerst, R., & Seale, B. (1950). Free 7-aminobutyric acid in brain. *Journal of Biological Chemistry, 187*, 35–39.

Baer, K., Essrich, C., Benson, J.A., Benke, D., Bluethmann, H., Fritschy, J.M., et al. (1999). Postsynaptic clustering of γ-aminobutyric acid type A receptors by the γ$_3$ subunit in vivo. *Proceedings of the National Academy of Sciences, 96*, 12860–12865.

Balakrishnan, V., Becker, M., Lohrke, S., Nothwang, H. G., Guresir, E., & Friauf, E. (2003). Expression and function of chloride transporters during development of inhibitory neurotransmission in the auditory brainstem. *Journal of Neuroscience, 23*, 4134–4145.

Barnard, E. A., Skolnick, P., Olsen, R. W., Mohler, H., Sieghart, W., Biggio, G., et al. (1998). International union of pharmacology. XV. Subtypes of γ-aminobutyric acid$_A$ receptors: Classification on the basis of subunit structure and receptor function. *Pharmacological Reviews, 50*, 291–313.

Bartho, P., Payne, J. A., Freund, T. F., & Acsady, L. (2004). Differential distribution of the KCl cotransporter KCC2 in thalamic relay and reticular nuclei. *European Journal of Neuroscience, 20*, 965–975.

Bartos, M., Vida, I., & Jonas P. (2007). Synaptic mechanisms of synchronized gamma oscillations in inhibitory interneuron networks. *Nature Reviews Neuroscience, 8*, 45–56.

Behar, T. N., Li, Y. X., Tran, H. T., Ma, W., Dunlap, V., Scott, C., et al. (1996). GABA stimulates chemotaxis and chemokinesis of embryonic cortical neurons via calcium-dependent mechanisms. *Journal of Neuroscience, 16*, 1808–1818.

Belelli, D., Peden, D. R., Rosahl, T. W., Wafford, K. A., & Lambert, J. J. (2005). Extrasynaptic GABA$_A$ receptors of thalamocortical neurons: A molecular target for hypnotics. *Journal of Neuroscience, 25*, 11513–11520.

Ben-Ari, Y. (2001). Developing networks play a similar melody. *Trends in Neurosciences, 24*(6), 353–360.

Ben-Ari, Y. (2002). Excitatory actions of GABA during development: The nature of the nurture. *Nature Reviews Neuroscience, 3*, 728–739.

Ben-Ari, Y., Cherubini, E., Corradetti, R., & Gaiarsa, J.L. (1989). Giant synaptic potentials in immature rat CA3 hippocampal neurones. *Journal of Physiology, 416*, 303–325.

Benke, D., Fakitsas, P., Roggenmoser, C., Michel, C., Rudolph, U., & Mohler, H. (2004). Analysis of the presence and abundance of GABA$_A$ receptors containing two different types of α subunits in murine brain using point-mutated α subunits. *Journal of Biological Chemistry, 279*, 43654–43660.

Bennett, V., & Baines, A. J. (2001). Spectrin and ankyrin-based pathways: Metazoan inventions for integrating cells into tissues. *Physiological Reviews, 81*, 1353–1392.

Berninger, B., Marty, S., Zafra, F., da Penha Berzaghi, M., Thoenen, H., & Lindholm, D. (1995). GABAergic stimulation switches from enhancing to repressing BDNF expression in rat hippocampal neurons during maturation in vitro. *Development. 121*(8), 2327–2335.

Binder, D. K., Croll, S. D., Gall, C. M., & Scharfman, H. E. (2001). BDNF and epilepsy: Too much of a good thing? *Trends in Neurosciences, 24*, 47–53.

Birnir, B., Everitt, A. B., Lim, M. S., & Gage, P. W. (2000). Spontaneously opening GABA(A) channels in CA1 pyramidal neurones of rat hippocampus. *Journal of Membrane Biology, 174*, 21–29.

Blaesse, P., Airaksinen, M. S., Rivera, C., & Kaila, K. (2009). Cation-chloride cotransporters and neuronal function. *Neuron, 61*, 820–838.

Blaesse, P., Guillemin, I., Schindler, J., Schweizer, M., Delpire, E., Khiroug, L., et al. (2006) Oligomerization of KCC2 correlates with development of inhibitory neurotransmission. *Journal of Neuroscience, 26*, 10407–10419.

Boettger, T., Rust, M. B., Maier, H., Seidenbecher, T., Schweizer, M., Keating, D. J., et al. (2003). Loss of K-Cl co-transporter KCC3 causes deafness, neurodegeneration and reduced seizure threshold. *EMBO Journal, 22*, 5422–5434.

Boistel, J., & Fatt, P. (1958). Membrane permeability change during inhibitory transmitter action in crustacean muscle. *Journal of Physiology, 144*, 176–191.

Bolea, S., Avignone, E., Berretta, N., Sanchez-Andres, J. V., & Cherubini, E. (1999). Glutamate controls the induction of GABA-mediated giant depolarizing potentials through AMPA receptors in neonatal rat hippocampal slices. *Journal of Neurophysiology, 81*, 2095–2102.

Bormann, J. (2000). The "ABC" of GABA receptors. *Trends in Pharmacological Sciences, 21*, 16–19.

Bormann, J., Hamill, O. P., & Sakmann, B. (1987). Mechanism of anion permeation through channels gated by glycine and gamma-aminobutyric acid in mouse cultured spinal neurones. *Journal of Physiology, 385*, 243–286.

Bragin, A., Jando, G., Nadasdy, N., Hetke, J., Wise, K., & Buzsaki, G. (1995). Gamma (40–100 Hz) oscillation in the hippocampus of the behaving rat. *Journal of Neuroscience, 15*, 47–60.

Brickley, S. G., Cull-Candy, S. G., & Farrant, M. (1996). Development of a tonic form of synaptic inhibition in rat cerebellar granule cells resulting from persistent activation of GABAA receptors. *Journal of Physiology, 497*, 753–759.

Brickley, S. G., Revilla, V., Cull-Candy, S. G., Wisden, W., & Farrant, M. (2001). Adaptive regulation of neuronal excitability by a voltage-independent potassium conductance. *Nature, 409*, 88–92.

Bright, D. P., Aller, M. I., & Brickley, S. G. (2007). Synaptic release generates a tonic GABA(A) receptor-mediated conductance that modulates burst precision in thalamic relay neurons. *Journal of Neuroscience, 27*, 2560–2569.

Brussaard, A. B., Kits, K. S., & de Vlieger, T. A. (1996). Postsynaptic mechanism of depression of GABAergic synapses by oxytocin in the supraoptic nucleus of immature rat. *Journal of Physiology, 497*, 495–507.

Buhl, D. L., & Buzsaki, G. (2005). Developmental emergence of hippocampal fast-field "ripple" oscillations in the behaving rat pups. *Neuroscience, 134*(4), 1423–1430.

Buzsaki, G. (1986). Hippocampal sharp waves: Their origin and significance. *Brain Research, 398*, 242–252.

Buzsaki, G. (2002). Theta oscillations in the hippocampus. *Neuron, 33*, 325–340.

Buzsaki, G. (2006). *Rhythms of the brain*, New York: Oxford University Press.

Buzsaki, G., & Draguhn, A. (2004). Neuronal oscillations in cortical networks. *Science, 304*, 1926–1929.

Buzsaki, G., Leung, L. W., & Vanderwolf, C. H. (1983). Cellular bases of hippocampal EEG in the behaving rat. *Brain Research, 287*, 139–171.

Cammack, J. N., Rakhilin, S. V., & Schwartz, E. A. (1994). A GABA transporter operates asymmetrically and with variable stoichiometry. *Neuron, 13*, 949–960.

Campo-Soria, C., Chang, Y., & Weiss, D. S. (2006). Mechanism of action of benzodiazepines on GABA$_A$ receptors. *British Journal of Pharmacology, 148*, 984–990.

Cancedda, L., Fiumelli, H., Chen, K., & Poo, M. M. (2007). Excitatory GABA action is essential for morphological maturation of cortical neurons in vivo. *Journal of Neuroscience, 27*, 5224–5235.

Capsoni, S., Tongiorgi, E., Cattaneo, A., & Domenici, L. (1999) Dark rearing blocks the developmental downregulation of brain-derived neurotrophic factor messenger RNA expression in layers IV and V of the rat visual cortex. *Neuroscience, 88*, 393–403.

Caraiscos, V. B., Elliott, E. M., You-Ten, K. E., Cheng, V. Y., Belelli, D., Newell, J.G., et al. (2004). Tonic inhibition in mouse hippocampal CA1 pyramidal neurons is mediated by alpha$_5$ subunit-containing gamma-aminobutyric acid type A receptors. *Proceedings of the National Academy of Sciences, 101*, 3662–3667.

Casula, S., Shmukler, B. E., Wilhelm, S., Stuart-Tilley, A. K., Su, W., Chernova, M. N., et al. (2001). A dominant negative mutant of the KCC1 K-Cl cotransporter: Both N- and C-terminal cytoplasmic domains are required for K-Cl cotransport activity. *Journal of Biological Chemistry, 276*, 41870–41878.

Chabot, C., Bernard, J., Normandin, M., Ohayon, M., Baudry, M., & Massicotte, G. (1996). Developmental changes in depolarization-mediated AMPA receptor modifications and potassium-induced long-term potentiation. *Brain Research, 93*, 70–75.

Chadderton, P., Margrie, T. W., & Hausser, M. (2004) Integration of quanta in cerebellar granule cells during sensory processing. *Nature, 428*, 856–860.

Chandra, D., Jia, F., Liang, J., Peng, Z., Suryanarayanan, A., Werner, D. F., et al. (2006). GABA$_A$ receptor alpha 4 subunits mediate extrasynaptic inhibition in thalamus and dentate gyrus and the action of gaboxadol. *Proceedings of the National Academy of Sciences, 103*(41), 15230–15235.

Chang, Y., & Weiss, D. S. (1999). Allosteric activation mechanism of the alpha$_1$beta$_2$gamma$_2$ gamma-aminobutyric acid type A receptor revealed by mutation of the conserved M2 leucine. *Biophysical Journal, 77*, 2542–2551.

Chebib, M., & Johnston, G. A. (2000) GABA-Activated ligand gated ion channels: Medicinal chemistry and molecular biology. *Journal of Medical Chemistry, 43*, 1427–1447.

Chesler, M. (2003). Regulation and modulation of pH in the brain. *Physiological Reviews, 83*, 1183–1221.

Chiu, C. S., Brickley, S., Jensen, K., Southwell, A., Mckinney, S., Cull-Candy, S., et al. (2005). GABA transporter deficiency causes tremor, ataxia, nervousness, and increased GABA-induced tonic conductance in cerebellum. *Journal of Neuroscience, 25*, 3234–3245.

Chudotvorova, I., Ivanov, A., Rama, S., Hubner, C. A., Pellegrino, C., Ben-Ari, Y., et al. (2005). Early expression of KCC2 in rat hippocampal cultures augments expression of functional GABA synapses. *Journal of Physiology, 566,* 671–679.

Clancy, B., Darlington, R. B., & Finlay, B. L. (2001). Translating developmental time across mammalian species. *Neuroscience, 105,* 7–17.

Clausen, T. (1986). Regulation of active Na K transport in skeletal muscle. *Physiological Reviews, 66,* 542–580.

Cohen, I., Navarro, V., Le Duigou, C., & Miles, R. (2003). Mesial temporal lobe epilepsy: A pathological replay of developmental mechanisms? *Biology of the Cell, 95,* 329–333.

Collingridge, G. L. (1992). The Sharpey–Schafer Prize Lecture. The mechanism of induction of NMDA receptor-dependent long-term potentiation in the hippocampus. *Experimental Physiology, 77,* 771–797.

Colonnese, M. T., Phillips, M. A., Constantine-Paton, M., Kaila, K., & Jasanoff, A. (2008) Emergence of hemodynamic responses and functional connectivity during development of rat somatosensory cortex. *Nature Neuroscience, 11,* 72–79.

Cope, D. W., Hughes, S. W., & Crunelli, V. (2005). GABA$_A$ receptor-mediated tonic inhibition in thalamic neurons. *Journal of Neuroscience, 25,* 11553–11563.

Cutting, G. R., Curristin, S., Zoghbi, H., O'Hara, B., Seldin, M. F., & Uhl, G. R. (1992). Identification of a putative gamma-aminobutyric acid (GABA) receptor subunit rho$_2$ cDNA and colocalization of the genes encoding rho$_2$ (GABRR2) and rho$_1$ (GABRR1) to human chromosome 6q14–q21 and mouse chromosome 4. *Genomics, 12,* 801–806.

Danglot, L., Triller, A., & Marty, S. (2006). The development of hippocampal interneurons in rodents. *Hippocampus, 16,* 1032–1060.

Dasen, J. S., Tice, B. C., Brenner-Morton, S., & Jessell, T. M. (2005). A Hox regulatory network establishes motor neuron pool identity and target-muscle connectivity. *Cell, 123,* 477–491.

DeFazio, R. A., Keros, S., Quick, M. W., & Hablitz, J. J. (2000). Potassium-coupled chloride cotransport controls intracellular chloride in rat neocortical pyramidal neurons. *Journal of Neuroscience, 20,* 8069–8076.

Deisz, R. A., & Lux, H. D. (1982). The role of intracellular chloride in hyperpolarizing post-synaptic inhibition of crayfish stretch receptor neurones. *Journal of Physiology, 326,* 123–138.

de Jong, J. C., Willems, P. H., Mooren, F. J., van den Heuvel, L. P., Knoers, N. V., & Bindels, R. J. (2003). The structural unit of the thiazide-sensitive NaCl cotransporter is a homodimer. *Journal of Biological Chemistry, 278,* 24302–24307.

Delpire, E., & Gagnon, K. B. (2006). SPAK and OSR1, key kinases involved in the regulation of chloride transport. *Acta Physiologica, 187,* 103–113.

Demarque, M., Represa, A., Becq, H., Khalilov, I., Ben-Ari, Y., & Aniksztejn, L. (2002). Paracrine intercellular communication by a Ca^{2+}- and SNARE- independent release of GABA and glutamate prior to synapse formation. *Neuron, 36,* 1051–1061.

Denker, S. P., & Barber, D. L. (2002). Ion transport proteins anchor and regulate the cytoskeleton. *Current Opinion in Cell Biology, 14,* 214–220.

Diamond, J. M. (1993). Evolutionary physiology. In D. Noble & C.A.R. Boyd (Eds.), *Logic of life: The challenge of integrative physiology* (pp. 89–111). Oxford: Oxford University Press.

Ding, R., Asada, H., & Obata, K. (1998). Changes in extracellular glutamate and GABA levels in the hippocampal CA3 and CA1 areas and the induction of glutamic acid decarboxylase-67 in dentate granule cells of rats treated with kainic acid. *Brain Research, 800,* 105–113.

Duebel, J., Haverkamp, S., Schleich, W., Feng, G., Augustine, G. J., Kuner, T., et al. (2006). Two-photon imaging reveals somatodendritic chloride gradient in retinal ON-type bipolar cells expressing the biosensor Clomeleon. *Neuron, 49,* 81–94.

Dunning, D. D., Hoover, C. L., Soltesz, I., Smith, M. A., & O'Dowd, D. K. (1999). GABA(A) receptor-mediated miniature postsynaptic currents and alpha-subunit expression in developing cortical neurons. *Journal of Neurophysiology, 82,* 3286–3297.

Dupont, E., Hanganu, I. L., Kilb, W., Hirsch, S., & Luhmann, H. J. (2006). Rapid developmental switch in the mechanisms driving early cortical columnar networks. *Nature, 439,* 79–83.

Erecinska, M., Cherian, S., & Silver, I. A. (2004). Energy metabolism in mammalian brain during development. *Progress in Neurobiology, 73,* 397–445.

Esposito, M. S., Piatti, V. C., Laplagne, D. A., Morgenstern, N. A., Ferrari, C. C., Pitossi, F. J., et al. (2005). Neuronal differentiation in the adult hippocampus recapitulates embryonic development. *Journal of Neuroscience, 25,* 10074–10086.

Essrich, C., Lorez, M., Benson, J. A., Fritschy, J. M., & Luscher, B. (1998). Postsynaptic clustering of major GABA$_A$ receptor subtypes requires the γ_2 subunit and gephyrin. *Nature Neuroscience, 1,* 563–571.

Farrant, M., & Kaila, K. (2007). The cellular, molecular and ionic basis of GABA(A) receptor signalling. *Progress in Brain Research, 160,* 59–87.

Farrant, M., & Nusser, Z. (2005). Variations on an inhibitory theme: Phasic and tonic activation of GABA$_A$ receptors. *Nature Reviews Neuroscience, 6,* 215–229.

Feller, M. B. (1999). Spontaneous correlated activity in developing neural circuits. *Neuron, 22,* 653–656.

Fitzgerald, M. (1987). Spontaneous and evoked activity of fetal primary afferents in vivo. *Nature, 326,* 603–605.

Fiumelli, H., Cancedda, L., & Poo, M. M. (2005) Modulation of GABAergic transmission by activity via postsynaptic Ca^{2+}-dependent regulation of KCC2 function. *Neuron, 48,* 773–786.

Flagella, M., Clarke, L. L., Miller, M. L., Erway, L. C., Giannella, R. A., Andringa, A., et al. (1999). Mice lacking the basolateral Na-K-2Cl cotransporter have impaired epithelial chloride secretion and are profoundly deaf. *Journal of Biological Chemistry, 274,* 26946–26955.

Freund, T. F. (2003). Rhythm and mood in perisomatic inhibition. *Trends in Neurosciences, 26,* 489–495.

Freund, T. F., & Buzsaki, G. (1996) Interneurons of the hippocampus. *Hippocampus, 6,* 347–470.

Fritschy, J. M., & Brunig, I. (2003). Formation and plasticity of GABAergic synapses: Physiological mechanisms and pathophysiological implications. *Pharmacology and Therapeutics, 98,* 299–323.

Fritschy, J. M., & Mohler, H. (1995). GABA$_A$-receptor heterogeneity in the adult-rat brain—Differential regional and cellular-distribution of 7 major subunits. *Journal of Comparative Neurology, 359,* 154–194.

Fritschy, J. M., Paysan, J., Enna, A., & Mohler, H. (1994). Switch in the expression of rat GABAA-receptor subtypes during postnatal development: An immunohistochemical study. *Journal of Neuroscience, 14,* 5302–5324.

Fujiwara-Tsukamoto, Y., Isomura, Y., Imanishi, M., Fukai, T., & Takada, M. (2007). Distinct types of ionic modulation of GABA actions in pyramidal cells and interneurons during electrical induction of hippocampal seizure-like network activity. *European Journal of Neuroscience, 25,* 2713–2725.

Fukuda, A., Muramatsu, K., Okabe, A., Shimano, Y., Hida, H., Fujimoto, I., et al. (1998). Changes in intracellular Ca²⁺ induced by GABA_A receptor activation and reduction in Cl⁻ gradient in neonatal rat neocortex. *Journal of Neurophysiology, 79,* 439–446.

Gaiarsa, J. L., Corradetti, R., Cherubini, E., & Ben-Ari, Y. (1991). Modulation of GABA-mediated synaptic potentials by glutamatergic agonists in neonatal CA3 rat hippocampal neurons. *European Journal of Neuroscience, 3,* 301–309.

Galanopoulou, A. S. (2005) GABA receptors as broadcasters of sexually differentiating signals in the brain. *Epilepsia, 46*(Suppl 5), 107–112.

Gamba, G. (2005). Molecular physiology and pathophysiology of electroneutral cation-chloride cotransporters. *Physiological Reviews, 85,* 423–493.

Gao, X. B., & van den Pol, A. N. (2000). GABA release from axonal growth cones. *Journal of Physiology, 523,* 629–637.

Gao, X. B., & van den Pol, A. N. (2001). GABA, not glutamate, a primary transmitter driving action potentials in developing hypothalamic neurons. *Journal of Neurophysiology, 85,* 425–434.

Garaschuk, O., Hanse, E., & Konnerth, A. (1998). Developmental profile and synaptic origin of early network oscillations in the CA1 region of rat neonatal hippocampus. *Journal of Physiology, 507,* 219–236.

Garaschuk, O., Linn, J., Eilers, J., & Konnerth, A. (2000). Large-scale oscillatory calcium waves in the immature cortex. *Nature Neuroscience, 3,* 452–459.

Ge, S., Goh, E. L., Sailor, K. A., Kitabatake, Y., Ming, G. L., & Song, H. (2006). GABA regulates synaptic integration of newly generated neurons in the adult brain. *Nature, 439,* 589–593.

Geal-Dor, M., Freeman, S., Li, G., & Sohmer, H. (1993). Development of hearing in neonatal rats: Air and bone conducted ABR thresholds. *Hearing Research, 69,* 236–242.

Glykys, J., & Mody, I. (2007). The main source of ambient GABA responsible for tonic inhibition in the mouse hippocampus. *Journal of Physiology, 582,* 1163–1178.

Glykys, J., Peng, Z., Chandra, D., Homanics, G. E., Houser, C. R., & Mody, I. (2006). A new naturally occurring GABA_A receptor subunit partnership with high sensitivity to ethanol. *Nature Neuroscience, 10*(1), 40–48.

Grover, L. M., Lambert, N. A., Schwartzkroin, P. A., & Teyler, T. J. (1993). Role of HCO₃⁻ ions in depolarizing GABA_A receptor-mediated responses in pyramidal cells of rat hippocampus. *Journal of Neurophysiology, 69,* 1541–1555.

Gulacsi, A., Lee, C. R., Sik, A., Viitanen, T., Kaila, K., Tepper, J. M., et al. (2003). Cell type-specific differences in chloride-regulatory mechanisms and GABA_A receptor-mediated inhibition in rat substantia nigra. *Journal of Neuroscience, 23,* 8237–8246.

Gulledge, A. T., & Stuart, G. J. (2003). Excitatory actions of GABA in the cortex. *Neuron, 37,* 299–309.

Gulyas, A. I., Sik, A., Payne, J. A., Kaila, K., & Freund, T. F. (2001). The KCl cotransporter, KCC2, is highly expressed in the vicinity of excitatory synapses in the rat hippocampus. *European Journal of Neuroscience, 13,* 2205–2217.

Gummer, A. W., & Mark, R. F. (1994). Patterned neural activity in brain stem auditory areas of a prehearing mammal, the tammar wallaby (*Macropus eugenii*). *Neuroreport, 5,* 685–688.

Hamann, M., Rossi, D. J., & Attwell, D. (2002). Tonic and spillover inhibition of granule cells control information flow through cerebellar cortex. *Neuron, 33,* 625–633.

Hamburger, V. (1963). Some aspects of the embryology of behavior. *Quarterly Review of Biology 38,* 342–365.

Hanganu, I. L., Staiger, J. F., Ben-Ari, Y., & Khazipov, R. (2007). Cholinergic modulation of spindle bursts in the neonatal rat visual cortex in vivo. *Journal of Neuroscience, 27,* 5694–5670.

Harris, K. M., & Teyler, T. J. (1984). Developmental onset of long-term potentiation in area CA1 of the rat hippocampus. *Journal of Physiology, 346,* 27–48.

Haydar, T. F., Wang, F., Schwartz, M. L., & Rakic, P. (2000). Differential modulation of proliferation in the neocortical ventricular and subventricular zones. *Journal of Neuroscience, 20,* 5764–5774.

Heck, N., Kilb, W., Reiprich, P., Kubota, H., Furukawa, T., Fukuda, A., et al. (2007). GABA-A receptors regulate neocortical neuronal migration in vitro and in vivo. *Cerebral Cortex, 17,* 138–148.

Hensch, T. K. (2005). Critical period plasticity in local cortical circuits. *Nature Reviews Neuroscience, 6,* 877–888.

Hering, H., & Sheng, M. (2001). Dendritic spines: Structure, dynamics and regulation. *Nature Reviews Neuroscience, 12,* 880–888.

Hilgenberg, L. G., Su, H., Gu, H., O'Dowd, D. K., & Smith, M. A. (2006). Alpha₃Na⁺/K⁺-ATPase is a neuronal receptor for agrin. *Cell, 125,* 359–369.

Hinde, R. A. (1970). *A synthesis of ethology and comparative psychology.* New York: McGraw-Hill.

Ho, S.M., & Waite, P.M. (1999). Spontaneous activity in the perinatal trigeminal nucleus of the rat. *Neuroreport 10,* 659–664.

Hollrigel, G. S., & Soltesz, I. (1997). Slow kinetics of miniature IPSCs during early postnatal development in granule cells of the dentate gyrus. *Journal of Neuroscience, 17,* 5119–5128.

Hollrigel, G. S., Ross, S. T., & Soltesz, I. (1998). Temporal patterns and depolarizing actions of spontaneous GABA_A receptor activation in granule cells of the early postnatal dentate gyrus. *Journal of Neurophysiology, 80,* 2340–2351.

Howard, M. A., Burger, R. M., & Rubel, E. W. (2007). A developmental switch to GABAergic inhibition dependent on increases in Kv1-type K+ currents. *Journal of Neuroscience 27,* 2112–2123.

Huang, Z. J., Di Cristo, G., & Ango, F. (2007) Development of GABA innervation in the cerebral and cerebellar cortices. *Nature Reviews Neuroscience, 8,* 673–686.

Huang, E. J., & Reichardt, L. F. (2001). Neurotrophins: Roles in neuronal development and function. *Annual Review of Neuroscience, 24,* 677–736.

Huang, E. J., & Reichardt, L. F. (2003). Trk receptors: Roles in neuronal signal transduction. *Annual Reviews of Biochemistry, 72,* 609–642.

Hubner, C. A., Stein, V., Hermans-Borgmeyer, I., Meyer, T., Ballanyi, K., & Jentsch, T. J. (2001). Disruption of KCC2 reveals an essential role of K-Cl cotransport already in early synaptic inhibition. *Neuron, 30,* 515–524.

Inoue, K., Ueno, S., & Fukuda, A. (2004). Interaction of neuron-specific K+-Cl- cotransporter, KCC2, with brain-type creatine kinase. *FEBS Letters, 564,* 131–135.

Jacobs, S., Hunt, R., Tarnow-Mordi, W., Inder, T., & Davis, P. (2007). Cooling for newborns with hypoxic ischaemic encephalopathy. *Cochrane Database of Systematic Reviews, 17,* CD003311.

Jackson, P. S., Suppes, T., & Harris, K. M. (1993). Stereotypical changes in the pattern and duration of long-term potentiation expressed at postnatal days 11 and 15 in the rat hippocampus. *Journal of Neurophysiology, 70,* 1412–1419.

Jarolimek, W., Lewen, A., & Misgeld, U. (1999) A furosemide-sensitive K+-Cl- cotransporter counteracts intracellular Cl-accumulation and depletion in cultured rat midbrain neurons. *Journal of Neuroscience, 19,* 4695–4704.

Jean-Xavier, C., Mentis, G. Z., O'Donovan, M. J., Cattaert, D., & Vinay, L. (2007). Dual personality of GABA/glycine-mediated depolarizations in immature spinal cord. *Proceedings of the National Academy of Sciences, 104,* 11477–11482.

Ji, F., Kanbara, N., & Obata, K. (1999). GABA and histogenesis in fetal and neonatal mouse brain lacking both the isoforms of glutamic acid decarboxylase. *Neuroscience Research, 33,* 187–194.

Jia, F., Pignataro, L., Schofield, C. M., Yue, M., Harrison, N. L., & Goldstein, P. A. (2005). An extrasynaptic GABA$_A$ receptor mediates tonic inhibition in thalamic VB neurons. *Journal of Neurophysiology, 94,* 4491–4501.

Jonas, P., Bischofberger, J., Fricker, D., & Miles, R. (2004). Interneuron Diversity series: Fast in, fast out—Temporal and spatial signal processing in hippocampal interneurons. *Trends in Neuroscience, 27,* 30–40.

Jones, B. L., Whiting, P. J., & Henderson, L. P. (2006). Mechanisms of anabolic androgenic steroid inhibition of mammalian epsilon-subunit-containing GABA$_A$ receptors. *Journal of Physiology, 573,* 571–593.

Kahle, K. T., Rinehart, J., Ring, A., Gimenez, I., Gamba, G., Hebert, S. C., et al. (2006). WNK protein kinases modulate cellular Cl- flux by altering the phosphorylation state of the Na-K-Cl and K-Cl cotransporters. *Physiology, 21,* 326–335.

Kaila, K. (1994). Ionic basis of GABA$_A$ receptor channel function in the nervous system. *Progress in Neurobiology, 42,* 489–537.

Kaila, K., Lamsa, K., Smirnov, S., Taira, T., & Voipio, J. (1997). Long-lasting GABA-mediated depolarization evoked by high-frequency stimulation in pyramidal neurons of rat hippocampal slice is attributable to a network-driven, bicarbonate-dependent K$^+$ transient. *Journal of Neuroscience, 17,* 7662–7672.

Kaila, K., Saarikoski, J., & Voipio, J. (1990). Mechanism of action of GABA on intracellular pH and on surface pH in crayfish muscle fibres. *Journal of Physiology, 427,* 241–260.

Kaila, K., & Voipio, J. (1987). Postsynaptic fall in intracellular pH induced by GABA-activated bicarbonate conductance. *Nature, 330,* 163–165.

Kaila, K., Voipio, J., Paalasmaa, P., Pasternack, M., & Deisz, R. A. (1993). The role of bicarbonate in GABA$_A$ receptor-mediated IPSPs of rat neocortical neurones. *Journal of Physiology, 464,* 273–289.

Kandler, K. (2004). Activity-dependent organization of inhibitory circuits: Lessons from the auditory system. *Current Opinion in Neurobiology, 14,* 96–104.

Kanold, P. O., & Shatz, C. J. (2006). Subplate neurons regulate maturation of cortical inhibition and outcome of ocular dominance plasticity. *Neuron, 51(5),* 627–638.

Kapur, J., & Macdonald, R. L. (1999). Postnatal development of hippocampal dentate granule cell gamma-aminobutyric acid$_A$ receptor pharmacological properties. *Molecular Pharmacology, 55,* 444–452.

Karlsson, K. A., & Blumberg, M. S. (2003). Hippocampal theta in the newborn rat is revealed under conditions that promote REM sleep. *Journal of Neuroscience, 23,* 1114–1118.

Karlsson, K. A., Mohns, E. J., di Prisco, G. V., & Blumberg, M. S. (2006) On the co-occurrence of startles and hippocampal sharp waves in newborn rats. *Hippocampus, 16,* 959–965.

Katagiri, H., Fagiolini, M., & Hensch, T. K. (2007). Optimization of somatic inhibition at critical period onset in mouse visual cortex. *Neuron, 53,* 805–812.

Katz, B. (1966). *Nerve, muscle and synapse.* New York: McGraw-Hill.

Katz, L. C., & Crowley, J. C. (2002). Development of cortical circuits: Lessons from ocular dominance columns. *Nature Reviews Neuroscience, 3,* 34–42.

Khalilov, I., Dzhala, V., Ben-Ari, Y., & Khazipov, R. (1999). Dual role of GABA in the neonatal rat hippocampus. *Developmental Neuroscience, 21,* 310–319.

Khazipov, R., Esclapez, M., Caillard, O., Bernard, C., Khalilov, I., Tyzio, R., et al. (2001). Early development of neuronal activity in the primate hippocampus in utero. *Journal of Neuroscience, 21,* 9770–9781.

Khazipov, R., Khalilov, I., Tyzio, R., Morozova, E., Ben-Ari, Y., & Holmes, G. L. (2004a). Developmental changes in GABAergic actions and seizure susceptibility in the rat hippocampus. *European Journal of Neuroscience, 19,* 590–600.

Khazipov, R., Leinekugel, X., Khalilov, I., Gaiarsa, J. L., & Ben-Ari, Y. (1997). Synchronization of GABAergic interneuronal network in CA3 subfield of neonatal rat hippocampal slices. *Journal of Physiology, 498,* 763–772.

Khazipov, R., Sirota, A., Leinekugel, X., Holmes, G. L., Ben-Ari, Y., & Buzsaki, G. (2004b). Early motor activity drives spindle bursts in the developing somatosensory cortex. *Nature, 432,* 758–761.

Khirug, S., Huttu, K., Ludwig, A., Smirnov, S., Voipio, J., Rivera, C., et al. (2005). Distinct properties of functional KCC2 expression in immature mouse hippocampal neurons in culture and in acute slices. *European Journal of Neuroscience, 21,* 899–904.

Khirug, S., Yamada, J., Afzalov, R., Voipio, J., Khiroug, L., & Kaila, K. (2008). GABAergic depolarization of the axon initial segment in cortical principal neurons is caused by the Na-K-2Cl cotransporter NKCC1. *Journal of Neuroscience, 28,* 4635–4639.

Kilb, W., & Luhmann, H. J. (2003). Carbachol-induced network oscillations in the intact cerebral cortex of the newborn rat. *Cerebral Cortex, 13,* 409–421.

Kittler, J. T., McAinsh, K., & Moss, S. J. (2002). Mechanisms of GABA$_A$ receptor assembly and trafficking—Implications for the modulation of inhibitory neurotransmission. *Molecular Neurobiology, 26,* 251–268.

Kittler, J. T., & Moss, S. J. (2003). Modulation of GABA$_A$ receptor activity by phosphorylation and receptor trafficking:

Implications for the efficacy of synaptic inhibition. *Current Opinion in Neurobiology, 13*, 341–347.

Klausberger, T., Magill, P. J., Marton, L. F., Roberts, J. D., Cobden, P. M., Buzsaki, G., et al. (2003). Brain-state- and cell-type-specific firing of hippocampal interneurons in vivo. *Nature, 421*, 844–848.

Krnjevic, K. (2004). How does a little acronym become a big transmitter? *Biochemical Pharmacology, 68*, 1549–1555.

Krnjevic, K., & Schwartz, S. (1967). The action of ff-aminobutyric acid on cortical neurones. *Experimental Brain Research, 3*, 320–336.

Korpi, E. R., Grunder, G., & Luddens, H. (2002). Drug interactions at GABA_A receptors. *Progress in Neurobiology, 67*, 113–159.

Kuffler, S. W., & Edwards, C. (1958). Mechanism of gamma aminobutyric acid (GABA) action and its relation to synaptic inhibition. *Journal of Neurophysiology, 21*, 589–610.

Kullmann, D. M., Ruiz, A., Rusakov, D. M., Scott, R., Semyanov, A., & Walker, M. C. (2005). Presynaptic, extrasynaptic and axonal GABA_A receptors in the CNS: Where and why? *Progress in Biophysics and Molecular Biology, 87*, 33–46.

Kuntz, A., Clement, H. W., Lehnert, W., van Calker, D., Hennighausen, K., Gerlach, M., et al. (2004). Effects of secretin on extracellular amino acid concentrations in rat hippocampus. *Journal of Neural Transmission, 111*, 931–939.

Kyrozis, A., & Reichling, D. B. (1995). Perforated-patch recording with gramicidin avoids artifactual changes in intracellular chloride concentration. *Journal of Neuroscience Methods, 57*, 27–35.

Lahtinen, H., Palva, J. M., Sumanen, S., Voipio, J., Kaila, K., & Taira, T. (2002). Postnatal development of rat hippocampal gamma rhythm in vivo. *Journal of Neurophysiology, 88*, 1469–1474.

Lamsa, K., Palva, J. M., Ruusuvuori, E., Kaila, K., & Taira, T. (2000). Synaptic GABA(A) activation inhibits AMPA-kainate receptor-mediated bursting in the newborn (P0–P2) rat hippocampus. *Journal of Neurophysiology, 83*, 359–366.

Laurie, D. J., Wisden, W., & Seeburg, P. H. (1992). The distribution of thirteen GABA_A receptor subunit mRNAs in the rat brain. III. Embryonic and postnatal development. *Journal of Neuroscience, 12*, 4151–4172.

Leblanc, M. O., & Bland, B. H. (1979). Developmental aspects of hippocampal electrical activity and motor behavior in the rat. *Experimental Neurology, 66*, 220–237.

Lee, H. H., Walker, J. A., Williams, J. R., Goodier, R. J., Payne, J. A., & Moss, S. J. (2007). Direct protein kinase c-dependent phosphorylation regulates the cell surface and activity of the potassium chloride cotransporter KCC2. *Journal of Biological Chemistry, 282*, 28777–28784.

Leinekugel, X., Khalilov, I., Ben-Ari, Y., & Khazipov, R. (1998). Giant depolarizing potentials: The septal pole of the hippocampus paces the activity of the developing intact septohippocampal complex in vitro. *Journal of Neuroscience, 18*, 6349–6357.

Leinekugel, X., Khazipov, R., Cannon, R., Hirase, H., Ben-Ari, Y., & Buzsaki, G. (2002). Correlated bursts of activity in the neonatal hippocampus in vivo. *Science, 296*, 2049–2052.

Lerma, J., Herranz, A. S., Herreras, O., Abraira, V., & Martin del Rio, R. (1986). In vivo determination of extracellular concentration of amino acids in the rat hippocampus.

A method based on brain dialysis and computerized analysis. *Brain Research, 384*, 145–155.

Lessmann, V., Gottmann, K., & Malcangio, M. (2003). Neurotrophin secretion: Current facts and future prospects. *Progress in Neurobiology, 69*, 341–374.

Lester, H. A., Dibas, M. I., Dahan, D. S., Leite, J. F., & Dougherty, D. A. (2004). Cys-loop receptors: New twists and turns. *Trends in Neurosciences, 27*, 329–336.

Li, H., Khirug, S., Cai, C., Ludwig, A., Blaesse, P., Kolikova, J., et al. (2007). KCC2 interacts with the dendritic cytoskeleton to promote spine development. *Neuron, 56*, 1019–1033.

Li, H., Tornberg, J., Kaila, K., Airaksinen, M. S., & Rivera, C. (2002). Patterns of cation-chloride cotransporter expression during embryonic rodent CNS development. *European Journal of Neuroscience, 16*, 2358–2370.

Liang, M., Tian, J., Liu, L., Pierre, S., Liu, J., Shapiro, J., et al. (2007). Identification of a pool of non-pumping Na/K-ATPase. *Journal of Biological Chemistry, 282*, 10585–10593.

Liu, Z., Neff, R. A., & Berg, D. K. (2006). Sequential interplay of nicotinic and GABAergic signaling guides neuronal development. *Science, 314*, 1610–1613.

Liu, Q. Y., Schaffner, A. E., Chang, Y. H., Maric, D., & Barker, J. L. (2000). Persistent activation of GABA(A) receptor/Cl(-) channels by astrocyte- derived GABA in cultured embryonic rat hippocampal neurons. *Journal of Neurophysiology, 84*, 1392–1403.

Liu, X., Wang, Q., Haydar, T. F., & Bordey, A. (2005). Nonsynaptic GABA signaling in postnatal subventricular zone controls proliferation of GFAP-expressing progenitors. *Nature Neuroscience, 8*, 1179–1187.

LoTurco, J. J., Owens, D. F., Heath, M. J., Davis, M. B., & Kriegstein, A. R. (1995). GABA and glutamate depolarize cortical progenitor cells and inhibit DNA synthesis. *Neuron, 15*, 1287–1298.

Lu, J., Karadsheh, M., & Delpire, E. (1999). Developmental regulation of the neuronal-specific isoform of K-Cl cotransporter KCC2 in postnatal rat brains. *Journal of Neurobiology, 39*, 558–568.

Luscher, B., & Keller, C. A. (2004). Regulation of GABA_A receptor trafficking, channel activity, and functional plasticity of inhibitory synapses. *Pharmacology and Therapeutics, 102*, 195–221.

Ma, W., & Barker, J. L. (1995). Complementary expressions of transcripts encoding GAD67 and GABAA receptor alpha 4, beta 1, and gamma 1 subunits in the proliferative zone of the embryonic rat central nervous system. *Journal of Neuroscience, 15*, 2547–2560.

Maffei, L., & Galli-Resta, L. (1990). Correlation in the discharges of neighboring rat retinal ganglion cells during prenatal life. *Proceedings of the National Academy of Sciences, 87*, 2861–2864.

Maguire, J., & Mody, I. (2007). Neurosteroid synthesis-mediated regulation of GABA(A) receptors: Relevance to the ovarian cycle and stress. *Journal of Neuroscience, 27*, 2155–2162.

Marchionni, I., Omrani, A., & Cherubini, E. (2007). In the developing rat hippocampus a tonic GABAA-mediated conductance selectively enhances the glutamatergic drive of principal cells. *Journal of Physiology, 581*, 515–528.

McCartney, M. R., Deeb, T. Z., Henderson, T. N., & Hales, T. G. (2007). Tonically active GABA_A receptors in hippocampal pyramidal neurons exhibit constitutive

GABA-independent gating. *Molecular Pharmacology, 71,* 539–548.

Marshall, F. H., Jones, K. A., Kaupmann, K., & Bettler, B. (1999). GABA$_B$ receptors—the first 7TM heterodimers. *Trends in Pharmacological Sciences, 20,* 396–399.

Martina, M., Royer, S., & Pare, D. (2001). Cell-type-specific GABA responses and chloride homeostasis in the cortex and amygdala. *Journal of Neurophysiology, 86,* 2887–2895.

Marty, S., Berninger, B., Carroll, P., & Thoenen, H. (1996). GABAergic stimulation regulates the phenotype of hippocampal interneurons through the regulation of brain-derived neurotrophic factor. *Neuron, 16,* 565–570.

Marty, A., & Llano, I. (2005). Excitatory effects of GABA in established brain networks. *Trends in Neurosciences, 28,* 284–289.

Marty, S., Wehrle, R., & Sotelo, C. (2000). Neuronal activity and brain-derived neurotrophic factor regulate the density of inhibitory synapses in organotypic slice cultures of postnatal hippocampus. *Journal of Neuroscience, 20,* 8087–8095.

McBain, C. J., & Fisahn, A. (2001). Interneurons unbound. *Nature Reviews Neuroscience, 2,* 11–23.

McKernan, R. M., & Whiting, P. J. (1996). Which GABA$_A$-receptor subtypes really occur in the brain? *Trends in Neurosciences, 19,* 139–143.

Meister, M., Wong, R. O., Baylor, D. A., & Shatz, C. J. (1991). Synchronous bursts of action potentials in ganglion cells of the developing mammalian retina. *Science, 252,* 939–943.

Menendez de la Prida, L., Bolea, S., & Sanchez-Andres, J. V. (1996). Analytical characterization of spontaneous activity evolution during hippocampal development in the rabbit. *Neuroscience Letters, 218,* 185–187.

Menendez de la Prida, L., Bolea, S., & Sanchez-Andres, J. V. (1998). Origin of the synchronized network activity in the rabbit developing hippocampus. *European Journal of Neuroscience, 10,* 899–906.

Menendez de la Prida, L., & Sanchez-Andres, J. V. (2000). Heterogeneous populations of cells mediate spontaneous synchroneous bursting in the developing hippocampus through a frequency-dependent mechanism. *Neuroscience, 97,* 227–241.

Mercado, A., Mount, D. B., & Gamba, G. (2004). Electroneutral cation-chloride cotransporters in the central nervous system. *Neurochemical Research, 29,* 17–25.

Michels, G., & Moss, S. J. (2007). GABA$_A$ receptors: Properties and trafficking. *Critical Reviews in Biochemistry and Molecular Biology, 42,* 3–14.

Minichiello, L., Casagranda, F., Tatche, R. S., Stucky, C. L., Postigo, A., Lewin, G.R., et al. (1998). Point mutation in trkB causes loss of NT4-dependent neurons without major effects on diverse BDNF responses. *Neuron, 21,* 335–345.

Minlebaev, M., Ben-Ari, Y., & Khazipov, R. (2007). Network mechanisms of spindle-burst oscillations in the neonatal rat barrel cortex in vivo. *Journal of Neurophysiology, 97,* 692–700.

Misgeld, U., Bijak, M., & Jarolimek, W. (1995). A physiological role for GABA$_B$ receptors and the effects of baclofen in the mammalian central nervous system. *Progress in Neurobiology, 46,* 423–462.

Misgeld, U., Deisz, R. A., Dodt, H. U., & Lux, H. D. (1986). The role of chloride transport in postsynaptic inhibition of hippocampal neurons. *Science, 232,* 1413–1415.

Mizoguchi, Y., Ishibashi, H., & Nabekura, J. (2003). The action of BDNF on GABA(A) currents changes from potentiating to suppressing during maturation of rat hippocampal CA1 pyramidal neurons. *Journal of Physiology, 548,* 703–709.

Mody, I. (2001). Distinguishing between GABAA receptors responsible for tonic and phasic conductances. *Neurochemical Research, 26,* 907–913.

Mody, I (2008). Extrasynaptic GABA(A) receptors in the crosshairs of hormones and ethanol. *Neurochemistry International, 52,* 60–64.

Mohajerani, M. H., & Cherubini, E. (2006). Role of giant depolarizing potentials in shaping synaptic currents in the developing hippocampus. *Critical Reviews in Neurobiology, 18,* 13–23.

Mohajerani, M. H., Sivakumaran, S., Zacchi, P., Aguilera, P., & Cherubini, E. (2007). Correlated network activity enhances synaptic efficacy via BDNF and the ERK pathway at immature CA3 CA1 connections in the hippocampus. *Proceedings of the National Academy of Sciences, 104,* 13176–13181.

Mohns, E. J., Karlsson, K., & Blumberg, M. S. (2007). Developmental emergence of transient and persistent hippocampal events and oscillations and their association with infant seizure susceptibility. *European Journal of Neuroscience, 26*(10), 2719–2730.

Moody, W. J, & Bosma, M. M. (2005). Ion channel development, spontaneous activity, and activity-dependent development in nerve and muscle cells. *Physiological Reviews, 85,* 883–941.

Moore-Hoon, M. L., & Turner, R. J. (2000). The structural unit of the secretory Na+-K+-2Cl- cotransporter (NKCC1) is a homodimer. *Biochemistry, 39,* 3718–3724.

Muller, D., Oliver, M., & Lynch, G. (1989). Developmental changes in synaptic properties in hippocampus of neonatal rats. *Brain Research. 49,* 105–114.

Nabekura, J., Ueno, T., Okabe, A., Furuta, A., Iwaki, T., Shimizu-Okabe, C., et al. (2002). Reduction of KCC2 expression and GABAA receptor-mediated excitation after in vivo axonal injury. *Journal of Neuroscience, 22,* 4412–4417.

Nusser, Z., Sieghart, W., & Somogyi, P. (1998) Segregation of different GABA$_A$ receptors to synaptic and extrasynaptic membranes of cerebellar granule cells. *Journal of Neuroscience, 18,* 1693–1703.

Obata, K., Oide, M., & Tanaka, H. (1978) Excitatory and inhibitory actions of GABA and glycine on embryonic chick spinal neurons in culture. *Brain Research, 144,* 179–184.

O'Donovan, M. J. (1999). The origin of spontaneous activity in developing networks of the vertebrate nervous system. *Current Opinion in Neurobiology, 9,* 94–104.

O'Donovan, K. J., Tourtellotte, W. G., Millbrandt, J., & Baraban, J. M. (1999). The EGR family of transcription-regulatory factors: Progress at the interface of molecular and systems neuroscience. *Trends in Neuroscience, 22,* 167–173.

Owens, D. F., & Kriegstein, A. R. (2002). Is there more to GABA than synaptic inhibition? *Nature Reviews Neuroscience, 3,* 715–727.

Owens, D. F., Liu, X., & Kriegstein, A. R. (1999). Changing properties of GABA$_A$ receptor-mediated signaling during early neocortical development. *Journal of Neurophysiology, 82,* 570–583.

Pan, Y., & Qian, H. (2005) Interactions between ρ and γ2 sub-units of the GABA receptor. *Journal of Neurochemistry, 94,* 482–490.

Pangratz-Fuehrer, S., Rudolph, U., & Huguenard, J. R. (2007). Giant spontaneous depolarizing potentials in the developing thalamic reticular nucleus. *Journal of Neurophysiology, 97,* 2364–2372.

Parker, M. D., & Boron, W. B. (2008). Sodium-coupled bicarbonate transporters. In R. Alpern & S. Hebert (Eds.), *Seldin & Giebisch's The Kidney* (pp. 1481–1498). Amsterdam: Elsevier.

Pasternack, M., Voipio, J., & Kaila, K. (1993). Intracellular carbonic anhydrase activity and its role in GABA-induced acidosis in isolated rat hippocampal pyramidal neurones. *Acta Physiologica Scandinavica, 148,* 229–231.

Pastorekova, S., Parkkila, S., Pastorek, J., & Supuran, C. T. (2004). Carbonic anhydrases: Current state of the art, therapeutic applications and future prospects. *Journal of Enzyme Inhibition and Medical Chemistry, 19,* 199–229.

Payne, J. A. (1997). Functional characterization of the neuronal-specific K-Cl cotransporter: Implications for $[K^+]_o$ regulation. *American Journal of Physiology, 273,* C1516–C1525.

Payne, J. A., Rivera, C., Voipio, J., & Kaila, K. (2003). Cation-chloride co-transporters in neuronal communication, development and trauma. *Trends in Neurosciences, 26,* 199–206.

Payne, J. A., Stevenson, T. J., & Donaldson, L. F. (1996). Molecular characterization of a putative K-Cl cotransporter in rat brain. A neuronal-specific isoform. *Journal of Biological Chemistry, 271,* 16245–16252.

Pedersen, S. F., O'Donnell, M. E., Anderson, S. E., & Cala, P. M. (2006). Physiology and pathophysiology of Na^+/H^+ exchange and Na^+ -K^+ -$2Cl^-$ cotransport in the heart, brain, and blood. *American Journal of Physiology-Regulatory Integrative and Comparative Physiology, 291,* R1–R25.

Penn, A. A., & Shatz, C. J. (1999). Brain waves and brain wiring: The role of endogenous and sensory-driven neural activity in development. *Pediatric Research, 45,* 447–458.

Perrot-Sinal, T. S., Sinal, C. J., Reader, J. C., Speert, D. B., & McCarthy, M. M. (2007). Sex differences in the chloride cotransporters, NKCC1 and KCC2, in the developing hypothalamus. *Journal of Neuroendocrinology, 19,* 302–308.

Pirker, S., Schwarzer, C., Wieselthaler, A., Sieghart, W., & Sperk, G. (2000). $GABA_A$ receptors: Immunocytochemical distribution of 13 subunits in the adult rat brain. *Neuroscience, 101,* 815–850.

Plotkin, M. D., Kaplan, M. R., Peterson, L. N., Gullans, S. R., Hebert, S. C., & Delpire, E. (1997). Expression of the Na^+-K^+-$2Cl^-$ cotransporter BSC2 in the nervous system. *American Journal of Physiology, 272,* C173–C183.

Pouille, F., & Scanziani, M. (2001). Enforcement of temporal fidelity in pyramidal cells by somatic feed-forward inhibition. *Science, 293,* 1159–1163.

Prenosil, G. A., Schneider Gasser, E. M., Rudolph, U., Keist, R., Fritschy, J. M., & Vogt, K. E. (2006). Specific subtypes of $GABA_A$ receptors mediate phasic and tonic forms of inhibition in hippocampal pyramidal neurons. *Journal of Neurophysiology, 96,* 846–857.

Qian, H., & Ripps, H. (1999). Response kinetics and pharmacological properties of heteromeric receptors formed by coassembly of GABA ρ- and γ2-subunits. *Proceedings of the Royal Society B—Biological Sciences, 266,* 2419–2425.

Represa, A., & Ben-Ari, Y. (2005). Trophic actions of GABA on neuronal development. *Trends in Neurosciences, 28*(6), 278–283.

Richerson, G. B., & Wu, Y. M. (2003). Dynamic equilibrium of neurotransmitter transporters: Not just for reuptake anymore. *Journal of Neurophysiology, 90,* 1363–1374.

Rivera, C., Li, H., Thomas-Crusells, J., Lahtinen, H., Viitanen, T., Nanobashvili, A., et al. (2002). BDNF-induced TrkB activation down-regulates the K^+-Cl^- cotransporter KCC2 and impairs neuronal Cl^- extrusion. *Journal of Cell Biology, 159,* 747–752.

Rivera, C., Voipio, J., & Kaila, K. (2005). Two developmental switches in GABAergic signalling: The K^+-Cl^- cotransporter KCC2 and carbonic anhydrase CAVII. *Journal of Physiology, 562,* 27–36.

Rivera, C., Voipio, J., Payne, J. A., Ruusuvuori, E., Lahtinen, H., Lamsa, K., et al. (1999). The K^+/Cl^- co-transporter KCC2 renders GABA hyperpolarizing during neuronal maturation. *Nature, 397,* 251–255.

Rivera, C., Voipio, J., Thomas-Crusells, J., Li, H., Emri, Z., Sipilä, S., et al. (2004). Mechanism of activity-dependent downregulation of the neuron-specific K-Cl cotransporter KCC2. *Journal of Neuroscience, 24,* 4683–4691.

Roberts, E., & Frankel, S. (1950). γ-Aminobutyric acid in brain: Its formation from glutamic acid. *Journal of Biological Chemistry, 187,* 55–63.

Romero, M. F., Fulton, C. M., & Boron, W. F. (2004). The SLC4 family of HCO_3-transporters. *Pflugers Archives, 447,* 495–509.

Roos, A., & Boron, W. F. (1981). Intracellular pH. *Physiological Reviews, 61,* 296–434.

Rudolph, U., & Mohler, H. (2004). Analysis of $GABA_A$ receptor function and dissection of the pharmacology of benzodiazepines and general anesthetics through mouse genetics. *Annual Reviews of Pharmacology and Toxicology, 44,* 475–498.

Russell, J. M. (2000). Sodium-potassium-chloride cotransport. *Physiological Reviews, 80,* 211–276.

Ruusuvuori, E., Li, H., Huttu, K., Palva, J. M., Smirnov, S., Rivera, C., et al. (2004). Carbonic anhydrase isoform VII acts as a molecular switch in the development of synchronous γ-frequency firing of hippocampal CA1 pyramidal cells. *Journal of Neuroscience, 24,* 2699–2707.

Safiulina, V. F., Kasyanov, A. M., Giniatullin, R., & Cherubini, E. (2005). Adenosine down-regulates giant depolarizing potentials in the developing rat hippocampus by exerting a negative control on glutamatergic inputs. *Journal of Neurophysiology, 94*(4), 2797–2804.

Saier, M. H. Jr., Tran, C. V., & Barabote, R. D. (2006) TCDB: The Transporter Classification Database for membrane transport protein analyses and information. *Nucleic Acids Research, 34* (Database issue): D181–D186.

Scimemi, A., Semyanov, A., Sperk, G., Kullmann, D. M., & Walker, M. C. (2005). Multiple and plastic receptors mediate tonic $GABA_A$ receptor currents in the hippocampus. *Journal of Neuroscience, 25,* 10016–10024.

Semyanov, A., Walker, M. C., Kullmann, D. M., & Silver, R. A. (2004). Tonically active $GABA_A$ receptors: Modulating gain and maintaining the tone. *Trends in Neurosciences, 27,* 262–269.

Senatorov, V. V., Stys, P. K., & Hu, B. (2000). Regulation of Na, K ATPase by persistent sodium accumulation in adult rat thalamic neurones. *Journal of Physiology, 525,* 343–353.

Serafini, R., Valeyev, A. Y., Barker, J. L., & Poulter, M. O. (1995). Depolarizing GABA-activated Cl⁻ channels in embryonic rat spinal and olfactory bulb cells. *Journal of Physiology, 488*, 371–386.

Shannon, C. E., & Weaver, W. (1949). *The mathematical theory of communication.* Chicago: University of Illinois Press.

Sieghart, W., & Ernst, M. (2005). Heterogeneity of GABA$_A$ receptors: Revived interest in the development of subtype-selective drugs. *Current Medicinal Chemistry—Central Nervous System Agents, 5*, 217–242.

Simard, C. F., Bergeron, M. J., Frenette-Cotton, R., Carpentier, G. A., Pelchat, M. E., Caron, L., et al. (2007). Homooligomeric and heterooligomeric associations between K+-Cl- cotransporter isoforms and between K⁺-Cl⁻ and Na⁺-K⁺-Cl⁻ cotransporters. *Journal of Biological Chemistry, 282*(25), 18083–18093.

Simon, J., Wakimoto, H., Fujita, N., Lalande, M., & Barnard, E. A. (2004). Analysis of the set of GABA$_A$ receptor genes in the human genome. *Journal of Biological Chemistry, 279*, 41422–41435.

Sine, S. M., & Engel, A. G. (2006). Recent advances in Cys-loop receptor structure and function. *Nature, 440*, 448–455.

Sipilä, S. T., Huttu, K., Soltesz, I., Voipio, J., & Kaila, K. (2005). Depolarizing GABA acts on intrinsically bursting pyramidal neurons to drive giant depolarizing potentials in the immature hippocampus. *Journal of Neuroscience, 25*, 5280–5289.

Sipilä, S., Huttu, K., Voipio, J., & Kaila, K., (2004). GABA uptake via GABA transporter-1 modulates GABAergic transmission in the immature hippocampus. *Journal of Neuroscience, 24*, 5877–5880.

Sipilä, S. T., Huttu, K., Voipio, J., & Kaila, K. (2006a). Intrinsic bursting of immature CA3 pyramidal neurons and consequent giant depolarizing potentials are driven by a persistent Na⁺ current and terminated by a slow Ca²⁺-activated K⁺ current. *European Journal of Neuroscience, 23*, 2330–2338.

Sipilä, S. T., Huttu, K., Yamada, J., Afzalov, A., Voipio, J., Blaesse, P., et al. (2009). Compensatory enhancement of intrinsic spiking upon NKCC1 disruption in neonatal hippocampus. *Journal of Neuroscience, 29*, 6982–6988.

Sipilä, S. T., Kaila, K. (2008). GABAergic control of CA3-driven network events in the developing hippocampus. *Results and Problems in Cell Differentiation, 44*, 99–121.

Sipilä, S. T., Schuchmann, S., Voipio, J., Yamada, J., & Kaila, K. (2006b). The cation-chloride cotransporter NKCC1 promotes sharp waves in the neonatal rat hippocampus. *Journal of Physiology, 573*(Pt 3), 765–773.

Sipilä, S. T., Voipio, J., & Kaila, K. (2007). GAT-1 acts to limit a tonic GABA(A) current in rat CA3 pyramidal neurons at birth. *European Journal of Neuroscience, 25*(3), 717–722.

Smirnov, S., Paalasmaa, P., Uusisaari, M., Voipio, J., & Kaila, K. (1999). Pharmacological isolation of the synaptic and nonsynaptic components of the GABA-mediated biphasic response in rat CA1 hippocampal pyramidal cells. *Journal of Neuroscience, 19*, 9252–9260.

Somogyi, P., & Klausberger, T. (2005). Defined types of cortical interneurone structure space and spike timing in the hippocampus. *Journal of Physiology, 562*(Pt 1), 9–26.

Starremans, P. G., Kersten, F. F., van den Heuvel, L. P., Knoers, N. V., & Bindels, R. J. (2003). Dimeric architecture of the human bumetanide-sensitive Na-K-Cl Co-transporter. *Journal of the American Society of Nephrology, 14*, 3039–3046.

Stasheff, S. F., Mott, D. D., & Wilson, W. A. (1993). Axon terminal hyperexcitability associated with epileptogenesis in vitro. II. Pharmacological regulation by NMDA and GABA$_A$ receptors. *Journal of Neurophysiology, 70*(3), 976–984.

Stein, V., Hermans-Borgmeyer, I., Jentsch, T. J., & Hubner, C. A. (2004) Expression of the KCl cotransporter KCC2 parallels neuronal maturation and the emergence of low intracellular chloride. *Journal of Comparative Neurology, 468*, 57–64.

Stell, B. M., Brickley, S. G., Tang, C. Y., Farrant, M., & Mody, I. (2003). Neuroactive steroids reduce neuronal excitability by selectively enhancing tonic inhibition mediated by delta subunit-containing GABA$_A$ receptors. *Proceedings of the National Academy of Sciences, 100*, 14439–14444.

Szabadics, J., Varga, C., Molnar, G., Olah, S., Barzo, P., & Tamas, G. (2006). Excitatory effect of GABAergic axo-axonic cells in cortical microcircuits. *Science, 311*, 233–235.

Takeuchi, A., & Takeuchi, N. (1971). Variations in the permeability properties of the inhibitory post-synaptic membrane of the crayfish neuromuscular junction when activated by different concentrations of GABA. *Journal of Physiology, 217*, 341–358.

Taira, T., Lamsa, K., & Kaila, K. (1997). Posttetanic excitation mediated by GABA(A) receptors in rat CA1 pyramidal neurons. *Journal of Neurophysiology, 77*(4), 2213–2218.

Taylor, J., & Gordon-Weeks, P. R. (1991). Calcium-independent gamma-aminobutyric acid release from growth cones: Role of gamma-aminobutyric acid transport. *Journal of Neurochemistry, 56*(1), 273–280.

Thompson, S. M., Deisz, R. A., & Prince, D. A. (1988a). Relative contributions of passive equilibrium and active transport to the distribution of chloride in mammalian cortical neurons, *Journal of Neurophysiology, 60*, 105–124.

Thompson, S. M., Deisz, R. A., & Prince, D. A. (1988b). Outward chloride/cation co-transport in mammalian cortical neurons. *Neuroscience Letters, 89*, 49–54.

Thompson, S. M., & Gähwiler, B. (1989). Activity-dependent disinhibition. II. Effects of extracellular potassium, furosemide and membrane potential on Ecl- in hippocampal CA3 neurons. *Journal of Neurophysiology, 61*, 512–523.

Tornberg, J., Voikar, V., Savilahti, H., Rauvala, H., & Airaksinen, M. S. (2005). Behavioural phenotypes of hypomorphic KCC2-deficient mice. *European Journal of Neuroscience, 21*(5), 1327–1337.

Tossman, U., & Ungerstedt, U. (1986). Microdialysis in the study of extracellular levels of amino acids in the rat brain. *Acta Physiologica Scandinavica, 128*(1), 9–14.

Toyoda, H., Ohno, K., Yamada, J., Ikeda, M., Okabe, A., Sato, K., et al. (2003). Induction of NMDA and GABA$_A$ receptor-mediated Ca²⁺ oscillations with KCC2 mRNA downregulation in injured facial motoneurons. *Journal of Neurophysiology, 89*, 1353–1362.

Tozuka, Y., Fukuda, S., Namba, T., Seki, T., & Hisatsune, T. (2005). GABAergic excitation promotes neuronal differentiation in adult hippocampal progenitor cells. *Neuron, 47*(6), 803–815.

Tretter, V., Ehya, N., Fuchs, K., & Sieghart, W. (1997). Stoichiometry and assembly of a recombinant GABA$_A$ receptor subtype. *Journal of Neuroscience, 17*, 2728–2737.

Tukker, J. J., Fuentealba, P., Hartwich, K., Somogyi, P., & Klausberger, T. (2007). Cell type-specific tuning of hippocampal interneuron firing during gamma oscillations in vivo. *Journal of Neuroscience, 27*(31), 8184–8189.

Tyzio, R., Cossart, R., Khalilov, I., Minlebaev, M., Hubner, C.A., Represa, A., et al. (2006). Maternal oxytocin triggers a transient inhibitory switch in GABA signaling in the fetal brain during delivery. *Science, 314*, 1788–1792.

Tyzio, R., Ivanov, A., Bernard, C., Holmes, G. L., Ben-Ari, Y., & Khazipov, R. (2003). Membrane potential of CA3 hippocampal pyramidal cells during postnatal development. *Journal of Neurophysiology, 90*(5), 2964–2972.

Tyzio, R., Represa, A., Jorquera, I., Ben-Ari, Y., Gozlan, H., & Aniksztejn, L. (1999). The establishment of GABAergic and glutamatergic synapses on CA1 pyramidal neurons is sequential and correlates with the development of the apical dendrite. *Journal of Neuroscience, 19*, 10372–10382.

Unwin, N. (2005). Refined structure of the nicotinic acetylcholine receptor at 4 Å resolution. *Journal of Molecular Biology, 346*, 967–989.

Uvarov, P., Ludwig, A., Markkanen, M., Pruunsild, P., Kaila, K., Delpire, E., et al. (2007) A novel N-terminal isoform of the neuron-specific K-Cl cotransporter KCC2. *Journal of Biological Chemistry 282*(42), 30570–30576.

Uvarov, P., Ludwig, A., Markkanen, M., Rivera, C., & Airaksinen, M. S. (2006). Upregulation of the neuron-specific K^+/Cl^- cotransporter expression by transcription factor early growth response 4. *Journal of Neuroscience, 26*, 13463–13473.

Vale, C., Caminos, E., Martinez-Galan, J. R., & Juiz, J. M. (2005). Expression and developmental regulation of the K^+-Cl^- cotransporter KCC2 in the cochlear nucleus. *Hearing Research, 206*(1–2), 107–115.

Valeyev, A. Y., Cruciani, R. A., Lange, G. D., Smallwood, V. S., & Barker, J. L. (1993). Cl- channels are randomly activated by continuous GABA secretion in cultured embryonic rat hippocampal neurons. *Neuroscience Letters, 155*(2), 199–203.

Vanhatalo, S., & Kaila, K. (2006). Development of neonatal EEG activity: From phenomenology to physiology. *Seminars in Fetal and Neonatal Medicine, 11*(6), 471–478.

Vanhatalo, S., Palva, J. M., Andersson, S., Rivera, C., Voipio, J., & Kaila, K. (2005). Slow endogenous activity transients and developmental expression of K^+-Cl^- cotransporter 2 in the immature human cortex. *European Journal of Neuroscience, 22*, 2799–2804.

Vanhatalo, S., Tallgren, P., Andersson, S., Sainio, K., Voipio, J., & Kaila, K. (2002). DC-EEG discloses prominent, very slow activity patterns during sleep in preterm infants. *Clinical Neurophysiology, 113*, 1822–1825.

van Praag, H., Shinder, A. F., Christie, B. R., Toni, N., Palmer, T. D., & Gage, F. H. (2002). Functional neurogenesis in the adult hippocampus. *Nature, 415*(6875), 1030–1034.

Vardi, N., Zhang, L. L., Payne, J. A., & Sterling, P. (2000). Evidence that different cation chloride cotransporters in retinal neurons allow opposite responses to GABA. *Journal of Neuroscience, 20*, 7657–7663.

Varoqueaux, F., Sigler, A., Rhee, J. S., Brose, N., Enk, C., Reim, K., et al. (2002). Total arrest of spontaneous and evoked synaptic transmission but normal synaptogenesis in the absence of Munc13-mediated vesicle priming. *Proceedings of the National Academy of Sciences, 99*, 9037–9042.

Verhage, M., Maia, A. S., Plomp, J. J., Brussaard, A. B., Heeroma, J. H., Vermeer, H., et al. (2000). Synaptic assembly of the brain in the absence of neurotransmitter secretion. *Science, 287*, 864–869.

Verheugen, J. A., Fricker, D., & Miles, R. (1999). Noninvasive measurements of the membrane potential and GABAergic action in hippocampal interneurons. *Journal of Neuroscience, 19*, 2546–2555.

Vida, I., Bartos, M., & Jonas, P. (2006). Shunting inhibition improves robustness of gamma oscillations in hippocampal interneuron networks by homogenizing firing rates. *Neuron, 49*, 107–117.

Vilen, H., Eerikäinen, S., Tornberg, J., Airaksinen, M. S., & Savilahti, H. (2001). Construction of gene-targeting vectors: A rapid Mu in vitro DNA transposition-based strategy generating null, potentially hypomorphic, and conditional alleles. *Transgenic Research, 10*(1), 69–80.

Voipio, J., & Kaila, K. (2000). GABAergic excitation and K(+)-mediated volume transmission in the hippocampus. *Progress in Brain Research, 125*, 329–338.

Voipio, J., Pasternack, M., Rydqvist, B., & Kaila, K. (1991). Effect of gamma-aminobutyric acid on intracellular pH in the crayfish stretch-receptor neurone. *Journal of Experimental Biology, 156*, 349–360.

Vullo, D., Voipio, J., Innocenti, A., Rivera, C., Ranki, H., Scozzafava, A., et al. (2005). Carbonic anhydrase inhibitors. Inhibition of the human cytosolic isozyme VII with aromatic and heterocyclic sulfonamides. *Bioorganic and Medicinal Chemistry Letters, 15*, 971–976.

Wake, H., Watanabe, M., Moorhouse, A. J., Kanematsu, T., Horibe, S., Matsukawa, N., et al. (2007). Early changes in KCC2 phosphorylation in response to neuronal stress result in functional downregulation. *Journal of Neuroscience, 27*(7), 1642–1650.

Wall, M. J., & Usowicz, M. M. (1997). Development of action potential-dependent and independent spontaneous GABA$_A$ receptor-mediated currents in granule cells of postnatal rat cerebellum. *European Journal of Neuroscience, 9*, 533–548.

Wang, C. T., Blankenship, A. G., Anishchenko, A., Elstrott, J., Fikhman, M., Nakanishi, S., et al. (2007). GABA(A) receptor-mediated signaling alters the structure of spontaneous activity in the developing retina. *Journal of Neuroscience, 27*, 9130–9140.

Wardle, R. A., & Poo, M. M. (2003). Brain-derived neurotrophic factor modulation of GABAergic synapses by postsynaptic regulation of chloride transport. *Journal of Neuroscience, 23*, 8722–8732.

Wei, W., Zhang, N., Peng, Z., Houser, C. R., & Mody, I. (2003). Perisynaptic localization of d subunit-containing GABA$_A$ receptors and their activation by GABA spillover in the mouse dentate gyrus. *Journal of Neuroscience, 23*, 10650–10661.

Welker, W. I. (1964) Analysis of sniffing of the albino rat. *Behaviour, 12*, 223–244.

Wells, J. E., Porter, J. T., & Agmon, A. (2000). GABAergic inhibition suppresses paroxysmal network activity in the neonatal rodent hippocampus and neocortex. *Journal of Neuroscience, 20*(23), 8822–8830.

Whittington, M. A., & Traub, R. D. (2003). Interneuron diversity series: Inhibitory interneurons and network oscillations in vitro. *Trends in Neurosciences, 26*, 676–682.

Williams, J. R., & Payne, J. A. (2004). Cation transport by the neuronal K(+)-Cl(-) cotransporter KCC2: Thermodynamics and kinetics of alternate transport modes. *American Journal of Physiology—Cell Physiology, 287*(4), C919–C931.

Williams, J. R., Sharp, J. W., Kumari, V. G., Wilson, M., & Payne, J.A. (1999). The neuron-specific K-Cl cotransporter, KCC2. Antibody development and initial characterization of the protein. *Journal of Biological Chemistry, 274,* 12656–12664.

Wisden, W., Laurie, D. J., Monyer, H., & Seeburg, P. H. (1992). The distribution of 13 $GABA_A$ receptor subunit mRNAs in the rat brain. I. Telencephalon, diencephalon, mesencephalon. *Journal of Neuroscience, 12,* 1040–1062.

Wojcik, S. M., Katsurabayashi, S., Guillemin, I., Friauf, E., Rosenmund, C., Brose, N., et al. (2006). A shared vesicular carrier allows synaptic corelease of GABA and glycine. *Neuron, 50*(4), 575–587.

Wolff, J. R., Joo, F., & Dames, W. (1978). Plasticity in dendrites shown by continuous GABA administration in superior cervical ganglion of adult rat. *Nature, 274,* 72–74.

Woo, N. S., Lu, J., England, R., McClellan, R., Dufour, S., Mount, D. B., et al. (2002). Hyperexcitability and epilepsy associated with disruption of the mouse neuronal-specific K-Cl cotransporter gene. *Hippocampus, 12,* 258–268.

Wotring, V. E., Chang, Y., & Weiss, D. S. (1999). Permeability and single channel conductance of human homomeric rho1 $GABA_C$ receptors. *Journal of Physiology, 521,* 327–336.

Wooltorton, J. R. A., Whiting, P., & Smart, T. G. (1995). Anion permeability of human recombinant $GABA_A$-gated chloride channels expressed in Xenopus oocytes. *Journal of Physiology, 489,* 80–81.

Yamada, J., Okabe, A., Toyoda, H., Kilb, W., Luhmann, H. J., & Fukuda, A. (2004) Cl- uptake promoting depolarizing GABA actions in immature rat neocortical neurones is mediated by NKCC1. *Journal of Physiology, 557,* 829–841.

Ylinen, A., Bragin, A., Nadasdy, Z., Jando, G., Szabo, I., Sik, A., et al. (1995b). Sharp wave-associated high-frequency oscillation (200 Hz) in the intact hippocampus: Network and intracellular mechanisms. *Journal of Neuroscience, 15,* 30–46.

Ylinen, A., Soltesz, I., Bragin, A., Penttonen, M., Sik, A., & Buzsaki, G. (1995a). Intracellular correlates of hippocampal theta rhythm in identified pyramidal cells, granule cells, and basket cells. *Hippocampus, 5,* 78–90.

Yuste, R., & Katz, L. C., (1991). Control of postsynaptic Ca^{2+} influx in developing neocortex by excitatory and inhibitory neurotransmitters. *Neuron, 6,* 333–344.

Yuste, R., Peinado, A., & Katz, L. C. (1992). Neuronal domains in developing neocortex. *Science, 257,* 665–669.

Zhou, Q., & Poo, M. M. (2004). Reversal and consolidation of activity-induced synaptic modifications. *Trends in Neurosciences, 27*(7), 378–383.

Neural Activity and Visual System Development

Tony del Rio *and* Marla B. Feller

Abstract

The connections that comprise the mature visual system are remarkably precise, forming spatial representations, or "maps," of various features of visual space. Maps emerge during development from initially diffuse and poorly ordered projections in a manner that is dependent upon molecular interactions and neural activity. Prior to the onset of vision, neural activity in the retina is spontaneously generated, exhibiting a correlated, propagating pattern termed retinal waves. At the same time, the retina, superior colliculus, thalamus, and visual cortex express guidance molecules that influence the final connectivity pattern. This chapter describes the relative role of neural activity and molecular guidance factors in the process of refinement of both retinotopic and ocular dominance maps in the visual system.

Keywords: spatial representations, maps, visual space, neural activity, retina, colliculus, thalamus, visual cortex

Introduction

Precise connectivity both within the retina and between the retina and brain was described over a century ago by Ramon y Cajal (Figure 7.1). Since that time, the visual system has become a classic model for studying the development of neural circuitry. One central question concerning visual system development is whether connections are specified from the outset, or whether precise connections are formed by a dynamic process through which inappropriate inputs are eliminated and appropriate ones are stabilized. Roger Sperry (1963) first proposed the notion that the orderly topographic projections of nerve fibers are mediated by molecular cue gradients. Experimentally, Sperry and colleagues found that by severing the optic trunk and selectively removing half of the retina of a fish, nerve fibers from remaining halves of the retina regrew into specific, predesignated

target zones in the midbrain (Figure 7.2). Based on this work and other studies of regeneration, a chemoaffinity hypothesis was proposed in which map specification was attributed to the presence of chemical tags distributed as gradients along different axes. In regeneration experiments, the chemical gradients would be present in both the midbrain and retina, with innervating axons presenting the gradient information from the retina. According to this hypothesis, any given location within two or more gradients will possess a unique chemical code that can then be matched between innervating axons and the target.

In the 1960s and 1970s, experiments by Hubel and Wiesel demonstrated the flexibility present within the developing visual system. They found that the representation of the inputs of the two eyes in primary visual cortex could be altered in response to closing one eye (Hubel & Wiesel, 1963; Wiesel

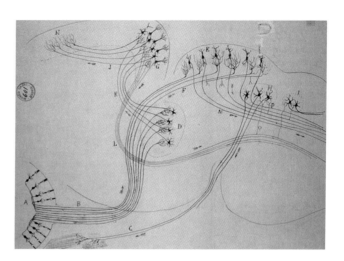

Figure 7.1 Schematic of pathways of the optic centers. (Drawing by S.R. y Cajal, 1901. Cajal Institute, CSIC [Consejo Superior de Investigaciones Científicas], Madrid, Spain.)

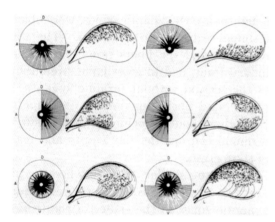

Figure 7.2 The regeneration and targeting of regions of the retina to the midbrain in fish reveals map specification. After removal of half of the retina and severance of the optic nerve, retinal projections regenerate in the fish tectum. The diagram is a summary of regeneration experiments performed by Roger Sperry and colleagues around 1960. The data demonstrate that patterns of nerve fibers from retinal halves of different regions in the eye target to predesignated zones in the midbrain tectum. (Image from Sperry, 1963.)

& Hubel, 1965a). This was a powerful demonstration of how altering neural activity by changing sensory experience could alter functional circuits of the brain.

These classic experiments have have led to investigations that are the focus of modern day developmental neurobiology—what are the relative roles of molecular cues and activity in the development of precisely connected neural circuits? The primary model is that the initial establishment of visual circuits, such as axons projecting to their correct target structures, is determined by molecular cues and that later stages of refinement are mediated by visual activity. However, there has been growing evidence that even before vision is possible, spontaneous activity in the retina plays a role in several aspects of the formation of early visual circuits.

Visual experience begins a few days prior to eye-opening, when light-evoked responses can be elicited in the retina (Akerman, Smyth, & Thompson, 2002; Tian & Copenhagen, 2003). Prior to this development, intrinsically photosensitive retinal ganglion cells (RGCs) have matured and circadian rhythms are detected (Tu et al., 2005). This chapter will focus on the period of visual system development prior to eye-opening, which represents the onset of normal visual experience. We review experiments that contribute to the current understanding of how visual system development is mediated by a combination of molecular cues and spontaneous retinal activity.

Organization of the Visual System

An important function of vision is to rapidly encode and distribute environmental signals perceived by the visual sensory organ to processing centers deep in the brain. At birth, mammalian vision can be poor or not possible, and the visual system continues to develop for weeks thereafter. The RGCs are the readout cells of the retina in that they are the sole transmitters of visual information to the brain. As the retina and brain develop, axonal projections from RGCs enter the optic stalk, the predecessor to the optic nerve, and later reach the visual centers in the brain. In general, an enormous amount of visual circuit development occurs between when RGC projections first innervate their primary targets in the brain and the onset of normal visual experience at eye-opening, a period that lasts several weeks in rodents, one-and-a-half months in cat and ferret, and several months in primates. (Table 7.1). This period in visual development is the topic of review here.

The primary targets of retinal projections are the superior colliculus (SC), which mediates visuomotor reflexes; the lateral geniculate nucleus (LGN) of the thalamus, which projects to primary visual cortex and is part of the pathway that mediates conscious visual experience (Figure 7.3); and the suprachiasmatic nucleus (SCN), involved in circadian rhythm control. While subclasses of RGCs project to several targets in the brain that mediate circadian rhythms, this will not be covered in this chapter. Primary visual cortex, also referred to as V1 or striate cortex, is where more complex receptive fields are formed, such as stimulus orientation, movement, and binocularity. In nonmammalian vertebrates, the SC is referred to as the optic tectum (OT). In many mammals such as rodents and primates, both the SC and LGN in each hemisphere of the brain receive direct inputs from both eyes.

A key feature of visual circuitry is that it is organized to convey spatial information in a visual field from the retina to the brain. Neighboring RGCs in the retina project to neighboring cells in the brain and form a continuous topographic map in the target. When retinal axons initially innervate the LGN and SC, they are unordered and intermingle.

Over time, and prior to eye-opening, retinotopic maps emerge.

In addition to forming topographic maps, retinal axon terminations in the LGN develop into eye-specific layers. Eye-specific layers are a physical segregation of projections from the two eyes within the dorsal LGN (dLGN) such that target neurons receive input exclusively from one or the other eye. In carnivores, such as ferrets and cats, ipsilateral eye inputs segregate into distinct cellular layers within the dLGN. In rodents, where less than 10% of the RGCs project ipsilaterally, the eye-specific regions are less well defined—ipsilateral inputs segregate into a small region surrounded by a larger, continuous layer of contralateral inputs. Eye-specific segregation is maintained in thalamic projections to visual cortex. The axons from the eye-specific layers in the dLGN segregate into ocular dominance columns (ODCs) within layer 4 in carnivores. In rodents, axons from eye-specific layers project to the binocular region where they intermingle, though individual layer 4 neurons receive input from one eye or the other. The first binocular cells are detected in layer 2/3.

In contrast to eye-specific layers in the dLGN, eye-specific patches form in the SC. The retinal projections to the SC are predominantly from the contralateral eye, but ipsilateral projections form patches in the rostral part of the SC. In rodents, an individual RGC projection to the dLGN is a collateral branch of the same projection to the SC, while in several other species, including cats, ferrets, and primates, distinct populations of RGCs project to either the dLGN or SC.

Table 7.1 A Comparison of the Relative Time Period of Early Visual Circuit Development Prior To Visual Stimulation Across Model Species and Humans

Species	RGC Birth	RGC Axons Innervate the Visual Centers	Eye Opening	Time Between Innervation/ Visual Stimulation (Post Birth)
Human	G38	G75 (60)	G160 (182)	12.1w (17.4)[a]
Monkey[b]	G31 (30)	G60	G126 (123)	9.4w [a]
Ferret	G20 (21)	G30.5 (26)	G75 (72)	6.4w (6.6)
Cat	G21.5 (19.5)	G33 (32)	G82 (72)	7w (5.7)
Rabbit	G13 (13)	G18.5	G43 (43)	3.5w
Rat	G11 (11.5)	G16 (15)	G36 (36)	2.9w (3)
Mouse	G10 (10.5)	G14 (15.5)	G30 (30)	2.3w (2.1)

Data adapted from Clancy, Darlington, and Finlay (2001) where a model was used to standardize the developmental time of neural events across species. When possible, empirically derived data was included in parenthesis (see Clancy et al., 2001 for references).
G = gestational day, w = weeks.
[a] Based on visual stimulation on the day of birth at G270 for human, and G165 for monkey.
[b] Macaque monkey.

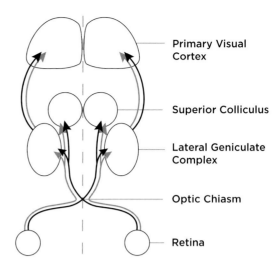

Figure 7.3 Simplified diagram of the retinocollicular and retinogeniculocortical pathways in mammals. Axons from the retina cross at the optic chiasm such that the visual centers in both the left and right hemispheres of the brain receive input from both left and right eyes. The primary visual centers include the lateral geniculate nucleus (LGN) and superior colliculus (SC). The LGN projects to the primary visual cortex, which also receives eye-specific input from both eyes.

Primary Visual Cortex

Superior Colliculus

Lateral Geniculate Complex

Optic Chiasm

Retina

Molecular Cues and Gradients

As mentioned above, the notion that the formation of orderly topographic projections of RGC axons is mediated by chemical tags was originally proposed by Sperry. It is now well accepted that molecular cues distributed in gradients can direct the formation of visual maps in the brain. Perhaps the best characterized guidance molecules include members of the ephrin family of ligands and receptors, and numerous studies on these molecules largely support Sperry's chemoaffinity hypothesis. The first ephrin receptor was identified in 1987 in a cancer-related screen, and termed "Eph" after the erythopoeitin-producing hepatocellular carcinoma cell line where its expression was found to be elevated (Hirai, Maru, Hagiwara, Nishida, & Takaku, 1987). The Ephs are receptor tyrosine kinases, with an extracellular domain that binds to ephrin ligands, a single transmembrane domain, and cytoplasmic homology to tyrosine kinase. The receptors are organized into subclasses A or B based on relative homology to each other, and their ligands, in turn, are divided into ephrin-A or -B classes based on binding preference to the receptor. While ephrin-B ligands are transmembrane molecules, ephrin-As are membrane associated via a glycosylphosphatidylinositol (GPI) anchor, a glycolipid, or carbohydrate-attached lipid modification, which inserts or anchors into membrane. Ephs can signal intracellularly once they are bound by their appropriate ligand, and there is evidence that both ephrin-A and ephrin-B ligand molecules can signal intracellularly (Flanagan, 2006; McLaughlin & O'Leary, 2005). At least 16 receptors (EphsA1–10, EphB1–6) and 9 ligands (ephrinA1–6, ephrinB1–3) have been discovered in vertebrates, providing the building blocks for a complex array of molecular cues in just the ephrin class of guidance molecules alone. Many of these ephrins and Ephs are found in gradients in both the retina and developing visual centers in the brain (Flanagan, 2006; McLaughlin & O'Leary, 2005).

Guidance Molecules and Retinocollicular Map Development

Retinotopic refinement within the SC is a classic example of how gradients of guidance molecules can mediate precise axon targeting during development. In the adult, the intersection of multiple molecular cue gradients identify a unique position within a colliculus, akin to a biological zip code composed of a unique concentration of different molecular cues. The question remains as to how these gradients function to generate the retinotopic maps during development.

In frogs and fish, RGC axons innervate the tectum and stop at the appropriate location, uniquely defined by the chemotropic signaling of guidance molecules, such as the ephrins. Once RGCs reach their locations, the tip of the axon sprouts many branches to generate the final target zone of the projection. However, in chicks and rodents, axons overshoot their appropriate location. They then undergo a process of refinement that involves increases in axonal branching along the axon shaft in the appropriate location and withdrawal of the overshooting part of the axon. How can a stationary gradient contribute to this dynamic process?

Here we review the evidence that supports the hypothesis that signaling between ephrins and Ephs contribute to this refinement process. Gradients of ephrins and their receptors, Ephs, from both subclasses (A and B) are found in the SC and retina (Flanagan, 2006; McLaughlin & O'Leary, 2005). One of the first in vivo reports of complementary molecular gradients showed that EphA3 is expressed in a low nasal to high temporal gradient in the chick retina, while its ligand ephrin-A2 is expressed low anterior to high posterior in the tectum (the nonmammalian SC) (Cheng, Nakamoto, Bergemann, & Flanagan, 1995). Since the temporal retina projects to the anterior region of the tectum, retinal axons expressing high amounts of EphA map to target regions expressing low levels of ephrin-A ligand, indicative of a repulsive guidance cue. Similar gradients were reported in mouse, with a low nasal to high temporal gradient of EphA5 in the retina and low anterior to high posterior ephrin-A2 and ephrin-A5 in the SC (Feldheim et al., 1998).

An important technique in the study of retinotopic map refinement is the visualization of termination zones (TZ) formed by a small group of neighboring RGCs in the retina. The axons of a small cluster of RGCs can be visualized by focal injection and subsequent anterograde labeling with the fluorescent lipophilic dye DiI (1,1'-dioctadecyl-3,3,3',3'-tetramethylindocarbocyanine perchlorate) (Thanos & Bonhoeffer, 1987). Using this technique, it was found that chick and rodent RGC axons initially overshoot their appropriate TZs in the tectum or SC along the anterior–posterior axis, extending posterior to their future TZ (Simon & O'Leary, 1992a; Yates, Roskies, McLaughlin, & O'Leary, 2001).

Importantly, targeted gene knockouts in mice have been coupled with DiI labeling of TZs to demonstrate a requirement for ephrins in proper retinal axon guidance in the midbrain. Mice lacking ephrin-A5 develop a subset of topographically incorrect RGC terminations consistent with the loss of the repellent cue in the posterior SC (Frisen et al., 1998). Anterior–posterior (A-P) patterning remains largely normal in ephrin-A5-null mice, but ectopically localized RGC terminations in these mutant mice appear to target regions of low ephrin-A2 expression along the A-P axis, suggesting that multiple cues work in concert to create continuous repulsive gradients. Indeed, truncation mutants of mouse EphA3 or chick EphA5, in which the membrane receptors have been truncated

by removal of intracellular regions containing the tyrosine kinase domain, demonstrated similar targeting defects (Feldheim et al., 2004). Furthermore, ephrin-A2/A5 double null mice exhibit more severe mistargeting than mice lacking either ephrin-A2 or ephrin-A5 alone (Feldheim et al., 2004). When four different retinal axes positions of ephrin-A2/A3/A5 triple knockout mice are labeled by DiI injection, multiple ectopic TZs are evident but are still targeted to the SC (Pfeiffenberger, Yamada, & Feldheim, 2006).

Gain-of-function experiments, in which isolated genes are expressed exogenously, have confirmed the repulsive cue nature of ephrins and Ephs in vivo. For example, virus-induced overexpression of ephrin-A2 in the chick tectum causes temporal, but not nasal retinal axons to avoid localized patches of elevated ephrin-A2 (Nakamoto et al., 1996). Interestingly, while EphA3 is expressed in chick but not mouse RGCs, its ectopic expression in a subset of mouse RGCs by a gene targeting approach caused RGC axons with high receptor expression to avoid regions of SC with high ephrin levels (Brown et al., 2000). Numerous in vitro stripe assays further demonstrate that mouse or chick RGCs avoid membrane stripes containing high levels of ephrin-As (Drescher et al., 1995; Feldheim et al., 1998; Nakamoto et al., 1996) or EphA-containing substrates (Rashid et al., 2005), but not those with low levels of these molecules. However, RGCs demonstrate a graded responsiveness to ephrin-A2 based on retinal position, where, in general, high amounts of ephrins are repulsive and low amounts attractive (Hansen, Dallal, & Flanagan, 2004). The transitional point, where the concentration of ephrin-A2 changes from an attractive to a repulsive cue and the net effect is neutral, appears to specify the target location for a given RGC within this gradient. By targeting their respective transitional or neutral points within gradients in the SC, neighboring RGCs are able to project a topographic map of their relative position in the retina. This is consistent with Sperry's chemoaffinity hypothesis proposed decades earlier.

Thus far, we have described the ingrowth and refinement of axons originating from the nasal–temporal (N–T) axis of the retina and described the role of ephrin-A/EphA signaling. The ingrowth and refinement of axons originating from the dorsal–ventral (D–V) axis of the retina relies on a different class of guidance molecules, ephrin-/EphB. Upon ingrowth into the SC, axons that emerge along the D–V retinal axis exhibit a broad distribution along the lateral–medial (L–M) axis (Simon & O'Leary, 1992a, 1992b). Axons from a given D–V location in the retina form interstitial branches that establish order along the L–M axis. Expression analysis shows that ephrin-Bs and their EphB receptors are expressed in countergradients in the OT/SC and retina in a way that could mediate mapping along the L–M axis. EphBs-2,3,4 are expressed in a low dorsal to high ventral gradient in the retina while ephrinB1 ligand is expressed low lateral to high medial in the SC (Hindges, McLaughlin, Genoud, Henkemeyer, & O'Leary, 2002) and OT (Braisted et al., 1997). The D–V retinal axis projects onto the L–M SC axis such that retinal axons that express high levels of EphBs map to target regions that express high levels of ephrinBs.

Mice lacking both EphB2 and EphB3 exhibit D–V mapping defects in the SC, thus directly demonstrating a role for EphB/ephrinB gradients in L–M axis mapping (Hindges et al., 2002). These mutant mice form lateral ectopic TZs, similar to mice expressing kinase-inactive EphB2 (Hindges et al., 2002). Gain-of-function experiments in chicks demonstrate that the ectopic expression of high ephrin-B1 levels repels RGC axon interstitial branches along the L–M axis, while the primary RGC axons are unaffected (McLaughlin, Hindges, Yates, & O'Leary, 2003a). Thus, at high concentration, ephrin-B1 may act as a repellant for interstitial branches and an attractant at lower concentrations although the presence of other repellant cues along the L–M axis cannot be eliminated.

Though ephrin gradients have been well-studied, there is a growing list of factors including morphogens (e.g., bone morphogenetic protein [BMP]; Chandrasekaran, Plas, Gonzalez, & Crair, 2005), chemoattractants (e.g., semaphorins; Halloran & Wolman, 2006; Komiyama, Sweeney, Schuldiner, Garcia, & Luo, 2007; Liu et al., 2004; Wolman, Liu, Tawarayama, Shoji, & Halloran, 2004), and transcription factors (e.g., Wnt3 and Engrailed-2; Brunet et al., 2005; Schmitt et al., 2006) whose expression as gradients in either the retina or the SC make them intriguing candidates for influencing the formation of retinotopic maps.

Guidance Molecules and Retinogeniculate Eye-Specific Map Development

Though there is tremendous evidence supporting the idea that guidance molecules contribute to retinotopic refinement, are they also involved in eye-specific refinement of retinogeniculate axons? Ipsilateral projecting axons emerge from lateral retina while contralateral projecting axons emerge from nasal retina. Hence, "eye-specific" layers may also represent a segregation of axons from two distinct topographic regions in the retina.

Gradients of ephrins exist in the thalamus of the developing brain, though in a somewhat more complicated pattern than in the SC. For example, ephrin-A2 and ephrin-A5 are expressed in a high ventro-lateral-anterior to low dorsal-medial-posterior gradient in the mouse dLGN and vLGN (Feldheim et al., 1998; Pfeiffenberger et al., 2005). Using a probe that detects multiple ephrin-A molecules, a high lateral to low medial gradient distribution was observed in the ferret LGN (Huberman, Murray, Warland, Feldheim, & Chapman, 2005). Furthermore, EphA molecules were found in a high center to low periphery gradient in the ferret retina. This indicates that the LGN receives contralateral inputs with higher EphA levels and ipsilateral inputs with lower EphA levels. The outer LGN (with high ephrinA) appears to repel contralateral axons (with high EphA), with targeting of contralateral inputs to layer A in the inner LGN (with low ephrinA). Therefore, as with RGC axons in the SC/tectum, high ephrin-A and EphA concentrations are repulsive while low ephrin-A and EphA pairings are attractive. A balance of attractive and repulsive cues in the LGN likely target RGC projections to a neutral point within gradients and can allow for the continuous mapping of retinal projections, resulting in topography.

In a loss-of-function experiment, focal injections of DiI in the developing retina of ephrin-A5-null mice reveal broader terminal arborizations to the dLGN that were scattered along the nasotemporal axis (Feldheim et al., 1998). In contrast to focal labeling in the retina, eye-specific layers in the LGN are readily visualized by the bulk labeling of RGCs in opposite eyes with anterograde tracers. Such tracers include [3H]-leucine, horseradish peroxidase–conjugated wheat germ agglutinin (WGA-HRP), and fluorophore-conjugated cholera toxin subunit B (Angelucci, Clasca, & Sur, 1996; Huberman, Stellwagen, & Chapman, 2002; Rakic, 1976; Shatz, 1983). Using bulk axonal labeling, it was shown that eye-specific layers are disrupted in mice lacking multiple ephrin ligands. In the combined absence of ephrins-A2/A5 or ephrins-A2/A3/A5 (but not single or other double mutants), eye-specific patches, and not intact layers, form along the entire dorsoventral axis of the dLGN (Pfeiffenberger et al., 2005). Although the triple mutant exhibits more severe ectopic patch formation in the thalamus, eye-specific inputs still segregate in the dLGN, showing that additional factors contribute to eye-specific segregation.

Efficient gene transfer by in vivo electroporation (the application of electric current to living cells to create a transient permeability of the cell surface) has allowed for new approaches to gene function analysis. This technique utilizes pulsed electrical fields to directly introduce DNA into animal cells and target ectopic expression of genes of interest (Swartz, Eberhart, Mastick, & Krull, 2001). Using binocular in vivo electroporation of ferret eyes well before eye-opening, ectopic overexpression of EphA3 or EphA5 in postnatal RGCs results in severe eye-specific targeting errors and the intermingling of ipsilateral and contralateral projections (Huberman et al., 2005). This overexpression phenotype is age-dependent since electroporation of ferret eyes at postnatal day (P) 1 misdirects RGC axons, while overexpression beginning at P5 or older has no effect on eye-specific segregation. Since ephrin-A expression in the ferret LGN is markedly reduced by P5, EphA overexpression in the retina appears able to disrupt eye-specific segregation only when the appropriate ligand is present (Huberman et al., 2005).

Spontaneous Activity Before Eye-Opening—the Phenomenon of Retinal Waves

There is abundant evidence that neural activity is necessary for the proper development of neural circuits in the brain (Zhang & Poo, 2001). In general, neural activity during development can be sensory-evoked, occurring later in circuit development, or spontaneous, beginning early in circuit formation and well before sensory experience is possible. One feature common to developing neural circuits in the hippocampus, spinal cord, and retina is the presence of rhythmic bursts of spontaneous action potentials in neurons (Feller, 1999). Such bursts are highly correlated across many neighboring neurons and occur prior to experience or sensory stimulation.

Spontaneous Patterned Activity in the Retina

Various techniques have contributed to the understanding of the phenomenon of retinal waves. Bursts of action potentials in individual RGCs in the developing retina were first recorded electrophysiologically in acutely isolated rabbit retina shortly after birth (Masland, 1977). The existence of spontaneous bursts in RGCs was later demonstrated in vivo by electrophysiological recordings in

fetal rats (Galli & Maffei, 1988; Maffei & Galli-Resta, 1990). However, the highly correlated and wavelike nature of spontaneous retinal activity was first described in isolated fetal cat and newborn ferret retina using multielectrode recordings (Meister, Wong, Baylor, & Shatz, 1991; Wong, Meister, & Shatz, 1993). Optical imaging of Ca^{2+} indicator dyes, such as fluorescent acetoxymethyl (AM) ester derivatives, allows for measuring the activity in neurons over larger regions of isolated retina. Although such imaging is an indirect measure of bursts of action potentials in neurons, the observation of changing Ca^{2+} levels by this means has been demonstrated to reflect Ca^{2+} influx during retinal neuron depolarization (Feller, Wellis, Stellwagen, Werblin, & Shatz, 1996; Wong, Chernjavsky, Smith, & Shatz, 1995). Imaging using fura2-AM reveals a spontaneous propagating wavefront of activity that synchronizes the firing of hundreds to thousands of neurons in the developing retina. These waves of correlated activity tile across the retina over spatially restricted domains with a refractory period of approximately 1–2 min (Feller et al., 1996; Wong et al., 1993) (Figure 7.4). The average wavefront velocity of retinal waves is approximately 100–300 µm/s (Feller, Butts, Aaron, Rokhsar, & Shatz, 1997; Meister et al., 1991; Wong et al., 1993).

Retinal waves have been found during early development in many vertebrate species, including chickens, turtles, and monkeys (Warland et al., 2006; Wong, 1999), in addition to mouse, rat, rabbit, ferret, and cat.

Mechanisms Underlying Retinal Waves

Retinal waves are mediated by transient retinal circuits that change during development. The circuits that mediate retinal waves have been divided into three stages (Table 7.2), which are remarkably similar across species, though there are some differences between species (Firth, Wang, & Feller, 2005; Sernagor, Eglen, & Wong, 2001; Wong, 1999).

Stage I waves emerge before conventional synaptogenesis in the retina in rabbits (embryonic day (E) 22–23) and mice (E16–P0) (Bansal et al., 2000; Syed, Lee, Zheng, & Zhou, 2004). The inner retina consists of a network of RGCs and interneurons called amacrine cells. Amacrine (which means "without axons") cells are specialized cells in the retina with neural processes that function as both axons and dendrites. Gap junction blockers are able to inhibit stage I rabbit retinal waves (Syed et al., 2004), whereas blockade of nicotinic acetylcholine

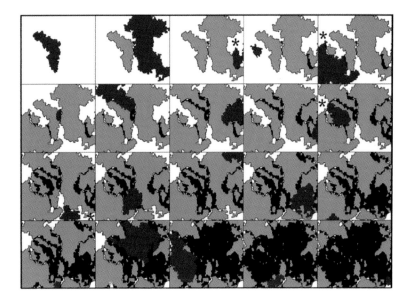

Figure 7.4 Spontaneous retinal waves propagate within spatial domains. Spontaneous retinal activity in P2 ferrets visualized with fura-2AM dye reveals a mosaic of domains. Red indicates the domain of a new wave of spontaneous activity, whereas shown in black are regions where more than one wave occurred during imaging. Over time, the entire retina surface has exhibited retinal waves. (Image taken from Feller et al., 1997.) The field of view is 1.2 mm × 1.4 mm; images were captured over 2 min.

receptor (nAChR) inhibits some, but not all of these early waves (Bansal et al., 2000).

Stage II waves emerge before birth in rabbits and around the time of birth in mice and are observed during the first and second postnatal weeks (Bansal et al., 2000; Syed et al., 2004). The cholinergic circuit that mediates stage II waves is the most well understood (for reviews, see Firth et al., 2005; Zhou, 1998). Application of nAChR antagonists blocks these retinal waves. The only source of acetylcholine (ACh) in the retina is from a subset of amacrine cells called starburst amacrine cells (SACs). Indeed, a cholinergic network of densely overlapping SACs exists in the retina (Tauchi & Masland, 1984; Vaney, 1984) and mediates recurrent excitation and spontaneous stage II

wave propagation in rabbits (Zheng, Lee, & Zhou, 2004). Thus, it was proposed that a cholinergic network of SACs initiates and propagates waves (Feller et al., 1997). Modeling of two retinal cell layers, one containing ganglion cells and the other amacrine cells, recreates the spatiotemporal aspects of waves when initiated by spontaneous depolarizations in the amacrine layer (Feller et al., 1997).

Mice carrying a null mutation for the β2-subunit of neuronal nAChRs are physiologically viable (Xu et al., 1999) and do not exhibit stage II retinal waves (Bansal et al., 2000; Muir-Robinson, Hwang, & Feller, 2002). As a result, the β2-nAChR-null mouse has become a major model system for studying the role of waves in visual system development (Bansal et al., 2000; Cang et al.,

Table 7.2 Timeline of Staged Development of Retinal Waves

Species	Stage I	Stage II	Stage III	Eye Opening
Mouse	E16–P0	P0–P11	P11–14	P13–14
Rabbit	E22–23	E23–P3	P3–7	P10–11
Ferret	?	<P2->P12	<P17-P30	P30–33
Cat	?	?	?	P7–9

E = embryonic, P = postnatal. Stage I waves are mediated by a non-chemical synaptic mechanism circuit. Stage II waves are mediated by activation of nicotinic acetylcholine receptors. Stage III retinal waves are mediated by activation of ionotropic glutamate receptors. While spontaneous activity is evident in the cat retina before eye opening, a detailed study of retinal wave propagation is lacking in this species. See text for references.

2005; Chandrasekaran et al., 2005; Feldheim et al., 2004; Grubb, Rossi, Changeux, & Thompson, 2003; McLaughlin, Torborg, Feller, & O'Leary, 2003b; Muir-Robinson et al., 2002; Pfeiffenberger et al., 2006; Rossi et al., 2001; Torborg, Hansen, & Feller, 2005; Torborg, Wang, Muir-Robinson, & Feller, 2004).

But what is the catalyst for the initiation of stage II waves? SACs function as pacemaker cells during stage II waves in rabbit retina (Zheng et al., 2006) and have been previously shown to propagate waves by corelease of ACh and γ-aminobutryic acid (GABA) onto RGCs and adjacent SACs (Zheng, Lee, & Zhou, 2004). Voltage-gated Ca^{2+} currents underlie the bursting spikes in SACs and tetrodotoxin (TTX) application does not block the compound bursts of SACs observed during waves (Zheng et al., 2006), supporting previous experiments where stage II waves still propagate during Na^+ channel blockade (Stellwagen, Shatz, & Feller, 1999). After a burst of calcium spikes, rabbit SACs exhibit a long-lasting after-hyperpolarization (AHP) that dictates the refractory period of spontaneous retinal waves (Zheng et al., 2006). This pacemaker property may not be unique to starburst cells. Indeed, several classes of amacrine cells immunoreactive for GABA have also been identified as pacemaker cells in dissociated rat retina cultures (Firth & Feller, 2006). However, stimulating a single-rabbit SAC is not sufficient to generate a wave, suggesting that wave initiation may depend upon the coordinated firing of a critical mass of neighboring SACs.

Stage III waves are mediated by ionotropic glutamate receptors and are not blocked by nAChR antagonists (Bansal et al., 2000; Wong, Myhr, Miller, & Wong, 2000; Zhou & Zhao, 2000). The neurotransmitter propagating the waves switches from ACh (stage II waves) to glutamate (stage III waves) and is coincident with the maturation of bipolar cell terminals as the source of glutamate (Miller, Tran, Wong, Oakley, & Wong, 1999; Wong et al., 2000). Bipolar cells are the primary source of glutamatergic input to RGCs. Waves persist in rabbits and ferrets until just before eye-opening (Syed et al., 2004; Wong et al., 1993) and can be observed in mice through eye-opening (Bansal et al., 2000) in which they persist for up to a few days after open-eye visual experience (Demas, Eglen, & Wong, 2003). GABA and glycine play a modulatory role in stage III waves (Fischer, Lukasiewicz, & Wong, 1998; Syed et al., 2004; Zhou & Zhao, 2000). The mechanisms underlying stage III wave

initiation and the source of coupling responsible for correlating glutamate transmission are not known.

Gap junctions have also been implicated in retinal wave propagation. Gap junctions are intercellular connections composed of two hemichannels that allow small molecules and ions to pass between cells. These chemical junctions can coordinate calcium transients and bursts of actions potentials in developing neurons (Roerig & Feller, 2000). Gap junction blockers exhibit variable effects on stage II waves, ranging from no effect to total blockade (Fischer et al., 1998; Singer, Mirotznik, & Feller, 2001; Stacy, Demas, Burgess, Sanes, & Wong, 2005; Syed et al., 2004).

Which gap junction proteins participate in stage II waves? Two gap junction proteins, connexins (Cx) 36 and 45, have been localized to the inner layers of the mammalian retina (Guldenagel et al., 2000; Sohl, Degen, Teubner, & Willecke, 1998; Sohl, Guldenagel, Traub, & Willecke, 2000). However, connexin 36 (Cx36) expression is weak at the beginning of the first postnatal week and increases through P14 (Hansen, Torborg, Elstrott, & Feller, 2005). RGCs in mice lacking Cx36 exhibit nearly normal firing patterns in the first postnatal week (at P4), but many more uncorrelated action potentials than wild-type mice in the second week (at P10) (Torborg et al., 2005). Both correlated and asynchronous action potentials in P10 Cx36-null RGCs are inhibited by bath application of an ionotropic glutamate receptor antagonist, a stage III blocker, demonstrating that the asynchronous action potentials are synaptically mediated (Hansen et al., 2005). Therefore, while Cx36-containing gap junctions do not mediate wave propagation, they may contribute to the suppression of RGC firing between waves. The role of Cx45 in retinal waves is, at present, unknown.

While connexins are likely to form at least some of the gap junctions involved in retinal waves, members of the pannexin family of gap junction proteins are expressed in the central nervous system (CNS) and are capable of forming functional intercellular channels (Bruzzone, Hormuzdi, Barbe, Herb, & Monyer, 2003). Expression of Pannexin 1 and 2 is observed in RGCs (Dvoriantchikova, Ivanov, Panchin, & Shestopalov, 2006), but their role in wave propagation is unknown. A combination of connexins and pannexins may be involved in stages I and II wave propagation, but their exact role is unclear.

Retinal wave patterns can be modulated by several factors. Elevation of cAMP increases wave frequency while inhibition of the cAMP/protein kinase A (PKA) pathway abolishes stage II waves, demonstrating a role for cAMP in wave regulation (Stellwagen et al., 1999). Interestingly, there is some evidence that the activity generated during retinal waves may be homeostatically regulated. By this, we mean that long-term inhibition of the circuitry that normally mediates waves leads to changes in functional circuits. For example, shortly after the appearance of stage II waves, several hours of blockade with nAChR antagonists causes a reversal to stage I waves (Syed et al., 2004). In addition, transgenic mice lacking choline acetyltransferase in the retina do not initiate stage II waves and, a few days after, waves reappear mediated by a novel circuit (Stacy et al., 2005). Though the appearance of a novel form of retinal waves in the absence of normal stage II waves is not immediate, as would be expected in a purely homeostatic system, the reemergence of waves does suggest some aspect of homeostatic regulation in the underlying circuitry, similar to that observed in the developing spinal cord (Milner & Landmesser, 1999; Myers et al., 2005; O'Donovan, 1999).

Axonal Refinement of Retinal Projections
Activity-dependent Mechanisms of Retinotopic Refinement—Permissive or Instructive?

A contentious debate in the field of retinotopic refinement centers on the extent of influence of intrinsic factors (molecular cues) versus neural activity (spontaneous activity of retinal waves). Sperry's experiments supporting his chemoaffinity hypothesis, and more current investigations of ephrin/Eph gradients clearly demonstrate an important role for matching molecular cues. But what role does neural activity have?

A popular model of how activity alters synaptic connectivity is provided by Hebb's neurophysiological postulate which, in part, states that: "When an axon of cell A is near enough to excite cell B and repeatedly or persistently takes part in firing of it, some growth process or metabolic change takes place in one or both cells such that A's efficiency, as one of the cells firing B, is increased" (Hebb, 1949). The idea that synaptic strength is enhanced by the correlated firing of two neurons is often summarized by the phrase, "neurons that fire together, wire together." The hypothesis has been expanded to include the complementary action where a neuron that repeatedly fails to excite another results in a weakening of synaptic strength between the two

(Stent, 1973). Thus, Hebbian learning rules permit the bidirectional alteration of synapses by the strengthening or weakening of synaptic strengths depending upon the rate of coincidence of pre- and postsynaptic activity (Lisman, 1989).

Activity-dependent mechanisms in retinotopic refinement are most often described in terms of Hebbian learning since spontaneous retinal waves appear to be well suited for such a model of axonal refinement (Butts, 2002; Eglen, 1999). One hypothesis is that spatiotemporal features of spontaneous retinal waves can drive synaptic remodeling of early, diffuse retinotopic connections in immature circuits, contributing to the formation of precise connections characteristic of adult neural circuits (Shatz, 1996). Retinal waves correlate spatial information of neighboring RGCs. Since waves occur independently in the two eyes with a recurrence of 1 to 2 min in a given location, the firing of cells in corresponding locations between two retinae is uncorrelated. Eye-specific information may be transmitted to targets in the brain, such as the LGN, where afferents from the two eyes are initially intermingled (Cucchiaro & Guillery, 1984; Linden, Guillery, & Cucchiaro, 1981; Penn, Riquelme, Feller, & Shatz, 1998; Shatz, 1983; Sretavan & Shatz, 1986). Therefore, it has been proposed that retinal waves are "instructive" in that nearby RGCs cells are more correlated in their firing than distant cells. This is in contrast to synchronous oscillation or random firing during which nearby and distant cells would exhibit the same correlation of activity. Hence, retinal waves encode information regarding the relative position of RGCs, which is the relevant information for driving retinotopic refinement, perhaps via a Hebbian competitive mechanism (Crair, 1999; Katz & Shatz, 1996). A competing idea is that spontaneous activity is "permissive" such that some minimal amount of activity is required to allow for the matching of molecular cues in a genetically predetermined environment for subsequent retinotopic refinement. For example, it was recently demonstrated that spontaneous activity in a RGC is necessary for growth cone collapse in the presence of ephrins (Nicol et al., 2007). In this case, activity is permissive in that it is required, but the relevant information for driving map refinement is contained in the ephrin gradients. Though it is generally accepted that spontaneous retinal activity is required for proper retinotopic refinement, the relative role of instructive versus permissive roles for activity in retinotopic refinement remains controversial.

Manipulations That Eliminate or Alter Retinal Wave Transmission in Animals

For decades, researchers have approached the study of retinal wave function in vivo by blocking retinal wave transmission or manipulating its spatiotemporal properties. While TTX application does not block retinal wave propagation (Stellwagen et al., 1999), TTX can effectively block retinal wave transmission by preventing action potentials in RGCs (Meister et al., 1991; Shatz & Stryker, 1988; Stryker & Harris, 1986). Concerns of toxicity due to TTX delivery in vivo have spurred the use of drugs that more specifically target receptors involved in transmitting retinal waves. For example, epibatidine is a potent cholinergic agonist that binds to nAChRs (Badio & Daly, 1994; Kittila & Massey, 1997) and, through receptor desensitization, blocks activity in the retina by eliminating stage II retinal waves (Cang et al., 2005; Huberman et al., 2002; Penn et al., 1998). However, following epibatidine injections, studies in ferrets demonstrate a complete block of retinal activity in addition to wave elimination (Huberman et al., 2002; Penn et al., 1998), while another study in mice shows a partial block, with some neurons becoming silent and others firing tonically (Cang et al., 2005). Therefore, a limitation of epibatidine blockade is the inability to assess the concentration and exposure to neurons in vivo across different experiments. In contrast to blockade, other manipulations have been used to increase the frequency of retinal wave initiations. Intraocular administrations of forskolin, an adenylate cyclase activator, or cpt-cAMP, a nonhydrolyzable analog of cAMP, elevate intracellular levels of cAMP and increase the frequency (waves per minute) of spontaneous retinal waves (Stellwagen & Shatz, 2002).

Another approach has been to eliminate SACs, the source of actylcholine during stage II waves. By intraocular injection of saporin, a ribosome-inactivating protein, conjugated to antivesicular acetylcholine transporter (VAChT) antibody, cholinergic SACs can be selectively ablated in vivo (Gunhan, Choudary, Landerholm, & Chalupa, 2002). Injection of this immunotoxin into the eyes of newborn ferrets results in a depletion of approximately 80%–90% of SACs during the next few days (Huberman et al., 2003). Interestingly, although immunotoxin-treated and -untreated RGCs exhibit similar average firing rates, treatment alters the periodic bursts of action potentials characteristic of stage II retinal waves and greatly reduces nearest neighbor correlations (Huberman et al., 2003).

A different method of manipulating retinal waves is through the use of transgenic mice in which genes that contribute to waves have been altered. Mutant mice null for the β2-subunit of the nAChR (β2-null) lack retinal waves during the first postnatal week and precociously develop stage III waves at P8 rather than P11 (Bansal et al., 2000). The glutamate-driven waves in the second postnatal week of β2-null mice propagate at about half the velocity of wild-type stage III waves and appear similar to early stage II waves in this regard (Muir-Robinson et al., 2002). However, the average firing rate of RGCs in β2-null mice is similar to wild-type during both the first and second postnatal weeks (Torborg et al., 2005).

Activity and Retinocollicular Map Development

At the time of birth, retinal projections to the rodent colliculus innervate both the superior and inferior colliculus. At this time, the majority of these are contralateral projections while a relative minority are ipsilateral in origin. During the first 2 weeks of postnatal development in rodents, the ipsilateral projections become restricted to the rostral part of the colliculus (Fawcett, O'Leary, & Cowan, 1984; O'Leary, Fawcett, & Cowan, 1986; Thompson & Holt, 1989). The restriction is activity-dependent since the refinement of ipsilateral projections are sensitive to blockade of neural activity. Repeated monocular or binocular intraocular injection of TTX during the first 2 postnatal weeks causes ipsilateral projections of the treated eye to become diffuse and overlap with contralateral projections in the rostral SC in rats and Syrian hamsters, respectively (Fawcett et al., 1984; Thompson & Holt, 1989).

Since TTX administration blocks all activity in RGCs, its administration does not address whether spatiotemporal features of activity, such as the correlated nature of retinal waves, is necessary for proper retinocollicular map refinement. β2-null mice exhibit uncorrelated RGC activity, and as a consequence, do not segregate into eye-specific areas in the SC where they innervate an extended territory compared to wild-type (Rossi et al., 2001). Indeed, the TZs of β2-null retinal projections are larger than normal in the SC and form broadly distributed arbors by the second postnatal week (Chandrasekaran et al., 2005; McLaughlin et al., 2003b). The presence of glutamatergic waves or visual activity during the second postnatal week cannot rescue the defect, demonstrating that the earlier presence of cholinergic-driven waves is critical for normal refinement.

Activity and Retinogeniculate Map Development

Eye-specific projections to the thalamus are initially intermingled in the dLGN of rodents (Godement, Salaun, & Imbert, 1984) and layers A/C and A1 of carnivores (Figure 7.5) (Cucchiaro & Guillery, 1984; Linden et al., 1981; Penn et al.,

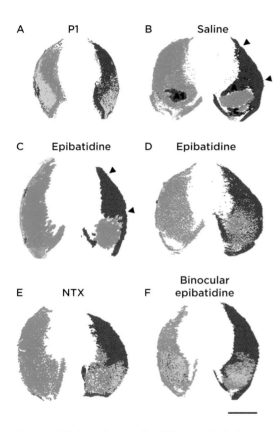

Figure 7.5 Prolonged intraocular cholinergic blockade in newborn ferrets disrupts eye-specific projections. Retinal projections in the LGN were visualized by anterograde transport of 3H-leucine (green, right eye) and WGA-HRP (red, left eye). Shortly after birth, significant overlap of projections from the two eyes is evident (A, yellow), from which eye-specific layers develop in the LGN by P9 (B, green and red). Prolonged monocular blockade of cholinergic activity by intraocular administration of epibatidine or nereistoxin (NTX) from P0 to P9 disrupts eye-specific segregation (C–E). The territory occupied by projections from the unaffected eye (green) expands in the binocular region during treatment, whereas the territory of the treated eye (red) decreases. The ipsilateral projection from the treated eye (red) is severely disrupted and nearly disappears. Following binocular blockade, the projections from both eyes expand and significantly overlap by P9 (F, yellow). Therefore, competition based on retinal activity drives the relative amount of territory occupied by eye-specific projections. Image from Penn et al. (Penn et al., 1998.)

1998; Shatz, 1983; Sretavan & Shatz, 1986). It is well accepted that neural activity is required for the segregation of RGC axons into eye-specific layers in the LGN. An early set of experiments demonstrated that repeated intracranial infusion of TTX for 2 weeks beginning at E42 in cats leads to a complete blockade of eye-specific segregation (Shatz & Stryker, 1988). Since then, more refined tests of the role of activity have been performed in other model animals, such as mice and ferrets, where spontaneous retinal waves are better studied. The segregation of eye-specific layers in the LGN occurs during stage II waves and is complete by P8 in mice (Godement et al., 1984; Upton et al., 1999) and P9 in ferrets (Cucchiaro & Guillery, 1984; Hutchins & Casagrande, 1990; Linden et al., 1981; Penn et al., 1998). Intraocular administration of stage II wave blockers that bind nAChRs, alters eye-specific patterning in ferrets (Penn et al., 1998) or mouse LGN (Rossi et al., 2001), demonstrating that blocking retinal activity alone is sufficient to alter segregation. Monocular cholinergic blockade in ferret from P0 to P9 causes contralateral projections from the untreated eye to fill the entire LGN, while ipsilateral projections from the untreated eye expand territory in the binocular region (Figure 7.5). In contrast, binocular cholinergic blockade causes projections from both eyes to fill and overlap in the binocular portion of the LGN in ferrets and mice (Penn et al., 1998; Rossi et al., 2001), similar to intracranial TTX blockade in cat (Shatz & Stryker, 1988).

Since monocular blockade results in an expansion of untreated eye territory in the LGN, it was proposed that competition based on relative levels of retinal activity drives eye-specific connections. A similar intraocular study using slow release of TTX in ferrets during the first postnatal week reports only a limited blockade of eye-specific segregation in the LGN, but still demonstrates some anomalous segregation (Cook, Prusky, & Ramoa, 1999). However, the idea that competitive spontaneous activity in the retina drives eye-specific segregation is bolstered by experiments where neural activity is monocularly elevated, rather than blocked. The elevation of intracellular levels of cAMP in the retina in vivo, via CPT-cAMP or forskolin, results in an increase in the treated eye territory at the expense of the untreated eye (Stellwagen & Shatz, 2002). Therefore, it was proposed that relative levels of neural activity between retinae determine the amount of LGN territory that is to be occupied by projections from each eye.

The ability to generate mutant mice lacking single nAChR subunits has provided an alternative to pharmacological studies that cannot target specific receptor subunits. However, genetic studies, in turn, have not allowed for eye-specific manipulations, which are easily accomplished with intraocular injection of drugs. Nevertheless, the study of β2-null mice has revealed a requirement for the β2-subunit of nAChRs for cholinergic-driven stage II waves (Bansal et al., 2000) and the proper development of retinal projections (Rossi et al., 2001). While retinal waves are absent in the first postnatal week of β2-null mice, glutamate-mediated stage III waves are present during the second postnatal week. The effect on retinogeniculate axon segregation is that these mutant mice never develop eye-specific layers in the LGN (Muir-Robinson et al., 2002; Rossi et al., 2001). However, the presence of stage III waves is sufficient to drive retinal axon segregation into eye-specific territories in the form of intermingled patches rather than layers. Focal DiI retinal injections reveal that β2-null projections target the correct region of the dLGN but form more diffuse TZs in comparison to normal mice (Grubb et al., 2003). In addition, intraocular epibatidine blockade in ferrets, during the period when stage II waves are normally present, followed by a prolonged recovery, results in variable and disorganized eye-specific patches instead of layers in the LGN (Huberman et al., 2002). Therefore, cholinergically driven retinal wave activity appears to be required for fine topographic refinement in addition to eye-specific layering. However, injection of an antibody specific for cholinergic neurons and conjugated to the toxin saporin leads to a significant depletion of SACs and does not disrupt eye-specific layering in the ferret LGN (Huberman et al., 2003). Why do both of these manipulations, which disrupt retinal wave circuitry, lead to different results? One proposed reason is the extent to which endogenous activity pattern in the retina is disrupted. For example, epibatadine application significantly decreases the firing of all RGCs, while the immunotoxin treatment reduces nearest neighbor correlations between RGCs but retains higher baseline firing. The exact reason for this disparity is unclear, but perhaps certain spatiotemporal features of retinal activity, present in one manipulation but not the other, can direct eye-specific layering.

To begin to address features of patterned activity that may be required for eye-specific segregation, the RGC firing patterns of several mutant mouse lines with different levels of eye-specific segregation were analyzed. Mice lacking the β2 subunit of nAChR do not exhibit retinal waves in the first postnatal week (Bansal et al., 2000), but individual RGCs continue to fire uncorrelated action potentials. Since β2-null mice do not form eye-specific layers, it appears that there is some feature in the endogenous firing pattern that is critical for eye-specific segregation. A second transgenic mouse, which lacks the gap junction protein Cx36, continues to exhibit retinal waves but exhibits a significant increase in the number of asynchronous action potentials. These additional action potentials introduce into the firing patterns a noise, which significantly reduces the nearest neighbor correlation observed in normal mice (Torborg et al., 2005). In contrast to β2-null mice, Cx36 null mice develop normal eye-specific segregation of retinogeniculate axons.

If both β2-null mice and Cx36 null mice exhibit altered spontaneous firing patterns, why do only the β2-null mice develop abnormal eye-specific layers? The answer to this question is likely that some features of retinal waves may be critical for eye-specific layer formation while others may not. By comparing the firing patterns of normal mice and Cx36-null mice (which develop normal eye-specific segregation) to β2-null mice (which lack eye-specific segregation), a list of firing pattern properties that may be critical for driving segregation were obtained. Based on this analysis, it was hypothesized that high-frequency bursts synchronized across RGCs is correlated with eye-specific segregation, while additional asynchronous spikes do not inhibit segregation (Torborg et al., 2005). However, any mechanistic changes driven by high-frequency activity, such as synaptic alteration, remain undefined.

Several other mutant mouse strains that develop altered eye-specific layers have been described and are reviewed elsewhere (Torborg & Feller, 2005). In addition to the mutants described in this review, it has recently been demonstrated that members of the neuronal pentraxin (NP) family of proteins, which share homology to pentraxin proteins that function in the immune system, are required for proper eye-specific refinement (Bjartmar et al., 2006).

Evidence for Synaptic Competition in RGC Axonal Refinement

What are the cellular mechanisms that translate neural activity into axonal refinement? A prevalent model is that activity drives a process of synaptic competition. In this model, cells that fire in a correlated manner are more likely to form stable synaptic contact with their postsynaptic partners than axons that are firing in an uncorrelated manner. In frogs and fish, in vivo recordings have given key insights into molecular factors that influence axonal refinement. These experiments have been reviewed elsewhere (Ruthazer & Cline, 2004).

Physiological studies of retinogeniculate synaptic refinement during development in mammals are technically difficult in vivo due the deep location in the brain. Brain slice preparations of mouse, rat, or ferret LGN that contain part of the optic nerve have proven useful since they maintain the retinogeniculate synapse and allow the study of a developing postsynaptic response to optic tract stimulation (Chen & Regehr, 2000; Mooney, Madison, & Shatz, 1993; Ziburkus & Guido, 2006). Indeed, bursts of high-frequency stimulation of the optic tract induces long-term synaptic enhancement at the retinogeniculate synapse in slices prepared from ferrets prior to eye-opening (Mooney et al., 1993). Mouse brain slices with optic tract, optic nerve, and retina still connected exhibit periodic bursts of spontaneous activity from retinal neurons (Mooney, Penn, Gallego, & Shatz, 1996). Such spontaneous activity in the retina drives LGN neurons to fire bursts of action potentials, suggesting that retinal input, in the form of waves, can shape synaptic modification in the thalamus (Mooney et al., 1996).

Developmental refinement at the retinogeniculate synapse is characterized by a reduction of retinal input onto individual LGN cells. In rat preparations, a dramatic reduction of retinal inputs onto single dLGN neurons is observed, but not until well after eye-opening (by P18) (Ziburkus & Guido, 2006). Prior to eye-opening in mice, geniculate neurons receive weak synaptic input from more than 20 RGCs and this is reduced to one to three inputs by P28, again well after eye-opening (Chen & Regehr, 2000). Since the segregation of eye-specific layers in the mouse LGN is complete by P8 in mice (Godement et al., 1984; Upton et al., 1999), retinal inputs are segregated to the correct region of the thalamus before eye-opening, but do not mature synaptically until later. There is some in vivo evidence that synaptic transmission at this stage may be important for retinotopic refinement. Activation of NMDA receptors is critical for the normal loss of inappropriate synapses (Colonnese & Constantine-Paton, 2006; Colonnese, Shi, & Constantine-Paton, 2003).

Is spontaneous retinal activity around eye-opening involved in the synaptic refinement process? Retinal waves are detected until 1 week after eye-opening (P21) (Demas et al., 2003) while photoreceptor-mediated light responses are evoked a few days before (at P10). Hence, there is a significant period of time during which retinal waves and sensory-driven activity in the retina coexist (Demas et al., 2003). Several days of in vivo activity blockade by intravitreal TTX release, beginning at P11 and spanning eye-opening, retards synaptic strengthening and inhibits retinal input reduction onto LGN neurons when assayed in slices (Hooks & Chen, 2006). But, is the synaptic refinement process involved in eye-specific layering in the LGN? While activity blockade during the first postnatal week of mice disrupts eye-specific layering, an in vitro preparation that recapitulates eye-specific segregation and allows for synaptic physiology studies at the same time is presently lacking.

Concerted Action of Molecular Cues and Neural Activity

Both molecular cues and neural activity are required for the formation of topographic maps. However, it has long been generally believed that there is a separation of action of molecular cues and retinal activity in topographic map formation. Ephrin-A2/A3/A5 triple knockout mice have ectopic projections to the LGN and SC but these ectopic projections undergo normal refinement. Mice lacking retinal wave activity do not refine but are targeted correctly and β2-null mice develop appropriately targeted projections but retain their immature overarborization. When ephrin-A2/A3/A5 triple knockout mice are combined with a β2-null background, the result is a near absence of topographic order in retinocollicular and retinogeniculate projections (Pfeiffenberger et al., 2006). Furthermore, the combination of β2-null mice with overexpression of the bone morphogenic protein (BMP), which causes ventral RGCs to take a dorsal fate resulting in disturbed axon guidance of ventral RGCs, results in a cumulative defect in retinotopic map formation in the SC (Chandrasekaran et al., 2005).

More recently, the notion of separate but cumulative mechanisms of action for patterned activity and guidance molecules has been challenged by experiments, demonstrating that manipulating neural activity can lead to alterations in molecular cue surface presentation. For example, in chicks, decreasing the frequency of rhythmic activity in spinal cord neurons can result in the downregulation of molecules that contribute to dorsoventral (D-V) pathfinding, including but not limited to polysialic acid (PSA) on neural cell adhesion molecule (NCAM) and ephrin receptor A4 (EphA4) (Hanson & Landmesser, 2004). Indeed, the precise frequency of rhythmic bursting activity appears to be critical for early pathfinding decisions of motoneurons in chick (Hanson & Landmesser, 2006).

In the developing visual system, rhythmic activity has been linked to intracellular signaling molecules known to modulate topographic refinement. This includes calcium-stimulated adenylate cyclases (AC), which synthesize intracellular cAMP upon activation and also play a role in topographic map refinement. During the first postnatal week in mice, expression of AC1 is localized to the dLGN, is strong in RGCs and the superficial layers of the SC, while the AC8 isoform is readily detected in the SC but not in RGCs or the dLGN (Plas, Visel, Gonzalez, She, & Crair, 2004; Ravary et al., 2003). The loss of AC1 in mice results in reduced eye-specific segregation of retinal projections in the dLGN and reduced retinotopic refinement in the SC, resulting in a larger TZs of retinal projections (Plas et al., 2004; Ravary et al., 2003). Cocultures of the retina and midbrain that recapitulate topographic specificity in the SC have determined a presynaptic role for AC1 in retinal axons (Nicol, Muzerelle, Rio, Metin, & Gaspar, 2006). In retinal explants lacking AC1, the defect in retinocollicular refinement is due to a lack of retinal axon retraction in response to ephrin-A5 signaling (Nicol et al., 2006). Importantly, periodic uncaging of cAMP is permissive for ephrin-A5-induced retinal axon retraction during activity blockade in retinocollicular cocultures (Nicol et al., 2007).

One hypothesis as to how retinal activity mediates visual system development is that retinal waves drive cAMP oscillations in RGC axons, which play a direct role in axon guidance mechanisms. Indeed, using fluorescent dyes, oscillations in cAMP and cAMP-dependent PKA can be visualized in RGCs in dissociated rat retina cultures (DiPilato, Cheng, & Zhang, 2004; Dunn et al., 2006). However, it is still unclear whether such oscillations occur in RGC axons or whether they are driven by retinal waves in vivo. Nevertheless, these observations demonstrate the presence of mechanisms in retinotopic refinement, which may be dependent on activity, but do not require coordinated firing among cells.

Activity and the Formation of Ocular Dominance Columns
Formation of Ocular Dominance Columns

ODCs were first described by Hubel and Wiesel in the early 1960s. They used in vivo extracellular recordings in cat primary visual cortex to show that one eye, independent of the other, can differentially activate a subset of cortical neurons and that this response appeared to be organized into discrete columns perpendicular to the cortical surface (Hubel & Wiesel, 1959, 1962). They termed these structures "ocular dominance columns." In subsequent seminal experiments, Hubel and Wiesel demonstrated that monocular eye closure followed by recovery in young kittens shifts eye-specific activation of neurons in the primary visual cortex in favor of the open eye (Wiesel & Hubel, 1963, 1965a).

By using monocular eye closure followed by recovery with visual stimulation in cats of different ages, the results of activity recordings began to define a critical period for ODC plasticity in the visual cortex (Hensch, 2004). Susceptibility to monocular closure is greatest during P28–35, where a few days of deprivation are sufficient to induce a maximal shift in receptive field properties (Hubel & Wiesel, 1970; Wiesel & Hubel, 1965a, 1965b). These experiments applied the concept of "critical periods" to visual system development (Hensch, 2004). In cats, eye opening occurs at P7–9 and the critical period occurs later during a time of visual experience, long after retinal waves have passed. A similar finite critical period is also found by using electrophysiology in ferrets after eye-opening, with the peak susceptibility to ODC shift toward the open eye occurring between P35 and P60 (Issa, Trachtenberg, Chapman, Zahs, & Stryker, 1999). Whereas 2 days of monocular deprivation (MD) during the peak critical period is sufficient to shift ocular dominance in young cats, immature ferrets require approximately 7 days of MD for a maximal shift in ocular dominance cortical response (Issa et al., 1999), demonstrating a species difference in ODC plasticity.

The use of transneuronal tracers in visual pathways in the 1970s enabled an anatomical assessment of ODC formation. Intraocular administration of 3H-glucose and/or 3H-proline, for example, was employed to visualize ocular dominance columns in monkey striate cortex (Rakic, 1976; Wiesel, Hubel, & Lam, 1974). In very young cats, intraocular radioactive amino acid injection results in a homogenous band of label in layer 4 of the visual cortex. Using this labeling method, distinct ODCs first appear during the third and fourth weeks in cats (P22–33), around the onset of the critical period, and gradually begin to develop into adult-like patterns of radioactive label during the fifth week (P39) (LeVay, Stryker, & Shatz, 1978).

Since increased binocular input is observed physiologically at the early age when there is broad transneuronal labeling in layer 4 (Hubel & Wiesel, 1963), it was proposed that ODCs initially overlap at the onset of the critical period of plasticity. Radioactive transynaptic labeling in ferret reveals a similar relationship between function and anatomy. Eye-opening in the ferret normally occurs around P30–33 and ODCs are not discernible at P30. Transynaptic labeling indicative of ODC formation begins to emerge around P37, is clearly present at P50, and becomes adult-like by P63 (Ruthazer, Baker, & Stryker, 1999). As with cats, the anatomical development in ferret visual cortex correlates well with the critical period defined by physiology. Based on these correlations, a Hebbian-based model of activity-dependent competition between eye-specific inputs was invoked to explain the emergence of ODCs. This became a classic paradigm for sensory-evoked circuit maturation in the developing central nervous system.

One limitation of using radioactive amino acids for eye-specific input labeling in the developing visual cortex is that radioactive label may not be confined to a single retinogeniculate synapse but may spill over to neighboring synapses. The level of spillover is noted in cat and ferret studies and while it does account for some aberrant signal, it is not responsible for a lack of eye-specific segregation in layer 4 at young ages (LeVay et al., 1978; Ruthazer et al., 1999; Stryker & Harris, 1986).

More recently, the results from different anatomical tracing methods have challenged the observation that geniculate projections representing inputs from the two eyes significantly overlap in layer 4 prior to ODC formation. In cats, anterograde tracing of fluorescent dextran or cholera toxin B subunit from the LGN to the visual cortex together with thin section analysis of transneuronal labeled visual cortex shows the emergence of ODCs between P7 and P14, at least a week earlier than previously reported (Crair, Horton, Antonini, & Stryker, 2001). Similar anterograde tracing from the ferret LGN clearly reveals segregated eye-specific patches in the visual cortex as early as P16, weeks before ODCs were believed to emerge and only shortly after geniculate axons first reach layer 4 (Crowley & Katz, 2000). The use of newer physiological techniques, such as intrinsic optical imaging and targeted multielectrode penetration recordings, confirm monocular responses in layer 4 of the visual cortex by P14 in cats (Crair, Gillespie, & Stryker, 1998; Crair et al., 2001). Therefore,

monocular response is evident in cats by 1 week after eye-opening (i.e., P14), which is 1 week prior to the critical period for monocular deprivation (Olson & Freeman, 1980). In ferrets, anatomical segregation of geniculocortical axons occurs 2 to 3 weeks prior to eye-opening, well before visual stimulation, several weeks prior to the critical period of monocular deprivation.

These recent discoveries have led to the definition of a "precritical period," which corresponds to the period of visual system development after the onset of visual experience and prior to the critical period for monocular deprivation (Feller & Scanziani, 2005). During the precritical period, cortical responses are dominated by contralateral input (Crair et al., 1998). Hence, any activity-dependent rearrangements of eye-specific inputs during the precritical period would not likely rely on a purely Hebbian-based model of competition.

Spontaneous Activity Influences Early Cortical Column Development

Do ODCs emerge through an activity-dependent refinement process or are they genetically predetermined? The strongest evidence that retinal activity, either spontaneous or visually evoked, is not involved comes from enucleation studies. In ferrets, neither monocular (Crowley & Katz, 2000) nor binocular enucleation (Crowley & Katz, 1999) at any time between P0 and P15 affects the clustering of thalamic axons. Based on these findings, it was hypothesized that retinal activity is not required for thalamocortical axons to cluster into eye-specific domains. However, after enucleation, the spontaneous activity patterns that persist in the dLGN have similar spatial and temporal patterns to those induced by retinal waves. These persisting patters could instruct sorting of thalamocortical axons in the absence of retinal activity, making it difficult to assess the role of retinal activity (Weliky & Katz, 1999). More recent experiments have implicated spontaneous retinal activity in the formation of both retinotopic and eye-specific maps in primary visual cortex. Recently, it was demonstrated that retinotopic refinement is altered in the β2-null mouse, which lacks retinal waves but exhibits uncorrelated firing of RGCs (Cang et al., 2005). In β2-null mice, the binocular region is also enlarged (Rossi et al., 2001). In addition, pharmacological blockade of nAChRs in vivo in ferrets prevents the formation of ocular dominance columns throughout life despite the recovery of normal vision in these animals (Huberman, Speer,

& Chapman, 2006). All of these results are consistent with the notion that spontaneous retinal activity plays a critical role in retinotopic and eye-specific refinement in early cortical development.

Conclusions

After 20 years of research, the visual system continues to provide important insights into how neural activity, whether spontaneous or sensory driven, influences the development of mature connectivity. Perhaps one of the most important concepts that has emerged from recent research is that the developmental mechanisms that underlie the construction of neural circuits are not easily broken into activity-dependent versus activity-independent. Rather, new questions and concepts are emerging. For example, how does the pattern of activity alter signaling events that, in turn, regulate cell function at levels ranging from transcription to posttranslational modifications? Is there a general feature of homeostasis in developing circuits such that they alter their connectivity and excitability to maintain certain levels of spontaneous activity? Are there non-Hebbian mechanisms by which activity can change the synaptic strength? Study of the visual system has revealed that "nature" versus "nurture" may be a false dichotomy and that true insights will arise only by understanding the detailed mechanisms that underlie the emergence of functional visual circuits during development.

References

Akerman, C. J., Smyth, D., & Thompson, I. D. (2002). Visual experience before eye-opening and the development of the retinogeniculate pathway. *Neuron, 36*(5), 869–879.

Angelucci, A., Clasca, F., & Sur, M. (1996). Anterograde axonal tracing with the subunit B of cholera toxin: A highly sensitive immunohistochemical protocol for revealing fine axonal morphology in adult and neonatal brains. *Journal of Neuroscience Methods, 65*(1), 101–112.

Badio, B., & Daly, J. W. (1994). Epibatidine, a potent analgetic and nicotinic agonist. *Molecular Pharmacology, 45*(4), 563–569.

Bansal, A., Singer, J. H., Hwang, B. J., Xu, W., Beaudet, A., & Feller, M. B. (2000). Mice lacking specific nicotinic acetylcholine receptor subunits exhibit dramatically altered spontaneous activity patterns and reveal a limited role for retinal waves in forming ON and OFF circuits in the inner retina. *Journal of Neuroscience, 20*(20), 7672–7681.

Bjartmar, L., Huberman, A. D., Ullian, E. M., Renteria, R. C., Liu, X., Xu, W., et al. (2006). Neuronal pentraxins mediate synaptic refinement in the developing visual system. *Journal of Neuroscience, 26*(23), 6269–6281.

Braisted, J. E., McLaughlin, T., Wang, H. U., Friedman, G. C., Anderson, D. J., & O'Leary D, D. (1997). Graded and lamina-specific distributions of ligands of EphB receptor tyrosine kinases in the developing retinotectal system. *Developmental Biology, 191*(1), 14–28.

Brown, A., Yates, P. A., Burrola, P., Ortuno, D., Vaidya, A., Jessell, T. M., et al. (2000). Topographic mapping from the retina to the midbrain is controlled by relative but not absolute levels of EphA receptor signaling. *Cell, 102*(1), 77–88.

Brunet, I., Weinl, C., Piper, M., Trembleau, A., Volovitch, M., Harris, W., et al. (2005). The transcription factor Engrailed-2 guides retinal axons. *Nature, 438*(7064), 94–98.

Bruzzone, R., Hormuzdi, S. G., Barbe, M. T., Herb, A., & Monyer, H. (2003). Pannexins, a family of gap junction proteins expressed in brain. *Proceedings of the National Academy of Sciences USA, 100*(23), 13644–13649.

Butts, D. A. (2002). Retinal waves: Implications for synaptic learning rules during development. *Neuroscientist, 8*(3), 243–253.

Cang, J., Renteria, R. C., Kaneko, M., Liu, X., Copenhagen, D. R., & Stryker, M. P. (2005). Development of precise maps in visual cortex requires patterned spontaneous activity in the retina. *Neuron, 48*(5), 797–809.

Chandrasekaran, A. R., Plas, D. T., Gonzalez, E., & Crair, M. C. (2005). Evidence for an instructive role of retinal activity in retinotopic map refinement in the superior colliculus of the mouse. *Journal of Neuroscience, 25*(29), 6929–6938.

Chen, C., & Regehr, W. G. (2000). Developmental remodeling of the retinogeniculate synapse. *Neuron, 28*(3), 955–966.

Cheng, H. J., Nakamoto, M., Bergemann, A. D., & Flanagan, J. G. (1995). Complementary gradients in expression and binding of ELF-1 and Mek4 in development of the topographic retinotectal projection map. *Cell, 82*(3), 371–381.

Clancy, B., Darlington, R. B., & Finlay, B. L. (2001). Translating developmental time across mammalian species. *Neuroscience, 105*(1), 7–17.

Colonnese, M. T., & Constantine-Paton, M. (2006). Developmental period for N-methyl-D-aspartate (NMDA) receptor-dependent synapse elimination correlated with visuotopic map refinement. *Journal of Comparative Neurology, 494*(5), 738–751.

Colonnese, M. T., Shi, J., & Constantine-Paton, M. (2003). Chronic NMDA receptor blockade from birth delays the maturation of NMDA currents, but does not affect AMPA/kainate currents. *Journal of Neurophysiology, 89*(1), 57–68.

Cook, P. M., Prusky, G., & Ramoa, A. S. (1999). The role of spontaneous retinal activity before eye opening in the maturation of form and function in the retinogeniculate pathway of the ferret. *Visual Neuroscience, 16*(3), 491–501.

Crair, M. C. (1999). Neuronal activity during development: Permissive or instructive? *Current Opinion in Neurobiology, 9*(1), 88–93.

Crair, M. C., Gillespie, D. C., & Stryker, M. P. (1998). The role of visual experience in the development of columns in cat visual cortex. *Science, 279*(5350), 566–570.

Crair, M. C., Horton, J. C., Antonini, A., & Stryker, M. P. (2001). Emergence of ocular dominance columns in cat visual cortex by 2 weeks of age. *Journal of Comparative Neurology, 430*(2), 235–249.

Crowley, J. C., & Katz, L. C. (1999). Development of ocular dominance columns in the absence of retinal input. *Nature Neuroscience, 2*(12), 1125–1130.

Crowley, J. C., & Katz, L. C. (2000). Early development of ocular dominance columns. *Science, 290*(5495), 1321–1324.

Cucchiaro, J., & Guillery, R. W. (1984). The development of the retinogeniculate pathways in normal and albino ferrets. *Proceedings of the Royal Society of London B: Biological Sciences, 223*(1231), 141–164.

Demas, J., Eglen, S. J., & Wong, R. O. (2003). Developmental loss of synchronous spontaneous activity in the mouse retina is independent of visual experience. *Journal of Neuroscience, 23*(7), 2851–2860.

DiPilato, L. M., Cheng, X., & Zhang, J. (2004). Fluorescent indicators of cAMP and Epac activation reveal differential dynamics of cAMP signaling within discrete subcellular compartments. *Proceedings of the National Academy of Sciences USA, 101*(47), 16513–16518.

Drescher, U., Kremoser, C., Handwerker, C., Loschinger, J., Noda, M., & Bonhoeffer, F. (1995). In vitro guidance of retinal ganglion cell axons by RAGS, a 25 kDa tectal protein related to ligands for Eph receptor tyrosine kinases. *Cell, 82*(3), 359–370.

Dunn, T. A., Wang, C. T., Colicos, M. A., Zaccolo, M., DiPilato, L. M., Zhang, J., et al. (2006). Imaging of cAMP levels and protein kinase a activity reveals that retinal waves drive oscillations in second-messenger cascades. *Journal of Neuroscience, 26*(49), 12807–12815.

Dvoriantchikova, G., Ivanov, D., Panchin, Y., & Shestopalov, V. I. (2006). Expression of pannexin family of proteins in the retina. *FEBS Letters, 580*(9), 2178–2182.

Eglen, S. J. (1999). The role of retinal waves and synaptic normalization in retinogeniculate development. *Philosophical Transactions of the Royal Society: Biological Sciences (London), 354*(1382), 497–506.

Fawcett, J. W., O'Leary, D. D., & Cowan, W. M. (1984). Activity and the control of ganglion cell death in the rat retina. *Proceedings of the National Academy of Sciences USA, 81*(17), 5589–5593.

Feldheim, D. A., Nakamoto, M., Osterfield, M., Gale, N. W., DeChiara, T. M., Rohatgi, R., et al. (2004). Loss-of-function analysis of EphA receptors in retinotectal mapping. *Journal of Neuroscience, 24*(10), 2542–2550.

Feldheim, D. A., Vanderhaeghen, P., Hansen, M. J., Frisen, J., Lu, Q., Barbacid, M., et al. (1998). Topographic guidance labels in a sensory projection to the forebrain. *Neuron, 21*(6), 1303–1313.

Feller, M. B. (1999). Spontaneous correlated activity in developing neural circuits. *Neuron, 22*(4), 653–656.

Feller, M. B., Butts, D. A., Aaron, H. L., Rokhsar, D. S., & Shatz, C. J. (1997). Dynamic processes shape spatiotemporal properties of retinal waves. *Neuron, 19*(2), 293–306.

Feller, M. B., & Scanziani, M. (2005). A precritical period for plasticity in visual cortex. *Current Opinion in Neurobiology, 15*(1), 94–100.

Feller, M. B., Wellis, D. P., Stellwagen, D., Werblin, F. S., & Shatz, C. J. (1996). Requirement for cholinergic synaptic transmission in the propagation of spontaneous retinal waves. *Science, 272*(5265), 1182–1187.

Firth, S. I., & Feller, M. B. (2006). Dissociated GABAergic retinal interneurons exhibit spontaneous increases in intracellular calcium. *Visual Neuroscience, 23*(5), 807–814.

Firth, S. I., Wang, C. T., & Feller, M. B. (2005). Retinal waves: Mechanisms and function in visual system development. *Cell Calcium, 37*(5), 425–432.

Fischer, K. F., Lukasiewicz, P. D., & Wong, R. O. (1998). Age-dependent and cell class-specific modulation of retinal ganglion cell bursting activity by GABA. *Journal of Neuroscience, 18*(10), 3767–3778.

Flanagan, J. G. (2006). Neural map specification by gradients. *Current Opinion in Neurobiology, 16*(1), 59–66.

Frisen, J., Yates, P. A., McLaughlin, T., Friedman, G. C., O'Leary, D. D., & Barbacid, M. (1998). Ephrin-A5 (AL-1/RAGS) is essential for proper retinal axon guidance and topographic mapping in the mammalian visual system. *Neuron, 20*(2), 235–243.

Galli, L., & Maffei, L. (1988). Spontaneous impulse activity of rat retinal ganglion cells in prenatal life. *Science, 242*(4875), 90–91.

Godement, P., Salaun, J., & Imbert, M. (1984). Prenatal and postnatal development of retinogeniculate and retinocollicular projections in the mouse. *Journal of Comparative Neurology, 230*(4), 552–575.

Grubb, M. S., Rossi, F. M., Changeux, J. P., & Thompson, I. D. (2003). Abnormal functional organization in the dorsal lateral geniculate nucleus of mice lacking the beta 2 subunit of the nicotinic acetylcholine receptor. *Neuron, 40*(6), 1161–1172.

Guldenagel, M., Sohl, G., Plum, A., Traub, O., Teubner, B., Weiler, R., et al. (2000). Expression patterns of connexin genes in mouse retina. *Journal of Comparative Neurology, 425*(2), 193–201.

Gunhan, E., Choudary, P. V., Landerholm, T. E., & Chalupa, L. M. (2002). Depletion of cholinergic amacrine cells by a novel immunotoxin does not perturb the formation of segregated on and off cone bipolar cell projections. *Journal of Neuroscience, 22*(6), 2265–2273.

Halloran, M. C., & Wolman, M. A. (2006). Repulsion or adhesion: Receptors make the call. *Current Opinion in Cell Biology, 18*(5), 533–540.

Hansen, K. A., Torborg, C. L., Elstrott, J., & Feller, M. B. (2005). Expression and function of the neuronal gap junction protein connexin 36 in developing mammalian retina. *Journal of Comparative Neurology, 493*(2), 309–320.

Hansen, M. J., Dallal, G. E., & Flanagan, J. G. (2004). Retinal axon response to ephrin-as shows a graded, concentration-dependent transition from growth promotion to inhibition. *Neuron, 42*(5), 717–730.

Hanson, M. G., & Landmesser, L. T. (2004). Normal patterns of spontaneous activity are required for correct motor axon guidance and the expression of specific guidance molecules. *Neuron, 43*(5), 687–701.

Hanson, M. G., & Landmesser, L. T. (2006). Increasing the frequency of spontaneous rhythmic activity disrupts pool-specific axon fasciculation and pathfinding of embryonic spinal motoneurons. *Journal of Neuroscience, 26*(49), 12769–12780.

Hebb, D. O. (1949). *The organization of behavior: A neuropsychological theory.* New York: Wiley.

Hensch, T. K. (2004). Critical period regulation. *Annual Review of Neuroscience, 27*, 549–579.

Hindges, R., McLaughlin, T., Genoud, N., Henkemeyer, M., & O'Leary, D. D. (2002). EphB forward signaling controls directional branch extension and arborization required for dorsal-ventral retinotopic mapping. *Neuron, 35*(3), 475–487.

Hirai, H., Maru, Y., Hagiwara, K., Nishida, J., & Takaku, F. (1987). A novel putative tyrosine kinase receptor encoded by the eph gene. *Science, 238*(4834), 1717–1720.

Hooks, B. M., & Chen, C. (2006). Distinct roles for spontaneous and visual activity in remodeling of the retinogeniculate synapse. *Neuron, 52*(2), 281–291.

Hubel, D. H., & Wiesel, T. N. (1959). Receptive fields of single neurones in the cat's striate cortex. *Journal of Physiology, 148*, 574–591.

Hubel, D. H., & Wiesel, T. N. (1962). Receptive fields, binocular interaction and functional architecture in the cat's visual cortex. *Journal of Physiology, 160*, 106–154.

Hubel, D. H., & Wiesel, T. N. (1963). Receptive fields of cells in striate cortex of very young, visually inexperienced kittens. *Journal of Neurophysiology, 26*, 994–1002.

Hubel, D. H., & Wiesel, T. N. (1970). The period of susceptibility to the physiological effects of unilateral eye closure in kittens. *Journal of Physiology, 206*(2), 419–436.

Huberman, A. D., Murray, K. D., Warland, D. K., Feldheim, D. A., & Chapman, B. (2005). Ephrin-As mediate targeting of eye-specific projections to the lateral geniculate nucleus. *Nature Neuroscience, 8*(8), 1013–1021.

Huberman, A. D., Speer, C. M., & Chapman, B. (2006). Spontaneous retinal activity mediates development of ocular dominance columns and binocular receptive fields in v1. *Neuron, 52*(2), 247–254.

Huberman, A. D., Stellwagen, D., & Chapman, B. (2002). Decoupling eye-specific segregation from lamination in the lateral geniculate nucleus. *Journal of Neuroscience, 22*(21), 9419–9429.

Huberman, A. D., Wang, G. Y., Liets, L. C., Collins, O. A., Chapman, B., & Chalupa, L. M. (2003). Eye-specific retinogeniculate segregation independent of normal neuronal activity. *Science, 300*(5621), 994–998.

Hutchins, J. B., & Casagrande, V. A. (1990). Development of the lateral geniculate nucleus: Interactions between retinal afferent, cytoarchitectonic, and glial cell process lamination in ferrets and tree shrews. *Journal of Comparative Neurology, 298*(1), 113–128.

Issa, N. P., Trachtenberg, J. T., Chapman, B., Zahs, K. R., & Stryker, M. P. (1999). The critical period for ocular dominance plasticity in the Ferret's visual cortex. *Journal of Neuroscience, 19*(16), 6965–6978.

Katz, L. C., & Shatz, C. J. (1996). Synaptic activity and the construction of cortical circuits. *Science, 274*(5290), 1133–1138.

Kittila, C. A., & Massey, S. C. (1997). Pharmacology of directionally selective ganglion cells in the rabbit retina. *Journal of Neurophysiology, 77*(2), 675–689.

Komiyama, T., Sweeney, L. B., Schuldiner, O., Garcia, K. C., & Luo, L. (2007). Graded expression of semaphorin-1a cell autonomously directs dendritic targeting of olfactory projection neurons. *Cell, 128*(2), 399–410.

LeVay, S., Stryker, M. P., & Shatz, C. J. (1978). Ocular dominance columns and their development in layer IV of the cat's visual cortex: A quantitative study. *Journal of Comparative Neurology, 179*(1), 223–244.

Linden, D. C., Guillery, R. W., & Cucchiaro, J. (1981). The dorsal lateral geniculate nucleus of the normal ferret and its postnatal development. *Journal of Comparative Neurology, 203*(2), 189–211.

Lisman, J. (1989). A mechanism for the Hebb and the anti-Hebb processes underlying learning and memory. *Proceedings of the National Academy of Sciences USA, 86*(23), 9574–9578.

Liu, Y., Berndt, J., Su, F., Tawarayama, H., Shoji, W., Kuwada, J. Y., et al. (2004). Semaphorin 3D guides retinal axons along the dorsoventral axis of the tectum. *Journal of Neuroscience, 24*(2), 310–318.

Maffei, L., & Galli-Resta, L. (1990). Correlation in the discharges of neighboring rat retinal ganglion cells during prenatal life. *Proceedings of the National Academy of Sciences USA, 87*(7), 2861–2864.

Masland, R. H. (1977). Maturation of function in the developing rabbit retina. *Journal of Comparative Neurology, 175*(3), 275–286.

McLaughlin, T., Hindges, R., Yates, P. A., & O'Leary, D. D. (2003a). Bifunctional action of ephrin-B1 as a repellent and attractant to control bidirectional branch extension in dorsal-ventral retinotopic mapping. *Development, 130*(11), 2407–2418.

McLaughlin, T., & O'Leary, D. D. (2005). Molecular gradients and development of retinotopic maps. *Annual Review of Neuroscience, 28*, 327–355.

McLaughlin, T., Torborg, C. L., Feller, M. B., & O'Leary, D. D. (2003b). Retinotopic map refinement requires spontaneous retinal waves during a brief critical period of development. *Neuron, 40*(6), 1147–1160.

Meister, M., Wong, R. O., Baylor, D. A., & Shatz, C. J. (1991). Synchronous bursts of action potentials in ganglion cells of the developing mammalian retina. *Science, 252*(5008), 939–943.

Miller, E. D., Tran, M. N., Wong, G. K., Oakley, D. M., & Wong, R. O. (1999). Morphological differentiation of bipolar cells in the ferret retina. *Visual Neuroscience, 16*(6), 1133–1144.

Milner, L. D., & Landmesser, L. T. (1999). Cholinergic and GABAergic inputs drive patterned spontaneous motoneuron activity before target contact. *Journal of Neuroscience, 19*(8), 3007–3022.

Mooney, R., Madison, D. V., & Shatz, C. J. (1993). Enhancement of transmission at the developing retinogeniculate synapse. *Neuron, 10*(5), 815–825.

Mooney, R., Penn, A. A., Gallego, R., & Shatz, C. J. (1996). Thalamic relay of spontaneous retinal activity prior to vision. *Neuron, 17*(5), 863–874.

Muir-Robinson, G., Hwang, B. J., & Feller, M. B. (2002). Retinogeniculate axons undergo eye-specific segregation in the absence of eye-specific layers. *Journal of Neuroscience, 22*(13), 5259–5264.

Myers, C. P., Lewcock, J. W., Hanson, M. G., Gosgnach, S., Aimone, J. B., Gage, F. H., et al. (2005). Cholinergic input is required during embryonic development to mediate proper assembly of spinal locomotor circuits. *Neuron, 46*(1), 37–49.

Nakamoto, M., Cheng, H. J., Friedman, G. C., McLaughlin, T., Hansen, M. J., Yoon, C. H., et al. (1996). Topographically specific effects of ELF-1 on retinal axon guidance in vitro and retinal axon mapping in vivo. *Cell, 86*(5), 755–766.

Nicol, X., Muzerelle, A., Rio, J. P., Metin, C., & Gaspar, P. (2006). Requirement of adenylate cyclase 1 for the ephrin-A5-dependent retraction of exuberant retinal axons. *Journal of Neuroscience, 26*(3), 862–872.

Nicol, X., Voyatzis, S., Muzerelle, A., Narboux-Neme, N., Sudhof, T. C., Miles, R., et al. (2007). cAMP oscillations and retinal activity are permissive for ephrin signaling during the establishment of the retinotopic map. *Nature Neuroscience, 10*(3), 340–347.

O'Donovan, M. J. (1999). The origin of spontaneous activity in developing networks of the vertebrate nervous system. *Current Opinion in Neurobiology, 9*(1), 94–104.

O'Leary, D. D., Fawcett, J. W., & Cowan, W. M. (1986). Topographic targeting errors in the retinocollicular projection and their elimination by selective ganglion cell death. *Journal of Neuroscience, 6*(12), 3692–3705.

Olson, C. R., & Freeman, R. D. (1980). Profile of the sensitive period for monocular deprivation in kittens. *Experimental Brain Research, 39*(1), 17–21.

Penn, A. A., Riquelme, P. A., Feller, M. B., & Shatz, C. J. (1998). Competition in retinogeniculate patterning driven by spontaneous activity. *Science, 279*(5359), 2108–2112.

Pfeiffenberger, C., Cutforth, T., Woods, G., Yamada, J., Renteria, R. C., Copenhagen, D. R., et al. (2005). Ephrin-As and neural activity are required for eye-specific patterning during retinogeniculate mapping. *Nature Neuroscience, 8*(8), 1022–1027.

Pfeiffenberger, C., Yamada, J., & Feldheim, D. A. (2006). Ephrin-As and patterned retinal activity act together in the development of topographic maps in the primary visual system. *Journal of Neuroscience, 26*(50), 12873–12884.

Plas, D. T., Visel, A., Gonzalez, E., She, W. C., & Crair, M. C. (2004). Adenylate cyclase 1 dependent refinement of retinotopic maps in the mouse. *Vision Research, 44*(28), 3357–3364.

Rakic, P. (1976). Prenatal genesis of connections subserving ocular dominance in the rhesus monkey. *Nature, 261*(5560), 467–471.

Rashid, T., Upton, A. L., Blentic, A., Ciossek, T., Knoll, B., Thompson, I. D., et al. (2005). Opposing gradients of ephrin-As and EphA7 in the superior colliculus are essential for topographic mapping in the mammalian visual system. *Neuron, 47*(1), 57–69.

Ravary, A., Muzerelle, A., Herve, D., Pascoli, V., Ba-Charvet, K. N., Girault, J. A., et al. (2003). Adenylate cyclase 1 as a key actor in the refinement of retinal projection maps. *Journal of Neuroscience, 23*(6), 2228–2238.

Roerig, B., & Feller, M. B. (2000). Neurotransmitters and gap junctions in developing neural circuits. *Brain Research and Brain Research Reviews, 32*(1), 86–114.

Rossi, F. M., Pizzorusso, T., Porciatti, V., Marubio, L. M., Maffei, L., & Changeux, J. P. (2001). Requirement of the nicotinic acetylcholine receptor beta 2 subunit for the anatomical and functional development of the visual system. *Proceedings of the National Academy of Sciences USA, 98*(11), 6453–6458.

Ruthazer, E. S., Baker, G. E., & Stryker, M. P. (1999). Development and organization of ocular dominance bands in primary visual cortex of the sable ferret. *Journal of Comparative Neurology, 407*(2), 151–165.

Ruthazer, E. S., & Cline, H. T. (2004). Insights into activity-dependent map formation from the retinotectal system: A middle-of-the-brain perspective. *Journal of Neurobiology, 59*(1), 134–146.

Schmitt, A. M., Shi, J., Wolf, A. M., Lu, C. C., King, L. A., & Zou, Y. (2006). Wnt–Ryk signalling mediates medial–lateral retinotectal topographic mapping. *Nature, 439*(7072), 31–37.

Sernagor, E., Eglen, S. J., & Wong, R. O. (2001). Development of retinal ganglion cell structure and function. *Progress in Retina and Eye Research, 20*(2), 139–174.

Shatz, C. J. (1983). The prenatal development of the cat's retinogeniculate pathway. *Journal of Neuroscience, 3*(3), 482–499.

Shatz, C. J. (1996). Emergence of order in visual system development. *Proceedings of the National Academy of Sciences USA, 93*(2), 602–608.

Shatz, C. J., & Stryker, M. P. (1988). Prenatal tetrodotoxin infusion blocks segregation of retinogeniculate afferents. *Science, 242*(4875), 87–89.

Simon, D. K., & O'Leary, D. D. (1992a). Development of topographic order in the mammalian retinocollicular projection. *Journal of Neuroscience, 12*(4), 1212–1232.

Simon, D. K., & O'Leary, D. D. (1992b). Influence of position along the medial–lateral axis of the superior colliculus on the topographic targeting and survival of retinal axons. *Brain Research and Developmental Brain Research, 69*(2), 167–172.

Singer, J. H., Mirotznik, R. R., & Feller, M. B. (2001). Potentiation of L-type calcium channels reveals nonsynaptic mechanisms that correlate spontaneous activity in the developing mammalian retina. *Journal of Neuroscience, 21*(21), 8514–8522.

Sohl, G., Degen, J., Teubner, B., & Willecke, K. (1998). The murine gap junction gene connexin36 is highly expressed in mouse retina and regulated during brain development. *Federation of European Biochemical Societies (FEBS) Letters, 428*(1–2), 27–31.

Sohl, G., Guldenagel, M., Traub, O., & Willecke, K. (2000). Connexin expression in the retina. *Brain Research and Brain Research Reviews, 32*(1), 138–145.

Sperry, R. W. (1963). Chemoaffinity in the orderly growth of nerve fiber patterns and connections. *Proceedings of the National Academy of Sciences USA, 50*, 703–710.

Sretavan, D. W., & Shatz, C. J. (1986). Prenatal development of retinal ganglion cell axons: Segregation into eye-specific layers within the cat's lateral geniculate nucleus. *Journal of Neuroscience, 6*(1), 234–251.

Stacy, R. C., Demas, J., Burgess, R. W., Sanes, J. R., & Wong, R. O. (2005). Disruption and recovery of patterned retinal activity in the absence of acetylcholine. *Journal of Neuroscience, 25*(41), 9347–9357.

Stellwagen, D., & Shatz, C. J. (2002). An instructive role for retinal waves in the development of retinogeniculate connectivity. *Neuron, 33*(3), 357–367.

Stellwagen, D., Shatz, C. J., & Feller, M. B. (1999). Dynamics of retinal waves are controlled by cyclic AMP. *Neuron, 24*(3), 673–685.

Stent, G. S. (1973). A physiological mechanism for Hebb's postulate of learning. *Proceedings of the National Academy of Sciences USA, 70*(4), 997–1001.

Stryker, M. P., & Harris, W. A. (1986). Binocular impulse blockade prevents the formation of ocular dominance columns in cat visual cortex. *Journal of Neuroscience, 6*(8), 2117–2133.

Swartz, M., Eberhart, J., Mastick, G. S., & Krull, C. E. (2001). Sparking new frontiers: Using in vivo electroporation for genetic manipulations. *Developmental Biology, 233*(1), 13–21.

Syed, M. M., Lee, S., Zheng, J., & Zhou, Z. J. (2004). Stage-dependent dynamics and modulation of spontaneous waves in the developing rabbit retina. *Journal of Physiology, 560*(Pt 2), 533–549.

Tauchi, M., & Masland, R. H. (1984). The shape and arrangement of the cholinergic neurons in the rabbit retina. *Proceedings of the Royal Society of London B: Biological Sciences, 223*(1230), 101–119.

Thanos, S., & Bonhoeffer, F. (1987). Axonal arborization in the developing chick retinotectal system. *Journal of Comparative Neurology, 261*(1), 155–164.

Thompson, I., & Holt, C. (1989). Effects of intraocular tetrodotoxin on the development of the retinocollicular pathway in the Syrian hamster. *Journal of Comparative Neurology, 282*(3), 371–388.

Tian, N., & Copenhagen, D. R. (2003). Visual stimulation is required for refinement of ON and OFF pathways in postnatal retina. *Neuron, 39*(1), 85–96.

Torborg, C., Wang, C. T., Muir-Robinson, G., & Feller, M. B. (2004). L-type calcium channel agonist induces correlated depolarizations in mice lacking the beta2 subunit nAChRs. *Vision Research, 44*(28), 3347–3355.

Torborg, C. L., & Feller, M. B. (2005). Spontaneous patterned retinal activity and the refinement of retinal projections. *Progress in Neurobiology, 76*(4), 213–235.

Torborg, C. L., Hansen, K. A., & Feller, M. B. (2005). High frequency, synchronized bursting drives eye-specific segregation of retinogeniculate projections. *Nature Neuroscience, 8*(1), 72–78.

Tu, D. C., Zhang, D., Demas, J., Slutsky, E. B., Provencio, I., Holy, T. E., et al. (2005). Physiologic diversity and development of intrinsically photosensitive retinal ganglion cells. *Neuron, 48*(6), 987–999.

Upton, A. L., Salichon, N., Lebrand, C., Ravary, A., Blakely, R., Seif, I., et al. (1999). Excess of serotonin (5-HT) alters the segregation of ispilateral and contralateral retinal projections in monoamine oxidase A knock-out mice: Possible role of 5-HT uptake in retinal ganglion cells during development. *Journal of Neuroscience, 19*(16), 7007–7024.

Vaney, D. I. (1984). "Coronate" amacrine cells in the rabbit retina have the "starburst" dendritic morphology. *Proceedings of the Royal Society of London B: Biological Sciences, 220*(1221), 501–508.

Warland, D. K., Huberman, A. D., & Chalupa, L. M. (2006). Dynamics of spontaneous activity in the fetal macaque retina during development of retinogeniculate pathways. *Journal of Neuroscience, 26*(19), 5190–5197.

Weliky, M., & Katz, L. C. (1999). Correlational structure of spontaneous neuronal activity in the developing lateral geniculate nucleus in vivo. *Science, 285*(5427), 599–604.

Wiesel, T. N., & Hubel, D. H. (1963). Single-cell responses in striate cortex of kittens deprived of vision in one eye. *Journal of Neurophysiology, 26*, 1003–1017.

Wiesel, T. N., & Hubel, D. H. (1965a). Comparison of the effects of unilateral and bilateral eye closure on cortical unit responses in kittens. *Journal of Neurophysiology, 28*(6), 1029–1040.

Wiesel, T. N., & Hubel, D. H. (1965b). Extent of recovery from the effects of visual deprivation in kittens. *Journal of Neurophysiology, 28*(6), 1060–1072.

Wiesel, T. N., Hubel, D. H., & Lam, D. M. (1974). Autoradiographic demonstration of ocular-dominance columns in the monkey striate cortex by means of transneuronal transport. *Brain Research, 79*(2), 273–279.

Wolman, M. A., Liu, Y., Tawarayama, H., Shoji, W., & Halloran, M. C. (2004). Repulsion and attraction of axons by semaphorin3D are mediated by different neuropilins in vivo. *Journal of Neuroscience, 24*(39), 8428–8435.

Wong, R. O. (1999). Retinal waves and visual system development. *Annual Review of Neuroscience, 22*, 29–47.

Wong, R. O., Chernjavsky, A., Smith, S. J., & Shatz, C. J. (1995). Early functional neural networks in the developing retina. *Nature, 374*(6524), 716–718.

Wong, R. O., Meister, M., & Shatz, C. J. (1993). Transient period of correlated bursting activity during development of the mammalian retina. *Neuron, 11*(5), 923–938.

Wong, W. T., Myhr, K. L., Miller, E. D., & Wong, R. O. (2000). Developmental changes in the neurotransmitter regulation of correlated spontaneous retinal activity. *Journal of Neuroscience, 20*(1), 351–360.

Xu, W., Orr-Urtreger, A., Nigro, F., Gelber, S., Sutcliffe, C. B., Armstrong, D., et al. (1999). Multiorgan autonomic dysfunction in mice lacking the beta2 and the beta4 subunits of neuronal nicotinic acetylcholine receptors. *Journal of Neuroscience, 19*(21), 9298–9305.

Yates, P. A., Roskies, A. L., McLaughlin, T., & O'Leary, D. D. (2001). Topographic-specific axon branching controlled by ephrin-As is the critical event in retinotectal map development. *Journal of Neuroscience, 21*(21), 8548–8563.

Zhang, L. I., & Poo, M. M. (2001). Electrical activity and development of neural circuits. *Nature Neuroscience,* 1207–1214.

Zheng, J., Lee, S., & Zhou, Z. J. (2006). A transient network of intrinsically bursting starburst cells underlies the generation of retinal waves. *Nature Neuroscience, 9*(3), 363–371.

Zheng, J. J., Lee, S., & Zhou, Z. J. (2004). A developmental switch in the excitability and function of the starburst network in the mammalian retina. *Neuron, 44*(5), 851–864.

Zhou, Z. J. (1998). Direct participation of starburst amacrine cells in spontaneous rhythmic activities in the developing mammalian retina. *Journal of Neuroscience, 18*(11), 4155–4165.

Zhou, Z. J., & Zhao, D. (2000). Coordinated transitions in neurotransmitter systems for the initiation and propagation of spontaneous retinal waves. *Journal of Neuroscience, 20*(17), 6570–6577.

Ziburkus, J., & Guido, W. (2006). Loss of binocular responses and reduced retinal convergence during the period of retinogeniculate axon segregation. *Journal of Neurophysiology, 96*(5), 2775–2784.

Early Patterns of Electrical Activity in the Developing Cortex

Rustem Khazipov *and* Gyorgy Buzsáki

Abstract

Early in development, spontaneous neuronal activity is believed to play an important role in the formation of neuronal networks. The dominant pattern of electrical activity in humans during the second half of gestation is "delta-brush," an intermittent, spatially confined oscillation at 5–25 Hz. A homologous pattern in the postnatal rodent neocortex is a spindle-burst. Delta-brushes and spindle-bursts are self-organized events that can be triggered in the somatosensory cortex by sensory feedback resulting from myoclonic twitches in a somatotopic manner. In the visual cortex, spindle-bursts are often driven by spontaneous retinal waves. Under the control of sensory inputs, these patterns provide ideal conditions to imprint metric information of the environment onto the synaptic connectivity of the developing brain.

Keywords: neonate, human, rat, cortex, hippocampus, EEG, delta-brush, spindle-bursts

During development, neurons establish specific synaptic connections to produce highly organized functional neuronal networks. While the general map of neuronal connections is encoded in genes, spontaneous and sensory-driven activities are thought to be equally important for cortical development. Considerable evidence indicates that early electrical activity controls a number of developmental processes including neuronal differentiation, migration, synaptogenesis, and synaptic plasticity (for reviews, see Ben-Ari, Khazipov, Leinekugel, Caillard, & Gaïarsa, 1997; Feldman, Nicoll, & Malenka, 1999; Feller & Scanziani, 2005; Fox, 2002; Henley & Poo, 2004; Katz & Crowley, 2002; Katz & Shatz, 1996; Rakic & Komuro, 1995; Zhou & Poo, 2004). Because electrical patterns are central to the hypothesis of specific synaptic connectivity, it is critical to explore the emergence of

the earliest patterns during development. In this chapter, we review what is currently known about the in vivo patterns of early cortical activity in humans and other animals.

Early Cortical Activity in Humans: *Tracé Discontinu, Tracé Alternant,* and "Delta-Brushes"

One of the most remarkable features of early cortical activity in humans and other animals is its *discontinuous temporal organization*. The first reports on the discontinuous nature of early cortical activity were made in human preterm neonates using scalp electrographic recordings by Dreyfus-Brisac, Monod, and their colleagues. They had analyzed electroencephalograms (EEGs) from preterm neonates, during the second half of gestation (Dreyfus-Brisac, 1962; Dreyfus-Brisac et al.,

1956; Dreyfus-Brisac & Larroche, 1971). They noted that cortical EEG was organized in intermittent bursts separated by periods of isoelectric EEG that could last for seconds or even tens of seconds. This temporal organization was named *tracé discontinu*. With maturation, flat periods between the bursts became shortened and starting from about 30 weeks of postconceptional age, *tracé discontinu* evolves to *tracé alternant* with low-voltage activity between the bursts. At term, some discontinuity is still evident (Lamblin et al., 1999; Stockard-Pope, Werner, & Bickford, 1992).

Variations of these basic patterns have been described by others. Patterns of human EEG in premature infants include transient periods of rhythmic activity and intermittent sharp events that are expressed during certain periods of fetal development (Anderson, Torres, & Faoro, 1985; Lamblin et al., 1999; Scher, 2006; Stockard-Pope et al., 1992). At mid-gestation, the activity is dominated by intermittent delta waves from 0.3 to 2 Hz. By the 7th month, slow oscillations are intermixed with rapid rhythms. Nevertheless, the dominant EEG pattern is the delta-brush (Figure 8.1; Anderson et al., 1985; Lamblin et al., 1999; Scher, 2006; Stockard-Pope et al., 1992). This basic pattern has also been described as spindle-shaped bursts of fast activity (Ellingson, 1958), rapid rhythm (Dreyfus-Brisac, 1962; Nolte, Schulte, Michaelis, Weisse, & Gruson, 1969; Parmelee, Akiyama, Stern, & Harris, 1969), rapid bursts (Dreyfus-Brisac, 1962), spindle-like fast rhythms (Watanabe & Iwase, 1972), fast activity at 14–24 Hz (Goldie, Svedsen-Rhodes, Easton, & Roberton, 1971), and ripples of prematurity (Engel, 1975). Delta-brush consists of 8–25 Hz spindle-like, rhythmic activity superimposed on delta waves. Recent studies using direct current (DC) recordings revealed that the delta wave component observed in the EEG is mainly due to the high-pass (0.5–1 Hz) filtering of an underlying larger amplitude (up to 800 μV) DC shift ("slow activity transient" [SAT]) (Vanhatalo et al., 2002, 2005). Delta-brushes are expressed in all cortical areas and they disappear in waking subjects near term. Thus, although some similarities exist between spindles and delta patterns in the premature and adult brains, their behavioral correlates often differ.

Besides delta-brushes, other patterns expressed in the premature brain may include neonatal "delta crest" (isolated frontopolar delta waves with superimposed fast activity), midline frontal theta/alpha burst, EEG spikes and sharp transients, anterior slow dysrhythmia, temporal sawtooth, or temporal theta bursts (Anderson et al., 1985; Lamblin et al., 1999; Scher, 2006; Stockard-Pope et al., 1992). Because nearly all information about the earliest cortical patterns in humans derive from scalp-recorded EEG of premature infants, these observations alone do not inform us whether they represent pathological activity of the immature brain or the normal physiological patterns of developing neuronal networks. Also, isoelectric epochs separating delta-brushes can represent temporally uncoordinated activity of neurons or absence of excitability of all neurons. Addressing these issues requires simultaneous recording of neuronal spiking and EEG activity in intact developing tissue.

Early Cortical Patterns In Vitro

Numerous patterns of correlated activity have been described in the developing cortical networks using reduced models such as slices, neuronal cultures, or largely intact preparations in vitro. These patterns include synchronized, gap junction–mediated neuronal domains (Kandler & Katz, 1995, 1998a, 1998b; Yuste, Nelson, Rubin, & Katz, 1995; Yuste, Peinado, & Katz, 1992), waves (Peinado, 2000, 2001), acetylcholine-dependent alpha/beta or beta/gamma oscillations (Dupont, Hanganu, Kilb, Hirsch, & Luhmann, 2006), and early network oscillations driven by intracortical glutamatergic and excitatory GABAergic connections (Garaschuk, Linn, Eilers, & Konnerth, 2000). Correlated neuronal activity was also observed in neonatal somatosensory cortex in the intact hemisphere preparation in vitro (Dupont et al., 2006; Schwartz et al., 1998). Parallel studies revealed significant developmental changes in the composition of ionic channels, synaptic connections, ionic transporters, and gap junctions. These developmental changes have a strong impact on the neuronal network activities and may explain the generation of particular patterns of activity in the immature networks (Ben-Ari, 2001, 2002; Ben-Ari et al., 1997; Moody & Bosma, 2005). Examples of discontinuous organization of activity are giant depolarizing potentials (GDPs) (Ben-Ari, Cherubini, Corradetti, & Gaïarsa, 1989) and early network oscillations (Adelsberger, Garaschuk, & Konnerth, 2005; Corlew, Bosma, & Moody, 2004; Garaschuk et al., 2000).

Similar intermittent and spatially confined patterns have been described in the spinal cord (O'Donovan, Chub, & Wenner, 1998), retina (Torborg & Feller, 2005), and tissue cultures of

Figure 8.1 Delta-brushes in human preterm neonate. (A) Representative example of three simultaneous EEG traces recorded in bipolar transversal montage (Frontal FP1-FP2, central C3-C4 and occipital O1-O2) during quiet sleep in a 30-weeks postconceptional age neonate. Bursts of delta waves alternate with periods of hypoactivity. Delta-brushes are characterized by alpha-beta oscillations superimposed on delta waves (gray squares). Traces show concomitant hand and foot movement recordings. (B) Wavelet analysis of bipolar EEG recordings shown in panel A. (Reproduced from Milh et al., 2006.)

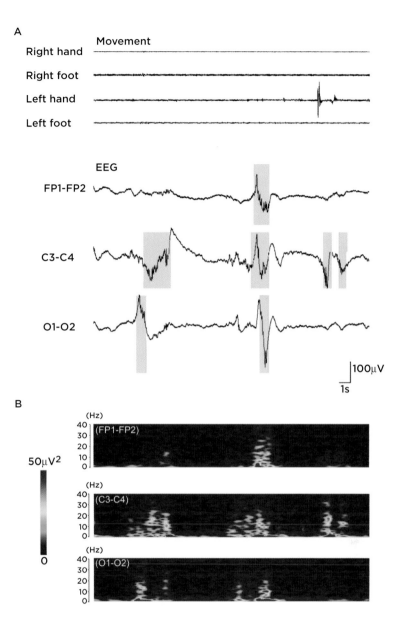

virtually all brain areas (van den Pol, Obrietan, & Belousov, 1996). Patterns resembling *tracé discontinu* were observed in recordings from fetal macaque hippocampal slices in vitro during the second half of gestation (Khazipov et al., 2001). The multitude of these in vitro patterns is in striking contrast to the relatively uniform and simple EEG patterns observed in preterm human babies. Nevertheless, a common underlying feature of all observations is that relatively long activity-free periods are regularly interrupted by transient, relatively uniform self-organized patterns (Figure 8.2). Although experiments using in vitro models have provided valuable information on the properties of developing networks, each of these patterns is different from the other in some important ways. Critically, it is not known whether the various patterns observed in different laboratories, preparations, and particular conditions correspond to distinct classes of naturally occurring patterns in the healthy developing brain or represent particular aspects of the same basic physiological pattern, as predicted by the observations in preterm humans.

First Organized Cortical Network Patterns in the Neonatal Rodent

The discontinuous mode of cortical function, *tracé discontinu* and *tracé alternant*—characteristic

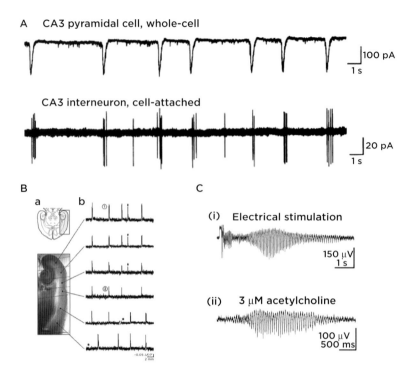

A   CA3 pyramidal cell, whole-cell

100 pA
1 s

CA3 interneuron, cell-attached

20 pA
1 s

B

a   b

–0.05 ΔF/F
2 min

C

(i)   **Electrical stimulation**

150 μV
1 s

(ii)   **3 μM acetylcholine**

100 μV
500 ms

Figure 8.2 Patterns of activity in the neonatal rodent cortex in vitro. (A) Giant depolarizing potentials (GDPs) in the neonatal rat hippocampal slice. Simultaneous whole-cell recordings from CA3 pyramidal cell (upper trace) and cell-attached recordings from CA3 interneuron (bottom trace) (Khazipov et al., 1997). (B) Early network oscillations (ENOs) in the neonatal rat neocortical slice. a, schematic drawing and microphotograph of the brain slice loaded with calcium-sensitive dye and b, changes in calcium-dependent fluorescence in various parts of the neocortex. (Reproduced from Garaschuk et al., 2000.) (C) Alpha-beta oscillations in the neonatal rat intact hemisphere preparation in vitro: field potential recordings from the neocortex in response to (i) electrical stimulation and (ii) application of 3 μM acetylcholine. (Reproduced from Dupont et al., 2006.)

temporal organizations of the cortical activity in humans during the second half of gestation—are present also in the postnatal rodent cortex after birth (Hanganu, Ben-Ari, & Khazipov, 2006; Khazipov et al., 2004b; Minlebaev, Ben-Ari, & Khazipov, 2007). This correspondence is consistent with the fact that the offspring of rats and mice are altricial, that is, they are born in an immature state (Clancy, Darlington, & Finlay, 2001).

Spindle-Bursts in Somatosensory Cortex

Extracellular and patch-clamp recordings from neonatal rat revealed that the dominant pattern of activity in the somatosensory neocortex is a spindle-burst (Khazipov et al., 2004b; Minlebaev et al., 2007). A spindle-burst is a transient burst of rhythmic, 5–25 Hz activity with duration of approximately 1 s (Figure 8.3). Spindle-bursts are reminiscent of adult sleep spindles (Steriade, 2001). However, in contrast to sleep spindles, neonatal spindle-bursts are local events with a limited

tendency to spread. Furthermore, spindle-bursts are present in the waking pup, even during walking and feeding, typically triggered by myoclonic twitches of isolated muscles or whole-body startles. Myoclonic twitches are one of the most remarkable developmental motor phenomena in the neonatal rat (Blumberg & Lucas, 1994; O'Donovan, 1999; Petersson, Waldenstrom, Fahraeus, & Schouenborg, 2003), human fetus, and premature neonate (Cioni & Prechtl, 1990; de Vries, Visser, & Prechtl, 1982; Hamburger, 1975; Prechtl, 1997). This particular type of motor activity results from the stochastic bursts of activity generated in the spinal cord under brainstem control (Blumberg & Lucas, 1994; Karlsson, Gall, Mohns, Seelke, & Blumberg, 2005; Kreider & Blumberg, 2000). Delay between the movements and cortical spindle-bursts, and the observation that spindle-bursts can be also induced by direct sensory stimulation indicate that spindle-bursts are triggered by sensory feedback initiated by spontaneous movements (Figure 8.4).

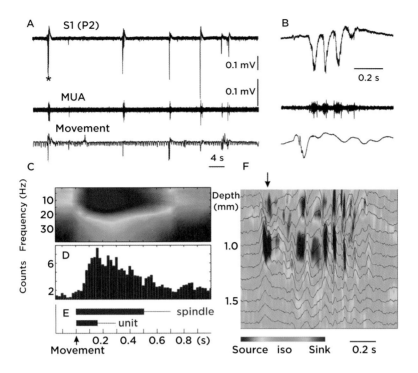

Figure 8.3 Movement-triggered spindle-bursts in primary somatosensory cortex (S1) of the newborn rat. (A) Wide-band recordings of extracellular activity and filtered (0.3–5 kHz) multiple unit activity (MUA) in S1 hind limb area of a P2 rat. Positivity is up. Bottom, movement of the contralateral hind limb. Continuous rhythm reflects respiration. Note that field events and synchronized unit bursts are associated with movements. The event marked by * is shown at expanded timescale in (B). (C) Averaged power spectrogram of field and (D) peri-event histogram of MUA, referenced to movement onset (0 s). Note increased power at 5–15 Hz (C, normalized color code) and MUA rate (D, normalized spikes per bin) between 50 and 550 ms. (E) Mean (+SD) delay between movement peak and peak of spindle power, and movement and unit firing. (F) Transcortical current source density of sharp potential (arrow) and spindle, recorded by a 16-site silicone probe in a P5 rat. (Reproduced from Khazipov et al., 2004b.)

Importantly, spindle-bursts persist after sensory deafferentation (e.g., spinal cord transection), although at a reduced frequency. These results suggested that spindle-bursts are endogenous—probably thalamocortical or intracortical—oscillations. However, external stimuli, for example, brought about by the thalamocortical afferents can trigger these oscillations in the somatosensory cortex in a somatotopic manner.

Spindle-Bursts in Visual Cortex

In the visual system, early stages of development are characterized by the presence of spontaneous waves of activity in the retina before it can respond to light. Retinal waves are generated in the network of retinal ganglion and amacrine cells and synchronize most of retinal activity (Galli & Maffei, 1988; Meister, Wong, Baylor, & Shatz, 1991; Torborg & Feller, 2005; Wong, Meister, & Shatz, 1993). Using an original in vitro preparation of the interconnected intact retina and lateral geniculate nucleus (LGN) of neonatal mouse it was demonstrated that spontaneous retinal activity is transmitted via the optic nerve to the LGN where it drives bursts of activity (Mooney, Penn, Gallego, & Shatz, 1996). Modulation of retinal waves during the first postnatal week results in alteration of retinal projections to their subcortical targets, suggesting an instructive role for retinal waves in the development of retinogeniculate connectivity (Chandrasekaran, Plas, Gonzalez, & Crair, 2005; Grubb, Rossi, Changeux, & Thompson, 2003; McLaughlin, Torborg, Feller, & O'Leary, 2003; Mrsic-Flogel et al., 2005; Muir-Robinson, Hwang, & Feller, 2002; Nicol et al., 2007; Penn, Riquelme, Feller, & Shatz, 1998; Shatz & Stryker, 1988; Stellwagen & Shatz, 2002). Evidence also exists for the contribution of retinal waves to cortical development. In monkeys, ocular dominance columns (ODCs) are formed already in utero before visual experience (Rakic, 1976). Although enucleation experiments suggest that retinal input may not be

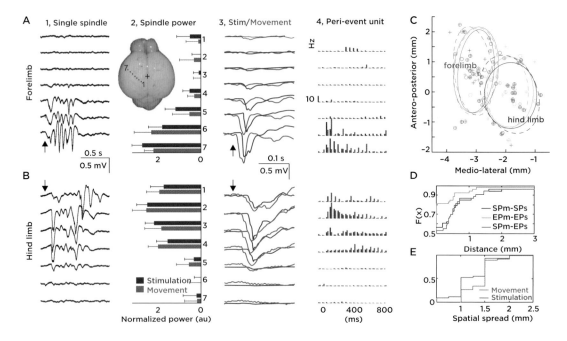

Figure 8.4 Cortical spindle-bursts are spatially confined. (A1) A single spindle event associated with contralateral forelimb jerk (arrow). (A2) Power of spindle events triggered by spontaneous forelimb movement ($n = 11$, blue) or by touch stimulation of the forelimb ($n = 34$, red). Inset: position of recording electrodes. +, bregma. (A3) Averaged field responses and (A4) peri-event time histograms of unit activity triggered by forelimb movement (blue) or touch stimulation (red). (B) Same as in A, but related to contralateral hind limb activity ($n = 20$ movements, $n = 90$ stimulations). (C) Spatial map (in stereotaxic coordinates) of maximal spindle power (crosses) and amplitude of field potentials (circles), triggered by movement (blue, red) or evoked by touch (green, orange), referenced to forelimb (blue-green) and hind limb (red-orange), based on 15 pups. Ellipsoids show 75% confidence intervals. (D) Cumulative probability density function of distances between locations of maximal spindle power triggered by movement or touch stimulation (SPm-SPs), maximal amplitude of evoked potential by movement or touch (EPm-EPs), maximal spindle power by movement or evoked potential by touch (SPm-EPs). (E) Cumulative probability density for effective spatial size of movement-triggered and touch stimulation–evoked spindles. (Reproduced from Khazipov et al., 2004b.)

required for the formation of ODCs (Crowley & Katz, 1999), complete blockade of retinal activity can disturb segregation of thalamocortical connections in ODCs (Stryker & Harris, 1986). In neonatal mice, suppression of retinal waves during the first postnatal week also results in imprecise geniculocortical mapping, suggesting that spontaneous retinal waves are also involved in the development of thalamic connections to the visual cortex (Cang et al., 2005).

These findings suggested the hypothesis that retinal waves are transmitted to and trigger activity in the developing visual cortex. This hypothesis has been tested in neonatal rats (Hanganu et al., 2006). Using extracellular and whole-cell recordings from visual cortex of neonatal rats in vivo, it was shown that, similar to the somatosensory cortex, the dominant pattern of activity in the immature visual cortex is a spindle-burst. Simultaneous recordings from the retina and V1 cortex revealed a strong

correlation between the spindle-bursts in visual cortex and spontaneous retinal waves (Figure 8.5). In addition, V1 spindle-bursts could be reliably evoked by direct stimulation of the optic nerve. Pharmacological modulation of retinal activity affected the rate of occurrence of V1 spindle-bursts; for instance, intraocular forskolin injection, known to increase the frequency and amplitude of retinal waves (Stellwagen et al., 1999), greatly increased the rate of occurrence of cortical spindle-bursts in the contralateral V1 cortex. On the other hand, blocking the propagation of retinal activity with local application of tetrodotoxin or removing the retina entirely resulted in a twofold reduction of V1 spindle-burst frequency, analogously to the reduction of somatosensory spindles after spinal cord transections. These results, therefore, support the hypothesis that spindle-bursts are self-organized patterns that are triggered by sensory feedback. The role of eye movements in the initiation of retinal

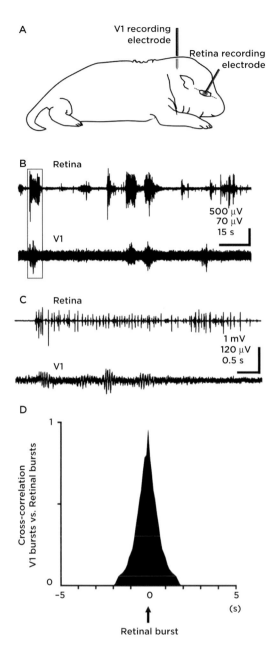

Figure 8.5 Correlation between retinal bursts and V1 cortical spindle-bursts. (A) Scheme of experimental setup for simultaneous cortical and retinal recordings. (B) Simultaneous extracellular local field potential recordings from retina and contralateral V1 in a P6 rat. (C) Strongly correlated retinal burst and V1 spindle-bursts from the traces shown in A and displayed at expanded timescale. (D) Cross-correlogram between the retinal bursts and V1 spindle-bursts. (Reproduced from Hanganu et al., 2006.)

waves or occipital spindle-bursts has not yet been studied.

Similar to neocortical activity in neonatal rats, spindle-bursts continue to be present at later stages of development when the retina becomes responsive to light. In postnatal day (P) 22–39 ferrets, V1 multiple unit activity (MUA) is organized in bursts with about 10 Hz intraburst MUA, and these bursts can be evoked by retinal light stimulation. When multielectrode arrays are used in the study, this bursting activity exhibited a patchy structure that reflects ODCs in visual cortex (Chiu & Weliky, 2001, 2002).

In parallel with electrophysiological discovery of spindle-bursts, a related pattern, termed early network oscillations (ENOs), has been described using calcium imaging of large neuronal populations in vivo (Figure 8.1B; Adelsberger et al., 2005). ENOs are characterized by synchronous intracellular calcium increases that last for about 1 s and recur at about 10-s intervals in P3–4 rats, similar to spindle-bursts. Recorded in temporal cortex, ENOs mainly occurred during movement-free resting periods and it remains unknown whether ENOs in somatosensory cortex are associated with movements. Nevertheless, optical ENOs appear similar to the electrographically defined spindle-bursts, including duration of events and interevent intervals. Although the dynamics of intracellular calcium increases during ENOs was rather smooth and no high-frequency component characteristic oscillation was evident, this may be due to slow dynamics of intracellular calcium and the limited temporal resolution of calcium imaging methods compared to electrophysiological recordings. Further experiments using simultaneous electrophysiological and imaging approaches are needed to determine whether or not spindle-bursts and ENOs reflect the same fundamental physiological patterns. Before speculation about the functional role of the early spontaneous patterns, we discuss the available observations that provide insights into their physiological mechanisms.

Mechanisms of Early Network Patterns
Glutamatergic Synapses

Whole-cell recordings from neonatal rat somatosensory (Khazipov et al., 2004b; Minlebaev et al., 2007) and visual (Hanganu et al., 2006) cortex revealed that spindle-bursts are mediated by both glutamatergic and GABAergic synaptic currents in neocortical neurons. Mechanisms of spindle-bursts were investigated in more detail in the neonatal rat barrel cortex (Minlebaev et al., 2007) using a superfused cortex preparation in vivo, enabling the application of drugs directly to the cortex.

Pharmacological analysis revealed that spindle-bursts are blocked by the AMPA/kainate receptor antagonist CNQX (Figure 8.6) but are little affected by N-*methyl-d-aspartate* (NMDA) receptor or gap junction antagonists. Because the glutamatergic synapses on cortical neurons are mainly provided by the intracortical connections and thalamocortical inputs, two nonexclusive models of spindle-burst oscillations can be proposed: intracortical and thalamocortical. In the intracortical model, the spindle-burst is a local oscillation generated by the network of interconnected cortical glutamatergic neurons. Each cycle of oscillation is set by synchronous excitation of cortical neurons via AMPA/kainate receptors at the corticocortical synapses. Because the GABA (A) receptor antagonists did not significantly affect the frequency of spindle-burst oscillations, neuronal inhibition

probably comes from an after-hyperpolarization mediated by voltage- and calcium-dependent potassium channels. In the thalamocortical model, spindle-bursts are generated by a rhythmic thalamocortical input provided by oscillations in thalamic neurons, similar to the mechanism of adult sleep spindles (Steriade, McCormick, & Sejnowski, 1993). The spatial confinement of spindle-bursts in the developing brain can be explained by the relative scarcity of long-range intracortical and corticothalamic connections early in development. Long-range intracortical projections have been shown to be critical for synchronization of sleep spindles over the entire cortex in adult cats (Contreras, Destexhe, Sejnowski, & Steriade, 1996). Locally emerging spindles in newborn rats may be aided by shunting surround inhibition of depolarizing GABA. We should stress that the two

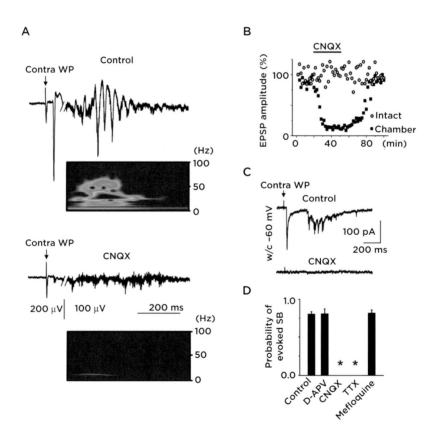

Figure 8.6 The effect of AMPA/kainate receptor antagonist CNQX on sensory-evoked spindle-bursts in barrel cortex. (A) Sensory evoked potentials and spindle-bursts in control conditions (above) and in the presence of CNQX (20 μM) (below). (B) Time course of the effect of CNQX on the amplitude of the sensory-evoked potentials in the superfused (squares) and intact barrel cortex (circles). (C) Whole-cell recordings of the sensory-evoked responses in control conditions and in the presence of CNQX (20 μM). (D) Summary plot on the effect of D-APV (*n* = 5 rats; P3–6), TTX (*n* = 3 rats; P4–6), CNQX (*n* = 7 rats; P2–7) and mefloquine (*n* = 5 rats; P1–3) on the probability of sensory-evoked spindle-bursts (* = *p* < 0.05). (Reproduced from Minlebaev et al., 2007.)

models are not incompatible: thalamic and cortical mechanisms may cooperate in the induction of spindle oscillations.

GABAergic Synapses

Blockade of GABA (A) receptors did not significantly affect the frequency of oscillation associated with spindle-bursts (Minlebaev et al., 2007). Therefore, it seems that GABAergic interneurons play only a minor role in pacing the rhythm of this neonatal oscillation, in contrast to major activity patterns in adults that are significantly influenced by interneurons (Freund & Buzsaki, 1996; Fuentealba & Steriade, 2005). GABAergic inhibition undergoes significant developmental changes during the first postnatal week in the rat; GABA acting via GABA (A) receptors depolarizes immature neocortical neurons because of elevated intracellular chloride concentration (LoTurco, Owens, Heath, Davis, & Kriegstein, 1995; Luhmann & Prince, 1991; Owens, Boyce, Davis, & Kriegstein, 1996; Tyzio et al., 2006; Yamada et al., 2004; Yuste & Katz, 1991). Elevated intracellular chloride in the immature neurons is a result of high activity of chloride loading cotransporter NKCC1 and delayed expression of the chloride extruder KCC2 (Rivera et al., 1999; Yamada et al., 2004). Interestingly, in the neonatal rat hippocampus, the dominant neuronal network patterns of activity (GDPs in vitro and sharp waves in vivo) are blocked by NKCC1 antagonist, bumetanide, which shifts the reversal potential of the GABA (A) receptor-mediated responses toward negative values (Dzhala et al., 2005; Sipila, Schuchmann, Voipio, Yamada, & Kaila, 2006; Tyzio et al., 2006). Although a similar effect of bumetanide on the GABA (A) reversal potential was found in neocortical neonatal neurons (Yamada et al., 2004), bumetanide did not significantly affect spindle-bursts. Therefore, it appears that early hippocampal patterns of sharp waves in vivo and GDPs in vitro are more dependent on the depolarizing actions of GABA than the neocortical pattern of spindle-bursts, consistent with observations in vitro (Garaschuk et al., 2000).

Although GABAergic interneurons may not be directly involved in setting the rhythm of spindle-burst oscillations, they play an important role in their horizontal compartmentalization. Blockade of GABA (A) receptors significantly increased the area of activation during spindle-bursts, as evidenced by increases in the amplitude and power of oscillations, duration of spindle-bursts, and their horizontal spread (Minlebaev et al., 2007).

Thus, compartmentalization of spindle-bursts is determined not only by the somatotopic glutamatergic excitation (Agmon, Hollrigel, & O'Dowd, 1996; Bureau, Shepherd, & Svoboda, 2004; Ferezou, Bolea, & Petersen, 2006; Higashi, Molnar, Kurotani, & Toyama, 2002; Khazipov et al., 2004b; Kidd & Isaac, 1999; Petersen & Sakmann, 2001), but also by surround GABAergic inhibition that prevents horizontal spread of the activity via long-range glutamatergic cortical connections, a pattern observed in the adult neocortex (Chagnac-Amitai & Connors, 1989; Fox, Wright, Wallace, & Glazewski, 2003; Sun, Huguenard, & Prince, 2006). The inhibitory action of depolarizing GABA at the network level is probably due to the shunting mechanisms amplified by the activation of the voltage-gated potassium channels and inactivation of sodium channels (Borg-Graham, Monier, & Fregnac, 1998; Gao, Chen, & van den Pol, 1998; Gulledge & Stuart, 2003; Lu & Trussell, 2001). These results are in general agreement with the finding that intraperitoneal administration of a GABA (A) antagonist, bicuculline, induces hypersynchronous seizure-like activity in the neocortex in vivo by P3 (Baram & Snead, 1990) and in vitro by P2 (Wells, Porter, & Agmon, 2000).

In Vivo versus In Vitro

As described earlier, numerous patterns of correlated activity have been described in postnatal rat neocortical slices in vitro (for review Moody & Bosma, 2005; Khazipov & Luhmann, 2006), including "synchronized-via-gap junctions neuronal domains" (Kandler & Katz, 1995, 1998a, 1998b; Yuste et al., 1992, 1995) and calcium waves (Peinado, 2000, 2001), gap junction and NMDA receptor–based cholinergic oscillations (Dupont et al., 2006), and GDPs and early network oscillations driven by glutamatergic and excitatory GABAergic synapses (Agmon et al., 1996; Ben-Ari et al., 1989; Garaschuk, Hanse, & Konnerth, 1998; Garaschuk et al., 2000; Khazipov, Leinekugel, Khalilov, Gaïarsa, & Ben-Ari, 1997; Leinekugel, Khalilov, Ben-Ari, & Khazipov, 1998; Leinekugel, Medina, Khalilov, Ben-Ari, & Khazipov, 1997). The large variability of neocortical in vitro patterns, we believe, can be largely explained by the diversity of experimental conditions, age differences, and other experimental variables. Studies using cortical preparations in vitro have emphasized the role of several developmentally regulated mechanisms of neuronal synchronization in the developing cortex including: (i) gap junctions (Dupont et al., 2006; Kandler & Katz, 1995, 1998a, 1998b;

Peinado, 2000, 2001; Yuste et al., 1992, 1995), (ii) NMDA receptors (Ben-Ari et al., 1989; Dupont et al., 2006; Leinekugel et al., 1997), and (iii) depolarizing GABA (Ben-Ari et al., 1989; Garaschuk et al., 1998, 2000; Khazipov et al., 1997, 2004a; Leinekugel et al., 1997; Sipila, Huttu, Soltesz, Voipio, & Kaila, 2005; Sipila et al., 2006). In contrast, pharmacological analysis of spindle-bursts in neonatal rat barrel cortex suggests that the generation of in vivo neocortical spindle-bursts relies on "mature" AMPA/kainate receptor-mediated synaptic transmission (Minlebaev et al., 2007). It should be noted that AMPA/kainate antagonists were also effective in suppressing some types of in vitro network activity during the neonatal period, including spontaneous—but not stimulation-evoked—GDPs (Ben-Ari et al., 1989; Bolea, Avignone, Berretta, Sanchez-Andres, & Cherubini, 1999; Khazipov et al., 1997; Lamsa, Palva, Ruusuvuori, Kaila, & Taira, 2000), polysynaptic events in barrel cortex evoked by thalamic stimulation (Agmon et al., 1996) and neocortical ENOs (Garaschuk et al., 2000).

Because the earliest in vivo patterns are congruent across cortical regions and species, including rats and humans, we believe that the various in vitro patterns described by various investigators all relate to certain aspects of a single physiological pattern: cortical spindle-bursts. Another fundamental difference between in vitro and in vivo population events is that whereas repetition of patterns in vitro are regular with intervals varying across preparations, in vivo patterns tend to be quite irregular. At least for the somatosensory cortical patterns, we can provide an explanation. Self-organized or spontaneous patterns emerge at every level of the neuraxis. In isolation, these patterns tend to be highly regular because the alternation of silent and active periods is determined by time constants intrinsic to the networks. However, relaxation oscillators with separable input and "duty cycle" (output) phases can be easily perturbed by external influences in the relaxation (input) periods (Buzsaki & Draguhn, 2004). In newborn rats, such effects arrive from sensory feedback from muscle twitches, limb jerks, and whole-body startles (Khazipov et al., 2004b). Because skeletal muscle activation is brought about by stochastic activity within the spinal cord and brain stem, the cortical spindles have an irregular appearance.

Why is Early Cortical Activity Discontinuous?

Although this question is important for understanding the mode of operation of the immature brain, it has received very little attention. Three important physiological changes in cortical activity should be emphasized during development. First, the long silent periods, characteristic of the immature cortical activity become systematically shorter with age. Second, the generalized silent periods become state-dependent. Third, the active and silent periods become temporally synchronized across large cortical domains. In the adult brain, generalized silent periods are short and present only during slow-wave sleep, marked by widely coherent delta waves. Similar to the immature brain, the adult neocortex "reboots" itself periodically after each delta wave ("down" state) event. However, the silent periods last only for 200–500 ms and can be synchronous over the entire neocortex–allocortex axis (Isomura et al., 2006; Steriade, 1993, 2001).

Mechanisms underlying discontinuity of activity in the immature cortex are largely unknown. At least five developmental factors may be involved:

1. *Intrinsic neuronal properties.* Although the resting membrane potential does not change with age (Tyzio et al., 2003), immature neurons fire few spontaneous action potentials, probably due to developmental changes in the expression of voltage-gated channels (Moody & Bosma, 2005). For instance, hyperpolarization-activated cationic channels that are important for spontaneous bursting of pyramidal cells are expressed late in development (Bender et al., 2005). In addition, immature neurons fail to maintain continuous firing upon depolarization (Luhmann, Reiprich, Hanganu, & Kilb, 2000). On the other hand, immature neurons have a very high input resistance—in the gigaohm range—and a small electrical capacitance (Luhmann et al., 2000; Tyzio et al., 2003) that makes them extremely sensitive to synaptic inputs.

2. *Synaptic connections* are very sparse at midgestation in primates and at birth in rodents and their numbers dramatically increase with maturation (Bannister & Larkman, 1995; Englisch, Kunz, & Wenzel, 1974; Khazipov et al., 2001; Minkwitz, 1976; Tyzio et al., 1999). For instance, up to 200 novel glutamatergic synapses are established on one CA1 pyramidal cell per day in macaque in utero to endow a pyramidal cell with about 7000 glutamatergic synapses at term (Khazipov et al., 2001). Not only the number, but also the properties of synaptic connections change during development including the depolarizing action of GABA (Ben-Ari, 2002; Ben-Ari et al., 1997; Cherubini, Gaïarsa, & Ben-Ari, 1991; Luhmann & Prince, 1991), presence of

silent NMDA receptor-based glutamatergic synapses that lack functional AMPA receptors in thalamocortical (Isaac, Crair, Nicoll, & Malenka, 1997) and intracortical synapses (Durand, Kovalchuk, & Konnerth, 1996), long openings of NMDA receptors (Carmignoto & Vicini, 1992; Hestrin, 1992; Khazipov, Ragozzino, & Bregestovski, 1995), activity-dependent depression in glutamatergic synapses (Burgard & Hablitz, 1993; Reyes & Sakmann, 1999), and lack of postsynaptic GABA (B)-mediated responses (Caillard, McLean, Ben-Ari, & Gaïarsa, 1998; Fukuda, Mody, & Prince, 1993) (for reviews, see Ben-Ari, 2002; Ben-Ari et al., 1997).

3. Maturation of the *generalized modulatory systems* (cholinergic, noradrenergic, etc.) that control cortical activity and determine the transitions between the vigilance states in adult (Jouvet, 1999; McCormick & Bal, 1997; Steriade, 2004).

4. *Corticothalamic* feedback and *intrathalamic connections* develop in parallel with the neocortex (Domich, Oakson, Deschenes, & Steriade, 1987; Warren & Jones, 1997).

5. *Intracortical excitatory feedback and especially long-range* connections are sparse at an early stage (Warren & Jones, 1997). Long-range connections, which arise from the superficial cortical layers, take particularly long time to develop in the postnatal time. In the absence of such regenerative feedback excitation, oscillatory phenomena can quickly dampen and remain local. In the adult brain, neuronal activity after a single stimulus may persist for a long time and involve large neuronal space with neuronal firing patterns, reflecting stimulus-specific features. In contrast, in the immature brain, the evoked activity remains largely localized.

Functions of Early Population Patterns

Numerous excellent reviews discuss the potential benefits provided by the earliest network patterns (Ben-Ari et al., 1997; Katz & Shatz, 1996; Moody & Bosma, 2005). Here, we will confine our speculations to the somatosensory cortex. Several lines of evidence indicate that spindle-bursts in the neonatal rat and preterm human delta-brushes are identical events (Khazipov & Luhmann, 2006; Khazipov et al., 2004b; Milh et al., 2006). This includes a similar spindle shape and oscillatory frequency, local nature, correlation with movements and the ability to be evoked by tactile stimulation in the somatosensory cortex, and occurrence within comparable developmental windows. Furthermore, DC recordings from the neonatal

rat somatosensory cortex revealed large NMDA and AMPA receptors mediated DC shifts (SATs) associated with spindle-bursts (Minlebaev, Ben Ari, & Khazipov 2009), similar to the underlying delta-brushes in human preterm babies (Vanhatalo et al., 2002, 2005). We therefore suggest that scalp-recorded delta-brushes and SATs in human babies and cortical spindle-bursts in rat pups are homologous events with likely identical cellular, synaptic, and other mechanisms.

The frequent occurrence of fetal movements or "baby kicks" in the later stages of pregnancy has been well-known to expectant mothers and physicians for long as an important indicator of the normal development of the fetus. The intermittent delta-brushes in the scalp-recorded EEG of preterm babies have also been known for several decades (Dreyfus-Brisac, 1962; Dreyfus-Brisac & Larroche, 1971; Lamblin et al., 1999; Stockard-Pope et al., 1992). Our studies in newborn rats and human preterm infants revealed an important link between these two lines of clinical observations (Khazipov et al., 2004b; Milh et al., 2006).

Analogous to human fetal movements, newborn rat pups also display muscle twitches, limb jerks, and whole-body startles, and stochastic motor patterns generated by the spinal cord even in the absence of the brain (Blumberg & Lucas, 1994; O'Donovan, 1999; Petersson et al., 2003). Importantly, our work has shown that each of these motor patterns has the ability to trigger a cortical S1 spindle-burst. Prompted by our findings in rat pups, we recently examined the relationship between delta-brushes in scalp-recorded EEG and spontaneous movements of premature human neonates of 29–31 weeks postconceptional age (Milh et al., 2006). In direct support of the observations in rats, sporadic hand and foot movements heralded the appearance of delta-brushes in corresponding areas of the cortex (lateral and medial regions of the contralateral central cortex, respectively). Furthermore, direct hand and foot stimulation also reliably evoked delta-brushes in the same areas (Figure 8.7). These results in humans demonstrate that sensory information derived from stochastic, spontaneous fetal movements can trigger delta-brush oscillations in the central cortex in a somatotopic manner. Based on the combined observations in rats and humans, we assume that a similar relationship exists in the human fetus in utero: spontaneous fetal movements provide sensory stimulation and drive delta-brush oscillations before the brain is exposed to the elaborated sensory input from the external world.

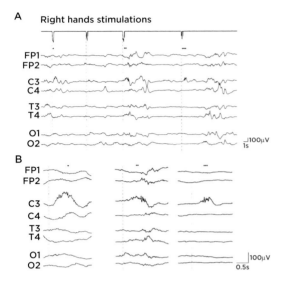

A
Right hands stimulations

FP1
FP2

C3
C4

T3
T4

O1
O2

⌐100μV
1s

B
FP1
FP2

C3
C4

T3
T4

O1
O2

|100μV
0.5s

C

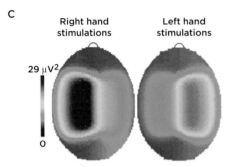

| Right hand stimulations | Left hand stimulations |

29 μV²

0

Figure 8.7 Sensory stimulation of the hand evokes contralateral central delta-brushes in the human premature neonate. (A) Simultaneous recordings of hand stimulation and monopolar recordings from eight recording sites (average as reference). Note that caressing the neonate's right hand (indicated by dashed line) reliably evokes deltabrushes in the left central region (C3). (B) Three examples of stimulation-evoked delta-brushes are shown on expanded timescale (dashed lines indicate the onset of stimulations). Wide band (0.16–96 Hz) recordings from 30-weeks postconceptional age neonate. (C) Cortical map of the responses evoked by right- and left-hand stimulation presented as alpha-beta power. Note that stimulation-evoked alpha-beta oscillations are predominant in the contralateral cortical areas. (Reproduced from Milh et al., 2006.)

From these recent findings, we conjectured that muscle activity–triggered cortical spindle-bursts may be critical for the development of the body map (Buzsaki, 2006; Khazipov et al., 2004b) (see also Blumberg & Lucas, 1996; Seelke, Karlsson, Gall, & Blumberg, 2005). Stretch sensors in muscles and tendons report the contractile state of the muscle to the spinal cord and eventually to the somatosensory cortex. In addition, twitches of

skeletal muscles increase the probability that the skin over the muscle may touch another pup in the litter or some other external objects, and the wall of the womb in case of human babies (Petersson et al., 2003). Uncoordinated induction of cortical activity by the several hundred skeletal muscles that move the mammalian body would be of very little relevance. However, due to the physical constraints of the bones and joints, only a limited number of muscle movement combinations can be realized out of the potentially very large degrees of freedom that would result from the unrestrained combination of muscle activity. Importantly, all these movement combinations are meaningful inputs to the somatosensory thalamus and cortex because these are the combinations that will be used later in life. We hypothesize that the coordination of movement–afferent feedback–cortical spindle-burst sequences serves to convert the initially abstract body representation in the sensory cortex to a concrete metric space. Such relationships cannot be achieved by a general genetic blueprint (Blumberg, 2005; Keller, 2000; Nijhout, 1990; Oyama, Griffiths, & Gray, 2001) since the metric relations among the body parts change dynamically as the body grows. We hypothesize that the "training" input from muscle combinations are translated into a synaptic organization in the somatosensory system by creating new connections and eliminating existing ones. The longlasting nature of the cortical spindle oscillation can sustain local activity so that activity patterns arising from other areas, mediated by the emerging intermediate and long-range corticocortical connections, can be temporally associated.

In parallel with the establishment of sensory-motor coordination, the thalamocortical circuit comes under the control of subcortical modulatory systems, which prevent the occurrence of spindles in the adult waking brain. Early development thus can be viewed as a "wakening" process of the forebrain from its dominantly sleep-like state. Nevertheless, the basic algorithms associated with the spindle mechanism may survive and may be utilized for other functions. Whereas in the premature brain, cortical spindles are explicitly triggered by body afferents, in adults they occur only during early stages of sleep. Sleep is generally thought of as a mechanism for the brain's separation from the environment and, to a large extent, from the body (Steriade et al., 1993). Nevertheless, spontaneous muscle twitches or even large startle motor patterns that seize the whole body continue to occur even in the adult at the transition to sleep and can trigger sleep spindles (Mello, Silva, Rueda, Poyares, & Tufik, 1997). We hypothesize that at least one physiological function of sleep spindles in the adult somatosensory cortex remains analogous to that of the early cortical spindles: assisting preservation of body representation.

References

Adelsberger, H., Garaschuk, O., & Konnerth, A. (2005). Cortical calcium waves in resting newborn mice. *Nature Neuroscience, 8*, 988–990.

Agmon, A., Hollrigel, G., & O'Dowd, D. K. (1996). Functional GABAergic synaptic connection in neonatal mouse barrel cortex. *Journal of Neuroscience, 16*, 4684–4695.

Anderson, C. M., Torres, F., & Faoro, A. (1985). The EEG of the early premature. *Electroencephalography and Clinical Neurophysiology, 60*, 95–105.

Bannister, N. J., & Larkman, A. U. (1995). Dendritic morphology of CA1 pyramidal neurones from the rat hippocampus: II. Spine distributions. *The Journal of Comparative Neurology, 360*, 161–171.

Baram, T. Z., & Snead, O. C. (1990). Bicuculline-induced seizures in infant rats: Ontogeny of behavioral and electrocortical phenomena. *Developmental Brain Research, 57*, 291–295.

Ben-Ari, Y. (2001). Developing networks play similar melody. *Trends in Neurosciences, 24*, 354–360.

Ben-Ari, Y. (2002). Excitatory actions of GABA during development: The nature of the nurture. *Nature Reviews Neuroscience, 3*, 728–739.

Ben-Ari, Y., Cherubini, E., Corradetti, R., & Gaïarsa, J. L. (1989). Giant synaptic potentials in immature rat CA3 hippocampal neurones. *The Journal of Physiology, 416*, 303–325.

Ben-Ari, Y., Khazipov, R., Leinekugel, X., Caillard, O., & Gaïarsa, J. L. (1997). GABA_A, NMDA and AMPA receptors: A developmentally regulated "ménage a trois." *Trends in Neurosciences, 20*, 523–529.

Bender, R. A., Galindo, R., Mameli, M., Gonzalez-Vega, R., Valenzuela, C. F., & Baram, T. Z. (2005). Synchronized network activity in developing rat hippocampus involves regional hyperpolarization-activated cyclic nucleotide-gated (HCN) channel function. *The European Journal of Neuroscience, 22*, 2669–2674.

Blumberg, M. S. (2005). *Basic instinct: The genesis of behavior.* New York: Thunder's Mouth Press.

Blumberg, M. S., & Lucas, D. E. (1994). Dual mechanisms of twitching during sleep in neonatal rats. *Behavioral Neuroscience, 108*, 1196–1202.

Blumberg, M. S., & Lucas, D. E. (1996). A developmental and component analysis of active sleep. *Developmental Psychobiology, 29*, 1–22.

Bolea, S., Avignone, E., Berretta, N., Sanchez-Andres, J. V., & Cherubini, E. (1999). Glutamate controls the induction of GABA-mediated giant depolarizing potentials through AMPA receptors in neonatal rat hippocampal slices (in process citation). *Journal of Neurophysiology, 81*, 2095–2102.

Borg-Graham, L. J., Monier, C., & Fregnac, Y. (1998). Visual input evokes transient and strong shunting inhibition in visual cortical neurons. *Nature, 393*, 369–373.

Bureau, I., Shepherd, G. M., & Svoboda, K. (2004). Precise development of functional and anatomical columns in the neocortex. *Neuron, 42*, 789–801.

Burgard, E. C., & Hablitz, J. J. (1993). Developmental changes in NMDA and non-NMDA receptor-mediated synaptic potentials in rat neocortex. *Journal of Neurophysiology, 69*, 230–240.

Buzsaki, G. (2006). *Rhythms of the brain.* New York: Oxford University Press.

Caillard, O., McLean, H. A., Ben-Ari, Y., & Gaïarsa, J. L. (1998). Ontogenesis of presynaptic GABA_B receptor-mediated inhibition in the CA3 region of the rat hippocampus. *Journal of Neurophysiology, 79*, 1341–1348.

Cang, J., Renteria, R. C., Kaneko, M., Liu, X., Copenhagen, D. R., & Stryker, M. P. (2005). Development of precise maps in visual cortex requires patterned spontaneous activity in the retina. *Neuron, 48*, 797–809.

Carmignoto, G., & Vicini, S. (1992). Activity-dependent decrease in NMDA receptor responses during development of the visual cortex. *Science, 258*, 1007–1011.

Chagnac-Amitai, Y., & Connors, B. W. (1989). Horizontal spread of synchronized activity in neocortex and its control by GABA-mediated inhibition. *Journal of Neurophysiology, 61*, 747–758.

Chandrasekaran, A. R., Plas, D. T., Gonzalez, E., & Crair, M. C. (2005). Evidence for an instructive role of retinal activity in retinotopic map refinement in the superior colliculus of the mouse. *Journal of Neuroscience, 25*, 6929–6938.

Cherubini, E., Gaïarsa, J. L., & Ben-Ari, Y. (1991). GABA: An excitatory transmitter in early postnatal life. *Trends in Neurosciences, 14*, 515–519.

Chiu, C., & Weliky, M. (2001). Spontaneous activity in developing ferret visual cortex in vivo. *Journal of Neuroscience, 21*, 8906–8914.

Chiu, C., & Weliky, M. (2002). Relationship of correlated spontaneous activity to functional ocular dominance columns in the developing visual cortex. *Neuron, 35*, 1123–1134.

Cioni, G., & Prechtl, H. F. (1990). Preterm and early post-term motor behaviour in low-risk premature infants. *Early Human Development, 23*, 159–191.

Clancy, B., Darlington, R. B., & Finlay, B. L. (2001). Translating developmental time across mammalian species. *Neuroscience, 105*, 7–17.

Contreras, D., Destexhe, A., Sejnowski, T. J., & Steriade, M. (1996). Control of spatiotemporal coherence of a thalamic oscillation by corticothalamic feedback. *Science, 274*, 771–774.

Corlew, R., Bosma, M. M., & Moody, W. J. (2004). Spontaneous, synchronous electrical activity in neonatal mouse cortical neurones. *The Journal of Physiology, 560*, 377–390.

Crowley, J. C., & Katz, L. C. (1999). Development of ocular dominance columns in the absence of retinal input. *Nature Neuroscience, 2*, 1125–1130.

de Vries, J. I., Visser, G. H., & Prechtl, H. F. (1982). The emergence of fetal behaviour. I. Qualitative aspects. *Early Human Development, 7*, 301–322.

Domich, L., Oakson, G., Deschenes, M., & Steriade, M. (1987). Thalamic and cortical spindles during early ontogenesis in kittens. *Brain Research, 428*, 140–142.

Dreyfus-Brisac, C. (1962). The electroencephalogram of the premature infant. *World Neurology, 3*, 5–15.

Dreyfus-Brisac, C., Fischgold, H., Samson-Dollfus, D., Saint-Anne Dargassies, S., Ziegler, T., Monod, N., & Blanc, C. (1956). Veille sommeil et reactivite sensorielle chez le premature et le nouveau-ne. *Electroencephalography and Clinical Neurophysiology, 6*, 418–440.

Dreyfus-Brisac, C., & Larroche, J. C. (1971). Discontinuous electroencephalograms in the premature newborn and at term. Electro-anatomo-clinical correlations. *Review of Electroencephalography and Clinical Neurophysiology, 1*, 95–99.

Dupont, E., Hanganu, I. L., Kilb, W., Hirsch, S., & Luhmann, H. J. (2006). Rapid developmental switch in the mechanisms driving early cortical columnar networks. *Nature, 439*, 79–83.

Durand, G. M., Kovalchuk, Y., & Konnerth, A. (1996). Long-term potentiation and functional synapse induction in developing hippocampus. *Nature, 381*, 71–75.

Dzhala, V. I., Talos, D. M., Sdrulla, D. A., Brumback, A. C., Mathews, G. C., Benke, T. A., Delpire, E., Jensen, F. E., & Staley, K. J. (2005). NKCC1 transporter facilitates seizures in the developing brain. *Nature Medicine, 11*, 1205–1213.

Ellingson, R. J. (1958). Electroencephalograms of normal, full-term newborns immediately after birth with observations on arousal and visual evoked responses. *Electroencephalography and Clinical Neurophysiology. Supplement, 10*, 31–50.

Engel, R. (1975). *Abnormal electroencephalograms in the neonatal period.* Springfield, IL: Charles C Thomas.

Englisch, H. J., Kunz, G., & Wenzel, J. (1974). Distribution of spines on the pyramidal neurons in the CA-1 region of the hippocampus in the rat. *Zeitschrift für Mikroskopisch-Anatomische Forschung, 88*, 85–102.

Feldman, D. E., Nicoll, R. A., & Malenka, R. C. (1999). Synaptic plasticity at thalamocortical synapses in developing rat somatosensory cortex: LTP, LTD, and silent synapses. *Journal of Neurobiology, 41*, 92–101.

Feller, M. B., & Scanziani, M. (2005). A precritical period for plasticity in visual cortex. *Current Opinion in Neurobiology, 15*, 94–100.

Ferezou, I., Bolea, S., & Petersen, C. C. H. (2006). Visualizing the cortical representation of whisker touch: Voltage-sensitive dye imaging in freely moving mice. *Neuron, 50*, 617–629.

Fox, K. (2002). Anatomical pathways and molecular mechanisms for plasticity in the barrel cortex. *Neuroscience, 111*, 799–814.

Fox, K., Wright, N., Wallace, H., & Glazewski, S. (2003). The origin of cortical surround receptive fields studied in the barrel cortex. *The Journal of Neuroscience, 23*, 8380–8391.

Freund, T., & Buzsaki, G. (1996). Interneurons of the hippocampus. *Hippocampus, 6*, 345–470.

Fuentealba, P., & Steriade, M. (2005). The reticular nucleus revisited: Intrinsic and network properties of a thalamic pacemaker. *Progress in Neurobiology, 75*, 125–141.

Fukuda, A., Mody, I., & Prince, D.A. (1993). Differential ontogenesis of presynaptic and postsynaptic GABA$_B$ inhibition in the rat somatosensory cortex. *Journal of Neurophysiology, 70*, 448–452.

Galli, L., & Maffei, L. (1988). Spontaneous impulse activity of rat retinal ganglion cells in prenatal life. *Science, 242*, 90–91.

Gao, X. B., Chen, G., & van den Pol, A. N. (1998). GABA-dependent firing of glutamate-evoked action potentials at AMPA/kainate receptors in developing hypothalamic neurons. *Journal of Neurophysiology, 79*, 716–726.

Garaschuk, O., Hanse, E., & Konnerth, A. (1998). Developmental profile and synaptic origin of early network oscillations in the CA1 region of rat neonatal hippocampus. *The Journal of Physiology, 507*, 219–236.

Garaschuk, O., Linn, J., Eilers, J., & Konnerth, A. (2000). Large-scale oscillatory calcium waves in the immature cortex. *Nature, 3*, 452–459.

Goldie, L., Svedsen-Rhodes, U., Easton, J., & Roberton, N. R. (1971). The development of innate sleep rhythms in short gestation infants. *Developmental Medicine and Child Neurology, 13*, 40–50.

Grubb, M. S., Rossi, F. M., Changeux, J. P., & Thompson, I. D. (2003). Abnormal functional organization in the dorsal lateral geniculate nucleus of mice lacking the beta 2 subunit of the nicotinic acetylcholine receptor. *Neuron, 40*, 1161–1172.

Gulledge, A. T., & Stuart, G. J. (2003). Excitatory actions of GABA in the cortex. *Neuron, 37*, 299–309.

Hamburger, V. (1975). Fetal behavior. In E. S. Hafez (Ed.), *The mammalian fetus: Comparative biology and methodology* (pp. 69–81). Springfield, IL: Charles C Thomas.

Hanganu, I. L., Ben-Ari, Y., & Khazipov, R. (2006). Retinal waves trigger spindle bursts in the neonatal rat visual cortex. *Journal of Neuroscience, 26*, 6728–6736.

Henley, J., & Poo, M. M. (2004). Guiding neuronal growth cones using Ca^{2+} signals. *Trends in Cell Biology, 14*, 320–330.

Hestrin, S. (1992). Developmental regulation of NMDA receptor-mediated synaptic currents at a central synapse. *Nature, 357*, 686–689.

Higashi, S., Molnar, Z., Kurotani, T., & Toyama, K. (2002). Prenatal development of neural excitation in rat thalamocortical projections studied by optical recording. *Neuroscience, 115*, 1231–1246.

Isaac, J. T. R., Crair, M. C., Nicoll, R. A., & Malenka, R. C. (1997). Silent synapses during development of thalamocortical inputs. *Neuron, 18*, 269–280.

Isomura, Y., Sirota, A., Ozen, S., Montgomery, S., Mizuseki, K., Henze, D. A., & Buzsaki, G. (2006). Integration and segregation of activity in entorhinal-hippocampal subregions by neocortical slow oscillations. *Neuron, 52*, 871–882.

Jouvet, M. (1999). Sleep and serotonin: An unfinished story. *Neuropsychopharmacology, 21*, 24S–27S.

Kandler, K., & Katz, L. C. (1995). Neuronal coupling and uncoupling in the developing nervous system. *Current Opinion in Neurobiology, 5*, 98–105.

Kandler, K., & Katz, L. C. (1998a). Coordination of neuronal activity in developing visual cortex by gap junction-mediated biochemical communication. *Journal of Neuroscience, 18*, 1419–1427.

Kandler, K., & Katz, L. C. (1998b). Relationship between dye coupling and spontaneous activity in developing ferret visual cortex. *Developmental Neuroscience, 20*, 59–64.

Karlsson, K. A., Gall, A. J., Mohns, E. J., Seelke, A. M., & Blumberg, M. S. (2005). The neural substrates of infant sleep in rats. *PLoS Biology, 3*, e143.

Katz, L. C., & Crowley, J. C. (2002). Development of cortical circuits: Lessons from ocular dominance columns. *Nature Reviews. Neuroscience, 3*, 34–42.

Katz, L. C., & Shatz, C. J. (1996). Synaptic activity and the construction of cortical circuits. *Science, 274*, 1133–1138.

Keller, E. F. (2000). *The century of the gene*. Cambridge, MA: Harvard University Press.

Khazipov, R., Esclapez, M., Caillard, O., Bernard, C., Khalilov, I., Tyzio, R., et al. (2001). Early development of neuronal activity in the primate hippocampus in utero. *Journal of Neuroscience*, *21*, 9770–9781.

Khazipov, R., Khalilov, I., Tyzio, R., Morozova, E., Ben-Ari, Y., & Holmes, G. L. (2004a). Developmental changes in GABAergic actions and seizure susceptibility in the rat hippocampus. *European Journal of Neuroscience*, *19*, 590–600.

Khazipov, R., Leinekugel, X., Khalilov, I., Gaïarsa, J. L., & Ben-Ari, Y. (1997). Synchronization of GABAergic interneuronal network in CA3 subfield of neonatal rat hippocampal slices. *The Journal of Physiology*, *498*, 763–772.

Khazipov, R., & Luhmann, H. J. (2006). Early patterns of electrical activity in the developing cerebral cortex of humans and rodents. *Trends in Neurosciences*, *29*, 414–418.

Khazipov, R., Ragozzino, D., & Bregestovski, P. (1995). Kinetics and Mg^{2+} block of *N*-methyl-D-aspartate receptor channels during postnatal development of hippocampal CA3 pyramidal neurons. *Neuroscience*, *69*, 1057–1065.

Khazipov, R., Sirota, A., Leinekugel, X., Holmes, G. L., Ben-Ari, Y., & Buzsaki, G. (2004b). Early motor activity drives spindle bursts in the developing somatosensory cortex. *Nature*, *432*, 758–761.

Kidd, F. L., & Isaac, J. T. (1999). Developmental and activity-dependent regulation of kainate receptors at thalamocortical synapses. *Nature*, *400*, 569–573.

Kreider, J. C., & Blumberg, M. S. (2000). Mesopontine contribution to the expression of active 'twitch' sleep in decerebrate week-old rats. *Brain Research*, *872*, 149–159.

Lamblin, M. D., Andre, M., Challamel, M. J., Curzi-Dascalova, L., d'Allest, A. M., De Giovanni, E., et al. (1999). Electroencephalography of the premature and term newborn. Maturational aspects and glossary. *Clinical Neurophysiology*, *29*, 123–219.

Lamsa, K., Palva, J. M., Ruusuvuori, E., Kaila, K., & Taira, T. (2000). Synaptic GABA(A) activation inhibits AMPA-kainate receptor-mediated bursting in the newborn (P0–P2) rat hippocampus. *Journal of Neurophysiology*, *83*, 359–366.

Leinekugel, X., Khalilov, I., Ben-Ari, Y., & Khazipov, R. (1998). Giant depolarizing potentials: The septal pole of the hippocampus paces the activity of the developing intact septohippocampal complex *in vitro*. *Journal of Neuroscience*, *18*, 6349–6357.

Leinekugel, X., Medina, I., Khalilov, I., Ben-Ari, Y., & Khazipov, R. (1997). Ca^{2+} oscillations mediated by the synergistic excitatory actions of GABA$_A$ and NMDA receptors in the neonatal hippocampus. *Neuron*, *18*, 243–255.

LoTurco, J. J., Owens, D. F., Heath, M. J., Davis, M. B., & Kriegstein, A. R. (1995). GABA and glutamate depolarize cortical progenitor cells and inhibit DNA synthesis. *Neuron*, *15*, 1287–1298.

Lu, T., & Trussell, L. O. (2001). Mixed excitatory and inhibitory GABA-mediated transmission in chick cochlear nucleus. *The Journal of Physiology*, *535*, 125–131.

Luhmann, H. J., & Prince, D. A. (1991). Postnatal maturation of the GABAergic system in rat neocortex. *Journal of Neurophysiology*, 247–263.

Luhmann, H. J., Reiprich, R. A., Hanganu, I., & Kilb, W. (2000). Cellular physiology of the neonatal rat cerebral cortex: Intrinsic membrane properties, sodium and calcium currents. *Journal of Neuroscience Research*, *62*, 574–584.

McCormick, D.A., & Bal, T. (1997). Sleep and arousal: Thalamocortical mechanisms. *Annual Review of Neuroscience*, *20*, 185–215.

McLaughlin, T., Torborg, C. L., Feller, M. B., & O'Leary, D. D. (2003). Retinotopic map refinement requires spontaneous retinal waves during a brief critical period of development. *Neuron*, *40*, 1147–1160.

Meister, M., Wong, R. O., Baylor, D. A., & Shatz, C. J. (1991). Synchronous bursts of action potentials in ganglion cells of the developing mammalian retina. *Science*, *252*, 939–943.

Mello, M. T., Silva, A. C., Rueda, A. D., Poyares, D., & Tufik, S. (1997). Correlation between K complex, periodic leg movements (PLM), and myoclonus during sleep in paraplegic adults before and after an acute physical activity. *Spinal Cord*, *35*, 248–252.

Milh, M., Kaminska, A., Huon, C., Lapillonne, A., Ben-Ari, Y., & Khazipov, R. (2006). Rapid cortical oscillations and early motor activity in premature human neonate. *Cerebral Cortex*, *17*(7), 1582–1594.

Minkwitz, H. G. (1976). Development of neuronal structure in the hippocampus during pre- and post-natal ontogenesis in the albino rat. III. Morphometric determination of ontogenetic changes in dendrite structure and spine distribution on pyramidal neurons (CA1) of the hippocampus. *Journal für Hirnforschung*, *17*, 255–275.

Minlebaev, M., Ben-Ari, Y., & Khazipov, R. (2007). Network mechanisms of spindle-burst oscillations in the neonatal rat barrel cortex in vivo. *Journal of Neurophysiology*, *97*, 692–700.

Minlebaev M, Ben Ari Y, & Khazipov R (2009) NMDA Receptors Pattern Early Activity in the Developing Barrel Cortex In Vivo. *Cerebral Cortex* 19: 688–696.

Moody, W. J., & Bosma, M. M. (2005). Ion channel development, spontaneous activity, and activity-dependent development in nerve and muscle cells. *Physiological Reviews*, *85*, 883–941.

Mooney, R., Penn, A. A., Gallego, R., & Shatz, C. J. (1996). Thalamic relay of spontaneous retinal activity prior to vision. *Neuron*, *17*, 863–874.

Mrsic-Flogel, T. D., Hofer, S. B., Creutzfeldt, C., Cloez-Tayarani, I., Changeux, J. P., Bonhoeffer, T., et al. (2005). Altered map of visual space in the superior colliculus of mice lacking early retinal waves. *Journal of Neuroscience*, *25*, 6921–6928.

Muir-Robinson, G., Hwang, B. J., & Feller, M. B. (2002). Retinogeniculate axons undergo eye-specific segregation in the absence of eye-specific layers. *Journal of Neuroscience*, *22*, 5259–5264.

Nicol, X., Voyatzis, S., Muzerelle, A., Narboux-Neme, N., Sudhof, T. C., Miles, R., et al. (2007). cAMP oscillations and retinal activity are permissive for ephrin signaling during the establishment of the retinotopic map. *Nature Neuroscience*, *10*, 340–347.

Nijhout, H. F. (1990). Metaphors and the role of genes in development. *Bioessays*, *12*, 441–446.

Nolte, R., Schulte, F. J., Michaelis, R., Weisse, U., & Gruson, R. (1969). Bioelectric brain maturation in small-for-dates infants. *Developmental Medicine and Child Neurology*, *11*, 83–93.

O'Donovan, M. J. (1999). The origin of spontaneous activity in developing networks of the vertebrate nervous system (in process citation). *Current Opinion in Neurobiology, 9*, 94–104.

O'Donovan, M. J., Chub, N., & Wenner, P. (1998). Mechanisms of spontaneous activity in developing spinal networks. *Journal of Neurobiology, 37*, 131–145.

Owens, D. F., Boyce, L. H., Davis, M. B., & Kriegstein, A. R. (1996). Excitatory GABA responses in embryonic and neonatal cortical slices demonstrated by gramicidin perforated-patch recordings and calcium imaging. *Journal of Neuroscience, 16*, 6414–6423.

Oyama, S., Griffiths, P. E., & Gray, R. D. (2001). *Cycles of contingency: Developmental systems and evolution.* Cambridge, MA: MIT Press.

Parmelee, A. H., Akiyama, Y., Stern, E., & Harris, M. A. (1969). A periodic cerebral rhythm in newborn infants. *Experimental Neurology, 25*, 575–584.

Peinado, A. (2000). Traveling slow waves of neural activity: A novel form of network activity in developing neocortex. *Journal of Neuroscience, 20*, RC54.

Peinado, A. (2001). Immature neocortical neurons exist as extensive synctial networks linked by dendrodendritic electrical connections. *Journal of Neurophysiology, 85*, 620–629.

Penn, A. A., Riquelme, P. A., Feller, M. B., & Shatz, C. J. (1998). Competition in retinogeniculate patterning driven by spontaneous activity. *Science, 279*, 2108–2112.

Petersen, C. C. H., & Sakmann, B. (2001). Functionally independent columns of rat somatosensory barrel cortex revealed with voltage-sensitive dye imaging. *Journal of Neuroscience, 21*, 8435–8446.

Petersson, P., Waldenstrom, A., Fahraeus, C., & Schouenborg, J. (2003). Spontaneous muscle twitches during sleep guide spinal self-organization. *Nature, 424*, 72–75.

Prechtl, H. F. (1997). State of the art of a new functional assessment of the young nervous system. An early predictor of cerebral palsy. *Early Human Development, 50*, 1–11.

Rakic, P., & Komuro, H. (1995). The role of receptor/channel activity in neuronal cell migration. *Journal of Neurobiology, 26*, 299–315.

Reyes, A., & Sakmann, B. (1999). Developmental switch in the short-term modification of unitary EPSPs evoked in layer 2/3 and layer 5 pyramidal neurons of rat neocortex. *Journal of Neuroscience, 19*, 3827–3835.

Rivera, C., Voipio, J., Payne, J. A., Ruusuvuori, E., Lahtinen, H., Lamsa, K., et al. (1999). The K+/Cl– co-transporter KCC2 renders GABA hyperpolarizing during neuronal maturation. *Nature, 397*, 251–255.

Scher, M. S. (2006). Electroencephalography of the newborn: Normal features. In G. L. Holmes, S. Moshe, & R. H. Jones (Eds.), *Clinical neurophysiology of infancy, childhood, and adolescence* (pp. 46–69). New York: Elsevier.

Schwartz, T. H., Rabinowitz, D., Unni, V., Kumar, V. S., Smetters, D. K., Tsiola, A., et al. (1998). Networks of coactive neurons in developing layer 1. *Neuron, 20*, 541–552.

Seelke, A. M., Karlsson, K. A., Gall, A. J., & Blumberg, M. S. (2005). Extraocular muscle activity, rapid eye movements and the development of active and quiet sleep. *European Journal of Neuroscience, 22*, 911–920.

Shatz, C. J., & Stryker, M. P. (1988). Prenatal tetrodotoxin infusion blocks segregation of retinogeniculate afferents. *Science, 242*, 87–89.

Sipila, S. T., Huttu, K., Soltesz, I., Voipio, J., & Kaila, K. (2005). Depolarizing GABA acts on intrinsically bursting pyramidal neurons to drive giant depolarizing potentials in the immature hippocampus. *Journal of Neuroscience, 25*, 5280–5289.

Sipila, S. T., Schuchmann, S., Voipio, J., Yamada, J., & Kaila, K. (2006). The Na-K-Cl cotransporter (NKCC1) promotes sharp waves in the neonatal rat hippocampus. *The Journal of Physiology, 573*(3), 765–773.

Stellwagen D, Shatz CJ & Feller MB (1999) Dynamics of retinal waves are controlled by cyclic AMP. *Neuron* 24: 673–685

Stellwagen, D., & Shatz, C.J. (2002). An instructive role for retinal waves in the development of retinogeniculate connectivity. *Neuron, 33*, 357–367.

Steriade, M. (2001). Impact of network activities on neuronal properties in corticothalamic systems. *Journal of Neurophysiology, 86*, 1–39.

Steriade, M. (2004). Acetylcholine systems and rhythmic activities during the waking–sleep cycle. *Progress in Brain Research, 145*, 179–196.

Steriade, M., McCormick, D. A., & Sejnowski, T. J. (1993). Thalamocortical oscillations in the sleeping and aroused brain. *Science, 262*, 679–685.

Stockard-Pope, J. E., Werner, S. S., & Bickford, R. G. (1992). *Atlas of neonatal electroencelography* (2nd ed.). New York: Raven Press.

Stryker, M. P., & Harris, W. A. (1986). Binocular impulse blockade prevents the formation of ocular dominance columns in cat visual cortex. *Journal of Neuroscience, 6*, 2117–2133.

Sun, Q. Q., Huguenard, J. R., & Prince, D. A. (2006). Barrel cortex microcircuits: Thalamocortical feed-forward inhibition in spiny stellate cells is mediated by a small number of fast-spiking interneurons. *Journal of Neuroscience, 26*, 1219–1230.

Torborg, C. L., & Feller, M. B. (2005). Spontaneous patterned retinal activity and the refinement of retinal projections. *Progress in Neurobiology, 76*, 213–235.

Tyzio, R., Cossart, R., Khalilov, I., Minlebaev, M., Hubner, C. A., Represa, A., et al. (2006). Maternal oxytocin triggers a transient inhibitory switch in GABA signaling in the fetal brain during delivery. *Science, 314*, 1788–1792.

Tyzio, R., Ivanov, A., Bernard, C., Holmes, G.L., Ben-Ari, Y., & Khazipov, R. (2003). Membrane potential of CA3 hippocampal pyramidal cells during postnatal development. *Journal of Neurophysiology, 90*, 2964–2972.

Tyzio, R., Represa, A., Jorquera, I., Ben-Ari, Y., Gozlan, H., & Aniksztejn, L. (1999). The establishment of GABAergic and glutamatergic synapses on CA1 pyramidal neurons is sequential and correlates with the development of the apical dendrite. *Journal of Neuroscience, 19*, 10372–10382.

van den Pol, A. N., Obrietan, K., & Belousov, A. (1996). Glutamate hyperexcitability and seizure-like activity throughout the brain and spinal cord upon relief from chronic glutamate receptor blockade in culture. *Neuroscience, 74*, 653–674.

Vanhatalo, S., Palva, J. M., Andersson, S., Rivera, C., Voipio, J., & Kaila, K. (2005). Slow endogenous activity transients and developmental expression of K+-Cl– cotransporter 2 in the immature human cortex. *European Journal of Neuroscience, 22*, 2799–2804.

Vanhatalo, S., Tallgren, P., Andersson, S., Sainio, K., Voipio, J., & Kaila, K. (2002). DC-EEG discloses prominent, very slow activity patterns during sleep in preterm infants. *Clinical Neurophysiology, 113*, 1822–1825.

Warren, R. A., & Jones, E. G. (1997). Maturation of neuronal form and function in a mouse thalamo-cortical circuit. *Journal of Neuroscience*, 17, 277–295.

Watanabe, K., & Iwase, K. (1972). Spindle-like fast rhythms in the EEGs of low-birth weight infants. *Developmental Medicine and Child Neurology*, 14, 373–381.

Wells, J. E., Porter, J. T., & Agmon, A. (2000). GABAergic inhibition suppresses paroxysmal network activity in the neonatal rodent hippocampus and neocortex. *Journal of Neuroscience*, 20, 8822–8830.

Wong, R. O., Meister, M., & Shatz, C. J. (1993). Transient period of correlated bursting activity during development of the mammalian retina. *Neuron*, 11, 923–938.

Yamada, J., Okabe, A., Toyoda, H., Kilb, W., Luhmann, H. J., & Fukuda, A. (2004). Cl– uptake promoting depolarizing GABA actions in immature rat neocortical neurones is mediated by NKCC1. *The Journal of Physiology Online*, 557, 829–841.

Yuste, R., & Katz, L. C. (1991). Control of postsynaptic Ca^{2+} influx in developing neocortex by excitatory and inhibitory neurotransmitters. *Neuron*, 6, 333–344.

Yuste, R., Nelson, D. A., Rubin, W. W., & Katz, L. C. (1995). Neuronal domains in developing neocortex: Mechanisms of coactivation. *Neuron*, 14, 7–17.

Yuste, R., Peinado, A., & Katz, L. C. (1992). Neuronal domains in developing neocortex. *Science*, 257, 665–669.

Zhou, Q., & Poo, M. M. (2004). Reversal and consolidation of activity-induced synaptic modifications. *Trends in Neurosciences*, 27, 378–383.

PART 2

Sensorimotor Systems

Experience in the Perinatal Development of Action Systems

Michele R. Brumley *and* Scott R. Robinson

Abstract

Explaining the emergence of behavioral organization and functional action patterns during ontogeny represents a challenge for developmental science. Using interlimb coordination in the fetal and neonatal rat as a model behavior, this chapter reviews central mechanisms and sensory regulation of spontaneous limb movement, pharmacological induction of locomotor-like behavior, motor learning and memory, and environmental factors that contribute to the construction of organized motor behavior during perinatal development. Recent experiments indicate that action systems in the fetus emerge under the joint influence of neural resources, biomechanical constraints, proprioceptive feedback, and contingencies posed by the intrauterine environment. This research suggests that experience accruing from feedback about motor performance may play a significant role in the perinatal construction of motor behavior.

Keywords: behavioral organization, fetus, newborn, ontogeny, locomotion, interlimb coordination, motor performance, limb movement, motor learning, L-DOPA, Quipazine

Introduction

Fetal and neonatal rats move and are capable of expressing behavioral organization immediately before and after birth. Yet functional patterns of motor coordination represent a challenge to the motor system, whereby different parts of the animal must move in rather specific spatial and temporal relationships to each other. Although motor activity expressed by the fetus often appears random, uncoordinated, and immature, quantitative approaches to examining motor behavior in the fetus have shown that fetal animals exhibit considerable movement organization, including examples of interlimb coordination, before birth (e.g., Kleven, Lane, & Robinson, 2004; Robinson & Smotherman, 1987; Smotherman & Robinson, 1987).

How the developing central nervous system (CNS) proceeds from initially expressing only spontaneous movement to shortly thereafter expressing functional patterns of motor behavior remains unresolved. Furthermore, how the developing animal continues to express functional patterns of movement with a continuously changing CNS and growing body is a remarkable challenge. This developmental challenge in motor control has been called the "calibration problem," implying that the developing animal must continually modify or recalibrate its motor execution strategy to satisfy the demands of the biomechanical and/or environmental context (Robinson & Kleven, 2005). Indeed, evidence is mounting that the developing animal can make use of sensory and movement-related feedback acquired during spontaneous movement to shape functional action patterns (Petersson, Waldenström, Fähraeus, & Schouenborg, 2003; Robinson, 2005; Robinson & Kleven, 2005; also see Khazipov & Buzsaki; Schouenborg; Chapter 20).

Understanding how coordinated movement is expressed and develops during the perinatal period requires characterization of the multiple factors that contribute to motor control: neural resources that must exist to generate organized movement, interactions between different parts of the animal—neural and biomechanical—that constrain and shape movement, and interactions between the animal and the environment in which movement is expressed. This multifactorial approach is complex, but essential for understanding perinatal motor development because these immature animals must maintain stability of motor performance in the face of dramatic changes in body and environment during the perinatal period (i.e., solving the calibration problem). From this approach, several tenets emerge: (1) much of fetal and neonatal behavior is continuous, (2) there are shared mechanisms of behavior during the perinatal period, (3) the developing motor system depends on sensory input to permit stable motor performance, and (4) contingencies in the environment contribute to perinatal behavioral development.

In this chapter, we review empirical evidence on the origins and determinants of motor coordination in the rat. We begin with a brief review of experimental demonstrations of action patterns in the fetus, followed by discussion of the mechanisms of motor coordination in the fetus and the newborn. Finally, we discuss evidence relating to the significance of early experience, plasticity, and interaction with the environment on motor behavior during perinatal development. We hope to promote a broader recognition of the multifactorial nature of motor behavior in the perinatal rat and highlight the role that the organism plays in influencing its own behavioral development.

Perinatal Behavioral Continuity: Moving Beyond the Fetal Freak Show

Anecdotes and descriptions of fetal behavior, obtained by opportunistic observations of human fetuses from prematurely terminated pregnancies (Hooker, 1952), in vivo preparations of animal fetuses (e.g., Angulo y Gonzalez, 1932; Narayanan, Fox, & Hamburger, 1971; Smotherman & Robinson, 1986), and most recently from real-time and 4D ultrasonic imaging of human fetuses (e.g., de Vries & Fong, 2006; de Vries, Visser & Prechtl, 1982; Kurjak et al., 2004), have provided important demonstrations of the ability of animal and human fetuses to express organized patterns of motor behavior. Such descriptive evidence has been instrumental in documenting that many patterns of functional postnatal behavior have their roots in the prenatal period. Developmental continuity between prenatal and postnatal behavior is a fact too often ignored in facile nativist interpretations of infant behavior (e.g., Marcus, 2001; Spelke & Newport, 1998). As a developmental concept, transnatal continuity is inherent in the principles of forward reference (Coghill, 1929) and anticipatory development (Carmichael, 1954; Oppenheim, 1981), which emphasize that behavior, like other functional systems, must begin to develop well before the behavior is needed to function. For example, developmental psychologists take for granted the expression of functional elements of suckling behavior (nipple search and attachment, organized sucking, and milk ingestion) by newborn infants. But the sudden expression of organized suckling behavior within minutes of birth does not imply instantaneous development or expression of a latent capacity constructed by genes; all these elements of suckling behavior are expressed before birth (Robinson et al., 1992; Robinson & Smotherman, 1992a; Smotherman & Robinson, 1992a) and can be evoked by stimuli available to the fetus in utero (Hepper, Wells & Lynch, 2005; Korthank & Robinson, 1998; Myowa-Yamakoshi & Takeshita, 2006; Ross & Nijland, 1998). Behavior is not a trivial aspect of prenatal life, nor is the prenatal period inconsequential for the expression of functional behavior after birth.

Mammalian fetuses are born after a period of physiological dependency on the mother, and because the fetus's life support derives from the placental connection to the mother's uterus, researchers face a significant challenge to gain experimental access to fetal subjects for behavioral study. Thus, in nearly all cases, proper experimental designs are feasible only with the use of nonhuman animals. The principal animal models in current use to study fetal development involve large domestic animals, such as sheep or pigs, which can support extensive chronic instrumentation and longitudinal research designs (Moore & Hanson, 1992), or laboratory rodents, such as rats and mice, that can be prepared for direct behavioral observation and permit efficient collection of statistical samples in cross-sectional experimental designs (Brumley & Robinson, 2005; Kleven & Ronca, 2009; Robinson & Smotherman, 1992b).

Our laboratories have concentrated attention on the rat fetus as a robust model of prenatal behavioral development. Experimental access to the rat fetus is provided by methods that permit exteriorization of the uterus and fetal subjects. The pregnant rat is prepared by chemical or pharmacological blockade of the spinal cord at the high lumbar level, obviating the need for general maternal anesthesia, which suppresses fetal activity (Smotherman & Robinson, 1991a). When immersed in a physiological saline bath at maternal body temperature (37.5°C), this maternal preparation provides clear visual and physical access to individual fetuses. Fetal rats can be observed through the semitransparent wall of the uterus (in utero), after delivery from the uterus into the saline bath while remaining within the amniotic sac (in amnion), or after removal of the amniotic and chorionic membranes that surround the fetus (ex utero). Each condition of observation presents different advantages: preparation in utero most closely approximates environmental conditions during normal pregnancy, while preparation in amnion and ex utero provide progressively clearer visualization and more direct experimental access to individual fetal subjects. These methods permit test sessions lasting up to 2 h that may include video recording of fetal motor behavior, experimental presentation of chemical or tactile stimuli, biomechanical constraint of movement, or manipulation of CNS function by peripheral or central drug administration, surgical lesion, or transection of the brainstem or spinal cord. Developmental changes in fetal behavior are measured by sampling from different pregnancies at different gestational ages from the inception of fetal movement on E16 (embryonic age 16 days postconception) through term (E22).

The advent of methods for studying the behavior of the exteriorized rodent fetus has provided a window on fetal development that has revealed an extensive repertoire of behavior that can be expressed before birth. Fetuses of all mammalian species exhibit spontaneous movement, but much of this motor activity superficially appears random, uncoordinated, and purposeless (Hamburger, 1973). However, application of statistical methods for quantifying temporal patterning (Kleven et al.,

2004; Robertson & Bacher, 1995; Robertson, Dierker, Sorokin, & Rosen, 1982; Robinson & Smotherman, 1992c), detailed video analysis of movement patterns (Bradley, Solanki, & Zhao, 2005; Chambers et al., 1995; Johnston & Bekoff, 1992; Robinson & Smotherman, 1991a; Watson & Bekoff, 1990), and experimental presentation of ecologically relevant sensory stimuli (Robinson & Smotherman, 1992a; Robinson et al., 1992; Ronca & Alberts, 1995) has uncovered behavioral organization that was not recognized in classic studies of fetal development (Carmichael, 1954; Hamburger, 1963). Some of these behavioral attributes are apparently unique to the fetus and may represent ontogenetic adaptations that promote survival and healthy development before birth (Oppenheim, 1982; Smotherman & Robinson, 1990). But most examples of fetal behavior—including simple reflexes, body orientation and posture, and components of locomotion, grooming, suckling, ingestive behavior, and species-typical reactions to appetitive and aversive stimuli—foreshadow functional action patterns of the infant or the adult. Many of the behavioral capacities that have been documented in this descriptive phase of behavioral research on the rat fetus have been the subject of previous reviews (Alberts & Ronca, 1996; Robinson & Brumley, 2005; Robinson & Smotherman, 1992d).

Basic identification of the range of phenomena to be explained is a necessary first step in any area of scientific inquiry, and characterization of the behavioral capacities of mammalian fetuses has been crucial to our beginning to understand principles of perinatal behavioral development. However, demonstration that a behavior pattern can be expressed by the fetus does not explain how that behavior develops before birth. Much of the attraction of classic and more recent descriptions of fetal behavior is the carnival-like novelty of revealing that a particular behavior can be expressed at such an early age. There is little doubt that such novelty can help draw attention to the theoretical implications of behavioral development before birth. But in themselves, mere demonstrations of behavioral expression in the fetus represent little more than a fetal freak show.

The existence of fetal behavior raises questions, generates hypotheses, and poses challenges for research, but it does not in itself provide an explanation for the development of behavior before birth. For instance, close examination of the expression of action patterns in immature animals is often fluid and variable, fragmented or incomplete, and far less coordinated or stereotyped than the same or similar action patterns expressed by the adult. Oral grasping of an artificial nipple in the rat fetus is not the same as functional suckling by the neonatal rat; facial wiping by the fetus is not identical to grooming by the adult rat; and stepping evoked by dopaminergic or serotonergic agonists is not isomorphic with walking locomotion. To move beyond simple descriptions and demonstration proofs of fetal competence, it is essential that investigators apply an experimental approach to study the determinants of perinatal behavioral development. Understanding how these early behavioral forms are related to and contribute to the development of functional adult behavior remains a largely unrealized challenge for future research.

Multiple Determinants of Action Systems in the Perinatal Rat

As in other aspects of fetal behavior, demonstration proofs of behavioral capacities before birth have been important for understanding the developmental trajectory of organized action. Their main contribution has been the identification of the age at which a measure of coordinated movement or an action pattern that resembles mature behavior can first be recognized to occur in the immature animal. Such demonstrations also indicate the developmental status of perceptual, motor, and/or neural systems that are necessary to initiate, coordinate, orient, and regulate organized action. With this information as a foundation, the broader field of fetal research can begin to turn its attention to identifying and explaining the causal mechanisms of behavioral development.

Here we offer a process-oriented developmental framework for understanding the development of action systems in the rat that is based on recognizing the multiple determinants of influence on motor performance. With this approach, we can move beyond mere demonstration proofs of behavioral capacities and begin to (1) provide a more mechanism-based and multifactorial explanation for the development of action systems and (2) reveal the role that experience and plasticity plays in shaping motor performance during perinatal behavioral development. This approach entails recognizing that motor organization is more loosely structured in the fetus and neonate and that the organism plays an active role in the development of coordinated movement. It also requires understanding the relationships among local neural resources, propriospinal interactions, kinesthetic feedback, biomechanical constraints, and environmental contingencies that the organism encounters during development and the expression of movement. Much of our effort to date has focused on interlimb coordination as a model system for addressing general problems in the development of action systems.

Endogenous Rhythmic Pattern Generators and Local Neural Mechanisms

In the rat, rudimentary forms of interlimb coordination are apparent during spontaneous motor activity expressed during the fetal period. Spontaneous movements are first expressed by the rat fetus on E16 and continue to occur at different rates and in different parts of the body throughout the prenatal and early postnatal periods (Corner, 1977; Gramsbergen, Schwartze, & Prechtl, 1970; Robinson, Blumberg, Lane, & Kreber, 2000; Seelke, Karlsson, Gall, & Blumberg, 2005; see Chapter 20). Early descriptions of fetal movement noted the nearly simultaneous movement of different parts of the body, variously referred to as "regional," "complex," or "synchronous" motor activity (Narayanan et al., 1971; Robinson & Smotherman, 1988; Smotherman & Robinson, 1986). Kleven et al. (2004) provided more quantitative measurement of the occurrence of synchronous limb movements during the period of fetal motility, from the inception of spontaneous movement to birth (E16–E22). At the inception of spontaneous movement, synchronous limb movements or interlimb synchrony was at chance levels for all limb pairs. Between E18 and E20, the occurrence of synchronous forelimb movements increased; thus, the forelimbs became more strongly coupled over this period. Synchrony profiles for the hindlimbs were significantly different from chance at E19, with the hindlimbs becoming more tightly coupled at E20. Intersegmental synchrony began to exhibit tight interlimb coupling at E20 as well. Thus, interlimb synchrony reveals that motor coordination may not be present when the rat fetus expresses its first spontaneous movements, but shows steady improvement as interlimb coupling increases during the late prenatal period (Kleven et al., 2004; Robinson & Smotherman, 1987).

From decades of research examining the neural mechanisms of spontaneous movement in various vertebrate species, it is clear that mechanisms within the spinal cord are a major determinant in initiating, modulating, and organizing spontaneous motor activity during the perinatal period. For instance, spontaneous movements in the embryonic chick are correlated with activity in the spinal cord (Provine, 1972), which continues to be expressed even after all afferent feedback has been eliminated (Narayanan & Malloy, 1974a, 1974b). In the rat fetus, spontaneous movement continues to be expressed and organized into multilimb bouts following a high cervical spinal transection (Robinson et al., 2000). Following a midthoracic spinal transection, both the forelimbs and hindlimbs continue to express spontaneous movement (Blumberg & Lucas, 1994), with activity continuing to show cyclic organization (Robertson & Smotherman, 1990). Thus, there is ample evidence showing that the earliest movements and forms of motor organization expressed by perinatal animals are generated by local mechanisms within the spinal cord.

In addition to its role in generating spontaneous movement, the spinal cord also houses the basic neural circuitry involved in the production of locomotion. In the in vitro spinal cord preparation, the spinal cord is extracted from the animal's body and pinned down in a bath chamber. Typically, all nerve processes are cut and recording electrodes are placed on select ventral roots (VRs). Variants of this preparation include leaving the brain stem intact with the spinal cord, leaving some nerve processes intact, and leaving the hindleg(s) attached to the spinal cord. Bath application of pharmacological agents, such as monoamines and excitatory amino acids, is effective in evoking locomotor-like activity in this preparation. Limb muscle, motor neuron, or VR recordings from the hindleg nerves show that the pattern of electrical activity induced by these agents is similar to that during locomotion—mainly extensor and flexor alternation on one side of the cord coupled with alternation on the contralateral side. Because the activity of the spinal cord generally corresponds to the pattern of hindleg activity during locomotion, alternation of motor neuron or VR activity between sides of the spinal cord is often referred to as "fictive locomotion."

Fictive locomotion can be induced in the developing rat spinal cord. Bath application of NMDA, 5-hydroxytryptamine (5-HT), acetylcholine, or dopamine to the in vitro perinatal spinal cord evokes alternated activity in contralateral hindlimb VRs and muscles of the hindlimbs (Atsuta, Abraham, Iwahara, Garcia-Rill, & Skinner, 1991; Cazalets, Grillner, Menard, Crémieux, & Clarac, 1990; Cazalets, Sqalli-Houssaini, & Clarac, 1992;

Cowley & Schmidt, 1994; Iizuka, Nishimaru, & Kudo, 1998; Kiehn & Kjaerulff, 1996; Kudo & Yamada, 1987; Smith, Feldman, & Schmidt, 1988; see also Chapter 10). These substances, however, do not evoke identical patterns of activity, indicating that the spinal mechanisms involved in locomotion can be modulated by the action of different neuroactive drugs. Recently, interneurons within specific spinal segments that mediate fictive locomotion of the hindlimbs have been identified in the isolated spinal cord of the neonatal rat in vitro (for review, see Kiehn & Butt, 2003).

Experiments with the isolated spinal cord of the rat fetus have shown that spinal locomotor networks undergo substantial developmental transitions, both in motor pattern output and in intrinsic properties, shortly before birth (Kudo, Nishimaru, & Nakayama, 2004). For instance, between E14.5 and E16.5, 5-HT induces rhythmic synchronization of extensor-dominant and flexor-dominant lumbar VRs (Iizuka et al., 1998; Nakayama, Nishimaru, & Kudo, 2001). The 5-HT pattern of VR discharge on E17 is highly variable (Nishimaru & Kudo, 2000). On E18.5, 5-HT induces alternation between the right and left hindlegs (Greer, Smith, & Feldman, 1992), although flexors and extensors are coactive in the same leg (Iizuka et al., 1998). By E20.5, 5-HT induces the fictive locomotor pattern (Iizuka et al., 1998). Coordinative changes in VR activity (from synchrony to alternation) are seen at the same ages during NMDA-induced VR activity as well (Ozaki, Yamada, Iizuka, Nishimaru, & Kudo, 1996).

Interestingly, there also is a switch from GABAergic to glycinergic inhibition during the prenatal period, with GABAergic synaptic transmission being prevalent in the spinal cord on E17/E18 and glycinergic transmission becoming more common during the neonatal period (Gao, Stricker, & Ziskind-Conhaim, 2001). During 5-HT-induced motor activity, glycine is an excitatory transmitter at E14.5/E15.5 (Nakayama et al., 2001). After E17.5/E18.5, glutamate becomes the main excitatory transmitter and glycine becomes the main inhibitory neurotransmitter during 5-HT-induced rhythmicity. Results from experiments that applied glycine receptor antagonists during 5-HT or NMDA-induced fictive locomotion suggest that glycine-mediated inhibition is responsible for changes in the pattern of motor output from synchrony on E16.5 to alternation on E20.5 (Iizuka et al., 1998; Nakayama et al., 2001; Ozaki et al., 1996).

In summary, experiments with the in vitro spinal cord preparation have shown that mechanisms that generate and coordinate locomotor-like activity are present and functional during the late fetal and early neonatal period in the rat (Clarac, Brocard, & Vinay, 2004). For a more comprehensive review of neural mechanisms involved in the development of locomotion, see Chapter 10.

Locomotor-like Behavior of the Perinatal Rat

Although the basic mechanisms for locomotion may be present at birth in the rat, behavioral experiments using whole animal preparations, such as the in vivo rat fetus and newborn, suggest that locomotor coordination is not crystallized in the spinal cord at this time. Because rats do not typically exhibit spontaneous episodes of quadrupedal walking until approximately 2 weeks postnatal (due to weak muscle strength and poor postural control), locomotor behavior is assessed in these young subjects in vivo by experimentally evoking locomotor-like patterns of limb coordination called "stepping" behavior.

Alternated stepping behavior is occasionally expressed during spontaneous motor activity in the near-term fetus (Bekoff & Lau, 1980). However, stepping can be reliably evoked in the newborn rat using pharmacological agents (i.e., serotonergic or catecholaminergic drugs) or strong sensory stimulation such as a tail-pinch (Norreel, Pflieger, Pearlstein, Simeoni-Alias, Clarac, & Vinay, 2003), placement of the pup on a cold surface (Altman & Sudarshan, 1975), or exposure to the scent of bedding and nesting materials (Fady, Jamon, & Clarac, 1998; Jamon & Clarac, 1998).

Presumably, pharmacological stimulation of neurotransmitter systems and forms of sensory-induced stepping in the immature rat either directly or indirectly impinge on spinal locomotor mechanisms. In the case of stepping behavior induced by serotonergic agonists, such as quipazine, it appears that 5-HT receptors directly activate spinal locomotor networks. Thus, a midthoracic spinal cord transection, which effectively eliminates communication between the brain and caudal levels of the spinal cord, does not eliminate quipazine-induced hindlimb stepping in the E20 rat fetus (Brumley & Robinson, 2005). This finding suggests that local 5-HT receptors in the spinal cord mediate 5-HT-induced stepping behavior in the young rat (Brumley & Robinson, 2005; McEwen, Van Hartesveldt, & Stehouwer, 1997).

Using quipazine to elicit stepping in fetal and newborn rats, we found that hindlimb stepping increased and coordination improved from E20 to P1 (postnatal day 1; 24 h after birth), though not in a strictly linear fashion (Figure 9.1). Stepping behavior also can be induced in perinatal rats by administration of the catecholamine precursor L-DOPA (Heberling & Robinson, 1997; McCrea, Stehouwer, & Van Hartesveldt, 1994; Van Hartesveldt, Sickles, Porter, & Stehouwer, 1991). Limb coordination during L-DOPA-induced stepping also is highly variable in E20 and E21 fetuses, but by P0 (day of birth), the stepping pattern is more constrained and rhythmically alternating (Robinson & Kleven, 2005). It should be noted that unlike 5-HT, which acts more directly at the level of spinal locomotor mechanisms, the effects of L-DOPA on stepping appear to depend on descending pathways from midbrain locomotor regions (McEwen et al., 1997).

The findings from 5-HT and L-DOPA-induced stepping provide convergent evidence that interlimb coordination during locomotor-like behavior is relatively immature and unstable during the perinatal period, but does exhibit developmental change (i.e., improvement). Such change is likely due to both central and peripheral influences on central locomotor generating circuitry. In conjunction with the results of in vitro spinal cord preparations and studies of spontaneous motor activity, studies of evoked locomotor-like activity suggest that the earliest forms of motor coordination are generated and regulated by the spinal cord, are expressed by the fetus and newborn, and show developmental change during both the prenatal and postnatal periods.

Proprioception and Interlimb Dynamics

One of the implications of the effectiveness of pharmacological probes, such as L-DOPA and 5-HT agonists, to activate locomotor behavior in perinatal animals is that local spinal networks are not completely autonomous, but are influenced by communication between different levels of the spinal cord and between the spinal cord and the brain. Accordingly, results from both behavioral and neurophysiological experiments, which involved performing surgical transection of the spinal cord, indicate that propriospinal projections influence interlimb coordination during spontaneous and locomotor activity. For instance, Robinson et al. (2000) showed that spontaneous limb activity in fetal and neonatal rats is organized into multilimb

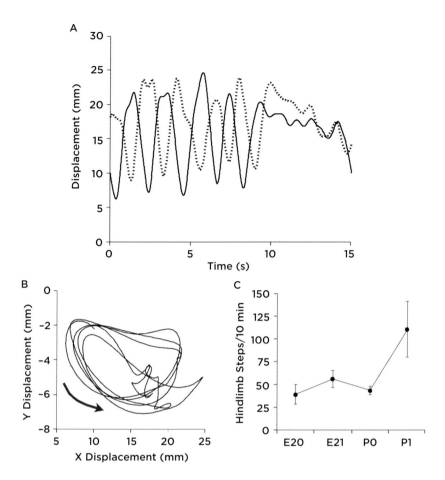

Figure 9.1 Quipazine-evoked hindlimb stepping in fetal and newborn rats. (A) Limb trajectories during a 15-s period of hindlimb stepping in an E20 rat fetus after administration of the serotonergic agonist quipazine (3.0 mg/kg i.p.). Lines depict toe displacements of the right (solid) and left (dashed) hindfoot in the rostral-caudal dimension; positive displacements indicate movement in the rostral direction (i.e., toward the head). This example depicts five clear cycles of alternated hindlimb stepping by the fetus. (B) Toe displacements of the right hindfoot depicting the cycle of limb motion in the sagittal plane (rostral toward the right; ventral toward the top) during the 15-s episode of stepping shown in A. (C) Developmental changes in alternated hindlimb stepping evoked by quipazine in the perinatal rat. Points display the mean number of alternated steps expressed in a 10-min test period in the fetus on E20 and E21 of gestation, and the newborn rat on P0 (day of birth) and P1; vertical lines show S.E.M.

bouts, whereby the probability of a limb movement occurring within 0.2 s of another limb movement is elevated until four limb movements have occurred. Thus, spontaneous limb activity in perinatal rats often involves reciprocal excitation among limbs coupled with a brief refractory period after each limb movement. Multilimb bout organization persists following cervical spinal transection, showing that descending influences from the brain are not necessary for this form of interlimb coordination (Robinson et al., 2000). This bout organization suggests a role for intraspinal connections as a regulating factor in the expression of spontaneous activity.

Additional evidence for functional propriospinal pathways in the perinatal rat comes from studies of fictive locomotion that have examined coordination between rostral and caudal spinal locomotor-generating circuitry (e.g., Ballion, Morin, & Viala, 2001; Juvin, Simmers, & Morin, 2005). Ballion and colleagues (2001) reported coordination between forelimb (C7–T1) and hindlimb (L2–L5) VRs during 5-HT/NMA-induced rhythmic activity in the P1–P4 rat in vitro brain stem–spinal cord preparation. In this study, fictive locomotion was evoked in each region of the cord separately (cervicothoracic and thoracolumbar), albeit at different burst frequencies. When the spinal cord was left intact, the slower rostral and faster caudal VR burst frequencies became coordinated and exhibited an intermediate burst frequency. Similarly, Robertson and Smotherman (1990) found that midthoracic spinal transection significantly slowed cyclic forelimb activity but did not slow cyclic hindlimb activity in the E20 rat fetus. Together, these studies suggest that propriospinal pathways entail ascending as well as descending influences on interlimb coordination in the perinatal rat.

Experiments with human infants and newborn rats in which an external weight has been applied to a single limb during spontaneous activity provide evidence that proprioceptive feedback influences the frequency and coordination of spontaneous movement. At 6 weeks of age, an external ankle weight attached to one leg of a human infant decreases the number of spontaneous kicks in the weighted leg but increases the number of kicks in the nonweighted leg (Thelen, Skala, & Kelso, 1987; Vaal, van Soest, & Hopkins, 2000). By 12–16 weeks of age, the kick rate of the nonweighted leg increases proportionally to the weight (25%–100% of the mass of the calf) added to the other leg (Ulrich, Ulrich, Angulo-Kinzler, & Chapman, 1997). These experiments show that human infants express compensatory changes in spontaneous kicking behavior in response to bilateral asymmetries in leg mass and suggest that proprioceptive feedback may serve to regulate the quantity and quality of movement during spontaneous motor activity.

We have tested the idea that proprioceptive feedback influences expression of spontaneous limb activity during the perinatal period in an experiment in which an external weight was added to one hindlimb of P1 rats (Hynes, Brumley, Oetken, & Robinson, 2003). Weights were calibrated to approximate 0%, 50%, or 100% of the average mass of a hindlimb and consisted of small lead disks attached to a strip of tape that was wrapped around the circumference of the limb at the ankle. As shown in Figure 9 2, the presence of the limb weight did not depress activity of the weighted limb. However, changes in the frequency of hindlimb movements were evident during the 30-min period during which the weight was attached. In subjects exposed to 50% or 100% limb weights, the nonweighted hindlimb showed more activity than the weighted limb (Figure 9.2B). These findings imply that neonatal rats compensate for a static load (weight) on a single limb, but as a result of this compensation, the nonweighted

limb in the same girdle is also affected. Thus, limb weighting is a useful experimental perturbation of the immature motor system that has been shown to reveal compensatory changes in limb movement as well as intrinsic dynamics between limbs during spontaneous activity. Whether the spinal cord mediates homeostatic-like regulation in spontaneous activity is unclear. But the evidence from studies discussed previously on the propriospinal mediation of interlimb coordination implies this may be plausible.

Behavioral experiments with human infants and newborn rabbits provide convergent support for the idea that proprioceptive feedback also may contribute to plasticity in the development of organized action patterns. Thelen (1994) probed the plasticity of the motor system in 3-month-old human infants in a variation on the well-known conjugate reinforcement learning paradigm. In its typical application, conjugate reinforcement takes advantage of the propensity of young infants to exhibit spontaneous kicking when lying in a supine posture; this kicking behavior typically involves movement synergies resembling stepping movements, including alternation between left and right legs (Thelen, 1985; Thelen & Fisher, 1983). To effect conjugate reinforcement, one end of a ribbon is attached to an ankle of the infant as it lies supine and the other end of the ribbon is attached to a mobile suspended overhead. Vigorous kicking of the tethered leg by the infant results in shaking of the mobile, which infants typically find reinforcing, resulting in an increase in the rate of kicking (Kraebel, Fable, & Gerhardstein, 2004; Rovee-Collier, Morrongiello, Aron, & Kupersmidt, 1978; Rovee & Rovee, 1969). In the variation of the above experiment performed by Thelen and colleagues, an elastic yoke was used to create a physical linkage between both ankles of the infant. A ribbon then was attached to one leg and the overhead mobile in the conventional manner. In this configuration, infants learned to kick both legs in a synchronous, in-phase pattern in order to vigorously shake the mobile (Thelen, 1994).

Comparable motor plasticity has been reported in the development of locomotion in newborn rabbits. Shortly after leaving the nest around 10 days after birth (P10), rabbit neonates exhibit an alternated quadrupedal walking gait. By P20, this alternated stepping is replaced by synchronized hopping. If the rabbit is prepared with a spinal transection at P10, the alternated hindlimb coordination persists, suggesting that the emergence of in-phase

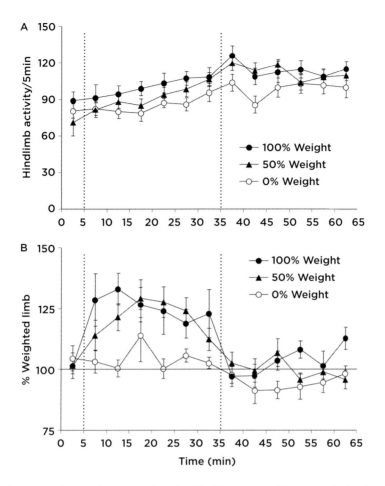

Figure 9.2 Hindlimb response of neonatal rats to a unilateral weight. The external weight was attached at the ankle with a small strip of tape and was calibrated to 50% or 100% of the average mass of the hindlimb; control subjects (0% weight) were exposed to the tape only. (A) Activity of the weighted hindlimb during and after exposure to a unilateral hindlimb weight. Points depict mean hindlimb movements per 5 min; vertical lines show S.E.M. Vertical dashed lines at 5 and 35 min indicate the times when the weight was added or removed from the hindlimb, respectively. (B) Activity of the nonweighted hindlimb expressed as a percentage of weighted hindlimb activity.

leg movements is dependent on intact supraspinal resources in the CNS. However, the developmental outcome was influenced by daily motor training between P10 and P20, which was accomplished by attaching the hindfeet of the rabbit to the pedals of a training device. When training consisted of in-phase rotation of the pedals, the rabbits learned a hopping gait, but when training was alternated (like a bicycle), they retained the immature, alternated walking pattern (Viala, 2006; Viala, Viala, & Fayein, 1986). As the authors concluded, these findings imply that proprioceptive feedback from the hindlimbs may have a structuring effect during early development on the spinal networks involved in controlling interlimb coordination during locomotion.

Kinesthetic Feedback in Prenatal Motor Development

Neuroembryological studies of motility in chicken embryos have clearly demonstrated that prenatal movements are not simple reflexive responses to random stimulation, but are the product of spontaneous activity in the CNS (Hamburger, Wenger, & Oppenheim, 1966), especially in brachial and lumbosacral regions of the spinal cord (Landmesser & O'Donovan, 1984; Narayanan & Hamburger, 1971). Although the expression of motility in the absence of proprioception implies that sensory feedback about movement is not important in neurobehavioral development before birth (Haverkamp & Oppenheim, 1986), evidence from nonmammalian embryos is divided in its implications for the role of experience in prenatal motor development. Classic and modern experiments in which amphibian larvae were raised in water containing an immobilizing drug found no lasting impairment in swimming behavior when the larvae were replaced in fresh water (Haverkamp & Oppenheim, 1986; Matthews & Detwiler, 1926), although these findings have been disputed by studies in which larval behavior was quantified more carefully (Fromme, 1941). In contrast, abundant evidence has emerged in recent years to support the opposite conclusion about the importance of proprioceptive feedback in early neuromotor development. Spontaneous activity of motor units (motor neurons and their associated muscle fibers) is necessary for the normal processes of cell death, synapse elimination, and restructuring of neuronal connectivity within the motor system that occur during perinatal development. Reduced neuronal activity results in sparing of supernumerary motor neurons, while externally applied stimulation accelerates the rate of cell death (Oppenheim, 1991; also see Chapter 5). Activity in the motor system also is thought to be responsible for the reduction of polysynaptic innervation of muscle fibers (Navarrete & Vrbova, 1993). Moreover, the amount of activity is not as important as the pattern of activity; bursts of electrical stimulation are more effective in promoting selective attrition of synapses than a steady rate of stimulation (Thompson, 1983). Knockout mice deficient in the gene for the trkC receptor exhibit gross motor deficits (Klein et al., 1994), which is likely due to the absence of muscle spindles at birth (Helgren et al., 1997; Hory-Lee, Russell, Linday & Frank, 1993; Kucera, Ernfors, Walros, & Jaenisch, 1995; Snider, 1994). These findings suggest that many functional properties of the motor system are shaped by proprioceptive feedback arising from patterned motor activity during prenatal development (Thompson, 1983).

Although earlier studies suggested that avian embryos, and by logical extension mammalian fetuses, are largely unresponsive to proprioceptive stimulation (Hamburger et al., 1966; Oppenheim, 1972), more recent experimental work has provided compelling evidence that embryonic behavior is strongly influenced by proprioceptive cues. For example, hatching behavior in the chick embryo is triggered by proprioceptive stimuli generated by the posture of the neck (Bekoff & Kauer, 1984). Changes in buoyancy associated with reduced amniotic fluid volume, or

experimental restraint of ankle movement, exert dramatic effects on the patterning of chick embryonic movement (Bradley, 1997, 2001; Bradley & Sebelski, 2000). Anatomical evidence suggests that muscle spindles begin to differentiate from primary myotubes within the period of fetal motility in the rat (E16–E18) and appear to be part of complete afferent circuits by E19 or E20 (Kucera, Walro, & Reichler, 1989). Electrical recording from primary afferent nerves in the fetal rat has provided more direct evidence that proprioceptors respond to changes in limb position as early as E18 (Fitzgerald, 1987), before sensory end organs are fully differentiated. These changes in neuroanatomy occur at the same time as dramatic changes in behavioral organization, including increases in motor activity (Smotherman & Robinson, 1986), expression of action patterns such as oral grasping of a nipple (Robinson et al., 1992), facial wiping (Robinson & Smotherman, 1991a), alternated stepping (Brumley & Robinson, 2005), and the capacity for motor learning (Robinson, Kleven, & Brumley, 2008).

INTERLIMB YOKE TRAINING: A MODEL OF MOTOR LEARNING IN THE PERINATAL RAT

The spontaneous movements expressed by the fetus and newborn rat often appear uncoordinated, yet coordinated action patterns that foreshadow functional patterns of adult behavior can be evoked by specific neurochemical or sensory stimulation. How do these action systems develop before birth, and what role may experience play in shaping their development? Although perinatal rats are less mature in their physical and neural development than 10-day-old rabbits or 3-month old human infants, the limb training methods pioneered by Viala et al. (1986) and Thelen (1994) discussed earlier presented an experimental opportunity to evaluate plasticity in interlimb coordination in immature rats. As adapted for fetal and neonatal rodents (Robinson, 2005), the yoke training paradigm involves use of an interlimb yoke fashioned from suture thread and polyethylene tubing to create a physical linkage between two limbs. With the yoke in place, active movement by one limb results in passive movement of the yoked limb, thereby altering kinesthetic feedback and producing gradual changes in interlimb coordination during spontaneous motor activity.

In the initial demonstration of yoke training in the rat fetus, E20 fetal subjects were fitted either with a thread that was immediately bisected (unyoked), or which remained in place for the first 30 min of a 60-min training and test session (yoked). Limb activity was scored from videotape records, taking care to record each instance of conjugate limb movement, which was defined as a movement in which both limbs initiated movement simultaneously and followed parallel spatial trajectories. Yoked subjects showed a pronounced increase in the occurrence of conjugate limb movements during the 30 min of yoke training. After the yoke was bisected with scissors, thereby removing the physical linkage between hindlimbs and marking the beginning of the test period, conjugate hindlimb movements continued to be expressed at rates well above those expressed by unyoked controls (Robinson, 2005).

Variations on this basic experimental design successfully demonstrated that E20 fetuses exhibited an increase in conjugate forelimb movements during training when both forelimbs were yoked,

and an increase in conjugate movements of an ipsilateral forelimb–hindlimb pair during yoke training of ipsilateral limbs. Transnatal continuity in yoke learning also was confirmed by testing neonatal rats in a similar yoke training situation (Figure 9.3). P1 rats were suspended in a harness from a horizontal support, which allowed all four legs to move freely without the constraints imposed by contact with a surface. In this posture, yoke training of the hindlimbs resulted in a nearly identical pattern of conjugate hindlimb activity during and after training as was originally reported in E20 fetuses (Figure 9.3A). To assess the specificity of the pattern of interlimb coordination enforced during training, P1 rats also were trained when both hindfeet were attached to a rigid arm that rotated around a central pivot. This "see-saw" training device enforced an antiphase (alternated) pattern of hindlimb movement during the 30-min training period, after which both feet were removed from the training device for the remainder of the

Figure 9.3 Motor learning in P1 rat pups exposed to hindlimb training with different enforced patterns of interlimb coordination. (A) Conjugate hindlimb movements during and after in-phase hindlimb training (yoked) or a control condition involving unconnected loops of thread (unyoked). (B) Alternated hindlimb movements during and after antiphase hindlimb training (yoked) or an unyoked control condition. Vertical dashed lines indicate the onset and termination of exposure to the interlimb yoke (yoked subjects) or unconnected loops of thread (unyoked). Note that both training regimes resulted in significant increases in the enforced pattern of interlimb coordination, but alternated hindlimb movements after antiphase training were expressed at a much higher rate.

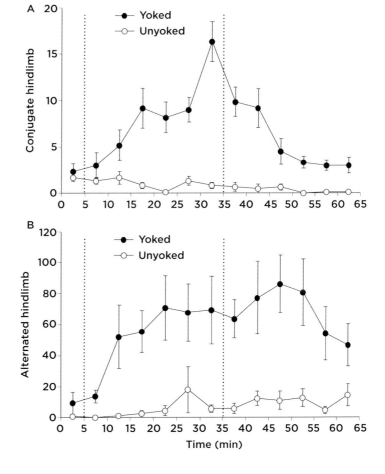

test session. Antiphase limb training resulted in a dramatic increase in alternated hindlimb movements in yoked pups, but no significant change in hindlimb alternation in unyoked controls (Figure 9.3B). The responsiveness of perinatal rats to different configurations and coordinative patterns of yoke training thus demonstrates that the E20 rat fetus and P1 rat pup can detect changes in proprioceptive feedback induced by the interlimb yoke, modify its interlimb coordination to adjust to specific patterns of movement constraint induced by the yoke, and continue to express changes in interlimb coordination for 15–30 min after the yoke is removed (Robinson, 2005). Notably, this type of learning appears to be mediated by feedback from spontaneous movements, and occurs without any form of explicit reinforcement.

Yoke training in the fetal and neonatal rat exhibits many of the essential features one would expect of true motor learning. (1) Changes in interlimb coordination occur gradually during the period of training and do not resemble a sudden stepwise increase as one might expect of a simple reflexive response to limb restraint (Robinson, 2005; Robinson & Kleven, 2005). (2) Trained patterns of limb activity persist at elevated levels after removal of the interlimb yoke, gradually returning to baseline levels within 20–30 min in E20 fetuses and P1 pups. Thus the effects of yoke training and removal of the yoke resemble conventional patterns of acquisition and extinction during associative learning (Robinson, 2005; Robinson et al., 2008). (3) Changes in interlimb coordination are specific to the limbs that experience yoke training. Conjugate forelimb movement does not increase when the hindlimbs are yoked, conjugate hindlimb movement does not increase when the forelimbs are yoked, and conjugate movement of left forelimb and hindlimb does not increase when the right forelimb and hindlimb are yoked (Robinson, 2005). (4) Changes in interlimb coordination are specific to the pattern of movement permitted during training. In-phase yoke training selectively promotes conjugate movements of the yoked limbs, whereas antiphase yoke training selectively promotes alternated limb movement (Marcano-Reik, Woller, & Robinson, 2005). (5) When tested in a second training session 30 min after initial conjugate yoke training, perinatal rats show a steeper increase of conjugate hindlimb activity (savings), indicating that yoke training results in effects that are longer lasting than the overt expression of conjugate hindlimb movements (Robinson, 2005).

(6) Savings is evident in P2 subjects when exposed to a second training session 24 h after initial training on P1 (Robinson, Woller, Khetarpal, Fromm, & Brumley, 2004). Savings after a 30-min or 24-h retention interval implies a simple form of motor memory that is established by yoke training.

SPINAL MEDIATION OF INTERLIMB YOKE LEARNING

In adults, motor learning is commonly assumed to be governed by brain regions such as the cerebellum or motor cortex, which have functional connections with spinal motor networks in human infants and rabbit kittens at the ages tested by Thelen (1994) and Viala et al. (1986), but are poorly developed in the newborn rat (Clancy, Darlington & Finlay, 2001; Lakke, 1997). To determine whether supraspinal sources are necessary for prenatal yoke learning, rat fetuses were prepared for in vivo study on E20 following complete midthoracic spinal transection (T6–9) or a sham spinal treatment (Figure 9.4). In a first experiment, spinally transected fetuses showed a 50% reduction in overall hindlimb activity relative to sham-treated controls. They nevertheless exhibited a significant increase in conjugate hindlimb movements during a 30-min period of conjugate yoke training. In a second experiment, the increase in conjugate hindlimb movement during training was replicated and conjugate movements continued to be expressed at high levels after the yoke was bisected (Figure 9.4A). In both experiments, although the incidence of conjugate hindlimb movement was reduced after spinal transection, spinal subjects showed no differences in performance relative to sham controls by the end of the 30-min training period when conjugate movements were expressed as a percentage of overall hindlimb activity. These results suggest that spinal cord circuitry alone is sufficient to support both acquisition and persistence of adaptive changes in interlimb coordination induced by yoke training.

Adaptive changes in interlimb coordination after spinal transection imply that the mechanisms for acquisition of yoke motor learning are localized in the spinal cord in the perinatal rat. But is the motor memory implicated by savings that occurs 30 min to 24 h after an initial training session also mediated by local networks in the spinal cord? To address this question, E20 fetal subjects were prepared for behavioral testing in a 95-min session. Following a 5-min baseline, subjects were exposed to conjugate hindlimb yoke training (yoked) or an unyoked control condition for 30 min. Half of

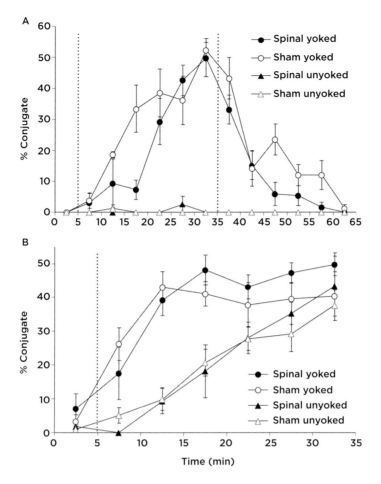

Figure 9.4 Yoke motor learning in the E20 rat fetus after midthoracic spinal transection. (A) Conjugate hindlimb movements, expressed as a percentage of total hindlimb activity, during and after yoke training. Fetal subjects were prepared by midthoracic spinal transection (spinal) or control treatment (sham) before the onset of the experimental session. Vertical dashed lines indicate the onset and termination of exposure to the interlimb yoke (yoked subjects) or unconnected loops of thread (Unyoked). (B) Conjugate hindlimb movements during a second training period 30 min after initial exposure to yoke training (yoked subjects) or control condition (unyoked). Half of the fetal subjects were prepared by midthoracic spinal transection (spinal) or sham treatment midway between the first and second training periods; all subjects received training with the interlimb yoke during the second training period. Note that intact (sham) and spinal subjects exposed to repeated yoke training exhibited savings in the rate of acquisition relative to fetuses exposed to yoke training for the first time (unyoked).

the subjects in each condition received a midthoracic spinal transection 15 min after training; the other half received a sham spinal treatment. After a 10-min delay, all subjects were exposed to a second training period consisting of a 5-min baseline and 30-min exposure to the interlimb yoke (Figure 9.4B). Conjugate hindlimb movements increased during the first training period in the yoked group and among all fetuses during the second training period. However, fetuses that were yoked during both periods exhibited a more rapid increase in conjugate activity than those yoked only in the second training period. Savings was evident in

spinal as well as sham subjects (Marcano-Reik & Robinson, 2004). This result confirmed that motor learning acquired during prior experience with the yoke, when the CNS was intact, could be retained and retrieved by the fetus after midthoracic spinal transection. Thus, the savings in motor learning expressed by fetuses after spinal transection implies a form of motor memory localized in the lumbosacral spinal cord.

Enhancement of conjugate limb coordination runs counter to the bias toward alternated coordination reported for perinatal rats both in vitro (as measured by VR activity in spinal cord explants stimulated with 5-HT or excitatory amino acids) and in vivo (as measured by 5-HT or L-DOPA-induced air-stepping). Yet both motor learning promoted by interlimb yoke training and locomotor-like behavior evoked pharmacologically can be supported by neural circuitry in the lumbosacral spinal cord alone. If motor experience influences the development of species-typical action systems, such as locomotion, one may expect motor learning to modulate, and perhaps shape the development of, spinal circuits involved in generating basic patterns of locomotor coordination.

To evaluate whether yoke training could influence interlimb coordination during species-typical behavior, stepping was evoked in P1 rats immediately after 30 min of yoke training in either an in-phase (conjugate) or antiphase (alternated) pattern (Marcano-Reik et al., 2005). The two training regimes produced expected results: in-phase yoke training increased conjugate hindlimb movements, while antiphase training promoted alternated hindlimb movements. As previously discussed, administration of quipazine, a serotonergic agonist, ordinarily is effective in evoking alternated stepping behavior in perinatal rats (Brumley & Robinson, 2005; McEwen et al, 1997). Therefore, quipazine was administered immediately after yoke training, and video recordings of hindlimb activity evoked by the 5-HT agonist were examined during reduced-speed playback to characterize interlimb coordination (Figure 9.5). Quipazine still promoted alternated stepping after yoke training in both training conditions. However, the 5-HT agonist evoked significantly more alternated steps in subjects exposed to antiphase training than subjects exposed to in-phase training (Figure 9.5A). Among subjects who received in-phase training, quipazine also promoted a significant increase in conjugate hindlimb movements, which were absent from subjects exposed to antiphase training (Figure 9.5B) (Marcano-Reik et al., 2005). Because in-phase training reduced quipazine-evoked alternated stepping and increased conjugate movements relative to both unyoked subjects and subjects that experienced antiphase training, the results of this experiment strongly suggest that kinesthetic feedback during hindlimb activity may help shape patterns of interlimb coordination in fetal and neonatal rats. More generally, the ability of a brief period of hindlimb yoke training to alter 5-HT-induced stepping implies experience-dependent plasticity in the prenatal development of central spinal networks that support basic patterns of locomotion.

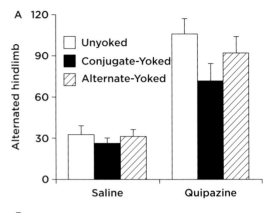

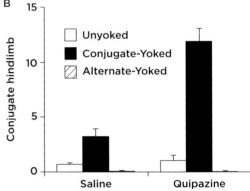

Figure 9.5 Quipazine-induced hindlimb coordination in neonatal rats after interlimb yoke training. P1 subjects received 30-min exposure to in-phase (conjugate) or antiphase (alternated) yoke hindlimb training (yoked groups) or unconnected thread loops (unyokeds) immediately before IP injection of Quipazine or saline control. (A) Number of alternated hindlimb movements by pups in 15-min test session after conjugate or alternated yoke training and administration of Quipazine or saline. (B) Number of conjugate hindlimb movements in test session after conjugate or alternated yoke training and injection of Quipazine or saline. All bars depict mean hindlimb movements (alternated or conjugate) per 5 min; vertical lines show S.E.M. Note that Quipazine induced more conjugate hindlimb movements and fewer alternated movements after in-phase training.

Biomechanical Influences and Embodied Development

Most developmental neuroscientists are accustomed to think of the primacy of the nervous system in the control and regulation of behavior. But behavior does not occur in a vacuum; it is produced by animals with a physical body moving in a physical environment. For the nervous system to produce coordinated movement, it must activate specific muscles with specific timing, which exert specific amounts of force on limb segments and other skeletal elements in a multijointed biomechanical system. In rapidly growing animals, the mass and dimensions of body segments undergo nonlinear change, necessitating different amounts and timing of muscular force to produce the same pattern of coordinated movement. The nervous system thus must continually adjust to maintain, let alone improve, functional motor performance in the face of changing physical dimensions. This "calibration problem" is recognized by a growing number of investigators interested in motor control and development (Adolph & Avolio, 2000; Adolph & Berger, 2006; Adolph, Vereijken, & Shrout, 2003; Carrier, 1996; Lam, Wolstenholme, & Yang, 2003; Myowa-Yamakoshi & Takeshita, 2006; Rieser, Pick, Ashmead, & Garing, 1995; Robinson & Kleven, 2005; Thelen, Corbetta, Kamm, Spencer, Schneider, & Zernicke, 1993; Thelen, Fisher, & Ridley-Johnson, 1984; Van Heijst, Vos, & Bullock, 1998). But it is difficult to imagine a solution to the calibration problem without neural plasticity and sensory feedback from actual motor performance.

The calibration problem may be most evident in the effects of changing body mass on motor development. Behavior occurs in a gravitational environment. In the womb, the fetus is immersed in amniotic fluid that provides buoyant support, which counters the effects of gravity on the motor system. But in the newborn, gravity constrains and alters motor performance. The effects of gravity on motor control and development are well illustrated by Thelen's reexamination of the stepping response of human newborns. Minutes after birth, human infants who are held upright can perform organized, alternated stepping movements that look remarkably like mature locomotion (Thelen et al., 1984). However, within a few weeks to months, infants no longer express the stepping response, and alternated stepping does not reappear until later in the first postnatal year with the emergence of cruising and walking. Neonatal stepping was well known to classic child developmentalists (e.g., McGraw, 1940) and its disappearance was traditionally explained as the suppression or "unlearning" of a primitive reflex with the maturation of cortical inhibitory mechanisms (Illingworth, 1966; Peiper, 1963). However, stepping disappears more quickly in infants with a higher body fat:muscle ratio (Thelen et al., 1984), and daily stepping practice extends the time that infants continue to show the stepping response (Zelazo, Zelazo, & Kolb, 1980). Finally, Thelen et al. (1984) demonstrated that applying external weights to the legs

suppressed the stepping response in 2–6-week-old infants, whereas immersing them to waist depth in water promoted the expression of stepping. Their conclusion was that early infant growth results in body mass increasing faster than muscle strength, eventually suppressing the performance of stepping until later ages. But reducing the gravitational load on the legs by providing buoyant support in water allows stepping to be expressed.

In the neonatal rat, which is born in a far less mature condition than humans, gravity severely restricts motor performance, and new action systems that function to maintain or modify body posture emerge, such as contact and vestibular righting responses (Pellis, Pellis, & Teitelbaum, 1991; Ronca & Alberts, 2000). Because behavior is expressed by whole animals, not disembodied nervous systems, behavioral performance is affected as the infant rat changes postures and encounters different effects of gravity on the motor system. Many investigators attempt to minimize the pervasive effects of gravity on motor performance by testing immature animals under conditions that free the limbs from contact with a surface. Newborn rats and mice, for instance, can perform facial wiping and grooming behavior if provided with external postural support or immersed in water (Fentress, 1978; Robinson & Smotherman, 1992d; Smotherman & Robinson, 1989). Like Thelen's case of neonatal stepping, facial wiping behavior disappears a few days after birth and then reappears late in the second postnatal week, when young rats begin to discover alternative strategies for maintaining postural support while freeing the forelimbs for paw–face contact (Smotherman & Robinson, 1989).

Stepping behavior also is expressed with much less constraint when rat pups are tested in a supine position (Brumley & Robinson, 2005), or when suspended in a harness in a prone posture (Fady et al., 1998; Van Hartesveldt et al., 1991). However, the effects of gravity on limb extension and flexion are not equivalent in different postures. In a suspended, prone position, gravitational loading promotes a resting posture in which the limbs are extended away from the body; in a supine posture, the limbs assume a more flexed position near the body; and in a lateral posture, the limbs on the side facing up are drawn toward the midline of the body, whereas the limbs on the side facing down are pulled away from the midline. We have examined the possibility that spontaneous motor activity in neonatal rats varies under different conditions of gravitational load by recording spontaneous limb movements of P0 or P1 rat pups in a prone, supine, or lateral posture (Brumley, Gregory & Robinson, 2002). Effects of posture on limb activity appeared to change during the first 24 h after birth. P0 subjects appeared insensitive to the three postural conditions. P1 subjects, however, showed almost twice as many hindlimb movements in the supine posture as in the other two postures and expressed fewer synchronized movements of both forelimbs or both hindlimbs when placed in a lateral posture (where gravity exerts differential effects on left and right limbs). Effects of initial posture also affect the specific motor patterns and efficiency of performing contact righting responses in newborn rats (Pellis et al., 1991). These findings provide evidence that limb movements during spontaneous and evoked activity in newborn rats are influenced by variations in vestibular or proprioceptive stimulation (cf., Clarac, Vinay, Cazalets, Fady & Jamon, 1998; Eilam & Smotherman, 1998; Ronca & Alberts, 2000). Furthermore, they suggest that experience with a gravitational environment affects the responsiveness of spontaneous motor activity to sensory feedback during perinatal development.

Could variation in physical forces, such as gravity, exert similar effects on behavior of fetuses in utero? Studies of chick embryos provide clues that gravitational loading may affect spontaneous motor activity. Reduction of amniotic fluid volume, which reduces buoyant support of the embryo in the egg, results in altered movement kinematics in the E9 chick embryo (Bradley, 1997). Limb activity increased after fluid reduction, as did intralimb coordination, particularly within the wings. But interlimb coordination decreased as patterns of movement expressed by wings and legs diverged: chicks ultimately showed synchronous, in-phase activity of the wings, and alternated, antiphase coordination of the legs. All three behavioral effects of diminished buoyancy, experimentally induced on E9 of incubation, resemble normal developmental trends correlated with reduced amniotic fluid volume and growth of the embryo from E9 to E13 (Hamburger, Balaban, Oppenheim, & Wenger, 1965; Provine, 1980; Sharp, Ma, & Bekoff, 1999).

Physical constraint of movement, associated with body growth within the egg or uterus, also creates biomechanical limitations for embryonic and fetal movement. As noted above, the chick embryo experiences sharply reduced free space within the egg during incubation, which likely contributes to increased motor activity and altered intralimb coordination from E9 to E13 and diminished motor

activity from E13 to hatching (E21) (Bradley, 2001). During the last few days of incubation, physical crowding within the egg is extreme as the embryo assumes a contorted body posture, with the head and neck tucked under one wing. Activity is sharply reduced at this stage and proprioceptive signals generated by the bending of the neck in this prehatching posture trigger the onset of hatching movements (Bekoff & Sabichi, 1987).

In contrast to birds, mammalian fetuses develop within an environment that expands as growth proceeds. Nevertheless, amniotic fluid volume reaches a peak in the rat fetus on E19 and diminishes sharply thereafter (Marsh, King, & Becker, 1963; Robinson & Smotherman, 1992b). Coupled with a nearly exponential rate of body growth (doubling mass every 1.4 days), the rat fetus is faced with a dramatic reduction in free space in utero late in gestation (Figure 9.6) (Robinson & Brumley, 2005). Spontaneous motor activity in utero increases steadily until the peak of amniotic fluid volume on E19, then levels off or diminishes over the last 2–3 days of gestation (Narayanan et al., 1971; Smotherman & Robinson, 1986), suggesting a suppressive effect of physical constraint similar to that seen in avian embryos. Indeed, one of the most robust effects reported on spontaneous motor activity in rodent fetuses is the difference in movement patterns when fetuses are observed in utero versus ex utero (externalized from the uterus and amniotic sac into the surrounding bath medium). Many studies agree that E20–21 rat fetuses show increased motor activity when released from intrauterine restraint (Bekoff & Lau, 1980; Narayanan et al., 1971; Robinson, 1989; Ronca, Kamm, Thelen, & Alberts, 1994; Smotherman, Richards, & Robinson, 1984; Smotherman & Robinson, 1986). Movements also become more temporally clustered in bouts, with briefer intervals between successive movement events (Robinson & Smotherman, 1988; Ronca et al., 1994), and movement synchrony and overall movement diversity increases ex utero (Robinson, 1989; Ronca et al., 1994; Smotherman & Robinson, 1987). Paradoxically, some forms of behavioral organization are facilitated when fetuses remain within the amniotic sac. Facial wiping behavior, for instance, involves forelimb and head coordination that is expressed in amnion and ex utero on E20, but occurs only when fetuses remain in amnion on E19. Video motion analysis suggests that the facilitative effect of the amniotic sac is a consequence of dampening lateral head movement, which promotes paw–face contact

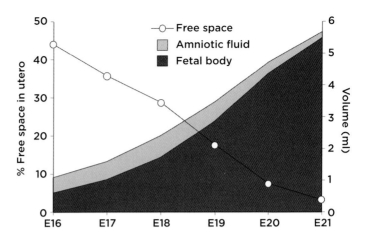

Figure 9.6 Developmental changes in fetal body volume and amniotic fluid volume (right axis), and resultant free space within the uterus (left axis) over the last six days of gestation in the rat. Fetal body volume is calculated from body mass; free space is expressed as the proportion of volume occupied by amniotic fluid (amniotic fluid / [fetal body + amniotic fluid]).

during sensory-evoked wiping responses in younger fetuses. The amniotic sac thus appears to serve as scaffolding, structuring the coordination of behavior (Robinson & Smotherman, 1991a).

Several explanations have been offered for the behavioral differences between fetuses in utero and ex utero. Early observers speculated that removal from the uterus might interfere with placental function and fetal oxygenation, resulting in hypoxia ex utero (Narayanan et al., 1971; Windle, Minear, Austin, & Orr, 1935). However, the behavior expressed by fetuses after externalization from the uterus does not resemble the effects of hypoxia induced by umbilical cord occlusion (Robinson & Smotherman, 1992b), and fetuses maintain stable levels of motor activity and sensory responsiveness for extended observation sessions (up to 2 h), suggesting that the enhanced behavioral organization evident ex utero is not due to general physiological impairment. Removal from the amniotic sac also eliminates fetal access to amniotic fluid and its complex assortment of chemical constituents (Ronca et al., 1994), some of which exert an influence on fetal behavior (e.g., Korthank & Robinson, 1998). But an alternative explanation is that fetuses either cannot move or inhibit movement under conditions of biomechanical restraint. It is possible that low-amplitude movements may be dampened by the restraining effects of the embryonic membranes and uterine wall, in effect filtering the expression of motor activity and preventing occurrence of fine movements. Or fetuses may detect the difference in physical restraint in utero and ex utero by cutaneous or proprioceptive sensation, and actively alter their motor behavior in the two conditions.

Additional evidence for the influence of the physical environment in utero has emerged from studies of posture and movement in human perinates. Free space in utero also diminishes sharply during the third trimester in humans (Almli, Ball, & Wheeler, 2001), which is associated with decreasing rates of fetal body movements in general (de Vries, Visser, & Prechtl, 1988; Edwards & Edwards, 1970; Roberts, Griffin, Mooney, Cooper, & Campbell, 1980), and leg movements in particular (Almli et al., 2001). Premature rupture of the amniotic sac and its concomitant reduction of amniotic fluid volume has been reported to decrease the amplitude and velocity of fetal movement (Sival, Visser, & Prechtl, 1990). Newborns exhibit dominance of flexor muscles and tightly flexed postures for weeks after birth, which has been interpreted as persistence of fetal accommodation to physical restraint during the last few months of gestation (Thelen et al., 1984).

Ultrasound assessment of human fetal posture and orientation in utero has confirmed a developmental trend toward increased limb flexion and lateralized head position during gestation (Ververs, de Vries, van Geijn, & Hopkins, 1994; Ververs, Van Gelder-Hasker, de Vries, Hopkins, & Van Geijn, 1998). Some aspects of arm flexion begin to develop as early as 12 weeks of gestation, when intrauterine space offers little restriction for fetal movement. But other aspects of arm posture (Ververs et al., 1998) and lateralized head orientation (Hopkins, Lems, Janssen, & Butterworth, 1987) are associated with diminishing free space in utero and may be less pronounced in breech body orientation, which provides more freedom for head and hand movement than typical cephalic/vertex (head down) body orientation (Fong, Buis, Saelsbergh, & de Vries, 2005). Breech orientation apparently has the opposite effect on coordinated leg movement, resulting in alterations in leg posture, reflexes, and walking coordination 12–18 months after birth (Sival, Prechtl, Sonder, & Touwen, 1993), and perhaps leading to different motor strategies in solving locomotor tasks at 2.5 years of age (Fong, Ledebt, Zwart, de Vries, & Savelsbergh, 2008). Finally, it is intriguing that the newborn stepping reflex also may be lateralized, with less intralimb coordination during left leg movement than right leg (Dömellof, Ronnqvist, & Hopkins, 2007), which in turn may be associated with lateralized head and body orientation in utero. The striking similarity of findings from studies of avian embryos, fetal and newborn rodents, and human perinates thus provides convergent support for the hypothesis that physical features of the intrauterine environment may enforce or reinforce postural and behavioral adaptation by the fetus.

Environmental Contingencies That Shape Movement and Task Demands

As discussed in the preceding section, the fetus develops in a physical environment surrounded by the concentric envelopes of the embryonic membranes (amnion and chorion), uterus (vascularized endometrium and muscular myometrium), and abdomen of the pregnant mother. For much of the early history of research in behavioral embryology, this physical environment was widely believed to be buffered from the continual bombardment of sensory stimuli available in the outside world. In recent decades, however, the intrauterine environment has been explored more thoroughly with recording instruments and experimental methods that have revealed a diverse sensory environment with stimuli penetrating from the outside world, which varies between pregnancies and across time within pregnancies. Foundational research on the embryology of sensory receptors and sensory regions of the brain (e.g., Bradley & Mistretta, 1975) revealed that all of the principal sensory systems begin to develop when the fetus resides in this environment, and functional sensation emerges in a lawful sequence across many species, beginning with the somatic senses and proprioception, proceeding with the chemical senses (main olfaction, vomeronasal olfaction, and gustation) and vestibular sensation, and culminating with audition and vision (Alberts, 1984; Gottlieb, 1971). In precocial species, such as sheep, primates and Guinea pigs,

all of these systems begin to transduce environmental stimuli and evoke fetal responses before birth; in less mature, altricial species, including rats and mice, only for audition and vision is the onset of function postponed until after birth. Investigators concerned with motor systems have long emphasized the nonreflexogenic nature of centrally generated motor patterns in the embryo and fetus, yet it is clear that the fetus is exposed to a rich array of sensory stimuli in multiple modalities that has the potential to evoke, modulate, and shape the development of motor responses.

The abilities of the fetus to detect and express organized responses to sensory stimulation, and to modify its responses as a consequence of sensory experience, have served as the major focus of experimental work in the field of prenatal behavioral research. Many of the distinctive, species-typical action patterns that can be expressed by the mammalian fetus or avian embryo were discovered during efforts to measure responsiveness to sensory stimulation (Robinson & Smotherman, 1992d; Smotherman & Robinson, 1987). This research also has revealed that fetal exposure to sensory stimuli under controlled experimental conditions can support nonassociative and associative learning, including habituation (Kisilevsky & Muir, 1991; Smotherman & Robinson, 1992b; van Heteren, Boekkooi, Jongsma, & Nijhuis, 2000), familiarity or preference learning through mere exposure (DeCasper & Spence, 1986; Hepper, 1988; Kisilevsky et al., 2003; Mennella, Jagnow, & Beauchamp, 2001; Mickley, Remmers-Roeber, Crouse, Walker, & Dengler, 2000; Smotherman, 1982a), and classical conditioning of general motor activity (Smotherman & Robinson, 1991b), as well as specific appetitive (Robinson, Arnold, Spear, & Smotherman, 1993), aversive (Kawai, Morokuma, Tomonaga, Horimoto, & Tanaka, 2004; Mickley et al., 2001; Smotherman, 1982b; Smotherman & Robinson, 1985), and physiological responses (Robinson et al., 1993). Indeed, some forms of prenatal learning can extend beyond the cesura of birth to influence sensory-mediated behavior into adulthood (Hepper, 1993; Smotherman, 1982a). Reviews are available that provide more complete summaries of research over the past 25 years on fetal sensation and learning capacities (Alberts & Ronca, 1993; Kisilevsky & Low, 1998; Lecanuet, Fifer, Krasnegor, & Smotherman, 1995; Lecanuet & Schaal, 1996; Lickliter, 2005; Robinson & Smotherman, 1991b; Schaal, 2005; Smotherman & Robinson, 1998).

The relevance of exteroceptive sensory function to the prenatal development of action systems is twofold. Methodologically, controlled sensory stimulation has made the study of coordinated action patterns possible in an experimental setting. Although descriptive studies have provided anecdotal information about species-typical action patterns in the fetus (e.g., Carmichael, 1954), detailed analysis of the causal mechanisms and development of action patterns has been greatly enhanced by the ability to evoke specific responses under controlled conditions. This is well illustrated by examples of fetal responses to appetitive and aversive chemosensory stimuli, such as the rat fetus's stretch response to milk (Robinson & Smotherman, 1992a) and facial wiping to lemon (Brumley & Robinson, 2004; Robinson & Smotherman, 1991a), respectively. The second source of relevance of prenatal sensory function is conceptual. Functional patterns of postnatal behavior are elicited and oriented with respect to sensory cues available in the environment. Although the fetus would seem to face few contingencies within the womb (cf. discussion in next section), the ability to distinguish sensory stimuli of biological relevance, express organized behavioral responses, orient motor responses relative to the spatial and temporal distribution of cues in the environment, modulate the expression, duration, and intensity of responses, and alter subsequent behavior as a result of sensory experience, all are defining characteristics of an integrated action system (Gallistel, 1980).

Much of the emphasis of research on fetal sensory competence has been devoted to understanding how stimuli in the world outside the mother may penetrate to the intrauterine environment, or how sensory stimuli may be mediated or generated by mother's own behavior and physiology. The best known examples include human fetal exposure to maternal speech sounds (DeCasper & Fifer, 1980; DeCasper & Spence, 1986; Fifer & Moon, 1995), and the parallel case of avian embryos hearing parental vocalizations in the egg (Gottlieb, 1997; Lickliter, 2005), and fetal exposure to complex olfactory and gustatory cues derived from the maternal diet (Hepper, 1988; Mennella et al., 2001; Mennella, Johnson & Beauchamp, 1995; Schaal, 2005; Schaal, Marlier, & Soussignan, 2000). Creative experimental techniques by Ronca and Alberts also have documented the range of maternal activities that may give rise to fetal cutaneous and vestibular stimulation in utero and the responsiveness of fetal rats to experimental stimuli that mimic those sensory qualities (Ronca & Alberts, 1994; Ronca, Lamkin, & Alberts, 1993). For example, pregnant rats produce rhythmic vibrational stimulation as they lick and groom their abdomen, and fetal rats are responsive to rhythmic tactile stimulation that simulates the frequency of maternal licking. Fetuses also are exposed to sources of sensory stimulation that are unique to the prenatal environment. However, the potential impact of these forms of prenatal sensory stimulation on early motor development has received comparatively little attention.

One example is the fetal response to occlusion of the umbilical cord, which results in a brief period of hypoxia. Gradual reduction of pO_2 levels in experimental preparations of large animal fetuses, such as fetal sheep, or in newborn rodents results in diminished motor activity until normoxic conditions are restored (Eden & Hanson, 1987). However, acute occlusion of the umbilical cord, which can be produced experimentally by applying a microvascular clamp, evokes a dramatic but transient increase in motor activity (Smotherman & Robinson, 1988). The form and developmental context of this motor activity suggest that fetal responses to hypoxia may be functional to remove the source of accidental cord compression. In rats and other rodents, the cord compression response can be elicited only during the last few days of gestation, as fetal growth begins to reduce free space in utero, perhaps making accidental occlusion of the cord more likely (Robinson & Smotherman, 1992b). Moreover, components of the motor response are vigorous and directed away from the body, including sudden lateral flexions of the trunk, dorsiflexion of the head and neck, and repeated kicking of the hindlimbs; in some experimental cases, these movements are sufficient to dislodge the clamp from the cord. If this interpretation is correct, then the fetal response to cord occlusion may represent an ontogenetic adaptation involving fetal behavior (Smotherman & Robinson, 1988). But it also is possible that the hypoxic reaction is the product of associative learning in utero. Odor cues associated with the onset of umbilical cord occlusion are effective in producing conditioned aversion to the odor (Hepper, 1991), whereas cues presented at the time of removal of the clamp and release from hypoxia result in conditioned preference for the odor (Hepper, 1993). These findings offer the intriguing possibility that fetal movements may be modified during normal development in response to naturally occurring contingencies in utero, such as transient fluctuations in oxygen availability resulting from torsion or compression of the umbilical cord.

Transient episodes of hypoxia and greatly increased pressure within the uterus occur in the form of nonlabor uterine contractions, also called contractures (Nathanielsz, 1995). Coordinated epochs of myometrical activity are a normal feature of the uterine environment throughout gestation, recurring 1–4 times per hour in sheep (Jenkin & Nathanielsz, 1994) and much more frequently in rats (Fuchs, 1969). During a contracture, fetal blood pressure rises as oxygen content decreases and the fetal thorax is significantly compressed (Harding & Poore, 1984). In the fetal sheep, contractures result in changes in behavioral state variables, such as eye movements, breathing activity, and high-amplitude electrocortical activity. The rhythmic occurrence of such myometrial activity during the last trimester may contribute to the development of normal sleep states (Nathanielsz, Bailey, Poore, Thorburn, & Harding, 1980; Robertson et al., 1996). In the rat fetus, simulation of moderate pressure changes during uterine contractions consistently evokes heart rate deceleration and increased motor activity (Ronca & Alberts, 1994). Because contractures are expressed in segments and not simultaneously throughout the uterus (Fuchs, 1969), siblings in different parts of the uterus are likely to be exposed to stimulation at different times, perhaps with different patterns or amounts of exposure that coincide with other sources of exteroceptive stimulation (e.g., from maternal activity). Yet the potential contribution of this ubiquitous feature of the prenatal sensory environment to individual differences in behavior, even among genetically similar siblings derived from the same pregnancy, has received scant attention.

A third source of cutaneous stimulation in utero (apart from maternal activity and uterine contractures) is available in animals that give birth to multiple offspring. In rats, mice, and other polytocous species, many fetuses develop within the two deeply divided horns of the duplex uterus. Because all of these fetuses express spontaneous motor activity, their movements serve as a potential source of stimulation for nearby siblings. The developmental consequences of hormonal and other chemical exchange between fetuses in utero (the vom Saal effect) has been well documented (Meisel & Ward, 1981; Ryan and Vandenbergh, 2002; vom Saal & Bronson, 1978), but the potential for direct behavioral interactions between fetuses has only recently been confirmed (Brumley & Robinson, 2002). In an initial analysis, we found that fetuses occupying contiguous positions in utero expressed synchronized movements more often than fetuses in noncontiguous positions or fetuses from different pregnancies (a control for coincidence). To assess sibling interactions experimentally, E20 fetal rats adjacent to focal subjects were immobilized by intraperitoneal injection of curare (10 mg/kg). Focal fetuses (not injected) that lay between two curarized siblings showed less activity than noninjected fetuses in other uterine positions. Conversely, noninjected focal subjects between two siblings that were injected with the kappa opioid agonist U50,488, which produces a four- to five-fold increase in fetal motor activity (Andersen, Robinson, & Smotherman, 1993), showed selective increases in motor behavior. In both pharmacological manipulations, drug-induced changes in the activity of adjacent siblings resulted in disproportionate changes in hindlimb movements of noninjected focal subjects (decreases when siblings were immobile; increases when siblings were activated). In some cases, subjects altered orientation within the uterus while expressing hindlimb movements that resembled alternated stepping. It is noteworthy in this context that chick embryos also exhibit alternated stepping movements of the legs as they rotate within the egg during hatching, between episodes of simultaneous leg extension as the eggshell is cracked (Bakhuis, 1974; Hamburger & Oppenheim, 1967). Real-time ultrasound recordings suggest that human fetuses may similarly employ step-like leg movements to turn to a vertex (head down) position within the uterus (Suzuki & Yamamuro, 1985). The implication of these comparative observations is that coordinated hindlimb behavior, perhaps stimulated by movements or changes in orientation by adjacent fetuses, may be functional before birth as a means of adjusting orientation in utero. More generally, these findings suggest that motor activity of nearby siblings may contribute to the prenatal sensory environment and thus to the motor and sensory development of the fetus.

Significance of Experience during Perinatal Development of Action Systems

The approach to understanding perinatal behavioral development that we are advocating attempts to relate the origin and development of behavioral competencies to mechanisms of perception and action and environmental resources that may functionally shape action systems. In the foregoing sections, we have presented evidence of (1) developmental continuity between prenatal and postnatal behavior, (2) overlapping mechanisms for different modes of action, (3) use of sensory feedback by perinatal animals to alter and learn new patterns of motor coordination, and (4) responsiveness of perinatal animals to features of the environment and the biomechanical context in which movement occurs. It is our view that consideration of all of these determinants of behavior is necessary to explain the development of action systems. Much of our discussion has focused on spontaneous and locomotor activity. In this final section, we speculate about a possible relationship between the development of these two types of behavior during perinatal ontogeny, while adopting a multifactorial approach whereby motor experience and environmental context both play significant roles in the shaping of these action systems.

In the few days before birth, spontaneous movement by the fetus changes in frequency and organization (de Vries et al., 1982, 1988; Kleven et al., 2004; Smotherman & Robinson, 1986) as the intrauterine environment changes markedly in terms of biomechanical constraints on movement (Almli et al., 2001; Robinson & Brumley, 2005). During this same period of time in which the fetus is essentially coming into more direct contact with the surrounding uterus, the neural mechanisms supporting locomotion are forming and changing in their pattern of evoked activity (Clarac et al., 2004; Kudo et al., 2004; Ozaki et al., 1996). Because there appears to be some sharing of neural resources between the mechanisms of spontaneous activity and locomotion (recall the experiment in which evoked stepping behavior was influenced by previous interlimb yoke training) (cf., Bradley et al., 2005; Bekoff, 1992), it is possible that contingencies in the fetal environment help to shape these neural resources and their behavioral expression.

Contingencies that are present during the last few days of gestation may provide conditional feedback during spontaneous fetal movement that helps to create an intrinsic bias in movement coordination (Robinson, Marcano-Reik, Brumley, & Kleven, 2006). For the fetus to move in utero, it must overcome resistance created by elasticity of the uterine myometrium. However, the force necessary to deform the uterus depends on the configuration and timing of leg extension during fetal movement. To measure the force necessary for limb extension in utero, a section of the uterus comprising uterine

endometrial and myometrial tissue was collected on E20 of gestation, opened along the mesometrial border, and stretched over a 3.5 cm diameter circular frame. One or two blunt probes (with 2-mm spheres at the tips) then were pressed against the center of the myometrial sheet, separated by varying distances, simulating the effects of fetal extension of one or two limbs. As shown in Figure 9.7, when the elastic membrane was deformed simultaneously at two contiguous points (0 mm separation), the total force required was less than twice the force involved in equal deformation at just one point. But when the membrane was deformed simultaneously at two points separated by 10 mm (the approximate distance between the two hindfeet of the rat fetus at term), more than twice the force was required than at a single point (Robinson et al., 2006).

The force relationships found in our deformation experiment are not unique to uterine tissue; they are intrinsic to all elastic membranes. The contingencies thus presented to fetuses surrounded by an elastic environment suggest that fetuses may expend less energy, or achieve greater limb extension for the same work, by extending one limb at a time (independently or by or alternated extension) rather than synchronously (conjugate extension) when pushing against the uterus. If these

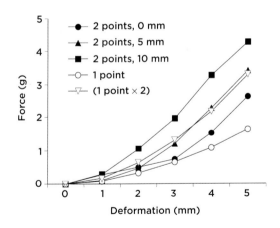

Figure 9.7 Contingent force required for deformation of myometrial tissue. Uterine tissue was collected on E20 of gestation. Each curve represents the force (vertical axis) necessary to deform a sample of myometrium to a specified extent (horizontal axis), when deformation occurs at one or two points on the myometrial sheet. Note that the force required when points of deformation are separated by 10 mm is more than twice that required to deform the tissue to the same extent at a single point. See text for further discussion.

contingent force relationships accurately reflect conditions in utero, the physics of moving within an elastic envelope created by the embryonic membranes, uterus, and maternal abdomen may provide an intrinsic form of reinforcement that would favor antiphase limb movements. Kinesthetic feedback gained from spontaneous movements made in such an environment therefore may serve to strengthen the developing bias of spinal circuits to exhibit alternated activity.

The suggestion that sensory feedback gained from spontaneous activity is used to help shape neural circuitry and functional behavior during ontogeny is not completely novel. In one of the best-studied examples, mallard duck embryos emerge from hatching with a predisposition to recognize and approach the source of a mallard maternal call. This predisposition was viewed by classical ethologists, such as Konrad Lorenz, as a definitive example of innate, instinctive behavior. However, Gottlieb showed in an elegant series of experiments (summarized in Gottlieb, 1997) that normal auditory perceptual development and preference for the mallard maternal call is dependent on auditory experience within the egg. Embryos that hear the mother through the shell, or other siblings vocalizing in nearby eggs, develop normally. But Gottlieb also showed that exposure to their own embryonic vocalizations in the egg is sufficient to establish the auditory bias. Thus, spontaneous vocal activity by embryos helps to tune the developing auditory system in ovo, establishing a perceptual bias that can develop when eggs are incubated in complete isolation (Gottlieb, 1997).

In the rat, Schouenborg and colleagues have discovered a similar experience-dependent pattern of development of the tail withdrawal reflex. The nociceptive withdrawal reflex, originally described by Sherrington (1910), is a fundamental mammalian action system that is governed by relatively simple neural circuitry located within the spinal cord (Schouenborg, 2002). In the newborn rat, however, application of a pain stimulus (such as heat) to a localized region of the tail results in erroneous flexion of the tail toward the stimulus in 50%–80% of trials (Waldenström, Thelin, Thimansson, Levinsson, & Schouenborg, 2003). Refinement of the tail withdrawal response occurs over the first few postnatal weeks as spontaneous tail movements, which occur during active sleep, result in localized contact of the tail with surrounding objects. By experimentally providing "incorrect" sensory feedback during tail twitches, Schouenborg and colleagues demonstrated that abnormal withdrawal responses develop, confirming that development of an efficient, functional nociceptive withdrawal response depends on specific cutaneous sensory feedback generated when different tail muscles are active (Petersson et al., 2003; Chapter 12). Examples of self-stimulation during development, such as the duckling auditory preference and nociceptive withdrawal response, highlight the active role of the organism as well as nonobvious sources of behavioral control and regulation in the developmental process of behavior construction.

In conclusion, there are multiple endogenous and exogenous factors that can influence behavioral performance in the fetus and newborn, and hence are likely to contribute to the developmental construction of perinatal action systems. This perspective is consistent with the principles of developmental systems theory (see Chapter 2), but it is not conceptually new. Many of the developmental resources that have been identified in psychobiological research in our laboratories and others were recognized as interacting participants in the developmental process by Zing Yang Kuo 75 years ago (Kuo, 1976). But such an experimental approach nevertheless is still needed to move perinatal research from "demonstration studies" of what the immature animal is capable of to explanations of the developmental process itself (Alberts, 2008).

References

Adolph, K. E., & Avolio, A. M. (2000). Walking infants adapt locomotion to changing body dimensions. *Journal of Experimental Psychology: Human Perception and Performance, 26,* 1148–1166.

Adolph, K. E., & Berger, S. A. (2006). Motor development. In W. Damon & R. Lerner (Series Eds.) & D. Kuhn & R. S. Siegler (Vol. Eds.), *Handbook of child psychology: Vol. 2: Cognition, perception, and language* (6th ed., pp. 161–216). New York: Wiley.

Adolph, K. E., Vereijken, B., & Shrout, P. E. (2003). What changes in infant walking and why. *Child Development, 74,* 475–497.

Alberts, J. R. (1984) Sensory-perceptual development in the Norway rat: A view toward comparative studies. In: R. Kail & N. Spear (Eds.), *Comparative perspectives on memory development* (pp. 65–101). New York: Plenum.

Alberts, J. R. (2008). Self-sensitivity in fetal development. *Infancy, 13,* 270–274.

Alberts, J. R., & Ronca, A. E. (1993). Fetal experience revealed by rats: Psychobiological insights. *Early Human Development, 35,* 153–166.

Alberts, J. R., & Ronca, A. E. (1996). Fetal behavior in developmental psychobiology. *Developmental Psychobiology, 29,* 185–190.

Almli, C. R., Ball, R. H., & Wheeler, M. E. (2001). Human fetal and neonatal movement patterns: Gender differences and fetal-to-neonatal continuity. *Developmental Psychobiology, 38*, 252–273.

Altman, J., & Sudarshan, K. (1975). Postnatal development of locomotion in the laboratory rat. *Animal Behaviour, 23*, 896–920.

Andersen, S. L., Robinson, S. R., & Smotherman, W. P. (1993). Ontogeny of the stretch response in the rat fetus: kappa opioid involvement. *Behavioral Neuroscience, 107*, 370–376.

Angulo y Gonzalez, A. W. (1932). The prenatal development of behavior in the albino rat. *Journal of Comparative Neurology, 55*, 395–442.

Atsuta, Y., Abraham, P., Iwahara, T., Garcia-Rill, E. & Skinner, R. D. (1991). Control of locomotion in vitro: II. chemical stimulation. *Somatosensory and Motor Research, 8*, 55–63.

Bakhuis, W. L. (1974). Observations on hatching movements in the chick (*Gallus domesticus*). *Journal of Comparative and Physiological Psychology, 87*, 997–1003.

Ballion, B., Morin, D., & Viala, D. (2001). Forelimb locomotor generators and quadrupedal locomotion in the neonatal rat. *European Journal of Neuroscience, 14*, 1727–1738.

Bekoff, A. (1992). Neuroethological approaches to the study of motor development in chicks: Achievements and challenges. *Journal of Neurobiology, 23*, 1486–1505.

Bekoff, A., & Kauer, J. A. (1984). Neural control of hatching: Fate of the pattern generator for the leg movements of hatching in posthatching chicks. *Journal of Neuroscience, 4*, 2659–2666.

Bekoff, A., & Lau, B. (1980). Interlimb coordination in 20-day-old rat fetuses. *Journal of Experimental Zoology, 214*, 173–175.

Bekoff, A., & Sabichi, A. L. (1987). Sensory control of the initiation of hatching in chicks: Effects of a local anesthetic injected into the neck. *Developmental Psychobiology, 20*, 489–495.

Blumberg, M.S., & Lucas, D.E. (1994). Dual mechanisms of twitching during sleep in neonatal rats. *Behavioral Neuroscience, 108*, 1196–1202.

Bradley, N. S. (1997). Reduction in buoyancy alters parameters of motility in E9 chick embryos. *Physiology & Behavior, 62*, 591–595.

Bradley, N. S. (2001). Age-related changes and condition-dependent modifications in distribution of limb movements during embryonic motility. *Journal of Neurophysiology, 86*, 1511–1522.

Bradley, R. M., & Mistretta, C. M. (1975). Fetal sensory receptors. *Physiological Reviews, 55*, 352–382.

Bradley, N. S., & Sebelski, C. (2000). Ankle restraint modifies motility at E12 in chick embryos. *Journal of Neurophysiology, 83*, 431–440.

Bradley, N. S., Solanki, D., & Zhao, D. (2005). Limb movements during embryonic development in the chick: Evidence for a continuum in limb motor control antecedent to locomotion. *Journal of Neurophysiology, 94*, 4401–4411.

Brumley, M. R., Gregory, D. J., & Robinson, S. R. (2002). Spontaneous limb movements and sensory feedback in the newborn rat. (Abstract). *Developmental Psychobiology, 41*, 301.

Brumley, M. R., & Robinson, S. R. (2002). Responsiveness of rat fetuses to sibling motor activity: communication in utero? (Abstract). *Developmental Psychobiology, 41*, 73.

Brumley, M. R., & Robinson, S. R. (2004). Effects of chemosensory stimulus parameters on the facial wiping response of the rat fetus. *Developmental Psychobiology, 44*, 219–229.

Brumley, M.R., & Robinson, S.R. (2005). The serotonergic agonists quipazine, CGS-12066A and ff-methylserotonin alter motor activity and induce hindlimb stepping in the intact and spinal rat fetus. *Behavioral Neuroscience, 119*, 821–833.

Carmichael, L. (1954). The onset and early development of behavior. In L. Carmichael (Ed.), *Manual of child psychology* (2nd ed., pp. 60–185). New York: Wiley.

Carrier, D. R. (1996). Ontogenetic limits on locomotor performance. *Physiological Zoology, 69*, 467–488.

Cazalets, J.-R., Grillner, P., Menard, I., Crémieux, J. & Clarac, F. (1990). Two types of motor rhythm induced by NMDA and amines in an in vitro spinal cord preparation of neonatal rat. *Neuroscience Letters, 111*, 116–122.

Cazalets, J. R., Sqalli-Houssaini, Y., & Clarac, F. (1992). Activation of the central pattern generators for locomotion by serotonin and excitatory amino acids in neonatal rat. *Journal of Physiology, 455*, 187–204.

Chambers, S. H., Bradley, N. S., & Orosz, M. D. (1995). Kinematic analysis of wing and leg movements for type I motility in E9 chick embryos. *Experimental Brain Research, 103*, 218–226.

Clancy, B., Darlington, R. B., & Finlay, B. L. (2001). Translating developmental time across mammalian species. *Neuroscience, 105*, 7–17.

Clarac, F., Brocard, F., & Vinay, L. (2004). The maturation of locomotor networks. *Progress in Brain Research, 143*, 57–66.

Clarac, F., Vinay, L., Cazalets, J.-R., Fady, J.-C., & Jamon, M. (1998). Role of gravity in the development of posture and locomotion in the neonatal rat. *Brain Research Reviews, 28*, 35–43.

Coghill, G. E. (1929). *Anatomy and the problem of behavior*. Cambridge: Cambridge University Press.

Corner, M. A. (1977). Sleep and the beginnings of behavior in the animal kingdom—Studies of ultradian motility cycles in early life. *Progress in Neurobiology, 8*, 279–295.

Cowley, K. C., & Schmidt, B. J. (1994). A comparison of motor patterns induced by *N*-methyl-D-aspartate, acetylcholine and serotonin in the in vitro neonatal rat spinal cord. *Neuroscience Letters, 171*, 147–150.

DeCasper, A.J., & Fifer, W.P. (1980). Of human bonding: Newborns prefer their mother's voices. *Science, 208*, 1174–1176.

DeCasper, A. J., & Spence, M. J. (1986). Prenatal maternal speech influences newborns' perception of speech sounds. *Infant Behavior and Development, 9*, 133–150.

de Vries, J. I. P., & Fong, B. F. (2006). Normal fetal motility: An overview. *Ultrasound in Obstetrics and Gynecology, 27*, 701–711.

de Vries, J. I. P., Visser, G. H. A., & Prechtl, H. F. R. (1982). The emergence of fetal behavior. I. Qualitative aspects. *Early Human Development, 7*, 301–322.

de Vries, J. I. P., Visser, G. H. A., & Prechtl, H. F. R. (1988). The emergence of fetal behavior. III. Individual differences and consistencies. *Early Human Development, 16*, 85–103.

Dömellof, E., Rönnqvist, L., & Hopkins, B. (2007). Functional asymmetries in the stepping response of the human newborn: A kinematic approach. *Experimental Brain Research, 177*, 324–335.

Eden, G. J., & Hanson, M. A. (1987). Maturation of the respiratory response to acute hypoxia in the newborn rat. *Journal of Physiology, 392*, 1–9.

Edwards, D. D., & Edwards, J. S. (1970). Fetal movement: Development and time course. *Science, 169*, 95–97.

Eilam, D., & Smotherman, W. P. (1998). How the neonatal rat gets to the nipple: Common motor modules and their involvement in the expression of early motor behavior. *Developmental Psychobiology, 32*, 57–66.

Fady, J.-C., Jamon, M., & Clarac, F. (1998). Early olfactory-induced rhythmic limb activity in the newborn rat. *Developmental Brain Research, 108*, 111–123.

Fentress, J. C. (1978). *Mus musicus*: The developmental orchestration of selected movement patterns in mice. In G. M. Burghardt & M. Bekoff (Eds.), *The development of behavior: Comparative and evolutionary aspects* (pp. 321–342). New York: Garland.

Fifer, W. P., & Moon, C. (1995). The effects of fetal experience with sound. In J.-P. Lecanuet, N. A. Krasnegor, W. P. Fifer, & W. P. Smotherman (Eds.), *Fetal development: A psychobiological perspective* (pp. 351–366). New York: Lawrence Erlbaum.

Fitzgerald, M. (1987). Spontaneous and evoked activity of primary afferents in vivo. *Nature, 326*, 603–605.

Fong, B. F., Buis, A. J. E., Savelsbergh, G. J. P., & de Vries, J. I. P. (2005). Influence of breech presentation on the development of fetal arm posture. *Early Human Development, 81*, 519–527.

Fong, B., Ledebt, A., Zwart, R., de Vries, J. I. P., & Savelsbergh, G. J. P. (2008). Is there an effect of prenatal breech position on locomotion at 2.5 years? *Early Human Development, 84*, 211–216.

Fromme, A. (1941). An experimental study of the factors of maturation and practice in the behavioral development of the embryo of the frog *Rana pipiens*. *Genetic Psychological Monographs, 24*, 219–256.

Fuchs, A.-R. (1969). Uterine activity in late pregnancy and during parturition in the rat. *Biology of Reproduction, 1*, 344–353.

Gallistel, C. R. (1980). *The organization of action: A new synthesis*. Hillsdale, NJ: Lawrence Erlbaum.

Gao, B. X., Stricker, C., & Ziskind-Conhaim, L. (2001). Transition from GABAergic to glycinergic synaptic transmission in newly formed spinal networks. *Journal of Neurophysiology, 86*, 492–502.

Gottlieb, G. (1971). Ontogenesis of sensory function in birds and mammals. In E. Tobach, L. Aronson, & E. Shaw (Eds.), *The biopsychology of development* (pp. 67–128). New York: Academic Press.

Gottlieb, G. (1997). *Synthesizing nature–nurture: Prenatal roots of instinctive behavior*. Mahwah, NJ: Lawrence Erlbaum.

Gramsbergen, A., Schwartze, P., & Prechtl, H. F. R. (1970). The postnatal development of behavioral states in the rat. *Developmental Psychobiology, 3*, 267–280.

Greer, J. J., Smith, J. C. & Feldman, J. L. (1992). Respiratory and locomotor patterns generated in the fetal rat brain stem–spinal cord in vitro. *Journal of Neurophysiology, 67*, 996–999.

Hamburger, V. (1963). Some aspects of the embryology of behavior. *Quarterly Review of Biology, 38*, 342–365.

Hamburger, V. (1973). Anatomical and physiological basis of embryonic motility in birds and mammals. In G. Gottlieb (Ed.), *Behavioral Embryology* (Vol. 1, pp. 51–76). New York: Academic Press.

Hamburger, V., Balaban, M., Oppenheim, R., & Wenger, E. (1965). Periodic motility of normal and spinal chick embryos between 8 and 17 days of incubation. *Journal of Experimental Zoology, 159*, 1–14.

Hamburger, V., & Oppenheim, R. (1967). Prehatching motility and hatching behavior in the chick. *Journal of Experimental Zoology, 166*, 171–204.

Hamburger, V., Wenger, E., & Oppenheim, R. W. (1966). Motility in the chick embryo in the absence of sensory input. *Journal of Experimental Zoology, 162*, 133–160.

Harding, R., & Poore, E. R. (1984). The effects of myometrial activity on fetal thoracic dimensions and uterine blood flow during late gestation in the sheep. *Biology of the Neonate, 45*, 244–251.

Haverkamp, L. J., & Oppenheim, R. W. (1986). Behavioral development in the absence of neural activity: Effects of chronic immobilization on amphibian embryos. *Journal of Neuroscience, 6*, 1332–1337.

Heberling, J. L., & Robinson, S. R. (1997). Kinematic analysis of L-DOPA-induced stepping in fetal and newborn rats [Abstract]. *Developmental Psychobiology, 32*, 150.

Helgren, M., Cliffer, K. D., Torrento, K., Cavnor, C., Curtis, R., Di Stefano, P. S., et al. (1997). Neurotrophin-3 administration attenuates deficits of pyridoxine-induced large-fiber sensory neuropathy. *Journal of Neuroscience, 17*, 372–382.

Hepper, P. G. (1988). Adaptive fetal learning: Prenatal exposure to garlic affects postnatal preferences. *Animal Behaviour, 36*, 935–936.

Hepper, P. G. (1991). Transient hypoxic episodes: A mechanism to support associative fetal learning. *Animal Behaviour, 41*, 477–480.

Hepper, P. G. (1993). In utero release from a single transient hypoxic episode: a positive reinforcer? *Physiology & Behavior, 53*, 309–311.

Hepper, P. G., Wells, D. L., & Lynch, C. (2005). Prenatal thumb sucking is related to postnatal handedness. *Neuropsychologia, 43*, 313–315.

Hooker, D. (1952). *The prenatal origin of behavior*. 18th Porter Lecture Series. Lawrence, KS: University of Kansas Press.

Hopkins, B., Lems, W., Janssen, B., & Butterworth, G. (1987). Postural and motor asymmetries in newlyborns. *Human Neurobiology, 6*, 153–156.

Hory-Lee, R., Russell, M., Linday, R. M., & Frank, E. (1993). Neurotrophin-3 supports the survival of developing muscle sensory neurons in culture. *Proceedings of the National Academy of Science, USA, 90*, 2613–2617.

Hynes, S. M., Brumley, M. R., Oetken, L. C., & Robinson, S. R. (2003). Probing the regulation of spontaneous motor activity with a proprioceptive hindlimb manipulation in the neonatal rat. (Abstract). *Developmental Psychobiology, 43*, 260.

Iizuka, M., Nishimaru, H., & Kudo, N. (1998). Development of the spatial pattern of 5-HT-induced locomotor rhythm in the lumbar spinal cord of rat fetuses in vitro. *Neuroscience Research, 31*, 107–111.

Illingworth, R. S. (1966). *The development of the infant and young child: Normal and abnormal* (3rd ed.). London: E&S Livingstone.

Jamon, M. & Clarac, F. (1998). Early walking in the neonatal rat: a kinematic study. *Behavioral Neuroscience, 112*, 1218–1228.

Jenkin, G., & Nathanielsz, P. W. (1994). Myometrial activity during pregnancy and parturition. In G. D. Thorburn & R. Harding (Eds.), *Textbook of fetal physiology* (pp. 405–414). Oxford: Oxford University Press.

Johnston, R.M. & Bekoff, A. (1992). Constrained and flexible features of rhythmical hindlimb movements in chicks: Kinematic profiles of walking, swimming and airstepping. *Journal of Experimental Biology, 171*, 43–66.

Juvin, L., Simmers, J. & Morin, D. (2005). Propriospinal circuitry underlying interlimb coordination in mammalian quadrupedal locomotion. *Journal of Neuroscience, 25*, 6025–6035.

Kawai, N., Morokuma, S., Tomonaga, M., Horimoto, N., & Tanaka, M. (2004). Associative learning and memory in a chimpanzee fetus: Learning and long-lasting memory before birth. *Developmental Psychobiology, 44*, 116–122.

Kiehn, O. & Butt, S. J. (2003). Physiological, anatomical and genetic identification of CPG neurons in the developing mammal spinal cord. *Progress in Neurobiology, 70*, 347–361.

Kiehn, O. & Kjaerulff, O. (1996). Spatiotemporal characteristics of 5-HT and dopamine-induced rhythmic hindlimb activity in the in vitro neonatal rat. *Journal of Neurophysiology, 75*, 1472–1482.

Kisilevsky, B. S., Hains, S. M. J., Lee, K., Xie, X. Huang, H. Ye, H. H., et al. (2003). Effects of experience on fetal voice recognition. *Psychological Science, 14*, 220–224.

Kisilevsky, B. S., & Low, J. A. (1998). Human fetal behavior: 100 years of study. *Developmental Review, 18*, 1–29.

Kisilevsky, B. S., & Muir, D. W. (1991). Human fetal and subsequent newborn responses to sound and vibration. *Infant Behavior and Development, 14*, 1–26.

Klein, R., Silos-Santiago, I., Smeyne, R. J., Lira, S., Brambilla, R., Bryant, S., et al. (1994). Disruption of the neurotrophin-3 receptor gene trkC eliminates Ia muscle afferents and results in abnormal movements. *Nature, 368*, 249–251.

Kleven, G. A., Lane, M. S., & Robinson, S. R. (2004). Development of interlimb movement synchrony in the rat fetus. *Behavioral Neuroscience, 118*, 833–844.

Kleven, G. A., & Ronca, A. E. (2009). Prenatal behavior of the C57BL/6J mouse: A promising model for human fetal movement during early to mid-gestation. *Developmental Psychobiology, 51*, 84–94.

Korthank, A. J., & Robinson, S. R. (1998). Effects of amniotic fluid on opioid activity and fetal responses to chemosensory stimuli. *Developmental Psychobiology, 33*, 235–248.

Kraebel, K. S., Fable, J., & Gerhardstein, P. (2004). New methodology in infant operant kicking procedures: Computerized stimulus control and computerized measurement of kicking. *Infant Behavior and Development, 27*, 1–18.

Kucera, J., Ernfors, P., Walro, J. and Jaenisch, R. (1995). Reduction in the number of spinal neurons in neurotrophin-3-deficient mice. *Neuroscience, 69*, 321–330.

Kucera, J., Walro, J. M., & Reichler, J. (1989). Role of nerve and muscle factors in the development of rat muscle spindles. *American Journal of Anatomy, 186*, 144–160.

Kudo, N., Nishimaru, H. & Nakayama, K. (2004). Developmental changes in rhythmic spinal neuronal activity in the rat fetus. *Progress in Brain Research, 143*, 49–55.

Kudo, N., & Yamada, T. (1987). *N*-Methyl-D,L-aspartate-induced locomotor activity in a spinal cord-hindlimb muscles preparation of the newborn rat studied in vitro. *Neuroscience Letters, 75*, 43–48.

Kuo, Z.-Y. (1967). *The dynamics of behavior development.* New York: Random House.

Kurjak, A., Stanojevic, M., Andonotopo, W., Salihagic-Kadic, A., Carrera, J. M., & Azumendi, G. (2004). Behavioral pattern continuity from prenatal to postnatal life—A study by four-dimensional (4D) ultrasonography. *Journal of Perinatal Medicine, 32*, 346–353.

Lakke, E. A. J. F. (1997). The projections to the spinal cord of the rat during development; a time-table of descent. *Advances in Anatomy, Embryology and Cell Biology, 135*, 1–143.

Lam, T., Wolstenholme, C., & Yang, J. F. (2003). How do infants adapt to loading of the limb during the swing phase of stepping? *Journal of Neurophysiology, 89*, 1920–1928.

Landmesser, L. T., & O'Donovan, M. J. (1984). Activation patterns of embryonic chick hindlimb muscles recorded in ovo and in an isolated spinal cord preparation. *Journal of Physiology, 347*, 189–204.

Lecanuet, J.-P., Fifer, W. P., Krasnegor, N. A., & Smotherman, W. P. (Eds.). (1995). *Fetal development: A psychobiological perspective.* Hillsdale, NJ: Lawrence Erlbaum.

Lecanuet, J.-P., & Schaal, B. (1996). Fetal sensory competencies. *European Journal of Obstetrics & Gynecology and Reproductive Biology, 68*, 1–23.

Lickliter, R. (2005). Prenatal sensory ecology and experience: Implications for perceptual and behavioral development in precocial birds. *Advances in the Study of Behavior, 35*, 235–274.

Marcano-Reik, A. J., & Robinson, S. R. (2004). Motor learning and memory after interlimb yoke training in the rat fetus is spinally mediated. Program No. 946.7. 2004 Abstract Viewer/Itinerary Planner. Washington, DC: Society for Neuroscience, 2004. Online.

Marcano-Reik, A. J., Woller, S. A., & Robinson, S. R. (2005). Hindlimb coordination after in-phase or antiphase yoke training in the infant rat: Developmental changes and effects of training on quipazine-induced stepping. Program No. 603.18. 2005 Abstract Viewer/Itinerary Planner. Washington, DC: Society for Neuroscience, 2005. Online.

Marcus, G. F. (2001). Plasticity and nativism: Towards a resolution of an apparent paradox. In S. Wermter, J. Austin & D. Willshaw (Eds.), *Emergent neural computational architectures based on neuroscience* (pp. 368–382). Heidelberg: Springer-Verlag.

Marsh, R. H., King, J. E., & Becker, R. F. (1963). Volume and viscosity of amniotic fluid in rat and guinea pig fetuses near term. *American Journal of Obstetrics & Gynecology, 85*, 487–492.

Matthews, S. A. & Detwiler, S. R. (1926). The reaction of Amblystoma embryos following prolonged treatment with chloretone. *Journal of Experimental Zoology, 45*, 279–292.

McCrea, A. E., Stehouwer, D. J., & Van Hartesveldt, C. (1994). L-DOPA-induced air-stepping in preweanling rats. I. Effects of dose and age. *Developmental Brain Research, 82*, 136–142.

McEwen, M. L., Van Hartesveldt, C., & Stehouwer, D. J. (1997). L-DOPA and quipazine elicit air-stepping in neonatal rats with spinal cord transections. *Behavioral Neuroscience, 111*, 825–833.

McGraw, M. B. (1940). Neuromuscular development of the human infant as exemplified in the achievement of erect locomotion. *Journal of Pediatrics, 17*, 747–771.

Meisel, R. L., & Ward, I. L. (1981). Fetal female rats are masculinized by male littermates located caudally in the uterus. *Science, 213*, 239–242.

Mennella, J. A., Jagnow, C. P., & Beauchamp, G. K. (2001). Prenatal and postnatal flavor learning by human infants. *Pediatrics, 107*, E88.

Mennella, J. A., Johnson, A., & Beauchamp, G. K. (1995). Garlic ingestion by pregnant women alters the odor of amniotic fluid. *Chemical Senses, 20*, 207–209.

Mickley, G.A., Remmers-Roeber, D. R., Crouse, C., Walker, C., & Dengler, C. (2000). Detection of novelty by perinatal rats. *Physiology & Behavior, 70*, 217–225.

Mickley, G.A., Remmers-Roeber, D. R., Dengler, C. M., Kenmuir, C. L., & Crouse, C. (2001). Paradoxical effects of ketamine on the memory of fetuses of different ages. *Developmental Brain Research, 127*, 71–76.

Moore, P. J., & Hanson, M. A. (1992). Animal investigations. In J. G. Nijhuis (Ed.), *Fetal behaviour: Developmental and perinatal aspects* (pp. 100–111). New York: Oxford University Press.

Myowa-Yamakoshi, M., & Takeshita, H. (2006). Do human fetuses anticipate self-oriented actions? A study by four-dimensional (4D) ultrasonography. *Infancy, 10*, 289–301.

Nakayama, K., Nishimaru, H., & Kudo, N. (2001). Developmental changes in 5-hydroxytryptamine-induced rhythmic activity in the spinal cord of the rat fetus in vitro. *Neuroscience Letters, 307*, 1–4.

Narayanan, C. H., Fox, M. W., & Hamburger, V. (1971). Prenatal development of spontaneous and evoked activity in the rat (*Rattus norvegicus*). *Behaviour, 40*, 100–134.

Narayanan, C. H., & Hamburger, V. (1971). Motility in chick embryos with substitution of lumbosacral by brachial and brachial by lumbosacral spinal cord segments. *Journal of Experimental Zoology, 178*, 415–432.

Narayanan, C. H. & Malloy, R. B. (1974a). Deafferentation studies on motor activity in the chick: I. Activity pattern of hindlimbs. *Journal of Experimental Zoology, 189*, 163–176.

Narayanan, C. H. & Malloy, R. B. (1974b). Deafferentation studies on motor activity in the chick: II. Activity pattern of wings. *Journal of Experimental Zoology, 189*, 177–188.

Nathanielsz, P. W. (1995). The effects of myometrial activity during the last third of gestation on fetal behavior. In J.-P. Lecanuet, N. A. Krasnegor, W. P. Fifer, & W. P. Smotherman (Eds.), *Fetal development: A psychobiological perspective* (pp. 369–382). New York: Lawrence Erlbaum.

Nathanielsz, P. W., Bailey, A., Poore, E. R., Thorburn, G. D., & Harding, R. (1980). The relationship between myometrial activity and sleep state and breathing in fetal sheep throughout the last third of gestation. *American Journal of Obstetrics and Gynecology, 138*, 653–659.

Navarrete, R., & Vrbova, G. (1993). Activity-dependent interactions between motoneurones and muscles: Their role in the development of the motor unit. *Progress in Neurobiology, 41*, 93–124.

Nishimaru, H., & Kudo, N. (2000). Formation of the central pattern generator for locomotion in the rat and mouse brain. *Brain Research Bulletin, 53*(5), 661–669.

Norreel, J.-C., Pflieger, J.-F., Pearlstein, E., Simeoni-Alias, J., Clarac, F. & Vinay, L. (2003). Reversible disorganization of the locomotor pattern after neonatal spinal cord transection in the rat. *Journal of Neuroscience, 23*, 1924–1932.

Oppenheim, R. W. (1972). An experimental investigation of the possible role of tactile and proprioceptive stimulation in certain aspects of embryonic behavior in the chick. *Developmental Psychobiology, 5*, 71–91.

Oppenheim, R. W. (1981). Ontogenetic adaptations and retrogressive processes in the development of the nervous system and behavior. In Connolly, K. & Prechtl, H., (Eds.), *Maturation and development: Biological and psychological perspectives* (pp. 198–215). Philadelphia: Lippincott.

Oppenheim, R. W. (1982). The neuroembryological study of behavior: Progress, problems, perspectives. *Current Topics in Developmental Biology, 17*, 257–309.

Oppenheim, R. W. (1991). Cell death during development of the nervous system. *Annual Review of Neuroscience, 14*, 453–501.

Ozaki, S., Yamada, T., Iizuka, M., Nishimaru, H., & Kudo, N. (1996). Development of locomotor activity induced by NMDA receptor activation in the lumbar spinal cord of the rat fetus studied in vitro. *Developmental Brain Research, 97*, 118–125.

Peiper, A. (1963). *Cerebral function in infancy and childhood*. New York: Consultants Bureau.

Pellis, V. C., Pellis, S. M., & Teitelbaum, P. (1991). A descriptive analysis of the postnatal development of contact-righting in rats (*Rattus norvegicus*). *Developmental Psychobiology, 24*, 237–263.

Petersson, P., Waldenström, A., Fåhraeus, C., & Schouenborg, J. (2003). Spontaneous muscle twitches during sleep guide spinal self-organization. *Nature, 424*, 72–75.

Provine, R. R. (1972). Ontogeny of bioelectric activity in the spinal cord of the chick embryo and its behavioral implications. *Brain Research, 22*, 365–378.

Provine, R. R. (1980). Development of between-limb movement synchronization in the chick embryo. *Developmental Psychobiology, 13*, 151–163.

Rieser, J. J., Pick, H. L., Ashmead, D. H., & Garing, A. E. (1995). Calibration of human locomotion and models of perceptual-motor organization. *Journal of Experimental Psychology: Human Perception and Performance, 21*, 480–497.

Roberts, A. B., Griffin, D., Mooney, R., Cooper, D. J., & Campbell, S. (1980). Fetal activity in 100 normal third trimester pregnancies. *British Journal of Obstetrics and Gynaecology, 87*, 480–484.

Robertson, S. S., & Bacher, L. F. (1995). Oscillation and chaos in fetal motor activity. In J.-P. Lecanuet, N. A. Krasnegor, W. P. Fifer, & W. P. Smotherman (Eds.), *Fetal development: A psychobiological perspective* (pp. 169–189). New York: Lawrence Erlbaum.

Robertson, S. S., Dierker, L. J., Sorokin, Y., & Rosen, M. G. (1982). Human fetal movement: Spontaneous oscillations near one cycle per minute. *Science, 218*, 1327–1330.

Robertson, S. S., Johnson, S. L., Bacher, L. F., Wood, J. R., Wong, C. H., Robinson, S.R., et al. (1996). Contractile activity of the uterus prior to labor alters the temporal organization of spontaneous motor activity in the fetal sheep. *Developmental Psychobiology, 29*, 667–683.

Robertson, S. S., & Smotherman, W. P. (1990). The neural control of cyclic activity in the fetal rat. *Physiology & Behavior, 47*, 121–126.

Robinson, S. R. (1989). *A comparative study of prenatal behavioral ontogeny in altricial and precocial murid rodents*. Unpublished doctoral dissertation, Oregon State University, Corvallis.

Robinson, S. R. (2005). Conjugate limb coordination after experience with an interlimb yoke: Evidence for motor learning in the rat fetus. *Developmental Psychobiology, 47,* 328–344.

Robinson, S. R., Arnold, H. M., Spear, N. E., & Smotherman, W. P. (1993). Experience with milk and an artificial nipple promotes conditioned opioid activity in the rat fetus. *Developmental Psychobiology, 26,* 375–387.

Robinson, S. R., Blumberg, M. S., Lane, M. S., & Kreber, L. (2000). Spontaneous motor activity in fetal and infant rats is organized into discrete multilimb bouts. *Behavioral Neuroscience, 114,* 328–336.

Robinson, S. R., & Brumley, M. R. (2005). Prenatal behavior. In I. Q. Whishaw & B. Kolb (Eds.), *The behavior of the laboratory rat: A handbook with tests* (pp. 257–265). New York: Oxford University Press.

Robinson, S. R., Hoeltzel, T. C. M., Cooke, K. M., Umphress, S. M., Murrish, D. E., & Smotherman, W. P. (1992). Oral capture and grasping of an artificial nipple by rat fetuses. *Developmental Psychobiology, 25,* 543–555.

Robinson, S. R., & Kleven, G. A. (2005). Learning to move before birth. In B. Hopkins & S. P. Johnson (Eds.), *Prenatal development of postnatal functions* (*Advances in Infancy Research series*) (pp. 131–175). Westport, CT: Praeger Publishers.

Robinson, S. R., Kleven, G. A., & Brumley, M. R. (2008). Prenatal development of interlimb motor learning in the rat fetus. *Infancy, 13,* 204–228.

Robinson, S. R., Marcano-Reik, A. J., Brumley, M. R., & Kleven, G. A. (2006). Development of interlimb coordination in the fetal rat: Do conditions in utero reinforce anti-phase movement? Program No. 638.3. 2006 Neuroscience Meeting Planner. Atlanta, GA: Society for Neuroscience. Online.

Robinson, S. R., & Smotherman, W. P. (1987). Environmental determinants of behavior in the rat fetus. II. The emergence of synchronous movement. *Animal Behaviour, 35,* 1652–1662.

Robinson, S. R. & Smotherman, W. P. (1988). Chance and chunks in the ontogeny of fetal behavior. In W. P. Smotherman & S. R. Robinson (Eds.), *Behavior of the fetus* (pp. 95–115). Caldwell, NJ: Telford Press.

Robinson, S. R., & Smotherman, W. P. (1991a). The amniotic sac as scaffolding: Prenatal ontogeny of an action pattern. *Developmental Psychobiology, 24,* 463–485.

Robinson, S. R., & Smotherman, W. P. (1991b). Fetal learning: Implications for the development of kin recognition. In P. G. Hepper (Ed.), *Kin recognition* (pp. 308–334). New York: Cambridge University Press.

Robinson, S. R., & Smotherman, W. P. (1992a). Organization of the stretch response to milk in the rat fetus. *Developmental Psychobiology, 25,* 33–49.

Robinson, S. R., & Smotherman, W. P. (1992b). Behavioral response of altricial and precocial rodent fetuses to acute umbilical cord compression. *Behavioral & Neural Biology, 57*(2), 93–102.

Robinson, S. R., & Smotherman, W. P. (1992c). The emergence of behavioral regulation during fetal development. In G. Turkewitz (Ed.), Developmental psychobiology. *Annals of the New York Academy of Sciences, 662,* 53–83.

Robinson, S. R., & Smotherman, W. P. (1992d). Fundamental motor patterns of the mammalian fetus. *Journal of Neurobiology, 23,* 1574–1600.

Robinson, S. R., Woller, S. A., Khetarpal, N., Fromm, D., & Brumley, M. R. (2004). 24-Hour retention of interlimb yoke training in the neonatal rat: Evidence for motor memory. Program No. 946.3. 2004 Abstract Viewer/Itinerary Planner. Washington, DC: Society for Neuroscience. Online.

Ronca, A. E., & Alberts, J. R. (1994). Sensory stimuli associated with gestation and parturition evoke cardiac and behavioral responses in fetal rats. *Psychobiology, 22,* 270–282.

Ronca, A. E., & Alberts, J. R. (1995). Maternal contributions to fetal experience and the transition from prenatal to postnatal life. In J.-P. Lecanuet, W. P. Fifer, N. A. Krasnegor, & W. P. Smotherman (Eds.), *Fetal development: A psychobiological perspective.* (pp. 331–350). Hillsdale, NJ: Lawrence Erlbaum.

Ronca, A. E., & Alberts, J. R. (2000). Effects of prenatal space-flight on vestibular responses in neonatal rats. *Journal of Applied Physiology, 89,* 2318–2324.

Ronca, A. E., Kamm, K., Thelen, E., & Alberts, J. R. (1994). Proximal control of fetal rat behavior. *Developmental Psychobiology, 27,* 23–38.

Ronca, A. E., Lamkin, C. A., & Alberts, J. R. (1993). Maternal contributions to sensory experience in the fetal and newborn rat (*Rattus norvegicus*). *Journal of Comparative Psychology, 107,* 61–74.

Ross, M. G., & Nijland, M. J. M. (1998). Development of ingestive behavior. *American Journal of Physiology, Regulatory Integrative Comparative Physiology, 274,* 879–893.

Rovee-Collier, C. K., Morrongiello, B. A., Aron, M., & Kupersmidt, J. (1978). Topographical response differentiation and reversal in 3-month-old infants. *Infant Behavior and Development, 1,* 323–333.

Rovee, C. K., & Rovee, D. T. (1969). Conjugate reinforcement of infant exploratory behavior. *Journal of Experimental Child Psychology, 8,* 33–39.

Ryan, B. C., & Vandenbergh, J. G. (2002). Intrauterine position effects. *Neuroscience and Biobehavioral Reviews, 26,* 665–678.

Schaal, B. (2005). From amnion to colostrum to milk: Odor bridging in early developmental transitions. In B. Hopkins & S. P. Johnson (Eds.), *Prenatal development of postnatal functions* (*Advances in Infancy Research series*) (pp. 51–102). Westport, CT: Praeger Publishers.

Schaal, B., Marlier, L., & Soussignan, R. (2000). Human foetuses encode odors from their pregnant mother's diet. *Chemical Senses, 25,* 729–737.

Schouenborg, J. (2002). Modular organisation and spinal somatosensory imprinting. *Brain Research Reviews, 40,* 80–91.

Seelke, A. M. H., Karlsson, K. A., Gall, A. J., & Blumberg, M. S. (2005). Extraocular muscle activity, rapid eye movements, and the development of active and quiet sleep. *European Journal of Neuroscience, 22,* 911–920.

Sharp, A. A., Ma, E., & Bekoff, A. (1999). Developmental changes in leg coordination in the chick at embryonic days 9, 11, and 13: Uncoupling of ankle movements. *Journal of Neurophysiology, 82,* 2406–2414.

Sherrington, C. S. (1910). Flexion-reflex of the limb, crossed extension reflex, and reflex stepping and standing. *Journal of Physiology, 40,* 28–121.

Sival, D. A., Prechtl, H. F., Sonder, G. H., & Touwen, B. C. (1993). The effect of intra-uterine breech position on post-natal motor functions of the lower limbs. *Early Human Development, 32,* 161–176.

Sival, D. A., Visser, G. H. A., & Prechtl, H. F. R. (1990). Does reduction of amniotic fluid affect fetal movements? *Early Human Development, 23*, 233–246.

Smith, J. C., Feldman, J. L. & Schmidt, B. J. (1988). Neural mechanisms generating locomotion studied in mammalian brainstem–spinal cord in vitro. *FASEB Journal, 2*, 2283–2288.

Smotherman, W. P. (1982a). In-utero chemosensory experience alters taste preferences and corticosterone respnsiveness. *Behavioral and Neural Biology, 36*, 61–68.

Smotherman, W. P. (1982b). Odor aversion learning by the rat fetus. *Physiology & Behavior, 29*, 769–771.

Smotherman, W. P., Richards, L. S., & Robinson, S.R. (1984). Techniques for observing fetal behavior in utero: A comparison of chemomyelotomy and spinal transection. *Developmental Psychobiology, 17*, 661–674.

Smotherman, W. P., & Robinson, S.R. (1985). The rat fetus in its environment: Behavioral adjustments to novel, familiar, aversive, and conditioned stimuli presented in utero. *Behavioral Neuroscience, 99*, 521–530.

Smotherman, W. P., & Robinson, S. R. (1986). Environmental determinants of behaviour in the rat fetus. *Animal Behaviour, 34*, 1859–1873.

Smotherman, W. P., & Robinson, S. R. (1987). Prenatal expression of species-typical action patterns in the rat fetus (*Rattus norvegicus*). *Journal of Comparative Psychology, 101*, 190–196.

Smotherman, W. P., & Robinson, S. R. (1988). The uterus as environment: The ecology of fetal experience. In E. M. Blass (Ed.), *Handbook of behavioral neurobiology, Vol. 9. Developmental psychobiology and behavioral ecology* (pp. 149–196). New York: Plenum Press.

Smotherman, W. P., & Robinson, S. R. (1989). Cryptopsychobiology: The appearance, disappearance and reappearance of a species-typical action pattern during early development. *Behavioral Neuroscience, 103*, 246–253.

Smotherman, W. P., & Robinson, S.R. (1990). The prenatal origins of behavioral organization. *Psychological Science, 1*, 97–106.

Smotherman, W. P., & Robinson, S. R. (1991a). Accessibility of the rat fetus for psychobiological investigation. In H. Shair, G. A. Barr, & M. A. Hofer (Eds.), *Developmental psychobiology: New methods and changing concepts* (pp. 148–166). New York: Oxford University Press.

Smotherman, W. P., & Robinson, S.R. (1991b). Conditioned activation of fetal behavior. *Physiology & Behavior, 50*, 73–77.

Smotherman, W. P., & Robinson, S. R. (1992a). Prenatal experience with milk: Fetal behavior and endogenous opioid systems. *Neuroscience & Biobehavioral Reviews, 16*(3), 351–364.

Smotherman, W. P., & Robinson, S.R. (1992b). Habituation in the rat fetus. *Quarterly Journal of Experimental Psychology, 44B*, 215–230.

Smotherman, W. P., & Robinson, S. R. (1998). Prenatal ontogeny of sensory responsiveness and learning. In G. Greenberg & M. Haraway (Eds.), *Comparative psychology: A handbook* (pp. 586–601). New York: Garland Publishing, Inc.

Snider, W. (1994) Functions of the neurotrophins during nervous system development: What the knockuts are teaching us. *Cell, 77*, 627–638.

Spelke, E. S., & Newport, E. L. (1998). Nativism, empiricism, and the development of knowledge. In W. Damon & R. M. Lerner (Eds.), *Handbook of child psychology. Volume 1:*

Theoretical models of human development (pp. 275–340). New York: John Wiley & Sons.

Suzuki, S., & Yamamuro, T. (1985). Fetal movement and fetal presentation. *Early Human Development, 11*, 255–263.

Thelen, E. (1985). Developmental origins of motor coordination: Leg movements in human infants. *Developmental Psychobiology, 18*, 1–22.

Thelen, E. (1994). Three-month-old infants can learn task-specific patterns of interlimb coordination. *Psychological Science, 5*, 280–285.

Thelen, E., Corbetta, D., Kamm, K., Spencer, J. P., Schneider, K., & Zernicke, R. F. (1993). The transition to reaching: Mapping intention and intrinsic dynamics. *Child Development, 64*, 1058–1098.

Thelen, E., & Fisher, D. M. (1983). From spontaneous to instrumental behavior: Kinematic analysis of movement changes during very early learning. *Child Development, 54*, 129–140.

Thelen, E., Fisher, D. M., & Ridley-Johnson, R. (1984). The relationship between physical growth and a newborn reflex. *Infant Behavior and Development, 7*, 479–493.

Thelen, E., Skala, K. D., & Kelso, J. A. (1987). The dynamic nature of early coordination: Evidence from bilateral leg movements in young infants. *Developmental Psychology, 23*, 179–186.

Thompson, W. (1983). Synapse elimination in neonatal rat muscle is sensitive to pattern of muscle use. *Nature, 302*, 614–616.

Ulrich, B., Ulrich, D., Angulo-Kinzler, R., & Chapman, D. (1997). Sensitivity of infants with and without down syndrome to intrinsic dynamics. *Research Quarterly for Exercise and Sport, 68*, 10–19.

Vaal, J., van Soest, A. J. K., & Hopkins, B. (2000). Spontaneous kicking behavior in infants: Age-related effects of unilateral weighting. *Developmental Psychobiology, 36*, 111–122.

Van Hartesveldt, C., Sickles, A. E., Porter, J. D., & Stehouwer, D. J. (1991). L-DOPA-induced air-stepping in developing rats. *Developmental Brain Research, 58*, 251–255.

Van Heijst, J. J., Vos, J. E., & Bullock, D. (1998). Development in a biologically inspired spinal neural network for movement control. *Neural Networks, 11*, 1305–1316.

van Heteren, C. F., Boekkooi, P. F., Jongsma, H. W., & Nihjuis, J. G. (2000). Fetal learning and memory. *Lancet, 356*, 1169–1170.

Ververs I. A. P., de Vries J. I. P., van Geijn H. P., & Hopkins B. (1994). Prenatal head position from 12–38 weeks. I. Developmental aspects. *Early Human Development, 39*, 83–91.

Ververs, I. A. P., Van Gelder-Hasker, M. R., DeVries, J. I. P., Hopkins, B., & van Geijn, H. P. (1998). Prenatal development of arm posture. *Early Human Development, 51*, 61–70.

Viala, D. (2006). Evolution and behavioral adaptation of locomotor pattern generators in vertebrates. *Comptes Rendus Palevol, 5*, 667–674.

Viala, D., Viala, G., & Fayein, N. (1986). Plasticity of locomotor organization in infant rabbits spinalized shortly after birth. In M. E. Goldberger, A. Gorio & A. Murray (Eds.), *Development and plasticity of the mammalian spinal cord* (pp. 301–310). New York: Springer-Verlag, New York.

vom Saal, F. S., & Bronson, F. H. (1978). In utero proximity of female mouse fetuses to males: Effects on reproductive performance during later life. *Biology of Reproduction, 19*, 842–853.

Waldenström, A., Thelin, J., Thimansson, E., Levinsson, A., & Schouenborg, J. (2003). Developmental learning in a pain-related system: Evidence for a cross-modality mechanism. *Journal of Neuroscience, 23,* 7719–7725.

Watson, S. J., & Bekoff, A. (1990). A kinematic analysis of hindlimb motility in 9-day-old and 10-day-old chick embryos. *Journal of Neurobiology, 21,* 651–660.

Windle, W. F., Minear, W. L., Austin, M. F., & Orr, D. W. (1935). The origin and early development of somatic behavior in the albino rat. *Physiological Zoology, 8,* 156–185.

Zelazo, P. R., Zelazo, N. A., & Kolb, S. (1980). "Walking" in the newborn. *Science, 176,* 314–315.

Development of Spinal Cord Locomotor Networks Controlling Limb Movements

Laurent Vinay, Edouard Pearlstein, *and* François Clarac

Abstract

This chapter compares the development of spinal cord locomotor networks controlling limb movements in precocial species, such as the chick, which are able to walk soon after birth, and altricial species, such as rodents and humans, which are quite immature at birth. Interestingly, both chicks and rodents undergo a 21-day embryonic period. The chapter starts by looking at the two kinds of motor patterns that spinal cord networks are able to generate in vitro: "fictive locomotion," which is similar to locomotion observed in vivo, and endogenously generated spontaneous activity, which plays a key role in motor development. The chapter then underscores some of the mechanisms that may account for the different locomotor abilities of precocial and altricial species at birth.

Keywords: spinal cord, locomotor networks, limb movements, precocial species, chick, altricial species, rodents, embryonic period, motor patterns, fictive locomotion

Introduction

The locomotor pattern in limb muscles is characterized in most cases (such as walking) by alternating flexion and extension of each limb and alternating movements of contralateral limbs. It is generated by spinal neuronal networks, referred to as central pattern generators (CPGs; Grillner, 1981; Kiehn, 2006; Kiehn & Butt, 2003; Rossignol, 1996). The locomotor pattern results from both the connectivity between the CPG interneurons and the intrinsic membrane properties of these neurons. The focus of this chapter is to examine the development of these networks controlling limb locomotor movements in a comparative perspective. Precocial species, such as the chick, are able to walk and run soon after birth or hatching, whereas altricial species, such as rodents and humans, are quite immature at birth and their locomotor pattern requires

weeks (rodents) or months (humans) to mature to the adult form (Muir, 2000). It is quite difficult to identify the reasons for these behavioral differences at birth when there are variations in the duration of prenatal development; given differences in rates of development, it is necessary to translate neurodevelopmental times across species (Clancy, Darlington, & Finlay, 2001). Interestingly, both chicks and rodents undergo a 21-day embryonic (E) period. The comparison between these species is therefore meaningful because it eliminates the duration of prehatching/prenatal development as a parameter that can account for differences in the locomotor abilities at birth (Muir, 2000).

A major advantage in comparing these two species is that both of them have been used for many years for in vitro preparations. Experiments on the spinal cord, isolated from immature chicks and rats, have offered some valuable insights into the mechanisms underlying the development of loco-motion and the organization of spinal cord loco-motor networks. Spinal cord networks are able to generate at least two kinds of motor patterns in these in vitro conditions. One activity recorded in vitro is called "fictive locomotion" because it shares several common features, in terms of period and phase relationships, with the locomotor move-ments observed in vivo. This fictive locomotor pat-tern is rarely observed spontaneously and its release requires pharmacological or electrical stimulation. A second endogenously generated activity observed in this preparation occurs *spontaneously*. Our chap-ter will first focus on these activities from both developmental and comparative perspectives. We will then review some of the data on the develop-ment of motoneurons (MNs) and their inputs from the periphery and the brain.

Locomotion and Spontaneous Motor Activities: Comparative Development in Precocial and Altricial Species

The chick and the rat are the two models in which the ontogeny of locomotion has been best studied both in vivo and in vitro. We will com-pare the early operation of spinal networks *in ovo* and in utero in these precocial and altricial species. Different types of movements have been described; their nature and role has long intrigued scientists. Although some of them appear to correspond to characteristic, alternating locomotor movements, others bear little resemblance to goal-directed behaviors. They have been named "spontaneous movements" because they are not "reflexogenic" and not organized by sensory inputs. They have been observed in all the species investigated so far. In humans, for instance, Prechtl (2001) dem-onstrated that any alteration of these spontaneous movements may be a good indicator of early brain dysfunction and subsequent cerebral palsy.

In Ovo Development of the Chick

Chick embryos become spontaneously active at E3.5 and escape the egg by the end of embry-onic development (E20–22). The pioneering stud-ies by Hamburger and colleagues (Hamburger & Balaban, 1963; Hamburger & Oppenheim, 1967) have described the development of this precocial motility (for detailed review see Bekoff, 2001). They distinguished three types of activity: types I, II, and III. From the beginning, the motility of the embryo is rhythmical; each cycle consists of a short

activity phase lasting 5–15 s, followed by a longer phase of complete quiescence, which lasts ~30–60 s. Type I motility begins at E3.5–4; the movements first consist of slight flexions of the neck to the left and the right. S-waves progressively extend with age to the base of the leg buds and the level of the tail (E5). Motility in wings and tail begins at E6.5. The limbs are most often integrated with total body movement. The waves are initiated at the level of the neck. However, motility may begin occasion-ally in the trunk, initiating two waves that spread simultaneously upward and downward. The limb movements are slight abductions and adductions in shoulder and hip, followed by slight up-and-down movements in wrist and ankle. Type I embryonic motility is observed throughout embryonic life. Electromyogram (EMG) recordings from leg mus-cles have revealed that the motor pattern consists of co-contraction of extensor muscles and flexor muscles, and alternation between these two syner-gies (Bekoff, 1976; Bekoff, Stein, & Hamburger, 1975; Bradley & Bekoff, 1990; Landmesser & O'Donovan, 1984). This is in line with the observa-tion that, when all three joints of the leg move, they extend and flex together (Watson & Bekoff, 1990). The coupling between the ankle and the other two leg joints decreases between E9 and E13, whereas the coordination between hip and knee increases (Bradley, Solanki, & Zhao, 2005; Sharp, Ma, & Bekoff, 1999). This was interpreted as an adaptive response to the spatial constraints of the egg as the size of the embryo increases. Uncoupling the ankle movements from the other two joints prevents the feet from hitting and likely damaging the shell. The coupling between wing and leg movements also decreases: this development may be a precursor to later behaviors in which these two limbs perform different functions (Bradley, 1999).

Type II motility consists of "startles" and "wrig-gles" and begins at E9–11. A joint abruptly flexes or extends and then rapidly returns to the initial posi-tion (Bradley, 1999). Type III motility, consisting of tucking, appears on day 17 and is linked to hatch-ing. Movements included in this type of motility appear to be smoother and more coordinated than those of the two other types of motility.

The isolated spinal cord/hind limb preparation exhibits spontaneous activity in vitro at E8–10 (Landmesser & O'Donovan, 1984). This activity consists of a series of 5–10 bursts lasting 15–30s and recurring every few minutes. Sequences are initiated by a short-duration, high-amplitude discharge that occurs nearly simultaneously in all muscles (Figure 10.1B, vertical arrows), closely resembling the synchronous discharge occurring *in ovo* (Figure 10.1A, arrows). Then, the bursts in the flexor muscles occur generally out of phase with that in the extensors (Figure 10.1B).

Exteroceptive reflexes start to be obtained at E7.5, demonstrating the nonreflexogenic spontaneous nature of the early type I behavior of the chick embryo, from the beginning of motility at E3.5–7.5 (Hamburger & Balaban, 1963). In addition, the patterned motor output can occur spontaneously in an isolated spinal cord preparation in vitro without afferent feedback (Landmesser & O'Donovan, 1984). Transection of the spinal cord at early stages does not preclude motility below the lesion, demonstrating that the spontaneous activity is generated in the spinal cord (Hamburger & Balaban, 1963). The periodicity is however different, indicating that the brain influences the intrinsic activity in the spinal cord.

Prenatal Development of Rodents

Perinatal behavioral development is considered in more detail in Chapter 9 by Robinson. We will therefore focus only on those aspects of motor behavior that are closely related to the development of locomotor coordination. In the 16–20-day-old (E16–20) rat fetus, there is a gradual extension of motility in rostrocaudal and proximodistal directions (Narayanan, Fox, & Hamburger, 1971). Movement of the different limbs occurs synchronously, that is, at nearly the same instant (Kleven, Lane, & Robinson, 2004). Although the alternating movements of left and right limbs within a girdle has been reported on E20 (Bekoff & Lau, 1980), they are not often seen in fetal rats (Robinson & Smotherman, 1992). High cervical spinal cord transection, which isolates the spinal cord from the brain, has little effect on early movements (Robinson, Blumberg, Lane, & Kreber, 2000). However, midthoracic spinal transection has been shown to reduce hind limb movements by 40%–50% in both fetal and infant rats (Blumberg & Lucas, 1994). Taken together, these data on the effects of cord transection on fetal movement demonstrate that descending influences from the brain play little or no role in generating these early behavioral patterns, but communication among various segments of the spinal cord is necessary to produce the exact patterns of spontaneous movement observed during early perinatal development (Robinson et al., 2000).

Developmental changes in the spontaneous activity along the rostrocaudal extent of the spinal cord were investigated using in vitro spinal cord preparations isolated from rodent fetuses (Nakayama, Nishimaru, Iizuka, Ozaki, & Kudo, 1999; Ren & Greer, 2003; Yvert, Branchereau, & Meyrand, 2004). There are age-dependent changes in the segmental location at which the rhythmic discharge starts and the timing of activity on cervical, thoracic, and lumbar roots (Nakayama et al., 1999; Ren & Greer, 2003). At E13.5 (younger fetuses not examined), rhythmic activity is restricted to thoracic and cervical ventral roots (VRs) (Figure 10.1C). At E14.5, the rhythmic motor pattern appears on thoracic VRs first and radiates in rostral and caudal directions to cervical and lumbar segments (Figure 10.1C, bottom left traces). By E16.5, the rhythmic activity appears on lumbar VRs first and radiates rostrally (Figure 10.1C, bottom right traces). Transection experiments demonstrated that cervical, thoracic, and lumbar segments are all capable of generating spontaneous rhythmic patterns (Ren & Greer, 2003). However, the dominant neuronal circuit initiating the spontaneous bursts shifts from cervical to lumbar region during this period. In the mouse, sequences of left–right alternation are observed only occasionally at the lumbar level at E14.5 (Yvert et al., 2004). In the rat, bursts at a given segmental level are present either synchronously on both sides or on one side without clear sequences of left–right alternation (Nakayama et al., 1999). When present, the motor bursts in the L3 and L5 VRs on the same side are not in antiphase (Fellippa-Marques, Vinay, & Clarac, 2000) as it is the case when the CPG for locomotion is active (Cazalets, Sqalli-Houssaini, & Clarac, 1992; Kiehn & Kjaerulff, 1996).

Fictive locomotion can be induced in vitro by perfusing pharmacological compounds (*N*-methyl-D-aspartate [NMDA], serotonin, etc.) on the spinal cord isolated from neonatal rodents (e.g., Bonnot & Morin, 1998; Bracci, Beatto, & Nistri, 1998; Cazalets et al., 1992; Kiehn & Kjaerulff, 1996; Kudo & Yamada, 1987b; Smith & Feldman, 1987; Taccola & Nistri, 2004, 2006; Whelan, Bonnot, & O'Donovan, 2000). The locomotor pattern in the lumbar enlargement is characterized by alternation both between the motor bursts on the left and right sides of the spinal cord, and between the activities recorded from L2/L3 and L5 VRs on one side (Cazalets et al., 1992; Kiehn & Kjaerulff, 1996). L2/L3 and L5 have been shown to represent the flexor–extensor alternation (Kiehn & Kjaerulff, 1996). The same kind of experiments made on E16 (i.e., 5 days prior to birth) have revealed a motor

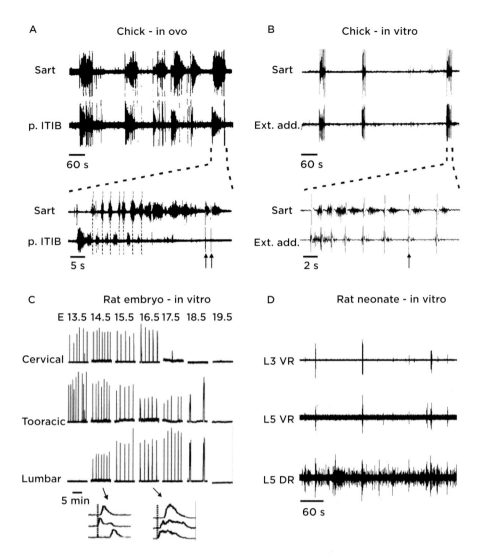

Figure 10.1 Spontaneous motor activity in the chick. (A) *In ovo* EMG recordings from the sartorius (Sart, flexor) and posterior iliotibialis (p. ITIB, extensor) muscles. (B) Spontaneous EMG activity recorded from the Sart and external adductor (Ext. add, extensor) muscles in the in vitro isolated spinal cord/hind limb preparation. The burst sequence on the right is displayed below on an expanded time base in both A and B. Note the spontaneously occurring alternation between flexor and extensor bursts. In addition, large-amplitude discharges of short duration were observed to occur synchronously in both muscles (arrows). (A and B adapted from Landmesser & O'Donovan, 1984.) (C) Development of spontaneous activity in the in vitro spinal cord isolated from embryonic rats. Activity is recorded from VRs at cervical, thoracic, and lumbar levels. At E13.5, rhythmic activity was restricted to thoracic and cervical VRs. At E14.5, the rhythmic motor pattern appeared on thoracic VRs first and radiated in rostral and caudal directions to cervical and lumbar segments (bottom traces). By E16.5, the rhythmic activity appeared on lumbar VRs first and radiated rostrally, demonstrating that lumbar segments become the site of initiation of the activity. By E18.5, the spontaneous bursting progressively disappeared starting at the C level. One can notice that the interburst intervals and burst durations increase with embryonic age. (Adapted from Ren & Greer, 2003.) (D) Spontaneous activity in the in vitro spinal cord isolated from neonatal rats. Bursting is occasionally recorded from VRs. Note that L3VR (flexors) and L5VR (extensors) are bursting synchronously, in contrast to the fictive locomotor activity recorded at the same age (Figure 10.2). The most striking feature of spontaneous activity in postnatal rats is observed in dorsal roots (DRs): action potentials (APs) resulting from $GABA_A$ receptor–mediated primary afferent depolarizations reaching firing threshold are conducted antidromically toward the periphery (Fellippa-Marques et al., 2000). (Adapted from Fellippa-Marques et al., 2000 and Vinay et al., 2000b.)

pattern with all bursts in phase (Iizuka, Nishimaru, & Kudo, 1998). The transition from left–right synchrony to alternation occurs at E18 (Iizuka et al., 1998) and is due to the maturation of reciprocal inhibitory connections between the two sides, more precisely to the shift of glycine-evoked potentials from excitation to inhibition (Nakayama, Nishimaru, & Kudo, 2002; see below). Alternation between L3 and L5 motor bursts appears at E20, shortly before birth (Figure 10.2B).

Besides the lumbar locomotor pattern, two other rhythms have been described (Figure 10.2C): one at the cervical level associated with forelimb movements (flexor MNs are recorded on C5 and C6, and extensors on C7, C8, and T1; Ballion, Morin, & Viala, 2001) and another in the sacrococcygeal spinal cord associated with tail movements (Lev-Tov, Delvolve, & Kremer, 2000). A strong mutual coupling exists between these different CPGs.

Are Spontaneous Activities the First Steps of the Central Pattern Generators for Locomotion?

The spontaneous rhythmic motor activity recorded in the developing spinal cord is often considered to be produced by the immature

CPGs for locomotion. As stated earlier, spontaneous bursting occurs synchronously on both sides of the spinal cord in the rat fetus at E15.5, a stage at which chemically induced rhythmic bursting is also synchronous in the left and right VRs as well as in the L2 and L5 VRs on the same side (Kudo & Nishimaru, 1998). However, the chemically induced activity is alternating at birth (Figure 10.2A,B), whereas the spontaneous motor activity is still in phase in L3 and L5 VRs. This, therefore, suggests that the networks generating spontaneous and locomotor activities are, at least partly, different. The situation is less clear in the chick embryo spinal cord, which exhibits sequences of flexion–extension alternations in vitro (Figure 10.1B). Even in this preparation, Chub and O'Donovan (1998) challenged the assumption that spontaneous activity is the product of an immature locomotor

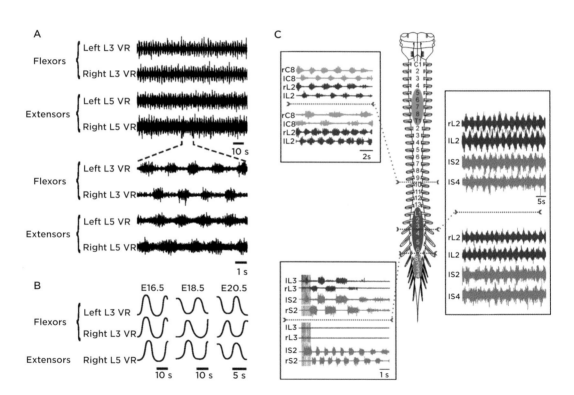

Figure 10.2 Pharmacologically and electrically evoked rhythms in the in vitro rodent spinal cord. (A) Fictive locomotion evoked at birth by bath application of excitatory amino acids (*N*-methyl-D,L-aspartate [NMA]) is characterized by the alternating bursting in the left and right VR and in the 3rd (flexors) and 5th (extensors) VRs on the same side. (B) Similar experiment performed at E16.5 evokes a synchronous bursting in all VRs. Left–right alternation appears at E18.5. (Redrawn from Iizuka et al., 1998.) (C) Rhythms evoked at the different levels of the spinal cord (C: cervical, L: lumbar, S: sacral). Top left panel: NMA-/5-HT-induced activity in the cervicothoracic and lumbar spinal cord before (top traces), and after (bottom traces) thoracic 9-10 spinal cord transection (SCT). (Adapted from Ballion et al., 2001.) Right panel: NMA-/5-HT-induced activity in to the lumbosacral spinal cord before (top traces), and after (bottom traces) L3–L4 SCT. (Adapted from Cazalets & Bertrand, 2000.) Bottom left panel: Sacrocaudal afferent (S4 dorsal root)–induced activity in the lumbosacral spinal cord before (top traces), and after (bottom traces) L6–S1 SCT. (Adapted from Lev-Tov et al., 2000.)

pattern generator. The main reason for this argument is provided by experiments aimed at blocking selectively the action of various neurotransmitters, which revealed that spontaneous rhythmic activity can be produced by very different spinal networks, comprising predominantly glutamatergic/cholinergic or alternatively GABAergic/glycinergic connections (see below). This is not in agreement with the detailed and specific synaptic connections that are often assumed to underlie central pattern-generating circuits. It is therefore proposed that, rather than representing the antecedent of locomotion, spontaneous rhythmic motor activity in the spinal cord reflects the general rhythmogenic property of developing networks (for reviews, see Ben-Ari, 2001; Feller, 1999; O'Donovan, 1999; Vinay et al., 2002; Vinay, Brocard, Pflieger, Simeoni-Alias, & Clarac, 2000b). This property has been described in other parts of the central nervous system (CNS) such as the trigeminal system (Ho & Waite, 1999), the hippocampus (Ben-Ari, Cherubini, Corradetti, & Gaiarsa, 1989), and the visual system (Wong, 1999). Because the networks generating these two types of activities likely share some common connectivity, spontaneous activity may subserve developmental functions (Vinay et al., 2000b, 2002). It is accompanied by Ca^{2+} oscillations (Wenner & O'Donovan, 2001), which play a key role in different developmental processes (for review, see Vinay et al., 2000b, 2002). *In ovo* pharmacological manipulation of the early activity has shown that early motor axon pathfinding events are highly dependent on the normal pattern of bursting activity (see Hanson, Milner, & Landmesser, 2008, for recent review). A modest decrease in episode frequency results in dorsal–ventral pathfinding errors by lumbar MNs, and in the downregulation of several molecules required to successfully execute this guidance decision (Hanson & Landmesser, 2004). Although increasing the episode frequency is without effect on dorsal–ventral pathfinding, it strongly perturbs the anteroposterior (A-P) pathfinding process by which MNs fasciculate into pool-specific fascicles at the limb base and then selectively grow to muscle targets (Hanson & Landmesser, 2006). Resumption of normal frequency allows axons to correct the A-P pathfinding errors by altering their trajectories distally, indicating the dynamic nature of this process and its continued sensitivity to patterned activity.

In addition, spontaneous activities and associated muscle twitches may contribute to an activity-dependent synaptic plasticity and thereby to the refinement of synaptic connections within the different modules of the locomotor pattern generator, as previously shown for the withdrawal reflex system (Petersson, Waldenstrom, Fahraeus, & Schouenborg, 2003; Schouenborg, 2004).

Late Development of Bipedal and Quadrupedal Locomotion

The differences between precocial and altricial species are quite important at birth. In the chick, locomotion starts shortly after hatching. CPG networks are already sufficiently robust to face perturbations. The locomotor EMG pattern has been described by Jacobson and Hollyday (1982a, 1982b) who demonstrated that the step cycle of the chick hind limb consists of three phases of movement (triphasic pattern): during the swing, the joints are flexed and the foot is lifted off the ground; this is followed by a swing extension when the foot is swung forward, the hip and ankle being kept flexed and the stance when the three joints are extended to support and propel the chick forward. Although the chick is able to walk at birth, some significant motor improvements occur throughout the first postnatal weeks. A comparative kinetic and kinematic walking and running analysis in the chick between posthatching (P) days 1–2 and 14 revealed that young birds (<P5) can run in an adult-like manner, but walk inefficiently. They are less competent than older birds in maintaining single leg support while walking and take shorter steps to compensate (Muir, Gosline, & Steeves, 1996). In contrast to young birds, P14 chicks are able to conserve energy within each walking stride by exploiting the exchange between potential and kinetic energy (Figure 10.3A). Chickens exhibit a characteristic locomotor-related behavior consisting of repetitive horizontal head movements while walking, referred to as head bobbing or head nystagmus (Figure 10.3C). This is an optokinetic response involving structures of the accessory optic system and functions to stabilize the visual world on the retina as the animal walks. Importantly, this behavior only occurs during walking and not while running. The role of experience in the development of locomotor and locomotor-related behaviors was addressed by manipulating the amount of locomotor experience that chicks receive during early posthatching and subsequently quantifying the changes in their locomotor pattern using kinematic measures (Muir & Chu, 2002). Chicks were randomly assigned to one of the three groups receiving either increased locomotor experience

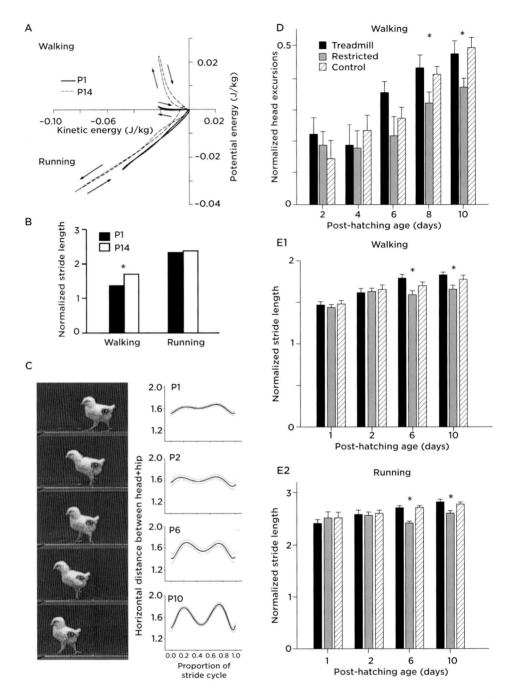

Figure 10.3 Posthatching development of locomotion in the chick. (A) Potential energy as a function of kinetic energy for a single step of walking and running at two ages (P1 and P14). Both potential and kinetic energy have been normalized for body weight and initial values have been set to zero to facilitate comparison between ages. The data fall only in the left quadrants because kinetic energy decreases in the first half of each stance phase and subsequently increases during the last half of the stance phase for both walking and running. Walking data fall in the upper left quadrant because potential energy first rises, then falls during each walking stance phase. Running data fall in the lower left quadrant because potential energy first decreases and then increases during each stance phase of running. While the data for running are quite similar at the two ages, differences appear for walking (P1 chicks have a slope close to zero. (Adapted from Muir et al., 1996.) (B) Mean stride length during walking and running for P1 and P14 chicks. *, P<.001. (Adapted from Muir et al., 1996.) (C) Development of head bobbing. The left panel displays video frame sequence showing head bobbing (horizontal head excursions) during walking. During a stride, the head excursions undergo two cycles. The graphs on the right panel show that the head–hip horizontal distance during stride increases with postnatal age. (Redrawn from Muir & Chu, 2002.) (D) Maximum head excursions as a function of age for

(i.e., treadmill exercise), decreased locomotor experience (i.e., decreased housing space), or no alteration in locomotor experience. Animals subject to exercise restriction for at least 6 days moved with shortened stride lengths (Figure 10.3E) and smaller horizontal head excursions (Figure 10.3D) compared with age-matched, treadmill-exercised or control animals, a change that was maintained for the duration of the study. Although the chick is able to walk right away after hatching, these data demonstrate that maturation of locomotor behavior depends on locomotor experience.

At birth, the rat is quite immature and sleeps most (70%) of the time (Jouvet-Mounier, Astic, & Lacote, 1970). A newborn rat has the limbs slightly extended away from the main axis of the body. When the pup is placed on its back, it is able to right itself (Altman & Sudarshan, 1975). Maturation occurs along a rostrocaudal gradient. At P2, at rest, the neonatal rat is able to make some pivoting movements of the head and to initiate some crawling sequences. During the first postnatal week, only the front part of the body exhibits a consistent postural control (elevation of the shoulders) but there are some sporadic postural reactions of the hind limbs (Brocard, Vinay, & Clarac, 1999). At P5, the pup can raise its head. During the second week, the pelvis region begins to support the body weight and by P10, the pup is able to have a raised quadruped posture, the belly being elevated above the ground. At P12–13, walking starts and eyes are opened. However, the leg movements are slow with a poor control of the trunk. At P15, rearing appears, the animal being able to use its forepaws for manipulations when sitting on its hind limbs. After P15, all complex behaviors such as walking on a turning rod, traversing paths of different lengths and widths, ascending and descending on a ladder, and climbing up a rope, are fluent and much more efficient (Westerga & Gramsbergen, 1990).

This period involves a sudden acceleration in the functional maturation of the hind limbs. Walking becomes digitigrade. Step cycle duration decreases from more than 1400 ms at P11–14 to ~600 ms at P15–16.

Development of posture is the limiting factor with regard to locomotor performance during the first postnatal week. Both air-stepping (with the rat suspended) and swimming can be obtained at P0, that is, when postural constraints are reduced. Air-stepping usually requires a pharmacological activation with L-Dopa and 5-HT agonists (McEwen & Stehouwer, 2001; McEwen, Van Hartesveldt, & Stehouwer, 1997; Staup & Stehouwer, 2006; Stehouwer & Van Hartesveldt, 2000; Tucker & Stehouwer, 2000) or a strong olfactory stimulus, such as the odor of the mother (Fady, Jamon, & Clarac, 1998). Note further that the olfactory stimulus used by this latter study can elicit plantigrade walking at P3–9 (Jamon & Clarac, 1998). Both air-stepping and swimming have a similar evolution from about 1 Hz at P0 to 4 Hz at P20. During the first day, only the front legs are used for swimming; within the next 24 h, all four legs are rhythmically activated with an alternation between ipsilateral and contralateral limbs, whereas diagonal limbs are in synchrony. Although movements of the two hind limbs are always alternating, the variability of the phase value decreases with age (Cazalets, Menard, Crémieux, & Clarac, 1990). The adult swimming pattern, which involves only the hind limbs, is observed from P12/15 onward, the forelimbs being involved in directing the behavior. Fady et al. (1998) investigated the olfaction-induced air-stepping with pups held in a harness, the limbs hanging on each side (Figure 10.2A). Regular alternating limb movements are observed between P0 and P4 when the mother's odor is presented in a tube in front of the nose of the animal (Figure 10.2C). In such a situation, long sequences of 30–50 air-stepping cycles can be obtained. The gait pattern at P0 is consistent with the diagonal gait observed at P5 in

---

treadmill-exercised, restricted exercise, and control groups of animals. Maximum head excursions are normalized to neck length to control size differences among different ages of animals. Older animals undergo significantly larger head excursions compared with younger animals ($P < .001$). Asterisks indicate the ages at which animals in the restricted exercise group had significantly smaller head excursions compared with treadmill-exercised or control animals ($P < .05$). E1–2, Stride lengths as a function of age during walking (E1) and running (E2) for treadmill-exercised, restricted exercise, and control groups of animals. Stride lengths have been normalized to hip height to control size differences between different ages of animals. Older animals walk with significantly longer stride lengths compared with younger birds ($P < .001$). Asterisks indicate the ages at which animals in the restricted exercise group had significantly shorter stride lengths compared with treadmill-exercised or control animals ($P < .05$).

swimming. A proximodistal gradient is observed in the hind limbs, the movements involving mainly the hip joint at P0 and all three joints at P4 (Figure 10.4B). EMG recordings during L-DOPA-induced air-stepping in the rat revealed that the activity of biceps femoris, vastus lateralis, gastrocnemius (GM), and tibialis anterior (TA) occurs in discrete bursts, which occur in a one-to-one relationship with the step cycle observed kinematically (Tucker & Stehouwer, 2000). Extensors are activated very briefly as compared with the duration of extension of the associated joints, with very little muscle activity between bursts. The temporal pattern of EMGs recorded from hind limb extensors remains constant between P5 and P20. The delay between muscle activation and overt movement of the hip and ankle increased during ontogeny. Together, these results suggest that changes in coordination during air-stepping result from biomechanical factors or changes in the output to flexor muscles, that is, peripheral maturation plays

a greater role than central maturation in the development of intralimb coordination.

In summary, both air-stepping and swimming demonstrate that the CPGs for locomotion are functional at birth but their expression is limited by postural immaturity. The adult walking in rats requires appropriate force generation in limb extensor muscles and sufficient stiffness between body segments such that these forces can be transmitted through the limb to the ground. The development of postural control of hind limbs has been investigated during the first postnatal week in the rat (Brocard et al., 1999). The whole body was tilted in a vertical plane with the nose up. The proportion of animals producing a complete extension of both hind limbs increased with age until the end of the first postnatal week. Motor responses at birth consisted of a slight extension of the hips, the knees, and the ankles remaining bent in most cases. The extension produced at the ankle level increased gradually during the first postnatal week.

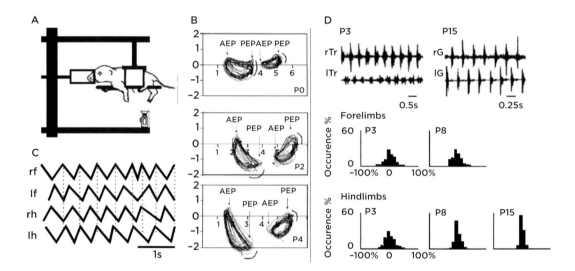

Figure 10.4 Air-stepping and swimming activities in the neonatal rat. (A) Air-stepping. The animal is held in a sling with the limbs hanging on each side. The nose is inserted in a tube containing nest-bedding materials. (B) Examples of left lateral views of typical leg movements induced by olfactory stimulation at P0 (top), P2 and P4 (bottom). The horizontal line shows the plane of the body support. Distances are in centimeters. The movements of the fore- and hind limbs are shown in the diagrams, with the swing phase in the upper part (from PEP to AEP) and stance in the lower part (from AEP to PEP). The curve segments at the end of the stance phase underline the slow movement phase. (C) Examples of stepping patterns with stable coordination. Stride amplitude is normalized. Maxima correspond to AEP and minima to PEP with opposite phase in contralateral forelimbs (right and left forelimbs: rf, lf), hind limbs (rh, lh), and a diagonal phase coupling. The dotted lines highlight the coordination between right and left hind limbs (rh, lh): left–right and ipsilateral anteroposterior alternations. Even if occasional failures appear in the coordination, the CPG is able to restore interlimb coordination from the day of birth onward. (Redrawn from Fady et al., 1998.) (D) Top: EMG recordings of the forelimb left and right trapezius muscles (rTr, lTr, on the left) at P3 and of hind limb left and right gastrocnemius (rG, lG, on the right) at P15 during swimming. Bottom: Distribution histograms of the percentage of variation between successive periods for hind limbs and forelimbs, established during swimming at three different ages (P3, P8, and P15). While there is no improvement in the forelimb beating stability between P3 and P8, the hind limb paddling becomes more stable with age. (Redrawn from Cazalets et al., 1990.)

This was correlated with a change in the EMG activity recorded from the triceps surae muscles (ankle extensors) during this postural reaction. There was a gradual acquisition of a tonic pattern. Characteristics of EMG responses changed significantly with age, demonstrating an important increase in the use of triceps surae muscles in this postural task. These data demonstrate that the first postnatal week is a critical period for the development of postural reactions in the hind limbs. They also suggest the existence of a proximodistal gradient in the maturation of postural control.

The pattern of postnatal development of hind limb extensor muscles such as soleus and gastrocnemius muscles has been investigated further over the second postnatal week (Westerga & Gramsbergen, 1990). It correlates with the appearance of the mature form of locomotion at P15. The development of the EMG of TA and medial GM during locomotion has been studied in normal rats from the onset of quadruped walking (postnatal day 10, P10) until P42 (Westerga & Gramsbergen, 1993). Both the EMG characteristics and the activation pattern show marked changes with age. Initially, the EMG bursts are irregular and protracted. The activity level in the two muscles, in particular, in GM, is low. Until P14, the motor units of GM show a tendency toward synchronization. The EMG of TA consists of an adult-like interference pattern from the youngest age studied. Although co-contraction of TA and GM is sometimes observed until P14, reciprocal activation of the muscles is evident at all ages. The timing of the alternating pattern becomes more accurate with age. The activity level in both muscles increases markedly from P15. The time course of these changes bears a close temporal relationship to the development of locomotion. These results suggest that the degree of muscle activation is a decisive factor with respect to locomotor development. The EMG of the soleus muscle was recorded by the same authors in rats aged 10–30 days (Westerga & Gramsbergen, 1994). EMG activity is closely related to motor behavior and posture. At P11, soleus is only phasically active during movements. Tonic EMG activity appears with age, and by P16, the activity pattern is similar to that of the adult. This is paralleled by a change in hind limb posture.

Maturation of the Lumbar Spinal Cord during the Perinatal Period

During the perinatal period, spinal neurons undergo marked changes in their morphology, electrical properties, and sensitivity to neurotransmitters. Although many characteristics evolve in a similar way in altricial and precocial species, the timescale of these changes slightly differ between these species.

Changes in the Somatodendritic Morphology and Gap Junctions

MNs are produced on E13–14 in the lumbosacral cord in the rat and about 1 week earlier in the chick (Altman & Bayer, 1984). Roughly, half of the MNs produced degenerate and die prior to birth (Bennett, McGrath, Davey, & Hutchinson, 1983; Curfs, Gribnau, & Dederen, 1993; Nurcombe, NcGrath, & Bennett, 1981; Oppenheim, 1986; Rootman, Tatton, & Hay, 1981). There is a fourfold increase in the soma area of soleus (ankle extensor) MNs during the first 3 weeks after birth, with the greatest rate of growth occurring during the second postnatal week (Kerai, Greensmith, Vrbova, & Navarrete, 1995; Tanaka, Mori, & Kimura , 1992; Westerga & Gramsbergen, 1992). At P21, soleus MNs reach 70% of their adult size. The range of soma areas increases with postnatal age over this period, and the distribution becomes bimodal, which may reflect a differential growth of alpha and gamma MNs (at around P7 for quadriceps femoris MNs [Tanaka et al., 1992] and at around P21 for soleus MNs [Kerai et al., 1995; Westerga & Gramsbergen, 1992]).

The dendritic tree of MNs develops predominantly postnatally. Although the number of primary dendrites does not change postnatally (Dekkers, Becker, Cook, & Navarrete, 1994), dendritic branches gradually increase in length during the first two postnatal months. At birth, the somatodendritic surface of the TA and extensor digitorum longus MNs is covered by growth-associated, spiny, or hair-like appendages (Dekkers et al., 1994; see also Cummings & Stelzner, 1984). These disappear in a somatofugal direction, on the soma before P4 and on most proximal dendrites by P7, whereas they persist until the second postnatal week on distal dendrites (Cummings & Stelzner, 1984). The complex longitudinal dendritic bundles of some MN pools, such as the one innervating the soleus muscle, start to develop by P10 (Westerga & Gramsbergen, 1992; see also Bellinger & Anderson, 1987a, 1987b). A period of dendritic retraction has been described to follow the period of dendritic extension during the development of MNs, supplying flexor and extensor muscles of the forelimb (Curfs et al., 1993).

A transient widespread electrotonic coupling is found between MNs in the perinatal spinal cord (Walton & Navarrete, 1991). Graded VR stimulation after blocking the antidromic action potential (AP) elicits electrotonic junctional potentials in lumbar MNs (Figure 10.5A). Electrotonic coupling is quite specific and restricted to MNs innervating the same skeletal muscle (Walton & Navarrete, 1991). Up to 18 (mean: 6) dye-labeled cells are observed, following the injection of neurobiotin into a single MN at P0 (Chang, Gonzalez, Pinter, & Balice-Gordon, 1999). However, electrical and dye coupling decrease with age and are no longer present after the first postnatal week (Figure 10.5B). MNs express five connexins: Cx36, Cx37, Cx43, Cx40, and Cx45 (Chang et al., 1999). Although the latter two connexins are downregulated during development, the other gap junction proteins are expressed by a large proportion of adult MNs. Therefore, the disappearance of electrical and dye coupling may be due to a modulation (and not the loss) of junctional communication among MNs, by unknown mechanisms that would affect gap junction assembly, permeability, or open state (Chang et al., 1999). This coupling may be reestablished in certain circumstances, for example, following nerve injury (Chang, Pereda, Pinter, & Balice-Gordon, 2000).

Tresch and Kiehn (2000) investigated the contribution of electrical coupling through gap junctions in neuronal coordination in the in vitro spinal cord preparation isolated from immature rats. They reported that motor pattern generation, induced by bath application of excitatory amino acids and serotonin persists in this preparation after eliminating information transmitted by chemical, action potential–dependent synapses to spinal MNs (Figure 10.5C, "control"; note the existence of fast synchronous oscillations in both VR and MN). These motor patterns are mediated by neuronal coordination across gap junctions as they are blocked by the gap junction inhibitor carbenoxolone (Figure 10.5C, right traces). Only slow large-amplitude oscillations resulting from the pacemaker properties of the neuron remained in the presence of carbenoxolone. These data suggest that gap junctions play an important role in motor pattern generation in the immature mammalian spinal cord (Taccola & Nistri, 2004; Tresch & Kiehn, 2000). In agreement with these inferences, we observed that carbenoxolone reduces the frequency of spontaneous bursting recorded in both dorsal roots (DRs) and

VRs (Figure 10.2D; Chaland & Vinay, unpublished; see also Hanson & Landmesser, 2003, in the mouse, and Milner & Landmesser, 1999, in the chick).

Several roles for electrical coupling through gap junctions have been proposed. An important contribution is related to specification of synapse formation. During late embryonic and early postnatal life, skeletal muscle fibers are initially innervated by several different motor axons. This is followed by synapse elimination, resulting in innervation by a single motor axon (Personius & Balice-Gordon, 2002; Wyatt & Balice-Gordon, 2003). This mature pattern of innervation enables gradual recruitment of muscle fibers as a result of gradually increased inputs to MNs. Synapse elimination is modulated by patterns of MN activity. Electrical coupling ensures that a common pattern of activity spreads among MNs of a given motor pool (see below); the synchronous activity helps to establish the initial polyneuronal innervation. Age-dependent reduction of spinal neuronal gap junctional coupling decreases correlated MN activity that, in turn, mediates synaptic competition and elimination of polyneuronal innervation of myofibers (Busetto, Buffelli, Tognana, Bellico, & Cangiano, 2000; Personius, Chang, Mentis, O'Donovan, & Balice-Gordon, 2007).

Maturation of Electrical Properties

The input resistance (R_i) of spinal MNs decreases during the perinatal period. This decrease starts around E18 in the rat (Gao & Ziskind-Conhaim, 1998) and persists after birth (Bonansco, Fuenzalida, & Roncagliolo, 2004; Fulton & Walton, 1986); in the chick there is a gradual decrease in R_i from E12 to E18 (Muramoto et al., 1996). This decrease likely results from the increased size and causes a reduction of MN excitability.

DEVELOPMENT OF SODIUM CURRENTS

In almost all terrestrial species, the AP properties of leg MNs undergo profound modifications during development (Figure 10.6A; Gao & Ziskind-Conhaim, 1998; Kellerth, Mellstrom, & Skoglund, 1971; McCobb, Best, & Beam, 1990; Naka, 1964). The AP threshold shifts toward more hyperpolarized values during the embryonic life in the rat, from −35 mV at E15–16 to −47 mV at P1–3 and remains stable after birth (Gao & Ziskind-Conhaim, 1998). In the chick, it shifts from −39 mV at E12 to −42 mV at E15 (Muramoto et al., 1996) and −49 mV at E18 (McCobb et al., 1990;

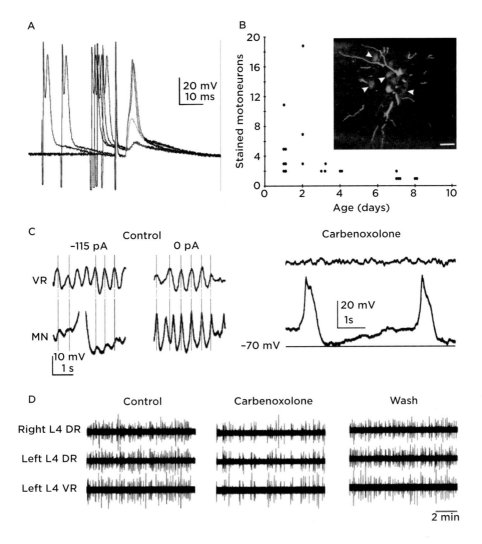

Figure 10.5 Electrical coupling in the immature rodent spinal cord. (A) Left traces show electrical coupling among developing rat motoneurons (MNs). Coupling potentials are characterized in P0–2 MNs by antidromic VR stimulation. An AP (blue) is elicited in the recorded MN by intracellular current injection during antidromic stimulation. By reducing the interval between the intracellular current pulse and antidromic stimulation, the antidromic AP (purple) fails to invade the soma, revealing an initial segment spike (pink). Reducing the interval further induces a collision between antidromically and intracellularly evoked actions potentials. The remaining depolarizing potential (red) is a coupling potential. (Redrawn from Chang et al., 1999.) (B) Number of neurobiotin-stained MNs (inset, arrowheads; scale bar, 10 μm) after injection of the dye in a single cell is shown plotted against postnatal age. The age-related reduction in the number of stained neurons between P0 and P8 is due to the disappearance of gap junctions during this period. (C) Simultaneous recording of a MN and a VR in the presence of NMDA/5-HT and tetrodoxin. When hyperpolarized around –60 mV (left) the MN displays two types of oscillations: fast and small ones occurring in phase (red dotted lines) with those recorded in the VR, and slow and large ones that are not observed on the VR recording and are due to intrinsic properties. When the MN is depolarized around –30 mV (right) the intrinsic oscillations disappear but not the fast ones. In the presence of carbenoxolone (a gap junction blocker) at –70 mV, only the slow oscillations persist, the fast ones disappear both in the MN and on the VR recording. This demonstrates that there is a network coordination in the absence of APs, which is mediated by gap junctions. (Redrawn from Tresch & Kiehn, 2000.) (D) Involvement of electrical coupling in spontaneous activity. The frequency of spontaneous activities recorded is strongly slowed down by application of carbenoxolone (middle traces) and is restored when the gap junction blocker is washed out (right traces). This indicates that electrical coupling has a major role in the expression of spontaneous activity. (L. Vinay, unpublished data.)

Muramoto et al., 1996). In the rat, this evolution results from the hyperpolarization with age of the activation threshold for the Na$^+$ current (I_{Na}; from –40 mV to –50 mV before and after birth,

respectively); such a change in voltage dependency has not been identified in the chick (McCobb et al., 1990). Other striking changes in AP properties are observed during development (Gao &

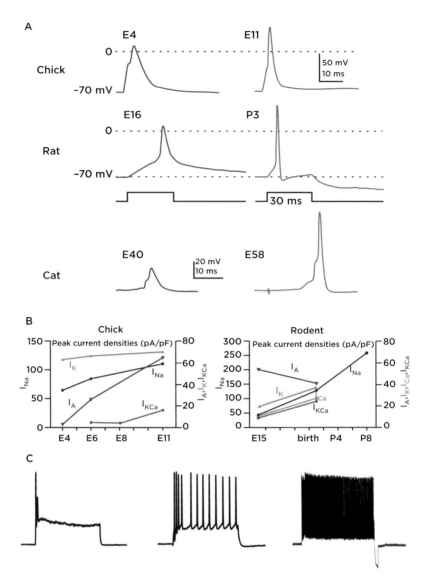

Figure 10.6 Development of electrical properties. (A) Development of APs in MNs. In all species, the size of the AP increases during development, whereas its duration shortens markedly. (Traces are redrawn from McCobb et al., 1990, for the chick; Gao & Ziskind-Conhaim, 1998, for the rat; and Naka, 1964, for the cat.) (B) Maturation of ionic currents. The evolution of current densities for the different ionic currents is quite comparable in the chick and the rat, but these modifications take place earlier in the chick. Chick data are from McCobb et al. (1989, 1990), and Martin-Caraballo and Dryer (2002); rodent data are from Gao and Ziskind-Conhaim (1998, for rat), and Garcia, Sprunger, Meisler, and Beam (1998, for mouse, only I_{Na} density at P8). (C) Gradual postnatal development of MN discharge properties. Most of the immature MNs (left traces) produce a single AP in response to a 500 ms depolarizing current pulse, whereas postnatal MNs (middle traces) display a sustained discharge in the same conditions. The last step in this maturation likely consists of the acquisition of plateau potential and bistability properties (cat MN, in the presence of serotonin, Perrier & Hounsgaard, 2000). (Redrawn from Vinay et al., 2002.)

Ziskind-Conhaim, 1998; Krieger & Sears, 1988; McCobb et al., 1990; Naka, 1964). The AP amplitude increases from 54 mV at E12 to 60 mV at E15 and 67 mV at E18 in the chick (Muramoto et al., 1996), and from 70 mV at E15–16 to 110 mV at P1–3 in the rat (Gao & Ziskind-Conhaim, 1998). This results from an increase in density of I_{Na} (Figure 10.6B; Gao & Ziskind-Conhaim, 1998; McCobb et al., 1990). The developmental shortening of the AP—from 9.3 ms at E15–16 to 3.4 ms at P1–3 in the rat and from 2.6 ms at E12 to 1.3 ms at E18 in the chick—is due, at least in part, to an increase in the rate of the depolarization (shorter time to peak I_{Na}) and repolarization phases.

DEVELOPMENT OF POTASSIUM CURRENTS

During development, there is an increase in the density of K⁺ currents that leads to a shortening of the AP duration and to the appearance of the AP afterhyperpolarization (AHP; Figure 10.6B; Gao & Ziskind-Conhaim, 1998; McCobb et al., 1990). Nevertheless the different K⁺ currents do not all develop in a similar fashion. While the AP in embryonic rat MNs is followed by an afterdepolarization (ADP, the membrane potential remains more positive than the resting membrane potential), the AP in neonatal MNs is followed by an AHP, the amplitude of which increases with age (Gao & Ziskind-Conhaim, 1998). By contrast, AP in embryonic chick MNs does not exhibit ADP and the AHP amplitude remains roughly constant over the E12–E18 period (Muramoto et al., 1996). The duration of the AHP decreases with age after birth in rat lumbar MNs, whereas it increases in slow—not fast—alpha MNs in kittens (Huizar, Kuno, & Miyata, 1975).

The fast transient outward K⁺ current (I_A) in chick lumbar MNs is absent or very small at E4 and is then strongly upregulated (16-fold increase) to reach a maximum at E11 (Figure 10.6B; McCobb et al., 1990). This current is relatively large in rat and mouse embryonic MNs and does not increase afterward (Gao & Ziskind-Conhaim, 1998; Safronov & Vogel, 1995). A recent study (Huang, Liao, Chen, & Tsaur, 2006) has shown that the $K_v4.2$ subunit, which is one of the two major I_A-expressing subunits in mammalian CNS (with $K_v4.3$), is detectable from E13.5 in spinal somatic MNs. It reaches a peak of expression around E17.5 and then starts to decrease until it becomes undetectable (around P14 and in adulthood). These data together with the fact that this K⁺ current is absent from adult cat, turtle, and frog MNs (Perrier & Hounsgaard, 2000) suggest that I_A is transiently expressed in somatic MNs during development.

In both chick and rat, the noninactivating, delayed rectifier K⁺ current (I_K) is upregulated during development (Figure 10.6B). Similarly, the amplitude of $I_{K(Ca)}$ strongly increases during development in rat (twofold increase from E15–16 to P1–3) and chick (sixfold increase from E8 to E13; Martin-Caraballo & Dryer, 2002).

DEVELOPMENT OF CALCIUM CURRENTS

Calcium currents are particularly robust in the very first postnatal days in rat and underlie stimulation-induced tetrodotoxin-resistant spikes (Walton & Fulton, 1986). By contrast, weak calcium-mediated AP can be triggered only when potassium conductances are reduced at the end of the first postnatal week. The high-voltage-activated (HVA) calcium current increases during development (Gao & Ziskind-Conhaim, 1998; McCobb, Best, & Beam, 1989). In the chick, N- and L-type currents undergo a threefold increase during the E4–11 period. In the rat, the HVA Ca²⁺ current is mediated by N-type (about 70%), P/Q-type (about 20%), and L-type (10%) Ca²⁺ channels. The relative contribution of the L-type Ca²⁺ channels to the HVA currents may be upregulated during postnatal development, as suggested by the fact that blocking these channels at P2–5 does not modify the chemically induced rhythmic activity in the isolated mouse spinal cord, whereas it reduces the motor output in animals older than P7 (Jiang et al., 1999). In agreement with these observations, immunostaining of the α1C and α1D subunits of the L-type Ca²⁺ channels increases with age, reaching the adult pattern by P18 (Jiang et al., 1999). This increase may be critical for the development of posture and locomotion since L-type calcium channels have been shown to mediate plateau potentials (Figure 10.6C, right trace, Guertin & Hounsgaard, 1998; Hounsgaard & Kiehn, 1989; see also for review Heckman, Lee, & Brownstone, 2003; Hultborn, Brownstone, Toth, & Gossard, 2004).

In chick and mouse, the T-type calcium channels, responsible for the low-voltage-activated (LVA) current, are present in spinal MNs at embryonic ages (E4 and E11 respectively). However, the current density rapidly decreases with age (75% reduction at E6 in the chick) and T-current is no more detectable at E11 (McCobb et al., 1989). Most of embryonic rat (E15, Scamps, Valentin, Dayanithi, & Valmier, 1998) and functionally mature mouse MNs (P9–16; Carlin, Jiang, & Brownstone, 2000) do not express this current.

DEVELOPMENT OF FIRING PROPERTIES

As a result of the development of the different ionic currents, MN discharge properties undergo important changes during embryonic (Hayashi, Mendelson, Phelan, Skinner, & Garcia-Rill, 1997) and postnatal life (Gao & Ziskind-Conhaim, 1998; Vinay, Brocard, & Clarac, 2000a; Vinay et al., 2000b). In the chick, at E12, almost all MNs display an adapting firing during which the AP frequency steadily decreases, whereas at E18, the great majority of MNs showed high frequency tonic firing (Hayashi et al., 1997). The same development is found in rat lumbar MNs. Prolonged depolarizations of MNs generate an afterdepolarizing potential at E16 and a sustained AP firing at P3 (Figure 10.6C, left and middle traces, respectively; Gao & Ziskind-Conhaim, 1998). Vinay, Brocard, and Clarac (2000a) have shown that the maturation of firing properties of extensor (E) and flexor (F) MNs does not occur at the same rate: 82% of F-MNs and only 48% of E-MNs are able to fire repetitively at P2–3; these proportions rise to 100% and 71%, respectively, two days later. Furthermore, considering only the MNs able to fire a sustained discharge during a comparable prolonged depolarization, F-MNs discharged at a higher steady-state frequency than E-MNs. This difference is likely due, at least partly, to a shorter AHP in F-MNs. These differences in repetitive firing behavior between the two groups of MNs demonstrate that, at birth, the maturation process of E-MNs lags behind that of F-MNs. This differential maturation may be responsible, at least partly, for the posture in flexion of neonates and for the gradual development of posture (see above).

Developmental Regulation of Synaptic Transmission

SEROTONERGIC TRANSMISSION

The action of some neurotransmitters, the expression of the receptors to which they bind, and the subunit composition of these receptors change during the perinatal period. 5-HT, via the activation of 5-HT_1 and 5-HT_2 receptors, hyperpolarizes spinal MNs and decreases their R_i in the E12 chick, and evokes opposite responses at E18 (Hayashi et al., 1997). As a consequence, 5-HT reduces and increases the discharge frequency of MNs at E12 and E18. In rat lumbar MNs, 5-HT induces long-lasting depolarizations associated with an increase in R_i as early as E16–17 (Gao & Ziskind-Conhaim, 1993; Ziskind-Conhaim, Seebach, & Gao, 1993). However, this response markedly increases during development from about 1–2 mV at E17 to 6–7 mV at E20–22. These effects increase further after birth (P1–3). The distribution of the different 5-HT receptor subtypes is also regulated during development. In the rat, there is a strong (three- to four-fold) decrease in the expression of 5-HT_{1A} receptor mRNA in facial, hypoglossal, cervical, and lumbar MNs between P7 and P28 (Talley & Bayliss, 2000). By contrast, the expression of 5-HT_{2A} receptors is upregulated during postnatal development. This increase is higher for slow extensor (soleus) than for fast flexor (extensor digitorum longus) MNs (Vult von Steyern & Lomo, 2005). This differential

development is interesting since the activation of 5-HT_2 receptors in MNs facilitates the expression of plateau properties (Harvey, Li, Li, & Bennett, 2006; Li, Murray, Harvey, Ballou, & Bennett, 2007; Perrier & Delgado-Lezama, 2005), which have been implicated in postural regulation (Kiehn & Eken, 1998). Monoamine depletion in the spinal cord indeed changes the EMG activity in the soleus muscle from a tonic to a phasic pattern (Kiehn, Erdal, Eken, & Bruhn, 1996) and affects posture in the rat (Pflieger, Clarac, & Vinay, 2002b). Plateau potentials are no longer observed shortly after the spinal cord has been transected in the cat, unless 5-HT agonists are injected (Hounsgaard, Hultborn, Jespersen, & Kiehn, 1988).

EXCITATORY AMINO ACIDS

The expression of receptors to excitatory amino acids is regulated during development. In rodents as well as in humans, NMDA and non-NMDA receptors are transiently expressed at high levels during the early postnatal period in the ventral horn (Gonzalez, Fuchs, & Droge, 1993; Kalb & Fox, 1997; Kalb, Lidow, Halsted, & Hockfield, 1992). In the rat, the level of NMDA receptors falls during the second and third postnatal weeks (Kalb et al., 1992). A similar developmental pattern is described in humans with a high level of expression of NMDA, kainate (KA), and AMPA receptors (Akesson, Kjaeldgaard, Samuelsson, Seiger, & Sundstrom, 2000) throughout the spinal gray matter at late fetal ages, followed by a decrease during postnatal period. The adult pattern of distribution of these receptors is mainly restricted to the substantia gelatinosa in the dorsal horn with very low levels of expression in the remaining spinal gray matter (Kalb & Fox, 1997). However, this decline in NMDA receptor has been shown to differ across spinal motor nuclei in the rat (Verhovshek, Wellman, & Sengelaub, 2005). The composition of the different NMDA, KA, and AMPA receptors changes with age in rat, the highest levels of expression being observed during the first two postnatal weeks for all subunits (Brown, Wrathall, Yasuda, & Wolfe, 2002; Stegenga & Kalb, 2001). Since these are important factors determining the functional properties and the Ca^{2+} permeability of AMPA receptors (Jonas & Burnashev, 1995), it has been suggested that the non-NMDA receptors expressed by neonatal rat MNs show greater sensitivity to agonists (i.e., produce higher levels of depolarization) and allow Ca^{2+} entry (Jakowec, Fox, Martin, & Kalb, 1995) as shown in cultured Xenopus spinal neurons (Gleason

& Spitzer, 1998; Rohrbough & Spitzer, 1999). This may provide a maturational mechanism by which MNs acquire mature properties through activity-dependent processes (Kalb et al., 1992). The high level of glutamate receptors in the perinatal period may also be responsible for a higher vulnerability to excitotoxic mechanisms of injury.

INHIBITORY AMINO ACIDS

Glycine and GABA are the major inhibitory transmitters in the adult mammalian spinal cord. The inhibitory systems undergo marked developmental changes (see also Chapter 6). The frequency and amplitude of glycine- and $GABA_A$-receptor-mediated miniature inhibitory postsynaptic currents (mIPSCs) increase significantly during the perinatal period in the rat (i.e., from E17–18 to

P1–3; Gao, Stricker, & Ziskind-Conhaim, 2001; Gao & Ziskind-Conhaim, 1995). Two populations of pharmacologically distinct mIPSCs can be recorded in the presence of glycine- or $GABA_A$-receptor antagonists: bicuculline-resistant, fast-decaying GlyR-mediated mIPSCs, and strychnine-resistant, slow-decaying $GABA_A$ receptor-mediated mIPSCs (Figure 10.7A). The frequency of $GABA_A$ receptor-mediated mIPSCs is fourfold higher than that of GlyR-mediated mIPSCs at E17–18 (Figure 10.7A, histograms), indicating that GABAergic synaptic sites are functionally dominant at early stages of neural network formation. A developmental shift from primarily long-duration GABAergic mIPSCs to short-duration glycinergic mIPSCs is evident after birth, when the frequency and amplitude of GlyR-mediated mIPSCs increase

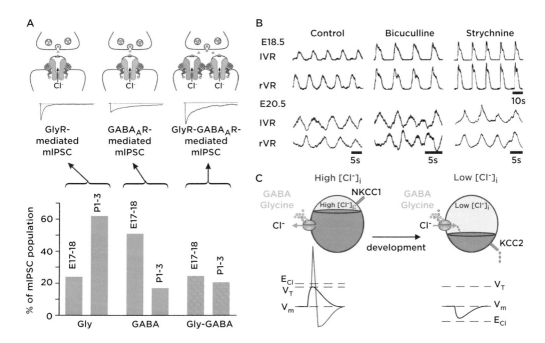

Figure 10.7 Development of inhibitory aminoacid transmission in the rat spinal cord. (A) Developmental switch from predominantly GABAergic synaptic sites at E17–18 to glycinergic sites at P1–3. Pure $GABA_A$R-mediated mIPSCs constitute 51.4% of mIPSC population at E17–18, whereas the contributions of pure GlyR-mediated mIPSCs and mixed GlyR–$GABA_A$R-mediated mIPSCs were 23.8% and 24.8% respectively. The contribution of GlyR-mediated mIPSCS to the total population increased to 62.0% at P1–3, whereas $GABA_A$R-mediated mIPSCs and the mixed GlyR–$GABA_A$R-mediated mIPSCs constituted only 17.0% and 21.0% respectively. (Adapted from Gao, Stricker, & Ziskind-Conhaim, 2001.) (B) In vitro application of 5-HT ("control") induces a rhythmic activity alternating between left ventral root (lVR) and right ventral root (rVR). Both $GABA_A$- and glycine-receptor antagonists (bicuculline and strychnine, respectively) switch the pattern from synchrony to alternation at E18.5, whereas blocking $GABA_A$ receptors has no effect at E20.5, demonstrating that glycine becomes the major neurotransmitter involved in left–right alternation. (Redrawn from Nakayama et al., 2002.) (C) Cation-chloride cotransporters are responsible for the regulation of intracellular chloride concentration ($[Cl^-]_i$). In immature neurons, $[Cl^-]_i$ is high and the equilibrium potential of Cl^- (E_{Cl}) is above the resting membrane potential (V_m). Activation of $GABA_A$ and glycine receptors may even trigger cell firing, when E_{Cl} is above AP threshold (V_T). Na^+, K^+, Cl^- cotransporters NKCC1 are responsible for intracellular Cl^- accumulation. $[Cl^-]_i$ decreases with age because of the upregulation of K^+, Cl^- cotransporters KCC2; E_{Cl} shifts to values below V_m. As a result, the strength of inhibitory connections increases. (Adapted from Vinay & Jean-Xavier, 2008, schemes for Cl^- regulation adapted from Price, Cervero, & de, 2005.)

ten- and twofold, respectively (Figure 10.7A). These data indicate that there is a switch from GABA to glycine during perinatal development. This can be due to an increase in the number of glycinergic synapses and/or in the probability in vesicular release (Gao et al., 2001). The hypothesis of an increase in glycinergic synapses is in agreement with results obtained in the cat demonstrating that, during the postnatal period, the increase in the number of glycine-containing nerve terminals contacting the dendritic compartment of MNs is more important than that of GABA-containing terminals (Simon & Horcholle-Bossavit, 1999). The age-related switch from GABA to glycine observed at the cellular level has some correlates at the level of locomotor network operation. The left–right alternation at E18.5 in the rat relies on both GABA and glycinergic reciprocal inhibition, whereas GABA plays a little role, if any, in the alternation after birth (Figure 10.7B; see also below; Hinckley, Seebach, & Ziskind-Conhaim, 2005; Nakayama et al., 2002; Pflieger, Clarac, & Vinay, 2002a).

The most striking difference in the development of inhibitory amino acid transmission is related to chloride (Cl⁻) homeostasis. The activation of GABA$_A$- and glycine-receptor-gated Cl⁻ channels results in an inward flux of Cl⁻ and membrane potential hyperpolarization in the adult spinal cord (Figure 10.7C). Therefore, the inhibitory action of glycine and GABA consists of both shunting incoming excitatory currents and moving the membrane potential away from the AP threshold. This "classical" hyperpolarizing inhibition is not observed in immature spinal neurons; inhibitory postsynaptic potentials (IPSPs) as well as glycine- and GABA-evoked potentials are instead depolarizing and often excitatory (Gao & Ziskind-Conhaim, 1995; Takahashi, 1984; Wu, Ziskind-Conhaim, & Sweet, 1992; Ziskind-Conhaim, 1998), because of a high intracellular chloride concentration ($[Cl^-]_i$), which favors Cl⁻ efflux through GABA$_A$- or glycine-operated Cl⁻ channels. GABA- and glycine-mediated depolarizations lead to activation of voltage-dependent Ca^{2+} channels and Ca^{2+} oscillations play a key role in neuronal maturation and synaptogenesis (Ben-Ari, 2002). With development, $[Cl^-]_i$ decreases, leading to a shift of the Cl⁻ equilibrium potential toward further negative values, and thereby, to a change in glycine- and GABA-evoked potentials from depolarization to hyperpolarization (Gao & Ziskind-Conhaim, 1995; Jean-Xavier, Pflieger, Liabeuf, & Vinay, 2006; Takahashi, 1984; Vinay

& Jean-Xavier, 2008). Upregulation of a transporter that regulates $[Cl^-]_i$, the neuron-specific K-Cl cotransporter, KCC2, underlies this shift (Delpire & Mount, 2002; Payne, Rivera, Voipio, & Kaila, 2003; Rivera et al., 1999; Rivera, Voipio, & Kaila, 2004; Stein, Hermans-Borgmeyer, Jentsch, & Hubner, 2004).

Mechanisms Underlying Spontaneous Activity

O'Donovan and coworkers (O'Donovan & Chub, 1997; O'Donovan & Rinzel, 1997) have proposed a conceptual model to account for the production of rhythmic episodes of spontaneous activity. In this model, an interneuronal network made of functionally excitatory connections is subject to a periodic variation in excitability. An episode of network activity results in a synaptic depression in active terminals (Fedirchuk et al., 1999) and a hyperpolarization of active cells. Some cells begin to fire as they recover from the depression and their membrane spontaneously depolarizes (Figure 10.8A). Once a critical number of neurons begin to fire, excitation rapidly propagates throughout the network. An important element in this propagation is the activation of the intraspinal target of MNs (R-interneurons; Figure 10.8B; Wenner & O'Donovan, 2001), which appear to be the avian homologue of the mammalian Renshaw cells (Wenner & O'Donovan, 1999). R-interneurons then excite the rest of the network. Synaptic depression and membrane hyperpolarization progressively then act to terminate the episode. Modeling studies confirmed that rhythmicity (0.1–2 Hz) within the episodes of spontaneous activity can arise from the interplay between excitatory connectivity and fast synaptic depression. A slow activity-dependent synaptic depression can account for the recurrence of episodes every 2–30 min.

The neuropharmacological mechanisms underlying spontaneous activity were investigated in the E10–11 embryonic chick (Chub & O'Donovan, 1998). Considering that GABA and glycine are excitatory at early developmental stages (Chapter 6; see above), they investigated the relative importance of different neurotransmitters in generating spontaneous rhythmic activity. They showed that spontaneous activity can still be expressed after blocking glycine and GABA connections or glutamatergic and nicotinic cholinergic connections. In the latter case, the activity transiently disappears and recovers, whereas in the presence of glycine- and GABA$_A$-receptor antagonists, the activity persists at a lower

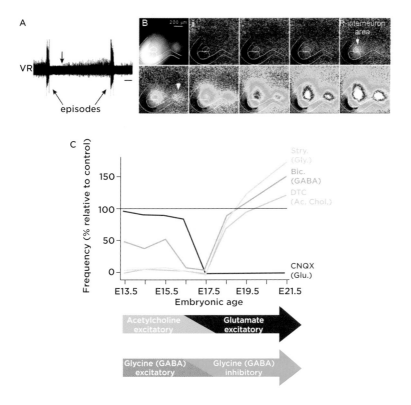

Figure 10.8 Mechanisms generating spontaneous activity in the immature spinal cord. (A) Recording from a VR showing that spike activity stops for several minutes after an episode and then resumes (vertical arrow) and progressively intensifies during the last 2/3 of the interepisode interval. (Adapted from Wenner & O'Donovan, 2001.) (B) Individual frames of the normalized fluorescence changes at the onset episodes of spontaneous activity shown and displayed in sequence showing the onset of spontaneous activity beginning in the R-interneuron region. The activity then propagates throughout the ventral spinal cord. (Adapted from Wenner & O'Donovan, 2001.) (C) Percentage of frequency changes of the spontaneous activity at different ages after blocking glycine (strychnine), or GABA$_A$ (bicuculline), or nicotinic acetylcholine (D-tubocurarine, DTC) or non-NMDA glutamate (CNQX) receptors. (Redrawn from Ren & Greer, 2003.)

frequency. Recovery is not observed when all these connections are blocked. These observations led to the conclusion that the output of developing spinal networks is homeostatically regulated.

In rats, the neuropharmacological control of the spontaneous activity can be divided into three periods (Ren & Greer, 2003). At E13.5–15.5, the spinal networks comprising cholinergic and glycinergic synaptic interconnections are capable of generating rhythmic activity, whereas GABAergic synapses play a role in supporting this activity. At a later stage (E16.5–17.5), the spontaneous activity results from the combination of synaptic drive acting via non-NMDA glutamatergic, nicotinic acetylcholine, glycine, and GABA$_A$ receptors. Closer to birth (E18.5–21.5), glutamate drive acting via non-NMDA receptors is primarily responsible for the rhythmic activity (Figure 10.8C). There is a switch in the contribution to spontaneous activity by chloride-mediated conductances

from excitatory to inhibitory during late gestation (Figure 10.8C).

In mice, a rhythmic spontaneous activity can be recorded in vitro as early as E12–13, when many lumbar MNs are still migrating and extending their peripheral projections (Hanson & Landmesser, 2003). This study provided evidence that electrical transmission plays a significant role in the generation of episodes since blockade of gap junction coupling by carbenoxolone abolishes the rhythmic episodes. In addition, these authors confirmed the key role of acetylcholine from E12.5 to E14.5. Stimulation of MNs at this stage elicits episodes of activity that propagate through the lumbar spinal cord, suggesting that MNs make excitatory connections on each other and on glycine/GABAergic interneurons via nicotinic receptors. From E15.5 onward, the glutamatergic neurotransmission becomes necessary for spontaneous motor activity, whereas blocking the cholinergic transmission has little effect (Myers et al., 2005). Application of strychnine to block glycine receptors markedly reduces and increases the bursting frequency in early and late embryos, respectively, suggesting that glycine switches from an excitatory to an inhibitory contribution to spontaneous activity. This transition occurs at about the same time as the switch from cholinergic to glutamatergic transmission. The contribution of acetylcholine was investigated further using a mouse model lacking the choline acetyltransferase (ChAT), the rate-limiting enzyme for acetylcholine biosynthesis. ChAT mutant embryos exhibit markedly reduced levels of activity compared to controls, even after E14.5, when acetylcholine is not essential to generate the activity.

The observation that network activity is essentially unchanged in the presence of glutamatergic and cholinergic transmitter antagonists suggests the importance of chloride-mediated transmission (Chub & O'Donovan, 1998). The fact that the classical inhibitory neurotransmitters can be functionally excitatory moves the balance between excitatory and inhibitory drives toward excitation. This renders developing networks hyperexcitable. $[Cl^-]_i$ undergoes significant changes during spontaneous activity in the chick spinal cord (Chub & O'Donovan, 2001). After an episode, the Cl^- equilibrium potential falls by ~10 mV, corresponding to a decline of intracellular Cl^- by ~15 mV. This reduces the excitatory contribution of GABA and glycine, and hence, network excitability. The $[Cl^-]_i$ is restored during the interepisode interval, as a result presumably of inward Cl^- pumping via cation-chloride cotransporters, leading to a progressive increase in network excitability. The importance of Cl^- dynamics in the genesis of spontaneous activity in the in vitro chick spinal cord between E9 and E11 was confirmed by the use of a model (Marchetti, Tabak, Chub, O'Donovan, & Rinzel, 2005).

Development of Inputs to Lumbar Networks and Motoneurons
Development of Inputs from the Brain

The development of electrical properties of neurons is dependent upon a multitude of factors. Among these factors, the glial environment plays an important role. Bonansco, Fuenzalida, and Roncagliolo (2004) have indeed shown that the postnatal (P4–10) maturation of electrical properties of spinal MN is strongly affected in the "taiep" mutant rat, which exhibits an abnormal glial development. The authors showed that neurons in

this model displayed no age-dependent change in membrane input resistance or AP characteristics, in contrast to control animals in which MN rheobase increased with age, associated with an increase of the AP amplitude and a reduction of its duration. Another factor that we will develop thereafter is the arrival of projections descending from supraspinal structures. They start to reach the lumbar spinal cord during the fetal period and their development is completed within the weeks that follow birth. However, the timetable of this development varies across species. Furthermore, the efficiency and the action of these pathways on the lumbar CPG also depend on the maturation of the receptors to the different neurotransmitters.

In many species (chick, opossum, rat, and mouse), the first detectable supraspinal projections that reach the lumbar spinal cord originate from the lateral vestibular nucleus, and the medullary and pontine formation (raphe magnus nucleus and gigantocellular reticular nucleus; Cabana, 2000; de Boer-van Huizen & ten Donkelaar, 1999; Kudo, Furukawa, & Okado, 1993; Lakke, 1997; Okado & Oppenheim, 1985; see for review, Vinay et al., 2000b). However, the development of this descending innervation occurs earlier in the chick since the first neurons can be retrogradely stained in the brain stem from the cervical and lumbar spinal cord by E4 and E5, respectively (Okado & Oppenheim, 1985). This corresponds to E16–17 in the rat. Such staining appears also during the prenatal period in the opossum *Monodelphis domestica*. Because birth occurs only 14–15 days after conception in this marsupial, the development of descending projections to the lumbar spinal cord is therefore faster in the opossum (Cabana, 2000).

Descending fibers containing serotonin (5-HT) and noradrenaline (NA) are considered to play important roles not only in the regulation of spinal cord function and in the modulation of spinal reflexes in the adult but also in the maturation of neurons and networks. At birth, in the North American opossum (12 days after conception, i.e., E12) serotonergic neurons are already present in almost all the brain stem areas where they are found in adult (Martin, Ghooray, Ho, Pindzola, & Xu, 1991). The first 5-HT neurons appear in the raphe nuclei at around E4 in the chick (Sako, Kojima, & Okado, 1986a, 1986b) and at E12–14 in the rat (Aitken & Tork, 1988; Wallace & Lauder, 1983). Although noradrenergic (NA) neurons in the locus coeruleus (LC) are detected earlier (E6 in the chick and E10–13 in the the rat), the first descending projections observed in the lumbar spinal cord are serotonergic. They are present in the marginal layer of the chick lumbar spinal cord at around E8; after a waiting period, these fibers start to penetrate into the gray matter and are first detected in the lamina VII at E10 (Sako et al., 1986b). The different laminae are then gradually innervated by these projections, which start to contact MNs (lamina IX) between E10 and E16. The development of raphespinal projections continues until P5 (Sako et al., 1986b). In the North American opossum, projections from neurons located in the caudal raphe and adjacent reticular formation can be detected in the lumbosacral spinal cord as early as P1 (that would correspond to E13 in the rat) and all areas providing a serotonergic innervation of the lumbar spinal cord can be retrogradely stained at P3 by dye injections at this level (Martin et al., 1991). In the rat, the first 5-HT projections to the lumbar region are first observed in the ventrolateral white matter at E15 (de Boer-van Huizen & ten Donkelaar, 1999; Rajaofetra, Sandillon, Geffard, & Privat, 1989) and in the gray matter at E18. Thereafter, the 5-HT innervation develops gradually to reach an adult pattern at P21.

NA projections reach the different spinal cord levels shortly after the serotonergic ones: they are detectable in the rat at E17 and E18 in the upper thoracic and lumbar levels, respectively (Lakke, 1997). They are likely originating first from the subcoeruleus nucleus (SCN) and then from the LC, which projects to the upper lumbar segments from E20 onward. NA innervation increases after birth up to a peak at P14, and then decreases to reach the adult pattern by P30 (Commissiong, 1983). In the cervical and lumbar spinal cord in the chick, the first projections from the SCN are seen at E5 and E7, respectively; those originating from the LC arrive at these same levels one day later. It is worth mentioning that 5-HT and NA fibers arrive shortly before the first spontaneous limb movements (chick) and left–right alternation (rat) are observed.

In the rat, projections descending from other brain stem nuclei reach the upper lumbar cord slightly before birth and the lower lumbar cord during the first postnatal days. The number of axons reaching the lumbar cord then increases gradually until the end of the second postnatal week when most descending pathways are fully developed (Leong, Shieh, & Wong, 1984). The first corticospinal projections can be detected only at the end of the first postnatal week in the rat (Donatelle, 1977; Schreyer & Jones, 1982). The expression of the growth-associated protein GAP-43 is detected by immunocytochemistry in the white matter areas of the corticospinal tracts of the lumbar spinal cord until P29 (Fitzgerald, Reynolds, & Benowitz, 1991).

The role of supraspinal descending projections in the development of spinal neurons and networks has been studied mostly in the case of monoaminergic pathways because they are among the earliest axonal systems to invade the developing spinal cord (Commissiong, 1983; Kudo et al., 1993; Lakke, 1997); they may therefore act as developmental signals (Whitaker-Azmitia, 1991; Whitaker-Azmitia, Druse, Walker, & Lauder, 1996). In addition, the contribution of nonmonoaminergic descending pathways (acetylcholine, excitatory amino acids, and inhibitory amino acids) to the maturation of networks is more difficult to evaluate because of the presence of spinal interneurons utilizing the same neurotransmitters. The possible contribution of descending pathways to spinal cord maturation has been studied by means of spinal cord section, removing all supraspinal influences, or inhibition of 5-HT synthesis during the perinatal period. In rat, depletion in 5-HT by injections of PCPA (an inhibitor of 5-HT synthesis) from the day of birth onward induces locomotor deficits (Myoga, Nonaka, Matsuyama, & Mori, 1995) and an impaired posture (Figure 10.9A; lesser flexion at the knee and ankle levels and lesser extension of the hip; Pflieger et al., 2002b). At the level of MNs, Pflieger, Clarac, and Vinay (2002) have shown that the PCPA treatment alters the development of electrical properties. The authors observed an increase in conduction velocity associated to a decreased excitability (higher rheobase and input conductance); these changes affected the hip extensor/knee flexor MNs more than the ankle extensor ones, which is in accordance with postural observations. Furthermore the maturation of MN repetitive firing properties was stopped by the PCPA treatment. We have shown (Pearlstein, Ben-Mabrouk, Pflieger, & Vinay, 2005) that the locomotor pattern recorded in vitro on a spinal cord isolated from PCPA-treated neonate rats was strongly impaired when compared with sham-treated animals (Figure 10.9B). These results indicated a deficit in interlimb coordination in agreement with the observations made in vivo (Myoga et al., 1995; Pflieger et al., 2002b). Interlimb coordinations at P6 are lost after a transection made on the day of birth (Figure 10.9C,D; Norreel et al., 2003). Intraperitoneal injections of a

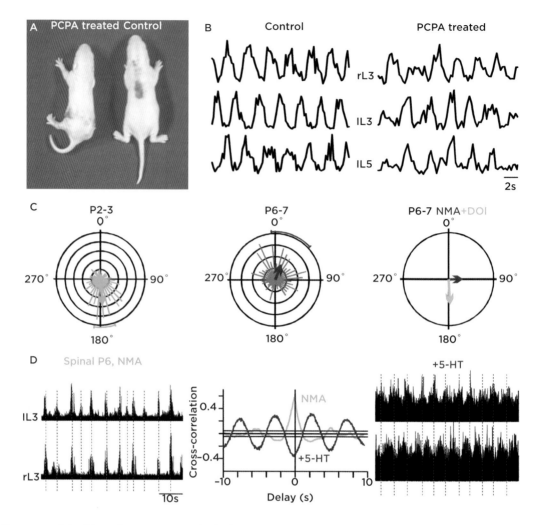

Figure 10.9 Role of descending projections in the development of posture and locomotion. (A) Dorsal view of PCPA-treated and sham-injected rats (P6) showing the postural impairment induced by the absence of 5-HT during development. (Adapted from Pflieger et al., 2002.) (B) Serotonergic control of locomotor pattern. In vitro, application of NMA (control) on an isolated rat (P4) spinal cord, in vitro, induces a fictive locomotor activity. However, in a rat treated with a 5-HT synthesis inhibitor (PCPA), daily, from the day of birth, the same application induces an activity with worse left–right and L3/L5 coordinations. This suggests that 5-HT descending projections play an important role in finely tuning the organization of the locomotor pattern. (Adapted from Pearlstein et al., 2005.) (C) The role of descending projections in the control of the locomotor pattern is explored by studying the effects of a spinal cord transection made at P0, on the locomotor pattern recorded during air-stepping. While the activities of the left and right ankle extensors muscles are still alternating at P2–3 (left diagram, the mean phase relationship is around 180°, light green arrow), at P6 (middle diagram) the coordinations are markedly disorganized: the mean phase relationship is close to zero and the variability is higher. Peritoneal injection of DOI (a 5-HT$_2$ receptor agonist) in a P6 cord-transected animal restores the alternating pattern (right, blue arrow). (Redrawn from Norreel et al., 2003.) (D) In vitro, application of NMA on an isolated spinal cord of a transected animal induced a synchronous rhythmic activity (red dotted lines) in left and right L3 VRs, the cross-correlation coefficient is positive (NMA, green trace on the graph). Addition of 5-HT reestablishes a left–right alternating pattern, the cross-correlation coefficient a $t = 0$ switches to a negative value (red trace). (Adapted from Norreel et al., 2003.)

5-HT$_2$ agonist to operated animals (Figure 10.9C), or in vitro application of 5-HT (in both spinal and PCPA-treated rats; Figure 10.9D) enables a recovery of locomotor alternations. In a recent study, we (Jean-Xavier et al., 2006) demonstrated that the postnatal upregulation of the K-Cl cotransporter, KCC2, which is responsible for the hyperpolarizing shift of the Cl⁻ equilibrium potential and thereby to the change in glycine and GABA-evoked potentials from depolarization to hyperpolarization, was absent after neonatal spinal cord transection. As a consequence, the hyperpolarizing shift of the IPSP reversal potential (E_{IPSP}) that normally takes place during the first postnatal week was not observed in those animals. These results demonstrate that, during the perinatal period, brain stem projections (and especially the serotonergic ones) exert a critical role in the maturation of spinal neurons and networks that control locomotion.

Maturation and Role of Sensory Afferents during Development

Collaterals from DR fibers in the rat start to reach the dorsal part of the dorsal horn at E15.5, the intermediate region at E16.5, and the motor nuclei at E17.5 (Kudo & Yamada, 1987a; Snider, Zhang, Yusoof, Gorukanti, & Tsering, 1992; Ziskind-Conhaim, 1990). The number of collaterals entering the ventral horn then increases with age (Kudo & Yamada, 1987a). The percentage of collaterals exhibiting growth cones decreases from 75% at E17.5 to 15% at around birth. DR stimulation evokes long-latency excitatory postsynaptic potentials (EPSPs) conveyed by polysynaptic pathways at E15 (Ziskind-Conhaim, 1990). Short-latency EPSPs, which are likely monosynaptic, are evoked in most MNs at E17, that is, 1–2 days after the formation of long-latency polysynaptic connections (Ziskind-Conhaim, 1990). The stretch reflex appears at E19–20 (Kudo & Yamada, 1985). The magnitude of the monosynaptic response increases until P2 (Kudo & Yamada, 1987a). Although the monosynaptic stretch reflex is present at birth, muscle spindles appear to be fully mature much later (at P12/15; Navarrete & Vrbova, 1983). The percentage of units in DR filaments exhibiting a repetitive firing in response to a 5-s stretch of the triceps surae muscles increases with age from 50% at P0 to 80% and 90% at P5 and P10, respectively (Vejsada, Hnik, Payne, Ujec, & Palecek, 1985). In the chick, monosynaptic connections appear at around E7 (Davis, Frank, Johnson, & Scott, 1989; Lee, Koebbe, & O'Donovan, 1988; Lee & O'Donovan, 1991; Maier, 1993).

A prominent feature of the transmission in the monosynaptic pathway in both the rat and the chick is a substantial depression in the amplitude of the monosynaptic EPSP during low rates of stimulation (Kudo & Yamada, 1985; Lee et al., 1988; Lee & O'Donovan, 1991; Lev-Tov & Pinco, 1992; Pinco & Lev-Tov, 1993a, 1993b). The prolonged depression of synaptic potentials in the neonatal rat is not due to failure of spike invasion of the afferent terminals (Lee et al., 1988) but instead reflects decreased transmitter release from the activated afferent terminals (Lev-Tov & Pinco, 1992). This decrease may be due to immature properties of the transmitter release machinery in developing synapses.

Recordings from single cutaneous primary afferent units in the DR ganglion showed that all the major cutaneous receptor types are developed at birth in the rat, although peak firing frequency and ability to follow high frequency electrical stimulation are low (Fitzgerald, 1987). However, recordings from dorsal horn cells showed that the synaptic coupling between cutaneous afferents and central cells is quite immature in the early postnatal period (Fitzgerald, 1985). Receptive field areas are large at birth and nociceptive withdrawal reflexes are often misdirected, bringing the stimulated area of the skin toward the stimulus instead of taking it away (Holmberg & Schouenborg, 1996). The size of receptive fields decreases with age, and from the third postnatal week, adequate withdrawal reflexes can be elicited, suggesting that some inappropriate connections become depressed or eliminated.

In all the species considered in this chapter, it is clear that different rhythmic activities emerge before the first sensory inputs are functional. Left–right and flexor–extensor alternations are present in vitro in the isolated spinal cord preparation indicating that they are produced by the CPGs. This, however, does not mean that sensory inputs do not play any role in the development of spinal cord networks and MNs. By means of EMG activities, Bekoff, Nusbaum, Sabichi, and Clifford (1987) examined the effect of removing sensory feedback from the legs on the production of the distinctive leg motor patterns. The temporal characteristics and interlimb coordination of hatching and walking are little affected. However, major changes in intralimb motor output patterns are seen when compared to records from normal chicks. In general, the walking pattern becomes more like hatching after deafferentation, which suggests that the hatching pattern is a more basic function. These data demonstrated that hatching and walking share some common basic neural circuits and that sensory inputs play a major role in refining the walking pattern.

Conclusion

What can account for the different locomotor abilities of precocial and altricial species at birth/hatching? A necessary but not sufficient requirement for locomotion is obviously that CPGs be functional. The spinal circuitry responsible for locomotion develops relatively early in both precocial and altricial species. CPGs are roughly functional (on the basis of their ability to produce left–right and flexor–extensor alternations) about 2 weeks prior to weight-supported locomotion, which occurs 1 day after hatching in the chick and within the second postnatal week in the rat (Figure 10.10). The fact that CPGs are functional at birth in rats does not mean that they are fully mature. For instance, further maturation of postsynaptic inhibition occurs postnatally: the Cl⁻ equilibrium potential continues to shift toward more hyperpolarized values during the first postnatal week in rats. This likely increases the strength of inhibitory synaptic connections within the network, thereby improving left–right and flexor–extensor coordinations.

An important difference between chicks and rats is the development of posture, a limiting factor with regard to locomotor performance, which occurs postnatally in the latter species. Postural development results from many factors including the development of electrical properties of MNs and their inputs from both the periphery and the brain. A stretch reflex can be elicited prior to birth in the rat and some descending connections are already established at that time. These projections are sufficient to activate the CPGs as demonstrated by the fact that olfactory stimulation can trigger air-stepping in neonates. However, it appears that only half of the units sensitive to stretch are mature and about 40% of the descending projections are reaching the lumbar cord at birth. The development of inputs therefore continues further postnatally. The first sensory and supraspinal connections to MNs are established earlier in the chick than in the rat. Although developmental data, at different stages, are lacking in chicks, it is likely that inputs to MNs are closer to the adult form at birth/hatching in this species.

Spontaneous activity plays a key role in many activity-dependent aspects of motor development. The first signs of spontaneous motility are observed as early as the first week of the embryonic period in the chick; spontaneous activity starts much later in the rat. This 10-day difference in the onset of spontaneous motility may account for a delay in the maturation of activity-dependent mechanisms in rodents, compared to chicks. A well-known mechanism that has been demonstrated to be closely dependent upon the pattern of spontaneous activity is the switch from polyneuronal innervation to monoinnervation of myofibers. This is an important event with regard to the acquisition of a gradual control of muscle force, a requirement for the development of posture. Elimination of polyneuronal innervation occurs prior to hatching in chicks and after birth in rats. Myelination is responsible for the

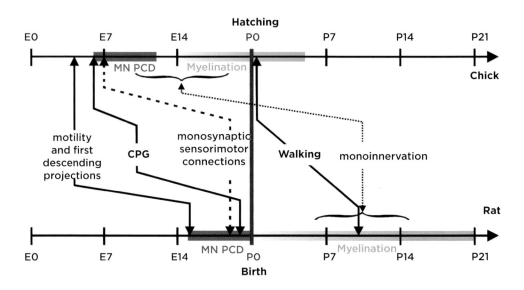

Figure 10.10 Comparison of the development of different components of the locomotor system between a precocial (chick) and an altricial species (rat). While the onset of walking occurs shortly after hatching in the chick, it is delayed by about 10 days in the rat due to the late development of the major components of the locomotor system. MN PCD (motoneuron programmed cell death) data from Yamamoto & Henderson, 1999; myelination data from Ziskind-Conhaim, 1988, for rats; and Uyemura, Horie, Kitamura, Suzuki, & Uehara, 1979, for chicks. (Redrawn from Clarac, Brocard, Pflieger, & Vinay, 2001.)

increase in conduction velocity in axons, a requirement for rapid adaptations of locomotor behavior to any change in the environment. Here again, there is a gap between chicks and rats; myelination occurs during the perinatal period in the former and only postnatally in the latter.

To conclude, each species has its own developmental time window, which results from a complex combination of genetic and environmental factors. All developmental events occur about 10–15 days later in rats, compared to chicks. This can account for the difference in the onset of locomotor behavior in these two species. The development of the chick occurs in a shorter time window in the protected environment of the egg; the shift of maturation toward the postnatal period in rodents likely make them be more vulnerable than chicks, with regard to environmental constraints.

References

Aitken, A. R., & Tork, I. (1988). Early development of serotonin-containing neurons and pathways as seen in whole-mount preparations of the fetal rat brain. *The Journal of Comparative Neurology, 274*, 32–47.

Akesson, E., Kjaeldgaard, A., Samuelsson, E. B., Seiger, A., & Sundstrom, E. (2000). Ionotropic glutamate receptor expression in human spinal cord during first trimester development. *Brain Research. Developmental Brain Research, 119*, 55–63.

Altman, J., & Bayer, S. A. (1984). The development of the rat spinal cord. *Advances in Anatomy, Embryology, and Cell Biology, 85*, 1–164.

Altman, J., & Sudarshan, K. (1975). Postnatal development of locomotion in the laboratory rat. *Animal Behaviour, 23*, 896–920.

Ballion, B., Morin, D., & Viala, D. (2001). Forelimb locomotor generators and quadrupedal locomotion in the neonatal rat. *European Journal of Neuroscience, 14*, 1727–1738.

Bekoff, A. (1976). Ontogeny of leg motor output in the chick embryo: A neural analysis. *Brain Research, 106*, 271–291.

Bekoff, A. (2001). Development of motor behaviour in chick embryos. In A. F. Kalverboer & A. Gramsbergen (Eds.), *Handbook of brain and behaviour in human development* (pp. 429–446). Dordrecht: Kluwer.

Bekoff, A., & Lau, B. (1980). Interlimb coordination in 20-day-old rat fetuses. *The Journal of Experimental Zoology, 214*, 173–175.

Bekoff, A., Nusbaum, M. P., Sabichi, A. L., & Clifford, M. (1987). Neural control of limb coordination. I. Comparison of hatching and walking motor output patterns in normal and deafferented chicks. *The Journal of Neuroscience, 7*, 2320–2330.

Bekoff, A., Stein, P. S., & Hamburger, V. (1975). Coordinated motor output in the hind limb of the 7-day chick embryo. *Proceedings of the National Academy of Sciences, USA, 72*, 1245–1248.

Bellinger, D. L., & Anderson, W. J. (1987a). Postnatal development of cell columns and their associated dendritic bundles in the lumbosacral spinal cord of the rat. I. The ventrolateral cell column. *Developmental Brain Research, 35*, 55–67.

Bellinger, D. L., & Anderson, W. J. (1987b). Postnatal development of cell columns and their associated dendritic bundles in the lumbosacral spinal cord of the rat. II. The ventromedial cell column. *Developmental Brain Research, 35*, 69–82.

Ben-Ari, Y. (2001). Developing networks play a similar melody. *Trends in Neurosciences, 24*, 353–360.

Ben-Ari, Y. (2002). Excitatory actions of GABA during development: The nature of the nurture. *Nature Reviews. Neuroscience, 3*, 728–739.

Ben-Ari, Y., Cherubini, E., Corradetti, R., & Gaiarsa, J. L. (1989). Giant synaptic potentials in immature rat CA3 hippocampal neurones. *The Journal of Physiology, 416*, 303–325.

Bennett, M. R., McGrath, P. A., Davey, D. F., & Hutchinson, I. (1983). Death of motorneurons during the postnatal loss of polyneuronal innervation of rat muscles. *The Journal of Comparative Neurology, 218*, 351–363.

Blumberg, M. S., & Lucas, D. E. (1994). Dual mechanisms of twitching during sleep in neonatal rats. *Behavioral Neuroscience, 108*, 1196–1202.

Bonansco, C., Fuenzalida, M., & Roncagliolo, M. (2004). Altered synaptic and electrical properties of lumbar motoneurons in the neurological glial mutant taiep rat. *Experimental Brain Research, 156*, 104–110.

Bonnot, A., & Morin, D. (1998). Hemisegmental localisation of rhythmic networks in the lumbosacral spinal cord of neonate mouse. *Brain Research, 793*, 136–148.

Bracci, E., Beatto, M., & Nistri, A. (1998). Extracellular K+ induces locomotor-like patterns in the rat spinal cord in vitro: Comparison with NMDA or 5-HT induced activity. *Journal of Neurophysiology, 79*, 2643–2652.

Bradley, N. S. (1999). Transformations in embryonic motility in chick: Kinematic correlates of type I and II motility at E9 and E12. *Journal of Neurophysiology, 81*, 1486–1494.

Bradley, N. S., & Bekoff, A. (1990). Development of coordinated movement in chicks: I. Temporal analysis of hind limb muscle synergies at embryonic days 9 and 10. *Developmental Psychobiology, 23*, 763–782.

Bradley, N. S., Solanki, D., & Zhao, D. (2005). Limb movements during embryonic development in the chick: Evidence for a continuum in limb motor control antecedent to locomotion. *Journal of Neurophysiology, 94*, 4401–4411.

Brocard, F., Vinay, L., & Clarac, F. (1999). Development of hind limb postural control during the first postnatal week in the rat. *Developmental Brain Research, 117*, 81–89.

Brown, K. M., Wrathall, J. R., Yasuda, R. P., & Wolfe, B. B. (2002). Quantitative measurement of glutamate receptor subunit protein expression in the postnatal rat spinal cord. *Brain Research. Developmental Brain Research, 137*, 127–133.

Busetto, G., Buffelli, M., Tognana, E., Bellico, F., & Cangiano, A. (2000). Hebbian mechanisms revealed by electrical stimulation at developing rat neuromuscular junctions. *The Journal of Neuroscience, 20*, 685–695.

Cabana, T. (2000). The development of mammalian motor systems: The opossum *Monodelphis domestica* as a model. *Brain Research Bulletin, 53*, 615–626.

Carlin, K. P., Jiang, Z., & Brownstone, R. M. (2000). Characterization of calcium currents in functionally mature mouse spinal motoneurons. *European Journal of Neuroscience, 12*, 1624–1634.

Cazalets, J. R., & Bertrand, S. (2000). Coupling between lumbar and sacral motor networks in the neonatal rat spinal cord. *European Journal of Neuroscience, 12*, 2993–3002.

Cazalets, J. R., Menard, I., Crémieux, J., & Clarac, F. (1990). Variability as a characteristic of immature motor systems: An electromyographic study of swimming in the newborn rat. *Behavioural Brain Research, 40*, 215–225.

Cazalets, J. R., Sqalli-Houssaini, Y., & Clarac, F. (1992). Activation of the central pattern generators for locomotion by serotonin and excitatory amino acids in neonatal rat. *The Journal of Physiology, 455*, 187–204.

Chang, Q., Gonzalez, M., Pinter, M. J., & Balice-Gordon, R. J. (1999). Gap junctional coupling and patterns of connexin expression among neonatal rat lumbar spinal motor neurons. *The Journal of Neuroscience, 19*, 10813–10828.

Chang, Q., Pereda, A., Pinter, M. J., & Balice-Gordon, R. J. (2000). Nerve injury induces gap junctional coupling among axotomized adult motor neurons. *The Journal of Neuroscience, 20*, 674–684.

Chub, N., & O'Donovan, M. J. (1998). Blockade and recovery of spontaneous rhythmic activity after application of neurotransmitter antagonists to spinal networks of the chick embryo. *The Journal of Neuroscience, 18*, 294–306.

Chub, N., & O'Donovan, M. J. (2001). Post-episode depression of GABAergic transmission in spinal neurons of the chick embryo. *Journal of Neurophysiology, 85*, 2166–2176.

Clancy, B., Darlington, R. B., & Finlay, B. L. (2001). Translating developmental time across mammalian species. *Neuroscience, 105*, 7–17.

Clarac, F., Brocard, F., Pflieger, J. F., & Vinay, L. (2001). Maturation of locomotion in the neonate rat. Comparisons with another higher vertebrate. In N. Gantchev (Ed.), *From basic motor control to functional recovery II. Towards an understanding of the role of motor control from simple systems to human performance* (pp. 3–10). Sofia, Bulgaria: Professor Marin Drinov Academic Publishing House.

Commissiong, J. W. (1983). Development of catecholaminergic nerves in the spinal cord of the rat. *Brain Research, 264*, 197–208.

Cummings, J. P., & Stelzner, D. J. (1984). Prenatal and postnatal development of lamina IX neurons in the rat thoracic spinal cord. *Experimental Neurology, 83*, 155–166.

Curfs, M. H., Gribnau, A. A., & Dederen, P. J. (1993). Postnatal maturation of the dendritic fields of motoneuron pools supplying flexor and extensor muscles of the distal forelimb in the rat. *Development, 117*, 535–541.

Davis, B. M., Frank, E., Johnson, F. A., & Scott, S. A. (1989). Development of central projections of lumbosacral sensory neurons in the chick. *The Journal of Comparative Neurology, 279*(4), 556–566.

de Boer-van Huizen, R., & ten Donkelaar, J. H. (1999). Early development of descending supraspinal pathways: A tracing study in fixed and isolated rat embryos. *Anatomy and Embryology, 199*, 539–547.

Dekkers, J., Becker, D. L., Cook, J. E., & Navarrete, R. (1994). Early postnatal changes in the somatodendritic morphology of ankle flexor motoneurons in the rat. *European Journal of Neuroscience, 6*, 87–97.

Delpire, E., & Mount, D. B. (2002). Human and murine phenotypes associated with defects in cation-chloride cotransport. *Annual Review of Physiology, 64*, 803–843.

Donatelle, J. M. (1977). Growth of the corticospinal tract and the development of placing reactions in the postnatal rat. *The Journal of Comparative Neurology, 175*, 207–232.

Fady, J. C., Jamon, M., & Clarac, F. (1998). Early olfactory-induced rhythmic limb activity in the newborn rat. *Developmental Brain Research, 108*, 111–123.

Fedirchuk, B., Wenner, P., Whelan, P. J., Ho, S., Tabak, J., & O'Donovan, M. J. (1999). Spontaneous network activity transiently depresses synaptic transmission in the embryonic chick spinal cord. *The Journal of Neuroscience, 19*, 2102–2112.

Feller, M. B. (1999). Spontaneous correlated activity in developing neural circuits. *Neuron, 22*, 653–656.

Fellippa-Marques, S., Vinay, L., & Clarac, F. (2000). Spontaneous and locomotor-related GABAergic input onto primary afferents in the neonatal rat. *European Journal of Neuroscience, 12*, 155–164.

Fitzgerald, M. (1985). The post-natal development of cutaneous afferent fibre input and receptive field organization in the rat dorsal horn. *The Journal of Physiology, 364*, 1–18.

Fitzgerald, M. (1987). Cutaneous primary afferent properties in the hind limb of the neonatal rat. *The Journal of Physiology, 383*, 79–92.

Fitzgerald, M., Reynolds, M. L., & Benowitz, L. I. (1991). GAP-43 expression in the developing rat lumbar spinal cord. *Neuroscience, 41*(1), 187–199.

Fulton, B. P., & Walton, K. (1986). Electrophysiological properties of neonatal rat motoneurones studied in vitro. *The Journal of Physiology, 370*, 651–678.

Gao, B. X., Stricker, C., & Ziskind-Conhaim, L. (2001). Transition from GABAergic to glycinergic synaptic transmission in newly formed spinal networks. *Journal of Neurophysiology, 86*, 492–502.

Gao, B. X., & Ziskind-Conhaim, L. (1993). Development of chemosensitivity in serotonin-deficient spinal cords of rat embryos. *Developmental Biology, 158*, 79–89.

Gao, B. X., & Ziskind-Conhaim, L. (1995). Development of glycine- and GABA-gated currents in rat spinal motoneurons. *Journal of Neurophysiology, 74*, 113–121.

Gao, B. X., & Ziskind-Conhaim, L. (1998). Development of ionic currents underlying changes in action potential waveforms in rat spinal motoneurons. *Journal of Neurophysiology, 80*, 3047–3061.

Garcia, K. D., Sprunger, L. K., Meisler, M. H., & Beam, K. G. (1998). The sodium channel Scn8a is the major contributor to the postnatal developmental increase of sodium current density in spinal motoneurons. *The Journal of Neuroscience, 18*, 5234–5239.

Gleason, E. L., & Spitzer, N. C. (1998). AMPA and NMDA receptors expressed by differentiating *Xenopus* spinal neurons. *Journal of Neurophysiology, 79*, 2986–2998.

Gonzalez, D. L., Fuchs, J. L., & Droge, M. H. (1993). Distribution of NMDA receptor binding in developing mouse spinal cord. *Neuroscience Letters, 151*, 134–137.

Grillner, S. (1981). Control of locomotion in bipeds, tetrapods, and fish. In J. M. Brookhart & V. B. Mountcastle (Eds.), *Handbook of physiology—The nervous system II* (pp. 1179–1236). Bethesda, MD: American Physiological Society.

Guertin, P. A., & Hounsgaard, J. (1998). NMDA-Induced intrinsic voltage oscillations depend on L-type calcium channels in spinal motoneurons of adult turtles. *Journal of Neurophysiology, 80*, 3380–3382.

Hamburger, V., & Balaban, M. (1963). Observations and experiments on spontaneous rhythmical behavior in the chick embryo. *Developmental Biology, 7*, 533–545.

Hamburger, V., & Oppenheim, R. (1967). Prehatching motility and hatching behavior in the chick. *The, Journal of Experimental Zoology, 166*, 171–203.

Hanson, M. G., & Landmesser, L. T. (2003). Characterization of the circuits that generate spontaneous episodes of activity in the early embryonic mouse spinal cord. *The Journal of Neuroscience, 23*, 587–600.

Hanson, M. G., & Landmesser, L. T. (2004). Normal patterns of spontaneous activity are required for correct motor axon guidance and the expression of specific guidance molecules. *Neuron, 43*, 687–701.

Hanson, M. G., & Landmesser, L. T. (2006). Increasing the frequency of spontaneous rhythmic activity disrupts pool-specific axon fasciculation and pathfinding of embryonic spinal motoneurons. *The Journal of Neuroscience, 26*, 12769–12780.

Hanson, M. G., Milner, L. D., & Landmesser, L. T. (2008). Spontaneous rhythmic activity in early chick spinal cord influences distinct motor axon pathfinding decisions. *Brain Research Reviews, 57*, 77–85.

Harvey, P. J., Li, Y., Li, X., & Bennett, D. J. (2006). Persistent sodium currents and repetitive firing in motoneurons of the sacrocaudal spinal cord of adult rats. *Journal of Neurophysiology, 96*, 1141–1157.

Hayashi, T., Mendelson, B., Phelan, K. D., Skinner, R. D., & Garcia-Rill, E. (1997). Developmental changes in serotonergic receptor-mediated modulation of embryonic chick motoneurons in vitro. *Brain Research. Developmental Brain Research, 102*, 21–33.

Heckman, C. J., Lee, R. H., & Brownstone, R. M. (2003). Hyperexcitable dendrites in motoneurons and their neuromodulatory control during motor behavior. *Trends in Neurosciences, 26*, 688–695.

Hinckley, C., Seebach, B., & Ziskind-Conhaim, L. (2005). Distinct roles of glycinergic and GABAergic inhibition in coordinating locomotor-like rhythms in the neonatal mouse spinal cord. *Neuroscience, 131*, 745–758.

Ho, S. M., & Waite, P. M. (1999). Spontaneous activity in the perinatal trigeminal nucleus of the rat. *Neuroreport, 10*, 659–664.

Holmberg, H., & Schouenborg, J. (1996). Postnatal development of the nociceptive withdrawal reflexes in the rat: A behavioural and electromyographic study. *The Journal of Physiology, 493*, 239–252.

Hounsgaard, J., Hultborn, H., Jespersen, B., & Kiehn, O. (1988). Bistability of alpha-motoneurones in the decerebrate cat and in the acute spinal cat after intravenous 5-hydroxytryptophan. *The Journal of Physiology, 405*, 345–367.

Hounsgaard, J., & Kiehn, O. (1989). Serotonin-induced bistability of turtle motoneurones caused by a nifedipine-sensitive calcium plateau potential. *The Journal of Physiology, 414*, 265–282.

Huang, H. Y., Liao, C. W., Chen, P. H., & Tsaur, M. L. (2006). Transient expression of A-type K channel alpha subunits Kv4.2 and Kv4.3 in rat spinal neurons during development. *European Journal of Neuroscience, 23*, 1142–1150.

Huizar, P., Kuno, M., & Miyata, Y. (1975). Differentiation of motoneurones and skeletal muscles in kittens. *The Journal of Physiology, 252*, 465–479.

Hultborn, H., Brownstone, R. B., Toth, T. I., & Gossard, J. P. (2004). Key mechanisms for setting the input-output gain across the motoneuron pool. *Progress in Brain Research, 143*, 77–95.

Iizuka, M., Nishimaru, H., & Kudo, N. (1998). Development of the spatial pattern of 5-HT-induced locomotor rhythm in the lumbar spinal cord of rat fetuses in vitro. *Neuroscience Research, 31*, 107–111.

Jacobson, R. D., & Hollyday, M. (1982a). A behavioral and electromyographic study of walking in the chick. *Journal of Neurophysiology, 48*, 238–256.

Jacobson, R. D., & Hollyday, M. (1982b). Electrically evoked walking and fictive locomotion in the chick. *Journal of Neurophysiology, 48*, 257–270.

Jakowec, M. W., Fox, A. J., Martin, L. J., & Kalb, R. G. (1995). Quantitative and qualitative changes in AMPA receptor expression during spinal cord development. *Neuroscience, 67*, 893–907.

Jamon, M., & Clarac, F. (1998). Early walking in the neonatal rat. A kinematic study. *Behavioral Neuroscience, 112*, 1218–1228.

Jean-Xavier, C., Pflieger, J. F., Liabeuf, S., & Vinay, L. (2006). Inhibitory post-synaptic potentials in lumbar motoneurons remain depolarizing after neonatal spinal cord transection in the rat. *Journal of Neurophysiology, 96*, 2274–2281.

Jiang, Z., Rempel, J., Li, J., Sawchuk, M. A., Carlin, K. P., & Brownstone, R. M. (1999). Development of L-type calcium channels and a nifedipine-sensitive motor activity in the postnatal mouse spinal cord. *European Journal of Neuroscience, 11*, 3481–3487.

Jonas, P., & Burnashev, N. (1995). Molecular mechanisms controlling calcium entry through AMPA-type glutamate receptor channels. *Neuron, 15*, 987–990.

Jouvet-Mounier, D., Astic, L., & Lacote, D. (1970). Ontogenesis of the states of sleep in rat, cat, and guinea pig during the first postnatal month. *Developmental Psychobiology, 2*, 216–239.

Kalb, R. G., & Fox, A. J. (1997). Synchronized overproduction of AMPA, kainate, and NMDA glutamate receptors during human spinal cord development. *The Journal of Comparative Neurology, 384*, 200–210.

Kalb, R. G., Lidow, M. S., Halsted, M. J., & Hockfield, S. (1992). *N*-Methyl-D-aspartate receptors are transiently expressed in the developing spinal cord ventral horn. *Proceedings of the National Academy of Sciences, USA, 89*, 8502–8506.

Kellerth, J. O., Mellstrom, A., & Skoglund, S. (1971). Postnatal excitability changes of kitten motoneurones. *Acta Physiologica Scandinavica, 83*, 31–41.

Kerai, B., Greensmith, L., Vrbova, G., & Navarrete, R. (1995). Effect of transient neonatal muscle paralysis on the growth of soleus motoneurones in the rat. *Developmental Brain Research, 85*, 89–95.

Kiehn, O. (2006). Locomotor circuits in the mammalian spinal cord. *Annual Review of Neuroscience, 29*, 279–306.

Kiehn, O., & Butt, S. J. (2003). Physiological, anatomical and genetic identification of CPG neurons in the developing mammalian spinal cord. *Progress in Neurobiology, 70,* 347–361.

Kiehn, O., & Eken, T. (1998). Functional role of plateau potentials in vertebrate motor neurons. *Current Opinion in Neurobiology, 8,* 746–752.

Kiehn, O., Erdal, J., Eken, T., & Bruhn, T. (1996). Selective depletion of spinal monoamines changes the rat soleus EMG from a tonic to a more phasic pattern. *The Journal of Physiology, 492* (Pt. 1), 173–184.

Kiehn, O., & Kjaerulff, O. (1996). Spatiotemporal characteristics of 5-HT and dopamine-induced rhythmic hindlimb activity in the in vitro neonatal rat. *Journal of Neurophysiology, 75,* 1472–1482.

Kleven, G. A., Lane, M. S., & Robinson, S. R. (2004). Development of interlimb movement synchrony in the rat fetus. *Behavioral Neuroscience, 118,* 835–844.

Krieger, C., & Sears, T. A. (1988). The development of voltage-dependent ionic conductances in murine spinal cord neurones in culture. *Canadian Journal of Physiology and Pharmacology, 66,* 1328–1336.

Kudo, N., Furukawa, F., & Okado, N. (1993). Development of descending fibers to the rat embryonic spinal cord. *Neuroscience Research, 16,* 131–141.

Kudo, N., & Nishimaru, H. (1998). Reorganization of locomotor activity during development in the prenatal rat. *Annals of the New York Academy of Sciences, 860,* 306–317.

Kudo, N., & Yamada, T. (1985). Development of the monosynaptic stretch reflex in the rat: An in vitro study. *The Journal of Physiology, 369,* 127–144.

Kudo, N., & Yamada, T. (1987a). Morphological and physiological studies of development of the monosynaptic reflex pathway in the rat lumbar spinal cord. *The Journal of Physiology, 389,* 441–459.

Kudo, N., & Yamada, T. (1987b). *N*-Methyl-D,L-aspartate-induced locomotor activity in a spinal cord-hindlimb muscles preparation of the newborn rat studied in vitro. *Neuroscience Letters, 75,* 43–48.

Lakke, E. A. J. F. (1997). The projections to the spinal cord of the rat during development: A time-table of descent. *Advances in Anatomy, Embryology, and Cell Biology, 135,* 1–143.

Landmesser, L. T., & O'Donovan, M. J. (1984). Activation patterns of embryonic chick hind limb muscles recorded in ovo and in an isolated spinal cord preparation. *The Journal of Physiology, 347,* 189–204.

Lee, M. T., Koebbe, M. J., & O'Donovan, M. J. (1988). The development of sensorimotor synaptic connections in the lumbosacral cord of the chick embryo. *The Journal of Neuroscience, 8,* 2530–2543.

Lee, M. T., & O'Donovan, M. J. (1991). Organization of hindlimb muscle afferent projections to lumbosacral motoneurons in the chick embryo. *The Journal of Neuroscience, 11,* 2564–2573.

Leong, S. K., Shieh, J. Y., & Wong, W. C. (1984). Localizing spinal-cord-projecting neurons in neonatal and immature albino rats. *The Journal of Comparative Neurology, 228,* 18–23.

Lev-Tov, A., Delvolve, I., & Kremer, E. (2000). Sacrocaudal afferents induce rhythmic efferent bursting in isolated spinal cords of neonatal rats. *Journal of Neurophysiology, 83,* 888–894.

Lev-Tov, A., & Pinco, M. (1992). In vitro studies of prolonged synaptic depression in the neonatal rat spinal cord. *The Journal of Physiology, 447,* 149–169.

Li, X., Murray, K., Harvey, P. J., Ballou, E. W., & Bennett, D. J. (2007). Serotonin facilitates a persistent calcium current in motoneurons of rats with and without chronic spinal cord injury. *Journal of Neurophysiology, 97,* 1236–1246.

Maier, A. (1993). Development of chicken intrafusal muscle fibers. *Cell Tissue Research, 274,* 383–391.

Marchetti, C., Tabak, J., Chub, N., O'Donovan, M. J., & Rinzel, J. (2005). Modeling spontaneous activity in the developing spinal cord using activity-dependent variations of intracellular chloride. *The Journal of Neuroscience, 25,* 3601–3612.

Martin, G. F., Ghooray, G., Ho, R. H., Pindzola, R. R., & Xu, X. M. (1991). The origin of serotoninergic projections to the lumbosacral spinal cord at different stages of development in the North American opossum. *Brain Research. Developmental Brain Research, 58,* 203–213.

Martin-Caraballo, M., & Dryer, S. E. (2002). Activity- and target-dependent regulation of large-conductance Ca^{2+}-activated K^+ channels in developing chick lumbar motoneurons. *The Journal of Neuroscience, 22,* 73–81.

McCobb, D. P., Best, P. M., & Beam, K. G. (1989). Development alters the expression of calcium currents in chick limb motoneurons. *Neuron, 2,* 1633–1643.

McCobb, D. P., Best, P. M., & Beam, K. G. (1990). The differentiation of excitability in embryonic chick limb motoneurons. *The Journal of Neuroscience, 10,* 2974–2984.

McEwen, M. L., & Stehouwer, D. J. (2001). Kinematic analyses of air-stepping of neonatal rats after mid-thoracic spinal cord compression. *Journal of Neurotrauma, 18,* 1383–1397.

McEwen, M. L., Van Hartesveldt, C., & Stehouwer, D. J. (1997). A kinematic comparison of L-DOPA-induced air-stepping and swimming in developing rats. *Developmental Psychobiology, 30,* 313–327.

Milner, L. D., & Landmesser, L. T. (1999). Cholinergic and GABAergic inputs drive patterned spontaneous motoneuron activity before target contact. *The Journal of Neuroscience, 19,* 3007–3022.

Muir, G. D. (2000). Early ontogeny of locomotor behaviour: A comparison between altricial and precocial animals. *Brain Research Bulletin, 53,* 719–726.

Muir, G. D., & Chu, T. K. (2002). Posthatching locomotor experience alters locomotor development in chicks. *Journal of Neurophysiology, 88,* 117–123.

Muir, G. D., Gosline, J. M., & Steeves, J. D. (1996). Ontogeny of bipedal locomotion: Walking and running in the chick. *The Journal of Physiology, 493* (Pt. 2), 589–601.

Muramoto, T., Mendelson, B., Phelan, K. D., Garcia-Rill, E., Skinner, R. D., & Puskarich-May, C. (1996). Developmental changes in the effects of serotonin and *N*-methyl-D-aspartate on intrinsic membrane properties of embryonic chick motoneurons. *Neuroscience, 75,* 607–618.

Myers, C. P., Lewcock, J. W., Hanson, M. G., Gosgnach, S., Aimone, J. B., Gage, F. H., et al. (2005). Cholinergic input is required during embryonic development to mediate proper assembly of spinal locomotor circuits. *Neuron, 46,* 37–49.

Myoga, H., Nonaka, S., Matsuyama, K., & Mori, S. (1995). Postnatal development of locomotor movements in normal and para-chlorophenylalanine-treated newborn rats. *Neuroscience Research, 21*, 211–221.

Naka, K. (1964). Electrophysiology of the fetal spinal cord. I. Action potentials of the motoneuron. *The Journal of General Physiology, 47*, 1003–1022.

Nakayama, K., Nishimaru, H., Iizuka, M., Ozaki, S., & Kudo, N. (1999). Rostrocaudal progression in the development of periodic spontaneous activity in fetal rat spinal motor circuits in vitro. *Journal of Neurophysiology, 81*, 2592–2595.

Nakayama, K., Nishimaru, H., & Kudo, N. (2002). Basis of changes in left-right coordination of rhythmic motor activity during development in the rat spinal cord. *The Journal of Neuroscience, 22*, 10388–10398.

Narayanan, C. H., Fox, M. W., & Hamburger, V. (1971). Prenatal development of spontaneous and evoked activity in the rat (Rattus Norvegicus Albinus). *Behaviour, 40*, 100–135.

Navarrete, R., & Vrbova, G. (1983). Changes of activity patterns in slow and fast muscles during postnatal development. *Developmental Brain Research, 8*, 11–19.

Norreel, J. C., Pflieger, J. F., Pearlstein, E., Simeoni-Alias, J., Clarac, F., & Vinay, L. (2003). Reversible disorganization of the locomotor pattern after neonatal spinal cord transection in the rat. *The Journal of Neuroscience, 23*, 1924–1932.

Nurcombe, V., NcGrath, P. A., & Bennett, M. R. (1981). Postnatal death of motor neurons during the development of the brachial spinal cord of the rat. *Neuroscience Letters, 27*, 249–254.

O'Donovan, M. J. (1999). The origin of spontaneous activity in developing networks of the vertebrate nervous system. *Current Opinion in Neurobiology, 9*, 94–104.

O'Donovan, M. J., & Chub, N. (1997). Population behavior and self-organization in the genesis of spontaneous rhythmic activity by developing spinal networks. *Seminars in Cell & Developmental Biology, 8*, 21–28.

O'Donovan, M. J., & Rinzel, J. (1997). Synaptic depression: A dynamic regulator of synaptic communication with varied functional roles. *Trends in Neurosciences, 20*, 431–433.

Okado, N., & Oppenheim, R. W. (1985). The onset and development of descending pathways to the spinal cord in the chick embryo. *The Journal of Comparative Neurology, 232*, 143–161.

Oppenheim, R. W. (1986). The absence of significant postnatal motoneuron death in the brachial and lumbar spinal cord of the rat. *The Journal of Comparative Neurology, 246*, 281–286.

Payne, J. A., Rivera, C., Voipio, J., & Kaila, K. (2003). Cation-chloride co-transporters in neuronal communication, development, and trauma. *Trends in Neurosciences, 26*, 199–206.

Pearlstein, E., Ben-Mabrouk, F., Pflieger, J. F., & Vinay, L. (2005). Serotonin refines the locomotor-related alternations in the *in vitro* neonatal rat spinal cord. *European Journal of Neuroscience, 21*, 1338–1346.

Perrier, J. F., & Delgado-Lezama, R. (2005). Synaptic release of serotonin induced by stimulation of the raphe nucleus promotes plateau potentials in spinal motoneurons of the adult turtle. *The Journal of Neuroscience, 25*, 7993–7999.

Perrier, J. F., & Hounsgaard, J. (2000). Development and regulation of response properties in spinal cord motoneurons. *Brain Research Bulletin, 53*, 529–535.

Personius, K. E., & Balice-Gordon, R. J. (2002). Activity-dependent synaptic plasticity: Insights from neuromuscular junctions. *Neuroscientist., 8*, 414–422.

Personius, K. E., Chang, Q., Mentis, G. Z., O'Donovan, M. J., & Balice-Gordon, R. J. (2007). Reduced gap junctional coupling leads to uncorrelated motor neuron firing and precocious neuromuscular synapse elimination. *Proceedings of the National Academy of Sciences, USA, 104*, 11808–11813.

Petersson, P., Waldenstrom, A., Fahraeus, C., & Schouenborg, J. (2003). Spontaneous muscle twitches during sleep guide spinal self-organization. *Nature, 424*, 72–75.

Pflieger, J. F., Clarac, F., & Vinay, L. (2002a). Picrotoxin and bicuculline have different effects on lumbar spinal networks and motoneurons in the neonatal rat. *Brain Research, 935*, 81–86.

Pflieger, J. F., Clarac, F., & Vinay, L. (2002b). Postural modifications and neuronal excitability changes induced by a short-term serotonin depletion during neonatal development in the rat. *The Journal of Neuroscience, 22*, 5108–5117.

Pinco, M., & Lev-Tov, A. (1993a). Modulation of monosynaptic excitation in the neonatal rat spinal cord. *Journal of Neurophysiology, 70*, 1151–1158.

Pinco, M., & Lev-Tov, A. (1993b). Synaptic excitation of α-motoneurons by dorsal root afferents in the neonatal rat spinal cord. *Journal of Neurophysiology, 70*, 406–417.

Prechtl, H. F. (2001). Prenatal and early postnatal development of human motor behaviour. In A. F. Kalverboer & A. Gramsbergen (Eds.), *Handbook of brain and behaviour in human development* (pp. 415–427). Great Britain: Kluwer Academic.

Price, T. J., Cervero, F., & de, K. Y. (2005). Role of cation-chloride-cotransporters (CCC) in pain and hyperalgesia. *Current Topics in Medicinal Chemistry, 5*, 547–555.

Rajaofetra, N., Sandillon, F., Geffard, M., & Privat, A. (1989). Pre- and post-natal ontogeny of serotonergic projections to the rat spinal cord. *The Journal of NeuroscienceResearch, 22*, 305–321.

Ren, J., & Greer, J. J. (2003). Ontogeny of rhythmic motor patterns generated in the embryonic rat spinal cord. *Journal of Neurophysiology, 89*, 1187–1195.

Rivera, C., Voipio, J., & Kaila, K. (2004). Two developmental switches in GABAergic signalling: The K-Cl cotransporter KCC2, and carbonic anhydrase CAVII. *The Journal of Physiology, 562*, 27–36.

Rivera, C., Voipio, J., Payne, J. A., Ruusuvuori, E., Lahtinen, H., Lamsa, K., et al. (1999). The K^+/Cl^- co-transporter KCC2 renders GABA hyperpolarizing during neuronal maturation. *Nature, 397*, 251–255.

Robinson, S. R., Blumberg, M. S., Lane, M. S., & Kreber, L. A. (2000). Spontaneous motor activity in fetal and infant rats is organized into discrete multilimb bouts. *Behavioral Neuroscience, 114*, 328–336.

Robinson, S. R., & Smotherman, W. P. (1992). Fundamental motor patterns of the mammalian fetus. *Journal of Neurobiology, 23*, 1574–1600.

Rohrbough, J., & Spitzer, N. C. (1999). $Ca^{(2+)}$-permeable AMPA receptors and spontaneous presynaptic transmitter release at developing excitatory spinal synapses. *The Journal of Neuroscience, 19,* 8528–8541.

Rootman, D. S., Tatton, W. G., & Hay, M. (1981). Postnatal histogenetic death of rat forelimb motoneurons. *The Journal of Comparative Neurology, 199,* 17–27.

Rossignol, S. (1996). Neural control of stereotypic limb movements. In L. B. Rowell & J. T. Sheperd (Eds.), *Handbook of Physiology, Section 12. Exercise: Regulation and integration of multiple systems* (1st ed., pp. 173–216). American Physiological Society.

Safronov, B. V., & Vogel, W. (1995). Single voltage-activated Na⁺ and K⁺ channels in the somata of rat motoneurones. *The Journal of Physiology, 487* (Pt. 1), 91–106.

Sako, H., Kojima, T., & Okado, N. (1986a). Immunohistochemical study on the development of serotoninergic neurons in the chick: I. Distribution of cell bodies and fibers in the brain. *The Journal of Comparative Neurology, 253,* 61–78.

Sako, H., Kojima, T., & Okado, N. (1986b). Immunohistochemical study on the development of serotoninergic neurons in the chick: II. Distribution of cell bodies and fibers in the spinal cord. *The Journal of Comparative Neurology, 253,* 79–91.

Scamps, F., Valentin, S., Dayanithi, G., & Valmier, J. (1998). Calcium channel subtypes responsible for voltage-gated intracellular calcium elevations in embryonic rat motoneurons. *Neuroscience, 87,* 719–730.

Schouenborg, J. (2004). Learning in sensorimotor circuits. *Current Opinion in Neurobiology, 14,* 693–697.

Schreyer, D. J., & Jones, E. G. (1982). Growth and target finding by axons of the corticospinal tract in prenatal and postnatal rats. *Neuroscience, 7,* 1837–1853.

Sharp, A. A., Ma, E., & Bekoff, A. (1999). Developmental changes in leg coordination of the chick at embryonic days 9, 11, and 13: Uncoupling of ankle movements. *Journal of Neurophysiology, 82,* 2406–2414.

Simon, M., & Horcholle-Bossavit, G. (1999). Glycine- and GABA-immunoreactive nerve terminals apposed to alpha-motoneurons during postnatal development in kittens: A quantitative study using the dissector. *Experimental Brain Research, 129,* 229–240.

Smith, J. C., & Feldman, J. L. (1987). In vitro brainstem-spinal cord preparations for study of motor systems for mammalian respiration and locomotion. *Journal of Neuroscience Methods, 21,* 321–333.

Snider, W. D., Zhang, L., Yusoof, S., Gorukanti, N., & Tsering, C. (1992). Interactions between dorsal root axons and their target motor neurons in developing mammalian spinal cord. *The Journal of Neuroscience, 12*(9), 3494–3508.

Staup, M. A., & Stehouwer, D. J. (2006). Ontogeny of L-DOPA-induced locomotion: Expression of c-Fos in the brainstem and basal ganglia of rats. *Brain Research, 1068,* 56–64.

Stegenga, S. L., & Kalb, R. G. (2001). Developmental regulation of *N*-methyl-D-aspartate- and kainate-type glutamate receptor expression in the rat spinal cord. *Neuroscience, 105,* 499–507.

Stehouwer, D. J., & Van Hartesveldt C. (2000). Kinematic analyses of air-stepping in normal and decerebrate preweanling rats. *Developmental Psychobiology, 36,* 1–8.

Stein, V., Hermans-Borgmeyer, I., Jentsch, T. J., & Hubner, C. A. (2004). Expression of the KCl cotransporter KCC2 parallels neuronal maturation and the emergence of low intracellular chloride. *The Journal of Comparative Neurology, 468,* 57–64.

Taccola, G., & Nistri, A. (2004). Low micromolar concentrations of 4-aminopyridine facilitate fictive locomotion expressed by the rat spinal cord in vitro. *Neuroscience, 126,* 511–520.

Taccola, G., & Nistri, A. (2006). Fictive locomotor patterns generated by tetraethylammonium application to the neonatal rat spinal cord in vitro. *Neuroscience, 137,* 659–670.

Takahashi, T. (1984). Inhibitory miniature synaptic potentials in rat motoneurons. *Proceedings of the Royal Society of London B, Biological Sciences, 221,* 103–109.

Talley, E. M., & Bayliss, D. A. (2000). Postnatal development of 5-HT(1A) receptor expression in rat somatic motoneurons. *Brain Research. Developmental Brain Research, 122,* 1–10.

Tanaka, H., Mori, S., & Kimura, H. (1992). Developmental changes in the serotoninergic innervation of hindlimb extensor motoneurons in neonatal rats. *Developmental Brain Research, 65,* 1–12.

Tresch, M. C., & Kiehn, O. (2000). Motor coordination without action potentials in the mammalian spinal cord. *Nature Neuroscience, 3,* 593–599.

Tucker, L. B., & Stehouwer, D. J. (2000). L-DOPA-induced air-stepping in the preweanling rat: Electromyographic and kinematic analyses. *Behavioral Neuroscience, 114,* 1174–1182.

Uyemura, K., Horie, K., Kitamura, K., Suzuki, M., & Uehara, S. (1979). Developmental changes of myelin proteins in the chick peripheral nerve. *Journal of Neurochemistry, 32,* 779–788.

Vejsada, R., Hnik, P., Payne, R., Ujec, E., & Palecek, J. (1985). The postnatal functional development of muscle stretch receptors in the rat. *Somatosensory Research, 2,* 205–222.

Verhovshek, T., Wellman, C. L., & Sengelaub, D. R. (2005). NMDA receptor binding declines differentially in three spinal motor nuclei during postnatal development. *Neuroscience Letters, 384,* 122–126.

Vinay, L., Brocard, F., & Clarac, F. (2000a). Differential maturation of motoneurons innervating ankle flexor and extensor muscles in the neonatal rat. *European Journal of Neuroscience, 12,* 4562–4566.

Vinay, L., Brocard, F., Clarac, F., Norreel, J. C., Pearlstein, E., & Pflieger, J. F. (2002). Development of posture and locomotion: An interplay of endogenously generated activities and neurotrophic actions by descending pathways. *Brain Research Reviews, 40,* 118–129.

Vinay, L., Brocard, F., Pflieger, J., Simeoni-Alias, J., & Clarac, F. (2000b). Perinatal development of lumbar motoneurons and their inputs in the rat. *Brain Research Bulletin, 53,* 635–647.

Vinay, L., & Jean-Xavier, C. (2008). Plasticity of spinal cord locomotor networks and contribution of cation-chloride cotransporters. *Brain Research Reviews, 57,* 103–110.

Vult von Steyern, F., & Lomo, T. (2005). Postnatal appearance of 5-HT2A receptors on fast flexor and slow extensor rat motor neurons. *Neuroscience, 136,* 87–93.

Wallace, J. A., & Lauder, J. M. (1983). Development of the serotonergic system in the rat embryo: An immunocytochemical study. *Brain Research Bulletin, 10,* 459–479.

Walton, K., & Fulton, B. P. (1986). Ionic mechanisms underlying the firing properties of rat neonatal motoneurons studied in vitro. *Neuroscience, 19,* 669–683.

Walton, K., & Navarrete, R. (1991). Postnatal changes in motoneurone electrotonic coupling studied in the in vitro rat lumbar spinal cord. *The Journal of Physiology, 433,* 283–305.

Watson, S. J., & Bekoff, A. (1990). A kinematic analysis of hindlimb motility in 9- and 10-day-old chick embryos. *Journal of Neurobiology, 21,* 651–660.

Wenner, P., & O'Donovan, M. J. (1999). Identification of an interneuronal population that mediates recurrent inhibition of motoneurons in the developing chick spinal cord. *The Journal of Neuroscience, 19,* 7557–7567.

Wenner, P., & O'Donovan, M. J. (2001). Mechanisms that initiate spontaneous network activity in the developing chick spinal cord. *Journal of Neurophysiology, 86,* 1481–1498.

Westerga, J., & Gramsbergen, A. (1990). The development of locomotion in the rat. *Developmental Brain Research, 57*(2), 163–174.

Westerga, J., & Gramsbergen, A. (1992). Structural changes of the soleus and the tibialis anterior motoneuron pool during development in the rat. *The Journal of Comparative Neurology, 319*(3), 406–416.

Westerga, J., & Gramsbergen, A. (1993). Changes in the electromyogram of two major hindlimb muscles during locomotor development in the rat. *Experimental Brain Research, 92*(3), 479–488.

Westerga, J., & Gramsbergen, A. (1994). Development of the EMG of the soleus muscle in the rat. *Brain Research. Developmental Brain Research, 80(1–2),* 233–243.

Whelan, P., Bonnot, A., & O'Donovan, M. J. (2000). Properties of rhythmic activity generated by the isolated spinal cord of the neonatal mouse. *Journal of Neurophysiology, 84,* 2821–2833.

Whitaker-Azmitia, P. M. (1991). Role of serotonin and other neurotransmitter receptors in brain development: Basis for developmental pharmacology. *Pharmacological Reviews, 43,* 553–561.

Whitaker-Azmitia, P. M., Druse, M., Walker, P., & Lauder, J. M. (1996). Serotonin as a developmental signal. *Behavioural Brain Research, 73,* 19–29.

Wong, R. O. (1999). Retinal waves and visual system development. *Annual Review of Neuroscience, 22,* 29–47.

Wu, W. L., Ziskind-Conhaim, L., & Sweet, M. A. (1992). Early development of glycine- and GABA-mediated synapses in rat spinal cord. *The Journal of Neuroscience, 12,* 3935–3945.

Wyatt, R. M., & Balice-Gordon, R. J. (2003). Activity-dependent elimination of neuromuscular synapses. *Journal of Neurocytology, 32,* 777–794.

Yamamoto, Y., & Henderson, C. E. (1999). Patterns of programmed cell death in populations of developing spinal motoneurons in chicken, mouse, and rat. *Developmental Biology, 214,* 60–71.

Yvert, B., Branchereau, P., & Meyrand, P. (2004). Multiple spontaneous rhythmic activity patterns generated by the embryonic mouse spinal cord occur within a specific developmental time window. *Journal of Neurophysiology, 91,* 2101–2109.

Ziskind-Conhaim, L. (1988). Physiological and morphological changes in developing peripheral nerves of rat embryos. *Developmental Brain Research, 42,* 15–28.

Ziskind-Conhaim, L. (1990). NMDA receptors mediate poly- and monosynaptic potentials in motoneurons of rat embryos. *The Journal of Neuroscience, 10,* 125–135.

Ziskind-Conhaim, L. (1998). Physiological functions of GABA-induced depolarizations in the developing rat spinal cord. *Perspectives on Developmental Neurobiology, 5,* 279–287.

Ziskind-Conhaim, L., Seebach, B. S., & Gao, B. X. (1993). Changes in serotonin-induced potentials during spinal cord development. *Journal of Neurophysiology, 69,* 1338–1349.

Development of Spinal Motor Networks Controlling Axial Movements

Keith Sillar

Abstract

Neuronal circuits generating rhythmic activation of the muscles during vertebrate swimming are assembled *in ovo*. Close similarities exist between these immature motor networks in fish and amphibian tadpoles despite clear differences in locomotor behaviors. The swimming network comprises excitatory interneurons that sustain swimming and reciprocal inhibitory interneurons coupling the two sides in alternation. After hatching, the properties of spinal neurons, their synaptic connectivity, and the motor output pattern are modified to accommodate changes in locomotion. In metamorphosing anuran amphibians, the axial system is superseded by a new network controlling the limbs. At intermediate stages, circuits for both axial and limbed locomotion coexist. The limb circuit initially expresses a rhythm coupled to the tail beat, before adopting its own independent cadence.

Keywords: *in ovo*, fish, amphibian tadpoles, locomotor behaviors, excitatory interneurons, anuran amphibians, axial system

Introduction

The tasks facing vertebrates with respect to the development of flexible and efficient locomotor systems needed for survival are exceedingly complex. First, the neurons that will eventually compose the central motor control networks of the spinal cord and brain stem must differentiate from embryonic progenitor cells. Second, the functional specializations and anatomical identities of the component neurons must be specified via the expression of genes for numerous neurotransmitters, transmembrane receptors, and ion channels that will confer upon them cell type–specific intrinsic response properties. Third, a complex web of synaptic interactions must be completed to form a central pattern–generating (CPG) network that produces coordinated rhythmic discharge patterns in the various motorneuron pools. Fourth,

the network must also allow for the integration of proprioceptive sensory information resulting from movements as well as exteroceptive sensory information. Finally, to endow these spinal networks with flexibility and to place their output in an appropriate behavioral context in relation to the developmental stage of the organism, the networks must incorporate the projections of numerous descending control pathways. Many of these pathways are fast-acting and involved in the initiation, modification, or termination of locomotion, but other systems are modulatory in function, changing motor activity in the longer term. Neither the precise mechanisms underlying how each of these tasks is accomplished nor how the completion of the different tasks is sequenced during ontogeny is fully understood for any organism. However, significant progress has recently been made using simpler vertebrate preparations, in particular the *Xenopus* tadpole and the zebrafish.

To what extent are the mechanisms contributing to each of these tasks evolutionarily conserved or, alternatively, representative of species-specific deviations from a common vertebrate developmental template? This important question can probably be resolved only through comparative study. At certain levels, for example at the level of CPG network organization, there is compelling evidence across a wide range of vertebrate species that the elementary organization of the CPG is similar, comprising a rhythm-generating "core" based on excitatory, predominantly glutamatergic transmission. Overlying this network of mutually excitatory cells are inhibitory glycinergic interneurons, which appear to play a coordinating role, coupling functionally antagonistic motorneurons in alternation. Many additional species- and developmental stage–specific components are, of course, integral to the operation of locomotor networks, so that both the behavioral repertoire and the way it unfolds during development match both the prevailing body format and the environmental and ecological constraints placed upon that species.

One feature that consistently appears across major phylogenetic boundaries is that the neuronal networks for locomotion are assembled and become functional extremely early in development, before birth or hatching, and prior to the emergence of the behaviors that they will eventually control, so that by the time of emergence, the central nervous system (CNS) alone can generate a basic rhythmic motorneuronal output (Sillar, 1994). This has been shown to occur in a diverse range of vertebrate species including fish, amphibian tadpoles, chicken embryos, and prenatal mammals such as the rat and mouse (for a series of reviews: McClellan, 2001; see also Chapter 10 by Vinay). Whether the same is true in humans is not known, but there is some evidence based on real-time ultrasonography in utero, for example, that as early as 10 weeks of gestation, the human fetus can make rhythmic locomotor-like movements of the legs (De Vries, Visser, & Prechtl, 1984). Since these movements presumably occur prior to the functional innervation of the spinal cord by descending systems of the brain, they may well reflect the output of immature spinal rhythm-generating networks.

An extended period of maturation follows during which the output of the network adapts to often profound changes both in the host organism and its behavioral repertoire. One framework that may facilitate thinking about how this challenge might be met is to reduce the need for change to two fundamentally different components. On the one hand, the network output must adapt to changes in body size and in the constraints thereby imposed on the locomotor system; that is, the network must accommodate quantitative change in biomechanical components. On the other hand, at least in certain cases, entirely new behaviors or body parts appear, necessitating functional reconfiguration of existing networks or even the assembly of completely new circuits. The emergence of limb circuitry during metamorphosis in the anuran amphibian, *Xenopus laevis*, serves not only as an example of how such transitions occur but also as a useful interface between this and the subsequent chapter on limb networks in developing mammals.

Ontogeny of Locomotor Behavior

Motor behaviors emerge in a precisely timed and species-specific sequence often beginning with spontaneous non-locomotor movements occurring within the egg. For example, in zebrafish (Figure 11.1A), the first embryonic movements are detected a mere 17 h after fertilization and involve spontaneous side-to-side coiling movements (reviewed in Drapeau et al., 2002). Four hours later, the embryos become responsive to mechanical stimulation and just 27 h after fertilization, they will swim away in response to touch. The frequency of early swimming movements is generally low (10 Hz) and the episodes of swimming are brief. Average swim frequency then increases approximately linearly to ca. 30 Hz after 36 h. Newly hatched larvae (hatching is at 52 h) are normally silent but will generate burst-swimming at 40 Hz or more when stimulated. By four days, the larvae switch to a beat-and-glide mode of swimming. The axially based swimming system is utilized throughout the life of the organism.

Xenopus frog embryos on the other hand are mainly silent *in ovo* although the first movements, flexions in response to touch, can be triggered when they are released from the egg membranes at developmental stage 26 (ca. 30 h after fertilization when reared at 23°C; Nieuwkoop & Faber, 1956). *Xenopus* embryos can swim when released from the egg after 32 h, around stage 28 (Van Mier, Armstrong, & Roberts, 1989), long before the time they normally hatch (Figure 11.1B). At hatching, they are normally silent, like zebrafish, but when touched, will swim at frequencies of 10–20 Hz.

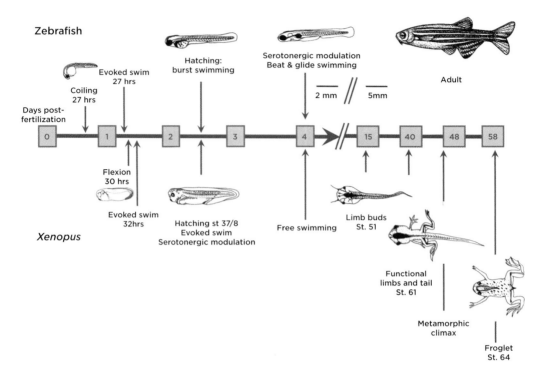

Figure 11.1 Behavioral landmarks in the development of *Xenopus* and zebrafish locomotor systems. In zebrafish the first movements, called coiling, occur *in ovo* after 17 h. Swimming can be evoked 27 h after fertilization. At hatching, burst-swimming occurs and by day 4, beat-and-glide swimming develops, In *Xenopus*, early spontaneous movements are rare, but trunk flexions can be evoked by tactile stimulation around 30 h after fertilization at stage 26. Approximately 2 h later, propulsive swimming can be evoked. At hatching, a robust self sustaining swimming behavior can be triggered by sensory stimulation. Continuous free-swimming occurs later once the yolk sac has been consumed, by stage 45 at around 4 days postfertilization. The fore- and hind limb buds are visible from around stage 50, approximately 16 days after fertilization, but the hind limbs only begin to contribute to locomotion at or around stage 58 (not illustrated). By stage 61, the hind limbs are powerful and generate synchronous extension/flexion thrusts, which assist in propulsion (see also Figure 11.2). At stage 64, around 58 days after fertilization, the tail has degenerated and the froglet locomotes using extension/flexion kick cycles. (For more details on zebrafish see Drapeau et al., 2002. For more details on *Xenopus* see Combes et al., 2004; Nieuwkoop & Faber, 1956; Van Mier et al., 1989.)

The range of swimming frequency increases during embryonic (Van Mier et al., 1989) and early larval life (Sillar, Wedderburn, & Simmers, 1991), but remains episodic and triggered by sensory stimulation until about 3 days after hatching. At this time, around stage 45, the tadpoles become continuously free-swimming. In a closely related species of anuran, the common frog *Rana temporaria*, hatchling embryos are more "reluctant" to swim when stimulated despite being capable of doing so (Soffe & Sillar, 1991) and instead normally only generate spontaneous lashing movements. It is possible that the most appropriate movement at the time of hatching in this species is to wriggle free from the gelatinous egg mass prior to swimming away (Merrywest, McLean, Buchanan, & Sillar, 2003).

Network Output Development

In parallel with, and presumably underlying these modifications in motor behavior, profound and rapid changes in the output of the newly developed networks occur after hatching in both fish and tadpoles. In *Xenopus* tadpoles, the motor pattern switches from one in which brief, relatively constant duration ventral root impulses occur in each cycle of swimming at the point of hatching (stage 37/38) to one in which bursts of more variable duration are recorded in young larvae (stage 42, Figure 11.2A,B; Sillar et al., 1991). This transition is relatively rapid (ca. 26.5 h at 23°C; Nieuwkoop & Faber, 1956), and it follows a rostrocaudal path such that at intermediate stage 40, the rostral ventral roots generate larval-like bursts, but the caudal ones retain the brief discharge typical

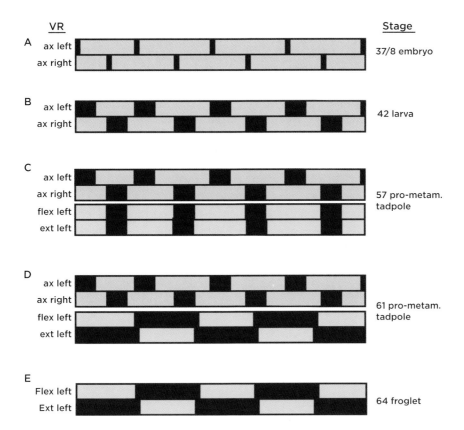

Figure 11.2 Ontogeny of CPG output in *Xenopus*. A, Around the time of hatching. stage 37/38 embryos generate a 10–20 Hz swimming rhythm with ventral root (VR) activity (black vertical bars) to the myotomal muscles (blue background) comprising brief bursts that alternate between the left and right sides. B, Approximately 1 day later, at stage 42, larvae generate ventral root bursts that are longer and more variable in duration. C, By stage 58, when the limbs have become motile, the axial (AX) rhythm persists, but in addition ventral roots innervating the hind limbs (beige background) also generate rhythmic bursts. Notably, these bursts are synchronous between flexor and extensor motorneurons and coactivate with the contralateral axial bursts. D, By stage 61, not only have the extensors and flexors switched coordination to become alternating, the limb rhythm frequency is now distinct and far slower than the axial rhythm. Although the limb and axial patterns are usually active together there is no obvious coupling between them. E, after metamorphosis, at stage 64, the tail has degenerated and only the limb CPGs remain. Fictive swimming at stages 37/38 and 42 (A,B) are compared in Sillar et al. (1991, 1992). In vitro patterns from metamorphic stages (C,D,E) are compared in Combes et al. (2004). Scale bars are approximate and used for illustration only.

of earlier embryonic swimming. The behavioral consequences of this transition are not well understood, but from the perspective of rhythm generation and its flexibility, the larval bursts provide a suitable "substrate" for altering burst duration and intensity and this may be an important prelude to the free-swimming lifestyle that is about to ensue. In zebrafish, the ontogeny of rhythm generation over the equivalent time period follows a rather different course of change (see above). A significant difference compared to *Xenopus* is that zebrafish larvae engage in "burst-and-glide" swimming from day 3–4, a behavior that becomes sustained at day 4–5 (Figure 11.1A). In *Xenopus*, free-swimming is a continuous activity, and although the reasons for

these interspecific differences are not known, it is tempting to speculate that they relate to the different needs of a predatory (zebrafish) versus a filter-feeding (*Xenopus*) lifestyle.

Assembly of Motor Networks during Embryogenesis
Specification of Neuronal Identity

Recently, there has been an explosion of new knowledge on how motor networks of the spinal cord are specified at the molecular level during development (for reviews, see Gordon & Whelan, 2006; Goulding & Pfaff, 2005; Kiehn & Kullander, 2004; Lewis, 2006). While much of this new information derives from work on the mouse, parallel experiments on lower vertebrates, notably the zebrafish (Lewis, 2006), have also yielded important data for comparison. What has already emerged from the implementation of these powerful new molecular genetic approaches is a remarkable conservation of neural network design across the vertebrate class. For example, the differentiation of various neuron types along the dorsoventral axis of the spinal cord is controlled by sonic hedgehog, retinoic acid, and bone morphogenic protein (BMP), which regulate the expression of several neuron-specific transcription factors. In this way, distinct populations of spinal neurons are determined by their position and the way differentiating precursor cells are influenced by gradients of surrounding signaling molecules. Cells destined to become neurons involved in controlling movements and in integrating movement-related sensory feedback are located in the ventral spinal cord; they differentiate into motorneurons and four classes of molecularly defined populations of postmitotic interneurons, called V0–V3. A detailed description of how this differentiation occurs is beyond the scope of the present chapter but the reader is referred to some excellent recent reviews on this general topic (Goulding & Pfaff, 2005; Kiehn & Kullander, 2004; Lewis, 2006).

This combinatorial pattern in turn determines the subsequent expression of cell type–specific transcription factors. In brief, motorneurons arise from precursors that are Hb9, Lhx3, and Isl1 transcription factor–positive. V0 interneurons express the transcription factor Evx2 and will ultimately become primarily inhibitory commissural interneurons with contralaterally projecting axons. The V1 group of postmitotic cells express En1, Pax2, and Foxd3 and in mammals differentiates into a population that processes proprioceptive information and fine tunes motorneuron activity (e.g., Renshaw cells, 1a and 1b interneurons). V2 interneurons express a number of transcription factors including Chx10 (called alx in zebrafish; Kimura, Okamura, & Higashijima, 2006); they possess ipsilaterally projecting processes and their fate is to become the excitatory interneurons responsible for generating the drive to motorneurons during locomotion. Thus, a very precise, phylogenetically conserved pattern of gene expression is involved in the production of the different neuron types that will populate the spinal CPG networks controlling movement.

Role of Spontaneous Activity

The pattern of transcription factor expression is certainly not, however, the only factor involved in determining the transmitter phenotype of the components of spinal locomotor networks during their assembly. For example, as in many other neural systems at early stages of development, notably in the retina (Katz & Shatz, 1996; see Wong, 1999 for a review), spontaneous activity is thought to play an essential role in the refinement of motor network connectivity. Recent experiments on *Xenopus* embryos have provided compelling evidence that levels of spontaneous activity are also important in defining the complement of neuron types in the spinal cord during the early development of locomotor circuitry (Borodinsky et al., 2004; Spitzer, Root, & Borodinsky, 2004). Shortly after neural tube closure, *Xenopus* spinal neurons generate spontaneous patterned activity in the form of calcium spikes (Spitzer, 1994). When this spontaneous activity is experimentally enhanced or suppressed, the transmitter phenotype of different spinal neuron classes changes. This activity-dependent specification of transmitter phenotype occurs in a homeostatic manner, as if the spinal circuitry recalibrates the weighting of synaptic interactions in order to maintain a particular level of network excitability. Thus, experimentally induced suppression of spontaneous activity results in an increased number of neurons expressing excitatory transmitters with a corresponding reduction in the number of inhibitory interneurons. The reverse occurs when activity is enhanced. Hence activity and gene expression interact in the specification of neuronal phenotype during the developmental assembly of the adult CNS.

The appropriate specification of neurotransmitter phenotype may not only be important in the later generation of rhythmic locomotor activity by CPG networks, it may also play a critical formative role much earlier in development when the neurons that form the networks are themselves differentiating. Thus, recent evidence suggests that neurotransmitters can act as signaling molecules in the developing nervous system even prior to synaptogenesis; immature neurons express functional receptors for various transmitters and can respond to them electrically. This form of "noncanonical" signaling, which is distinct from conventional synaptic transmission, is present in many regions of the developing CNS. Glutamate, glycine, GABA, and acetylcholine, which are some familiar players in motor network function during locomotion, have all been implicated in noncanonical signaling, but the details of how neurotransmitters and their receptors act as developmental signaling molecules before synapses have formed is not well understood. One possibility is that the membrane depolarization (and calcium entry) they produce triggers a cascade of intracellular changes, which in turn alter gene expression. In the case of glycine and GABA, traditionally fast inhibitory neurotransmitters, the earliest neuronal responses can be depolarizing due to the fact that chloride transporter expression is lacking, so the chloride gradients are the opposite of normal (e.g., Rohrburgh & Spitzer, 1996; Wu, Ziskind-Conhaim, & Smeet, 1992). Thus, when glycine or GABA binds to its receptor and the associated ion channel opens, chloride ions flow out of the neuron and this extrusion of negative charge leads to membrane potential depolarization.

Direct evidence for glycine regulating the assembly of networks via regulation of interneuron differentiation derives from studies on the zebrafish in which the function of glycine receptors is perturbed by targeted knockdown of the α2-subunit using morpholino techniques (McDearmid, Liao, & Drapeau, 2006). When the receptors are impaired from the onset of development, locomotor rhythm generation is subsequently severely disrupted. The cause of the disruption seems to be that activation of glycine receptors prior to the establishment of network synaptic connectivity regulates interneuron (but not motor or sensory neuron) differentiation. When the α2-subunits of glycine receptors are knocked down, fewer cells exit the cell cycle to become interneurons, so the resulting locomotor network is deficient in interneuronal numbers.

Mechanisms of Swimming Rhythm Generation
Coordination of Locomotor Output

Once the neurons have differentiated and a network of synaptic connectivity has been established, how do the interactions between cellular properties and synaptic physiology generate a rhythm of motorneuron firing appropriate for propulsive locomotion? In order to generate forward propulsion during swimming, the myotomal muscles of fish and amphibian tadpoles must be activated in a precise temporal sequence: muscles on opposite sides contract in alternation to set up local area of body curvature that oscillates between the left and right sides, while muscles on the same side contract in a head-to-tail sequence to propel the region of body curvature rearward. Although species-specific differences inevitably exist, there is a growing consensus that the basic cellular components of spinal sensory and motor circuitry are almost identical in *Xenopus* and zebrafish at equivalent stages of developments (Table 11.1; Roberts, 2000). Perhaps not surprisingly, then, the elementary mechanisms of rhythm generation are also largely conserved, supporting the view that vertebrate spinal cord development and evolution converged on a simple functional network that is retained in some form

Table 11.1 Comparison of Neuron Types, Transmitter Phenotype, and Function of Spinal Classes around the Time of Hatching in *Xenopus* and Zebrafish

	Xenopus	*Zebrafish*	
Glutamatergic			Function
	Rohon-Beard (RB)	RB	Primary mechanosensory
	Dorsolateral commissural (dlc)	Commissural primary ascending (CoPA) Commissural secondary ascending (CoSA)	Sensory interneuron
	Descending (dIN)	Circumferential descending (CiD)	Premotor excitatory
Glycinergic			
	Commissural (cIN)	Commissural bifurcating longitudinal (CoBL)	Reciprocal inhibition
	Ascending (aIN)	Commissural secondary ascending (CoSA) Circumferential ascending (CiA)	Sensory interneuron
GABAergic			
	Kolmer-Agdhur (KA)	KA	Not known
	Dorsolateral ascending (dla)	Dorsal longitudinal ascending (DoLA)	Sensory interneuron

For more details on *Xenopus* see Roberts (2000); Li et al. (2004, 2006); Soffe, Clarke, and Roberts (1984). For more details on zebrafish see Bernhardt et al. (1990); Hale et al. (2001); Higashijima et al. (2004).

throughout the class. This network comprises excitatory interneurons that primarily release glutamate (although other transmitters such as acetylcholine may also be involved; Li, Soffe, & Roberts, 2004) to generate drive to the motorneurons, and reciprocal glycinergic inhibition to help ensure that functional antagonists on the left and right sides are coupled in alternation. It bears remarkable similarities to the spinal network–generating swimming activity in the adult lamprey (Grillner, 2003), and also that generating fictive locomotion in the mammalian spinal cord (Kiehn & Butt, 2003).

Location of the Central Pattern Generator

Much of our knowledge on the neuronal mechanisms underlying the generation of swimming at early stages of development has been derived from studies of swimming in the hatching stage (37/38; Nieuwkoop & Faber, 1956) *Xenopus* embryo (for reviews see: Roberts, 2000; Roberts, Soffe, & Perrins, 1997). The simplicity of this organism and the accessibility of its nervous system to detailed study have greatly facilitated answers to some basic questions such as where in the nervous system is swimming activity produced? Rhythm generation persists after immobilization (e.g., in α-bungarotoxin or curare), indicating that swimming activity is driven by a CPG, and since activity can also be recorded after spinalization, there is clearly sufficient neural machinery to produce swimming located within the spinal cord. However, the ability to sustain swimming is severely compromised by spinalization at progressively more caudal levels (Roberts & Alford, 1986), in turn suggesting that the rhythm-generating machinery extends some way into the brain stem. Indeed recent evidence, based on careful lesioning experiments, points to a small region of caudal hindbrain and rostral spinal cord that is sufficient to generate prolonged swimming bouts in response to a brief sensory trigger (Li, Soffe, Wolf, & Roberts, 2006).

Origins of the Synaptic Drive

Initial studies showed that broad-spectrum excitatory amino acid receptor antagonists like kynurenic acid severely compromise or completely abolish rhythm generation (Dale & Roberts, 1985). During swimming, both AMPA and NMDA-type glutamate receptors are activated, with the latter glutamate receptors being responsible for producing long-duration excitatory postsynaptic potentials (EPSPs), which summate from one cycle to the next to generate a tonic excitatory drive during

swimming (Dale & Roberts, 1985). These data supported the conclusion that glutamatergic interneurons are essential for rhythm generation. However, glutamate transmission is not the only excitatory drive to motorneurons. In fact, there are at least three additional sources of excitation: firstly, the glutamatergic interneurons corelease both acetylcholine and glutamate (Li et al., 2004); secondly, the motorneurons may release acetylcholine not only at peripheral neuromuscular junctions but also at synapses made centrally onto other motorneurons and also onto interneurons (Perrins & Roberts, 1995a, 1995b, 1995c); and thirdly, there is extensive electrical coupling between neurons of the *Xenopus* embryo locomotor network (Perrins & Roberts, 1995a, 1995b). Clearly, rhythm generation in the hatchling *Xenopus* embryo does not rely on a single excitatory mechanism and is therefore very robust.

What role does inhibition play in the production of swimming? Glycinergic inhibition deriving from commissural interneurons presumably plays a role in coupling the two sides of the spinal cord in alternation (Soffe et al., 1984); motorneurons receive mid-cycle glycinergic inhibition during swimming and the commissural glycinergic interneurons are rhythmically active during swimming (Dale, 1985). However, reciprocal glycinergic transmission cannot be essential for rhythm generation, which persists after longitudinal sections through the cord (i.e., a single side can produce rhythmic activity; Soffe, 1989) or after the block of glycine receptors by strychnine (Reith & Sillar, 1999; Soffe, 1989; see, however, Roberts et al., 1986). Curiously, it has proven difficult to interfere with the cross-cord coupling by manipulating the strength of glycinergic transmission in the tadpole; strychnine application, for example, does not abolish left–right alternation during fictive swimming (Soffe, personal communication and unpublished observations). Assuming that strychnine is an effective blocker of glycine receptors, this may indicate that additional, as yet undiscovered mechanisms contribute to left–right coordination during swimming in *Xenopus* embryos. Left–right alternation in the zebrafish at approximately equivalent stages of development also involves glycinergic transmission from CoBL interneurons (homologues of commissural interneurons in *Xenopus*; Table 11.1). In this system, strychnine applied to NMDA-induced fictive swimming switches alternating activity to a rhythm with left–right synchrony (McDearmid & Drapeau, 2006). Glycinergic inhibition is clearly important in both *Xenopus* embryos and zebrafish in the left–right coordination of swimming (although unresolved issues clearly remain) but it also plays additional roles, for instance, in the coordination of activity along the rostrocaudal axis (Tunstall & Roberts, 1994; Tunstall & Sillar, 1993) and in the gating of cutaneous sensory inputs during swimming (Li, Soffe, & Roberts, 2002; Sillar & Roberts, 1988).

An important and, until recently, unresolved issue concerns the mechanisms that sustain swimming. Once initiated by a brief trigger input, swimming is self-sustaining and will continue often for many hundreds of cycles, far outlasting the immediate effects of sensory stimulation. Initial computer simulations of the *Xenopus* swim network pointed to the importance of rebound from inhibition at mid-cycle and to the requirement of positive feedback among the excitatory interneurons in order to sustain activity (Roberts & Tunstall, 1990). Until recently, direct experimental evidence for mutual excitation was not forthcoming, but Li and colleagues (2006) have reported that a population of hindbrain interneurons are rhythmically active during swimming and make excitatory synaptic connections not only with spinal CPG neurons but also with each other. This network of mutually excitatory interneurons produces a reverberating positive feedback excitation that allows swimming to be self-sustaining once started.

Regulation of Locomotor Output Frequency

The locomotor movements of animals vary extensively in speed and strength, from relatively slow and weak to fast and intense behavior. Presumably, opposite ends of this spectrum of behavioral outputs are produced by changes in the operation of a single underlying motor control network. If so, how is this network adapted to accommodate changes in output frequency and intensity? At the level of the output stage, the size principle of motorneuron recruitment (Henneman, 1957) provides a plausible mechanism for incorporating previously silent, higher threshold units into the production of more rigorous movements. However, this does not necessarily provide a good explanation for how changes in rhythm frequency occur; particularly, in *Xenopus* embryos where the majority of motorneurons tends to fire a single action potential is each cycle of locomotion. One possibility is that the number of interneurons that are active in a given cycle determines the cycle period, raising the possibility that interneuron recruitment underlies increases in locomotor frequency (Sillar & Roberts, 1993). An alternative possibility is that interneurons that are already active increase their discharge, for which supportive evidence from the zebrafish has recently been forthcoming (Bhatt, McLean, Hale, & Fetcho, 2007). Using a combination of electrophysiology and calcium imaging, it has been shown that circumferential descending interneurons (CiDs), presumed homologues of descending interneurons in *Xenopus*, discharge during swims evoked by tactile stimulation of the tail but discharge even more in response to stimuli applied to the head, which require more energetic escape maneuvers. The activity of inhibitory interneurons and the strength of inhibitory synapses is also an important determinant of the cycle period during swimming in tadpoles (Dale, 1985; Reith & Sillar, 1999) and zebrafish (McDearmid & Drapeau, 2006) since blocking the inhibition accelerates (but does not abolish) swimming activity. Computer simulation of the *Xenopus* embryo swimming network suggests that low inhibitory conductances lead to fast swimming, whereas large inhibitory conductances produce slow swimming (Dale, 1995).

In summary, it is most probably the fine balance between excitatory and inhibitory synaptic strengths that sets the cycle period, in part by determining the number of interneurons that are active and by setting their discharge rates. The inherent ability of the swimming network to vary the frequency and intensity of output is a property that is accessed by intrinsic mechanisms including modulatory influences that become incorporated into the spinal locomotor networks as development proceeds. Interestingly, evidence from the *Xenopus* tadpole points to inhibitory synapses as the main targets for neuromodulation (Sillar, McLean, Fischer, & Merrywest, 2002; see below).

Postembryonic Maturation of Spinal Cord and Brain Stem Networks
Ontogeny of Cellular and Synaptic Properties

In many networks, the complement of ion channels expressed in the membranes of component neurons changes markedly and indeed is inextricably linked with network development. In the *Xenopus* embryo, ion channels in the membrane of spinal neurons and their contribution to swimming have been well characterized (Dale & Kuenzi, 1997), providing a useful starting point for studies of how this changes during development. Corresponding with the appearance of the more adaptable larval rhythm in posthatching *Xenopus* tadpoles, there is a shift in the balance of cationic currents in spinal neurons;

at stage 37/38, outward currents are dominated by delayed rectifiers, with calcium-dependent potassium (K_{Ca}) channels contributing little to burst termination. However, by stage 42, the presence and contribution of K_{Ca} to swimming increases markedly; blocking of K_{Ca} with iberiotoxin increases the firing of spinal neurons and delays the termination of motor bursts during swimming (Sun & Dale, 1998). Presumably, this developmental alteration in ion channel distribution contributes to the maturation of swimming, as described earlier.

Significant developmental changes also occur in the way that spinal neurons respond following activation of certain neurotransmitter receptors, changes which exert a powerful influence on the rhythmic locomotor output for swimming. In particular, spinal motorneurons acquire the ability to generate NMDA receptor–mediated oscillations in membrane potential during the first day of larval life (Scrymgeour-Wedderburn, Reith, & Sillar, 1997). These oscillations are slow (ca. 0.5 Hz) relative to the cycle periods attained during larval swimming (10–30 Hz), but evidence suggests that the oscillations modify swimming over many consecutive cycles with the plateau phase representing a boost of excitation, which leads to an acceleration of the swimming rhythm (Reith & Sillar, 1998). The induction of the oscillations, which are tetrodoxin-resistant and hence, intrinsic properties of the neurons, not only requires activation of the NMDA receptor but also coactivation of 5-HT receptors. In this respect, the oscillations resemble those described at the hatching stage of *R. temporaria* (Sillar & Simmers, 1994). There is also evidence that similar NMDA oscillations are expressed in neonatal rat spinal neurons (reviewed in Schmidt, Hochman, & MacLean, 1998), which also closely resemble those initially reported in adult lamprey neurons (Wallen & Grillner, 1987). There is no evidence for NMDA oscillations in motorneurons at the hatching stage 37/38 in *Xenopus* (Scrymgeour-Wedderburn et al., 1997) or in zebrafish larvae (McDearmid & Drapeau, 2006), even in the presence of 5-HT. It is possible that the induction of oscillations in *Xenopus* relies on the activation of 5-HT receptors on spinal neurons during the invasion of the spinal cord by serotonergic projections emanating from the raphe system of the brain stem (Reith & Sillar, 1998).

Brain Stem Modulatory Control of Network Maturation

The progressive changes in locomotor output that occur during development are thus due, at least in part, to a precisely sequenced set of modifications in the properties of neurons and their synaptic interconnections. But what activates the switch? There is considerable evidence from a variety of different model systems that neuromodulatory inputs to the spinal cord from the brain are involved and in some cases there is evidence for a causal link between the integration of these inputs into the spinal circuitry and the maturation of locomotor behavior. In *Xenopus* tadpoles, the transition from the embryonic to the larval pattern fails to occur when developing 5-HT projections are ablated during development using a neurotoxin (Sillar, Woolston, & Wedderburn, 1995). In zebrafish, locally restricted populations of aminergic neurons and their projections, including those from the serotonergic raphe, appear in the hindbrain and spinal cord of larvae after hatching, by day 4 (McLean & Fetcho, 2004). In contrast to the situation in *Xenopus* tadpoles, 5-HT only affects the swimming pattern from day 4 onward, once sustained episodes of spontaneous swimming have developed (Brustein, Chong, Holmqvist, & Drapeau, 2003; Drapeau et al., 2002). However, 5-HT has no significant effects on the properties of swim episodes, such as their duration or swim frequency, or on the properties of motorneurons (e.g., neuronal input resistance, rheobasic current, and resting potential). Instead, there is evidence from the zebrafish that serotonin modulates chloride homeostasis to exert its effects on the frequency of swimming episodes during development (Brustein & Drapean, 2006). Taken together, these results suggest that 5-HT neuromodulation becomes integrated early in development of the zebrafish locomotor network to increase its output by reducing periods of inactivity with little effect on the activity periods, in contrast to the neuromodulatory effects of 5-HT in the tadpoles (see below) and in neonatal mammalian preparations (see Chapter 10 by Vinay). Given that the basic rhythm-generating networks of *Xenopus* and zebrafish larvae are constructed similarly, from neuron populations that appear to be close homologues (Table 11.1; Roberts, 2000), it is tempting to suggest that the overt differences that exist in the way that motor system and locomotor behavior are expressed may be due to the differential time of arrival and subsequent cellular influences of modulatory systems, originating primarily in the brain stem.

Modulation, Metamodulation, and Spinal Network Reconfiguration

A primary function of brain stem systems, as they become incorporated in the spinal cord, may be the developmental maturation of motor control networks. However, the same modulatory systems also remain during development and into adulthood where they continue to be involved in short-term network reconfiguration. In *Xenopus* larvae 5-HT, as in other locomotor systems, affects locomotor output (Sillar, Wedderburn, & Simmers, 1992). In contrast to zebrafish at equivalent stages of development (Drapeau et al., 2002; see above), the effect of 5-HT is to increase motor burst duration both in real time and in relation to the duty cycle. The opposite effect is mediated by a second biogenic amine, noradrenaline (NA), in that swimming becomes slower and weaker. Thus the two amines sculpt opposite extremes of network performance (McDearmid, Scrymgeour-Wedderburn, & Sillar, 1997), but how is this regulation achieved? Both 5-HT and NA have direct effects on the properties of spinal neurons, but they also affect the strength of specific synaptic connections within the spinal network. In particular, they have opposing effects on glycinergic transmission—5-HT weakens these connections, whereas NA strengthens them. Since these effects occur presynaptically via modulation of the glycine release machinery, it can be concluded that 5-HT and NA receptors are located on terminals of commissural interneurons in the spinal cord. It is as if 5-HT and NA control these glycinergic synapses rather like a rheostat with profound consequences on the form of locomotor activity that results.

What regulates the activity of modulatory systems that have such differential influences on network activity? "Metamodulation" or, the modulation of modulatory systems, offers a possible answer to this question. In the context of spinal locomotor networks, one metamodulator that has recently been studied is the free radical molecule nitric oxide (NO; McLean & Sillar, 2001, 2004). The role of NO in tadpole swimming is complex and the mechanisms in which it is involved occur on many different levels. On the level of the network output, NO has two main effects; it produces shorter bouts of swimming and leads to reduced swimming frequencies. This net inhibitory influence on motor activity involves parallel effects directly on the membrane properties of spinal motorneurons (McLean & Sillar, 2002) and on the strength of GABAergic inputs to motorneurons with the latter effect serving to reduce swimming episode durations. In addition, however, NO slows down swimming by potentiating reciprocal glycinergic inhibition. This effect is similar to that produced by NA, described earlier (McDearmid et al., 1997). It is the relationship between the NO and the NA effects that place NO higher up in the modulatory hierarchy because the way that NO affects glycinergic inhibition is by potentiating the effects of NA. Thus, NO effects on glycine release are occluded by NA receptor antagonists, whereas in the presence of an NO scavenger, NA can still slow swimming (McLean & Sillar, 2004).

Interspecific Variation in Network Development in Relation to Niche: Neuroecology

Remarkable homologies exist between the networks of vertebrates at early stages of development at the molecular, cellular, and network levels. For example, in both lower vertebrates and mammals, glutamate is an important excitatory amino acid transmitter, which generates much of the synaptic drive required to take neurons above threshold during locomotion. However, these comparisons seem to be at odds with the overt interspecific differences in the way that the behavioral repertoires unfold, using very similar molecular and cellular components of locomotor networks. This dichotomy highlights an important challenge, namely to bridge the gap between molecular, cellular, and circuit properties and how these link with behavior, how these behaviors appear during development, and how behavior interfaces with the animal's environmental niche. There must be critical species-specific differences in the locomotor systems that diverge as the developmental timetable unfolds to provide for divergent behavioral repertoires that are tuned to the organism's environmental constraints. The design, operation, and ontogeny of neural circuits that control behavior must ultimately match the functional demands imposed by an organism's niche, an idea encapsulated by the term "neuroecology" (Robertson, 2004).

The role of neuromodulators in the control of movement at early stages of development is one example of the way in which neurobiology and ecology are beginning to converge. For example, comparative studies on two closely related amphibians (*X. laevis* and *R. temporaria;* reviewed in Merrywest et al., 2004) have revealed species-specific roles for NO in motor control at the time of hatching from the egg. *Xenopus* eggs are laid singly on surfaces in the environment, such as the underside of leaves, and although normally silent, the emerging tadpole can swim efficiently when stimulated. In this species, at the time of hatching, NO has a metamodulatory effect, slowing down swimming (McLean & Sillar, 2000, 2004; see above). In *Rana*, by contrast, a species in which the eggs are laid in large gelatinous clumps, the emerging tadpole does not usually swim but slowly and intermittently lashes its trunk and tail from side to side as if to wriggle free from the egg mass. In this species, NO does not affect swimming but instead triggers the expression of this hatching motor pattern. Interestingly, the neuronal source of NO in the two species appears to be from broadly homologous groups of neurons located in the brain stem (McLean, McDearmid & Sillar, 2001). It seems, therefore, that the species-specific differences in behavior at the point of hatching are partly related to the way in which NO activates downstream targets in the respective motor systems. For each species, the effects of NO are indistinguishable from the effects of NA, suggesting a link between the two modulatory systems. In the case of *Xenopus*, both NO and NA lead to a slow form of rhythmic swimming and in this case, the link has been established with NO acting as a metamodulator to facilitate the effects of NA rather than vice versa. In hatchling *Rana* tadpoles, NO and NA both trigger the hatching motor program, although it is not yet known whether NO functions in this system as a metamodulator with its effects being mediated through the noradrenergic system.

Evolutionary and Developmental Interface between Axial and Limb Networks

Amphibians are an important and diverse group, which provide an opportunity to explore the evolutionary and developmental transition from axial- to limb-based locomotor strategies in vertebrates. For example, many salamanders retain both strategies as adults, switching between the axial system for swimming and the limb system for terrestrial locomotion. The caecilians possess only rudimentary limbs and retain an axial-based locomotor system throughout their lives. In contrast, in anuran frogs and toads, the switch from tail-swimming to limbed locomotion occurs during development. Metamorphosis in anurans is a remarkable transformation involving the simultaneous remodeling of almost every organ in the body (Fox, 1991), including the gut, associated with a switch in diet from filter-feeder to predator, and the visual system, from laterally directed monocular to forward-directed binocular fields of view (Hoskins, 1990). In the context of locomotion, there is the complete loss of the tail, the main structure involved in

generating thrust during swimming in larvae, and the acquisition of the limbs, which produce coordinated contractions of extensor and flexor muscles during swimming, walking, and jumping. During the intervening stages of development, the neuromuscular machinery for the limbs must develop, whereas the tail-based system is still present and functional. Thus, during the metamorphic period, a complete complement of spinal circuitry for the limbs must differentiate de novo within the anatomical framework of an existing network controlling the axial musculature. The entire transition is controlled by two thyroid hormones, T3 and its precursor T4, but the intervening steps between activation of nuclear thyroid hormone (TH) receptors and the simultaneous formation of the limb network and destruction of the tail network remain very poorly understood.

Recent experiments on metamorphosis in *X. laevis* have begun to address this issue via the development of new in vitro preparations of the brain stem and spinal cord, which are capable of spontaneously generating motor rhythms in the limb and/or tail ventral roots appropriate to drive the movements of the host organism's developmental stage (Combes, Merrywest, Simmers, & Sillar, 2004; reviewed in Sillar et al., 2007). The data show that early in its formation, the limb network output adopts the coordination of the tail CPG, supporting the conclusion that the latter forms a functional scaffold for the former (Combes et al., 2004; Figure 11.2C). Only later, once the limbs are fully functional, does the limb network "break free" to produce left–right synchrony of limb motorneuron bursting, with a different, slower cadence than the tail-based system (Figure 11.2D,E). The two systems coexist and are functional, often simultaneously, such that the slower limb kicks assist the faster tail oscillations in generating the forward thrust of the animal. The development of these physiologically viable in vitro preparations offers opportunities to address a suite of hitherto intractable issues. One avenue relates to the way in which thyroid hormones orchestrate the appearance and integration of the limb motor circuitry in specific regions of the spinal cord. One possibility is that thyroid hormones trigger the expression of nitric oxides synthase (the enzyme that manufactures NO from L-arginine) in the spinal cord in a regionally and temporally specific pattern and that NO then engages an ensemble of subordinate developmental and modulatory pathways that in turn regulate the emergence of the limb circuit and the disappearance of the axial system (Ramanathan, Combes, Molinari, Simmers, & Sillar, 2006).

Conclusions

It is tempting to speculate that early in the evolution of the vertebrates, nature settled upon a simple neuronal network capable of generating a basic locomotor rhythm involving alternating activation of functionally antagonistic muscles and that elements of this network have been retained by higher forms as the group radiated. The version of the network that operates across a wide range of vertebrates today is primarily based upon glutamatergic excitation and reciprocal glycinergic inhibition, although many additional components and mechanisms exist and new ones are still being discovered. Nevertheless, the basic circuitry for *Xenopus* tadpole and zebrafish larval swimming shares common operational principles not only with swimming in adult fish such as the lamprey, but also with the limb-based systems of mammals. Variations upon a common design, with layers of additional control pathways appended onto the basic network, provide the phylogenetic richness visible in the diversity of locomotor systems displayed by vertebrates. During evolution and development, major differences in the control of overtly different body parts can, in principle, be accomplished by relatively small and subtle changes in the organization and function of the underlying circuitry.

The two simple and amenable systems offered by *Xenopus* tadpoles and zebrafish have, in combination, yielded important new advances in motor control research and no doubt they will continue to do so. However, more comparative data is needed because sampling just two members of a large and diverse phylogenetic group will provide only a sketchy picture of network design from the perspectives of neuroecology and evolution. Therefore, an important avenue to pursue in future exploration of the ontogeny and phylogeny of locomotor systems is the comparative approach that identifies differences in how the same basic network is modified by the incorporation of layers of complexity in higher and adult forms. If we are to appreciate interspecific differences in the development and evolution of motor control pathways, the devil will lie in the detail.

Acknowledgments
I am grateful to Royal Society, the Wellcome Trust, the BBSRC, and the Leverhulme Trust for supporting work in my laboratory. I thank Jon Issberner, HongYan Zhang, Micol Molinari, David McLean and Gareth Miles for comments on the manuscript and Steve Soffe for helpful discussions.

References

Bhatt, D. H., McLean, D. L., Hale, M. E., & Fetcho, J. R. (2006). Grading movement strength by changes in firing intensity versus recruitment. *Neuron, 53,* 91–102.

Borodinsky, L. N., Root, C. M., Cronin, J. A., Sann, S. R. Gu, X., & Spitzer, N. C. (2004). Activity-dependent homeostatic expression of transmitter expression in embryonic neurons. *Nature, 429,* 523–530.

Brustein, E., Chong, M., Holmqvist, B., & Drapeau, P. (2003). Serotonin patterns locomotor network activity in the developing zebrafish by modulating quiescent periods. *Journal of Neurobiology, 57,* 303–322.

Brustein, E., & Drapeau, P. (2006). Serotoninergic modulation of chloride homeostasis during maturation of the locomotor network in zebrafish. *Journal of Neuroscience, 25,* 10607–10616.

Combes, D., Merrywest, S. D., Simmers, J., & Sillar, K. T. (2004). Developmental segregation of spinal networks driving axial- and hind limb-based locomotion in metamorphosing *Xenopus laevis.* *The Journal of Physiology, 559,* 17–24.

Dale, N. (1985). Reciprocal inhibitory interneurones in the *Xenopus* embryo spinal cord. *The Journal of Physiology, 363,* 61–70.

Dale, N. (1995). Experimentally derived model for the locomotor pattern generator in the *Xenopus* embryo. *The Journal of Physiology, 489,* 489–510.

Dale, N., & Kuenzi, F. M. (1997). Ion channels and the control of swimming in the *Xenopus* embryo. *Progress in Neurobiology, 53,* 729–756.

Dale, N., & Roberts, A. (1985). Dual component excitatory amino acid-mediated synaptic potentials: Excitatory drive for swimming in *Xenopus* embryos. *The Journal of Physiology, 365,* 35–59.

De Vries, J. I. P., Visser, G. H. A., & Prechtl, H. F. R. (1984). Fetal motility in the first half of pregnancy. In H. F. R. Prechtl (Ed.), *Continuity of neural functions from prenatal to postnatal life, clinic in developmental medicine* (Vol. 94, pp. 46–64). Oxford: Spastics International Publications.

Drapeau, P., Saint-Amant, L., Buss, R. R., Chong, M., McDearmid, J. R., & Brustein, E. (2002). Development of the locomotor network in zebrafish. *Progress in Neurobiology, 68,* 85–111.

Fox, H. (1981). Cytological and morphological changes during amphibian metamorphosis. In L. I. Gilbert & E. Frieden (Eds.), *Metamorphosis. A problem in developmental biology* (pp. 327–363). New York: Plenum Press.

Gordon, I. T., & Whelan, P. J. (2006). Deciphering the organization and modulation of spinal locomotor central pattern generators. *Journal of Experimental Biology, 209,* 2007–2014.

Goudling, M., & Pfaff, S. L. (2005). Development of circuits that generate simple rhythmic behaviors in vertebrates. *Current Opinion in Neurobiology, 15,* 14–20.

Grillner, S. (2003). The motor infrastructure: From ion channels to neuronal networks. *Nature Reviews. Neuroscience, 4,* 573–586.

Henneman, E. (1957). Relationship between size of neurons and their susceptibility to discharge. *Science*, *126*, 1347–1347.

Hoskins, S. G. (1990). Metamorphosis of the amphibian eye. *Journal of Neurobiology*, *21*, 970–989.

Katz, L. C., & Shatz, C. J. (1996). Synaptic activity and the construction of cortical circuits. *Science*, *274*, 1133–1138.

Kiehn, O., & Butt, S. J. (2003). Physiological, anatomical and genetic identification of CPG neurons in the developing mammalian spinal cord. *Progress in Neurobiology*, *70*, 347–361.

Kiehn, O., & Kullander, K (2004). Central pattern generators deciphered by molecular genetics. *Neuron*, *41*, 317–321.

Kimura, Y., Okamura, Y., & Higashijima, S. (2006). Alx, a zebrafish homolog of Chx10, marks ipsilateral descending excitatory interneurones that participate in the regulation of spinal locomotor circuits. *Journal of Neuroscience*, *26*, 5684–5697.

Lewis, K. (2006). How do genes regulate simple behaviours? Understanding how different neurons in the spinal cord are genetically specified. *Philosophical transactions of the Royal Society B*, *361*, 45–66.

Li, W. C., Soffe, S. R., & Roberts, A. (2002). Spinal inhibitory neurons that modulate modulate cutaneous sensory pathways during locomotion in a simple vertebrate. *Journal of Neuroscience*, *22*, 10924–10934.

Li, W. C., Soffe, S. R., & Roberts, A. (2004). Glutamate and acetylcholine corelease at developing synapses. *Proceedings of the National Academy of Science*, *101*, 15488–15493.

Li, W. C., Soffe, S. R., Wolf, E., & Roberts, A. (2006). Persistent responses to brief stimuli: Feedback excitation among brainstem neurons. *Journal of Neuroscience*, *26*, 4026–4035.

McClellan, A. (2001). Special issue: Neural development of motor behaviour. *Brain Research Reviews*, *53*, 471–719.

McDearmid, J. R., & Drapeau, P. (2006). Rhythmic motor activity evoked by NMDA in the spinal zebrafish larva. *Journal of Neurophysiology*, *95*, 401–4017.

McDearmid, J. R., Liao, M., & Drapeau, P. (2006). Glycine receptors regulate interneuron differentiation during spinal network development. *Proceedings of the National Academy of Sciences*, *25*, 9679–9684.

McDearmid, J. R., Scrymgeour-Wedderburn, J. F., & Sillar, K. T. (1997). Aminergic modulation of glycine release in a spinal network controlling swimming in *Xenopus laevis*. *The Journal of Physiology*, *503*, 111–117.

McLean, D. L., & Fetcho, J. R. (2004). Ontogeny and innervation patterns of dopaminergic, noradrenergic and serotonergic neurons of larval zebrafish. *Journal of Comparative Neurology*, *480*, 38–56.

McLean, D. L., McDearmid, J. R., & Sillar, K. T. (2001). Induction of a non-rhythmic motor pattern by nitric oxide in *Rana temporaria* frog embryos. *Journal of Experimental Biology*, *204*, 1307–1317.

McLean, D. L., & Sillar, K. T. (2000). The distribution of NADPH-diaphorase-labelled interneurons and the role of nitric oxide in the swimming system of *Xenopus laevis* larvae. *Journal of Experimental Biology*, *203*, 705–713.

McLean, D. L., & Sillar, K. T. (2001). Spatiotemporal pattern of nicotinamide adenine dinucleotide phosphate-diaphorase reactivity in the developing central nervous system of premetamorphic *Xenopus laevis* tadpoles. *Journal of Comparative Neurology*, *437*, 350–362.

McLean, D. L., & Sillar, K. T. (2002). Nitric oxide selectively tunes inhibitory synapses to modulate vertebrate locomotion. *The Journal of Neuroscience*, *22*, 4175–4184.

McLean, D. L., & Sillar, K. T. (2004). Metamodulation of a spinal locomotor network by nitric oxide. *The Journal of Neuroscience*, *24*, 9561–9571.

Merrywest, S. D., McLEan, D. L., Buchanan, J. T., & Sillar, K. T. (2004). Evolutionary divergence in developmental strategies and neuromodulatory control systems of two amphibian locomotor networks. *Integrative and Comparative Biology*, *44*, 47–56.

Nieuwkoop, P. D., & Faber, J. (1956). *Normal tables for Xenopus laevis*. Amsterdam: North Holland Publishing.

Perrins, R., & Roberts, A. (1995a). Cholinergic and electrical synapses between synergistic spinal motoneurons in the *Xenopus laevis* embryo. *The Journal of Physiology*, *485*, 135–144.

Perrins, R., & Roberts, A. (1995b). Cholinergic and electrical motoneuron-to-motoneuron synapses contribute to on-cycle excitation during swimming in *Xenopus* embryos. *Journal of Neurophysiology*, *73*, 1013–1019.

Perrins, R., & Roberts, A. (1995c). Cholinergic contribution to excitation in a spinal locomotor central pattern generator in *Xenopus* embryos. *Journal of Neurophysiology*, *73*, 1015–1012.

Ramanathan, S., Combes, D., Molinari, M., Simmers, J., & Sillar, K. T. (2006). Developmental and regional expression of NADPH-diaphorase/nitric oxide synthase in spinal cord neurons correlates with the emergence of limb motor networks in metamorphosing *Xenopus laevis*. *European Journal of Neuroscience*, *24*, 1907–1922.

Reith, C. A., & Sillar, K. T. (1998). A role for slow NMDA receptor-mediated intrinsic neuronal oscillations in the control of fast fictive swimming in *Xenopus laevis* larvae. *European Journal of Neuroscience*, *10*, 1329–1340.

Reith, C. A., & Sillar, K. T. (1999). Development and role of GABA$_A$ receptor-mediated synaptic potentials during swimming in postembryonic *Xenopus laevis* tadpoles. *Journal of Neurophysiology*, *82*, 3175–3187.

Roberts, A. (2000). Early functional organization of spinal neurons in developing lower vertebrates. *Brain Research Bulletin*, *53*, 585–593.

Roberts, A., & Alford, S. T. (1986) Descending projections and excitation during fictive swimming in *Xenopus* embryos—neuroanatomy and lesion experiments. *Journal of Comparative Neurology*, *250*, 253–261.

Roberts, A., Soffe, S. R., & Perrins, R. (1997). Spinal networks controlling swimming in hatchling *Xenopus* tadpoles. In P. S. G. Stein, S. Grillner, A. I. Selverston, & D. G. Stuart (Eds.), *Neurons, networks and motor behavior* (Chapter 7, pp. 83–89). Cambridge, MA: MIT Press.

Roberts, A., & Tunstall, M. J. (1990). Mutual-reexcitation with post-inhibitory rebound: A simulation study on the mechanisms for locomotor rhythm generation in the spinal cord of *Xenopus* embryos. *European Journal of Neuroscience*, *2*, 11–23.

Robertson, R. M. (2004). Neuroecology. In G. Adelman & B. Smith (Eds.), *Encyclopedia of neuroscience* (3rd ed.). Amsterdam: Elsevier Science.

Rohrburgh, J., & Spitzer, N. C. (1996). Regulation of intracellular Cl$^-$ levels by Na$^+$-dependent-Cl$^-$cotransport distinguishes depolarizing from hyperpolarizing GABA$_A$ receptor-mediated responses in spinal neurons. *Journal of Neuroscience*, *16*, 82–91.

Schmidt, B. J., Hochman, S., & MacLean, J. N. (1998). NMDA receptor-mediated oscillatory properties: Potential role in rhythm generation in the mammalian spinal cord. In O. Kiehn, R. M. Harris-Warrick, L. M. Jordan, H. Hultoborn, & N. Kudo (Eds.), *Neuronal mechanisms for generating locomotor activity* (Vol. 860, pp. 189–202). New York: Annals of the New York Academy of Sciences.

Scrymgeour-Wedderburn, J. F., Reith, C. A., & Sillar, K. T. (1997). Voltage oscillations in *Xenopus* spinal cord neurons: Developmental onset and dependence on co-activation of NMDA and 5-HT receptors. *European Journal of Neuroscience, 9,* 1473–1482.

Sillar, K. T. (1994). Synaptic specificity: Development of locomotor rhythmicity. *Current Opinion in Neurobiology, 4,* 101–107.

Sillar, K. T., Combes, D., Ramanathan, S., Molinari. M., & Simmers, A. J. (2007) Neuromodulation and developmental plasticity in the locomotor system of anuran amphibians during metamorphosis. *Brain Research Reviews.* Special Issue on "Networks in Motion," *57,* 94–102.

Sillar, K. T., McLean, D. L., Fischer, H., & Merrywest, S. D. (2002). Fast inhibitory synapses: Targets for neuromodulation and development of vertebrate motor behaviour. *Brain Research Reviews, 40,* 130–140.

Sillar, K. T., & Roberts, A. (1993). Control of frequency during swimming in *Xenopus* embryos: a study on interneuronal recruitment in a spinal rhythm generator. *Journal of Physiology, 472,* 557–572.

Sillar, K. T., & Roberts, A. (1988). A neuronal mechanism for sensory gating during locomotion in a vertebrate. *Nature, 331,* 262–265.

Sillar, K. T., & Simmers, A. J. (1994). 5HT induces NMDA receptor-mediated intrinsic oscillations in embryonic amphibian spinal neurones. *Proceedings of the Royal Society, Series B, 255,* 139–145.

Sillar, K. T., Wedderburn, J. F. S., & Simmers, A. J. (1991). The development of swimming rhythmicity in post-embryonic *Xenopus laevis. Proceedings of the Royal Society of London B, 246,* 147–153.

Sillar, K. T., Wedderburn, J. F. S., & Simmers, A. J. (1992). Modulation of swimming rhythmicity by 5-hydroxytryptamine during post-embryonic development in *Xenopus laevis. Proceedings of the Royal Society of London B, 250,* 107–114.

Sillar, K. T., Woolston, A. M., & Wedderburn, J. F. S. (1995). Involvement of brainstem serotonergic interneurons in the development of a spinal locomotor circuit. *Proceedings of the Royal Society of London B, 259,* 63–70.

Soffe, S. R. (1989). Roles of glycinergic inhibition and *N*-Methyl-D-Aspartate receptor mediated excitation in the locomotor rhythmicity of one half of the *Xenopus* embryo central nervous system. *European Journal of Neuroscience, 1,* 561–571.

Soffe, S. R., Clarke, J. D., & Roberts, A. (1984). Activity of commissural interneurons in spinal cord of *Xenopus* embryos. *Journal of Neurophysiology, 51,* 1257–1267.

Soffe, S. R., & Sillar, K. T. (1991). Patterns of synaptic drive to ventrally located neurons in Rana temporaria embryos during rhythmic and non-rhythmic motor responses. *Journal of Experimental Biology, 156,* 101–118.

Spitzer, N. (1994). Spontaneous Ca^{2+} spikes and waves in embryonic neurons—signaling systems for differentiation. *Trends in Neurosciences, 17,* 115–118.

Spitzer, N., Root, C. M., & Borodinsky, L. N. (2004). Orchestrating neuronal differentiation: Patterns of Ca2+ spikes specify transmitter choice. *Trends in Neurosciences, 27,* 415–421.

Sun, Q. Q., & Dale, N. (1998). Developmental changes in the expression of ion currents accompany maturation of locomotor pattern in frog tadpoles. *The Journal of Physiology, 507*(1), 257–264.

Tunstall, M. J., & Roberts, A. (1994). A longitudinal gradient of synaptic drive in the spinal cord of *Xenopus* embryos and its role in coordination of swimming. *The Journal of Physiology, 474,* 393–405.

Tunstall, M. J., & Sillar, K. T. (1993). Physiological and developmental aspects of intersegmental coordination in *Xenopus* embryos and tadpoles. *Seminars in the Neurosciences, 5,* 29–40.

Van Mier, P., Armstrong, J., & Roberts, A. (1989). Development of early swimming in *Xenopus laevis* embryos: Myotomal musculature, its innervation and activation. *Neuroscience, 32,* 113–126.

Wallen, P., & Grillner, S. (1987). N-methyl-D-aspartate receptor-induced inherent oscillatory activity in neurons active during fictive locomotion in the lamprey. *Journal of Neuroscience, 7,* 2745–2755.

Wong, R. O. (1999). Retinal waves and visual system development. *Annual Review of Neuroscience, 22,* 29–47.

Wu, W. L., Ziskind-Conhaim, L., & Smeet, M. A. (1992). Early development of glycine-and GABA-mediated synapses in rat spinal cord. *Journal of Neuroscience, 12,* 3935–3945.

Role of Spontaneous Movements in Imprinting an Action-based Body Representation in the Spinal Cord

Jens Schouenborg

Abstract

During development, an action-dependent body representation is engraved at the network level through learning-dependent mechanisms termed "somatosensory imprinting." Somatosensory imprinting depends on the tactile input that arises as a consequence of spontaneous movements during sleep and results in elimination of erroneous connections and establishment of appropriate weighting of correct connections. Spontaneous movements thus provide a key mechanism for adapting sensorimotor circuits to the body anatomy and biomechanics. More recently, data have been accumulating that indicate a role of N-methyl-D-aspartate (NMDA) receptors in somatosensory imprinting. Given that spontaneous movements are a ubiquitous phenomenon during embryonic development in all vertebrates, probing the sensory consequence on spontaneous interneuronal activity in interneurons may be a general strategy employed by the nervous system during developmental self-organization.

Keywords: somatosensory imprinting, spontaneous movements, correct connections, sensorimotor circuits, NMDA receptors, interneurons

Introduction

To be useful in motor control, somatosensory information must be encoded (weighted) with respect to body anatomy and movement patterns produced by the sensorimotor circuits. This is a computationally demanding task since the multi-sensory information (nociception, pressure, temperature, joint angles, muscle force, and length) arises from a complex body constitution. Understanding how the basic sensorimotor spinal circuits are organized and adapted to the body anatomy and biomechanics during development is therefore of great importance. In this chapter, I will review the evidence for a modular organization of spinal sensorimotor networks and then discuss the role of spontaneous movements in functionally adapting these networks during development.

Modular Organization of Sensorimotor Circuits in the Spinal Cord

During the last 15 years, the concept of a modular organization of the spinal cord has grown stronger. The idea of a modular organization of motor circuits in central nervous system (CNS) is not new and this organization was proposed for the spinal cord already in 1981 by Grillner for locomotor circuits ("unit bursters" causing rhythmic activity around a joint) and later for circuits controlling scratch reflexes in the turtle (Berkowitz, 2001; Mortin, Keifer, & Stein, 1985; Stein, McCullough, & Currie, 1998). However, although a modular organization is conceivable, it is not yet clear what constitutes a module in these rhythm-generating systems, the extent to which the different modules overlap, and how sensory information is related to the function of these modules (Tresch, Saltiel, D'Avella, & Bizzi, 2002).

A modular type of reflex organization in the mammalian spinal cord was first demonstrated for the nociceptive withdrawal reflex (NWR) system in the rat (Schouenborg, Holmberg, & Weng, 1992; Schouenborg & Kalliomäki, 1990), but subsequently also in cats (Levinsson, Garwicz, & Schouenborg, 1999), mice (Thelin & Schouenborg, 2002), and humans (Sonnenborg, Andersen, & Arendt-Nielsen, 2002). Here, the word "modular" is used synonymously with the term "functional unit" of a system (i.e., it does not allude to the existence of different motor systems, such as stepping, standing, scratching, or withdrawal reflex systems). For the NWR system, each excitatory module preferentially acts on a single muscle and performs a detailed sensorimotor transformation, resulting in a graded withdrawal of the limb (or part of the limb) from its receptive field. For each excitatory NWR module, the input strength has a characteristic pattern on the skin that mimics the pattern of withdrawal efficacy in a standing position when the principal output muscle of the module contracts (Figure 12.1; Schouenborg & Weng, 1994). In a sense, the pattern of withdrawal (or unloading) efficacy is "imprinted" on the receptive field of the module. It may be worth noting that the sensory modalities converging onto the NWR include receptors that are unloaded (i.e., whose activity decrease) on contraction in the output muscle of the module (Weng & Schouenborg 1998). That temperature receptors do not contribute to the NWR is consistent with this view.

Neurons that encode sensory input in this motor frame of reference, termed reflex encoders (REs; Levinsson, Holmberg, Broman, Zhang, & Schouenborg, 2002; Schouenborg, Weng, Kalliomäki, & Holmberg, 1995), are located mainly in deep dorsal horn laminae IV–VI. These neurons receive and weight the multisensory input from both tactile Ab and nociceptive Ad and C afferent fibers in proportion to the withdrawal/unloading action of the modules in a standing position (Figure 12.2). In fact, a large proportion of the wide-dynamic-range neurons (i.e., neurons receiving a convergent input from tactile and nociceptive receptors), often referred to as wide-dynamic-range neurons, in the deep layers of the fifth lumbar segment appear to be of the RE type (Levinsson et al., 2002; Schouenborg et al., 1995). Within the L4–5 segments, REs for the interossei, flexor digitorum longus, gastrocnemius, peronei, and extensor digitorum longus muscles are located in a mediolateral sequence reminiscent of the corresponding topographical organization of the motoneuron columns in the ventral horn. Hence, the REs appear to be located in discrete pools that have a "musculotopic" organization (see below). It is worth noting that REs of the interossei are located most medially. Since interossei receptive fields are located on the central pads, this explains why this skin area (and not the skin on the digits) is "represented" most medially in the dorsal horn. A corresponding set of inhibitory reflex modules also exists. However, their receptive fields instead correspond to the graded movement of the skin area toward external stimulation (i.e., increase in load) on contraction of

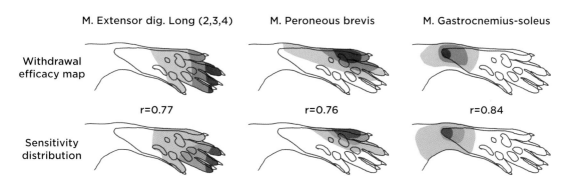

Figure 12.1 Action-based sensory encoding in rats. Typical distributions of sensitivity and corresponding withdrawal action for three muscles are shown. Low-, medium-, and high-dot density indicates areas of the skin on which the withdrawal action and from which the evoked responses on mechanical stimulation were 0%–30%, 30%–70%, and 70%–100% of maximum, respectively. Withdrawal reflexes were evoked by mechanical noxious stimulation. Withdrawal action was defined as the movement vector perpendicular to the skin surface and measured using a 3D motion analysis system. (Modified from Schouenborg & Weng, 1994.)

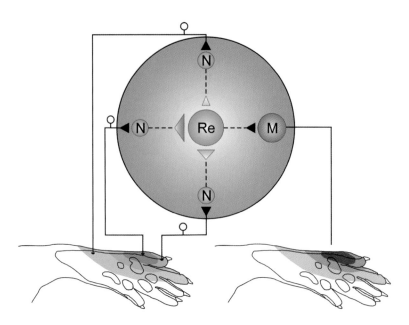

Figure 12.2 Schematic circuitry organization of a withdrawal reflex module. Nociceptive afferents from the receptive field (right) synapse with nociceptive neurons (N) in the superficial laminae of the dorsal horn. Reflex encoder (RE) neurons receive a weighted nociceptive input from superficially located neurons. REs project either directly or indirectly to motoneurons essentially controlling the action of a single muscle. Withdrawal efficacy of the module is shown to the left. Sensitivity in strength of primary afferent input and sensitivity in receptive fields is coded by color intensity. Tactile input is omitted for clarity.

the muscle in the module (Weng & Schouenborg, 1996). As a result of this organization, the excitatory and inhibitory modules are engaged to a degree that is proportional to their respective withdrawal/loading efficacy on skin stimulation. The same principles of sensorimotor transformation in the NWR have been found in rats, cat, mice, and humans (Levinsson et al., 1999; Sonnenborg et al., 2002; Thelin & Schouenborg, 2002).

Based on microstimulation in the dorsal horn of the spinal cord, a somewhat different modular organization of sensorimotor circuits acting on synergistic muscle groups was later proposed in frogs and rats (Bizzi, Tresch, Saltiel, & d'Avella, 2000; Saltiel, Wyler-Duda, D'Avella, Tresch, & Bizzi, 2001; Tresch & Bizzi, 1999). According to these authors, electrical and glutamatergic stimulation of the deep dorsal horn often results in a movement toward an equilibrium point, independent of the starting position of the limb. Here the output of a module would include activity in two or more different muscles. Whether these findings reflect the existence of a fundamentally different type of reflex system than that of the withdrawal reflex system or the outcome of a combined stimulation of many withdrawal reflex modules is not clear at present. In a study by Avella and colleagues, it was suggested

that, by analyzing electromyogram (EMG) in frog hind limbs during "kicking," a combination of a limited number of synergistic units were used for this behavior (Avella, Saltiel, & Bizzi, 2003).

Action-based Sensory Encoding

By mapping tactile input to the dorsal horn, longitudinal cigar-shaped zones that weight the monosynaptic cutaneous tactile input as a function of the unloading pattern caused by individual muscles was found (Figure 12.3; Levinsson et al., 2002). This finding indicates that tactile input to the spinal cord gets organized and weighted in a motor frame of reference already at the level of the first-order synapses and that there may, consequently, not be a true somatotopically organized "map" of the body in the spinal cord as previously thought (Brown, Koerber, & Millecchia, 1997; Mirnic & Koerber, 1995; Molander & Grant 1985; Silos-Santiago, Jeng, & Snider, 1995). Given that one main function of the spinal cord is to translate sensory information into movement corrections, action-based sensory encoding fulfills that function in an economical and fast way.

There are many reasons to think that action-based sensory encoding is fundamental also for higher-order motor systems. For example, the C1,

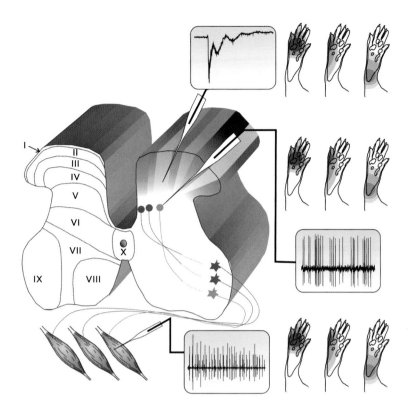

Figure 12.3 Schematic figure of proposed modular organization of the spinal cord. Columns of the dorsal horn receive a cutaneous input that has a specific weight distribution. This weight distribution is the same as that of nociceptive input to REs (interneurons that can encode the withdrawal reflex strength of individual modules) in deep dorsal horn. The REs are assumed to project to single muscles and weigh the input according to the withdrawal efficacy of the output muscle. Sensitivity in strength of primary afferent input and sensitivity in receptive fields is coded by color intensity. Upper recordings, receptive fields of monosynaptic tactile field potentials; middle recordings, receptive fields of REs; and bottom recordings, receptive fields of single muscles. Schematic indication of Rexed's laminae.

C3, and X zones in the anterior cerebellar lobe is divided into microzones, where each microzone is defined by its climbing fiber input from a specific receptive field on the skin (Apps & Garwicz, 2005; Ekerot, Garwicz, & Schouenborg, 1991a; Garwicz, 2002; Garwicz, Levinsson, & Schouenborg, 2002). These climbing fibers receive sensory input that is encoded in the same way as individual spinal modules (i.e., as a function of the unloading pattern caused by single muscle contraction). In cats, it is known that the postsynaptic dorsal column pathway mediates this input to the climbing fibers (Ekerot, Garwicz, & Schouenborg, 1991b). Hence, this pathway appears to signal the evoked activity in spinal reflex modules.

It can be speculated that spinal reflex modules are used by higher order motor centers when executing motor commands to load or unload the skin. If this notion proves to be true, the sensory encoding of the NWR may work as a simple error measurement of the action of the corresponding spinal modules. This notion would be consistent with the assumed role of climbing fibers in mediating motor error signals to the cerebellar cortex. Taken together, the sensory encoding performed by the NWR circuits may prove fundamental for understanding how sensory information is used in motor control.

Functional Adaptation of Sensorimotor Circuits during Development

Given that the adult sensorimotor transformations performed by the spinal withdrawal reflex circuits reflect precisely weighted connections in modules—how can this weighting be achieved during development? While the gross topographical organization of interneurons of the spinal cord is likely to be guided by gradients of trophic substances during development (Albright, Jessell, Kandel, & Posner, 2000; Chen et al., 2006b; Chen, de Nooij, & Jessell, 2006; Kramer et al., 2006), it is difficult to see how such mechanisms could encode the detailed and action-based strength of every connection in a network. The results from the NWR system provide some clues to this problem. The sensorimotor transformations performed by its modules are functionally adapted during the first postnatal weeks in rats (Holmberg & Schouenborg, 1996a). During this time, the strength of the erroneous connections becomes weaker, whereas the strength of the adequate connections becomes proportional to the unloading effect on the skin of muscle contraction. Moreover, during this time, NWR can adapt to both altered innervation of the skin caused by nerve sections (Holmberg & Schouenborg, 1996b) and to altered movement patterns caused by tendon transfer in the neonatal rat (Holmberg, Schouenborg, Yu, & Weng, 1997). Blocking the sensory input during the time of functional adaptation abolishes the learning (Waldenström, Thelin, Thimansson, Levinsson, & Schouenborg, 2003), thus indicating a role for sensory input. Notably, a selective block of the nociceptive input by EMLA salve, a topical analgesic composed of 50%

lidocaine and 50% prilociane (note that EMLA did not block tactile sensitivity), did not have an effect as compared to vehicle treatment. The functional adaptation is not blocked unless tactile input is also blocked indicating a key role for tactile input in tuning nociceptive connections (Figure 12.4A). This conclusion is supported by the finding that tactile feedback ensuing on spontaneous motility in spinal sensorimotor circuits alters the nociceptive connection strengths in NWR modules during postnatal development (Figure 12.4B,C; Petersson, Waldenström, Fåhreaus, & Schouenborg, 2003). Thus, the pattern of tactile inputs arriving in conjunction with the spontaneous movements has an instructive role in the functional adaptation of the reflex modules. Uncorrelated input (given at random time points) does not cause a learning effect. Since this learning process results in an imprint of the withdrawal efficacy on the reflex modules, it was termed "somatosensory imprinting" (Holmberg et al., 1997; Petersson et al., 2003).

The finding that the strength of the nociceptive connections to the NWR network can be functionally adapted by tactile input discloses a hitherto unknown form of cross-modality learning in the spinal cord that solves the puzzle of how a

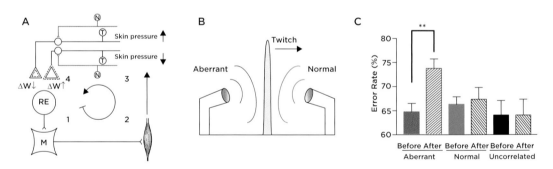

Figure 12.4 Somatosensory imprinting. (A) Proposed learning cycle underlying somatosensory imprinting. A learning cycle consists of the following chain of events: (1) Spontaneous bursts in REs. (2) Motoneuron (M) activation leading to a muscle twitch that causes skin movement. (3) Increased or decreased skin pressure resulting in altered sensory input to pre-RE interneurons. Black lines (T) represent afferents from skin areas from where an increase and decrease, respectively, in low-threshold mechanoreceptor input would occur. Red lines (N) symbolize nociceptive afferents. (4) The strengths of erroneous connections (receiving increased tactile input) between pre-RE interneurons and REs are weakened and that of appropriate ones (receiving reduced tactile input) is strengthened (Dw = change in connection strength). (Modified from Waldenström et al, 2003.) (B) Behavioral experiments. Schematic training setup depicting aberrant and normal training protocol. Distal tail of a sleeping rat pup is shown. Air puffs directed to the skin surface moving toward or away from the air stream is termed aberrant or normal conditioning, respectively. One session of conditioning stimulation lasted for 2 h. Arrow indicates direction of spontaneous tail flick. (Modified from Petersson et al, 2003.) (C) The NWR error rate (%) before and after aberrant or normal tactile stimulation (mean SE). The NWR error rate was significantly increased (Kruskal-Wallis and Dunnett's test, $P < .01$) in rats given aberrant tactile feedback for 2 h (47 training sessions). Normal air-puff stimulation (53 training sessions) had no effect. Control experiments, using random air-puff stimulation (23 training sessions) or no stimulation (23 training sessions) did not affect NWR adaptation (Wilcoxon signed rank test, $P = .65$ and $P = .37$, respectively), ruling out direct effects of the setup, test stimulations, or of uncorrelated stimulation. (Modified from Petersson et al., 2003.)

pain-related system can be learned during post-natal development despite the rare occurrence of noxious events. Notably, this novel form of unsupervised learning occurs during active sleep, characterized by atonia in the skeletal musculature (see Chapter 20) and, usually, with the plantar skin in contact with the ground. The atonic state may be particularly advantageous for learning since the sensory feedback on muscle contraction stands out from a more or less silent background.

A hitherto neglected problem is how the myriad of different types of somatosensory primary afferents, conveying information from different sensory modalities and locations, get organized in the dorsal horn so that spinal multisensory modules receive topographically ordered information. Considering the apparent lack of somatotopic organization in the dorsal root ganglia and that different nerve fiber types enter the spinal cord by different routes and at different times during development, this is not a trivial problem. Indeed, recent data indicate that the adult body representation in the dorsal horn arises from an initially "floating" and plastic organization with many inappropriate connections through profound activity-dependent rewiring, involving both sprouting and elimination of afferent connections. In this process, tactile input seems to guide the alignment of tactile and nociceptive termination since disturbed tactile input patterns results in disturbed termination patterns of both tactile and nociceptive afferent fibers (Granmo, Jensen, Lind, & Schouenborg, 2005; Granmo, Levinsson, & Schouenborg, 2002; Petersson, Mundt-Petersen, & Schouenborg, 2004). The activity-dependent changes in the organization of the primary afferent termination in the spinal cord, including changes in laminar termination patterns of tactile afferents, are paralleled in time by reflex sensorimotor transformations. This suggests that the emerging action-based body representation is at least partly imprinted on first-order synapses. Importantly, these findings suggest that the adult action-based sensory encoding emerges by sensorimotor circuits probing the patterns of tactile input that ensue on movements caused by the effector muscles.

Spontaneous movements are a ubiquitous phenomenon during embryonic development in all vertebrates and mammals (Blumberg & Lucas, 2000; Corner, 1977; De Vries, Visser, & Prechtl, 1982). While a role for spontaneous movements in maturation of motoneurons, motoneuronal axonal pathfinding, and contacts with skeletal muscles appears likely (Hanson & Landmesser, 2004,

2006), their role in the CNS and for sensorimotor learning in particular has, however, not been known. The activity appears to be caused by spontaneous endogenous activity in neuronal circuits in the spinal cord and brain stem (Blumberg & Lucas, 2000; Karlsson, Gall, Mohns, Seelke, & Blumberg, 2005; Kreider & Blumberg, 2000). Although present classifications tend to lump the spontaneous motility broadly into a few categories, detailed studies in humans distinguished 16 different types (De Vries et al., 1982). The prevalence and complexity of these movements lead us to suggest that all major spinal motor systems contribute to the spontaneous movements during development. Furthermore, since somatosensory imprinting is highly effective and precise, we have proposed that all major groups of spinal motor systems learn relevant aspects of the body anatomy and biomechanics during development by probing the sensory feedback after spontaneous endogenous activation. It has also been suggested that the sensory input arising after spontaneous movements guide the tuning of the somatotopic organization of the somatosensory cortex during development (see Chapter 8; Khazipov et al., 2004). It may thus be proposed that sensory input arising as a consequence of spontaneous movements during development also play a key role in the organization of higher-order sensorimotor systems (Seelke, Karlsson, Gall, & Blumberg, 2005; see also Chapter 20).

As yet, little is known about the molecular mechanisms underlying somatosensory imprinting. While calcium transients (Perrier & Hounsgaard, 2000; Russier, Carlier, Ankri, Fronzaroli, & Debanne, 2003) and/or spontaneous fluctuations of glutamate release (O'Donovan 1999; O'Donovan, Wenner, Chub, Tabak, & Rinzel, 1998) have been suggested to play a role for the initiation of spontaneous movements, NMDA receptors may also be involved in the learning mechanisms since the rewiring of the tactile afferent fiber termination in the dorsal horn during development is blocked by topically applied MK-801 (Beggs, Torsney, Drew, & Fitzgerald, 2002; Granmo et al, 2002, 2005; Mendelson, 1994). Moreover, mice that have difficulty expressing hippocampal long-term potentiation (LTP) exhibit disturbed receptive fields of NWR, thus suggesting that LTP-like mechanisms in the spinal cord may be involved in somatosensory imprinting (Thelin, 2005). Unraveling the molecular mechanisms that underlie somatosensory imprinting is clearly an important goal for future research.

Concluding Remarks

Taken together, these findings indicate that sensory feedback ensuing on spontaneous movements has a key role in the functional adaptation of spinal sensorimotor circuits and in engraving an action-based body representation in the spinal cord. It may also be worth noting that the emerging view of the spinal cord as a highly adaptive body–brain interface, translating sensory information into functionally meaningful signals that can be used by the brain in motor control contrasts with the common notion of the spinal cord as a primitive and stereotypic "old" structure.

Acknowledgment

This research was supported by Swedish MRC project no. 01013 and a 'Linne' grant, Knut and Alice Wallenbergs Foundation, and Kocks Foundation.

References

Albright, T. D., Jessell, T. M., Kandel, E. R., & Posner, M. I. (2002). Neural science: A century of progress and the mysteries that remain. *Neuron, 25*(Suppl.), S1–S55.

Apps, R., & Garwicz, M. (2005). Anatomical and physiological foundations of cerebellar information processing. *Nature Reviews. Neuroscience, 6*(4), 297–311.

Avella, A., Saltiel, P., & Bizzi, E. (2003). Combinations of muscle synergies in the construction of a natural motor behavior. *Nature Neuroscience, 6,* 300–308.

Beggs, S., Torsney, C., Drew, L. J., & Fitzgerald, M. (2002). The postnatal reorganization of primary afferent input and dorsal horn cell receptive fields in the rat spinal cord is an activity-dependent process. *European Journal of Neuroscience, 16,* 1249–1258.

Berkowitz, A. (2001). Broadly tuned spinal neurons for each form of fictive scratching in spinal turtles. *Journal of Neurophysiology, 86,* 1017–1025.

Bizzi, E., Tresch, M. C., Saltiel, P., & d'Avella, A. (2000). New perspectives on spinal motor systems. *Nature Reviews. Neuroscience, 1,* 101–108.

Blumberg, M. S., & Lucas, D. E. (2000). Dual mechanisms of twitching during sleep in neonatal rats. *Behavioural Neuroscience, 108,* 1196–1202.

Brown, P. B., Koerber, H. R., & Millecchia, R. (1997). Assembly of the dorsal horn somatotopic map. *Somatosensory Motor Research, 14,* 93–106.

Chen, A. I., de Nooij, J. C., & Jessell, T. M. (2006a). Graded activity of transcription factor Runx3 specifies the laminar termination pattern of sensory axons in the developing spinal cord. *Neuron, 49,* 395–408.

Chen, C. L., Broom, D. C., Liu, Y., de Nooij, J. C., Li, Z., Jessell, T. M., et al. (2006b). Runx1 determines nociceptive sensory neuron phenotype and is required for thermal and neuropathic pain. *Neuron, 49,* 365–377.

Corner, M. A. (1977). Sleep and the beginnings of behavior in the animal kingdom—Studies of ultradian motility cycles in early life. *Progress in Neurobiology, 8,* 279–295.

De Vries, J. I., Visser, G. H., & Prechtl, H. F. (1982). The emergence of fetal behaviour. I. Qualitative aspects. *Early human Development, 7,* 301–322.

Ekerot, C. F., Garwicz, M., & Schouenborg, J. (1991a). Topography and nociceptive receptive fields of climbing fibres projecting to the cerebellar anterior lobe in the cat. *The Journal of Physiology, 441,* 257–274.

Ekerot, C. F., Garwicz, M., & Schouenborg, J. (1991b). The postsynaptic dorsal column pathway mediates nociceptive information to cerebellar climbing fibres. *The Journal of Physiology, 441,* 275–284.

Garwicz, M. (2002). Spinal reflexes provide motor error signals to cerebellar modules—Relevance for motor coordination. *Brain Research Reviews, 40,* 152–165.

Garwicz, M., Levinsson, A., & Schouenborg, J. (2002). Common principles of sensory encoding spinal reflex modules and cerebellar climbing fibres. *The Journal of Physiology, 540,* 1061–1069.

Granmo, G., Jensen, T., Lind, G., & Schouenborg, J. (2005). NMDA dependent changes in dorsal horn somatotopy in the developing rat [Abstract]. *IASP 11th World Congress on Pain,* Sydney.

Granmo, M., Levinsson, A., & Schouenborg, J. (2002). Postnatal changes in dorsal horn somatotopy in the rat [Abstract]. *IASP 10th World Congress on Pain,* P77–P73.

Grillner, S. (1981). Control of locomotion in bipeds, tetrapods, and fish. In V. B. Brooks (Ed.), *Handbook of physiology* (Vol. 2, Section 1, pp. 1179–1236). Bethesda, MD: American Physiological Society.

Hanson, M. G., & Landmesser, L. T. (2004). Normal patterns of spontaneous activity are required for correct motor axon guidance and the expression of specific guidance molecules. *Neuron, 43*(5), 687–701.

Hanson, M. G., & Landmesser, L. T. (2006, December 6). Increasing the frequency of spontaneous rhythmic activity disrupts pool-specific axon fasciculation and pathfinding of embryonic spinal motoneurons. *Journal of Neuroscience, 26*(49), 12769–12780.

Holmberg, H., & Schouenborg, J. (1996a). Postnatal development of the nociceptive withdrawal reflexes in the rat: A behavioural and electromyographic study. *The Journal of Physiology, 493,* 239–252.

Holmberg, H., & Schouenborg, J. (1996b). Developmental adaptation of withdrawal reflexes to early alteration of peripheral innervation in the rat. *The Journal of Physiology, 495,* 399–409.

Holmberg, H., Schouenborg, J., Yu, Y., & Weng, H. R. (1997). Developmental adaptation of rat nociceptive withdrawal reflexes after neonatal tendon transfer. *The Journal of Neuroscience, 17,* 2071–2078.

Karlsson, K. Æ., Gall, A. J., Mohns, E. J., Seelke, A. M. H., & Blumberg, M. S. (2005). The neural substrates of infant sleep in rats. *PLoS Biology, 3,* 891–901.

Khazipov, R., Sirota, A., Leinekugel, X., Holmes, G. L., Ben-Ari, Y., & Buzsaki, G. (2004). Early motor activity drives spindle bursts in the developing somatosensory cortex. *Nature, 432*(7018), 758–761.

Kramer, I., Sigrist, M., de Nooij, J. C., Taniuchi, I., Jessell, T. M., & Arber, S. (2006). A role for Runx transcription factor signaling in dorsal root ganglion sensory neuron diversification. *Neuron, 49,* 379–393.

Kreider, J. C., & Blumberg, M. S. (2000). Mesopontine contribution to the expression of active 'twitch' sleep in decerebrate week-old rats. *Brain Research, 872,* 149–159.

Levinsson, A., Garwicz, M., & Schouenborg, J. (1999). Sensorimotor transformation in cat nociceptive withdrawal reflex system. *European Journal of Neuroscience, 11,* 4327–4332.

Levinsson, A., Holmberg, H., Broman, J., Zhang, M., & Schouenborg, J. (2002). Spinal sensorimotor transformation: Relation between cutaneous somatotopy and a reflex network. *The Journal of Neuroscience, 22,* 8170–8182.

Mirnics, K., & Koerber, H. R. (1995). Prenatal development of rat primary afferent fibers: II. Central projections. *Journal of Comparative Neurology, 355,* 601–614.

Molander, C., & Grant, G. (1985). Cutaneous projections from the rat hind limb foot to the substantia gelatinosa of the spinal cord studied by transganglionic transport of WGA-HRP conjugate. *Journal of Comparative Neurology, 237,* 476–484.

Mortin, L. I., Keifer, J., & Stein, P. S. G. (1985).Three forms of the scratch reflex in the spinal turtle: Movement analyses. *Journal of Neurophysiology, 53,* 1501–1516.

O'Donovan, M. J. (1999). The origin of spontaneous activity in developing networks of the vertebrate nervous system. *Current Opinion in Neurobiology, 9,* 94–104.

O'Donovan, M. J., Wenner, P., Chub, N., Tabak, J., & Rinzel, J. (1998). Mechanisms of spontaneous activity in the developing spinal cord and their relevance to locomotion. *Annals of the New York Academy of Sciences, 860,* 130–141.

Perrier, J. F., & Hounsgaard, J. (2000). Development and regulation of response properties in spinal cord motoneurones. *Brain Research Bulletin, 53,* 529–535, 2000.

Petersson, P. Mundt-Petersen, K., & Schouenborg, J. (2004). Changes in primary afferent termination patterns accompany functional adaptation of nociceptive withdrawal reflexes [Abstract 177.3]. *Society for Neuroscience Congress.*

Petersson, P., Waldenström, A., Fåhreaus, C., & Schouenborg, J. (2003). Spontaneous muscle twitches during sleep guide spinal self-organization. *Nature, 424*(6944), 72–75.

Russier, M., Carlier, E., Ankri, N., Fronzaroli, L., & Debanne, D. (2003). A-, T-, and H-type currents shape intrinsic firing of developing rat abducens motoneurons. *The Journal of Physiology, 549,* 21–36.

Saltiel, P., Wyler-Duda, K., D'Avella, A., Tresch, M. C., & Bizzi, E. (2001). Muscle synergies encoded within the spinal cord: Evidence from focal intraspinal NMDA iontophoresis in the frog. *Journal of Neurophysiology, 85,* 605–619.

Schouenborg, J., Holmberg, H., & Weng, H. R. (1992). Functional organization of the nociceptive withdrawal reflexes. II. Changes of excitability and receptive fields after spinalization in the rat. *Experimental Brain Research, 90,* 469–478.

Schouenborg, J., & Kalliomäki, J. (1990). Functional organization of the nociceptive withdrawal reflexes. I. Activation of hind limb muscles in the rat. *Experimental Brain Research, 83,* 67–78.

Schouenborg, J., & Weng, H. R. (1994). Sensorimotor transformation in a spinal motor system. *Experimental Brain Research, 100,* 170–174.

Schouenborg, J., Weng, H. R., Kalliomäki, J., & Holmberg, H. (1995). A survey of spinal dorsal horn neurones encoding the spatial organization of withdrawal reflexes in the rat. *Experimental Brain Research, 106,* 19–27.

Seelke, A. M. H., Karlsson, K. Æ., Gall, A. J., & Blumberg, M. S. (2005). Extraocular muscle activity, rapid eye movements, and the development of active and quiet sleep. *European Journal of Neuroscience, 22,* 911–920.

Silos-Santiago, I., Jeng, B., & Snider, W. D. (1995). Sensory afferents show appropriate somatotopy at the earliest stage of projection to dorsal horn. *Neuroreport, 6,* 861–865.

Sonnenborg, F. A., Andersen, O. K., & Arendt-Nielsen, L. (2000). Modular organization of excitatory and inhibitory reflex receptive fields elicited by electrical stimulation of the foot sole in man. *Clinical Neurophysiology, 111*(12), 2160–2169.

Stein, P. S., McCullough, M. L., & Currie, S. N. (1998). Spinal motor patterns in the turtle. *Annals of the New York Academy of Sciences, 16,* 142–154.

Thelin, J. M. (2005). Plasticity in mice nociceptive spinal circuits—Role of cell adhesion molecules (Doctoral dissertation, Lund University, Faculty of Medicine, 2005). *Doctoral Dissertation Series, 94,* ISSN 1652–8220, ISBN 91–85439-95–9.

Thelin, J., & Schouenborg, J. (May 21, 2008). Spatial encoding in spinal sensorimotor circuits differs in different wild type mice strains. *BMC Neuroscience. 9,* 45.

Thelin, J. M., & Schouenborg, J. (2003). Postnatal learning in nociceptive withdrawal reflexes in different mouse strains [Abstract viewer/itinerary planner]. Program no. 260.18. Washington, DC: Society for Neuroscience Congress.

Tresch, M. C., & Bizzi, E. (1999). Responses to spinal microstimulation in the chronically spinalized rat and their relationship to spinal systems activated by low threshold cutaneous stimulation. *Experimental Brain Research, 129,* 401–416.

Tresch, M. C., Saltiel, P., D'Avella, A., & Bizzi, E. (2002). Coordination and localization in spinal motor systems. *Brain Research Reviews, 40,* 66–79.

Waldenström, A., Thelin, J., Thimansson, E., Levinsson, A., & Schouenborg, J. (2003). Developmental learning in a pain-related system: Evidence for a cross-modality mechanism. *The Journal of Neuroscience, 23,* 7719–7725.

Weng, H. R., & Schouenborg, J. (1996). Cutaneous inhibitory receptive fields of withdrawal reflexes in the decerebrate spinal rat. *The Journal of Physiology, 493,* 253–265.

Weng, H. R., & Schouenborg, J. (1998). On the cutaneous receptors contributing to withdrawal reflex pathways in the rat. *Experimental Brain Research, 118,* 71–77.

Development of Sound Localization Mechanisms

Daniel J. Tollin

Abstract

Decades of research has demonstrated anatomical, physiological, and behavioral consequences of manipulations of the acoustic sensory environment early in life. These manipulations, either naturally occurring in humans or experimentally induced in laboratory animals, deprive sounds to one or both ears. In this chapter, experience-dependent plasticity in the development of the auditory system is examined with an emphasis on the pathways that subserve binaural and spatial hearing—the coordinated use of information from the two ears for auditory perceptions such as sound location. A balance of inputs from the two ears is necessary for normal development of the central auditory system, and disruption of this balance early in life results in anatomical and physiological reorganization of the binaural auditory pathways and corresponding behavioral deficits.

Keywords: acoustic sensory environment, experience-dependent plasticity, auditory system, binaural hearing, spatial hearing, sound location

Introduction

Auditory-guided behavior depends on the ability of the nervous system to construct an accurate representation of the sounds in the environment. To this end, the auditory system must determine both "what" it was in the environment that produced a sound and "where" in space the sound occurred. Knowledge of both the position of a sound's source and what produced it facilitates the initiation of an appropriate behavioral response. For example, a predator like a cat might move toward the sound produced by a mouse rustling in the leaves while the mouse might freeze or move away from the sounds of the approaching cat.

Binaural hearing refers to the coordinated use of information from the two ears for auditory perceptions such as sound location. For humans, binaural hearing confers additional important perceptual benefits due to the ability to spatially separate and

selectively attend to a particular sound source, such as speech, in the presence of other competing sounds. A typical auditory environment, like an auditorium or classroom, involves multiple and concurrent sound sources. Often referred to as the "cocktail party" phenomenon, our spatial hearing ability substantially increases the comprehension of speech in such noisy and reverberant environments (Yost, 1997). When our binaural and spatial hearing mechanisms are disrupted or do not develop properly, auditory perception in such environments becomes impaired.

The ability to locate sensory stimuli is not unique to the auditory system as it is also shared by the visual and somatosensory systems. The locations of visual and tactile objects are encoded directly in these systems due to the topographic, spatial organization of the receptors, the rods and cones of the retina, and the mechanoreceptors of the skin.

In contrast, in the auditory system, the hair cells of the cochlea are designed to encode sound frequency and intensity and have no mechanisms to sense sound location directly (Yin, 2002). Therefore, sound location must be computed centrally in the auditory system based on the neural representations of the spectral and temporal characteristics of the acoustic stimuli arriving at the two ears. Yet the magnitudes of these acoustical cues to sound location and the manner in which they change with sound location are solely dependent on the physical size of the head and external ears. This creates a challenge during development where the growing size of the head and ears increase dramatically, thus also changing substantially the relationship between the acoustical cues and a particular sound location. The final mature size of the head and ears, and thus the final set of acoustical cues for sound location likely cannot be predicted. Therefore, the precise neural circuits mediating localization probably are also not likely to be genetically encoded. An attractive hypothesis, therefore, is that auditory experience early in life calibrates the neural circuits that process sound source location to the exact acoustical properties of the head and ears of each individual.

The terms "critical period" and "sensitive period" are often used to describe the influence of experience on the normal development of a sensory system, although sensitive period is the term most often used. As distinguished by Knudsen (2004), sensitive periods apply when there is an unusually strong influence of experience on brain development during a limited period of time, times during which important behavioral capabilities are easily shaped or altered by environmental influences. In general, the undesirable effects of abnormal experience during a sensitive period cannot be easily remediated by restoring typical experience later in life. But restoration of normal sensory input for brain functions subject to sensitive periods can potentially lead to a remediation of the problem. Naturally, it is of extreme interest to identify what developmental processes are subject to sensitive periods, and what the durations of those periods are so that appropriate clinical diagnoses and interventions can take place.

It has long been known that environmental sensory experience early in life can have profound and long-lasting impacts on behavior later in life. In this chapter, our understanding of experience-dependent plasticity in the developing mammalian auditory system is reviewed with a focus on the neural pathways and mechanisms that subserve binaural and spatial hearing, including sound localization. Experience-dependent refers to plasticity that is dependent upon the acoustical information available only from the interaction of the organism in its present environment. The chapter begins with a description of the basic mechanisms underlying sound localization including a discussion of the acoustical cues to location. The anatomical, physiological, and behavioral consequences of manipulations of the acoustic sensory environment in experimental animals that have been used to induce modifications in the developing auditory system are then examined. These manipulations include limiting or depriving acoustic input to one ear or to both ears. The results of these studies are beginning to paint a picture of a competitive interaction between the developing inputs from both ears. A balance of inputs from the left and right ears appears to be necessary for normal development of the central auditory system, and anything that disrupts this balance early in development results in substantial reorganization of the binaural auditory pathway, both the anatomy and physiology, synaptic structure, and ultimately behavior. Finally, some of the naturally occurring manipulations of the auditory systems in clinical populations are described that have indicated that there is indeed some form of experience-dependent plasticity in the human binaural auditory system.

Development of Sound Localization—A Model System for Experience-dependent Plasticity

Since the classic studies of the development of the binocular visual system by Hubel and Wiesel, it is now a firmly established tenet of developmental neuroscience that the relative sensitivity, or plasticity, of the nervous system to sensory inputs can be altered by manipulations of the sensory environment within some limited time period of early development (Wiesel, 1982). As the organism matures, the degree of plasticity generally diminishes. The results of these and many subsequent studies have shown that abnormal sensory input for a limited period of time early in life, often called the sensitive period (Wiesel & Hubel, 1965), can alter and modify the structure–function relationship of neural circuits, and can therefore have profound effects on perception and behavior and the capacity for such later in life. These findings likely apply to the development of the auditory system as well, although much less is known. This is ironic because one of the very first conclusive demonstrations of experience-dependent plasticity was in the auditory system, in which Levi-Montalcini (1949) found that depriving neonatal chickens of normal acoustic input resulted in substantial shrinkage, atrophy, and general reorganization in the central auditory pathways. Thus, auditory development is not driven exclusively by genetic factors. One of the goals of basic research in the neurosciences is to determine the relative importance of genetic and molecular mechanisms and experience-dependent influences on the development of neural function so that these findings can be translated into effective clinical interventions. The studies of the development of binaural auditory system focus on these areas of research.

Much in the same way that the binocular visual system provided a good model system for the experience-dependent developmental studies of Hubel and Weisel due to the ability to manipulate the sensory environment of each eye independently, the binaural auditory system also relies on interactions between sensory inputs from two spatially opposed sensory structures, the two ears. The ability to localize sounds results from computations in the central auditory system because the peripheral receptors in the cochlea of each ear have no mechanisms themselves to encode spatial location. In terms of the development of the auditory system, it is known that the structural and functional susceptibility to manipulations of the ear and to environmental influences is by measures of degeneration in at least some auditory nuclei, lost at a very early stage of development, well before the onset of hearing in many experimental animals (Moore & King, 2004). Yet for other auditory system pathways, particularly those subserving binaural interaction, there seems to be a much longer lasting susceptibility to manipulations of the ear and the acoustic environment. This may allow experience-dependent influences to sculpt the final disposition and information processing capabilities of these neural circuits for sound localization.

Sound Localization: The Acoustical Cues and Their Encoding
Acoustical Cues to Sound Source Location

Since the focus of this chapter is on the development and plasticity of the binaural auditory system, it is useful to review the acoustical cues to sound source location and the basic neural mechanisms by which the cues are encoded. There are

three primary acoustical characteristics of sounds, or cues, to the spatial position of a sound source (Figure 13.1) (Tollin & Koka, 2009): the interaural time differences (ITDs), interaural level differences (ILDs), and monaural spectral shape cues. The cues are created by three different ways by which the propagating sound waves from a source physically interact with and are modified by the head and external ear before entering the ear canal. The ITD cues result because the two ears are physically separated in space by the head. The direction-dependent differences in path lengths that sound must travel to reach each ear from the source will generate different times of arrival of the sound at the two ears, or ITDs (Figure 13.1B,E). The ILDs result from the fact that the two ears are separated by an obstacle, the head. For sounds of high frequency (or wavelengths shorter than the diameter of the head), the head casts an acoustic shadow. Consequently, the resulting sound arriving at the ear farthest from the source is attenuated (Figure 13.1B), thereby creating direction- and frequency-dependent differences in the amplitudes, or levels, of the sounds that reach the two ears (Figure 13.1C,D). The ITD and ILD cues are used primarily for localizing sounds varying in azimuth, but are not useful for localization in elevation because their values change little with variations in source elevation. The so-called monaural spectral shape cues, however, do change systematically with source elevation. Spectral shape cues arise from direction- and frequency-dependent reflection and diffraction of the pressure waveforms of sounds by the head, torso, and pinnae that result in broadband spectral patterns, or shapes, that change with location (e.g., the deep "notches" that occur at some locations, like 5.5 and 9.5 kHz for the left and right ear, respectively, in Figure 13.1C).

Neural Encoding of the Acoustical Cues to Sound Location

The three localization cues are initially extracted and encoded at a very early stage in the ascending auditory system. There are three parallel pathways through the brain stem that encode separately the ITD, ILD, and spectral cues. Figure 13.2 shows the pathways that are involved in the central processing of sound location from the cochlea through the auditory brain stem, midbrain, and finally to the primary auditory cortex; note that only one "half" of the ascending auditory pathway is represented in Figure 13.2. Sound entering the external ears ultimately stimulates the peripheral auditory receptors,

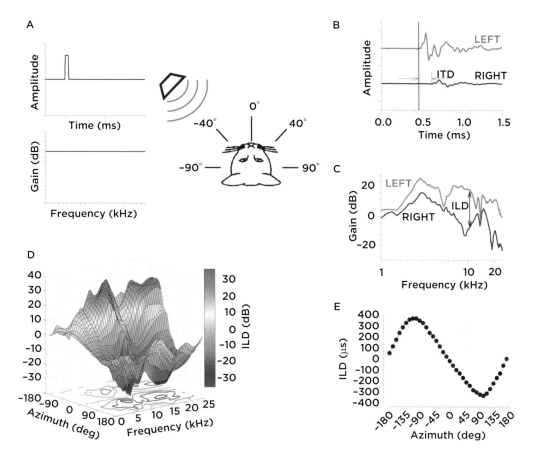

Figure 13.1 The acoustical cues to sound location. In the example, the cues are shown for the cat, but the same three cues are available in all species, although the magnitude of the cues will be different. (A) A broadband transient sound is presented from a loudspeaker at (−40°,0°). (B) The resulting acoustical responses to the transient near the eardrums in the left (red) and right (blue) ears. The difference in the onset times of the sounds at each ear yields the interaural time difference (ITD) cue and difference in amplitudes reflect the interaural level difference (ILD) cue. (C) The frequency spectrum of the acoustical responses in B. The spectral shape cues are captured by the changes in the patterns of the sound spectra as a function of source location. The ILD cue is the difference in sound level computed at each frequency. (D) The joint spatial and frequency dependence of ILDs for sources varying along the horizontal plane. ILDs are a complicated function of azimuth and frequency for high-stimulus frequencies. (E) The ITD plotted as a function of sound source azimuth. ITDs are minimal near the midline and maximal for sources to either side. For illustrative purposes, sources were restricted to the horizontal plane for frequencies between 1 and 25 kHz. (Data computed from Tollin & Koka, 2009.)

the hair cells, initiating the transduction of airborne sound into spatiotemporal patterns of neural activity in the array of auditory nerve fibers (ANFs; see Ruggero, 1992). As a result of the mechanical frequency analysis of sound by the cochlea, the ascending system is organized according to sound frequency. That is, there is tonotopic organization, which refers to the fact that the neurons within the nuclei depicted in Figure 13.2 are arranged according to their frequency selectivity.

Specific details of how each of these cues are encoded by these neural circuits are reviewed in great detail elsewhere (ITD: Yin, 2002; spectral cues: Young & Davis, 2002; ILD: Tollin, 2003;

Tollin, 2008). In short, spectral cues are thought to be encoded in the dorsal cochlear nucleus (DCN), which will not be discussed here. The ITD and ILD cues are encoded in two parallel circuits in the superior olivary complex (SOC). The SOC contains two nuclei, the lateral (LSO) and medial superior olive (MSO), which are the first major sites in the ascending auditory pathway to receive inputs from both ears. The SOC is essential for sound localization; cutting the afferents to the SOC (Masterton, Jane, & Diamond, 1967; Moore, Casseday, & Neff, 1974) or lesioning the cell bodies of the SOC itself (Kavanagh & Kelly, 1992) dramatically disrupts behavioral localization

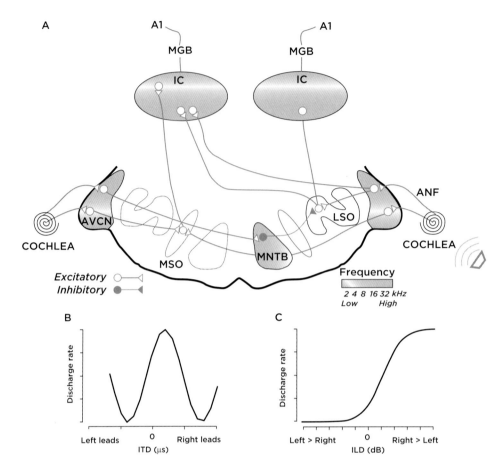

Figure 13.2 Illustration of a frontal section through the mammalian brain stem showing the ascending pathways from the cochlea through the primary auditory cortex (A1). (A) The pathways through the main binaural auditory nuclei when stimulated with a sound source on the right side are highlighted in this figure. The lateral superior olive (LSO), which is believed to be responsible for encoding interaural level differences (ILDs), receives bilateral inputs from both ears. The inputs from the ipsilateral ear (right) via the neurons of the anteroventral cochlear nucleus (AVCN, or just CN) are excitatory (open symbols) but the inputs from the contralateral ear (left) are inhibitory (filled symbols) due to the additional synapse in the ipsilateral medial nucleus of the trapezoid body (MNTB). AVCN neurons receive inputs from the auditory nerve fibers (ANFs) via the hair cells of the cochlea. The ipsilateral excitation and contralateral inhibition allows LSO neurons to encode ILDs (panel C). LSO neurons send excitatory projections to the contralateral inferior colliculus (IC) and dorsal nucleus of the lateral lemniscus (DNLL, not shown) and inhibitory projections to the ipsilateral IC and DNLL. Neurons of the medial superior olive (MSO) receive bilateral excitatory inputs from both ears via AVCN. MSO neurons encode the interaural time difference (ITD) cue (panel B). MSO neurons send an excitatory projection to the ipsilateral inferior colliculus (IC) and DNLL (not shown). Finally, neurons in the AVCN send excitatory projections primarily to the contralateral IC, but there is also a small projection to the ipsilateral IC (not shown). The auditory thalamus, the medial geniculate body (MGB), receives input primarily from the ipsilateral IC and sends projections to the ipsilateral A1. The color bar and shading indicates the tonotopic organization of these nuclei for the cat.

ability. The LSO and MSO separately extract the ILD and ITD cues, respectively. LSO and MSO neurons project to the inferior colliculus (IC), an obligatory relay site in the midbrain where virtually all the auditory circuits that have diverged into multiple streams in the brain stem by and large reconverge (Winer & Schreiner, 2005). In terms of sound localization, most IC neurons are sensitive to sound sources in the contralateral hemifield.

Reflecting the importance of the IC for localization, lesions of its output pathways or the IC itself results in severe deficits in localization performance in animals (Jenkins & Masterton, 1982; Kelly & Kavanagh, 1994) and humans (Litovsky, Fligor, & Tramo, 2002), particularly for sources in the hemisphere contralateral to the lesion.

Sensitivity to ILD cues in LSO neurons results because they are inhibited by sounds to the contralateral ear and excited by sounds to the ipsilateral ear (Figure 13.2A). The input from the ipsilateral ear (right ear in Figure 13.2) is conveyed via ANF projections to the cochlear nucleus (CN), which then sends an excitatory projection to the ipsilateral LSO. The afferent input from the contralateral ear (left ear in Figure 13.2) also comes from the CN, but in this case, the axons project across the midline to the medial nucleus of the trapezoid body (MNTB). MNTB neurons are glycinergic, so their projection to the LSO has an inhibitory effect. Because of the interplay of the ipsilateral excitation from the CN and contralateral inhibition from the MNTB, LSO neurons essentially compute the difference between the neural representations of the sound levels present at the two ears. Hence, LSO neurons encode ILDs. LSO neurons respond best to ipsilateral sound sources that produce ILDs favoring the excitatory ear (Figure 13.2C; Tollin & Yin, 2002; Tollin, Koka, & Tsai, 2008). LSO neurons project bilaterally to the IC. In order to achieve the contralateral representation of space that is a basic feature of higher sensory and motor areas of the brain, LSO neurons send excitatory projections to the contralateral IC and predominantly inhibitory projections to the ipsilateral IC. As a result, most neurons in the IC respond best to contralateral sound sources (e.g., sounds at the right ear in Figure 13.2A) as depicted in Figure 13.2C.

The MSO neurons receive excitatory inputs from the CN on both sides. Via a process called phase locking, the afferents to MSO from the CN on both sides encode the relative time differences (i.e., ITDs) in terms of the precise encoding of the ongoing sound waveform via the trains of action potentials. MSO neurons act as coincidence detectors, increasing their responses when action potentials arrive nearly simultaneously from the left and right ear afferents but decreasing their responses when they do not arrive simultaneously (Figure 13.2B). Although beyond the scope of this chapter (see Yin, 2002), as shown in the figure, the MSO encodes ITDs for sounds located primarily in the contralateral field (i.e., contralateral to the MSO). Unlike the LSO, the excitatory outputs from the MSO innervate only the ipsilateral IC. Consequently, IC neurons that are sensitive to ITDs encode sounds in the contralateral field (Figure 13.2B; Palmer & Kuwada, 2005).

Finally, the CN, including the DCN, which encodes the spectral shape cues to sound elevation, also projects to the IC, but the projection is highly asymmetric, with the IC receiving excitatory input predominantly from the contralateral CN and very little input from the ipsilateral CN (Figure 13.2; Winer & Schriner, 2005). Because of the large-scale convergence of these ascending inputs from the MSO, LSO, CN, and other brain stem nuclei to the IC, it is thought that the IC may represent a site in the auditory pathway that is particularly amenable to developmental and experience-dependent plasticity (Yu, Sanes, Aristizabal, Wadghiri, & Turnbull, 2007).

Why Should the Localization System Be Plastic? Developmental Challenges Faced by the Binaural Auditory System

Why should the neural circuits mediating sound localization and binaural hearing be plastic early in development? And why should auditory system pathways specifically subserving binaural interaction exhibit a longer lasting susceptibility to manipulations of the ear and the acoustic environment (Moore & King, 2004)? Some newborn mammals, including human infants (Muir & Field, 1979; Wertheimer, 1961), have some capability to make orienting movements to the location of sounds immediately at or shortly after birth. For example, kittens, a common animal model for the development of the auditory system, can reliably approach sounds by 24 days of age (~2 weeks after hearing onset), although with considerably less accuracy and precision than adult cats (Clements & Kelly, 1978).

The ability of humans, kittens, and other infant animals to make overt orienting responses to sounds suggests that the basic organization of the binaural system may be established early in development. But physiological and simple reflexive behavioral responses to sounds in general are typically seen much earlier, around the time of birth for cats and in utero for humans (Rubsamen & Lippe, 1998). Moreover, sound localization acuity in humans does not mature until 5 years of age or older (Litovsky & Ashmead, 1994). The apparent delay in directional responding and the long period until sound localization acuity is mature might be related to a slower rate of development of the binaural hearing mechanism, the specific cues for location, or simply motor control. Whatever the reason, a behavioral directional response to sound likely requires at least some development of the central auditory system beyond that needed to respond simply to general acoustic information. This is because accurate localization requires that the specialized binaural mechanisms discussed above (Figure 13.2) be in place to process the cues involved in sound localization (Figure 13.1) and ultimately make the correct association of these cues with the appropriate spatial locations.

Evidence from animal models confirms that the rough circuitry of the binaural auditory system appears to be in place and largely functional even while the peripheral auditory system is still developing. For example, neurons in the LSO (Sanes & Rubel, 1988) and IC (Blatchley & Brugge, 1990; Clopton & Silverman, 1977) are crudely sensitive to the ILD cue to sound localization (Figure 13.1) shortly after the onset of hearing. Developmental studies of ILD sensitivity of neurons in the IC, which receives input from the LSO (Figure 13.2), show some adult-like ILD sensitivity at the onset of hearing in the cat (Blatchley & Brugge 1990), but other studies do not report adult-like sensitivity until 31–40 days postnatal (Moore & Irvine, 1981). By adult-like, it is meant that individual neurons respond over a range of acoustic ILD cues (dynamic range) similar to that found in adult animals. Neurons in the IC of infant cats are also sensitive to ITDs (Blatchley & Brugge, 1990), with some neurons appearing adult-like in their ability to process ITD. Yet other important aspects of the responses are not even close to adult-like, such as the maximum discharge rate, the slopes of the functions relating the response of the neuron to the sound localization cues, and the neural response variance (Sanes & Rubel, 1988; Seidl & Grothe, 2005). These results indicate that while the subcortical neural circuits mediating sensitivity to ITD and ILD are in place and largely capable of some rudimentary function at a very early age, there are still considerable changes that take place during development. The early establishment of the binaural anatomy may allow auditory experience to exert its effects on the binaural system through experience-dependent plasticity. In precocial mammals, such as humans and chinchillas, some of this development likely takes place in utero through the sounds experienced there. However, since much of this early patterning of the auditory system occurs prior to the emergence of electrical activity in auditory neurons, the establishment of these circuits is likely guided by activity-independent factors (see Friauf, 2004). But the experience-dependent sculpting of these circuits later in development ultimately allows for the subtle variations in processing that are necessary to accommodate the organism in its current environment.

One of the purposes of a sensitive period in the development of binaural and spatial hearing might be to accommodate the large changes in the acoustical cues to location that are experienced during development due to growth of the head and ears. Plasticity during development would allow a precise calibration of the neural circuits for spatial hearing to the actual values of the cues associated with the individual. During development, the diameter of the human head nearly doubles (Clifton, Gwiazda, Bauer, Clarkson, & Held, 1988); the same is true for the cat (Tollin & Koka, 2009). That is, the two ears of an adult are not only twice as far apart but are also separated by a much larger obstacle than in an infant. Therefore, the values of ITD at any horizontal location will be roughly twice as large. The ILD values will not only be considerably larger at any one sound frequency due to the larger effect of the head shadow, but also be generated for lower frequencies. There seems to be little effect on behavior of the changing cues due to development since infant and juvenile animals and humans have at least some capacity to localize/orient to sound sources with a decent degree of accuracy (Clements & Kelly, 1978). This would not be possible if the animals were simply interpreting their immature acoustical cues in terms of a genetically predisposed adult mapping of cue values to location. Thus, sound localization behavior appears to be adapting as the cues themselves change.

Experience-dependent Development of the Binaural Auditory System

There are both activity-independent and activity-dependent processes in the development of the auditory system (Rubel, Parks, & Zirpel, 2004). For example, the development of the crude tonotopic organization of the auditory system (the topographic organization based on sound frequency) and the rough anatomical connections between appropriate nuclei and between the two ears is most likely determined via molecular markers that are controlled largely via activity-independent mechanisms (Rubel et al., 2004). Activity-dependent processes on the other hand are thought to exert their affects later in development to control cell growth and death, axonal and dendritic pruning and growth, synaptic strength, and thus the fine-tuning of the circuits. Because many neurons in the normal auditory system are spontaneously active in the absence of auditory input, activity-dependent processes are not necessarily the same as experience-dependent processes. In fact, there are spontaneous responses in the peripheral auditory system prior to hearing onset (Lippe, 1994). As discussed below, the competitive interactions necessary for the development of the binaural auditory system require at least some balanced activity from the two sides (left and right ears), be it due to evoked responses from normal acoustical input or from the spontaneous activity of afferent fibers. Development of sound localization capability, then, seems to be a joint product of genetics and experience-dependent plasticity.

In order to study the experience-dependent role of acoustic stimulation on development, experimental manipulations of the peripheral parts of the ear have been employed to deprive the system of acoustic inputs. Using acoustic sensory deprivation gives the experimenter some control over the acoustic environment that an animal is reared in. Studies in such animals have revealed a variety of changes in central auditory neurons following experimentally induced or naturally occurring deafness. Depriving experimental animals (or humans) of normal auditory input during restricted periods of early development alters the normal formation of neural circuits for sound localization in an often irreversible fashion. Based on such experiments, it has been hypothesized that in the development of binaural and spatial hearing, a competition between the two ears takes place for synaptic space on binaurally innervated neurons in the auditory brain stem (Moore, Hutchings, King, & Kowalchuk, 1989). This hypothesis is examined in the following section.

Acoustic Deprivation—Control of Sensory Experience

There are several different methods that have been used to modify the acoustic experience in experimental animals to study the experience-dependent aspects of auditory system development. Two techniques have been most commonly used: (1) conductive hearing losses that interfere mechanically with the normal acoustic input pathways to the inner ear and (2) sensorineural hearing losses that directly interfere with the neural transduction mechanisms, either by removing or damaging the cochlea, hair cells, and/or ANF array. The former modifies the acoustic input, which simply reduces, but does not eliminate, the overall level of sound-evoked activity in the peripheral auditory system. While conductive losses have no effect on spontaneous activity levels, sensorineural manipulation reduces or, in many cases, even abolishes both

sound-evoked and spontaneous activity (Tucci, Born, & Rubel, 1987). It has to be kept in mind that studies that have used these techniques to examine the sensitive period in the development of the auditory system have been complicated by the fact that most procedures used to deprive the experimental animals of normal auditory experience have been either irreversible (cochlear ablation, hair cell destruction, etc.), or if they were reversible (ear plugs, ear canal atresia, etc.), they do not provide sufficient deprivation of sound to eliminate all neural activity. Moreover, even with the latter, less invasive type of deprivation, it has typically not been demonstrated by the experimenter that some form of sensorineural hearing loss did not develop as an unintended consequence of the manipulation.

There are many good experimental and logical reasons for using both kinds of deprivation techniques. Conductive hearing losses are of interest because they are potentially reversible (e.g., ear plugs) and do not typically result in any peripheral neuron death (discussed below). Moreover, the spontaneous activity of peripheral neurons is preserved. With this technique, the auditory system can be tested for functionality at some time after the deprivation. For example, behavioral and/or neural responses to sounds of interest presented to the manipulated ear could be examined. Complete, but reversible auditory deprivation is difficult to achieve in experimental animals because simply occluding an ear to airborne sound does not preclude bone-conducted sound. The final advantage is that conductive hearing losses simulate known human hearing disorders. The sensorineural method induces complete irreversible damage of the inner ear (via ototoxic drug exposure, noise exposure, or ablation of the cochlea). This method has the advantage that it typically results in complete removal of not only sound-evoked but also spontaneous neural activity. Clearly the limitation of this technique is that it does not allow for the testing of the physiological or behavioral consequences of the manipulated ear at some later age because there is typically substantial peripheral neuron death (although such systems can be stimulated electrically). Moreover, sensorineural manipulations do not really simulate any common human hearing disorders (Moore & King, 2004). Therefore, the clinical value of such experiments may not be informative for human auditory pathology.

In the following discussion of the anatomical, physiological, and behavioral consequences of unilateral (one ear) and bilateral (both ears) sound deprivation, reference will not be made to what kind of experimental manipulation (conductive or sensorineural) was employed, unless it is critical for the interpretation of the data. However, there are two critically important differences in the outcomes of experiments using the two different techniques that should be kept in mind. These differences depend on the age of the animal. First, in altricial animals (which are born deaf), peripheral neurons (ANF, CN, etc.) are lost (neuron death) in massive numbers when cochlear ablation is induced *before* the onset of hearing function (Hashisaki & Rubel, 1989; Tierney, Russell, & Moore, 1997). This seems to be the result of abolishing the intrinsic spontaneous activity that is present in peripheral auditory neurons even before hearing onset (Lippe, 1994). It is known that destroying the cochlea (Koerber, Pfeiffer, Warr, & Kiang, 1966) or chemically silencing the electrical activity of hair cells (Pasic, Moore, & Rubel, 1994) abolishes spontaneous activity in central auditory neurons. Thus, there appears to be a correlation between hearing onset and neuron loss in response to a peripheral sensorineural hearing loss. If cochlear ablation or hair cell activity silencing occurs prior to hearing onset, there is neuron loss on a massive scale; if the

cochlear ablation or hair cell activity silencing is near hearing onset or after, there is no neuron loss, only soma shrinkage and a reduction in the volume of auditory nuclei (CN, LSO, etc., Figure 13.2) that receive excitatory input from the manipulated ear as well as other synaptic changes that will be discussed below. Conductive hearing losses induced at any point during development do not result in neuron death, but can result in substantial reduction in neuron size and nucleus volume and can lead to large-scale synaptic modifications. Finally, as stated earlier, experiments employing sensorineural hearing losses do not allow for functional assessment of the system, behaviorally or neurally, at a later time period.

Monaural Sound Deprivation—A Case of "Use It or Lose It?"

The studies reviewed here on the development of the auditory system suggest that early deprivation of auditory experience can produce structural and organizational changes in the auditory pathway. Here the anatomical, physiological, and then behavioral consequences of monaural sound deprivation are discussed, with an emphasis on how this manipulation affects binaural and spatial hearing. Figure 13.3A shows a simplified schematic of the

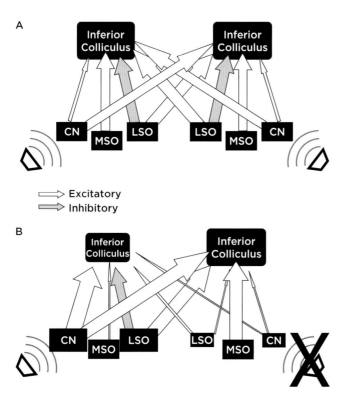

Figure 13.3 Illustration of the normal auditory pathways through the inferior colliculus (IC). See Figure 13.2 for details. (A) The inputs to the ICs of both sides are balanced in the normal auditory system. (B) After unilateral deprivation of the right ear, there are large-scale changes in the balance of the ascending pathways to the ICs. The auditory nerve (not shown), cochlear nucleus (CN), medial nucleus of the trapezoid body (MNTB, not shown), lateral superior olive (LSO), and IC all exhibit volume reductions, neuron shrinkage and/or death, and morphological and synaptic changes, as indicated by the smaller size of the nucleus in the figure. Moreover, the patterns and strengths of projections to the IC from the brain stem nuclei are altered, as indicated by increases or reductions in the widths of the projections relative to normal (panel A). After bilateral deprivation (not shown), the circuit resembles the normal-hearing circuit in A.

anatomical pathways from the CN through to the IC (see Figure 13.2 for details). The relative size of the arrows roughly indicates the number and strength of the neural projections between nuclei. The shading indicates excitatory (open) or inhibitory (shaded) connections. In the normally developed auditory system, the inputs from the two sides of the brain stem to the ICs on both sides are balanced. In the following, the changes that occur to this circuit due to altered auditory experience are examined.

ANATOMICAL CHANGES

Neonatal animals raised with a unilateral hearing loss (right ear, Figure 13.2B) of either type, conductive or sensorineural, show profound changes in the anatomy of the ascending auditory system. The auditory nerve shrinks or dies (not shown in Figure 13.2B; Hardie & Shepherd, 1999; Moore et al., 1989; Moore & Kowalchuk, 1988; Webster, 1983a, 1983b) and there is a large decrease in the size and density of neurons in the ipsilateral CN on the affected side, particularly in the ventral regions of the CN, whose neurons send projections to the MSO and LSO for sound localization (Figure 13.2B; Blatchley, Williams, & Coleman, 1983; Coleman, Blatchley, & Williams, 1982; Coleman & O'Connor, 1979; Hardie & Shepherd, 1999; Moore et al., 1989; Moore & Kowalchuk, 1988; Nordeen, Killackey, & Kitzes, 1983; Tierney et al., 1997; Trune, 1982a, 1982b; Webster, 1983a, 1983b, 1988; Webster & Webster, 1977, 1979). The cross-sectional area of the dendritic fields of CN neurons ipsilateral to the affected ear are reduced by half (Trune, 1982b). The auditory nerve and CN on the side of the unaffected ear are largely normal. These observed effects are illustrated in Figure 13.2B by the reduction in size of the CN on the side of the manipulated ear (right ear).

The effects of monaural deprivation on the morphology of these peripheral neurons tended to depend upon the age at which the deprivation occurred. In rats, Blatchley et al. (1983) found that neurons in the ventral cochlear nucleus (VCN) were most affected when the deprivation was initiated between 10 and 16 days after birth. As the deprivation was initiated later, the effects on the VCN were reduced. Webster (1983b) found a similar trend in mice were a unilateral conductive loss had the most effect on VCN cell size and volume if the loss spanned a restricted period from 12 to 24 days after birth. Deprivation ending before 12 days or initiated after 24 days resulted in little change in

the VCN. Other studies have shown little effect of conductive hearing losses on VCN neuron size or volume (Moore et al., 1989). The reasons for these discrepancies are not known.

The binaural nuclei are also affected by unilateral manipulations of the ear. Removing or reducing sound-evoked (and spontaneous) activity from one side clearly disrupts the balance of neural inputs to the MSO and LSO. The normal balance of inputs to these nuclei (Figure 13.3A) is reduced (conductive loss) or eliminated (sensorineural loss), and as such, the ability of MSO and LSO neurons to process the binaural cues to sound location, ITD and ILDs, respectively, will also be disrupted. Anatomically, unilateral cochlear ablation in adult cats produced shrinkage of neurons in ipsilateral LSO (right side, Figure 13.3B) and contralateral MNTB (not shown), but no loss of neurons (Powell & Erulkar, 1962). Conductive losses also produce substantial neuron shrinkage in contralateral MNTB (Moore, 1992; Webster, 1983a, 1983b). Pasic et al. (1994) reported substantial neuron shrinkage, but no loss of contralateral MNTB in response to chemical blockade of electrical activity in the cochleas of juvenile, but not infant, gerbils. Neurons in the LSO ipsilateral to the manipulated ear (Figure 13.3B) also exhibit profound shrinkage (conductive loss: Webster, 1983a, 1983b) and loss (sensorineural loss: Moore, 1992). There are also substantial morphological changes in the dendritic arbors of LSO neurons (Sanes, Markowitz, Bernstein, & Wardlow, 1992). Interestingly, LSO neurons contralateral to the manipulated ear (left side, Figure 13.3B) do not show shrinkage or loss. Recall that LSO receives inputs from both ears (Figure 13.2), that is, excitation from the ipsilateral and inhibition from the contralateral ear. The fact that LSO neurons ipsilateral but not contralateral to the manipulated ear show shrinkage and loss suggests that the contralateral inhibitory input to the LSO ipsilateral to the manipulation is not sufficient to maintain the LSO (Moore, 1992). Excitatory synapses appear to be required to strengthen and maintain synaptic connections, neuron size, and nucleus volume.

In support of this hypothesis, unilateral manipulations do not lead to neuron shrinkage or loss in the MSO of either side (Russell & Moore, 2002; Webster, 1983a, 1983b). MSO neurons receive predominantly excitatory inputs from each ear. There are, however, large-scale morphological changes in MSO neurons. MSO neurons have a bipolar morphology with dendrites extending medially and laterally in the brain stem. The medial dendrites receive input from the contralateral CN while the lateral dendrites from the ipsilateral CN (e.g., Figure 13.2A). In response to unilateral hearing loss (right ear, Figure 13.3B), changes occur in the MSO on both sides of the brain stem; the dendrites receiving inputs from the side of the manipulation degenerate while the dendrites receiving input from the normal ear expand (Feng & Rogowski, 1980; Perkin, 1973; Russell & Moore, 1999). There is also evidence that sensorineural losses before the onset of hearing can lead to the growth of novel neural connections between the CN, MNTB, LSO, and MSO (Kitzes, Kageyama, Semple, & Kil, 1995; Russell & Moore, 1995), but this topic is beyond the scope of this chapter (see Moore & King, 2004). Finally, neurons in the IC are also affected by unilateral hearing loss. Neurons in the IC contralateral to the manipulated ear (left side, Figure 13.3B) exhibit shrinkage (Webster, 1983a, 1983b). Such manipulations in adult animals do not result in shrinkage (Webster, 1983b). Moreover, unilateral deafness does not alter synaptic density in the IC on either side in cats (Hardie, Martsi-McClintock, Aitkin, & Shepherd, 1998).

In addition to the changes in neuron size and morphology resulting from unilateral manipulations of the ear, there are also substantial changes in the strength and magnitudes of the afferent projections from one nucleus to another. As reviewed earlier (e.g., Figure 13.2), the IC receives bilateral inputs from all brain stem nuclei, but in a highly asymmetric manner (Figure 13.3A). In normal-hearing animals (e.g., Figure 13.2 and 13.3A), the major afferent projection to the IC from the CN is contralateral with a very small ipsilateral projection (Moore et al., 1989; Nordeen et al., 1983; Oliver, 1987). Neonatal removal of the cochlea changes the CN neuron projections to the IC in dramatic ways. For example, the IC on the side of the unlesioned ear (Figure 13.3B, left side) receives 40% more inputs than normal from the ipsilateral CN (Moore & Kowalchuck, 1988; Nordeen et al., 1983), but the projections to the contralateral IC from the CN of the unlesioned ear remain normal (i.e., Figure 13.3B, left CN to right IC). In contrast, the IC contralateral to the lesioned ear receives 30% less inputs from the CN on the lesioned side (i.e., Figure 13.3B, right CN to left IC). Thus, unilateral cochlear removal in infancy results in a dramatic change in the anatomical balance of inputs to the IC from the CN. There is an increase of inputs to the IC of both sides from the CN on the unlesioned side and a concomitant decrease in the inputs to the IC on both sides from the CN on the lesioned side. Similar results were found in experiments in which a unilateral conductive hearing loss was simulated with ear plugs (Moore et al., 1989). Because unilateral deafness does not alter the synaptic density in IC (Hardie et al., 1998), these results are suggestive of a developing auditory system that competes for a limited and fixed amount of synaptic space in the IC. In terms of the development of the afferent input to the IC, there is a competitive interaction of inputs from the two ears during development, but only for a limited period of time. Cochlear removal after this time period (which is different for the different species studies) does not generally alter this anatomy.

PHYSIOLOGICAL CHANGES

The increased magnitude of the projections from the ipsilateral CN to ipsilateral IC following unilateral hearing loss is associated with significant changes in the physiological responses of IC neurons to sounds (Clopon & Silverman, 1977; Kitzes, 1984; Kitzes & Semple, 1985; McAlpine et al, 1997; Silverman & Clopton, 1977). These findings indicate that the observed anatomical changes reviewed above are associated with significant functional changes at the physiological level. After unilateral deafening as neonates, sound-evoked activity in neurons of the IC contralateral to the manipulation (i.e., Figure 13.3B, left IC) in response to sounds presented to the unmanipulated ear (i.e., Figure 13.3B, left ear) increased in adult animals to ~90% of responsive neurons from only ~30% in normal-hearing adults (Kitzes & Semple, 1985; McAlpine et al., 1997; Moore et al., 1993; Nordeen et al., 1983). Moreover, the activity levels of neurons (discharge rates) more than doubled, response thresholds decreased substantially, and the latency to first response decreased (Kitzes, 1984; Kitzes & Semple, 1985). These findings are suggestive of the development of a reduced amount of ipsilateral inhibition from the lesioned side. To test whether these inhibitory inputs were simply "unmasked" by the degeneration of CN neurons by cochlear removal, Moore and Kitzes (1986) lesioned the CN of adult animals. Lesions to the CN did not change the responsiveness of the IC ipsilateral to the intact ear, implying that the changes seen in the developmental experiments were not due to unmasking of inhibitory inputs, but were indeed limited to a developmental sensitive period.

In a very influential series of experiments, rats were raised with a unilateral conductive hearing loss beginning before the onset of hearing (Silverman & Clopton, 1977). The effect of the hearing loss on binaural interaction in neural responses in the IC (Figure 13.2A) was then assessed 3–5 months later. Figure 13.4A shows the Silverman and Clopton data schematically (not actual data). Figure 13.4A illustrates how the IC neurons on the left side responded in normal-hearing rats to monaural sound stimulation of the contralateral ear (right ear, dashed line) and to binaural stimulation of both ears (solid line). When stimulated monaurally, as the sound pressure level (SPL) of the stimulus was increased, the IC neurons increased their discharge rate accordingly. When stimulated binaurally, sounds were presented to both ears and the ILD of the stimulus was varied. Notice that when sounds were presented to both ears, there was a substantial reduction in the discharge rate of the neurons. That is, in the normal-hearing rats, IC neurons are excited by sounds presented to the contralateral (right) ear and inhibited by sounds presented to the ipsilateral (left) ear. This is most apparent at an ILD of 0 dB, where the sound levels at the two ears are identical, in that the responses of IC neurons are largely suppressed. Simply removing the stimulus from the inhibitory ipsilateral ear (i.e., the monaural condition) led to a large increase in neural responsiveness.

In the Silverman and Clopton (1977) experiments, unilateral occlusion in rats during development modified the binaural response properties of IC neurons in dramatic ways. First, the normal ipsilateral suppression of responses present in normal ears (e.g., Figure 13.4A) was largely absent after the deprivation (Figure 13.4B). Note, for example, that the binaural responses with an ILD of 0 dB were equivalent to the monaural responses from the contralateral ear (i.e., no ipsilateral suppression). Moreover, in the IC contralateral to the occlusion, there appeared to be an increase in the strength of inhibition (Figure 13.4C) ipsilaterally from the normal ear. In this case, for a binaural stimulus with an ILD of 0 dB, there was substantially more reduction in the response relative to the monaural contralateral ear than was seen in normal ears. In line with a sensitive period for the development of binaural interaction in the IC, these effects were most pronounced when rats were deprived early in development, and the effect was no longer present if adult rats were deprived (Clopton & Silverman, 1977). Moore and Irvine (1981) reported similar findings in the IC of cats raised with unilateral conductive hearing losses. Finally, both studies

attributed the changes in the physiology of IC neurons to central plasticity and not to peripheral changes in auditory sensitivity. In each study, physiological measures of the sensitivity of auditory neurons in the peripheral parts of the manipulated ear (e.g., cochlear microphonic or auditory nerve action potential thresholds) were normal. That is, the method of manipulation did not induce any peripheral sensorineural hearing loss.

These results together reveal that a unilateral conductive hearing loss during some early part of development can lead to substantial anatomical and synaptic reorganization, and this has profound consequences for the physiological responses to binaural stimuli at the level of the IC. These data are strongly consistent with the notion of a competition between converging ipsilateral and contralateral inputs to the IC from the two ears during development. The data are consistent with a general downregulation of synaptic activity in the auditory pathways that receive their major afferent input from the ear with the hearing loss. There might also be a compensatory upregulation of synaptic activity in pathways from the normal hearing ear in order to keep the synaptic density, or the overall responsiveness of the neurons, constant (e.g., Hardie et al., 1998). Similar changes in the binaural physiology might be apparent at earlier levels in the auditory pathway, like the MSO, LSO, and their projections to the IC (Figure 13.2), but studies have not yet looked systematically at this.

BEHAVIORAL CHANGES

Given the obvious importance of the effects of unilateral hearing loss on the development of basic auditory capabilities like sound localization, there is surprisingly very little experimental data on the behavioral deficits that animals reared under these conditions exhibit. In one study, Clements and Kelly (1978) reared guinea pigs with plugs in one or both ears for 11 days after birth and then tested them on a sound localization task for 21 days after that. Guinea pigs are precocial animals whose auditory systems begin to function well before birth. They can make orienting movement to sound sources shortly after birth, suggesting that the binaural circuitry for sound localization is largely in place at birth. Compared to normal animals, animals reared with a unilateral plug and then tested with the plug removed performed extremely poorly (in fact, at chance) and never regained the ability to localize sounds accurately. Knudsen, Esterly, and Knudsen (1984) reported a similar deficit in sound

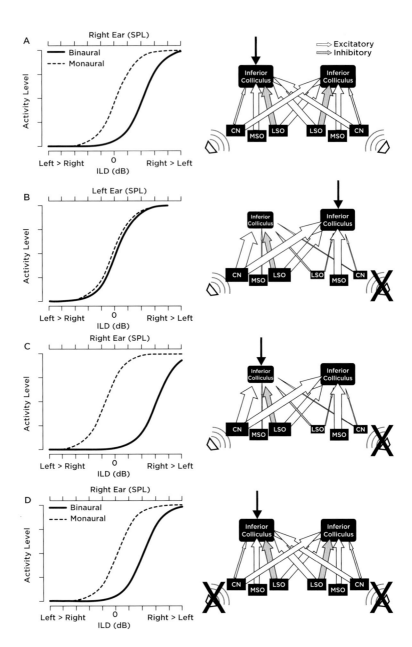

Figure 13.4 Functional physiological consequences of unilateral and bilateral auditory deprivation on the responses of neurons in the IC. (A) Normal hearing. Normal auditory pathways (right panel). Recordings from neurons in left IC (right, arrow). For sounds presented monaurally to the ear contralateral (right ear) to the IC being recorded from (left IC), as the sound level was increased the responses of the neurons increased accordingly (dashed line, left panel). When sounds were presented binaurally to both ears and the ILD was varied, the responses of the IC were suppressed relative to the monaural responses (solid line). That is, sounds presented to the ipsilateral ear are inhibitory and sounds to the contralateral ear excitatory, as in Figure 13.2. (B) For animals reared with unilateral conductive hearing loss (X, right ear), neurons in the IC ipsilateral to the loss (right IC) were still responsive to sounds presented monaurally to the normal left ear. But for sounds presented binaurally, the ipsilateral inhibition from the deprived ear (right ear) onto the right IC has been almost completely eliminated as a consequence of the unilateral deprivation. Right panel shows anatomical consequences of the deprivation, as in Figure 13.3. (C) For animals reared with a unilateral conductive hearing loss (right ear), neurons in the IC contralateral to the loss (left IC) respond normally to sounds presented monaurally to the deprived ear (right ear). But for sound presented binaurally, the ipsilateral inhibition from the undeprived ear has been strengthened leading to substantially more suppression of the neural responses relative to normal. Right panel shows anatomical consequences of the deprivation, as in Figure 13.3. (D) For animals reared with bilateral conductive hearing loss (both ears), the responses monaurally and binaurally were essentially the same as normals in A. Right panel shows anatomical consequences of the deprivation, as in Figure 13.3. (Data in left panels based on Silverman and Clopton, 1977.)

localization in barn owls reared with a unilateral conductive hearing loss, but these animals learned how to compensate for the unilateral loss and regain near-normal localization abilities; similar findings were reported for the ferret (King et al., 2001; King, Parsons, & Moore, 2000). It was speculated that the ferrets learned how to use the monaural spectral shape cues (e.g., Figure 13.1C) to localize sound accurately even though the binaural cues (ILD and ITD) were disrupted during development.

The results from unilateral deprivation during early development are supportive of a "use it or lose it" strategy. If the inputs to an auditory nucleus from one or both ears are not stimulated, they atrophy. And this atrophy has profound implications for the anatomy, physiology, and resultant behavior of the binaural auditory system.

Binaural Deprivation–Balanced and Competitive Interactions

Because bilateral auditory deprivation affects the inputs to the two ears in roughly equal ways (either sensorineural or conductive hearing loss), the central binaural neurons should be equally affected (e.g., neuron shrinkage, death, morphological and synaptic changes, etc.). That is, if "use it or lose it" is the method by which the auditory system develops, then depriving both ears should affect the pathways on both sides in equal ways. However, if a competitive interaction between the inputs from the two ears is necessary for normal development, then occluding both ears should lead to a somewhat "normal" binaural auditory system, since the balance is restored, albeit with less overall input (might only be spontaneous inputs). Unfortunately, there are surprisingly few experimental studies of the effects of binaural deprivation on the development of the anatomy, physiology, and behavior.

ANATOMICAL CHANGES

As might be expected, rearing animals with bilateral hearing losses leads to the same kinds of anatomical and morphological changes to peripheral auditory nuclei that receive input predominantly from one ear, such as the auditory nerve, CN, and MNTB (Figure 13.3B). But with binaural hearing losses, the changes occur equally on both sides (at least to the extent to which the magnitude of the hearing losses on each side is equal). For example, after bilateral cochlear lesion in infancy, there was near total atrophy of the auditory nerve cells on both sides, and there were also consequent reductions in CN volume (Hardie & Shepherd,

1999; Moore, 1990). Moreover, CN and MNTB neurons were significantly smaller than normal (Webster & Webster, 1977). However, at least one report indicates no significant CN neuron shrinkage after bilateral conductive deprivation (Coleman & O'Connor, 1979). More centrally, while LSO neurons exhibited shrinkage (Webster & Webster, 1977), MSO neurons of binaurally occluded rats had normal dendritic fields, with dendrites projecting equally both medially and laterally (Feng & Rogowski, 1980). Unlike for unilateral loss, where there is IC neuron shrinkage contralateral to the loss (Webster, 1983), after binaural loss, there was no (Webster & Webster, 1979) or minor (Nishiyama, Hardie, & Shepherd, 2000) neuron shrinkage. However, at the synaptic level, bilateral hearing loss in cats initiated near the onset of hearing results in a significant reduction in the number and density of synapses in the IC at adulthood compared to normal animals (Hardie et al., 1998). This latter finding suggests that auditory-evoked inputs are necessary to complete normal levels of synapse development in the central auditory system.

Several studies have also examined the projection patterns from the CN to the IC. Interestingly, bilateral cochlear ablation leads to no quantitative changes in these projections from normal; neither the absolute number nor the bilateral symmetry of the labeled neurons differed significantly from normal adult ferrets (Moore, 1990). Bilateral cochlear removal does not produce the same change in brain stem connections as unilateral removal or unilateral conductive hearing loss. Ferrets with bilateral cochlear lesions just before hearing onset experienced no reduction in the absolute number of IC neurons and the symmetry of the ICs was preserved, just as in normal binaural hearing controls (Moore, 1990).

Studies in the so-called deaf white cat (DWC) have also proven valuable to the investigation of the role of experience in the development of binaural hearing. The DWC has abnormal inner ear structure that causes complete sensorineural deafness at birth, with even a complete lack of spontaneous activity in the auditory nerve (Ryugo, Pongstaporn, Huchton, & Niparko, 1997). The DWC provides an opportunity to study equal binaural deprivation during development. Anatomical studies of the pathways subserving binaural hearing (Figure 13.2) show the binaural deprivation does not alter the normal development of the projection patterns in the brain stem. Early deafness binaurally had no effect on the basic projection patterns seen in normal controls. Congenital binaural deafness in the DWC did not show any significant effects on the connections within the auditory brain stem, and the projections of the LSO and MSO to the IC on both sides were normal. These results are in agreement with those in the ferret by Moore (1990).

PHYSIOLOGICAL CHANGES

There are even fewer studies that have examined the physiological consequences of binaural auditory deprivation. The reasons for this lack of data is due to the method of deprivation often used—cochlear ablation. Clearly, without the cochlea, there can be no assessment of the functional consequences of binaural deprivation. However, future research using bilateral cochlear implant stimulation of the two ears (e.g., Smith & Delgutte, 2007) in bilaterally deafened animals could provide valuable information on the plasticity of the developing binaural auditory system and the role of experience. The effects of bilateral conductive hearing losses during development were also examined in the seminal studies of Silverman and Clopton (1977) and Clopton and Silverman (1977). In agreement with the anatomical findings reviewed earlier, Silverman and Clopton (1977) found that binaural deprivation essentially resulted in normal patterns of binaural interaction in IC neurons (e.g., Figure 13.4D). In other words, the pattern of results in the normal rats (Figure 13.4A) was similar to the pattern for binaurally deprived rats (Figure 13.4D). These results are in agreement with the competition hypothesis of binaural auditory system development. Even when the input levels at each ear are severely depressed, provided that the inputs are still balanced, then normal anatomy and physiology emerges.

BEHAVIORAL CHANGES

Clements and Kelly (1978) reared guinea pigs with plugs in both ears for 11 days after birth and then tested them on a sound localization task. Animals reared with plugs in both ears performed as good as normal animals. As with the anatomical and physiological studies, these behavioral studies underscore the importance of balanced inputs from the two ears during the sensitive period of development. What seems to matter is not the overall level of the two inputs, but rather whether they are balanced.

Hebbian Processes and the Development of the Binaural Auditory System

In the case of the binaural nuclei of interest here, the MSO, LSO, and IC, it appears that somewhat normal development of the anatomy, physiology, and resultant behavior emerges even after bilateral hearing deprivation during a sensitive period of development. Unilateral deprivation is devastating to the development of the auditory system during the sensitive period. But in the discussions above, there was consideration of only whether there was a balanced amount of neural activity in the two ears. The temporal nature of that activity and whether or not it was correlated at the two ears was not considered. This latter point is important for the following reason: In normal environments, sounds reaching the two ears from any one source will be highly correlated (e.g., Figure 13.1A). As a consequence of this, the evoked neural activity at the two ears will also be highly correlated. One of the most common forms of synaptic plasticity is Hebb's hypothesis (Hebb, 1949) in which the temporal correlation between presynaptic and postsynaptic neural activity plays a pivotal role in the strengthening or weakening of synaptic contacts. In the binaural auditory system, another kind of Hebbian interaction can be envisioned in which inputs from the two ears onto binaural neurons (MSO, LSO, IC, etc.) are strengthened and maintained when inputs are correlated at the two ears, but reduced or eliminated when they are uncorrelated. There is evidence that this additional developmental mechanism is operating in the binaural auditory pathway.

To test whether correlated inputs from the two ears is an important component of competitive interactions of developmental connections, it is necessary to create an environment where the inputs to the two ears are uncorrelated, but the relative levels of activity remain the same. That is, each ear gets a normal, balanced set of auditory inputs, but the temporal relationships of the inputs are not normal. In one study, Withington-Wray et al. (1990) raised guinea pigs in an environment of so-called omnidirectional white noise. This procedure effectively makes the acoustic inputs to the two ears uncorrelated and unsynchronized, which would result in uncorrelated and unsynchronized neural activity in the two ears. Normally, a single sound source arriving at the two ears results in sound and neural activity that is highly correlated and synchronized, which is critical for the encoding of ITDs. However, such an environment would not necessarily alter the ILD cues. They demonstrated a sensitive period for the development of the so-called auditory space map in the superior colliculus, a multimodal midbrain structure that receives input from the IC. By rearing the animals in this environment at different ages and for different time periods, they concluded that during an approximately 4-day window from P26 to P30, normal auditory experience at both ears was necessary for the normal development of the space map. At this age, the peripheral auditory system, including the brain stem up to the IC, is largely adult-like in its responsiveness to sound. Hence, this result is particular to the development of binaural interactions. This study suggests that in addition to the normal balanced levels of input to the two ears, synchronized acoustic inputs (as would be experienced by sounds arriving at the two ears from a single sound source) are also necessary for the establishment and maintenance of neural structures that are involved in binaural and spatial hearing.

In another series of experiments, gerbils were raised in omnidirectional noise. In normal, binaural hearing adult gerbils, inhibitory inputs to the MSO (a projection not discussed in this chapter) are confined primarily to the soma, while excitatory inputs synapse the distal dendrites. The spatial distribution of glycinergic inputs to the gerbil MSO is initially diffuse and then undergoes a substantial refinement within the first few days after hearing onset. The refinement does not occur if binaural inputs are manipulated during this time by either unilateral or binaural cochlear lesions or raising the animals in omnidirectional noise (Kapfer et al., 2002). Both these manipulations eliminate the correlated inputs to the two ears necessary for binaural hearing based on time differences. Adults in this environment do not exhibit altered glycine distributions. Thus, there is an experience-dependent refinement of synapses from the two ears.

There are also corresponding physiological consequences of this altered experience. Seidl and Grothe (2005) examined the coding of ITDs (see Figures 13.1B,E, and 13.2B), which depend heavily on correlated inputs to the two ears, in the dorsal nucleus of the lateral lemniscus (DNLL). The DNLL is located between the SOC nuclei (MSO and LSO) and the IC, and receives strong inputs from the MSO and LSO. They examined DNLL neurons that presumably received direct inputs predominantly from MSO. In normal animals, no ITD-sensitive neurons were found at P14, but by P15, some neurons were ITD sensitive, but with very low responsiveness (i.e., low discharge rates). ITD sensitivity of neurons in omnidirectional noise-reared animals tested as adults was similar to that of the P15 juveniles, but not adult normals or adults that were exposed to the noise. Data from

the noise-reared animals shows that adult-like ITD sensitivity can be suppressed during a sensitive period right after hearing onset and that development of ITD tuning in the gerbil most likely occurs due to plasticity at the level of the ITD detector itself. It is possible that the posthearing onset refinement of glycinergic projections is based on temporal correlations of the naturally produced auditory activity, selectively eliminating inputs that are not contributing properly. These results suggest that the maturation of sound-localization encoding depends on patterned acoustic experience. Experience-dependent plasticity might be necessary for proper ITD tuning and may represent a mechanism of direct adjustment of neuronal processing to behaviorally relevant cues.

The results of binaural deprivation studies, although few, suggest that simple reduction in neural activity might be less detrimental to the development of the binaural circuits for sound localization than unilateral deprivation. At least for the binaural nuclei of interest in this chapter (MSO, LSO, and IC), there appears to be near-normal patterns of development of these binaural circuits. However, normal development of the nuclei that receive bilateral inputs seem to also require correlated acoustical inputs, and thus correlated neural activity, at the two ears. Brain stem development of the representation of both ears appears to start out equal, but is then sculpted and shaped by experience. Balance of inputs is retained in normal binaural hearing, but is substantially altered in monaurally deprived animals. This upsets the competitive balance necessary for normal development. The active ear obtains a competitive advantage and the main anatomical circuits from that ear begin to take over and possibly actively suppress synaptic contacts from the occluded ear. Many of these data, particularly those related to the IC, are consistent with a homeostatic plasticity hypothesis (see Burrone & Murthy, 2003) in which the number and strengths (or gains) of synapses from inputs from the two ears (e.g., CN inputs to the IC as in Figure 13.3A) is adjusted during development to maintain some fixed level of excitability of the neurons.

Evidence of Experience-dependent Plasticity in Human Sound Localization Development

In this section, evidence is considered from human populations that some form of experience-dependent plasticity exists in the development of the human binaural auditory system. A sensitive period for auditory system development is certainly an advantage because it allows for the organism to adapt to its unique acoustic environment. However, plasticity during these periods can also be problematic if the sensory environment is distorted or altered from normal. For example, relatively mild conductive hearing losses in infancy and early childhood may result in communication difficulties when children reach school age. But children whose hearing losses are identified and corrected prior to ~6 months of birth are much more likely to develop better language skills than children whose hearing loss is diagnosed and corrected later (Yoshinaga-Itano, Sedey, Coulter, & Mehl, 1998). Part of this progress is due to normal binaural hearing, since children with even mild unilateral hearing losses (one impaired and one normal hearing ear) also develop poorer language skills and have additional behavioral and educational problems (increased rates of grade failure) than their normal binaural hearing peers (Bess, Dodd-Murphy, & Parker, 1998). This likely occurs because children with unilateral loss require higher speech-to-noise ratios to understand speech in typical settings, like noisy, reverberant classrooms where the ability to hear speech is difficult.

There are many common diseases early in life that alter substantially the normal acoustic inputs to the two ears. In essence, these examples provide naturally occurring "experiments" on the effects of auditory deprivation during development. For example, chronic otitis media (ear infections), otosclerosis, and ear canal atresia all result in varying degrees of conductive hearing loss. Conductive hearing loss results from abnormalities in the outer and/or middle ear that impede the conduction of airborne sound to the inner ear; that is, the sounds that are ultimately transduced into neural impulses in the cochlea are not only attenuated but also delayed in time (Hartley & Moore, 2003). For example, the excessive fluid buildup in the middle ear in otitis media ultimately causes mechanical changes in the coupling of the eardrum to the inner ear, resulting in a conductive hearing loss. This is in contrast to sensorineural hearing loss in which there has been some form of damage or abnormality to the auditory receptors (hair cells), the auditory nerve, or more central parts of the auditory system, which disrupts the normal electrical functioning of the ascending system. There is strong evidence, discussed below, that even temporary hearing loss of any type, conductive or sensorineural, early in life can lead to permanent and wide ranging changes in the structure and function of the auditory system, with profound implications for behavior.

Children who either are born with bilateral or unilateral conductive hearing losses or incur them later (e.g., ear infections) provide important insights into the effects on human development of early deprivation and of uneven competition between the ears for brain stem development. Children with these deficits have been shown to have impairments in basic auditory functions even well after the cause of the conductive loss has passed (e.g., clearing up of ear infection) or surgically corrected and peripheral sensitivity to sound in each ear has returned to normal (Moore, Hutchings, & Meyer, 1991). This is particularly the case for binaural and spatial hearing, where poor performance relative to normal hearing peers may still be detected many years later (Hall & Derlacki, 1986; Hall, Grose, & Pillsbury, 1995; Moore et al., 1991; Pillsbury, Grose, & Hall, 1991). Children who have had higher than normal incidences of otitis media have been shown to often develop deficits in language, reading, and attentional tasks (Zinkus et al. 78). Moreover, children born with otosclerosis (Lucente & Sobol, 1988), ear canal atresia (Wilmington, Gray, & Jahrsdoerfer, 1984), or severe deafness (Beggs & Foreman, 1980) often perform poorly at tasks involving binaural hearing, even well after the problem has been corrected. Because language is often learned in noisy and reverberant acoustic environments, like classrooms, these deficits are believed to be a function of disrupted binaural hearing mechanisms as opposed to a simple attenuation of the sounds, and thus the sensitivity, of each ear (Moore, Hartley, & Hogan, 2003). Indeed, there are physiological correlates of these changes in children with conductive hearing impairment, where they consistently show increased latencies and other abnormalities in binaurally evoked auditory brain stem–evoked responses (Folsom, Weber, & Thompson, 1993; Gunnarson & Finitzo, 1991; Hall & Grose, 1993).

Plasticity is also evident in children born with congenital deafness or deaf children with little or no prior auditory experience. Although research in this area is just now emerging, many of these children have been shown to obtain significant benefit from electrical stimulation of the inner ear via cochlear implants, but only if the device is installed at a relatively young age (Harrison, Gordan, & Mount, 2005; Litovsky et al., 2006). Such results can be at least partially attributed to brain plasticity. The best candidates for cochlear implantation, in terms of outcomes, are very young children and infants or adults who have developed some linguistic skills prior to becoming deaf (Niparko, Cheng, & Francis, 2000; Waltzman, Cohen, & Shapiro, 1991). It is believed that sensory stimulation, whether natural or electrical via the cochlear implant, is necessary during early life to ensure the normal development of the central auditory system. Recent evidence suggests that the human binaural auditory system might be subject to a sensitive period; bilateral electrical stimulation has been shown to be beneficial in adults with post-linguistic onset hearing loss, while those who had little or no auditory experience early in life experience fewer benefits of bilateral cochlear implants (Litovsky et al., 2004, 2006). Clearly, the rationale behind early cochlear implantation is based upon the belief that there is a sensitive period of approximately 4–6 years after birth during which the loss of auditory input is especially detrimental to the development of speech and language abilities (Yoshinaga-Itano et al., 1998), important auditory cortical areas (Harrison et al., 2005; Kral, Tillein, Heid, Hartmann, & Klinke, 2005; Sharma, Dorman, & Kral, 2005), and binaural and spatial hearing (Litovsky et al., 2006). Together, these data support the hypothesis of a sensitive period for the development of binaural hearing in humans and establish this system as a potential model for experience-dependent plasticity.

Acknowledgments

Preparation of this chapter was supported in part by a grant from the NIH-NIDCD (DC006865). I am grateful to the members of my laboratory, Dr. Kanthaiah Koka, Dr. Jeff Tsai, Heath Jones, and Eric Lupo for their comments on and discussions about earlier versions of this chapter.

References

Beggs, W. E., & Foreman, D. L. (1980). Sound localization and early binaural experience in the deaf. *British Journal of Audiology, 14*, 41–48.

Bess, F. H., Dodd-Murphy, J., & Parker, R. A. (1998). Children with minimal sensorineural hearing loss: Prevalence, educational performance, and functional status. *Ear and Hearing, 19*, 339–354.

Blatchley, B. J., & Brugge, J. F. (1990). Sensitivity to binaural intensity and phase difference cues in kitten inferior colliculus. *Journal of Neurophysiology, 64*, 582–597.

Blatchley, B. J., Williams, J. E., & Coleman, J. R. (1983). Age-dependent effects of acoustic deprivation on spherical cells of the rat anteroventral cochlear nucleus. *Experimental Neurology, 80*, 81–93.

Burrone, J., & Murthy, V. N. (2003). Synaptic gain control and homeostasis. *Current Opinion in Neurobiology, 13*, 560–567.

Clements, M., & Kelly, J. B. (1978). Directional responses by kittens to an auditory stimulus. *Developmental Psychobiology, 11*, 505–511.

Clifton, R. K., Gwiazda, J., Bauer, J. A., Clarkson, M. G., & Held, R. (1988). Growth in head size during infancy: Implications for sound localization, *Developmental Psychology, 24*, 477–483.

Clopton, B. M., & Silverman, B. M. (1977). Plasticity of binaural interaction. II. Critical period and changes in midline response. *Journal of Neurophysiology, 40*, 1275–1280.

Coleman, J., Blatchley, B. J., & Williams, J. E. (1982). Development of the dorsal and ventral cochlear nuclei in rat and effects of acoustic deprivation. *Developmental Brain Research, 4*, 119–123.

Coleman, J. R., & O'Connor, P. (1979). Effects of monaural and binaural sound deprivation on cell development in the anteroventral cochlear nucleus of rats. *Experimental Neurology, 64*, 553–566.

Feng, A. S., & Rogowski, B. A. (1980). Effects of monaural and binaural occlusion on the morphology of neurons in the medial superior olivary nucleus of the rat. *Brain Research, 189*, 530–534.

Folsom, R. C., Weber, B. A., & Thompson, G. (1993). Auditory brainstem responses in children with early recurrent middle ear disease. *The Annals of Otology, Rhinology, and Laryngology, 92*, 249–253.

Friauf, E. (2004). Developmental changes and cellular plasticity in the superior olivary complex, In T. N. Parks, E. W. Rubel, R. R. Fay, & A. N. Popper (Eds.), *Development of the auditory system, Springer handbook of auditory research* (pp. 49–95). New York: Springer-Verlag.

Gunnarson, A. D., & Finitzo, T. (1991). Conductive hearing loss during infancy: Effects on later brainstem electrophysiology. *Journal of Speech and Hearing Research, 34*, 1207–1215.

Hall, J. W., & Derlacki, E. L. (1986). Effect of conductive hearing loss and middle ear surgery on binaural hearing. *The Annals of Otology, Rhinology, and Laryngology, 95*, 525–530.

Hall, J. W., & Grose, J. H. (1993). Short-term and long-term effects on the masking level difference following middle ear surgery. *Journal of the American Academy of Audiology, 4*, 307–312.

Hall, J. W., Grose, J. H., & Pillsbury, H. C. (1995). Long-term effects of chronic otitis media on binaural hearing in children. *Archives of Otolaryngology—Head and Neck Surgery, 121*, 847–852.

Hardie, N. A., Martsi-McClintock, A., Aitkin, L., & Shepherd, R. K. (1998). Neonatal sensorineural hearing loss affects synaptic density in the auditory midbrain. *Neuroreport, 9*, 2019–2022.

Hardie, N. A., & Shepherd, R. K. (1999). Sensorineural hearing loss during development: Morphological and physiological response of the cochlear and auditory brainstem. *Hearing Research, 128*, 147–165.

Harrison, R. V., Gordan, K. A., & Mount, R. J. (2005). Is there a critical period for cochlear implantation in congenitally deaf children? Analyses of hearing and speech perception performance after implantation. *Developmental Psychobiology, 46*, 252–261.

Hartley, D. E., & Moore, D. R. (2003). Effects of conductive hearing loss on temporal aspects of sound transmission through the ear. *Hearing Research, 177*, 53–60.

Hashisaki, G. T., & Rubel, E. W. (1989). Effects of unilateral cochlea removal on anteroventral cochlear nucleus neurons in developing gerbils. *The Journal of Comparative Neurology*, *283*, 465–473.

Hebb, D. O. (1949). *The organisation of behaviour*. New York: Wiley.

Jenkins, W. M., & Masterton, R. B. (1982). Sound localization: Effects of unilateral lesions in the central auditory system. *Journal of Neurophysiology*, *47*, 987–1016.

Kapfer, C., Seidl, A. H., Schweizer, H., & Grothe, B. (2002). Experience-dependent refinement of inhibitory inputs to auditory coincidence-detector neurons. *Nature Neuroscience*, *5*, 247–253.

Kavanagh, G. L., & Kelly, J. B. (1992). Midline and lateral field sound localization in the ferret (*Mustela putorius*): Contribution of the superior olivary complex. *Journal of Neurophysiology*, *67*, 1643–1658.

Kelly, J. B., & Kavanah, G. L. (1994). Sound localization after unilateral lesions of inferior colliculus in the ferret (*Mustela putorius*). *Journal of Neurophysiology*, *71*, 1078–1087.

King, A. J., Kacelnik, O., Mrsic-Flogel, T. D., Schnupp, J. W. H., Parsons, C. H., & Moore, D. R. (2001). How plastic is spatial hearing? *Audiology and Neuro-otology*, *6*, 182–186.

King, A. J., Parsons, C. H., & Moore, D. R. (2000). Plasticity in the neural coding of auditory space in the mammalian brain. *Proceedings of the National Academy of Sciences, USA*, *97*, 11821–11828.

Kitzes, L. M. (1984). Some physiological consequences of neonatal cochlear destruction in the inferior colliculus of the gerbil, *Meriones unguiculatus*. *Brain Research*, *306*, 171–178.

Kitzes, L. M., & Semple, M. N. (1985). Single-unit responses in the inferior colliculus: Effects of neonatal unilateral cochlear ablation. *Journal of Neurophysiology*, *53*, 1483–1500.

Kitzes, L. M., Kageyama, G. H., Semple, M. N., & Kil, J. (1995). Development of ectopic projections from the ventral cochlear nucleus to the superior olivary complex induced by neonatal ablation of the contralateral cochlea. *The Journal of Comparative Neurology*, *353*, 341–363.

Knudsen, E. I. (2004). Sensitive periods in the development of the brain and behavior. *Journal of Cognitive Neuroscience*, *16*, 1412–1425.

Knudsen, E. I., Esterly, S. D., & Knudsen, P. F. (1984). Monaural occlusion alters sound localization during a sensitive period in the barn owl. *The Journal of Neuroscience*, *4*, 1001–1011.

Koerber, K. C., Pfeiffer, R. R., Warr, W. B., & Kiang, N. Y. S. (1966). Spontaneous spike discharges from single units in the cochlear nucleus after destruction of the cochlea. *Experimental Neurology*, *16*, 119–130.

Kral, A., Tillein, J., Heid, S., Hartmann, R., & Klinke, R. (2005). Postnatal cortical development in congenital auditory deprivation. *Cerebral Cortex*, *15*, 252–562.

Levi-Montalcini R. (1949). Development of the acoustico-vestibular centers in the chick embryo in the absence of the afferent root fibers and of descending fiber tracts. *The Journal of Comparative Neurology*, *91*, 209–242.

Lippe, W. R. (1994). Rhythmic spontaneous activity in the developing avian auditory system. *The Journal of Neuroscience*, *14*, 1486–1495.

Litovsky, R. Y., & Ashmead, D. H. (1994). Development of binaural and spatial hearing in infants and children. In R. H. Gilkey & T. R. Anderson (Eds.), *Binaural and spatial hearing in real and virtual environments* (pp. 571–592). Mahwah, NJ: Erlbaum.

Litovsky, R. Y., Fligor, B., & Tramo, M. (2002). Functional role of the human inferior colliculus in binaural hearing. *Hearing Research*, *165*, 177–188.

Litovsky, R. Y., Parkinson, A., Arcaroli, J., Peters, R., Lake, J., Johnstone, P., et al. (2004). Bilateral cochlear implants in adults and children. *Archives of Otolaryngology—Head and Neck Surgery*, *130*, 648–655.

Litovsky, R. Y., Johnstone, P. M., & Godar, S. P. (2006). Benefits of bilateral cochlear implants and/or hearing aids in children. *International Journal of Audiology*, *45*(Suppl. 1), S78–S91.

Lucente, F. E., & Sobol, S. M. (1988). *Essentials of otolaryngology* (2nd ed.). New York: Raven.

Masterton, B., Jane, J. A., & Diamond, I. T. (1967). Role of brainstem auditory structures in sound localization. I. Trapezoid body, superior olive, and lateral lemniscus. *Journal of Neurophysiology*, *30*, 341–359.

McAlpine, D., Martin, R. L., Mossop, J. E., & Moore, D. R. (1997). Response properties of neurons in the inferior colliculus of the monaurally deafened ferret to acoustic stimulation of the intact ear. *Journal of Neurophysiology*, *78*, 767–779.

Moore, D. R. (1990). Auditory brainstem of the ferret: Bilateral cochlear lesions in infancy do not affect the number of neurons projecting from the cochlear nucleus to the inferior colliculus. *Developmental Brain Research*, *54*, 125–130.

Moore, D. R. (1992). Trophic influences of excitatory and inhibitory synapses on neurones in the auditory brainstem. *Neuroreport*, *3*, 269–272.

Moore, C. N., Casseday, J. H., & Neff, W. D. (1974). Sound localization: The role of the commissural pathways of the auditory system of the cat. *Brain Research*, *82*, 13–26.

Moore, D. R., Hartley, D. E. H., & Hogan, S. (2003). Effects of otitis media with effusion (OME) on central auditory function. *International Journal of Pediatric Otorhinolaryngology*, *67*(Suppl. 1), S63–S67.

Moore, D. R., Hutchings, M. E., King, A. J., & Kowalchuk, N. E. (1989). Auditory brainstem of the ferret: Some effects of rearing with a unilateral ear plug on the cochlea, cochlear nucleus, and projections to the inferior colliculus. *The Journal of Neuroscience*, *9*, 1213–1222.

Moore, D. R., Hutchings, M. E., & Meyer, S. E. (1991). Binaural masking level differences in children with a history of otitis media. *Audiology*, *30*, 91–101.

Moore, D. R., & Irvine, D. R. F. (1981). Development of responses to acoustic interaural intensity differences in the cat inferior colliculus. *Brain Research*, *208*, 198–202.

Moore, D. R., King, A. J., McAlpine, D., Martin, R. L., & Hutchings, M. E. (1993). Functional consequences of neonatal unilateral cochlear removal. *Progress in Brain Research*, *97*, 127–133.

Moore, D.R., & King, A. J. (2004). Plasticity of binaural systems, In T. N. Parks, E. W. Rubel, R. R. Fay, & A. N. Popper (Eds.), *Development of the auditory system, Springer handbook of auditory research* (pp. 96–172). New York: Springer-Verlag.

Moore, D. R., & Kitzes, L. M. (1986). Cochlear nucleus lesions in the adult gerbil: Effects on neurone responses in the contralateral inferior colliculus. *Brain Research*, *373*, 268–272.

Moore, D. R., & Kowalchuk, N. E. (1988). Auditory brainstem of the ferret: Effects of unilateral cochlear lesions on cochlear nucleus volume and projections to the inferior colliculus. *The Journal of Comparative Neurology, 272,* 503–515.

Muir, D., & Field, T. (1979). Newborn infants orient to sounds. *Child Development, 50,* 431–436.

Niparko, J. K., Cheng, A. K., & Francis, H. W. (2000). Outcomes of cochlear implantation: Assessment of quality of life impact and economic evaluation of the benefits of the cochlear implant in relation to costs. In J. Niparko, K. Kirk, N. Mellan, R. McKonkey, D. Tucci, & B. Wilson (Eds.), *Cochlear implants: Principles and practice* (pp. 269–287). Hagertown, MD: Lippincott, Williams and Wilkins.

Nishiyama, N., Hardie, N. A., & Shepherd, R. K. (2000). Neonatal sensorineural hearing loss affects neurone size in cat auditory midbrain. *Hearing Research, 140,* 18–22.

Nordeen, K. W., Killackey, H. P., & Kitzes, L. M. (1983). Ascending projections to the inferior colliculus following unilateral cochlear ablation in the neonatal gerbil, Meriones unguiculatus. *Journal of Comparative Neurology, 214,* 144–153.

Oliver, D. L. (1987). Projections to the inferior colliculus from the anteroventral cochlear nucleus in the cat: Possible substrates for binaural interaction. *The Journal of Comparative Neurology, 264,* 24–46.

Palmer, A. R., & Kuwada, S. (2005). Binaural and spatial coding in the inferior colliculus, In J. A. Winer & C. E. Schreiner (Eds.), *The inferior colliculus* (pp. 377–410). New York: Springer.

Pasic, T. R., Moore, D. R., & Rubel, E. W. (1994). Effect of altered neuronal activity on cells size in the medial nucleus of the trapezoid body and ventral cochlear nucleus of the gerbil. *The Journal of Comparative Neurology, 348,* 111–120.

Perkins, R. E. (1973). An electron microscopic study of synaptic organization in the medial superior olive of normal and experimental chinchillas. *The Journal of Comparative Neurology, 148,* 387–416.

Pillsbury, H. C., Grose, J. H., & Hall, J. W. (1991). Otitis media with effusion in children. Binaural hearing before and after corrective surgery. *Archives of Otolaryngology—Head and Neck Surgery, 117,* 718–723.

Powell, T. P. S., & Erulkar, S. D. (1962). Transneural cell degeneration in the auditory relay nuclei of the cat. *Journal of Anatomy, 96,* 249–268.

Rubel, E. W., Parks, T. N., & Zirpel, L. (2004). Assembling, connecting, and maintaining the cochlear nucleus, In T. N. Parks, E. W. Rubel, R. R. Fay, & A. N. Popper (Eds.), *Development of the auditory system, Springer handbook of auditory research* (pp. 8–47). New York: Springer-Verlag.

Rubsamen, R., & Lippe, W. R. (1998). Development of cochlear function, In E. W. Rubel, A. N. Popper, R. R. Fay (Eds.), *Development of the auditory system, Springer handbook of auditory research* (pp. 193–270). New York: Springer-Verlag.

Ruggero, M. A. (1992). Physiology and coding of sound in the auditory never. In A. N. Popper & R. R. Fay (Eds.), *The mammalian auditory pathway: Neurophysiology, Springer handbook of auditory research* (pp. 34–93). New York: Springer-Verlag.

Russell, F. A., & Moore, D. R. (1995). Afferent reorganisation within the superior olivary complex of the gerbil: Development and induction by neonatal, unilateral cochlear removal. *The Journal of Comparative Neurology, 352,* 607–625.

Russell, F. A., & Moore, D. R. (1999). Effects of unilateral cochlear removal on dendrites in gerbil medial superior olivary nucleus. *The European Journal of Neuroscience, 11,* 1379–1390.

Russell, F. A., & Moore, D. R. (2002). Ultrastructural effects of unilateral deafening on afferents to the gerbil medial superior olivary nucleus. *Hearing Research, 173,* 43–61.

Ryugo, D. K., Pongstaporn, T., Huchton, D. M., & Niparko, J. K. (1997). Ultrastructural analysis of primary endings in deaf white cats: Morphologic alterations in endbulbs of Held. *The Journal of Comparative Neurology, 385,* 230–244.

Sanes, D. H., & Rubel, E. W. (1988). The ontogeny of inhibition and excitation in the gerbil lateral superior olive. *The Journal of Neuroscience, 8,* 682–700.

Sanes, D. H., Markowitz, S., Bernstein, J., & Wardlow, J. (1992). The influence of inhibitory afferents on the development of postsynaptic dendritic arbors. *The Journal of Comparative Neurology, 321,* 637–644.

Seidl, A. H., & Grothe, B. (2005). Development of sound localization mechanisms in mammals is shaped by early acoustic experience. *Journal of Neurophysiology, 94,* 1028–1036.

Sharma, A., Dorman, M., & Kral, A. (2005). The influence of a sensitive period on central auditory development in children with unilateral and bilateral cochlear implants. *Hearing Research, 203,* 134–143.

Silverman, M. S., & Clopton, B. M. (1977). Plasticity of binaural interaction. I. Effect of early auditory deprivation. *Journal of Neurophysiology, 40,* 1266–1274.

Smith, Z. .M., & Delgutte, B. (2007). Sensitivity to interaural time differences in the inferior colliculus with bilateral cochlear implants. *Journal of Neuroscience, 27,* 6740–6750.

Tierney, R. S., Russell, F. A., & Moore, D. R. (1997). Susceptibility of developing cochlear nucleus neurons to deafferentation-induced death abruptly ends just before the onset of hearing. *The Journal of Comparative Neurology, 378,* 295–306.

Tollin, D. J. (2003). The lateral superior olive: A functional role in sound source localization. *The Neuroscientist, 9,* 127–143.

Tollin, D .J. (2008). Encoding of interaural level differences for sound localization, In: A.I. Basbaum, A. Kaneko, G.M. Shepherd & G. Westheimer (Eds.), *The senses: A comprehensive reference, Vol 3, Audition,* P. Dallos & D. Oertel (Eds.),. San Diego: Academic Press; 631–654.

Tollin, D. J., Koka, K., & Tsai, J. J. (2008) Interaural level difference discrimination thresholds for single neurons in the lateral superior olive. *The Journal of Neuroscience, 28,* 4848–4860.

Tollin, D. J., & Koka, K. (2009) Postnatal development of sound pressure transformations by the head and pinnae of the cat: Monaural characteristics. *Journal of the Acoustical Society of America, 125,* 980–994.

Tollin, D. J., & Yin, T. C. T. (2002). The coding of spatial location by single units in the lateral superior olive of the cat. I. Spatial receptive fields in azimuth. *The Journal of Neuroscience, 22,* 1454–1467.

Trune, D. R. (1982a). Influence of neonatal cochlear removal on the development of mouse cochlear nucleus: I. Number, size, and density of its neurons. *The Journal of Comparative Neurology, 209,* 409–424.

Trune, D. R. (1982b). Influence of neonatal cochlear removal on the development of mouse cochlear nucleus: II. Dendritic morphometry of its neurons. *The Journal of Comparative Neurology, 209,* 425–434.

Tucci, D. L., Born, D. E., & Rubel, E. W. (1987). Changes in spontaneous activity and CNS morphology associated with conductive and sensorineural hearing loss in chickens. *The Annals of Otology, Rhinology, and Laryngology, 96,* 343–350.

Waltzman, S. B., Cohen, N. L., & Shapiro, W. H. (1991). Effects of chronic electrical stimulation on patients using a cochlear prosthesis. *Otolaryngology—Head and Neck Surgery, 105,* 797–801.

Webster, D. B. (1983a). Auditory neuronal sizes after a unilateral conductive hearing loss. *Experimental Neurology, 79,* 130–140.

Webster, D. B. (1983b). A critical period during postnatal auditory development in mice. *International Journal of Pediatric Otorhinolaryngology, 6,* 107–118.

Webster, D. B. (1988). Conductive hearing loss affects the growth of the cochlear nuclei over an extended period of time. *Hearing Research, 32,* 185–192.

Webster, D. B., & Webster, M. (1977). Neonatal sound deprivation affects brain stem auditory nuclei. *Archives of Otolaryngology, 103,* 392–396.

Webster, D. B., & Webster, M. (1979). Effects of neonatal conductive hearing loss on brain stem auditory nuclei. *Annals of Otology, 88,* 684–688.

Wertheimer, M. (1961). Psychomotor coordination of auditory and visual space at birth, *Science, 134,* 1692.

Wiesel, T. N. (1982). Postnatal development of the visual cortex and the influence of environment, *Nature, 299,* 583–591.

Wiesel, T. N., & Hubel, D. H. (1965). Comparison of the effects of unilateral and bilateral eye closure on cortical unit responses in kittens. *Journal of Neurophysiology, 28,* 1029–1040.

Wilmington, D., Gray, L., & Jahrsdoerfer, R. (1994). Binaural processing after corrected congenital unilateral conductive hearing loss. *Hearing Research, 74,* 99–114.

Winer, J. A., & Schreiner, C. E. (2005). The central auditory system: A functional analysis, In J. A. Winer & C. E. Schreiner (Eds.), *The inferior colliculus* (pp. 1–68). New York: Springer.

Withington-Wray, D. J., Binns, K. E., & Keating, M. J. (1990). The developmental emergence of a map of auditory space in the superior colliculus of the guinea pig. *Brain Research. Developmental Brain Research, 51,* 225–236.

Yin, T. C. T. (2002). Neural mechanisms of encoding binaural localization cues in the auditory brainstem. In D. Oertel, R. R. Fay, & A. N. Popper (Eds.), *Integrative functions of the mammalian auditory pathway, Springer handbook of auditory research* (pp. 99–159). New York: Springer-Verlag.

Yoshinaga-Itano, C., Sedey, A. L., Coulter, D. K., & Mehl, A. L. (1998). Language of early- and later-identified children with hearing loss. *Pediatrics, 102,* 1161–1171.

Yost, W. A. (1997). The cocktail party problem: Forty years later, In R. H. Gilkey & T. R. Anderson (Eds.), *Binaural and spatial hearing in real and virtual environments* (pp. 329–347). Mahwah, NJ: Lawrence Erlbaum Associates.

Young, E. D., & Davis, K. A. (2002). Circuitry and function of the dorsal cochlear nucleus. In D. Oertel, R. R. Fay, & A. N. Popper (Eds.), *Integrative functions of the mammalian auditory pathway, Springer handbook of auditory research* (pp. 160–206). New York: Springer-Verlag.

Yu, X., Sanes, D. H., Aristizabal, O., Wadghiri, Y. Z., & Turnbull, D. H. (2007). Large-scale reorganization of the tonotopic map in mouse auditory midbrain revealed by MRI. *Proceedings of the National Academy of Sciences, USA, 104,* 12193–12198.

Zinkus, P. W., Gottlieb, M. I., & Shapiro, M. (1978). Developmental and psychoeducational sequelae of chronic otitis media. *Archives of Pediatrics and Adolescent Medicine, 132,* 1100–1104.

PART 4

Early Experience and Developmental Plasticity

Early Sensory Experience, Behavior, and Gene Expression in *Caenorhabditis elegans*

Evan L. Ardiel, Susan Rai, *and* Catharine H. Rankin

Abstract

The soil-dwelling nematode, *Caenorhabditis elegans*, is an ideal system to study developmental plasticity. Researchers are aided by a mapped and sequenced genome, a complete cell lineage, and a neural wiring diagram. The predictability with which these worms develop makes it possible to examine subtle alterations that occur as a result of early experience. Experiments show effects of early deprivation/enrichment on behavior, growth, and neural structure. Studies using genetic mutants have revealed activity-dependent structural plasticity in specific neurons and long-lasting impacts of early sensory input have been demonstrated using mechanical and olfactory stimuli. Such a thorough investigation of the complex interaction between the environment and the genome has not been possible in any other organism studied to date.

Keywords: *Caenorhabditis elegans*, developmental plasticity, neural structure, genetic mutants, activity-dependent structural plasticity

The role of early experience in sculpting the nervous system is one of the most intriguing questions in neurobiology. The long-held belief that nervous system development is governed by a hardwired genetic program uninfluenced by external factors has been shown to be incorrect in organisms across the phylogenetic tree. Research in this area has only begun to shed light on the ways in which sensory input influences development. These findings are not only of interest to biologists and psychologists, as they have important implications for public policy. For example, findings that show how to reverse the effects of sensory deprivation will be critical in developing strategies to best help individuals who have experienced early deprivation. A valuable step in understanding the ways in which the environment influences the human nervous system is to characterize the effects of early sensory experience in model organisms. The soil-dwelling nematode *Caenorhabditis elegans* is one such model.

There is very little variation in the nervous systems of individuals in a colony of self-fertilizing hermaphroditic *C. elegans*. Each worm has 959 cells, 302 of which are neurons, forming about 5000 chemical synapses, 600 gap junctions, and 2000 neuromuscular junctions (White, Southgate, Thomson, & Brenner, 1986). The number and variety of neurons are consistent among individuals. Axon morphology is predictable and synaptic connections are highly characteristic, with approximately 80%–90% of the synapses reproduced from one worm to the next. This seems to suggest that the nervous system of *C. elegans* is largely unaffected by experience and therefore not a useful model for developmental plasticity. However, *C. elegans* actually exhibits a considerable degree of plasticity and is thus an ideal system for study.

One of the most extreme forms of experience-dependent plasticity is an altered life cycle in response to environmental cues. Under certain conditions, *C. elegans* will enter larval diapause (cease developing) until favorable conditions return. As would be expected, this life stage change results in a considerable alteration of the nervous system. In addition to this extreme form of plasticity, *C. elegans* also displays more subtle forms of experience-dependent plasticity. For example, every sensory system (mechanosensation, thermosensation, and chemosensation) has shown a capacity for mediating learning and memory (Giles, Rose, & Rankin, 2006) and studies of mutant worms with altered neural functions suggest that normal sensory activity is necessary for normal growth and axon morphology (Fujiwara, Segupta, & McIntire, 2002; Peckol, Zallen, Yarrow, & Bargmann, 1999; Zhao & Nonet, 2000). Since there is a fully mapped and sequenced genome and a complete cell lineage history and neural wiring diagram, neuronal changes can be examined relatively easily in *C. elegans* at both cellular and molecular levels. Mutants with alterations in neural genes with known gene expression patterns are readily available to researchers and this organism's small, tractable nervous system means that the activity of individual neurons can be studied. The worm's small size (~1 mm in length) and short life cycle (<3 days) also make it amenable for laboratory manipulations. Above all, *C. elegans* is an exquisite model for plasticity studies because worms develop independently and predictably, leading to genetically identical colonies in which the influence of the environment can be assessed directly without worry of confounding biological factors.

This chapter examines the degree to which the nervous system of *C. elegans* is sculpted by early experience. The first section discusses the causes and consequences of larval diapause. This is followed by a review of research involving mutations that alter the level of neural activity in different circuits and lead to specific alterations of sensory and motor neuron morphology. The final section is a review of manipulations of the external environment that have predictable impacts on worm biology. In particular, this section of the chapter examines the effects of exposure to conspecifics and odorants. The depth of analysis possible with *C. elegans* is unrivalled by any other model system. As a result, rapid progress is currently being made

in understanding developmental plasticity at the behavioral, cellular, and molecular levels.

Larval Diapause

C. elegans has two distinct life cycles (Figure 14.1). If reared under optimal conditions, worms develop through four larval stages (L1, L2, L3, and L4) to become fully reproducing adults 3 days after fertilization. However, high population densities and limited food can lead to a developmental diversion into larval diapause, called "the dauer stage," at the end of L1. This is highly adaptive given the "boom and bust" strategy of habitat depletion employed by this soil nematode (Riddle & Albert, 1997). With a specialized biology for long-term survival and dispersal, dauer larvae appear thin and dense (Figure 14.2) and exhibit distinctly different behavioral patterns from developing larvae. Pharyngeal pumping (feeding) is suppressed (Cassada & Russell, 1975) and movement is limited in order to conserve energy. Worms do respond to touch, but do not exhibit chemotaxis (i.e., oriented movements toward or away from a chemical stimulus) toward food and unlike adult worms, dauer worms exhibit thermotaxis (i.e., oriented movements toward or away from heat) to novel ambient air temperatures (Hedgecock & Russell, 1975). Dauer larvae may also climb objects and wave their bodies in the air (Croll & Matthews 1977), a behavior that probably leads to insect-mediated dispersal in the natural environment. Restructuring of the sensory neurons is likely responsible for some of these dauer-specific behaviors (Albert & Riddle, 1983).

The amphid is the principal chemosensory organ of *C. elegans*. It is a prominent bilaterally symmetrical structure located at the side of the head (Figure 14.2iv) and is composed of 12 neurons, eight of which make direct contact with the environment through a pore in the cuticle (Ward, Thomson, White, & Brenner, 1975; Ware, Clark, Crossland, & Russel, 1975). In dauer larvae, amphid sensory neurons ASG, ASI, AWC, and AFD (see Table 14.1) adopt a dauer-specific shape or location (Albert & Riddle, 1983). Unlike the amphid pores, the channels of the inner labial sensilla are almost completely closed throughout larval diapause (Figure 14.2iii; Albert & Riddle, 1983). The six inner labial channels are arranged symmetrically around the mouth at the apex of the lips and each houses two neurons. In dauer worms, the dendritic tips of the two neurons switch position relative to each other, so that inner labial neuron

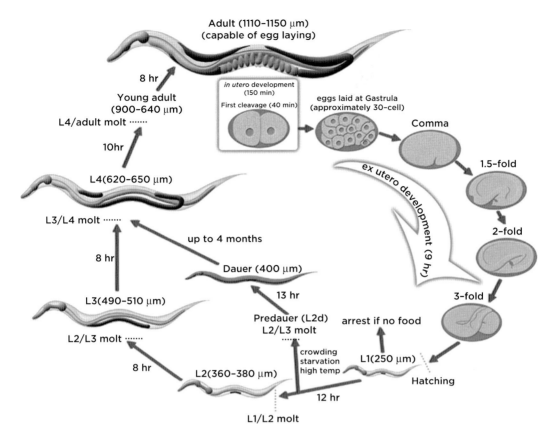

Figure 14.1 The life cycles of *C. elegans* indicating worm length and duration of developmental stage at 22°C. (Reprinted from www.wormatlas.org with permission.)

1, thought to be mechanosensory, becomes more anterior than inner labial neuron 2, thought to be chemosensory. In addition, the cilia of inner labial neuron 2 are markedly reduced as compared to the cilia of developing larvae (Figure 14.2v). In another sensory structure, the deirid, the mechanosensory neurons are also altered in structure and orientation in dauer larvae (Riddle & Albert, 1997). The dendritic tip of each neuron is attached to the body wall cuticle by a substructure not seen at any other life stage and is oriented parallel to the longitudinal axis of the body, as opposed to the perpendicular orientation seen in growing larvae. It is apparent, then, that dauer development leads to considerable reorganization of the sensory neurons. Changes in these neurons alter the worm's perception of the environment and are likely responsible for the changes in chemotactic behavior and recovery from the dauer state. Modification of the sensory endings may also serve to protect the neurons from the harsh environments often encountered by dauer worms.

As would be expected, metabolism in the developmentally arrested worms also changes to meet the demands of long-term survival in the absence of food. Decreased citric acid cycle activity relative to glyoxylate cycle activity and high phosphofructokinase activity suggests increased glycogen metabolism and lipid storage (O'Riordan & Burnell, 1989). The unique metabolic state of dauer larvae is underlined by a less acidic intracellular environment (Wadsworth & Riddle, 1988). Studies also suggest that transcriptional activity is reduced in this alternate larval stage (Dalley & Golomb, 1992; Snutch & Baillie, 1983) and oxidative damage is minimized by increased superoxide dismutase (Anderson, 1982; Larsen, 1993) and catalase (Vanfleteren & De Vreese, 1995) activity. It is evident that these two divergent life cycles necessitate profoundly different alterations to worm morphology, physiology, and behavior.

Whether a worm continues the normal course of development or becomes a dauer larva is dependent on three environmental factors: population

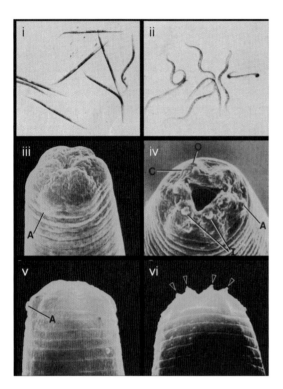

Figure 14.2 Dauer larvae with characteristic thin, dense appearance (i) versus same-age L3 developing larvae (ii). Scanning electron micrographs showing dauer (iii and v) and developing (iv and vi) larva head morphologies (11500x). Most of the anterior sensory structures visible in developing larvae (iv; subdorsal and subventral outer labial sensilla, O, cephalic sensilla, C, inner labial sensilla, I, and amphids, A) are obscured by the cuticle in dauer larvae (iii and v). Arrows indicate the protruding inner labial sensilla of a developing larva (vi) not present in dauer larvae (v). (Courtesy of John Wiley & Sons, Canada [i and ii] and Journal of comparative neurology [iii–vi].)

density, food supply (quality and quantity), and temperature. Population density is the most important factor and is measured indirectly by the worm through the concentration of dauer pheromone, a stable pheromone compound constitutively released by conspecifics (Golden & Riddle, 1984a). Food cues and temperature have an auxiliary role in promoting dauer formation. Food supply cues come in the form of volatile chemicals released by bacteria. Abundant food and low pheromone concentration promote "normal" development (Golden & Riddle, 1984b), while high temperatures promote dauer development (Golden & Riddle, 1984c). Once favorable conditions resume, dauer larvae recover to become "normal" fertile adults. Recovery is mediated by the same three environmental cues (Golden & Riddle, 1984b) and is more easily initiated in

older dauer larvae (Riddle & Albert, 1997). This environmentally induced change in phenotype provides a vivid example of early sensory experience shaping an organism's biology.

With so much riding on the developmental pathway, evolution has selected for optimal sensitivity of dauer formation to sensory inputs. Cell ablation studies have shown that under conditions favoring nondauer development, ADF, ASI, and ASG neurons promote "normal" development, while ASJ neurons promote dauer development (Bargmann & Horvitz, 1991). Mutant screens have identified more than 30 genes important for diversion to the dauer life cycle and many of these have a role in the development or function of the aforementioned sensory neurons. For example, *daf-1*, *daf-4*, *daf-7*, *daf-8*, and *daf-14* (see Table 14.1) are essential components of the signaling pathway for the polypeptide growth factor, TGF-β (Thomas, Birnby, & Vowels, 1993), through which sensory neurons promote nondauer development via regulated transcription of *daf-7* (Ren et al., 1996; Schackwitz, Inoue, & Thomas, 1996). It is hypothesized that DAF-7 is released by sensory neurons to bind to the receptors of other cells and promote nondauer development. An additional signaling pathway, mediated by a transmembrane guanylyl cyclase (encoded by *daf-11*), is thought to inhibit ASJ dauer-promoting activity

(Riddle & Albert, 1997). Complex, overlapping pathways speak to the exquisite sensitivity of larvae to environmental cues. Appropriate response to these cues is highly adaptive given the critical implications that life cycle choice has on the worm's reproductive survival.

Environmentally induced life cycle changes are the ultimate form of experience-dependent developmental plasticity and dauer formation certainly highlights the significant impact that sensory input can have on the biology of the worm, but plasticity is often much more subtle than a life cycle diversion and recent studies have begun to examine the extent to which this 302-neuron nervous system organizes itself in response to sensory input.

Activity-dependent Neuron Morphology

Peckol et al. (1999) demonstrated that normal axon morphology in several sensory neurons is dependent upon normal neural activity. They established an experimental paradigm for sensory deprivation using sensory transduction mutants with defective sensory cilia (i.e., *daf-6, osm-1, osm-5, osm-6, che-3,* and *che-11*) or ion channels (*unc-36, eat-12, tax-2,* and *tax-4*). All of these mutations resulted in the formation of ectopic or extra processes in the ASE, ASJ, ASI, and AWB chemosensory neurons (Figure 14.3), with the highest frequency of occurrence in the ASE and ASJ neurons. The abnormal processes were consistent with axons because of the accumulation of synaptic markers (vesicle-associated membrane proteins; Jorgensen et al., 1995) and the absence of dendritic markers. The fact that all of these signal transduction mutants had similar abnormal axon morphologies in the same subset of sensory neurons suggests that a lack of neuronal activity was responsible. It appears that sensory deprivation affected axon growth and not axon guidance because the ectopic processes did not appear until long after the wild-type axon had reached the nerve ring in late embryogenesis. Peckol et al. (1999) hypothesized that morphology of the axons of the ASE, ASJ, ASI, and AWB sensory neurons has two distinct phases of development, the activity-independent initial axon outgrowth and the activity-dependent maintenance of sensory neuron morphology.

The importance of activity for normal neural structure is not limited to sensory neurons. Zhao and Nonet (2000) demonstrated that *C. elegans* motor neurons also exhibit experience-dependent structural plasticity. They found that activity at the neuromuscular junction plays a role in remodeling the axons of three SAB motor neurons. SABVL, SABVR, and SABD project anteriorly to the head muscles, where they form cholinergic synapses. SAB axonal projections innervate the head muscles during embryogenesis and continually form synaptic varicosities throughout larval development. Acetylcholine (ACh) is the dominant neuromuscular neurotransmitter and complete loss of ACh synthesis or vesicular transport results in arrested

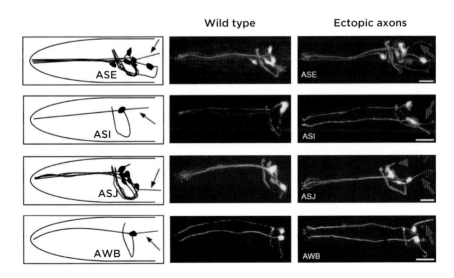

Figure 14.3 Wild type and mutant ASE, ASI, ASJ, and AWB neurons in the worm head. Arrows indicate the characteristic ectopic axons resulting from disturbance of activity in these neurons. Ventral is down and anterior is to the left. Bars = 10 μm. (Reproduced with permission of the Company of Biologists.)

development at L1. Each axon in the adult worm typically contains about 12 synaptic variscosities, but this morphology is sensitive to neuronal activity. Zhao and Nonet (2000) found that disruption of electrical activity or synaptic transmission resulted in the formation of abnormal axon sprouts in the SAB neurons (Figure 14.4; Zhao & Nonet, 2000). These sprouts contained several variscosities evenly distributed along a short single branch, with some sprouts displaying secondary branches. Less frequently, the axons of the mutant SAB neurons displayed a second phenotypic alteration, an abnormal extension of the axon that looped back toward the posterior. Based on these data, Zhao and Nonet (2000) concluded that reduced ACh activity in the neuromuscular junction generated sprouting in SAB axons. Remarkably, SAB axon morphology is not only influenced by its own activity, but is also affected by activity in the postsynaptic muscle cell (Zhao & Nonet, 2000), implicating a retrograde signal of some kind. Mutants with either defective nicotine ACh receptor subunits (*unc-29*) or reduced muscle cell excitability displayed axon sprouts similar to those produced by the disruption of presynaptic activity, although at a reduced frequency. From these data, Zhao and Nonet (2000) hypothesized that the postsynaptic muscle cell somehow communicates with the presynaptic motor neuron to influence its morphology.

Sculpting the nervous system in response to activity during critical periods is a key feature of

neurodevelopment and Zhao and Nonet (2000) used ACh synthesis temperature-sensitive mutants to demonstrate that the structural plasticity of SAB neurons is restricted to early larval stages. Larvae exposed to the nonpermissive temperature (22.5°C) in either L1 or L2 had a high incidence of axonal sprouting (Figure 14.4). Sprouting frequency dropped dramatically in worms exposed to the nonpermissive temperature in L3 and reached baseline levels in worms exposed in L4. Thus, SAB axonal morphology appears to be developmentally controlled, with larval stages L1 and L2 most sensitive to a reduction in ACh activity. Although the frequency of sprouting was maximal in worms exposed to the nonpermissive temperature for 12 h, it appeared in worms exposed for only 2 h. Fifteen percent of the sprouts formed during early exposure retracted after continued development at the permissive temperature. The conclusion from this observation is that sprouts are readily formed in inactive SAB neurons in L1 and L2 larvae, but the remodeling is not necessarily permanent.

Neural activity-dependent processes play a pivotal role in shaping the final patterns and strengths of many of the synaptic connections of the nervous system. The studies of Peckol et al. (1999) and Zhao and Nonet (2000) highlight the usefulness of *C. elegans* in studying these processes. For example, visualizing individual neuronal changes was aided considerably by the complete anatomical map, transparent cuticle, and lack of dendritic arbors. The presence of many well-characterized *C. elegans* mutants was also extremely valuable. In both studies, mutants were used to establish a simulated reduction in neural activity. The following studies examine how actually manipulating the developing worm's environment can impact its neurobiology.

Sensory Cues from Conspecifics and Mechanosensory Stimulation

A common method used to assess the effects of experience on development is to deprive the organism of the experience of interest. For example, rearing rats in isolation with little stimulation leads to thinner visual cortices (Volkmar & Greenough, 1972) and fewer synapses per neuron (Turner & Greenough, 1985). Similar results are observed in invertebrates: *Drosophila melanogaster* reared in isolation show 15% fewer Kenyon cell fibers in their mushroom bodies than flies reared in colonies (Heisenberg, Heusipp, & Wanke, 1995). The same types of effects have also been observed in *C. elegans*: Rose, Sangha, Rai, Norman, and Rankin

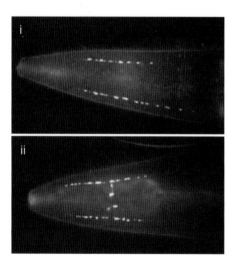

Figure 14.4 Lateral view of worm heads with normal (i) and sprouting (ii) SAB morphology. Sprout formation was induced by a reduction in cholinergic activity. Bar = 10 μm. (Reproduced with permission of the Company of Biologists.)

(2005) examined developmental plasticity in *C. elegans* using a paradigm in which worms were raised in isolation versus in groups. As noted earlier, *C. elegans* senses and responds to dauer pheromone released by other worms, but conspecifics are also a source of mechanosensory stimulation during development as they contact one another while they move through their environment. Rose et al. (2005) found that worms reared in isolation showed decreased adult responsiveness to mechanical stimuli, altered gene expression of both a pre- and a postsynaptic marker in the mechanosensory neural circuit, and slowed rates of physical development.

Forward swimming worms briefly reverse direction in response to a mechanical tap delivered to the side of the plastic Petri plate in which they reside. The neural circuit that mediates the response to this tap includes seven mechanosensory neurons (ALM (2), AVM (1), PLM (2), and PVD (2); Wicks & Rankin, 1995). These neurons synapse onto four pairs of command interneurons

(AVD, AVB, AVA, and PVC), which synapse onto a large cluster of motor neurons. In their study of activity-dependent plasticity during development, Rose et al. (2005) measured adult responsiveness to mechanical stimuli by tapping the worm's Petri plate and measuring the distance the worm swam backwards. They found that adult worms reared in isolation responded less than worms reared in groups (colony worms) (Figure 14.5i).

In a previous study, it was shown that adult worms can habituate (a nonassociative form of learning) to the tapping stimulus and that they are capable of forming both short- and long-term memory for this habituation (Rankin, Beck, & Chiba, 1990). In an attempt to locate the site of plasticity for habituation, Wicks and Rankin (1997) carried out a series of behavioral experiments that led them to conclude that the synapses between the mechanosensory neurons and the interneurons were the most likely sites for experience-dependent modification of the tap circuit. The neurons in the

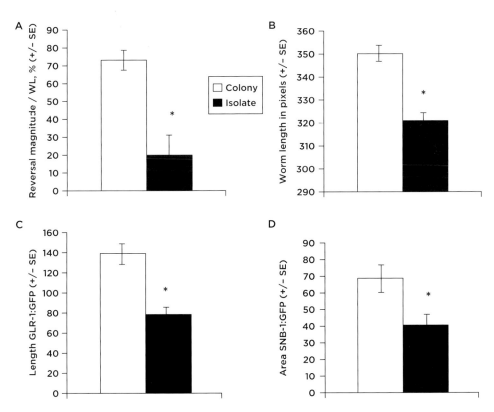

Figure 14.5 Effects of isolation on tap reversal response (i), worm length (ii), and glutamate receptor (iii) and vesicle expression (iv). Colony worms were significantly longer than isolate-reared worms (ii; p < 0.0001). Correcting for worm length, WL, reveals that the tap-induced reversal magnitude of isolate-reared worms was significantly less than that of colony worms (i; p ≤ 0.0002). The mean length of GLR-1:GFP expressing clusters in the ventral cord of isolate-reared worms was significantly less than the length of GFP expressing clusters in colony worms (iii; p ≤ 0.0001), as was the mean area of SNB-1:GFP expression (iv; p = 0.01).

tap circuit are glutamatergic and the command interneurons express GLR-1, a *C. elegans* homolog of a mammalian AMPA-/Kainate-type glutamatergic receptor subunit. In adult learning, strains of worms with mutations in *glr-1* show normal short-term habituation, but no long-term retention, suggesting that long-term memory requires activation of GLR-1 receptors. In the study of Rose et al. (2005), *glr-1* mutants also failed to show the effect of isolation on adult responsiveness to tap, thereby implicating glutamate neurotransmission in developmental plasticity.

Using confocal microscopy and transgenic worms expressing GLR-1 fused to a green fluorescent protein (GFP), Rose, Kaun, Chen, and Rankin (2003) quantified GLR-1:GFP expression along the posterior ventral nerve cord of *C. elegans*. They found that GLR-1:GFP expression was significantly reduced in worms that had received a long-term memory training protocol 24 h earlier. This reduction came in the form of smaller, but not fewer, GLR-1:GFP-expressing clusters. Because the GLR-1:GFP construct did not discriminate membrane-bound and intracellular GLR-1, the observed reduction in GLR-1 likely resulted from degradation or removal from the cell process, as opposed to the cytosolic internalization and repackaging seen in mammalian neurons. Thus long-term habituation appears to be mediated by a downregulation of glutamate receptors. Changes in glutamate receptor expression have been found to affect synaptic strength and may be a mechanism for the formation of memories in mammalian systems (Lüscher & Frerking, 2001; Malinow & Malenka, 2002).

Using the same strain of transgenic worms, Rose et al. (2005) showed that isolate-reared worms also had significantly less GLR-1:GFP expression than colony worms (Figure 14.5iii). Remember that both isolate-reared worms and habituated worms exhibit a reduction in response to tap as compared to colony and unhabituated worms, respectively. The concordance between the behavior and the expression patterns of GLR-1 receptors underscores the important role of glutamate receptor trafficking in the plasticity of the tap-withdrawal response. It is interesting to note that both the absence of mechanical stimulation (during isolation) and the persistence of mechanical stimulation (during habituation training) lead to a similar behavioral pattern mediated by the same mechanism, i.e., a downregulation of *glr-1*, which results in weaker synapses between the touch cells and/or the interneurons and a decreased responsiveness to tap.

Rearing condition also alters the presynaptic terminals of the mechanosensory neurons. *snb-1* encodes synaptobrevin, the synaptic vesicle protein that regulates vesicle fusion to the presynaptic terminal. SNB-1 levels in the neuron can be used as an indirect measure of the number of synaptic vesicles in the presynaptic terminal. Rose et al. (2005) were able to quantify SNB-1 expression in the six mechanosensory neurons of the tap withdrawal circuit using a SNB-1:GFP transgene under the control of the *mec-7* promoter. They found that isolate-reared worms had significantly smaller areas of fluorescence (Figure 14.5iv), suggesting that the amount of synaptobrevin (and by extension the number of synaptic vesicles) was determined by the amount of mechanosensory input received during development. This is in contrast to studies of adult plasticity where long-term habituated worms showed no change in SNB-1:GFP expression in the sensory neurons (Rose et al., 2003). Taken together, the data showing a decrease in the expression of both *glr-1* glutamate receptors in the interneurons and synaptobrevin in the sensory neurons suggest that the decrease in early mechanosensory experience leads to the development of a weaker synaptic connection between the sensory neurons and interneurons than in worms receiving normal stimulation. Thus, the amount of early stimulation appears to play a critical role in determining synaptic strength.

These studies also demonstrate that developmental experience can alter gene expression in the nervous system, leading to behavioral changes in adult worms. It appears as though the absence of mechanosensory input from interactions with conspecifics results in decreased activity in the mechanosensory neural circuit, causing the development of a weak synapse between the mechanosensory neurons and/or between the interneurons. However, it should be noted that worms reared in isolation are also deprived of the chemosensory cues of other worms. To address this issue, isolated worms were reared on plates that had once held a colony of worms. Isolated worms reared on these conditioned plates still showed a decreased response to tap, suggesting that chemosensory input from stable chemical cues had little to no influence on the strength of the mechanosensory synapse, but a role for chemosensory input could not be ruled out entirely because the conditioned plates lacked the volatile cues constitutively released by worms. However, colony worms with a mutation rendering them insensitive to chemosensory cues exhibited a greater response to tap than isolate-reared worms with the same mutation. Since these chemosensory mutants showed the isolate/colony effect on the response to tap, the requirement of chemosensory stimulation for normal development of the tap withdrawal response was ruled out.

A number of studies using rodents have reversed the effects of environmental deprivation by applying mechanosensory stimulation, such as the "stroking" of deprived rat pups. Stroking with a fine paintbrush mimics the touch stimulation normally provided to pups by the mother when she licks and grooms them (Lovic & Fleming, 2004; Schanberg & Field, 1987). If it was only the lack of mechanosensory stimulation during development that led to the decreased response to tap and the downregulation of the associated pre- and postsynaptic markers, snb-1 and glr-1, respectively, then we would predict that receiving supplemental mechanical stimuli during development could rescue the effects of isolation on the tap-withdrawal response. This was indeed the case. Rose et al. (2005) produced mechanical stimulation by putting all of the Petri plates housing isolated worms into a box and repeatedly dropping the box onto a flat surface from a height of about 2 in. Such stimulation rescued the effects of isolation on the worm's mechanosensory circuit. Brief stimulation (30 drops) anytime during development reversed the effects of isolation on tap reversal and glr-1 expression in adult worms (Rai & Rankin, 2007, in press). Low levels of stimulation early in development also rescued snb-1 expression in adults, but as the age at which stimulation was administered increased, so too did the amount of stimulation required to rescue snb-1 expression: 400 drops at L2 or L3 and 800 drops at L4 and YAD. This suggests that as the worm ages, snb-1 expression becomes less susceptible to environmental manipulation. The differing ability to rescue GLR-1 and SNB-1 suggests that there is no strong relationship between pre- and postsynaptic gene expression. This emphasizes the point that alleviating the effects of isolation on one aspect of development has in no way reversed the impact of isolation on the organism as a whole. Without rescuing both the pre- and postsynaptic markers, mechanosensory behavior is still deficient. For example, isolate-reared worms that were stimulated enough to rescue GLR-1, but not SNB-1, habituated to tap more rapidly than group-reared worms (Rose et al., 2005). It is worth noting that the ability to relate animal behavior to both pre- and postsynaptic elements of identified neurons has not been possible in any other organism.

Rose et al. (2005) found that worms reared in isolation were also delayed in physical development. Isolate-reared worms were shorter (Figure 14.5ii) and narrower than colony worms and showed a later onset of egg laying. Body size was not rescued using the 30–800 Petri plate drops that rescued responsiveness to tap, glr-1 expression, and snb-1 expression. Perhaps accelerated development is mediated by mechanosensory input resulting from specific interactions with other worms that are not reproduced by Petri plate drops, or more likely, from an integration of several different sensory inputs.

The effect of isolation on body size could be rescued by transferring worms to a colony plate within a critical period of development. Worms reared in isolation and then transferred to a colony either at the start of L1, L2, or L3 did not differ in body size from worms reared in colonies throughout development. However, if transferred to a colony condition at the start of L4 or later, worms remained significantly shorter than colony worms. In a complimentary study, worms reared in a colony condition were transferred to individual isolate plates. If the transfer occurred at the start of L1, L2, or L3, the worms remained significantly shorter than colony worms. In contrast, transferring colony worms to individual isolate plates at the start of L4 or later did not affect body size.

Fujiwara et al. (2002) showed that worms with defective chemosensory organs were smaller than wild-type worms, but not delayed in development. In this study, the rate of development was determined by gonad maturation. Perhaps the use of a similar marker will reveal that isolate-reared worms are delayed only in the onset of egg-laying, as opposed to all aspects of development. Fujiwara et al. (2002) found that the effect of defective chemosensory organs on body size was mediated by egl-4, a gene encoding a cGMP-dependent protein kinase. EGL-4 is expressed in several head neurons, some muscle cells, and in the intestine (Hirose et al., 2003). As a part of the DBL-1 TGF-β signaling cascade, egl-4 plays an important role in processing sensory information and regulating body size in C. elegans. Mutations in dbl-1 (TGF-β ligand) and sma-6 (TGF-β type I receptor) result in worms that are only about half the size of wild-types. dbl-1 is expressed in the neurons and appears to control transcription of genes regulating body size by activating a SMA-6 receptor in the hypodermis (Suzuki et al., 1999; Yoshida, Morita, Mochii, & Ueno, 1991). Genetic interaction studies performed by

Fujiwara et al. (2002) suggest that EGL-4 mediates body size by regulating *dbl-1*. Rose et al. (2005) showed that the effects of isolation on body size are also mediated by *egl-4*. Thus, isolation leads to decreased body size in a way somehow mediated by the cGMP-dependent kinase *egl-4*.

So far we have only discussed the developmental impacts of deprivation, but receiving extra mechanosensory stimulation also alters behavior and gene expression later in life. Ebrahimi and Rankin (2007) showed that distributed training (100 taps separated by 1 min and divided into five blocks separated by 1 h) early in development had long-term effects on worm biology and that these effects were not consistent across the life span. Following exposure to a distributed training paradigm in L1, 3-day-old worms showed increased responsiveness to tap as compared to untrained worms, while 5-day-old worms trained in L1 showed decreased responsiveness to tap. This effect was protein synthesis–dependent. It is quite striking to note that control worms responded more and more to tap as they aged from 3 to 4, and then to 5 days of age, but worms receiving just 100 taps in L1 showed the opposite trend. Interestingly, the patterned stimulation only led to an increase in reversal of magnitude in 3-day-old worms when it was administered in L1, suggesting a critical period for this developmental plasticity. In contrast, the depressed response seen in 5-day-old worms had no critical period and could be induced with patterned stimulation administered in L1, L2, or L4, but not L3. The lack of plasticity seen in worms stimulated in L3 may be due to the addition of the AVM neuron to the tap circuit during this stage. Consistent with other studies, *glr-1* was found to be critical for behavioral plasticity: worms with mutations in *glr-1* failed to show any effect of patterned stimulation on adult behavior. Once again, increased GLR-1:GFP expression and *glr-1* mRNA levels correlated with larger responses to tap and decreased GLR-1:GFP expression and *glr-1* mRNA levels correlated with smaller responses to tap. From these observations, we see that the timing and pattern of stimulation received as a juvenile (larva) plays a major role in adult worm behavior (Figure 14.6).

The depressed behavioral response observed in 5-day-old worms was similar to the 24-h long-term retention of habituation previously discussed in this chapter. To qualify as long-term habituation, the response decrement must be dependent on interstimulus interval (Beck & Rankin, 1997; Carew, Pinsker, & Kandler, 1972; Rose, Kaun, & Rankin,

2002), temporal pattern of stimulation (spaced vs. massed), activation of gene transcription, protein synthesis (Scharf et al., 2002), and glutamatergic activity (Rose et al., 2003). The depressed response seen in 5-day-old worms meets all of these criteria. It is also sensitive to reconsolidation blockade. Reconsolidation blockade occurs when a recalled memory becomes labile and is then eliminated by manipulations that interfere with memory consolidation (Rose & Rankin, 2006). In the long-term habituation paradigm, reconsolidation blockade is accomplished by first training the worms in L1, waiting for 24 h, and then administering 10 reminder taps followed by 40 min of heat shock at 32°C (heat shock halts protein synthesis and has been shown to block long-term retention of habituation in *C. elegans*; Rose et al., 2003). Under such treatment, the 3-day response enhancement was still present, but the 5-day response depression was lost. This seems to suggest that early training produces a memory for habituation that is not expressed until the worm is 5 days old. *glr-1* expression levels show no depression until day 5, thus some other mechanism must be encoding the earlier training for expression in 5-day-old adults. The adaptive advantage of this phenomenon is unclear. Future research in this area may provide some insight on the nature of latent memories.

Olfactory Imprinting

Memories allow animals to alter their behavior based on past experience. Holding a memory of habituation training for 5 days (Ebrahimi & Rankin, 2006) is an impressive feat for a worm that only lives about 2 weeks under laboratory conditions at 20°C. Another learning paradigm, known as sensory imprinting, also highlights this ability. An olfactory imprint is a long-lasting memory of an odor encountered during a sensitive period in the life of an organism. The sensitive period may be a specific developmental stage or physiological state (e.g., estrus). Olfactory imprinting is best known in Pacific salmon, which use olfactory imprints of their natal stream to aid in the home-stream migration (Hasler & Scholz, 1983). A study by Remy and Hobert (2005) showed that *C. elegans* are also capable of this form of learning. Worms exposed to an attractive odorant during the first larval stage (L1) changed their locomotive and egg-laying behavior in the presence of that odorant later in life, provided the cue was presented in combination with food or exogenous serotonin (which mimicked the presence of food; Remy & Hobert, 2005). When

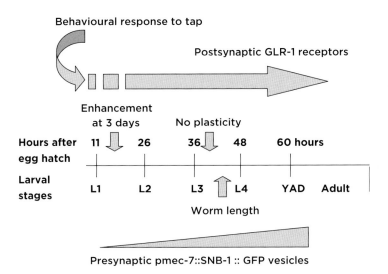

Figure 14.6 Summary of critical periods during *C. elegans* development. Brief mechanical stimulation at any point in development reversed the effect of isolation on the tap-withdrawal response and GLR:GFP expression, while rescuing SNB-1:GFP expression required progressively more stimulation as the worm developed. L3 was the critical period for an initially isolated worm to achieve a colony worm body size. L1 was the only stage at which patterned mechanical stimulation led to an enhanced tap-withdrawal response in 3-day old colony worms and L3 was the only stage at which patterned mechanical stimulation did not alter the adult behavior of colony worms.

preexposed worms encountered imprinted odorants as adults, they exhibited increased positive chemotaxis and laid twice as many eggs as control worms. Just as olfactory imprinting was restricted to a developmental stage, L1, the behavioral output was only expressed once worms reached reproductive maturity. These findings suggest that *C. elegans* use olfactory imprinting to locate nutrient-rich environments in which to lay their eggs, thereby permitting their progeny to benefit from the memory of a favorable growth site.

The use of *C. elegans* makes it possible to investigate the cellular and molecular mechanisms underlying sensory imprinting. Remy and Hobert (2005) found that only odorants with receptors in AWC sensory neurons are imprintable. Although each AWC sensory neuron displays multiple receptors (including those for benzaldehyde and isoamylalcohol), the memory appears to be odorant-specific. Benzaldehyde-imprinted worms did not show a preference for isoamylalcohol and vice versa. Furthermore, larval worms simultaneously imprinted with benzaldehyde and isoamylalcohol formed an imprint for each individual odorant. The researchers also showed that olfactory imprinting required the AIY interneurons and *sra-11*. SRA-11 is a G protein–coupled seven-transmembrane putative chemoreceptor expressed in several

interneurons throughout development. *sra-11* null mutants did not show olfactory imprinting, but still exhibited normal chemotaxis, egg-laying, and other behaviors associated with functioning AIY interneurons. This suggests that the SRA-11 protein is required for odorant-nonspecific imprinting. It is still unclear whether odorant exposure in L1 modifies the sensory neurons themselves or receptors downstream on the interneurons.

By now, it should be apparent that although worm colonies vary genetically very little from worm to worm, the developing nervous system of *C. elegans* is highly sensitive to early experience, with particular sensory experiences leading to neural changes that produce specific behavioral outcomes. *C. elegans* has proven to be an exquisite model for developmental plasticity. Despite the vast amount of information available on its behavior and cell biology, remarkably little is known about its ecology or natural history. Future work in these areas will give researchers the evolutionary perspective needed to better understand the significance of their laboratory findings.

Examining how stimulation of sensory neurons affects both the nervous system and the organism as a whole can help us understand child development and may aid in the formation of remedies for cases of early deprivation. However, before policies are drafted for practical application in humans, much research is needed on the underlying cellular and molecular mechanisms of developmental plasticity. The power of *C. elegans* as a model organism makes it an ideal system to explore these mechanisms.

References

Albert, P. S., & Riddle, D. L. (1983). Developmental alterations in sensory neuroanatomy of the Caenorhabditis elegans dauer larva. The Journal of Comparative Neurology, 219(4), 461–481.

Anderson, G. L. (1982). Superoxide dismutase activity in the dauer larvae of Caenorhabditis elegans. Canadian Journal of Zoology, 60(3), 288–291.

Bargmann, C. I., & Horvitz, H. R. (1991). Control of larval development by chemosensory neurons in Caenorhabditis elegans. Science, 251(4998), 1243–1246.

Beck, C. D. O., & Rankin, C. H. (1997). Long-term habituation is produced by distributed training at long ISIs and not by massed training at short ISIs in Caenorhabditis elegans. Animal Learning and Behavior, 25(4), 446–457.

Carew, T. J., Pinsker, H. M., & Kandler, E. R. (1972). Long-term habituation of a defensive withdrawal reflex in aplasia. Science, 175(4020), 451–454.

Cassada, R. C., & Russell, R. L. (1975). The dauer larva, a post-embryonic developmental variant of the nematode Caenorhabditis elegans. Developmental Biology, 46(2), 326–342.

Croll, N. A., & Matthews, B. E. (1977). Biology of nematodes. New York: John Wiley.

Dalley, B. K., & Golomb, M. (1992). Gene expression in the Caenorhabditis elegans dauer larva: Developmental regulation of Hsp90 and other genes. Developmental Biology, 151(1), 80–90.

Ebrahimi, C. M., & Rankin, C. H. (2007). Early patterned stimulation produces changes in adult behavior and gene expression in C. elegans. Genes, Brain, and Behavior, 6(6), 517–528.

Fujiwara, M., Segupta, P., & McIntire, S. L. (2002). Regulation of body size and behavioral state of C. elegans by sensory perception and the egl-4 cGMP-dependent protein kinase. Neuron, 366(6), 1091–1102.

Giles, A. C., Rose, J. K., & Rankin, C. H. (2006). Investigations of learning and memory in Caenorahabditis elegans. International Review of Neurobiology, 69, 37–71.

Golden, J. W., & Riddle, D. L. (1984a). A Caenorhabditis elegans dauer-inducing pheromone and an antagonistic component of the food supply. Journal of Chemical Ecology, 10(8), 1265–1280.

Golden, J. W., & Riddle, D. L. (1984b). The Caenorhabditis elegans dauer larva: Developmental effects of pheromone, food, and temperature. Developmental Biology, 102(2), 368–378.

Golden, J. W., & Riddle, D. L. (1984c). A pheromone-induced developmental switch in Caenorhabditis elegans: Temperature-sensitive mutants reveal a wild-type temperature-dependent process. Proceedings of the National Academy of Sciences, USA, 81(3), 819–823.

Hasler, A. D., & Scholz, A. T. (1983). Olfactory imprinting and homing in salmon. Berlin, New York: Springer-Verlag.

Hedgecock, E. M., & Russell, R. L. (1975). Normal and mutant thermotaxis in the nematode Caenorhabditis elegans. Proceedings of the National Academy of Sciences, USA, 72(10), 4061–4065.

Heisenberg, M., Heusipp, M., & Wanke, C. (1995). Structural plasticity in the Drosophila brain. The Journal of Neuroscience, 15(3), 1951–1960.

Hirose, T., Nakano, Y., Nagamatsu, Y., Misumi, T., Ohta, H., & Oshima, Y. (2003). Cyclic GMP-dependent protein kinase EGL-4 controls body size and lifespan in C. elegans. Development, 130(6), 1089–1099.

Jorgensen, E. M., Hartwieg, E., Schuske, K., Nonet, M. L., Jin, Y., & Horvitz, H. R. (1995). Defective recycling of synaptic vesicles in synaptotagmin mutants of Caenorhabditis elegans. Nature, 378(6553), 196–199.

Larsen, P. L. (1993). Aging and resistance to oxidative damage in Caenorhabditis elegans. Proceedings of the National Academy of Sciences, USA, 90(19), 8905–8909.

Lovic, V., & Fleming, A. S. (2004). Artificially-reared female rats show reduced prepulse inhibition and deficits in the attentional set shifting task-reversal of effects with maternal-like licking stimulation. Behavioural Brain Research, 148(1), 209–219.

Lüscher, C., & Frerking, M. (2001). Restless AMPA receptors: Implications for synaptic transmission and plasticity. Trends in Neurosciences, 24(11), 665–670.

Malinow, R., & Malenka, R. C. (2002). AMPA receptor trafficking and synaptic plasticity. Annual Review of Neuroscience, 25, 103–126.

O'Riordan, V., & Burnell, A. M. (1989). Intermediary metabolism in the dauer larva of the nematode C. elegans. I. Glycolysis, gluconeogenesis, oxidative phosphorylation and the tricarboxylic acid cycle. Comparative Biochemistry and Physiology, 92(2), 233–238.

Peckol, E. L., Zallen, J. A., Yarrow, J. C., & Bargmann, C. I. (1999). Sensory activity affects sensory axon development in C. elegans. Development, 126(9), 1891–1902.

Rai, S., & Rankin, C. H. (2007). Reversing the effects of early isolation on behavior, size and gene expression. Developmental Neurobiology, 67(11), 1443–1456..

Rankin, C. H., Beck, C., & Chiba, C. (1990). Caenorhabditis elegans: A new model system for the study of learning and memory. Behavioural Brain Research, 37(1), 89–92.

Remy, J. J., & Hobert, O. (2005). An interneural chemoreceptor required for olfactory imprinting in C. elegans. Science, 309(5735), 787–790.

Ren, P. F., Lim, C. S., Johnsen, R., Albert, P. S., Pilgrim, D., & Riddle, D. L. (1996). Control of C. elegans larval development by neuronal expression of a TGF-beta homolog. Science, 274(5291), 1389–1391.

Riddle, D. L., & Albert, P. S. (1997). Genetic and environmental regulation of dauer larva development. In D. L. Riddle, T. Blumenthal, B. J. Meyer, & J. R. Priess (Eds.), C. elegans II (pp. 739–768). New York: Cold Spring Harbor Laboratory Press.

Rose, J. K., Kaun, K. R., & Rankin, C. H. (2002). A new group training procedure for habituation demonstrates that presynaptic glutamate release contributes to long-term memory in C. elegans. Learning and Memory, 9(3), 130–137.

Rose, J. K., Kaun, K. R., Chen, S. H., & Rankin, C. H. (2003). Glutamate receptor trafficking underlies long-term memory in C. elegans, The Journal of Neuroscience, 23(29), 9595–9600.

Rose, J. K., & Rankin, C. H. (2006). Blocking memory reconsolidation reverses a cellular mechanism of memory. The Journal of Neuroscience, 26(45), 11582–11587.

Rose, J. K., Sangha, S., Rai, S., Norman, K., & Rankin, C. H. (2005). Decreased sensory stimulation reduces behavioral responding, retards development and alters neuronal connectivity in Caenorhabditis elegans. The Journal of Neuroscience, 25(31), 7159–7168.

Schackwitz, W. S., Inoue, T., & Thomas, J. H. (1996). Chemosensory neurons function in parallel to mediate a pheromone response in C. elegans. Neuron, 17(4), 719–728.

Schanberg, S. M., & Field, T. M. (1987). Sensory deprivation stress and supplemental stimulation in the rat pup and preterm human neonate. Child Development, 58(6), 1431–1447.

Scharf, M. T., Woo, N. H., Lattal, K. M., Young, J. Z., Nguyen, P. V., & Abe, T. (2002). Protein synthesis is required for the enhancement of long-term potentiation and long-term memory by spaced training. Journal of Neurophysiology, 87(6), 2770–2777.

Snutch, T. P., & Baillie, D. L. (1983). Alterations in the pattern of gene expression following heat shock in the nematode Caenorhabditis elegans. Canadian Journal of Biochemistry and Cell Biology, 61(6), 480–487.

Suzuki, Y., Yandell, M. D., Roy, P. J., Krishna, S., Savage-Dunn, C., Ross, R. M., et al. (1999). A BMP homolog acts as a dose-dependent regulator of body size and male tail patterning in Caenorhabditis elegans. Development, 126(2), 241–250.

Thomas, J. H., Birnby, D., & Vowels, J. (1993). Evidence for parallel processing of sensory information controlling dauer formation in Caenorhabditis elegans. Genetics, 134(4), 1105–1117.

Turner, A., & Greenough, W. (1985). Differential rearing effects on rat visual cortex synapses. Brain Research, 329(1–2), 195–203.

Vanfleteren, J. R., & DeVreese, A. (1995). The gerontogenes age-1 and daf-2 determine metabolic rate potential in aging Caenorhabdtis elegans. FASEB Journal, 9(13), 1355–1361.

Volkmar, F., & Greenough, W. (1972). Rearing complexity affects branching of dendrites in the visual cortex of the rat. Science, 176(42), 1145–1147.

Wadsworth, W. G., & Riddle, D. L. (1988). Acidic intracellular pH shift during Caenorhabditis elegans larval development. Proceedings of the National Academy of Sciences, USA, 85(22), 8435–8438.

Ward, S., Thomson, N., White, J. G., & Brenner, S. (1975). Electron microscopical reconstruction of the anterior sensory anatomy of the nematode Caenorhabditis elegans. The Journal of Comparative Neurology, 160(3), 313–337.

Ware, R. W., Clark, D., Crossland, K., & Russell, R. L. (1975). The nerve ring of the nematode Caenorhabditis elegans: Sensory input and motor output. The Journal of Comparative Neurology, 162(1), 71–110.

White, J. B., Southgate, E., Thomson, J. N., & Brenner, S. (1986). The structure of the nervous system of Caenorhabditis elegans. Philosophical Transactions of the Royal Society of London Series B, Biological Sciences, 314(1165), 1–340.

Wicks, S. R., & Rankin, C. H. (1995). Integration of mechanosensory stimuli in Caenorhabditis elegans. The Journal of Neuroscience, 15, 2434–2444.

Wicks, S. R., & Rankin, C. H. (1997). The effects of tap withdrawal response habituation on other withdrawal behaviors: The localization of habituation in the nematode Caenorhabditis elegans. Behavioral Neuroscience, 111(2), 342–353.

Yoshida, S., Morita, K., Mochii, M., & Ueno, N. (2001). Hypodermal expression of Caenorhabditis elegans TGF-beta type I receptor SMA-6 is essential for the growth and maintenance of body length. Developmental Biology, 240(1), 32–45.

Zhao, H., & Nonet, M. L. (2000). A retrograde signal is involved in activity-dependent remodeling at a C. elegans neuromuscular junction. Development, 127(6), 1253–1266.

Development of Central Visceral Circuits

Linda Rinaman *and* **Thomas J. Koehnle**

Abstract

This chapter is written from the perspective that central visceral and emotional neural circuits are largely coextensive. Mounting evidence supports the view that visceral functions are intimately associated with higher emotional and cognitive neurobehavioral systems. In laboratory rats, descending visceral motor output pathways and ascending visceral sensory feedback pathways undergo a significant amount of synaptic assembly and refinement during the first 2 weeks of postnatal life. A large experimental literature supports the view that maternally derived sensory stimulation of rat pups during the same developmental window can exert profound lifelong effects on adult stress responsiveness, emotionality, and temperament. These effects may involve experience-dependent modification of visceral circuit assembly during a sensitive postnatal period of circuit development.

Keywords: coextensive, visceral functions, synaptic assembly, rats, stress responsiveness, emotionality, temperament

Introduction

Sensory signals from within the body shape the behavioral, emotional, and physiological responses of animals to events in their environments. Such interoceptive feedback has a powerful impact on motivation and emotional learning, and allows animals to anticipate or flexibly respond to contingencies. Despite the importance of interoceptive and emotional circuits in both health and disease states, only limited research has been directed at understanding how these circuits are shaped by early experience.

In our view, the mother–infant relationship is conceived fundamentally as one of homeostatic regulation (Hofer, 1994). Newborn mammals are largely insulated from environmental demands. Adequate maternal care and their own limited mobility help to ensure that they are buffered against physiological insults. As the infant grows and becomes more independent, maternal buffering decreases, and young animals must increasingly rely on their own physiological systems and behavioral adjustments to survive. Smaller, younger animals are less able to buffer against novelty, shortage of resources, or illness, while older, larger animals have higher buffering capacities and can be more flexible in their responses to external and internal challenge. Therefore, the functional assembly of interoceptive circuits should be parallel to an organism's behavioral development: when reliance on maternal care begins to decrease, neural and behavioral systems should be in place to help the young animal cope with environmental challenges.

The brain exhibits a high degree of neural plasticity during early postnatal development. There likely is no manipulation during this period that would not have some impact on the developmental assembly of central nervous system (CNS) circuits, including circuits involved in the behavioral and physiological expression of emotion. Indeed, an ever-growing literature has repeatedly confirmed that early life experience impacts later emotion-ality and stress responsiveness in laboratory rats and other mammalian species, including humans (Maunder & Hunter, 2001) (also see Chapter 16). A central thesis of this literature is that the various changes in behavior, emotionality, and physiology that result from early life experience emerge from the interaction of maternal care and individual history: maternal care can be enhanced or disorga-nized, and the infant situated in that environment will react differently based on its prior history and its current physiological state.

From a developmental systems perspective (Ford & Lerner, 1992; Oyama, 1985), perturbations of the normal regulatory relationship between mother and offspring are expected to significantly alter infant development. Although the linkage between particular neural states and given behaviors is not clear-cut (Schall, 2004), a wealth of information has demonstrated the critical importance of vis-ceral sensory and motor circuits in supporting and shaping emotional experience. In rats, the progres-sive functional assembly of central visceral circuits during early postnatal life makes them ideal for the study of the effects of altered early life experience on emotional circuit development.

Visceral Circuits and Emotional Circuits Are Largely Coextensive

William James proposed that emotional feelings represent the perceptual consequences of somato- and viscerosensory feedback to the brain (James, 1884). James wrote:

> My thesis…is that the bodily changes follow directly the PERCEPTION of the exciting fact, and that our feeling of the same changes as they occur IS the emotion. (pp. 189–190)

The core of James' theory persists today amid mounting evidence that visceral functions are intimately associated with higher emotional and cognitive neurobehavioral systems. For the remainder of this chapter, we shall view emotions through the lens of systems theory, that is, as spe-cific bodily states that adaptively guide organisms toward goals and away from threats (Craig, 2002; Schulkin, Thompson, & Rosen, 2003; Thayer &

Lane, 2000). We shall focus on emotional states such as those related to fear and anxiety, which acutely restore homeostasis in the presence of a threat, but which can lead to behavioral and phys-iological dysfunction under chronic conditions. Descending limbs of visceral motor circuits serve to couple cognitive and emotional states with appropriate somatovisceral support. The hypothal-amus, central nucleus of the amygdala (CeA), bed nucleus of the stria terminalis (BNST), insular cortex (IC), and medial prefrontal cortex (mPFC) serve as principal gateways for septohippocampal and cortical influences over autonomic response components of emotional state (Crestani et al., 1999; Phillips & LeDoux, 1994; Pratt, 1992; Stein, 1998; Vouimba, Garcia, & Jaffard, 1998). Bodily reactions promote simultaneous interocep-tive feedback signals that are delivered to the same diencephalic and telencephalic regions; this feed-back is thought to bias emotional and cognitive states and thereby guide ongoing and future moti-vated behavior (Cameron, 2001; Craig, 2002). Accordingly, the state of the body is proposed to serve as the basis for mood, affect, and other com-ponents of emotional feelings in both reduction-ist and complex systems accounts of emotion (for review, see Damasio, 1999).

Emotional experiences are associated with altered visceral function. Evidence exists in humans that various physiological components of autonomic reactions are specific for six basic emotional cate-gories (i.e., anger, fear, sadness, disgust, happiness, and surprise; Levenson, 2003). Indeed, differences in measured autonomic outputs such as heart rate and skin temperature are strongly correlated with the specific category of experienced emotion. This specificity of emotional experience and emotional motor responses appears to be independent of cul-tural background, age, and social/professional sta-tus (Levenson, Ekman, Heider, & Friesen, 1992). Levenson and colleagues concluded that autonomic patterns are specific for different affective states, and that the physiological features of different emotional states may comprise adaptive functions that emerged during evolution. These observations are bolstered by findings that autonomic outputs are exquisitely and individually matched to meet specific environmental challenges, at least within the laboratory context (Pacak et al., 1998; Pacak & Palkovits, 2001; Palkovits, 1999).

Central visceral circuits receive continuous sen-sory feedback signals from the body. Thus, intero-ceptive circuits comprise the afferent limb of the visceral neuraxis, monitoring acute and chronic alterations in the organism's physiological state. Although interoceptive signals generally do not reach conscious awareness, they directly impact neural activity within behavioral and emotional output circuits. A.D. Craig makes the compelling argument that interoception should be defined as the sense of the physiological condition of the entire body, not just of the internal viscera (Craig, 2002). Interoceptive signals are conveyed to widespread regions of the CNS, including portions of the hypothalamus, thalamus, and limbic forebrain that are involved not only in modulating neuroendocrine and autonomic outflow, but also in generating motivated behavior, controlling mood, and shaping emotional learning (Mayer & Saper, 2000).

Overview of Central Visceral Circuits

Langley originally proposed the term "autonomic nervous system" to describe the motor innervation of essentially all body tissues except skeletal muscle (Langley, 1921). Visceral target tissues (i.e., cardiac muscle, smooth muscle, and glands) are innervated by neurons whose cell bodies reside in peripheral autonomic ganglia. Autonomic ganglia are innervated by cranial or spinal nerve branches that contain the axons of preganglionic autonomic neurons whose cell bodies reside in the caudal brain stem or intermediolateral spinal cord. Thus, brainstem and spinal cord preganglionic motor neurons represent the brain–body interface of the visceral motor system.

The visceral motor system modifies bodily functions to meet moment-to-moment demands of immediate or anticipated changes in the organism's internal and external environments. At their most basic level, central visceral pathways are organized for discrete sensory-motor reflex adjustments of specific end organ functions. Examples include micturition and defecation reflexes, the cardiovascular baroreceptor reflex, the gastric accommodation reflex, and the pupillary light reflex. Such reflex pathways involve relatively simple neural circuits contained entirely within the brainstem and/or spinal cord. Other central autonomic pathways are organized for integrative functions involving more complex changes that affect multiple organ systems. These visceral functions are integrated, coordinated, and modulated by descending neural projections from specific pontine, midbrain, and hypothalamic nuclei that target brain stem and spinal parasympathetic and sympathetic output neurons (Figure 15.1). Visceral motor outputs are

subject to further modulation by limbic forebrain sites that allow complex and nuanced visceral reactions to various threats and opportunities to which the organism is exposed. The involvement of cortical and limbic forebrain regions allows information to be retained over time, so that visceral reactions can be based on conscious or subconscious memory of past experience (Price, 2005). In all cases, adjustment of visceral motor outputs depends critically on interoceptive feedback signals delivered to the central nervous system. Indeed, visceromotor and viscerosensory pathways are highly reciprocal (Figure 15.1). Incoming sensory fibers carrying visceral sensations are involved in reflex modification of visceral target tissues and also contribute to ascending pathways responsible for more complex integrative functions. Some still undefined set or sets of executive neural circuits act to initiate, maintain, and terminate visceral motor outputs as a function of the integrated inputs received from interoceptive and exteroceptive sensory feedback. Executive circuits are responsible for the temporal patterning and sequencing of visceral motor outputs, and for determining and modulating the animal's overall behavioral state (i.e., asleep, aroused, quiescent). Thus, visceral neural circuits include (1) motor circuits for controlling autonomic output, (2) sensory circuits for monitoring interoceptive events, and (3) executive circuits that modulate the salience of interoceptive and exteroceptive signals in a context- and state-dependent manner, and which ultimately initiate, maintain, and terminate neural activity within the motor output circuits.

Physiological responses to stimuli that elicit strong emotions typically include significant alterations of cardiovascular, gastrointestinal, and other visceral functions. These altered functions are largely mediated through central neural circuits that include the medullary dorsal vagal complex (DVC), comprising the dorsal motor nucleus of the vagus, nucleus of the solitary tract (NST), and area postrema (Rinaman, 2003b). The DVC receives sensory feedback from the body on a moment-to-moment basis, and conveys these interoceptive signals to multiple brain stem and forebrain regions, including key components of emotional circuits. Thus, we have structured this chapter with a special focus on the functional organization and development of ascending and descending DVC neural circuits, theorizing that they provide a critical brain–body interface for emotion. DVC neurons receive direct and relayed synaptic input from

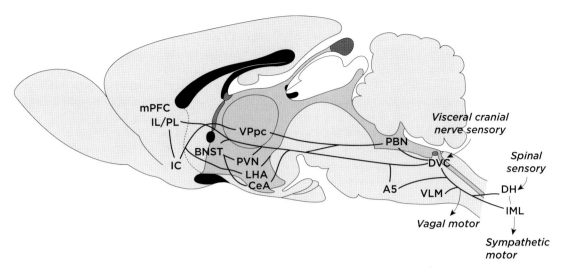

Figure 15.1 Schematic mid-saggital view of the adult rat brain depicting the approximate location of central visceral sensory and motor areas discussed in the text. Lines between areas represent reciprocal ascending and descending connections. Abbreviations as in the text.

olfactory, vagal, glossopharyneal, trigeminal, facial, and spinal somatosensory and viscerosensory afferents. The area postrema and a significant portion of the medial NST contain fenestrated capillaries, giving blood-borne factors (e.g., toxins, cytokines, hormones, and osmolytes) access to the local brain parenchyma to thereby affect neural activity. Vagal parasympathetic motor neurons regulate visceral secretory and motor functions throughout the thoracic and abdominal cavities. As detailed further below, direct and relayed reciprocal neural pathways exist between the DVC and higher pontine, diencephalic, and telencephalic emotional circuit components. In adult rats and other animals, reciprocal descending and ascending interactions of higher brain regions with the DVC allow emotional and cognitive events to modulate visceral motor function, and provide a route through which interoceptive feedback from the body can shape emotional and cognitive processing.

Descending Visceral Motor Control Pathways

Several excellent, comprehensive reviews are available that describe the anatomical organization of central visceral control circuits in adult rats and other mammalian species (Card & Sved, 2009; Janig, 2006; Loewy, 1990; Saper, 2002, 2004), and so only a brief discussion is presented here. Our current view of how central preautonomic visceral circuits are organized owes much to the results of studies using neurotropic alpha-herpesviruses for retrograde transneuronal tracing of multisynaptic pathways in rats (Card, 1998; Loewy, 1995; Strack & Loewy, 1990; Strack, Sawyer, Hughes, Platt, & Loewy, 1989). Such studies use attenuated strains of neurotropic pseudorabies virus (PRV) that move selectively across synapses in the retrograde direction. For example, the Bartha strain of PRV (Bartha, 1961) injected into the wall of the stomach (Card et al., 1993; Rinaman, Levitt, & Card, 2000; Yang, Card, Tirabassi, Miselis, & Enquist, 1999) or other visceral organs initially infects sympathetic and parasympathetic preganglionic motor neurons in the spinal cord and caudal medulla, respectively, and subsequently is transported retrogradely and transneuronally to infect preautonomic neurons within specific, circumscribed regions of the brainstem and forebrain. Retrograde transneuronal viral transport from visceral targets that receive only sympathetic inputs (e.g., adrenal medulla, kidney, spleen) identifies essentially the same sets of medullary, pontine, midbrain, and diencephalic structures as are labeled by retrograde transport of classical tracers from different spinal levels of the sympathetic preganglionic column (Cano, Card, Rinaman, & Sved, 2000; Cano, Sved, Rinaman, Rabin, & Card, 2001; Strack et al., 1989). These structures include several hypothalamic nuclei [i.e., paraventricular nucleus, retrochiasmatic nucleus, arcuate nucleus, and lateral hypothalamic area (LHA)], as well as the periaqueductal gray, locus coeruleus, Barrington's nucleus, ventromedial and ventrolateral pontine and medullary reticular formation, medullary raphe nuclei, and the caudal medial NST.

Retrograde transneuronal viral transport from viscera that receive both sympathetic and parasympathetic innervation (e.g., the wall of the stomach) identifies the same medullary, midbrain, and diencephalic preautonomic regions as mentioned above; however, the additional involvement of parasympathetic DVC circuits leads to additional early transneuronal infection of several subcortical and cortical telencephalic regions (Card et al., 1993; Rinaman et al., 2000; Yang et al, 1999). These regions include the CeA, BNST, IC, and mPFC. Other evidence that telencephalic regions provide relatively specific direct inputs to the DVC but not to sympathetic spinal neurons was obtained in adult rats in which virus was injected into the pancreas after its extrinsic sympathetic or parasympathetic innervation was surgically eliminated (Jansen, Hoffman, & Loewy, 1997; Loewy & Haxhiu, 1993). When virus was injected into the pancreas after removing its parasympathetic innervation, transneuronal viral transport labeled presympathetic neurons in the hypothalamus but not within limbic or cortical regions. Conversely, when sympathetic input to the pancreas was eliminated, transneuronal viral labeling of preparasympathetic neurons was observed within hypothalamic, limbic, and cortical regions. Studies using conventional anterograde and retrograde tract tracers also have demonstrated that hypothalamic nuclei project directly to both sympathetic and parasympathetic preganglionic neurons in adult rats, whereas autonomic-related regions of the telencephalon appear to target the DVC directly but not the sympathetic spinal cord (Loewy, 1991).

In rats, the CeA and BNST together form a reciprocally interconnected continuum of "prevagal" neurons (Schwaber, Kapp, Higgins, & Rapp, 1982) and are implicated in the expression of autonomic correlates of emotional arousal (LeDoux, Iwata, Cicchetti, & Reis, 1988). The amygdala is involved in affective processes, and amygdalo-cortical circuits are conceptualized as guiding behavior based on environmental and somatovisceral feedback (Bechara, Damasio, & Damasio, 2003). Amygdala lesions block the expression of conditioned fear responses, and direct descending projections from the CeA and BNST to the DVC represent a sufficient pathway for the regulation of visceral motor function by telencephalic structures (Bernston, Sarter, & Cacioppo, 1998). Results from anatomical and electrophysiological studies suggest that visceral activation accompanying emotional responses involves direct inhibition of GABAergic preautonomic NST neurons by GABAergic neurons in the medial CeA (Pickel, Bockstaele, Chan, & Cestari, 1996; Rogers & Hermann, 1992). Thus, stimulation of inhibitory CeA inputs to the DVC disinhibits vagal motor outflow and increases vagally mediated gastric motility in adult rats (Hermann, McCann, & Rogers, 1990).

The rat DVC also receives direct input from pyramidal neurons in the IC and mPFC (Saper, 1982; Terreberry & Neafsay, 1983; Van der Kooy, Koda, McGinty, Gerfen, & Bloom, 1984; Yasui, Itoh, Kaneko, Shigemoto, & Mizuno, 1991). These visceral cortex areas also project to preautonomic regions of the periaqueductal gray, hypothalamus, CeA, and BNST in rats, and are implicated in autonomic reactivity associated with anxiety and other affective processes (LeDoux et al., 1988; Vertes, 2004, 2006). Stimulation of visceral cortex potently alters autonomic outflow, producing an inhibition of gastrointestinal activity similar to the inhibition produced by exposure to fear-inducing stimuli (Aleksandrov, Bagaev, Nozdrachev, & Panteleev, 1996; Yasui, Breder, Saper, & Cechetto, 1991). The IC in rats, which corresponds to Brodmann's area 13 in humans, is reciprocally connected with "prelimbic" and "infralimbic" regions of the mPFC (Gabbott, Warner, Jays, & Bacon, 2003), which appear to be homologous to Brodmann's areas 32 and 25, respectively, in humans and nonhuman primates. In addition to its role in modulating autonomic functions, the mPFC subserves functions related to cognitive processing, working memory, social behavior, response learning, and the initiation and pursuit of goal-directed behavior (Vertes, 2004, 2006). Results from many functional magnetic resonance imaging (MRI) studies in humans have demonstrated that emotional experiences invariably increase activation of these visceral cortical regions, which have been shown to innervate central preautonomic neurons in nonhuman primates (Barbas, Saha, Rempel-Clower, & Ghashghaei, 2003).

Ascending Viscerosensory Pathways

Interoceptive information is relayed from body to brain along neural pathways that form largely reciprocal inputs to the same diencephalic and telencephalic regions that control visceral motor outflow.

Spinal Pathways

In mature rats, spinal viscerosensory afferents terminate in laminae I–VII of the dorsal horn and intermediate zone, and in lamina X around the central canal (Green & Dockray, 1987). Inputs from visceral and somatic afferents converge onto second-order spinal neurons, which also receive convergent inputs from visceral afferents serving separate viscera. The central terminals of spinal visceral afferents spread over more rostrocaudal segments than somatic afferents, possibly contributing to the vague localization of visceral stimuli. A subset of dorsal horn neurons convey convergent somato- and viscerosensory signals to the diencephalon via the spinothalamic tract. A separate spinal pathway appears to relay viscerosensory signals through lamina X, medial lamina VII, and the dorsal gray commissure, ascending at the junction of the gracile and cuneate fasciculi to terminate in the medullary dorsal column nuclei, which then project to the contralateral ventroposterior (VP) thalamic complex (Wang, Willis, & Westlund, 1999; Willis & Westlund, 2001). Collateral projections from the spinothalamic and dorsal column pathways also merge with other ascending sensory pathways that access the forebrain by relaying in the DVC (discussed further below), the ventromedial and ventrolateral reticular formation, and the pontine parabrachial nucleus (PBN) (Potts, Lee, & Anguelov, 2002). In fact, the large majority of lamina I spinothalamic axons in rats send collaterals to the PBN (Hylden, Anton, & Nahin, 1989). Thus, ascending spinal visceral sensory pathways converge with and are essentially identical to the classic spinoreticular and spinothalamic tracts, although direct spinal inputs to the hypothalamus and amygdala also have been reported (Menetrey & de Pommery, 1991). Bilateral damage to the spinothalamic tract blunts many autonomic reflex responses, including the abdominal visceromotor reflex response to colonic distension. However, spinothalamic tract lesions do not abolish responses of thalamic neurons to other visceral stimuli, likely due to neural transmission through the dorsal column pathway (Willis & Westlund, 2001; Wang et al., 1999).

Viscerosensory Signaling through the NST

As mentioned above, spinal visceral sensory pathways converge with cranial nerve visceral sensory pathways by virtue of collateralized spinal inputs to the medullary reticular formation and NST, and to the pontine PBN (Menetrey & Basbaum, 1987). Visceral sensory information also enters the NST directly via four cranial nerves (i.e., trigeminal, facial, glossopharyngeal, and vagal). Visceral afferents from these cranial nerves enter the dorsolateral medulla via multiple sensory rootlets and converge within the solitary tract, analogous to the spinal trigeminal tract or Lissauer's tract, which conveys visceral sensory fibers along the rostrocaudal length of the NST. A strong visceral topography is evident in the terminal arborizations of primary visceral afferents within the NST (Altschuler, Bao, Bieger, Hopkins, & Miselis, 1989; Shapiro & Miselis, 1985).

Since most visceral afferent pathways involve a synaptic relay within the NST, analysis of the central projections of NST neurons reveals the brainstem and higher-order targets of viscerosensory signaling pathways (Bailey, Hermes, Andresen, & Aicher, 2006; Horst, Boer, Luiten, & Willigen, 1989; Horst & Streefland, 1994). NST neurons project directly to multiple central regions, including the ventrolateral medulla, locus coeruleus, PBN, midline thalamic nuclei, PVN, LHA, tuberomammilary nuclei, arcuate nucleus, median preoptic area, subfornical organ, supraoptic nucleus, dorsomedial hypothalamus, CeA, and BNST. Of these projections, the most massive output from the NST is directed toward the pontine PBN. The PBN has at least 12 distinct subnuclei, many of which form reciprocated projections to multiple sites in the brain stem, hypothalamus, limbic forebrain (CeA, BNST), visceral sensory thalamus, and cerebral cortex (Fulwiler & Saper, 1984; Herbert, Moga, & Saper, 1990; Moga et al., 1990; Saper & Loewy, 1980). Spinal and NST inputs to the internal lateral PBN, which in turn provides a diffuse input to the intralaminar thalamic nuclei, may be involved in arousal responses to visceral stimuli, while inputs to the external medial PBN may contribute to conscious appreciation of visceral sensation via thalamic relay inputs to IC. Viscerosensory projections from the NST to pontine, diencephalic, and telencephalic target nuclei are primarily (although not exclusively) catecholaminergic, arising from noradrenergic A2 and adrenergic C2 neurons contained within the NST. Projections from the NST also recruit a parallel ascending viscerosensory projection arising from catecholaminergic neurons of the caudal ventrolateral medulla (A1/C1 cell groups) at the same rostrocaudal medullary levels.

Visceral Sensory Inputs to Cortex

Interoceptive signals can reach conscious awareness by engaging the visceral cortices. In addition to its component of pyramidal preautonomic output neurons, IC is visceral sensory cortex. Electrical stimulation of vagal afferents in humans activates the thalamus, hypothalamus, amygdala, and IC, and can trigger EEG cortical responses with a latency and morphology similar to those seen after visceral stimulation (Narayanan et al., 2002; Schachter & Saper, 1998). Signaling to regions of the IC (Brodmann's area 13) allows conscious appreciation of visceral sensation. Wilder Penfield's cortical stimulation studies revealed subjective sensations of oropharyngeal, esophageal, and gastrointestinal sensation organized in a topographic sensory homunculus running ventrally from the tongue sensory area into the operculum and insula (Penfield & Faulk, 1955). Cechetto and Saper reported a similar topographic pattern of visceral sensory responses in rats, involving regions of the dysgranular and granular IC that corresponded to viscerotopically organized inputs from the VP thalamus (Cechetto & Saper, 1987). Electrical stimulation of different VP thalamic regions in humans produces distinct visceral sensations (Lenz et al., 1997), suggesting a generally similar topographic thalamocortical organization. More recent functional human imaging studies have confirmed that visceral stimulation activates not only IC, but also mPFC and anterior cingulate cortex (Brodmann's areas 25 and 32, corresponding to the infralimbic and prelimbic cortical regions in rats), and, less consistently, primary somatosensory cortex (Derbyshire, 2003; Nicotra, Critchley, Mathias, & Dolan, 2006). Interestingly, human subjects with upper spinal cord injury demonstrate altered activation of these and other brain regions accompanied by altered autonomic responsiveness to emotive stimuli (Nicotra et al., 2006).

Although conscious perception of visceral stimuli requires engagement of cortical structures, most interoceptive signals never reach conscious awareness even when they activate the cortex (Bielefeldt, Christianson, & Davis, 2005). The LC, LHA, and midline thalamic nuclei each have direct but diffuse cortical projections that likely participate in arousal and overall cortical "tone," and each of these regions receives neural input relayed from the viscerosensory NST. The NST also projects directly and via the nucleus paragigantocellularis and LC to the basal forebrain corticopetal cholinergic system (Bernston et al., 1998;

Berntson, Sarter, & Cacioppo, 2003). The basal forebrain cholinergic system is implicated in cortical arousal, attention, and anxiety, and is considered a widespread regulatory modulator that serves to enhance or amplify cognitive processing. Thus, visceral sensory inputs can modify cortical functions and thereby exert control over behavior and affect even when they do not evoke conscious visceral perceptions.

Postnatal Development of Central Visceral Circuits

All of the various spinal, brain stem, hypothalamic, and limbic components of central visceral circuits are present at birth in newborn rats. However, much refinement of chemical signaling pathways and synaptic circuitry within and among these regions takes place after birth, even within relatively simple spinal and brainstem reflex arcs. For example, cardiac baroreceptor reflexes are decidedly immature during the first postnatal week, as evidenced by minimal cardiac sympathetic activation or vagal withdrawal following vasodilation (Quigley, Myers, & Shair, 2005), and by certain forms of cardiac phasic activity that are not present in adult rats (Hofer, 1984). Mature spinobulbospinal reflexes subserving micturition and defecation do not emerge until the third postnatal week in rats (Araki & Groat, 1997). During the same developmental period, descending corticobulbar projection systems become increasingly myelinated and continue to establish new synaptic connections with brainstem target neurons (Iriki, Nozaki, & Nakamura, 1988; Martin, Cabana, Culberson, Curry, & Tschismadia, 1980; Rinaman, Levitt, & Card, 2000; Sarnat, 1989). The PVN, CeA, BNST, IC, and infralimbic/prelimbic (IL/PL) cortices serve as principal gateways for septohippocampal and cortical influences over autonomic components of emotional motor responses (LeDoux, 1996; Phillips & LeDoux, 1994; Pratt, 1992; Vouimba et al., 1998). Thus, information about the ontogeny of descending projections from hypothalamic and limbic forebrain regions to autonomic output centers is of utmost importance for considering how epigenetic events might affect the assembly and maturation of central emotional circuits.

Early Development of the DVC

The peripheral axon terminals of preganglionic parasympathetic vagal motor neurons reach abdominal visceral targets by embryonic day 15 in developing rats, shortly after the central arrival of vagal sensory afferents and the first appearance of identifiable synapses within the presumptive NST (Rinaman & Levitt, 1993; Zhang & Ashwell, 2001; Figure 15.2). Contrary to what occurs in many other brain regions, there is no evidence for massive synapse overproduction and subsequent elimination within the DVC during embryonic or postnatal development in rats (Lachamp, Tell, & Kessler, 2002). Indeed, the organization of viscerosensory inputs to the DVC and vagal motor outputs to the gastrointestinal tract is remarkably adult-like at the time of birth (Rinaman & Levitt, 1993; Figure 15.2). However, synaptic density within the rat NST continues to increase over a protracted postnatal period that involves distinct successive episodes of synapse production. Morphologically immature synapses are prevalent transiently within medial visceral subnuclei of the NST a few days after birth, with a second wave of new immature synapses appearing near the end of the second postnatal week (Lachamp et al., 2002). Synaptic bouton density and synaptophysin expression increase markedly within the NST over the first 10 postnatal days (Miller, McKoon, Pinneau, & Silverstein, 1983; Rao, Jean, & Kessler, 1997). Dendritic spines and filopodia, which are likely involved in synapse formation, are transiently present on NST neurons after birth, with peak density occurring around P12 (Vincent & Tell, 1999). Significant changes in markers of glutamatergic neurotransmission within the NST occur during the first month of postnatal life, with especially robust changes during the first 9 postnatal days (Rao et al., 1997). Electrophysiological data also reveal significant reorganization of local network properties within the NST during the first postnatal week (Kawai & Senba, 2000). As reviewed in more detail below, descending inputs from the hypothalamus, CeA, BNST, and visceral cortices reach the DVC between birth and P6, depending on their origin, but do not immediately establish synaptic connections there (Rinaman et al., 2000). Instead, diencephalic and telencephalic synaptic inputs to DVC neurons emerge gradually over a relatively protracted postnatal period.

Postnatal Development of Forebrain Inputs to the DVC

Transneuronal viral labeling of preautonomic circuits in neonatal rats indicates that diencephalic and telencephalic inputs to gastric-related DVC

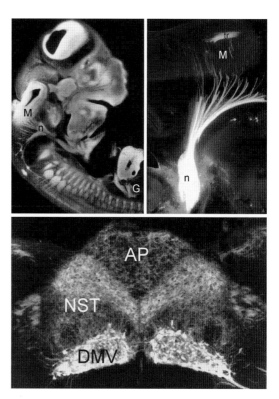

Figure 15.2 The upper left panel shows a photomicrograph of a thick vibratome section through a fixative-preserved rat embryo (E13–14). Crystals of the lipophilic carbocyanine dye (DiI) were placed into the stomach wall (G) of the fixed specimen (Rinaman & Levitt, 1993). The upper right panel shows resulting DiI labeling in the vagal sensory nodose ganglion (n), and sensory fibers in the presumptive tractus solitarius (tr) within the medulla (M). Labeled vagal rootlets also can be seen entering and leaving the medulla. The lower panel shows sensory and motor labeling within the DVC in a 2-day-old rat after tracer (CTb) was injected into both vagus nerves on the previous day. Abbreviations as in the text.

neurons are largely absent at birth and emerge gradually over the first 10 postnatal days (Rinaman et al., 2000; Rinaman, Roesch, & Card, 1999). In these two transneuronal viral tracing studies, stomach wall PRV inoculation parameters and postinjection survival times were kept constant for each postnatal age examined, and generated similar patterns of neuronal infection in the spinal cord and caudal brainstem of rats in each age group. A subset of hypothalamic PVN synaptic projections to gastric-related autonomic neurons already were present in rat pups injected with virus on P1 and examined 2.5 days later (Rinaman et al., 1999). However, the CeA, BNST, IC, mPFC, and LHA were not transneuronally infected in P1-injected pups. All of these regions except the visceral cortices

(IC and mPFC) were infected in pups injected with virus on P4 and examined 2.5 days later. All of the diencephalic and telencephalic regions, including the visceral cortices, were transneuronally infected in pups injected on P8 and examined 2.5 days later, similar to observations of transneuronal labeling from the stomach wall in adult rats (Rinaman et al., 1993; Yang et al., 1999). Thus, diencephalic and telencephalic preautonomic synaptic inputs to gastric-related DVC neurons emerge gradually over the first 10 days of postnatal life.

The cortex is quite undeveloped in newborn rats (Van Eden, Kros, & Uylings, 1990), in which visceral regions of the mPFC consist only of layer I, the cortical plate, and the subplate (Van Eden & Uylings, 1985). By P6, all cytoarchitectural cortical layers are distinguishable, although amygdala afferent fiber density still is diffuse and increasing in density as increasing numbers of amygdala neurons innervate the cortical zone (Verwer, Vulpen, & Uum, 1996). Anterograde and retrograde neural tracing demonstrates that projections from the amygdala to the mPFC develop postnatally in rats, with only a few scattered projection fibers visible between P0–4 (Verwer et al., 1996). The transition from an immature and diffuse fiber distribution to the adult-like bilaminar pattern occurs around P12–14 in the lateral and rostral medial PFC, paralleling the emergence of PFC cytoarchitectural organization. Given the protracted postnatal development of visceral cortex and its inputs from the amygdala, it is perhaps not surprising that efferent projections from the cortex and other limbic forebrain regions to DVC autonomic output neurons do not emerge until after the end of the first postnatal week.

The absence of transneuronal PRV labeling in the LHA, CeA, BNST, and cortex in the youngest rat pups examined was not due to an inability of neurons in those areas to take up or replicate virus. Many LHA, CeA, and BNST neurons (but not cortical neurons) were retrogradely labeled after injection of PRV directly into the medullary DVC on P1, evidence that at least some neurons within these forebrain regions already have axons in or near the DVC, and that the cellular mechanisms necessary for PRV neuronal invasion, retrograde transport, and replication are indeed functional shortly after birth. However, the LHA, CeA, and BNST neurons apparently do not yet form synaptic contacts with gastric-related DVC neurons at this early developmental time point. Further, cortical (i.e., IC and mPFC) neurons do not have axons

in or near the DVC in newborn rats, because no cortical labeling was observed 48–50 h after direct DVC injections of either PRV or a standard retrograde tracer (i.e., cholera toxin) on P1. However, DVC injections of cholera toxin on P6 produced retrograde labeling of neurons in both the IC and mPFC along with other diencephalic and telencephalic structures, as in adult rats, indicating that initial visceral cortex axonal inputs to the DVC first arrive at some time between P1 and P6.

These neural tracing results collectively demonstrate progressive postnatal increases in synaptic inputs from the limbic forebrain to medullary autonomic neurons. The number of transneuronally infected hypothalamic neurons also increased significantly in rats during the first 10 postnatal days. PVN and LHA neurons that project to the DVC are implicated in emotional and stress-related effects on autonomic function, including increased acid secretion and inhibition of gastric emptying (Ferguson, Marcus, Spencer, & Wallace, 1988; Taché, Martinez, Million, & Rivier, 1999). Approximately 6%–10% of PVN neurons that project to the DVC in adult rats are immunoreactive for oxytocin (OT) (Olson, Hoffman, Sved, Stricker, & Verbalis, 1992; Sofroniew & Schrell, 1981). Because OT inputs to the DVC arise exclusively from the PVN in rats, the presence of OT-positive fibers provides a useful proxy for estimating hypothalamic inputs to the DVC over the course of development. The cumulative length of OT-immunopositive fibers in the rat DVC increases markedly in rats between birth and the time of weaning (Rinaman, 1998), consistent with transneuronal viral tracing evidence that hypothalamic inputs to the DVC are only partially complete in newborn rats, with additional projections arriving postnatally.

Although OT-containing projections comprise only a subset of PVN inputs to the DVC, OT signaling pathways are critical for hypothalamic control over vagally mediated gastric functions (Rogers & Hermann, 1985, 1987, 1992). In adult rats, OT inputs to the DVC provide a tonic inhibition of vagally mediated gastric motility (Flanagan, Olson, Sved, Verbalis, & Stricker, 1992). More pronounced OT-mediated gastric inhibition follows various treatments that stimulate OT neurons, including systemic administration of hypertonic saline (HS) (Flanagan, Verbalis, & Stricker, 1989). HS treatment produces acute hypernatremia, which increases the effective osmotic pressure of extracellular fluid and draws water out of the intracellular compartment (Gilman, 1937). HS treatment also generates pronounced hypernatremia in neonatal rats accompanied by adult-like neural Fos activation patterns in osmosensitive regions of the basal forebrain and hypothalamus, including magnocellular and parvocellular PVN neurons. However, very little DVC Fos expression occurs in neonates after HS treatment, as opposed to marked DVC activation in HS-treated adult rats. Early functional immaturity of hypothalamic OT inputs to the DVC also is evidenced by findings that HS treatment fails to inhibit gastric emptying in neonatal rats (Callahan & Rinaman, 1998). Thus, the available anatomical and functional data indicate that the first 10 days of postnatal development in rats are characterized by significant temporally sequenced synapse formation occurring between neurons in diencephalic and telencephalic regions and autonomic output neurons. Highly specialized mechanisms are crucial for the initial establishment of postsynaptic specializations during synaptogenesis, and for activity-dependent changes in synaptic strength that underlie experience-dependent plasticity (Pérez-Otaño & Ehlers, 2005). By analogy to other CNS systems, the early postnatal period likely represents a sensitive period of development for neural circuits that underlie emotional interpretation and expression, during which time neural activity arising from internal and/or environmental events might participate in shaping ongoing synapse formation.

Postnatal Development of Central Viscerosensory Pathways

As mentioned above, viscerosensory projections from the NST to other central targets are primarily catecholaminergic (i.e., nor/adrenergic). Viscerosensory activation of nor/adrenergic projections from the NST and caudal VLM are implicated in recruiting neural activation of target neurons within the PVN, BNST, and CeA during stress responses and emotional learning in adult animals. Interestingly, however, the first 2–3 postnatal weeks in rats correspond to a so-called "stress hyporesponsive period" (SHRP) characterized by reduced or absent hypothalamic-pituitary-adrenal (HPA) axis responsiveness to certain types of stressful stimuli (Pihoker, Owens, Kuhn, Schanberg, & Nemeroff, 1993; Sapolsky & Meaney, 1986; Walker, Scribner, Cascio, & Dallman, 1991). Maternally derived factors appear to contribute importantly to maintaining this stress hyporesponsivity, because maternal separation (MS) for

periods longer than a few hours is able to restore HPA responsiveness to certain stimuli in neonatal rats (Levine, Huchton, Weiner, & Rosenfeld, 1991). Ample evidence in adult rats indicates that nor/adrenergic inputs provide critical control over the activity of stress-responsive PVN corticotropin releasing factor (CRF)-containing neurons at the apex of the HPA axis (Al-Damluji, 1988; Alonso, Szafarczyk, Balmefrezol, & Assenmacher, 1986; Gaillet, Lachuer, Malaval, Assenmacher, & Szafarczyk, 1991; Kiss & Aguilera, 1992; Liposits, Phelix, & Paull, 1986). Immaturity of ascending nor/adrenergic viscerosensory pathways may partially underlie the documented hyporesponsiveness of PVN neurosecretory cells to interoceptive stimuli in rats during the SHRP. To further examine this possibility, nor/adrenergic projection neurons and fibers were identified by immunocytochemical localization of dopamine beta-hydroxylase (DbH), the enzyme that converts dopamine to norepinephrine in all nor/adrenergic neurons (Rinaman, 2001). DbH fiber immunolabeling increased progressively in the PVN in rats between postnatal days (P)1 and P21, when adult-like levels were achieved. Similar observations were made regarding DbH immunolabeling within the BNST in rats during postnatal development (Koehnle & Rinaman, 2007).

The apparent neurochemical immaturity of nor/adrenergic inputs from the NST and VLM to the PVN and BNST in neonatal rats suggests that these ascending viscerosensory pathways may also be functionally immature. To test this hypothesis, immunocytochemical detection of the immediate-early gene protein product, Fos, was used to identify central neurons that are activated in P2 rats after systemic administration of cholecystokinin octapeptide (CCK) (Rinaman, Hoffman, Stricker, & Verbalis, 1994). Exogenous CCK stimulates gastrointestinal vagal afferents via a CCK-1 receptor-mediated mechanism (Day, McKnight, Poat, & Hughes, 1994; Schwartz & Moran, 1998), and is an effective pharmacological tool with which to stimulate central viscerosensory pathways (Rinaman et al., 1994, 1995; Rinaman, Verbalis, Stricker, & Hoffman, 1993). The ability of exogenous CCK to engage medullary DVC circuits (Rinaman et al., 1994) and thereby affect hindbrain feeding motor outputs in neonatal rats (Robinson, Moran, & McHugh, 1985, 1988) means that the necessary vagal afferent inputs and efferent outputs of the DVC already are functional at birth. Indeed, as reviewed above, anatomical tracing studies in fetal and newborn rats reveal a precocious development of DVC motor outputs to the gastrointestinal tract, and a correspondingly early development of viscerosensory inputs to the DVC. Hindbrain Fos expression was virtually identical in P2 and adult rats after CCK treatment, with activated neurons located in specific subregions of the DVC that receive gastric vagal sensory input. A similar pattern of DVC activation was reported in neonatal rats after milk ingestion via suckling (Hironaka, Shirakawa, Toki, Kinoshita, & Oguchi, 2000). However, in striking contrast to results in adult rats, CCK treatment at P2 did not activate cFos expression in the hypothalamus or other forebrain regions, and did not stimulate pituitary hormone release (Rinaman et al., 1994). Thus, viscerosensory activation of hindbrain circuits appears sufficient to mediate the inhibitory effects of exogenous CCK on independent ingestion in neonatal rats (see Figure 15.3). Experiments in decerebrate adult rats also support the view that the hypothalamus and other forebrain regions are unnecessary for CCK-induced hypophagia (Grill & Smith, 1988). The lack of hypothalamic activation in neonates after CCK treatment is consistent with other evidence for delayed postnatal maturation of ascending nor/adrenergic projections from the NST and ventrolateral medulla (Rinaman et al., 2000) that transmit viscerosensory information to the hypothalamus and other forebrain regions in adult rats (Ericsson, Kovacs, & Sawchenko, 1994; Rinaman et al., 1995; Sawchenko & Swanson, 1981, 1982). Indeed, our neurotoxic lesioning experiments in adult rats have demonstrated that ascending noradrenergic projections from the NST are critical for the ability of systemic CCK to activate Fos expression in CRF-positive PVN neurons that comprise the apex of the HPA axis (Rinaman, 2003a).

We have also investigated the postnatal maturation of central neural responses to interoceptive stimuli (Koehnle & Rinaman, 2007) by examining central neural activation patterns in rat pups after treatment with lithium chloride (LiCl), a malaise-inducing agent. Rat pups were injected i.p. with 0.15 M LiCl (2% BW) or control solution (0.15 M NaCl) at multiple time points between birth (P0) and P28. Compared to saline, LiCl increased Fos only slightly in the area postrema, NST, and lateral PBN in newborn rats. LiCl did not increase Fos above control levels in the CeA, BNST, or PVN on P0, but did on P7 and later. Maximal Fos responses

to LiCl were observed on P14 in all areas except the BNST, in which LiCl-induced Fos activation continued to increase through P28. Comparable results have been obtained by others examining central Fos responses to an acute lipopolysaccharide challenge in developing rats (Oladehin & Blatteis, 1995). These findings provide additional evidence that central interoceptive circuits in rats are not fully functional at birth, and show age-dependent increases in neural recruitment following viscerosensory stimulation.

Effects of Early Life Experience on Emotionality and Stress-Responsiveness

Most of the peripheral and central components of stress-responsive circuits are capable of being activated in neonatal rats, given sufficient experimental or natural conditions (Levine, 2001). However, stress responsiveness of the HPA axis in neonatal rats is mostly suppressed by behavioral interactions of the dam with her pups. These interactions generate interoceptive signals in the pup that include thermal, chemical, and mechanoreceptive components from throughout the body (Levine, 2001; Van Oers, de Kloet, Whelan, & Levine, 1998). The initial papers demonstrating the profound effects of early manipulation of dam–pup interactions on subsequent behavior and activity of the HPA stress axis of adult offspring were published 50 years ago (Levine, 1957; Levine, Chevalier, & Korchin, 1956). Several model systems have emerged in the intervening years in studies of early life experience on adult emotionality and cognition, including early enrichment paradigms (Benaroya-Milshtein et al., 2004; Moncek, Duncko, Johansson, & Jezova, 2004), acute and chronic treatment with toxic or inflammatory agents (Al-Chaer, Kawasaki, & Pasricha, 2000; Boissé, Mouihate, Ellis, & Pittman, 2004; Shanks, Larocque, & Meaney, 1995), early treatment with acute stressors (Wiedenmayer, 2004; Wiedenmayer & Barr, 2001; Wiedenmayer, Magarinos, McEwen, & Barr, 2005), and paradigms involving repeated episodes of brief handling coupled with brief or extended periods of maternal separation (H/MS). Of these divergent approaches to the study of experience-induced neural plasticity, we shall focus on the H/MS model, principally because the etiology and neuroendocrine results of the approach are so well described (see also Chapter 16).

Following the discovery of the effects of early H/MS on emotionality and stress responses in adult rats by Seymour Levine's group (Levine, 1957; Levine et al., 1956), Paul Plotsky, Michael Meaney, and others have developed a relatively standardized H/MS model for manipulating early postnatal interactions between mother rats and their pups (Huot, Gonzalez, Ladd, Thrivikraman, & Plotsky, 2004; Ladd et al., 2000; Plotsky & Meaney, 1993; Wigger & Neumann, 1999). Published results from large numbers of H/MS studies have generally confirmed that repeated daily handling coupled with brief (i.e., 10–15 min) MS and reunion of rat pups during the first 2 postnatal weeks results in adult rats that are less anxious in temperament and more behaviorally and physiologically resistant to laboratory stress paradigms. Conversely, a single 24-h MS or repeated daily 3–4-h MS over the first 10–14 days postnatal produces adult rats that generally are more anxious and are hyperresponsive to stress. Interestingly, it seems that dam–pup interactions within the highly artificial context of a completely stable environment with no MS results in offspring with relatively high adult HPA reactivity and fearfulness, which in many studies appears similar to the effects of prolonged daily repeated MS (Macrì & Wurbel, 2006). Conversely, moderately challenging environments (i.e., daily nest disruption and brief MS) produce offspring with significantly dampened HPA stress responsiveness. One group has reported that P10 (but not P3) rats show a pronounced bradycardia that persists for at least several minutes after nest disruption and pup removal from littermates (Hofer, 1984), suggesting that the physiological effects of these experimental manipulations appear early in development. Others also have demonstrated that H/MS effects on hypothalamic CRF signaling pathways are already demonstrable by P9 (Avishai-Eliner, Eghbal-Ahmadi, Tabatchnik, Brunson, & Baram, 2001; Fenoglio et al., 2005).

Accumulating evidence supports the view that the effects of early handling and H/MS are the joint product of experimentally induced alterations of both pups and dam (Denenberg, 1999; Denenberg, Ottinger, & Stephens, 1962; Macri, Mason, & Wurbel, 2004; Macrì & Wurbel, 2006). Rat pups normally huddle together and are protected in their nest whether or not the dam is present; thus, nest disruptions themselves are highly unusual. One study found that newborn rat pups spend as much as 85% of their time attached to a nipple, although only a subset of that time involves nutritive suckling (Stern & Johanson, 1989). Experimental disruption of the home cage environment during removal of the pups, their subsequent absence, and then their sudden return each present potentially stressful challenges to the dam. Separation from the pups disrupts normal maternal behavior and increases maternal anxiety (Kalinichev, Easterling, & Holtzman, 2000). Providing rat dams with surrogate litters during both 15-min and 3-h MS reversed the effects of the 15-min but not the 3-h MS treatment (Huot et al., 2004). In mice, treatment of the dam with anxiolytic drugs abolished the neuroendocrine and behavioral effects on the pups produced by 15-min MS (D'Amato, Cabib, Ventura, & Orsini, 1998). Thus, H/MS paradigms affect both pups and dam, and the relative impact of these effects is difficult to assess experimentally (Macrì & Wurbel, 2006).

It has long been assumed that the effect of early experience on lifelong emotionality and stress responsiveness involves epigenetic modification of CNS systems that regulate those responses (Caldji et al., 1998; Levine, 1957). The long-term consequences of early H/MS experience on behavioral and physiological responses to stress in the adult offspring are at least partially mediated by early experience-dependent alterations of central CRF signaling pathways and glucocorticoid receptors involved in negative feedback control over the HPA axis (Bhatnagar, Shanks, Plotsky, & Meaney, 1996; Levine, 2005; Meaney et al., 1996; Plotsky et al., 2005; Schwetz et al., 2005). Altered norepinephrine levels within the ventral striatum and serotoninergic raphe neurons also have been reported (Andersen, Lyss, Dumont, & Teicher, 1999). Though most studies using this model system have focused on the neuroendocrine effects of H/MS, particularly alterations in the HPA axis, there is a growing literature documenting how manipulation of maternal care alters adult visceral sensory-motor functions. For example, neonatal H/MS promotes sex-specific alterations in adult baseline mean arterial blood pressure and hypoxic ventilatory responses that are at least partly due to enhanced responsiveness of the phrenic and carotid sinus nerves (Ábrahám & Kovacs, 2000; Genest, Gulemetova, Laforest, Drolet, & Kinkead, 2004; Kinkead, Gulemetova, & Bairam, 2005; Kinkead, Joseph, Lajeunesse, & Bairam, 2005). Daily repeated MS (brief or prolonged) has been shown to alter adult behavioral responses (e.g., jumping and ultrasonic vocalization) to foot shock, and to alter context- and cue-dependent fear conditioning (Kosten, Lee, & Kim, 2006). While altered autonomic responses presumably would also be observed in these animals, this has not been specifically examined. Adult rats exposed to neonatal MS are more prone to display stress-induced intestinal mucosal dysfunction (including impaired host defense to luminal bacteria) and visceral hypersensitivity, including an exaggerated visceromotor response to an acute stress challenge (Coutinho et al., 2002; Gareau, Jury, Yang, MacQueen, & Perdue, 2006; Milde, Enger, & Murison, 2004; Schwetz et al., 2005; Welting, Wijngaard, Jonge, Holman, & Boeckxstaens, 2005). Other treatments in young pups that have been reported to increase adult visceromotor responses (e.g., repeated neonatal colonic irritation with mustard oil; Al-Chaer et al., 2000) can be interpreted as replicating aspects of the H/MS model.

Experience-dependent Modification of Visceral Circuit Assembly

As reviewed briefly above, laboratory rats that are repeatedly separated from their dam for brief or extended periods of time during early development exhibit altered behavioral, endocrine, and autonomic responses to stress during adolescence (Colorado, Shumake, Conejo, Gonzalez-Pardo, & Gonzalez-Lima, 2006) and adulthood. However, the extent to which repeated brief or prolonged MS alters the functional development of central neural circuits that underlie these responses is unknown. Autonomic and neuroendocrine circuits regulate visceral responses to stress and emotionally evocative stimuli. Central components of these emotional motor circuits include hypothalamic and limbic forebrain preautonomic nuclei that provide direct and powerful modulatory control over sympathetic and parasympathetic outflow to the viscera. Autonomic responses to stimuli that elicit fear, anxiety, or other strong emotions typically include significant alterations of autonomic outflow, including altered gastrointestinal function (Kaplan, Masand, & Gupta, 1996; Mayer, Naliboff, Chang, & Coutinho, 2001; Punyabati, Deepak, Sharma, & Dwivedi, 2000). As reviewed above, the majority of these preautonomic forebrain neurons first establish synaptic connections with hindbrain and spinal autonomic neurons after birth in rats (Rinaman et al., 2000). The PVN becomes integrated into preautonomic circuits relatively early, whereas the CeA, BNST, and visceral cortices become integrated at progressively later time points (Rinaman et al., 1999, 2000). Thus, this early developmental window represents

a potential "sensitive period" during which experience may influence the ongoing assembly of central circuits that modulate autonomic motor outflow and emotional expression.

We hypothesized that repeated MS of rat pups during early postnatal life might alter the developmental assembly of central autonomic circuits, thereby providing a potential structural correlate for early experience-dependent effects on later responsiveness to emotionally evocative stimuli. To test this hypothesis, we used the classic "Plotsky and Meaney" H/MS model (Plotsky & Meaney, 1993). As reviewed briefly above, this approach has revealed a sensitive period of postnatal development during which repeated brief or prolonged MS elicits persistent changes in stress responsiveness and emotionality. Circuit development was traced by synapse-dependent retrograde transneuronal transport of PRV from the stomach wall, as in our earlier studies. Control and H/MS rats were analyzed between P6 and P10, a period of rapid synaptic assembly among preautonomic circuit components. Pups in H/MS groups were removed from their dam daily for either 15 min or 3 h beginning on P1 and continuing through P10. The same pups were injected with virus on P8 and perfused on P10. Quantitative analyses of primary and trans-synaptic PRV immunolabeling confirmed the previously reported age-dependent assembly of hypothalamic, limbic, and cortical inputs to autonomic nuclei. Circuit assembly was significantly altered in H/MS pups, in which fewer neurons in the CeA, BNST, and visceral cortices were infected on P10 compared to infection in age-matched controls. In contrast, H/MS had little or no effect on the assembly of PVN inputs to gastric autonomic neurons. Rather surprisingly, reductions in limbic and cortical transneuronal infection were similar in pups exposed daily to either 15 min or 3 h of MS. These findings indicate that environmental events during early postnatal life can influence the formation of neural circuits that provide limbic and cortical control over autonomic components of emotional behavior. This result was unrelated to any effect of brief or prolonged daily H/MS on overall body growth; thus, it strongly implicates an experience-dependent effect on the developmental assembly of central neural circuits.

The significant reduction in transneuronal infection of limbic cell groups in H/MS rats cannot be attributed to a general treatment-related suppression of PRV replication and/or transport, because in the same animals there was little or no effect of

H/MS on transneuronal viral transport to the parvocellular PVN. Instead, the results are consistent with an experience-induced alteration of the assembly of specific limbic and cortical preautonomic circuits that normally undergo large-scale increases in synaptic connectivity during the same postnatal period. Independent support for this suggestion comes from a study in which repeated neonatal H/MS in a precocious South American rodent species (*Octodon degus*) was associated with a significant decrement in a chemically identified population of neurons within IL and PL regions of the adult mPFC (Poeggel et al., 1999). Conversely, the relative lack of treatment-related effects on the distribution and density of transneuronal infection within the PVN and within autonomic and preautonomic brain stem nuclei is consistent with evidence presented previously (Rinaman et al., 1999, 2000), and confirmed in the H/MS study, that these circuits are established earlier during development than the limbic and cortical circuits. The earlier assembly of brain stem and hypothalamic circuits may render them less susceptible to significant modification as a result of H/MS manipulations.

It is not clear why the 15-min and 3-h H/MS manipulations produced equivalent reductions in limbic forebrain transneuronal viral transport. Previous work using similar H/MS paradigms reported reliable differences in certain behavioral, molecular, and physiological parameters between adult rats that were daily handled and separated from their dam for 15 min versus 3 h during early postnatal life (Francis, Caldji, Champagne, Plotsky, & Meaney, 1999; Ladd et al., 2000; McIntosh, Anisman, & Merali, 1999; Meaney, 2001; Plotsky & Meaney, 1993). These studies, however, also report some significant effects of early experience that were of similar magnitude and direction in both 15 min and 3 h H/MS rats (Macrì & Wurbel, 2006). It is important to emphasize that our neuroanatomical analyses were limited to a single early time point (i.e., P8/P10) within the ongoing development of the circuits under study. It will be of considerable interest to determine whether these experience-induced alterations in circuit assembly are associated with long-lasting alterations of autonomic circuit connectivity in adult animals. It also is interesting that transneuronal labeling within the CeA and BNST was more variable in control P10 pups compared to labeling in pups from the 15-min and 3-h H/MS groups. Individual differences in behavioral and neuroendocrine responses to stress in rats are, in part, derived from naturally occurring variations in maternal care (Ladd et al., 2000; Meaney, 2001; Watts & Swanson, 2002). Therefore, it is possible that both 15-min and 3-h daily MS serves to reduce this natural variability.

The PVN is a phenotypically and functionally heterogeneous nucleus. In this regard, it is interesting that one subregion of the PVN, the posterior parvocellular, displayed a small but statistically significant treatment-related reduction in transneuronal viral labeling in the H/MS viral tracing study. This posterior subdivision demonstrated the largest increase in viral transneuronal labeling out of all four parvocellular subdivisions between P4/P6 and P8/P10 in control rats, evidence that a significant amount of synaptic connectivity normally emerges between posterior parvocellular PVN neurons and gastric-related autonomic neurons within that timeframe, and perhaps accounting for the observed treatment-related circuit plasticity. It will be important to determine whether the experience-dependent changes in circuit assembly are similarly restricted to effects exerted during the first postnatal week and, more importantly, whether these changes represent a permanent modification of the system as has been demonstrated for the HPA axis and for behavioral responses to stressful and emotionally evocative stimuli (Francis et al., 1999; Ladd et al., 2000; Meaney, 2001; Plotsky & Meaney, 1993).

Potential Impact of Interoception on the Postnatal Assembly of Central Visceral Circuits

Results of the H/MS virus tracing study support the view that the relatively late-developing components of central autonomic circuits exhibit plasticity in response to significant postnatal epigenetic events. It seems likely that repeated daily occurrence of brief or prolonged MS also affects ascending viscerosensory pathway development. Indeed, neonatal rearing conditions were reported to have a significant impact on stress-evoked norepinephrine release in the PVN, associated with altered alpha2 autoreceptor binding in the DVC (Liu, Caldji, Sharma, Plotsky, & Meaney, 2000). As discussed above, brain stem nor/adrenergic projections to the PVN provide a major source of ascending input to initiate and modulate HPA axis responses to stress. A subset of DVC nor/adrenergic neurons project directly to the PVN, and this projection undergoes significant postnatal maturation (Rinaman, 2001). Thus, alteration of nor/adrenergic signaling pathways from the DVC to the PVN could contribute to experience-dependent differences in stress-induced norepinephrine release in the PVN, and differences in HPA activity.

Despite the growing literature reporting altered neural control of visceral function in adult rats after early manipulation of maternal care, very little is known about how these alterations come about. Although the physiological effects of H/MS on rat pups have not been rigorously examined, the available evidence suggests that they occur rapidly. For example, growth hormone (GH) levels and ornithine decarboxylase activity (necessary for the production of polyamine compounds required for cell division) are reduced in pups within the first 15 min of MS (Kuhn, Pauk, & Schanberg, 1990). Normal cellular responses to GH are lost with longer periods of MS (Kuhn, Evoniuk, & Schanberg, 1979), although plasma corticosterone levels do not increase until pups have been isolated for several hours (Levine et al., 1991). While changes in pup plasma osmolality and glucose are unlikely within the 3-h window typical of most MS paradigms, hypovolemia sets in within 2–3 h, depending on pup age (Friedman, 1975).

Maternal touching and nursing behaviors promote particular rhythms of activity within developing somatosensory and visceral circuits of rat pups that are important for their physiological regulation. After 3 h of MS, pups have relatively distended bladders and colons due to the absence of anogenital stimulation that normally is provided by maternal licking and grooming. Certain experimental interventions—such as intragastric infusion of liquid nutrients and experimental simulation of anogenital licking and grooming of maternally deprived pups—can partially ameliorate the effects of prolonged MS (Van Oers, de Kloet, & Levine, 1999), but the mechanisms through which such interventions exert their effects are largely unknown. Relatively little has been reported regarding the effects of MS on other potentially critical variables such as plasma ketones and proteins or the amount and quality of milk delivered to pups upon resumption of nursing (but see Fukushima, Yokouchi, Kawagishi, & Moriizumi, 2006; Lau & Henning, 1984). Infant mammals must process large quantities of milk during early stages of rapid growth, and rat pups ingest as much as 30% of their body weight in milk every day. The upper gastrointestinal tract of rat pups after 3 h of MS contains significantly less milk compared to nonseparated pups (Lorenz, 1985). Hofer has demonstrated that the presence of milk in the gastrointestinal tract modulates the activity of cardiac visceral sensory and motor pathways in neonatal rats, supporting the view that milk is a physiological regulator of early autonomic activity (Hofer, 1984). In 1- to 2-week-old pups, high levels of tonic sympathetic tone set a baseline from which phasic vagally mediated bradycardia is evident in response to loss of milk from the gastrointestinal tract. The concurrent absence of tonic vagal restraint in pups of this age allows cardiac pumping rate to be closely controlled by the presence of milk in the gut. Cardiovascular responses to milk diminish markedly during the third and fourth postnatal weeks, as tonic cardiac vagal restraint develops (Hofer, 1984). Thus, tonic autonomic regulation in rat pups is under close maternal control, providing a means by which early pup–dam interactions might affect the development of autonomic balance.

Stimulus-evoked activation of interoceptive circuits during their developmental assembly initiates relatively simple somatovisceral and viscerovisceral reflexes (e.g., licking-induced urination and defecation). This early developmental period of circuit assembly comprises a sensitive period during which the nature and frequency of somatosensory and interoceptive stimuli presumably affect the establishment and strength of synaptic connections that shape visceral regulatory capacities. In addition to yielding water and nutrients, suckling exerts profound behavioral effects on newborn rats and human infants (Blass, 1994). Suckling calms the infant, reduces its heart rate and metabolic rate, and elevates its pain threshold. In this regard, the H/MS model in rats may re-create certain aspects of the classic studies by Harlow showing the importance of conspecific (i.e., maternal) contact for emotional development in nonhuman primates (Harlow, 1958). Repeated H/MS in experimental animals also may model aspects of the delay in growth and development observed in touch-deprived premature human infants. In rats, maternal licking and grooming (tactile stimulation) increase pup tissue levels of ornithine decarboxylase (Pauk, Kuhn, Field, & Schanberg, 1986) and plasma levels of GH (Kuhn & Schanberg, 1998) and lactate (Alasmi, Pickens, & Hoath, 1997). In premature incubator-isolated infants, supplementing tactile stimulation–promoted marked gains in body weight and behavioral development, improved habituation and motor control, and significantly enhanced sympathoadrenal maturation (Kuhn & Schanberg, 1998). Clinical studies also have demonstrated that providing human infants with active and passive touch, including skin-to-skin "kangaroo care" (Dodd, 2005; Feldman, Weller, Sirota, & Eidelman, 2002; McCain, Ludington-Hoe, Swinth, & Hadeed, 2005), alleviates many of the adverse effects of sensory neglect on physiological and emotional regulation.

How might maternal contact affect the developmental assembly of visceral circuits in neonatal rats? Neonatal rats exhibit a complex series of behaviors in response to a variety of salient stimuli such as the odor of maternal saliva, tactile stroking, and intraoral milk infusions (Specht, Burright, & Spear, 1996). Presumably some combination of these stimuli and/or the pup's responses to them is required for "normal" nervous system development. Where might these stimuli interact to produce their long-lasting effects? A consideration of interoceptive transmission through the medullary DVC may be illuminating. Recall that the DVC receives direct visceral sensory inputs as well as indirect somatosensory inputs relayed from the spinal cord. Within the DVC, neural and/or hormonal signals related to the presence of milk within the pup's gastrointestinal tract may interact with signals related to the amount and frequency of maternal licking and grooming received. Combined artificial feeding and stroking of rat pups during 24-h MS was remarkably effective in reversing MS-induced effects on adult HPA regulation, whereas stroking alone was ineffective (Van Oers et al., 1999). Gastrointestinal and somatosensory signals derived either directly or indirectly from maternal contact may synergize with increased or decreased levels of circulating factors such as GH and CCK. Plasma levels of GH and CCK fall during H/MS and increase during and after feeding and/or tactile stimulation (Kuhn et al., 1979; Weller et al., 1992), and both peptides are known to affect the behavior, growth, and physiology of developing rat pups. Interestingly, CCK alters GH secretion in adult male rats (Peuranen et al., 1995), suggesting the possibility that endogenous CCK levels in rat pups may influence GH levels during maternal care, MS, and after reunion. However, the specific maternally derived factor(s) that leads to increased levels of CCK and GH are not clear. Natural suckling after H/MS promotes increased plasma GH levels, but so does intragastric infusion or subcutaneous injection of milk (but not glucose or protein) in MS rat pups (Kacsoh, Terry, Meyers, Crowley, & Grosvenor, 1989). Although some biologically active component of rat milk is sufficient

to release GH from neonatal rat pituitary glands (Kacsoh et al., 1989), GH levels also increase when pups suckle dams with ligated milk ducts (Kacsoh, Meyers, Crowley, & Grosvenor, 1990). The ability of "dry suckling" to increase GH levels in the pups appears to depend on active maternal contact with pups while they are attached to the nipple, because GH levels do not increase in pups that suckle an anesthetized dam that has been treated with OT to enhance milk let-down (Kacsoh et al., 1990). A warm ambient nest temperature also appears to contribute importantly to the ability of active maternal care to promote increased GH levels in rat pups (Kacsoh et al., 1990).

In addition to its potential influence on GH levels in developing pups, CCK has other effects that can modify the physiology and behavior of infant mammals from the time of birth (see Figure 15.3). Nutrients transferred from stomach to small intestine stimulate CCK release from intestinal mucosal secretory cells (Liddle, 1995). CCK promotes growth of the gastrointestinal tact and pancreas, induces the release of nutrient-digesting enzymes, regulates gastric emptying, and increases the efficiency of insulin-mediated glucose utilization (Liddle, 1995; Raybould & Tache, 1988; reviewed by Weller, 2006). CCK also exerts a satiety effect via actions on CCK-1 receptors expressed in the gastrointestinal tract and along vagal afferent fibers (Moran, Baldessarini, Salorio, Lowery, & Schwartz, 1997; Schwartz & Moran, 1998) that activate vagal sensory inputs to the medullary DVC (Moran et al., 1997). CCK receptors are especially abundant and widely distributed in the upper gastrointestinal tract in newborn rats (Robinson et al., 1985; Robinson, Moran, Goldrich, & McHugh, 1987). Plasma CCK levels fall during MS and increase during suckling in rat pups (Weller et al., 1992). Plasma CCK levels also rapidly increase in human infants during suckling (Uvnäs-Moberg, Marchini, & Winberg, 1993). The rapid time course suggests that tactile or visceral stimulation contributes to the initial elevation of plasma CCK during suckling independent of postingestive nutrient effects, while nutrient effects later promote and sustain CCK release during and after the nursing bout (Uvnäs-Moberg et al., 1993).

Intragastric milk and exogenously administered CCK have calming effects in neonatal rats (Blass & Shide, 1993; Weller & Blass, 1988; Weller & Dubson, 1998), and functional antagonism of CCK receptors counteracts the calming effect of milk infusion or normal suckling (Blass & Shide,

1993; Weller & Dubson, 1998). It has been proposed that sustained contact with the dam supports calm, quiescent behavior in the pup, which may be maintained in the absence of the dam or augmented in her presence by milk-related CCK release (Blass, Fillion, Weller, & Brunson, 1990). At the termination of a nursing bout, rat pups' plasma CCK levels are high and the relatively sedated pups are unlikely to leave the nest or vocalize, thereby allowing the dam to leave the litter to forage for food (Blass & Shide, 1993). Unsatisfied pups remain more active at the end of a nursing bout, making it less likely that the dam will leave the litter and more likely that nursing will continue (Stern & Keer, 2002). Indeed, rat pups that congenitally lack CCK-1 receptors display more ultrasonic distress vocalizations during MS, spend more time nursing when the dam is present, and gain more body weight compared to pups that express CCK-1 receptors (Blumberg, Haba, Schroeder, Smith, & Weller, 2006; Weller, 2006; Weller & Feldman, 2003). Recent work supports the view that increased vocalization in rat pups is related to their need to sustain blood pressure in the face of homeostatic challenge, rather than being related to anxiety or distress per se (Blumberg, Johnson, & Middlemis-Brown, 2005; Blumberg, Sokoloff, Kirby, & Kent, 2000). A potentially similar syndrome in human infants is suggested by findings that plasma CCK levels are negatively correlated with excessive crying (Huhtala, Lehtonen, Uvnäs-Moberg, & Korvenranta, 2003).

How might CCK be differentially affected by repeated daily incidences of brief versus prolonged MS? In neonatal rats, anogenital licking by the dam stimulates colonic transit and defecation by the pups. When pups are separated from their dams for periods of 3 or 4 h, colonic distension due to accumulating fill would presumably inhibit gastric motility and emptying, which should decrease intestinal release of CCK below normal levels. Conversely, rat pups separated from their dams for brief periods (i.e., 15 min) should not experience any decrease in CCK. After maternal reunion, however, licking-induced reflexive gastrointestinal transit in both 15-min and 3-h MS pups may promote increased delivery of milk from the stomach to the duodenum, which may contribute to the observed spike in plasma CCK levels in MS pups after reunion with the dam. Plasma CCK levels increase more quickly and reach higher peak levels in calves that are allowed to suckle nonnutritively after a milk meal (Passille, Christopherson,

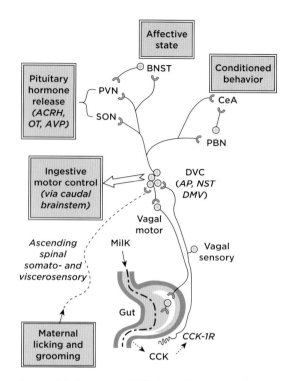

Figure 15.3 Endogenous CCK released from the gut during milk digestion in neonatal rats activates vagal sensory inputs to the caudal medulla (DVC) through a CCK-1 receptor-mediated mechanism. Within the DVC, vagal sensory signals can interact with other ascending somatosensory and visceral sensory signals, including those generated by maternal licking and grooming of the rat pup. These signals may thereby modulate the functional development of parellel ascending projections from the DVC to hypothalamic and limbic forebrain regions that modulate physiological and behavioral responses to the animal's internal and external environment. Abbreviations as in the text.

& Rushen, 1993), evidence for a role of continued tactile and/or visceral sensory-motor factors in promoting nutrient-induced CCK release. In human infants fed milk via a nasogastric tube, CCK levels increased by a markedly greater amount when infants were maintained in skin-to-skin contact with a caregiver during and after the feeding, compared to CCK levels in infants fed via nasogastric tube without concurrent contact (Tornhage, Serenius, Uvnäs-Moberg, & Lindberg, 1998). The increased maternal care received by 15-min H/MS pups should therefore increase their total exposure to CCK and thus increase gastrointestinal vagal sensory activation over the course of early postnatal development. Conversely, longer periods of MS should be associated with less pup exposure to endogenous CCK and less vagal sensory activation. Thus, CCK may provide a common pathway for the effects of maternal touch and milk to regulate visceral circuit development during early postnatal life (Figure 15.3).

Conclusions

Normal interactions between an infant and its mother (or primary caregiver) are critical for normal growth and development in mammalian species, and perturbations of these interactions can disrupt physiological and behavioral functions in the offspring. Neural systems that control visceral responsiveness overlap with those that regulate behavioral arousal, and the long-lasting influence of early epigenetic influences on later behavioral and physiological responses to emotional stimuli (Jordan, 1990) presumably is linked to altered formation of central limbic-autonomic circuits that underlie interoceptive interpretation and affective expression. In humans, visceral hypersensitivity and neuroendocrine dysfunctions are recognized as common symptoms of anxiety and depressive disorders, which feature inappropriate physiological responses to interoceptive and exteroceptive triggering stimuli. Aberrant activity within visceral circuits may also support the "vicious cycle" of reciprocal ascending/descending activity that underlies pathological conditions such as panic disorder, irritable bowel disorder, and other functional disorders (Berntson et al., 2003; Mayer et al., 2001). Aberrant neural activity may arise, at least in part, as a product of postnatal ontogenetic events that occur during neural circuit assembly. Evaluation of this hypothesis has proved difficult, because the normal developmental assembly of visceral and emotional neural circuits is largely undescribed in both human and nonhuman animals. Moreover, the specific regulatory interactions between mothers and offspring are only minimally understood. Despite these limitations in our current understanding, the extant literature and ongoing research continue to support an intimate association between viscerosensory circuit function and affective behavior. The challenges inherent in pushing the frontier outward in understanding the development of these systems under normal and abnormal conditions remain for us one of the prime attractions of this field of study.

References

Ábrahám, I. M., & Kovacs, K. J. (2000). Postnatal handling alters the activation of stress-related neuronal circuits. *European Journal of Neuroscience, 12*, 3003–3014.

Al-Chaer, E. D., Kawasaki, M., & Pasricha, P. J. (2000). A new model of chronic visceral hypersensitivity in adult rats induced by colon irritation during postnatal development. *Gastroenterology, 119*, 1276–1285.

Al-Damluji, S. (1988). Adrenergic mechanisms in the control of corticotropin secretion. *Journal of Endocrinology, 119*, 5–14.

Alasmi, M. M., Pickens, W. L., & Hoath, S. B. (1997). Effect of tactile stimulation on serum lactate in the newborn rat. *Pediatric Research, 41*(6), 857–861.

Aleksandrov, V. G., Bagaev, V. A., Nozdrachev, A. D., & Panteleev, S. S. (1996). Identification of gastric related neurones in the rat insular cortex. *Neuroscience Letters, 216*(1), 5–8.

Alonso, G., Szafarczyk, A., Balmefrezol, M., & Assenmacher, I. (1986). Immunocytochemical evidence of stimulatory control by the ventral noradrenergic bundle of parvicellular neurons of the paraventricular nucleus secreting corticotropin-releasing hormone and vasopressin in rats. *Brain Research, 397*, 297–307.

Altschuler, S. M., Bao, X., Bieger, D., Hopkins, D. A., & Miselis, R. R. (1989). Viscerotopic representation of the upper alimentary tract in the rat: Sensory ganglia and nuclei of the solitary and spinal trigeminal tracts. *Journal of Comparative Neurology, 283*, 248–268.

Andersen, S. L., Lyss, P. J., Dumont, N. L., & Teicher, M. H. (1999). Enduring neurochemical effects of early maternal separation on limbic structures. *Annals of the New York Academy of Sciences, 877*, 756–759.

Araki, I., & Groat, W. C. d. (1997). Developmental synaptic depression underlying reorganization of visceral reflex pathways in the spinal cord. *The Journal of Neuroscience, 17*(21), 8402–8407.

Avishai-Eliner, S., Eghbal-Ahmadi, M., Tabatchnik, E., Brunson, K. L., & Baram, T. Z. (2001). Downregulation of hypothalamic corticotropin-releasing hormone messenger ribonucleic acid precedes early-life hippocampal glucocorticoid receptor–mRNA changes. *Endocrinology, 142*, 89–97.

Bailey, T. W., Hermes, S. M., Andresen, M. C., & Aicher, A. A. (2006). Cranial visceral afferent pathways through the nucleus of the solitary tract to caudal ventrolateral medulla or paraventricular hypothalamus: Target-specific synaptic reliability and convergence patterns. *The Journal of Neuroscience, 26*(46), 11893–11902.

Barbas, H., Saha, S., Rempel-Clower, N., & Ghashghaei, T. (2003), *Serial pathways from primate prefrontal cortex to autonomic areas may influence emotional expression.* from http://www.biomedcentral.com/1471-2202/4/25

Bartha, A. (1961). Experimental reduction of virulence of Aujeszky's disease virus. *Magy Allotorv Lapja, 16*, 42–45.

Bechara, A., Damasio, H., & Damasio, A. R. (2003). Role of the amygdala in decision-making. *Annals of the New York Academy of Sciences, 985*, 356–369.

Benaroya-Milshtein, N., Hollander, N., Apter, A., Kulkulansky, T., Raz, N., Wilf, A., et al. (2004). Environmental enrichment in mice decreases anxiety, attenuates stress responses and enhances natural killer cell activity. *European Journal of Neuroscience, 20*(5), 1341–1347.

Berntson, G. G., Sarter, M., & Cacioppo, J. T. (1998). Anxiety and cardiovascular reactivity: The basal forebrain cholinergic link. *Behavioural Brain Research, 94*, 225–248.

Berntson, G. G., Sarter, M., & Cacioppo, J. T. (2003). Ascending visceral regulation of cortical affective information processing. *European Journal of Neuroscience, 18*, 2103–2109.

Bhatnagar, S., Shanks, N., Plotsky, P. M., & Meaney, M. J. (1996). Hypothalamic-pituitary-adrenal responses in neonatally handled and nonhandled rats: Differences in facilitatory and inhibitory neural pathways. In R. McCarthy, G. Agulara, E. Sabba & R. Kvetnansky (Eds.), *Stress: Molecular and neurobiological advances* (pp. 1–24). New York: Gordon & Breach.

Bielefeldt, K., Christianson, J. A., & Davis, B. M. (2005). Basic and clinical aspects of visceral sensation: Transmission in the CNS. *Neurogastroenterology and Motility, 17*, 488–499.

Blass, E. M. (1994). Behavioral and physiological consequences of suckling in rat and human newborns. *Acta Paediatrica Supplement, 397*, 71–76.

Blass, E. M., Fillion, T. J., Weller, A., & Brunson, L. (1990). Separation of opioid from nonopioid mediation of affect in neonatal rats: Nonopioid mechanisms mediate maternal contact influences. *Behavioral Neuroscience, 104*(4), 625–636.

Blass, E. M., & Shide, D. J. (1993). Endogenous cholecystokinin reduces vocalization in isolated 10-day-old rats. *Behavioral Neuroscience, 107*(3), 488–492.

Blumberg, M. S., Haba, D., Schroeder, M., Smith, G. P., & Weller, A. (2006). Independent ingestion and microstructure of feeding patterns in infant racks lacking CCK-1 receptors. *American Journal of Physiology—Regulatory, Integrative, and Comparative Physiology,, 290*(1), R208–R218.

Blumberg, M. S., Johnson, E. D., & Middlemis-Brown, J. E. (2005). Inhibition of ultrasonic vocalizations by beta-adrenoceptor agonists. *Developmental Psychobiology, 47*(1), 66–76.

Blumberg, M. S., Sokoloff, G., Kirby, R. F., & Kent, K. J. (2000). Distress vocalizations in infant rats: What's all the fuss about? *Psychological Science, 11*(1), 78–81.

Boissé, L., Mouihate, A., Ellis, S., & Pittman, Q. J. (2004). Long-term alterations in neuroimmune responses after neonatal exposure to lipopolysaccharide. *The Journal of Neuroscience, 24*, 4928–4934.

Caldji, C., Tanenbaum, B., Sharma, S., Francis, D., Plotsky, P. M., & Meaney, M. J. (1998). Maternal care during infancy regulates the development of neural systems mediating the expression of fearfulness in the rat. *Proceedings of the National Academy of Sciences, 95*, 5335–5340.

Callahan, J. B., & Rinaman, L. (1998). The postnatal emergence of dehydration anorexia in rats is temporally associated with the emergence of dehydration-induced inhibition of gastric emptying. *Physiology and Behavior, 64*, 683–687.

Cameron, O. G. (2001). Interoception: The inside story—A model for psychosomatic processes. *Psychosomatic Medicine, 63*, 697–710.

Cano, G., Card, J. P., Rinaman, L., & Sved, A. F. (2000). Connections of Barrington's nucleus to the sympathetic nervous system in rats. *Journal of the Autonomic Nervous System, 79*, 117–128.

Cano, G., Sved, A. F., Rinaman, L., Rabin, B. S., & Card, J. P. (2001). Characterization of the central nervous system innervation of the rat spleen using viral transneuronal tracing. *The Journal of Comparative Neurology, 439*, 1–18.

Card, J. P. (1998). Exploring brain circuitry with neurotropic viruses: New horizons in neuroanatomy. *The Anatomical Record (New Anatomy), 253*, 176–185.

Card, J. P., Rinaman, L., Lynn, R. B., Lee, B. –H., Meade, R. P., Miselis, R. R., et al. (1993). Pseudorabies virus infection of the rat central nervous system: Ultrastructural characterization of viral replication, transport, and pathogenesis. *The Journal of Neuroscience, 13*(6), 2515–2539.

Card, J. P., & Sved, A. F. (2009, in press). Central autonomic networks. In *Central regulation of autonomic function* (2nd ed.). New York: Oxford University Press.

Cechetto, D. F., & Saper, C. B. (1987). Evidence for a viscerotopic sensory representation in the cortex and thalamus in the rat. *The Journal of Comparative Neurology, 262*(1), 27–45.

Colorado, R. A., Shumake, J., Conejo, N. M., Gonzalez-Pardo, H., & Gonzalez-Lima, F. (2006). Effects of maternal separation, early handling, and standard facility rearing on orienting and impulsive behavior of adolescent rats. *Behavioural Processes, 71*(1), 51–58.

Coutinho, S. V., Plotsky, P. M., Sablad, M., Miller, J. C., Zhou, H., Bayati, A. I., et al. (2002). Neonatal maternal separation alters stress-induced responses to viscerosomatic nociceptive stimuli in rat. *American Journal of Physiology—Gastrointestinal and Liver Physiology, 282*, G307–G316.

Craig, A. D. (2002). How do you feel? Interoception: The sense of the physiological condition of the body. *Nature Reviews—Neuroscience, 2*, 655–666.

Crestani, F., Lorez, M., Baer, K., Essrich, C., Benke, D., Laurent, J. P., et al. (1999). Decreased GABAA-receptor clustering results in enhanced anxiety and a bias for threat cues. *Nature Neuroscience, 2*(9), 833–839.

D'Amato, F. R., Cabib, S., Ventura, R., & Orsini, C. (1998). Long-term effects of postnatal manipulation on emotionality are prevented by maternal anxiolytic treatment in mice. *Developmental Psychobiology, 32*, 225–234.

Damasio, A. (1999). *The feeling of what happens: Body and emotion in the making of consciousness.* New York: Harcourt Brace.

Day, H. E. W., McKnight, A. T., Poat, J. A., & Hughes, J. (1994). Evidence that cholecystokinin induces immediate early gene expression in the brainstem, hypothalamus and amygdala of the rat by a CCK$_A$ receptor mechanism. *Neuropharmacology, 33*(6), 719–727.

Denenberg, V. H. (1999). Commentary: Is maternal stimulation the mediator of the handling effect in infancy? *Developmental Psychobiology, 34*, 1–3.

Denenberg, V. H., Ottinger, D. R., & Stephens, M. W. (1962). Effects of maternal factors upon growth and behavior of the rat. *Child Development, 33*, 65–71.

Derbyshire, S. W. (2003). A systematic review of neuroimaging data during visceral stimulation. *The American Journal of Gastroenterology, 98*(1), 12–20.

Dodd, V. L. (2005). Implications of kangaroo care for growth and development in preterm infants. *Journal of Obstetric, Gynecologic, and Neonatal Nursing, 34*(2), 218–232.

Ericsson, A., Kovacs, K. J., & Sawchenko, P. E. (1994). A functional anatomical analysis of central pathways subserving the effects of interleukin-1 on stress-related neuroendocrine neurons. *The Journal of Neuroscience, 14*(2), 897–913.

Feldman, R., Weller, A., Sirota, L., & Eidelman, A. I. (2002). Skin-to-skin contact (kangaroo care) promotes self-regulation in premature infants: Sleep–wake cyclicity, arousal modulation, and sustained exploration. *Developmental Psychology, 38*(2), 194–207.

Fenoglio, K. A., Brunson, K. L., Avishai-Eliner, S., Stone, B. A., Kapadia, B. J., & Baram, T. Z. (2005). Enduring, handling-evoked enhancement of hippocampal memory function and glucocorticoid receptor expression involves activation of the corticotropin-releasing factor type 1 receptor. *Endocrinology, 146*(9), 4090–4096.

Ferguson, A. V., Marcus, P., Spencer, J., & Wallace, J. L. (1988). Paraventricular nucleus stimulation causes gastroduodenal mucosal necrosis in the rat. *American Journal of Physiology—Regulatory, Integrative, and Comparative Physiology,255*, R861–R865.

Flanagan, L. M., Olson, B. R., Sved, A. F., Verbalis, J. G., & Stricker, E. M. (1992). Gastric motility in conscious rats given oxytocin and an oxytocin antagonist centrally. *Brain Research, 578*, 256–260.

Flanagan, L. M., Verbalis, J. G., & Stricker, E. M. (1989). Effects of anorexigenic treatments on gastric motility in rats. *American Journal of Physiology—Regulatory, Integrative, and Comparative Physiology,, 256,*, R955–R961.

Ford, D. H., & Lerner, R. M. (1992). *Developmental systems theory: An integrative approach*. Newbury Park, CA: Sage Publications.

Francis, D. D., Caldji, C., Champagne, F., Plotsky, P. M., & Meaney, M. J. (1999). The role of corticotropin-releasing factor-norepinephrine systems in mediating the effects of early experience on the development of behavioral and endocrine responses to stress. *Biological Psychiatry, 46*, 1153–1166.

Friedman, M. I. (1975). Some determinants of milk ingestion in suckling rats. *Journal of Comparative and Physiological Psychology, 89*(6), 636–647.

Fukushima, N., Yokouchi, K., Kawagishi, K., & Moriizumi, T. (2006). Effect of maternal deprivation on milk intake in normal and bilaterally facial nerve-injured developing rats. *Neuroscience Research, 54*(2), 154–157.

Fulwiler, C. E., & Saper, C. B. (1984). Subnuclear organization of the efferent connections of the parabrachial nucleus in the rat. *Brain Research Reviews, 7*, 229–259.

Gabbott, P. L., Warner, T. A., Jays, P. R., & Bacon, S. J. (2003). Areal and synaptic interconnectivity of prelimbic (area 32), infralimbic (area 25) and insular cortices in the rat. *Brain Research, 993*(1–2), 59–71.

Gaillet, S., Lachuer, J., Malaval, F., Assenmacher, I., & Szafarczyk, A. (1991). The involvement of noradrenergic ascending pathways in the stress-induced activation of ACTH and corticosterone secretions is dependent on the nature of the stressors. *Experimental Brain Research, 87*, 173–180.

Gareau, M. G., Jury, J., Yang, P. C., MacQueen, G., & Perdue, M. H. (2006). Neonatal maternal separation causes colonic dysfunction in rat pups including impaired host resistance. *Pediatric Research, 59*(1), 83–88.

Genest, S. E., Gulemetova, R., Laforest, S., Drolet, G., & Kinkead, R. (2004). Neonatal maternal separation and sex-specific plasticity of the hypoxic ventilatory response in awake rat. *The Journal of Physiology, 554*(part 2), 543–557.

Gilman, A. (1937). The relation beween osmotic pressure, fluid distribution, and voluntary water intake. *American Journal of Physiology, 120*, 323–328.

Green, T., & Dockray, G. J. (1987). Calcitonin gene-related peptide and substance P in afferents to the upper gastrointestinal tract in the rat. *Neuroscience Letters, 76*(2), 151–156.

Grill, H. J., & Smith, G. P. (1988). Cholecystokinin decreases sucrose intake in chronic decerebrate rats. *American Journal of Physiology—Regulatory, Integrative, and Comparative Physiology, , 253*, R853–R856.

Harlow, H. F. (1958). The nature of love. *American Psychologist, 13*(573–685).

Herbert, H., Moga, M. M., & Saper, C. B. (1990). Connections of the parabrachial nucleus with the nucleus of the solitary tract and the medullary reticular formation in the rat. *The Journal of Comparative Neurology, 293*, 540–580.

Hermann, G. E., McCann, M. J., & Rogers, R. C. (1990). Activation of the bed nucleus of the stria terminalis increases gastric motility in the rat. *Journal of the Autonomic Nervous System, 30*(2), 123–128.

Hironaka, S., Shirakawa, T., Toki, S., Kinoshita, K., & Oguchi, H. (2000). Feeding-induced c-fos expression in the nucleus of the solitary tract and dorsal medullary reticular formation in neonatal rats. *Neuroscience Letters, 293*, 175–178.

Hofer, M. A. (1984). Early stages in the organization of cardiovascular control. *Proceedings of the Society for Experimental Biology and Medicine, 175*, 147–157.

Hofer, M. A. (1994). Early relationships as regulators of infant physiology and behavior. *Acta Paediatrica Supplement, 397*, 9–18.

Horst, G. J. T., Boer, P. D., Luiten, P. G. M., & Willigen, J. D. V. (1989). Ascending projections from the solitary tract nucleus to the hypothalamus. A *Phaseolus vulgaris* lectin tracing study in the rat. *Neuroscience, 31*, 785–797.

Horst, G. J. T., & Streefland, C. (1994). Ascending projections of the solitary tract nucleus. In I. R. A. Barraco (Ed.), *Nucleus of the solitary tract* (pp. 93–103). Boca Raton, FL: CRC Press.

Huhtala, V., Lehtonen, L., Uvnäs-Moberg, K., & Korvenranta, H. (2003). Low plasma cholecystokinin levels in colicky infants. *Journal of Pediatric Gastroenterology and Nutrition, 37*(1), 42–46.

Huot, R. L., Gonzalez, M. E., Ladd, C. O., Thrivikraman, K. V., & Plotsky, P. M. (2004). Foster litters prevent hypothalamic-pituitary-adrenal axis sensitization mediated by neonatal maternal separation. *Psychoneuroendocrinology, 29*, 279–289.

Hylden, J. L., Anton, F., & Nahin, R. L. (1989). Spinal lamina I projection neurons in the rat: Collateral innervation of parabrachial area and thalamus. *Neuroscience, 28*(1), 27–37.

Iriki, A., Nozaki, S., & Nakamura, Y. (1988). Feeding behavior in mammals: Corticobulbar projection is reorganized during conversion from sucking to chewing. *Brain Research, 44*, 189–196.

James, W. (1884). What is an emotion? *Mind, 9*, 188–205.

Janig, W. (2006). *The integrative action of the autonomic nervous system*. New York: Cambridge University Press.

Jansen, A. S. P., Hoffman, J. L., & Loewy, A. D. (1997). CNS sites involved in sympathetic and parasympathetic control of the pancreas: A viral tracing study. *Brain Research, 766*, 29–38.

Jordan, D. (1990). Autonomic changes in affective behavior. In A. D. Loewy & K. M. Spyer (Eds.), *Central regulation of autonomic functions*. New York: Oxford University Press.

Kacsoh, B., Meyers, J. S., Crowley, W. R., & Grosvenor, C. E. (1990). Maternal modulation of growth hormone secretion in the neonatal rat: Involvement of mother–offspring interactions. *The Journal of Endocrinology, 124*(2), 233–240.

Kacsoh, B., Terry, L. C., Meyers, J. S., Crowley, W. R., & Grosvenor, C. E. (1989). Maternal modulation of growth hormone secretion in the neonatal rat. I. Involvement of milk factors. *Endocrinology, 125*(3), 1326–1336.

Kalinichev, M., Easterling, K. W., & Holtzman, S. G. (2000). Periodic postpartum separation from the offspring results in long-lasting changes in anxiety-related behaviors and sensitivity to morphine in Long-Evans mother rats. *Psychopharmacology, 152*, 431–439.

Kaplan, D. S., Masand, P. S., & Gupta, S. (1996). The relationship of irritable bowel syndrome (IBS) and panic disorder. *Annals of Clinical Psychiatry, 8*(2), 81–88.

Kawai, Y., & Senba, E. (2000). Postnatal differentiation of local networks in the nucleus of the tractus solitarius. *Neuroscience, 100*(1), 109–114.

Kinkead, R., Gulemetova, R., & Bairam, A. (2005). Neonatal maternal separation enhances phrenic responses to hypoxia and carotid sinus nerve stimulation in the adult anesthetized rat. *Journal of Applied Physiology, 99*(1), 189–196.

Kinkead, R., Joseph, V., Lajeunesse, Y., & Bairam, A. (2005). Neonatal maternal separation enhances dopamine D_2-receptor and tyrosine hydroxylase mRNA expression levels in carotid body of rats. *Canadian Journal of Physiology and Pharmacology, 83*, 76–84.

Kiss, A., & Aguilera, G. (1992). Participation of alpha1-adrenergic receptors in the secretion of hypothalamic corticotropin-releasing hormone during stress. Neuroendocrinology, 56, 153–160.

Koehnle, T., & Rinaman, L. (2007). Progressive postnatal increases in Fos immunoreactivity in the forebrain and brainstem of rats after viscerosensory stimulation with lithium chloride. *American Journal of Physiology— Regulatory, Integrative, and Comparative Physiology,, 292*, R1212–R1223.

Kosten, T. A., Lee, H. J., & Kim, J. J. (2006). Early life stress impairs fear conditioning in adult male and female rats. *Brain Research, 1087*(1), 142–150.

Kuhn, C. M., Evoniuk, G., & Schanberg, S. M. (1979). Loss of tissue sensitivity to growth hormone during maternal deprivation in rats. *Life Science, 25*, 2090–2097.

Kuhn, C. M., Pauk, J., & Schanberg, S. M. (1990). Endocrine responses to mother–infant separation in developing rats. *Developmental Psychobiology, 23*(5), 395–410.

Kuhn, C. M., & Schanberg, S. M. (1998). Responses to maternal separation: Mechanisms and mediators. *International Journal of Developmental Neuroscience, 16*(3–4), 261–270.

Lachamp, P., Tell, F., & Kessler, J. P. (2002). Successive episodes of synapse production in the developing rat nucleus tractus solitarii. *Journal of Neurobiology, 52*(4), 336–342.

Ladd, C. O., Huot, R. L., Thriikraman, K. V., Nemeroff, C. B., Meaney, M. J., & Plotsky, P. M. (2000). Long-term behavioral and neuroendocrine adaptations to adverse early experience. In E. A. Mayer & C. B. Saper (Eds.), *Progress in brain research* (Vol. 122, pp. 81–103). Amsterdam: Elsevier.

Langley, J. N. (1921). *The autonomic nervous system*. Cambridge: Heffer and Sons.

Lau, C., & Henning, S. J. (1984). Regulation of milk ingestion in the infant rat. *Physiology and Behavior, 33*, 809–815.

LeDoux, J. E. (1996). *The emotional brain—The mysterious underpinnings of emotional life*. New York: Simon & Schuster.

LeDoux, J. E., Iwata, J., Cicchetti, P., & Reis, D. J. (1988). Different projections of the central amygdaloid nucleus mediate autonomic and behavioral correlates of conditioned fear. *The Journal of Neuroscience, 8*(7), 2517–2529.

Lenz, F. A., Gracely, R. H., Zirh, T. A., Leopold, D. A., Rowland, L. H., & Dougherty, P. M. (1997). Human thalamic nucleus mediating taste and multiple other sensations related to ingestive behavior. *Journal of Neurophysiology, 77*(6), 3406–3409.

Levenson, R. W. (2003). Blood, sweat, and fears: The autonomic architecture of emotion. *Annals of the New York Academy of Sciences, 1000*, 348–366.

Levenson, R. W., Ekman, P., Heider, K., & Friesen, W. V. (1992). Emotion and autonomic nervous system activity in the Minangkabau of west Sumatra. *Journal of Personality and Social Psychology, 62*(6), 972–988.

Levine, S. (1957). Infantile experience and resistance to stress. *Science, 126*, 405.

Levine, S. (2001). Primary social relationships influence the development of the hypothalamic-pituitary-adrenal axis in the rat. *Physiology and Behavior, 73*, 255–260.

Levine, S. (2005). Developmental determinants of sensitivity and resistance to stress. *Psychoneuroendocrinology, 30*(10), 939–946.

Levine, S., Chevalier, J. A., & Korchin, S. J. (1956). The effects of early handling and shock on later avoidance behavior. *Journal of Personality, 24*, 475–493.

Levine, S., Huchton, D. M., Weiner, S. G., & Rosenfeld, P. (1991). Time course of the effect of maternal deprivation on the hypothalamic-pituitary-adrenal axis in the infant rat. *Developmental Psychobiology, 24*, 547–558.

Liddle, R. A. (1995). Regulation of cholecystokinin secretion by intraluminal releasing factors. *American Journal of Physiology—Gastrointestinal and Liver Physiology, 269*, G319–G327.

Liposits, Z., Phelix, C., & Paull, W. K. (1986). Adrenergic innervation of corticotropin releasing factor (CRF)—Synthesizing neurons in the hypothalamic paraventricular nucleus of the rat. *Histochemistry, 84*, 201–205.

Liu, D., Caldji, C., Sharma, S., Plotsky, P. M., & Meaney, M. J. (2000). Influence of neonatal rearing conditions on stress-induced adrenocorticotropin responses and norepinephrine release in the hypothalamic paraventricular nucleus. *Journal of Neuroendocrinology, 12*, 5–12.

Loewy, A. D. (1990). Central autonomic pathways. In A. D. Loewy & K. M. Spyer (Eds.), *Central regulation of autonomic functions* (1st ed., pp. 88–103). New York: Oxford University Press.

Loewy, A. D. (1991). Forebrain nuclei involved in autonomic control. *Progress in Brain Research, 87*, 253–268.

Loewy, A. D. (1995). Pseudorabies virus: A transneuronal tracer for neuroanatomical studies. In A. D. Loewy & M. G. Kaplitt (Eds.), *Viral vectors. Gene therapy and neuroscience applications* (pp. 349–366). San Diego: Academic Press.

Loewy, A. D., & Haxhiu, M. A. (1993). CNS cell groups projecting to pancreatic parasympathetic preganglionic neurons. *Brain Research, 620*, 323–330.

Lorenz, D. N. (1985). Gastric emptying of milk in rat pups. *American Journal of Physiology—Regulatory, Integrative, and Comparative Physiology, , 248*, R732–R738.

Macri, S., Mason, G. J., & Wurbel, H. (2004). Dissociation in the effects of neonatal maternal separations on maternal care and the offspring's HPA and fear responses in rats. *European Journal of Neuroscience, 20*(4), 1017–1024.

Macrì S., & Wurbel, H. (2006). Developmental plasticity of HPA and fear responses in rats: A critical review of the maternal mediation hypothesis. *Hormones and Behavior, 50*(5), 667–680.

Martin, G. F., Cabana, T., Culberson, J. L., Curry, J. J., & Tschismadia, I. (1980). The early development of corticobulbar and corticospinal systems. Studies using the North American opossum. *Anatomy and Embryology, 161*(2), 197–213.

Maunder, R. G., & Hunter, J. J. (2001). Attachment and psychosomatic medicine: Developmental contributions to stress *Psychosomatic Medicine, 63*, 556–567.

Mayer, E. A., Naliboff, B. D., Chang, L., & Coutinho, S. V. (2001). Stress and the gastrointestinal tract. V. Stress and irritable bowel syndrome. *American Journal of Physiology—Gastrointestinal and Liver Physiology, 280*(4), G519–G524.

Mayer, E. A., & Saper, C. B. (Eds.). (2000). *The biological basis for mind body interactions* (Vol. 122). Amsterdam: Elsevier.

McCain, G. C., Ludington-Hoe, S. M., Swinth, J. Y., & Hadeed, A. J. (2005). Heart rate variability responses of a preterm infant to kangaroo care. *Journal of Obstetric, Gynecologic, and Neonatal Nursing, 34*(6), 689–694.

McIntosh, J., Anisman, H., & Merali, Z. (1999). Short- and long-periods of neonatal maternal separation differentially affect anxiety and feeding in adult rats: Gender-dependent effects. *Developmental Brain Research, 113*, 97–106.

Meaney, M. J. (2001). Maternal care, gene expression, and the transmission of individual differences in stress reactivity across generations. *Annual Review of Neuroscience, 24*, 1161–1192.

Meaney, M. J., Diorio, J., Francis, D., Widdowson, J., LaPlante, P., Caldji, C., et al. (1996). Early environmental regulation of forebrain glucocorticoid receptor gene expression: Implications for adrenocortical responses to stress. *Developmental Neuroscience, 18*, 49–72.

Menetrey, D., & Basbaum, A. I. (1987). Spinal and trigeminal projections to the nucleus of the solitary tract: A possible substrate for somatovisceral and viscerovisceral reflex activation. *The Journal of Comparative Neurology, 255*, 439–450.

Menetrey, D., & de Pommery, J. (1991). Origins of spinal ascending pathways that reach central areas involved in visceroception and visceronociception in the rat. *European Journal of Neuroscience, 3*, 249–259.

Milde, A. M., Enger, O., & Murison, R. (2004). The effects of postnatal maternal separation on stress responsivity and experimentally induced colitis in adult rats. *Physiology and Behavior, 81*(1), 71–84.

Miller, A. J., McKoon, M., Pinneau, M., & Silverstein, R. (1983). Postnatal synaptic development of the nucleus tractus solitarius (NTS) of the rat. *Developmental Brain Research, 8*, 205–213.

Moga, M. M., Herbert, H., Hurley, K. M., Yasui, Y., Gray, T. S., & Saper, C. B. (1990). Organization of cortical, basal forebrain, and hypothalamic afferents to the parabrachial nucleus in the rat. *The Journal of Comparative Neurology, 295*, 624–661.

Moncek, F., Duncko, R., Johansson, B. B., & Jezova, D. (2004). Effect of environmental enrichment on stress related systems in rats. *Journal of Neuroendocrinology, 16*(5), 423–431.

Moran, T. H., Baldessarini, A. R., Salorio, C. F., Lowery, T., & Schwartz, G. J. (1997). Vagal afferent and efferent contributions to the inhibition of food intake by cholecystokinin. *American Journal of Physiology—Regulatory, Integrative, and Comparative Physiology,, 272*, R1245–R1251.

Narayanan, J. T., Watts, R., Haddad, N., Labar, D. R., Li, P. M., & Filippi, C. G. (2002). Cerebral activation during vagus nerve stimulation: A functional MR study. *Epilepsia, 43*(12), 1509–1514.

Nicotra, A., Critchley, H. D., Mathias, C. J., & Dolan, R. J. (2006). Emotional and autonomic consequences of spinal cord injury explored using functional brain imaging. *Brain, 129*, 718–728.

Oladehin, A., & Blatteis, C. M. (1995). Lipopolysaccharide-induced fos expression in hypothalamic nuclei of neonatal rats. *Neuroimmunomodulation, 2*(5), 282–289.

Olson, B. R., Hoffman, G. E., Sved, A., Stricker, E. M., & Verbalis, J. G. (1992). Cholecystokinin induces cFos expression in hypothalamic oxytocinergic neurons projecting to the dorsal vagal complex. *Brain Research, 569*, 238–248.

Oyama, S. (1985). *The ontogeny of information*. Cambridge: Cambridge University Press.

Pacak, K., & Palkovits, M. (2001). Stressor specificity of central neuroendocrine responses: Implications for stress-related disorders. *Endocrine Reviews, 22*(4), 502–548.

Pacak, K., Palkovits, M., Yadid, G., Kvetnansky, R., Kopin, I. J., & Goldstein, D. S. (1998). Heterogeneous neurochemical responses to different stressors: A test of Selye's doctrine of nonspecificity. *American Journal of Physiology—Regulatory, Integrative, and Comparative Physiology,, 275*(44), R1247–R1255.

Palkovits, M. (1999). Interconnections between the neuroendocrine hypothalamus and the central autonomic system. *Frontiers in Neuroendocrinology, 20*, 270–295.

Passille, A. M. B. D., Christopherson, R., & Rushen, J. (1993). Non-nutritive sucking by the calf and postprandial secretion of insulin, CCK, and gastrin. *Physiology and Behavior, 54*, 1069–1073.

Pauk, J., Kuhn, C. M., Field, T. M., & Schanberg, S. M. (1986). Positive effects of tactile versus kinesthetic or vestibular stimulation on neuroendocrine and ODC activity in matenally-deprived rat pups. *Life Sciences, 39*, 2081–2087.

Penfield, W., & Faulk, M. E. (1955). The insula; further observations on its function. *Brain, 78*(4), 445–470.

Pérez-Otaño, I., & Ehlers, M. D. (2005). Homeostatic plasticity and NMDA receptor trafficking. *Trends in Neurosciences, 28*(5), 229–238.

Peuranen, E., Vasar, E., Koks, S., Volke, V., Lang, A., Rauhala, P., et al. (1995). Further studies on the role of cholecystokinin-A and B receptors in secretion of anterior pituitary hormones in male rats. *Neuropeptides, 28*(1), 1–11.

Phillips, R. G., & LeDoux, J. E. (1994). Lesions of the dorsal hippocampal formation interfere with background but not foreground contextual fear conditioning. *Learning and Memory, 1*(1), 34–44.

Pickel, V. M., Bockstaele, E. J. V., Chan, J., & Cestari, D. M. (1996). GABAergic neurons in rat nuclei of solitary tracts receive inhibitory-type synapses from amygdaloid efferents lacking detectable GABA-immunoreactivity. *Journal of Neuroscience Research, 44*, 446–458.

Pihoker, C., Owens, M. J., Kuhn, C. M., Schanberg, S. M., & Nemeroff, C. B. (1993). Maternal separation in neonatal rats elicits activation of the hypothalamic-pituitary-adren ocortical axis: A putative role for corticotropin-releasing factor. *Psychoneuroendocrinology, 18*(7), 485–493.

Plotsky, P. M., & Meaney, M. J. (1993). Early, postnatal experience alters hypothalamic corticotropin-releasing factor (CRF) mRNA, median eminence CRF content and stress-induced release in adult rats. *Molecular Brain Research, 18*, 195–200.

Plotsky, P. M., Thrivikraman, K. V., Nemeroff, C. B., Caldji, C., Sharma, S., & Meaney, M. J. (2005). Long-term consequences of neonatal rearing on central corticotropin-releasing factor systems in adult male rat offspring. *Neuropsychopharmacology, 30*(12), 2192–2204.

Poeggel, G., Lange, E., Hase, C., Metzger, M., Gulyaeva, N., & Braun, K. (1999). Maternal separation and early social deprivation in *Octodon degus*: Quantitative changes of nicotinamide adenine dinucleotide phosphate-diaphorase-reactive neurons in the prefrontal cortex and nucleus accumbens. *Neuroscience, 94*(2), 497–504.

Potts, J. T., Lee, S. M., & Anguelov, P. I. (2002). Tracing of projection neurons from the cervical dorsal horn to the medulla with the anterograde tracer biotinylated dextran amine. *Autonomic Neuroscience: Basic and Clinical, 98*, 64–69.

Pratt, J. A. (1992). The neuroanatomical basis of anxiety. *Pharmacology and Therapeutics, 55*(2), 149–181.

Price, J. L. (2005). Free will versus survival: Brain systems that underlie intrinsic constraints on behavior. *The Journal of Comparative Neurology, 493*, 132–139.

Punyabati, O., Deepak, K. K., Sharma, M. P., & Dwivedi, S. N. (2000). Autonomic nervous system reactivity in irritable bowel syndrome. *Indian Journal of Gastroenterology, 19*(3), 122–125.

Quigley, K. S., Myers, M. M., & Shair, H. N. (2005). Development of the baroreflex in the young rat. *Autonomic Neuroscience: Basic and Clinical, 121*(1–2), 26–32.

Rao, H., Jean, A., & Kessler, J.-P. (1997). Postnatal ontogeny of glutamate receptors in the rat nucleus tractus solitarii and ventrolateral medulla. *Journal of the Autonomic Nervous System, 65*(1), 25–32.

Raybould, H. E., & Tache, Y. (1988). Cholecystokinin inhibits gastric motility and emptying via a capsaicin-sensitive vagal pathway in rats. *American Journal of Physiology—Gastrointestinal and Liver Physiology, 255*, G242–G246.

Rinaman, L. (1998). Oxytocinergic inputs to the nucleus of the solitary tract and dorsal motor nucleus of the vagus in neonatal rats. *Journal of Comparative Neurology, 399*(1), 101–109.

Rinaman, L. (2001). Postnatal development of catecholamine inputs to the paraventricular nucleus of the hypothalamus in rats. *The Journal of Comparative Neurology, 438*, 411–422.

Rinaman, L. (2003a). Hindbrain noradrenergic lesions attenuate anorexia and alter central cFos expression in rats after gastric viscerosensory stimulation. *The Journal of Neuroscience, 23*(31), 10084–10092.

Rinaman, L. (2003b). Postnatal development of hypothalamic inputs to the dorsal vagal complex in rats. *Physiology and Behavior, 79*, 65–70.

Rinaman, L., Card, J. P., & Enquist, L. W. (1993). Spatiotemporal responses of astrocytes, ramified microglia, and brain macrophages to central neuronal infection with pseudorabies virus. *Journal of Neuroscience, 13*, 685–702.

Rinaman, L., Hoffman, G. E., Dohanics, J., Le, W. W., Stricker, E. M., & Verbalis, J. G. (1995). Cholecystokinin activates catecholaminergic neurons in the caudal medulla that innervate the paraventricular nucleus of the hypothalamus in rats. *The Journal of Comparative Neurology, 360*(2), 246–256.

Rinaman, L., Hoffman, G. E., Stricker, E. M., & Verbalis, J. G. (1994). Exogenous cholecystokinin activates cFos expression in medullary but not hypothalamic neurons in neonatal rats. *Developmental Brain Research, 77*(1), 140–145.

Rinaman, L., & Levitt, P. (1993). Establishment of vagal sensory-motor circuits during fetal development in rats. *Journal of Neurobiology, 24*, 641–659.

Rinaman, L., Levitt, P., & Card, J. P. (2000). Progressive postnatal assembly of limbic-autonomic circuits revealed by central transneuronal transport of pseudorabies virus. *The Journal of Neuroscience, 20*(7), 2731–2741.

Rinaman, L., Roesch, M. R., & Card, J. P. (1999). Retrograde transsynaptic pseudorabies virus infection of central autonomic circuits in neonatal rats. *Developmental Brain Research, 114*, 207–216.

Rinaman, L., Verbalis, J. G., Stricker, E. M., & Hoffman, G. E. (1993). Distribution and neurochemical phenotypes of caudal medullary neurons activated to express cFos following peripheral administration of cholecystokinin. *The Journal of Comparative Neurology, 338*(4), 475–490.

Robinson, P. H., Moran, T. H., Goldrich, M., & McHugh, P. R. (1987). Development of cholecystokinin binding sites in the rat upper gastrointestinal tract. *American Journal of Physiology—Gastrointestinal and Liver Physiology, 252*, G529–G534.

Robinson, P. H., Moran, T. H., & McHugh, P. R. (1985). Gastric cholecystokinin receptors and the effect of cholecystokinin on feeding and gastric emptying in the neonatal rat. *Annals of the New York Academy of Science, 448*, 627–629.

Robinson, P. H., Moran, T. H., & McHugh, P. R. (1988). Cholecystokinin inhibits independent ingestion in neonatal rats. *American Journal of Physiology—Regulatory, Integrative, and Comparative Physiology, 255*, R14–R20.

Rogers, R. C., & Hermann, G. E. (1985). Dorsal medullary oxytocin, vasopressin, oxytocin antagonist, and TRH effects on gastric acid secretion and heart rate. *Peptides, 6*(6), 1143–1148.

Rogers, R. C., & Hermann, G. E. (1987). Oxytocin, oxytocin antagonist, TRH, and hypothalamic paraventricular nucleus stimulation effects on gastric motility. *Peptides, 8*, 505–513.

Rogers, R. C., & Hermann, G. E. (1992). Central regulation of brainstem gastric vago-vagal control circuits. In S. Ritter, R. C. Ritter & C. D. Barnes (Eds.), *Neuroanatomy and Physiology of Abdominal Vagal Afferents* (pp. 99–134). Boca Raton, FL: CRC Press.

Saper, C. B. (1982). Convergence of autonomic and limbic connections in the insular cortex of the rat. *Journal of Comparative Neurology, 210*, 163–173.

Saper, C. B. (2002). The central autonomic nervous system: Conscious visceral perception and autonomic pattern generation. *Annual Review of Neuroscience, 25*, 433–469.

Saper, C. B. (2004). Central Autonomic System. In G. Paxinos (Ed.), *The rat nervous system* (3rd ed., pp. 761–796). San Diego: Elsevier Academic Press.

Saper, C. B., & Loewy, A. D. (1980). Efferent connections of the parabrachial nucleus in the rat. *Brain Research, 197*, 291–317.

Sapolsky, R. M., & Meaney, M. J. (1986). Maturation of the adrenocortical stress response: Neuroendocrine control mechanisms and the stress hyporesponsive period. *Brain Research Reviews, 4*, 65–76.

Sarnat, H. B. (1989). Do the corticospinal and corticobulbar tracts mediate functions in the human newborn? *Canadian Journal of Neurological Sciences, 16*(2), 157–160.

Sawchenko, P. E., & Swanson, L. W. (1981). Central noradrenergic pathways for the integration of hypothalamic neuroendocrine and autonomic responses. *Science, 214*, 685–687.

Sawchenko, P. E., & Swanson, L. W. (1982). The organization of noradrenergic pathways from the brainstem to the paraventricular and supraoptic nuclei in the rat. *Brain Research Reviews, 4*, 275–325.

Schachter, S. C., & Saper, C. B. (1998). Vagus nerve stimulation. *Epilepsia, 39*, 677–686.

Schall, J. D. (2004). On building a bridge between brain and behavior. *Annual Review of Psychology, 55*, 23–50.

Schulkin, J., Thompson, B. L., & Rosen, J. B. (2003). Demythologizing the emotions: Adaptation, cognition, and visceral representations of emotion in the nervous system. *Brain and Cognition, 52*, 15–23.

Schwaber, J. S., Kapp, B. S., Higgins, G. A., & Rapp, P. R. (1982). Amygdaloid and basal forebrain connections with the nucleus of the solitary tract and the dorsal motor nucleus. *Journal of Neuroscience, 2*, 1424–1438.

Schwartz, G. J., & Moran, T. H. (1998). Integrative gastrointestinal actions of the brain-gut peptide cholecystokinin in satiety. *Progress in Psychobiology and Physiological Psychology, 17*, 1–34.

Schwetz, I., McRoberts, J. A., Coutinho, S. V., Bradesi, S., Gale, G., Fanselow, M.,et al. (2005). Corticotropin-releasing factor receptor 1 mediates acute and delayed stress-induced visceral hyperalgesia in maternally separated Long-Evans rats. *American Journal of Physiology—Regulatory, Integrative, and Comparative Physiology, 289*, G704–G712.

Shanks, N., Larocque, S., & Meaney, M. J. (1995). Neonatal endotoxin exposure alters the development of the hypothalamic-pituitary-adrenal axis: Early illness and later responsivity to stress. *The Journal of Neuroscience, 15*, 376–384.

Shapiro, R. E., & Miselis, R. R. (1985). The central organization of the vagus nerve innervating the stomach of the rat. *Journal of Comparative Neurology, 238*, 473–488.

Sofroniew, M. V., & Schrell, U. (1981). Evidence for a direction projection from oxytocin and vasopressin neurons in the hypothalamic paraventricular nucleus to the medulla oblongata: Immunohistochemical visualization of both the horseradish peroxidase transported and the peptide produced by the same neurons. *Neuroscience Letters, 22*, 211–217.

Specht, S. M., Burright, R. G., & Spear, L. P. (1996). Behavioral components of milk-induced activation in neonatal rat pups. *Perceptual and Motor Skills, 83*(3 pt 1), 903–911.

Stein, M. B. (1998). Neurobiological perspectives on social phobia: From affiliation to zoology. *Biological Psychiatry, 44*(12), 1277–1285.

Stern, J. M., & Johanson, S. K. (1989). Ventral somatosensory determinants of nursing behavior in Norway rats. Effects of variations in the quality and quantity of pup stimuli. *Physiology and Behavior, 47*, 993–1011.

Stern, J. M., & Keer, S. E. (2002). Acute hunger of rat pups elicits increased kyphotic nursing and shorter intervals between nursing bouts: Implications for changes in nursing with time postpartum. *Journal of Comparative Psychology, 116*(1), 83–92.

Strack, A. M., & Loewy, A. D. (1990). Pseudorabies virus: A highly specific transneuronal cell body marker in the sympathetic nervous system. *Journal of Neuroscience, 10*, 2139–2147.

Strack, A. M., Sawyer, W. B., Hughes, J. H., Platt, K. B., & Loewy, A. D. (1989). A general pattern of CNS innervation of the sympathetic outflow demonstrated by transneuronal pseudorabies viral infections. *Brain Research, 491*, 156–162.

Strack, A. M., Sawyer, W. B., Platt, K. B., & Loewy, A. D. (1989). CNS cell groups regulating the sympathetic outflow to adrenal gland as revealed by transneuronal cell body labeling with pseudorabies virus. *Brain Research, 491*, 274–296.

Taché, Y., Martinez, V., Million, M., & Rivier, J. (1999). Corticotropin-releasing factor and the brain-gut motor response to stress. *Canadian Journal of Gastroenterology, 13*(Suppl. A), 18A–25A.

Terreberry, R. R., & Neafsay, E. J. (1983). Rat medial frontal cortex: A visceral motor region with a direct projection to the solitary nucleus. *Brain Research, 278*, 245–249.

Thayer, J. F., & Lane, R. D. (2000). A model of neurovisceral integration in emotional regulation and dysregulation. *Journal of Affective Disorders, 61*, 201–216.

Tornhage, C. J., Serenius, F., Uvnäs-Moberg, K., & Lindberg, T. (1998). Plasma somatostatin and cholecystokinin levels in preterm infants during kangaroo care with and without nasogastric tube-feeding. *Journal of Pediatric Endocrinology and Metabolism, 11*, 645–651.

Uvnäs-Moberg, K., Marchini, G., & Winberg, J. (1993). Plasma cholecystokinin concentrations after breast feeding in healthy 4-day-old infants. *Archives of Disease in Childhood, 68*, 46–48.

Van der Kooy, D., Koda, L. K., McGinty, J. F., Gerfen, C. R., & Bloom, F. E. (1984). The organization of projections from the cortex, amygdala, and hypothalamus to the nucleus of the solitary tract in rat. *The Journal of Comparative Neurology, 1984*, 1–24.

Van Eden, C. G., Kros, J. M., & Uylings, H. B. (1990). The development of the rat prefrontal cortex. Its size and development of connections with thalamus, spinal cord and other cortical areas. *Progress in Brain Research, 85*, 169–183.

Van Eden, C. G., & Uylings, H. B. (1985). Cytoarchitectonic development of the prefrontal cortex in the rat. *The Journal of Comparative Neurology, 241*(3), 253–267.

Van Oers, H. J. J., de Kloet, E. R., Whelan, T., & Levine, S. (1998). Maternal deprivation effect on the infant's neural stress markers is reversed by tactile stimulation and feeding but not by suppressing corticosterone. *Journal of Neuroscience, 18*, 10171–10179.

Van Oers, H. J. J., de Kloet, E. R.., & Levine, S. (1999). Persistent effects of maternal deprivation on HPA regulation can be reversed by feeding and stroking, but not by dexamethasone. *Journal of Neuroendocrinology, 11*(8), 581–588.

Vertes, R. P. (2004). Differential projections of the infralimbic and prelimbic cortex in the rat. *Synapse, 51*(32–58).

Vertes, R. P. (2006). Interactions among the medial prefrontal cortex, hippocampus and midline thalamus in emotional and cognitive processing in the rat. *Neuroscience, 142*, 1–20.

Verwer, R. W., Vulpen, E. H. V., & Uum, J. F. V. (1996). Postnatal development of amygdaloid projections to the prefrontal cortex in the rat studied with retrograde and anterograde tracers. *Journal of Comparative Neurology, 376*(1), 75–96.

Vincent, A., & Tell, F. (1999). Postnatal development of rat nucleus tractus solitarius neurons: Morphological and electrophysiological evidence. *Neuroscience, 93*, 293–305.

Vouimba, R. M., Garcia, R., & Jaffard, R. (1998). Opposite effects of lateral septal LTP and lateral septal lesions on contextual fear conditioning in mice. *Behavioral Neuroscience, 112*(4), 875–884.

Walker, C. D., Scribner, V. A., Cascio, C. S., & Dallman, M. F. (1991). The pituitary–adrenocortical system of neonatal rats is responsive to stress throughout development in a time dependent and stress-specific fashion. *Endocrinology, 128*, 1385–1396.

Wang, C.-C., Willis, W. D., & Westlund, K. N. (1999). Ascending projections from the area around the spinal cord central canal: A Phaseolus vulgaris leucoagglutinin study in rats. *The Journal of Comparative Neurology, 415*, 341–367.

Watts, A. G., & Swanson, L. W. (2002). Anatomy of motivational systems. In R. Gallistel (Ed.), Stevens' *handbook of experimental psychology* (3rd ed., pp. 563–631). New York: John Wiley & Sons.

Weller, A. (2006). The ontogeny of postingestive inhibitory stimuli: Examining the role of CCK. *Developmental Psychobiology, 48*, 368–379.

Weller, A., & Blass, E. M. (1988). Behavioral evidence for cholecystokin-opiate interactions in neonatal rats. *American Journal of Physiology—Regulatory, Integrative, and Comparative Physiology, 255*, R901–R907.

Weller, A., Corp, E. S., Tyrka, A., Ritter, R. C., Brenner, L., Gibbs, J., & Smith, G. P. (1992). Trypsin inhibitor and maternal reunion increase plasma cholecystokinin in neonatal rats. *Peptides, 13*, 939–941.

Weller, A., & Dubson, L. (1998). A CCK(A)-receptor antagonist administered to the neonate alters mother–infant interactions in the rat. *Pharmacology Biochemistry and Behavior, 59*(4), 843–851.

Weller, A., & Feldman, R. (2003). Emotion regulation and touch in infants: The role of cholecystokinin and opioids. *Peptides, 24*, 779–788.

Welting, O., Wijngaard, R. M. V. D., Jonge, W. J. D., Holman, R., & Boeckxstaens, G. E. (2005). Assessment of visceral sensitivity using radio telemetry in a rat model of maternal separation. *Neurogastroenterology and Motility, 17*(6), 838–845.

Wiedenmayer, C. P. (2004). Adaptations or pathologies? Long-term changes in brain and behavior after a single exposure to severe threat. *Neuroscience and Biobehavioral Reviews, 28*, 1–12.

Wiedenmayer, C. P., & Barr, G. A. (2001). Developmental changes in c-fos expression to an age-specific social stressor in infant rats. *Behavioural Brain Research, 126*, 147–157.

Wiedenmayer, C. P., Magarinos, A. M., McEwen, B. S., & Barr, G. A. (2005). Age-specific threats induce CRF expression in the paraventricular nucleus of the hypothalamus and hippocampus of young rats. *Hormones and Behavior, 47*, 139–150.

Wigger, A., & Neumann, I. D. (1999). Periodic maternal deprivation induces gender-dependent alterations in behavioral and neuroendocrine responses to emotional stress in adult rats. *Physiology and Behavior, 66*(2), 293–302.

Willis, W. D., & Westlund, K. N. (2001). The role of the dorsal column pathway in visceral nociception. *Current Pain and Headache Reports, 5*, 20–26.

Yang, M., Card, J. P., Tirabassi, R. S., Miselis, R. R., & Enquist, L. W. (1999). Retrograde, transneuronal spread of pseudorabies virus in defined neuronal circuitry of the rat brain is facilitated by gE mutations that reduce virulence. *Journal of Virology, 73*(5), 4350–4359.

Yasui, Y., Breder, C. D., Saper, C. B., & Cechetto, D. F. (1991). Autonomic responses and efferent pathways from the insular cortex in the rat. *The Journal of Comparative Neurology, 303*(3), 355–374.

Yasui, Y., Itoh, K., Kaneko, T., Shigemoto, R., & Mizuno, N. (1991). Topographical projections from the cerebral cortex to the nucleus of the solitary tract in the cat. *Experimental Brain Research, 85*, 75–84.

Zhang, L.-L., & Ashwell, K. W. S. (2001). The development of cranial nerve and visceral afferents to the nucleus of the solitary tract in the rat. *Anatomy and Embryology, 204*, 135–151.

Maternal Care as a Modulating Influence on Infant Development

Frances A. Champagne *and* **James P. Curley**

Abstract

The quality of maternal care provided to offspring can have long-term consequences on the offspring's development and behavior. This chapter reviews evidence for maternal modulation of offspring phenotype during preconceptual, prenatal and postnatal periods. In humans, primates, and rodents, previous animal model studies support the role of mother–infant interactions in serving as critical cue for infant development. This evidence comes from studies of the effects of maternal separation or deprivation and from study of natural variations in maternal care. Though the neurobiological changes associated with maternal care have been investigated in many species, the molecular substrates of these effects have primarily been explored in a rodent model and the studies implicate epigenetic mechanisms in maintaining the long-term effects of variations in mother–infant interaction.

Keywords: maternal care, maternal modulation, phenotype, mother–infant interactions, maternal separation, deprivation

In mammals, the quality of mother–infant interactions is one of the most salient aspects of the early environment. These interactions are initiated in many species by a complex interplay of physiological signals from the developing fetus, the response of the maternal endocrine and neuroendocrine system to these signals, and the behavioral consequences of these neuroendocrine changes. Though the importance of these interactions during both the prenatal and postnatal period in promoting growth and survival have certainly been appreciated, there is growing evidence for the long-term impact of maternal care on the neurobiology and behavior of offspring. This evidence comes from a variety of experimental paradigms including manipulations of the mother–infant relationship and from longitudinal studies in which aspects of maternal care are associated with phenotypic characteristics of offspring. These converging sources of evidence suggest that the quality of early experiences, conferred by the quality of the maternal environment, has a profound impact on stress responsivity and social behavior of offspring which are associated with region-specific changes in gene expression and receptor densities in the brain. In this chapter, we will review the evidence for the maternal modulation of offspring phenotype from human, primate, and rodent studies and explore possible mechanisms through which early experiences can exert a long-term impact on offspring development. In addition, we will discuss the potential for experiences at later periods of development to alter phenotype and will conclude with a discussion of the adaptive advantage conferred by allowing mother–infant interactions to shape offspring development.

Maternal Effects during the Preconceptional Period

Evidence that maternal condition even prior to conception can have long-term consequences for the neurobiology and behavior of offspring is not often considered when discussing maternal influences on development. Yet, the process of generation and maturation of the female gametes, which can occur over the course of decades (Bukovsky et al., 2005), provides opportunities for variations in the maternal environment at the cellular level to influence offspring. Developmental abnormalities as a consequence of maternal age (Hook, 1981; Tarin et al., 2003), maternal stress (Weinstock, Fride, & Hertzberg, 1988), exposure to toxins (Gal & Sharpless, 1984), and malnourishment (Symonds, Budge, Stephenson, & McMillen, 2001) during the preconception period are often attributed to genetic perturbations of the germ line cells that are inherited by offspring. However, reductions in levels of oocyte gene expression and protein synthesis can also exert effects on development, particularly during the postfertilization period. Prior to maturation, levels of transcription and translation in the oocyte are extremely high which serves to "stockpile" proteins and mRNA that will be needed in early zygotic development (Wassarman & Kinloch, 1992). Zygotic genes are silenced through chromatin-mediated suppression of transcription during the postfertilization phase and thus all protein synthesis is mediated by maternal mRNAs and enzymes alone until zygotic gene activation during the two-cell embryo stage (De Sousa, Caveney, Westhusin, & Watson, 1998; Nothias, Majumder, Kaneko, & DePamphilis, 1995). Moreover, it is the gradients of maternal mRNA present in the zygote that will serve to drive segmentation of the embryo and anterior–posterior polarity of the nervous system (Gavis & Lehmann, 1992; Scott, 2000). Oocyte gene expression has been found to be altered as a function of maternal age (Eichenlaub-Ritter, 1998; Janny & Menezo, 1996) and nutrition (Symonds, Budge, Stephenson, & Gardner, 2005), though the consequences of these particular disruptions on the neurobiology and behavior of the offspring have not been thoroughly investigated in mammals. It is likely that while these preconceptional maternal factors can alter development directly, there is also considerable interaction between preconceptional and gestational maternal condition on offspring development.

Maternal Influence during the Prenatal Period

Mothers invest in their offspring's development even before birth. Pregnancy is a period when many demands are made on maternal physiology to support the energetic needs of the developing fetus (Weissgerber & Wolfe, 2006). When these needs are not met or the maternal prenatal environment is disrupted, there can be long-term consequences for growth, metabolism, and behavior of the offspring. Low birth weight, particularly as a consequence of reduced maternal food intake during pregnancy such as occurs during famines or in areas of unpredictable food supply, is associated with a multitude of long-term health, metabolic, and physiological outcomes including cardiovascular disease, diabetes, elevated blood pressure, glucose intolerance, and obesity in the offspring (Painter, Roseboom, & Bleker, 2005; Roseboom, de Rooij, & Painter, 2006; Roseboom et al., 2000). These outcomes are explained in terms of the "developmental origins" hypothesis, which argues that when the fetus detects low-energy supplies from the mother, then changes in gene expression occur that prepare the organism for a nutritionally poor postnatal environment (Barker, 2004; McMillen & Robinson, 2005). These adaptive developmental changes allow for the storage of energy as fat in adulthood, which in an environment of adequate energy supply leads to obesity and other negative health consequences. Thus, the mismatch between prenatal and postnatal nutritional environments can have a profound impact on development (Gluckman, Hanson, & Pinal, 2005).

Other disruptions of the prenatal maternal environment can also have long-term effects on child development. Exposure to toxins during sensitive periods of brain development can lead to pathological outcomes; for instance, excess maternal consumption of alcohol produces fetal alcohol syndrome (Hoyseth & Jones, 1989; Olegard et al., 1979); increased smoking is associated with failure to thrive (Bernstein et al., 2005; Higgins, 2002); and prenatal exposure to cocaine and heroin are strong risk factors for pregnancy complications, infant mortality, infant drug dependency, and learning difficulties (Fulroth, Phillips, & Durand, 1989; Wagner, Katikaneni, Cox, & Ryan, 1998). Although data are difficult to obtain and vary by socioeconomic status (SES), maternal age, and ethnicity, recent large-scale studies estimate that in the United States up to 20% of mothers continue to smoke and use alcohol during pregnancy and

5% use illicit drugs (Statistics, 2005). Exposure to severe psychosocial stressors such as war, terrorist attacks, or natural disasters during pregnancy has also been associated with reduced birth weight, infant survival, and modified sex ratio (more males born in relation to females) (Catalano, Bruckner, Hartig, & Ong, 2005; Rondo et al., 2003; Saadat & Ansari-Lari, 2004; Zorn, Sucur, Stare, & Meden-Vrtovec, 2002). Even more common stressful life events, such as death in the family, starting a new job, or chronic exposure to daily hassles have been found to alter maternal and fetal physiology (Tambyrajia & Mongelli, 2000). The biological basis of these effects has been investigated in primates and rodents, and the studies investigating these effects suggest the role of increasing levels of maternal stress hormones (Weinstock, 2005). Psychosocial stress activates the maternal hypothalamic-pituitary-adrenal (HPA) axis, resulting in the release of glucocorticoids, which activate the parasympathetic nervous system (Steckler, Kalin, & Ruel, 2005). Though enzymes within the placenta, such as 11-β-hydroxysteroid dehydrogenase-2 (11-βHSD-2), can inactivate glucocorticoids and thus buffer the developing fetus from these steroid hormones, severe stress may overwhelm the capacity of the enzymatic conversion (Edwards, Benediktsson, Lindsay, & Seckl, 1996; Seckl, Nyirenda, Walker, & Chapman, 1999). Moreover, in cases of severe maternal undernutrition, the levels of expression of 11-βHSD-2 are decreased, thus exposing the fetus to an increased risk of both metabolic and stress-related disorders (Lesage, Blondeau, Grino, Breant, & Dupouy, 2001). Experimental work with rats suggests that prenatal stress, typically induced by long periods of physical restraint, induces a number of effects in offspring that can be observed in adulthood. Such offspring exhibit elevated plasma corticosterone (Stohr et al., 1998), increased CRH (corticotrophin releasing hormone) mRNA in the amygdala (Cratty, Ward, Johnson, Azzaro, & Birkle, 1995), and reduced monoamine and catecholamine turnover (Peters, 1982; Takahashi, Turner, & Kalin, 1992). Behaviorally, these offspring are more hyperactive, inhibited from exploring novelty, impaired on cognitive measures such as the Morris Water Maze, and display deficits in social behavior (Patin, Lordi, Vincent, & Caston, 2005; Weinstock et al., 1988). Though evidence certainly implicates fetal exposure to prenatal maternal glucocorticoid secretion as a mediator of these effects (Barbazanges, Piazza, Le Moal,

& Maccari, 1996), there is also the possibility that gestational maternal stress will compromise later postnatal maternal care, resulting in similar effects on offspring development (Champagne & Meaney, 2006; Moore & Power, 1986).

Maternal Deprivation as a Cue for Infant Development

Some children develop in the absence of any parental care. In many countries, particularly during tumultuous periods of history when war or any other event leads to loss of one or both parents, children have been institutionalized from birth. These children are at increased risk of suffering social, emotional, and cognitive deficits, and developing psychopathology (Goldfarb, 1943; Hodges & Tizard, 1989a, 1989b; Quinton, Rutter, & Liddle, 1984; Rutter, 2002; Veijola et al., 2004). In particular, children reared in institutions are consistently reported to have problems in forming social relationships as well as in understanding and responding appropriately to emotions throughout their life (Rutter, 2002; Sigal, Rossignol, & Perry, 1999; Vorria et al., 2006). These effects can be observed even after children are fostered into families of higher SES (Fisher, Armes, Chisholm, & Savoie, 1997; O'Connor & Rutter, 2000). Significantly, many studies report that the problem behavior of these children is highly correlated with the duration of time spent in institutions (Castle et al., 1999; Fisher, 1997; MacLean, 2003). There is evidence that the effects of parental deprivation can be sustained into adulthood. Studies by Sigal and colleagues found that adults over the age of 45 years who were separated from parents at birth or before the age of 5 years were significantly more socially isolated, suffered greater psychological distress, were more at risk of attempting suicide, had increased psychopathology, and were more susceptible to chronic illness (Sigal, 2004; Sigal et al., 1999; Sigal, Perry, Rossignol, & Ouimet, 2003).

In the 1950s and 1960s, Harlow examined the impact of complete maternal deprivation on the development of rhesus macaques. His work provided an influential experimental model for studying the causal influence of maternal care on infant behavior. Harlow implemented an artificial rearing paradigm in which infant rhesus monkeys were reared in complete social isolation for periods of 3–12 months (Seay & Harlow, 1965). Juveniles reared in this environment displayed marked deficits in play behavior, exhibited aggression when placed in social contact with peers, and showed learning impairments on cognitive discrimination tasks (Seay, Alexander, & Harlow, 1964; Seay & Harlow, 1965; Suomi, Harlow, & Kimball, 1971). Maternally deprived infants developed heightened fear-related behaviors, displayed behavioral inhibition, and reduced exploration of inanimate objects. Females who spent the first 6 months of postnatal life in isolated rearing conditions also displayed impairments in maternal behavior as adults (Arling & Harlow, 1967; Harlow & Suomi, 1971; Seay et al., 1964), including high rates of abuse, neglect, and infanticide. Though these effects could be attributed to the general isolation experienced by neonates rather than the specific effects of maternal deprivation, more recent studies have shown that peer-reared rhesus macaques that have been maternally deprived yet permitted to interact with same-age same-sex peers have an elevated behavioral and HPA response to stress and show significant impairments in learning and social behavior (Fahlke et al., 2000; Shannon, Champoux, & Suomi, 1998). In primates, maternal deprivation is associated with disruption of offspring serotonergic systems, which may account for these behavioral changes (Shannon et al., 2005). Recent positron emission tomography imaging studies comparing peer-reared and mother-reared rhesus macaques have found reduced serotonin transporter binding in multiple brain regions including the raphe, thalamus, striatum, and temporal cortex (Ichise et al., 2006) of the maternally deprived rhesus macaques. Decreases in oxytocin neuropeptide levels have also been detected in maternally deprived rhesus infants and may contribute to the deficits in social behavior observed under these rearing conditions (Winslow, 2005).

In rodents, the effects of complete maternal deprivation have been studied using an artificial rearing (AR) paradigm in which pups are removed from their mother on Day 3 postpartum and raised in complete social isolation (Hall, 1975). Adult offspring reared under these conditions are more fearful, engage in fewer open-arm entries in an elevated plus maze, display hyperactive locomotor activity and cognitive impairments related to attention-shifting, and are impaired on measures of social behavior, including maternal care (Gonzalez & Fleming, 2002; Gonzalez, Lovic, Ward, Wainwright, & Fleming, 2001; Lovic & Fleming, 2004). Females raised under these conditions display deficits in maternal licking/grooming (LG) and other forms of contact with their own pups

(Fleming et al., 2002) and may be less responsive to hormonal priming of maternal behavior (Novakov & Fleming, 2005b). Unlike primate studies, in which peer-reared infants exhibit similar behavioral and neuroendocrine deficits as infants who have no social or maternal contact, artificial rearing under social conditions in rats (in which pups are raised with one peer) can ameliorate the deficits normally observed (Melo et al., 2006).

Long-Term Consequences of Maternal Separation

Investigations of the effects of complete maternal deprivation on offspring development have provided useful insights concerning the importance of mother–infant interactions. However, a more common occurrence across mammalian species is not the complete removal of the mother, which would be fatal to offspring, but prolonged periods of separation between the mother and the infant. In humans, neglect can be thought of as prolonged periods of physical or psychological withdrawal and has been correlated with an increased sensitivity to stressors in adolescence, cognitive delays, and an increased risk of psychopathology (Ammerman, Cassisi, Hersen, & van Hasselt, 1986; Harkness, Bruce, & Lumley, 2006; Trickett & McBride-Chang, 1995). The neurobiological effects of these early experiences have been studied in primates and rodents using paradigms that reduce the contact between the mother and the infant early in development. In primates, reduced maternal contact has been accomplished by changing the foraging demand placed on mothers (Rosenblum & Paully, 1984). The most profound effects on offspring reared under these conditions are observed when using a variable foraging demand (VFD), a condition in which the effort required to acquire food fluctuates randomly across days and thus the time available for mother–infant interactions also fluctuates. Offspring reared under these conditions exhibit behavioral inhibition and reduced social behavior associated with increased HPA activity, reduced levels of growth factors, a compromised immune response, and altered neurotransmitter metabolite levels in the anterior cingulate and medial temporal lobes (Andrews & Rosenblum, 1991, 1994; Coplan et al., 1998, 2000, 2001, 2005; Rosenblum, Forger, Noland, Trost, & Coplan, 2001). The VFD methodology, in addition to creating prolonged maternal separation, has been show to reduce the maternal responsivity of mothers when they are in contact with the offspring (Rosenblum & Paully, 1984), suggesting that these effects may be manifested by changes in the quality rather than the simply the quantity of care received.

In rodents, there has been extensive use of maternal separation to study the long-term influences of early experiences. The maternal separation paradigm, involving hours of daily mother–infant separation, was initially used to manipulate the responsivity of the HPA axis (Plotsky & Meaney, 1993; Plotsky et al., 2005; Rosenfeld, Wetmore, & Levine, 1992). These rearing conditions lead to a multitude of behavioral and neurobiological changes including decreased exploration, behavioral inhibition, increased CRH mRNA in the paraventricular nucleus (PVN), increased corticosterone response to stress, and decreased levels of hippocampal glucocorticoid receptor (GR) mRNA (Lehmann, Pryce, Bettschen, & Feldon, 1999; Meaney et al., 1996; Plotsky & Meaney, 1993). Cognitive ability is also modified by this experience as indicated by increased latencies on the Morris Water Maze, decreased hippocampal synaptophysin levels, and increased apoptosis (Lehmann et al., 2002a). There is also growing evidence that maternal separation reduces social behavior in both infant males and females when they become adults. Females separated from their mothers for 5 h per day during the preweanling period showed later deficits in maternal LG toward their own offspring (Fleming et al., 2002).

The expression of separation effects is dependent on many factors including (1) the duration of the separation, (2) the condition of the pups during the separation, and (3) the condition of the mother during the separation. Brief periods of separation, in which pups are removed from the home cage for 10–20 min [a procedure referred to as neonatal handling (Levine, 1957)], typically shows effects opposite to those produced by longer periods of maternal separation. Such handling can result in an attenuated response to stress, increased hippocampal GR mRNA, improved cognitive ability, and increased levels of social behavior (Lehmann et al., 2002a; Meaney, Aitken, Bhatnagar, & Sapolsky, 1991; Meaney, Aitken, Viau, Sharma, & Sarrieau, 1989). These short-duration separations are thought to stimulate maternal care and thus increase the responsivity of dams when reintroduced to pups (Lee & Williams, 1974; Liu et al., 1997), whereas longer periods of separation are associated with increased pup corticosterone (Lehmann, Russig, Feldon, & Pryce, 2002b) and reduced maternal care following separation (Boccia et al., 2006).

However, if pups are treated with anxiolytic drugs during the period of separation, the long-term consequences are ameliorated. Thus, pups treated with oxytocin or allopregnalone exhibit an attenuated stress response and adults do not exhibit the behavioral and physiological stress reactivity associated with maternal separation (Pedersen & Boccia, 2002; Zimmerberg, Brunelli, & Hofer, 1994). These studies suggest that the quality of the mother–infant interaction is altered by long periods of maternal separation and this change in the quality of care may modulate offspring phenotype.

Influence of Mother–Infant Interactions in Humans

In humans, traditional approaches to studying the role of maternal care in shaping offspring development have focused on disruptions of this relationship through deprivation or separation as described in previous sections. There is substantial evidence, however, that natural variations in parental styles or behaviors modulate infant development. To reveal these relationships, studies must employ a longitudinal design in which the mother–infant relationship is characterized and infant development is monitored across a lengthy period of time. The practical restrictions of conducting this type of study have led to the development of retrospective questionnaires designed to assess the quality of the mother–infant relationship in adult respondents. One of the most commonly used retrospective tools is the Parental Bonding Instrument (PBI; Parker, Tupling, & Brown, 1979). This self-report questionnaire elicits reports from subjects about perceived rearing experiences during their first 16 years. Despite the response bias that might be predicted, subject reports correlate with independently assessed reports of parental care (Parker, 1981; Reti et al., 2002b), are consistent over time (Mackinnon, Henderson, Scott, & Duncan-Jones, 1989; Wilhelm, Niven, Parker, & Hadzi-Pavlovic, 2005; Wilhelm & Parker, 1990), and are not dependent on current psychological state of the adult respondent (Parker, 1993).

The 25 items of the PBI were originally construed to characterize the care and protection/control dimensions of parental behavior (Parker, 1990), though several studies have shown that the items from this questionnaire factor into three categories of perceived parenting: care, overprotection, and authoritarianism (Cox, Enns, & Clara, 2000; Heider et al., 2005; Murphy, Brewin, & Silka, 1997; Reti et al., 2002b; Sato et al., 1999).

Maternal care is related to the ability of the mother to be emotionally available, attentive, and interested in the child, while overprotection and authoritarianism are related to a parent's tendency to be manipulative, arbitrary, or harsh in disciplining the child. Maternal depression has consistently been associated with low scores for care and high scores for overprotection (Hickie, Parker, Wilhelm, & Tennant, 1991). Having a mother with low scores for maternal care and high scores for overprotection, a "style" referred to as "affectionless control," is a risk factor for depression (Parker, 1981, 1993; Sato et al., 1998; Wilhelm et al., 2005), antisocial personality traits (Reti et al., 2002a), anxiety disorders, drug use, obsessive-compulsive disorder, and attention-deficit disorders (Gerra et al., 2006; Parker, 1984; Parker, Kiloh, & Hayward, 1987; Torresani, Favaretto, & Zimmermann, 2000) in the adult. Of these two factors, it is maternal care that has the largest overall effect as a risk factor for the development of later psychopathology (Enns, Cox, & Clara, 2002; Heider, Matschinger, Bernert, Alonso, & Angermeyer, 2006; Mackinnon, Henderson, & Andrews, 1993; Parker, Hadzi-Pavlovic, Greenwald, & Weissman, 1995).

Associations between other parental styles and adult psychopathology have also been demonstrated. For instance, high maternal care and overprotection ("affectionate constraint" style) is specifically found to be higher among offspring with panic disorders (Silove, Parker, Hadzi-Pavlovic, Manicavasagar, & Blaszczynski, 1991). Low care and low constraint ("neglectful parenting") is associated with increased risk of pathological gambling disorder (Grant & Kim, 2002). Conversely, having a mother with high scores for maternal care and low scores for overprotection, a "style" referred to as "optimal bonding," is protective against psychopathology (Parker et al., 1987). While these associations are strong in selective clinical samples, in nonclinical populations, they are much weaker (Enns et al., 2002) and sometimes nonexistent (Mackinnon et al., 1989).

Parental bonding has also been associated with neurobiological measures associated with stress responsivity. Nonclinical subjects who reported high levels of maternal care on the PBI were found to have elevated self-esteem, reduced trait anxiety, and decreased salivary cortisol in response to stress (Pruessner, Champagne, Meaney, & Dagher, 2004). Elevated cortisol in the low maternal care subjects was associated with increased dopamine release in the ventral striatum in response to stress measured with [^{11}C] raclopride during a positron emission tomography scan (Pruessner et al., 2004). A significant linear negative correlation has also been found between cerebrospinal levels of CRH and reported levels of parental care (Lee, Gollan, Kasckow, Geracioti, & Coccaro, 2006). Thus, the PBI, when combined with brain imaging and physiological measures, can provide useful insights into the biological factors that mediate the increased risk of psychological disorder associated with the quality of maternal care.

Though retrospective indices of parental bonding provide an essential tool for studying long-term effects of the quality of the mother–infant relationship, these measures lack the level of behavioral detail that longitudinal studies of attachment behavior have provided. Attachment theory was developed by the work of John Bowlby (1988) who considered attachment as an emotional bond between the mother and the infant that is evidenced by the need for maintaining proximity, the perception of the mother as a secure base, and the experience of separation distress when the mother is absent. Patterns of attachment behavior are typically characterized during the *strange situation test* (Ainsworth & Wittig, 1969) in which the behavior of the child is observed in a laboratory setting during short separations and reunions with the caregiver. Although originally designed for 12-month-old infants, this test has been modified and can now be applied to children at 18 months as well to preschoolers (Feldman & Ingham, 1975; Radke-Yarrow, Cummings, Kuczynski, & Chapman, 1985). Significantly, at each age, it is not the frequency of behaviors observed but the overall organization of the infant's behavior in this situation that is used to classify the attachment relationship. Thus, the mother–child relationship can be recorded as secure (B), insecure resistant (C), insecure avoidant (A), or controlling (CN), all of which may be considered to be organized strategies to seek maximum comfort from the caregiver (Ainsworth, Blehar, Waters, & Wall, 1978). In a significant number of cases, however, there is no overall organization to the attachment behavior and infants are classified as disorganized (D). Across cultures, these attachment relationships have been reported as roughly 66% B, 10% C, 4% A, 5% CN, and 15% D (Ainsworth et al., 1978). These frequencies, however, may shift in relation to other factors; for example, low SES increases the frequency of insecure and disorganized cases (Sroufe, 2005).

Prospective studies have evidenced that maternal characteristics and behavior during the formation of the attachment relationship during the infant's first year, rather than child temperament, are the best predictors for the subsequent attachment relationship. This was first documented in Ainsworth's original study of mothers who were assessed during their interaction with their infants both in the home and the laboratory, and has been subsequently demonstrated by other studies in which detailed home observations followed by the Ainsworth Strange Situation (ASS) Test were conducted (Ainsworth et al., 1978). Mothers who rate high for maternal sensitivity (that is, mothers who respond appropriately toward the child and are psychologically aware of the signals and needs of their child) are more likely to have securely attached infants (Ainsworth et al., 1978; Egeland & Farber, 1984; Pederson & Moran, 1996). Mothers of secure infants also pace their interactions appropriately, are more relaxed with infants, and have more positive and less negative affect (Stevenson-Hinde & Shouldice, 1995). Conversely, lower maternal sensitivity is found in infants with insecure attachment. Resistant infant mothers also tend to be intrusive, seek interactions with the infant at inappropriate times, and interfere with their infant's exploration of the environment (Stevenson-Hinde & Shouldice, 1995). Moreover, high levels of maternal anxiety have been associated with an increased frequency of insecure resistant attachment. Mothers of insecure avoidant infants tend to have negative feelings about motherhood, are tense, irritable, psychologically unavailable, and perform perfunctory caregiving (Egeland & Farber, 1984; Egeland & Sroufe, 1981). In particular, mothers of avoidant infants, although distant to infants when they are in need of comfort, tend to be intrusive and overwhelming toward infants when they do interact with their infant (Ainsworth et al., 1978; Isabella, 1993; Isabella & Belsky, 1991). Disorganized and controlling attachment is highly predicted by caregiver intrusiveness, frightening behavior, and by both physical and psychological maltreatment, rather than by maternal insensitivity (Carlson, 1998; Jacobvitz, Leon, & Hazen, 2006; Schuengel, Bakermans-Kranenburg, & Van, 1999; van Ijzendoorn, Schuengel, & Bakermans-Kranenburg, 1999).

Thus, the type of attachment relationship that a child has with its mother is largely dependent upon maternal characteristics and behavior. Longitudinal studies have demonstrated that the type of mother–child relationship is crucial in shaping the cognitive, emotional, and social development of the child (Sroufe, 2005). Throughout childhood and adolescence, secure children are found to be more self-reliant and exhibit increased self-confidence and self-esteem than individuals classified as insecure at 12 and 18 months. Secure infants also have improved emotional regulation, are more ego-resilient, have greater positive emotion expression, and exhibit appropriate persistence and flexibility in response to stress. Compared to insecure infants, secure infants also exhibit higher social competence throughout development, are less frequently isolated, more socially active, are able to maintain friendships, and demonstrate quiet authority and social assurance. Infants classified as insecure resistant are frequently found during childhood to be more neophobic and easily frustrated by challenges. In social situations in middle childhood, resistant subjects attempt to interact with peers but find it difficult to initiate social situations or maintain friendships. Later in adolescence and as young adults, insecure resistant infants are at increased risk of having anxiety disorders (Sroufe, 2005; Sroufe, Egeland, Carlson, & Collins, 2005). Avoidant infants are found during middle childhood to be more challenged by social situations that required closeness, and teachers report that they are more isolated, asocial, and emotionally insulated (Shulman, Elicker, & Sroufe, 1994). Moreover, both insecure avoidant and resistant infants are found to be at increased risk of depression. Infant disorganized attachment has been associated with the highest risk of developing later psychopathology (van Ijzendoorn et al., 1999), including dissociative disorders (Carlson, 1998), aggressive behavior (Lyons-Ruth, Bronfman, & Parsons, 1999), and conduct disorder and self-abuse (Sroufe, 2005). Hence, natural variations in human caregiving are related to the quality of the mother–child attachment relationship. This nature of this relationship is then strongly associated with variations in social and emotional behavior of the child throughout infancy, adolescence, and into adulthood.

Natural Variations in the Quality of Maternal Care in Primates and Rodents

It is clear from both retrospective and longitudinal studies in human populations that variations in the quality of mother–infant interactions can have a profound influence on infant development (Figure 16.1). However, our understanding of how these interactions influence neurobiology and behavior has come primarily from

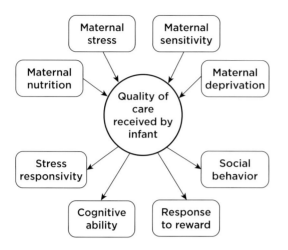

Figure 16.1 Illustration of potential maternal factors that may influence the care received by an infant and the possible consequences of this variation in care for infant development. In this context, care can be considered very broadly to include nutritional, hormonal, and behavioral aspects of the maternal/infant environment.

investigations of naturally occurring variations in maternal care in primates and rodents. Much like humans, primates display individual differences in behavior toward their offspring, which can be characterized early in development (Fairbanks, 1989; Fairbanks & McGuire, 1988). Observations of vervet monkeys in undisturbed social groups suggest that maternal behavior can be classified along two dimensions: protectiveness and rejection (Fairbanks & McGuire, 1988). Protectiveness consists of high levels of "contact-seeking" by the mother and includes high frequencies of making contact, restraining, approaching, and inspecting the infant whereas rejecting females are characterized by a high frequency of rejection associated with frequent attempts to break contact or to leave the infant. Increased behavioral inhibition toward novelty in 1- and 2-year-old infants is associated with increased maternal protectiveness as measured in the infant's first 6 months of postnatal life, providing further support for the developmental influence of early maternal care.

Abusive behavior exhibited by postpartum rhesus and pigtail macaques is also associated with changes in the behavioral and neurobiological characteristics of offspring (Maestripieri, Lindell, Ayala, Gold, & Higley, 2005; Maestripieri, Tomaszycki, & Carroll, 1999; Maestripieri, Wallen, & Carroll, 1997). Abuse is characterized by hitting, dragging, biting, and sitting on the infant and abusive females

exhibit high levels of controlling behavior and maternal rejection. Infant abuse occurring during the first 3 months is associated with an increased frequency of screaming, yawning, and other indices of infant distress at 4–6 months. The high level of maternal rejection exhibited by these females may have a particularly profound effect on offspring behavior and is correlated with increased solitary play and decreased cerebrospinal fluid (CSF) levels of 5-HIAA, implicating the role of serotonergic activity (Maestripieri et al., 2005, 2006). Cross-fostering of infants from abusive to nonabusive mothers indicates that these effects are indeed mediated by the quality of care received rather than by genetic transmission (Maestripieri, 2005).

Postpartum maternal care in rodents varies significantly between individuals and is as stable over time as human and primate care (Champagne, Francis, Mar, & Meaney, 2003a). During the first week postpartum, lactating female rats display high levels of nursing/contact with pups accompanied by bouts of LG. These behaviors serve to provide nutrients, heat, and stimulation to altricial young (Jans & Woodside, 1990; Sullivan, Shokrai, & Leon, 1988; Sullivan, Wilson, & Leon, 1988). The frequency of these behaviors varies both within and between strains and has been implicated in shaping offspring phenotype. Myers, Brunelli, Squire, Shindeldecker, and Hofer (1989) reported that spontaneously hypertensive (SHR) and Wistar Kyoto (WKY) rats exhibited differences in maternal behavior during the postpartum period and demonstrated that strain differences in adult blood pressure between offspring of SHR and WKY rats were related to differences in maternal LG, retrieval of pups, and nursing posture exhibited by these two strains. Furthering this finding, Myers, Brunelli, Shair, Squire, and Hofer (1989) demonstrated that pups cross-fostered from a WKY mother to a SHR mother exhibited a phenotype similar to that of the biological offspring of an SHR mother, suggesting that the behaviors exhibited by the mother were directly related to offspring development. Strain differences in maternal care of mice have also been implicated as an influence on offspring behavior (Francis, Szegda, Campbell, Martin, & Insel, 2003; Priebe et al., 2005). Balb/c mice have an elevated physiological and behavioral response to stress and perform poorly on learning and memory tasks compared to C57BL/6 mice. C57BL/6 embryos that are transferred prenatally to Balb/c dams and reared by a Balb/c female develop characteristics similar to Balb/c mice including decreased exploration of a novel environment (a presumed indicator of increased anxiety). Though the characteristics that differentiate the prenatal environment of these strains are unknown, Balc/c females display decreased levels of postpartum LG, which may contribute to the observed rearing effects (Francis et al., 2003).

The role of individual differences in maternal LG in modulating offspring gene expression, physiology, and behavior has been explored extensively in Long Evans rats (Meaney, 2001). Initial studies demonstrated an association between levels of LG and stress responsivity, with the adult male offspring of High LG dams, in relation to Low LG dams, being more exploratory in a novel environment, having reduced plasma adrenocorticotropin and corticosterone in response to stress, elevated hippocampal GR mRNA, decreased hypothalamic CRH mRNA, and increased density of benzodiazepine receptors in the amygdala (Caldji, Diorio, & Meaney, 2000; Francis, Caldji, Champagne, Plotsky, & Meaney, 1999a; Liu, Caldji, Sharma, Plotsky, & Meaney, 2000; Liu et al., 1997). Offspring of High LG dams also exhibit enhanced performance on tests of spatial leaning and memory, elevated hippocampal brain-derived neurotrophic factor (BDNF) mRNA, and increased hippocampal choline acetyltransferase and synaptophysin (Liu, Diorio, Day, Francis, & Meaney, 2000). GABA subunit expression is altered by maternal LG with implications for benzodiazepine binding (Caldji, Diorio, & Meaney, 2003). Neuronal survival in the hippocampus is increased and apoptosis decreased among the offspring of High LG dams associated with elevated levels of fibroblast growth factor (Bredy, Grant, Champagne, & Meaney, 2003a; Weaver, Grant, & Meaney, 2002). Dopaminergic release associated with stress responsivity in males and reward in females is also altered as a function of LG (Champagne et al., 2004; Zhang, Chretien, Meaney, & Gratton, 2005). Importantly, cross-fostering studies have demonstrated that these maternal effects are related to the level of postpartum care received rather that genetic or prenatal factors (Champagne et al., 2003a; Francis, Diorio, Liu, & Meaney, 1999b). Thus, the offspring of High LG dams cross-fostered to Low LG dams are indistinguishable in phenotype from the biological offspring of Low LG dams. Conversely, the offspring of Low LG dams when reared by High LG dams resemble the biological offspring of High LG dams on measures of both gene expression and behavior.

Epigenetic Mechanisms of Maternal Influence

Converging evidence supports the hypothesis that maternal care serves as a critical modulating influence on offspring phenotype and that this influence is mediated by changes in gene expression in brain regions implicated in stress responsivity and social behavior. How is it that the effects of an environmental experience occurring early in development can have this long-term impact on gene expression and behavior? One prediction might be that early rearing experiences results in altered niche selection, which serves to reinforce the maternal effects after the postpartum period. However, in the case of laboratory-reared rodents, the postmaternal environment is highly standardized and yet these maternal effects persist.

The answer to our question above may involve the same mechanisms that mediate long-term silencing of gene expression and thus generate phenotypic differentiation at a cellular level (Jones & Taylor, 1980; Taylor & Jones, 1985). DNA methylation is a modification to DNA structure that does not alter the nucleotide sequence. Within the DNA sequence, there are specific sites where a methyl group can attach to cytosine through an enzymatic reaction involving DNA methyltransferase. The sites where this can occur reside primarily within the regulatory regions of a gene, in the promoter area upstream from the transcription start site. At a functional level, methylation prevents access of transcription factors and RNA polymerase to DNA, resulting in silencing of the gene. In addition to the gene silencing that occurs in the presence of DNA methylation, these methyl groups attract other protein complexes that then promote histone deacetylation, further decreasing the likelihood of gene expression (Razin, 1998; Strathdee & Brown, 2002). The bond between the cytosine and methyl group is very strong, resulting in a stable yet potentially reversible change in gene expression. DNA methylation patterns are maintained after cell division and thus passed from parent to daughter cells and it is through this form of epigenetic modification that cellular differentiation occurs (Jones & Taylor, 1980). Though several examples of environmentally induced changes in DNA methylation have been demonstrated (Anway, Cupp, Uzumcu, & Skinner, 2005; Jaenisch & Bird, 2003; Waterland, 2006), the question is whether the changes in gene expression that have been associated with postnatal mother–infant interactions are associated with these epigenetic modifications.

The first investigation of epigenetic regulation of phenotypes associated with levels of maternal care focussed on the levels of hippocampal GR mRNA observed in the offspring of High and Low LG dams (Weaver et al., 2004a). Analysis of the level of DNA methylation within the GR 1_7 promoter region suggests that elevated levels of maternal LG are associated with decreased GR 1_7 methylation corresponding to the elevated levels of receptor expression observed in the hippocampus. Site-specific analysis of the methylation pattern in this region indicates that the binding site for nerve growth factor inducible-protein A (NGFI-A), a transcription factor involved in regulation of GR expression, is differentially methylated in the offspring of High and Low LG dams and subsequent analysis indicated that the binding of NGF1-A to this region is reduced in hippocampal tissue taken from the offspring of Low LG dams. A temporal analysis of the methylation of the GR 1_7 promoter indicates that differences between the offspring of High and Low LG dams emerge during the postpartum period and are sustained at weaning and into adulthood. Thus, the differences in gene expression and behavior that are observed in the adult offspring associated with the quality of maternal care received during the first week postpartum may be mediated by the long-term silencing of gene expression achieved through differential methylation. The mediating role of epigenetic modifications in sustaining these phenotypes is supported by findings that the increased anxiety, elevated stress-induced corticosterone, and decreased hippocampal GR mRNA expression observed in the offspring of Low LG dams can be altered by pharmacologically targeting the epigenome (Weaver et al., 2004a; Weaver, Diorio, Seckl, Szyf, & Meaney, 2004b; Weaver, Meaney, & Szyf, 2006). Central administration of trichostatin-A, a histone deacetylase inhibitor that promotes demethylation, to the adult offspring of Low LG dams reverses the effects associated with maternal care and produces a phenotype that is indistinguishable from that of the offspring of High LG dams (Weaver et al., 2004a). Conversely, central administration of methionine, a methyl donor that promotes methylation, to the adult offspring of High LG dams results in increased anxiety, increased corticosterone responses to stress, decreased GR mRNA, and decreased binding of NGF1-A to the hippocampal GR 1_7 promoter region (Weaver et al., 2005, 2006). Thus epigenetic regulation of gene expression is critical for shaping the brain and

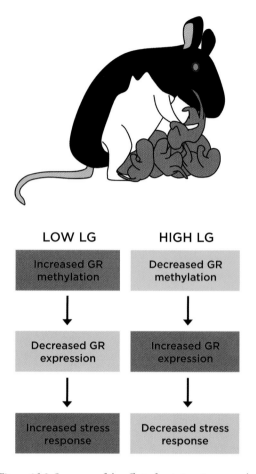

Figure 16.2 Summary of the effect of variations in maternal licking/grooming (LG) by rat dams on the methylation and expression of hippocampal glucocorticoid receptors (GR) and subsequent consequences for stress responsivity of offspring.

behavior and, moreover, maternal care experienced in infancy is associated with the epigenetic status of genes in adulthood (Figure 16.2). Though the relationship between maternal care and epigenetic regulation of gene expression has not been explored in the context of maternal deprivation, separation, or in humans and primates, such regulation is likely to play an important role in sustaining the effects of early experiences.

Transgenerational Effects of Maternal Care

The epigenetic modifications associated with maternal care illustrate the long-term effects of mother–infant interactions within one generation. However, there is increasing evidence that maternal care can also shape the phenotype of future generations. The transgenerational continuity of child abuse in humans is striking. It is currently estimated that up to 70% of abusive parents were themselves abused, whereas 20%–30% of abused infants are likely to become abusers (Chapman & Scott, 2001; Egeland, Jacobvitz, & Papatola, 1987). Women reared in institutional settings without experiencing parental care display less sensitivity and are more confrontational toward their own children (Dowdney, Skuse, Rutter, Quinton, & Mrazek, 1985). An intergenerational transmission of maternal care and overprotection as rated by the BPI has also been shown between women and their daughters (Miller, Kramer, Warner, Wickramaratne, & Weissman, 1997) and this transmission of parental style was found to be independent of SES, or maternal or daughter temperament or depression. A mother's own attachment to her mother, as assessed by the retrospective Adult Attachment Interview, is a good predictor of her infant's attachment, especially for secure and disorganized patterns of attachment (Benoit & Parker, 1994; Main & Hesse, 1990; Pederson, Gleason, Moran, & Bento, 1998; van Ijzendoorn, 1995). Sroufe and colleagues have also reported preliminary results from a prospective study suggesting transmission of attachment classifications as measured in the ASS from mother to daughter and to granddaughter (Sroufe et al., 2005).

The transmission of maternal behavior from mother to daughter has also been observed in primates. Dario Maestripieri and colleagues have demonstrated the influence of abusive parenting styles of rhesus macaques in modulating the subsequent maternal behavior of offspring. They found that over 50% of offspring who had received abusive parenting during the first 6 months of postnatal life would then exhibit abusive parenting themselves as adults (Maestripieri, 1998, 1999; Maestripieri & Carroll, 1998). Infants cross-fostered from an abusive female to a nonabusive female were not abusive to their own offspring, suggesting the role of the postnatal environment in mediating these effects (Maestripieri, 2005). Such transmission of abuse across generations has long been suspected from observational studies of rhesus and pigtail macaque social groups where infant abuse is highly concentrated within certain matrilines and among closely related females (Maestripieri & Carroll, 1998; Maestripieri et al., 1997). This generational transmission, however, is not limited to abusive behaviors. Among captive vervet monkeys, the best predictor of the frequency of mother–infant contact is the level of contact the female received from her mother during the first

6 postnatal months (Fairbanks, 1989). Matrilineal transmission of maternal rejection rates has also been observed amongst rhesus monkeys (Berman, 1990). Moreover, the overall frequency of maternal behaviors has been found to differ in rhesus matrilines, which may be passed intergenerationally (Simpson & Howe, 1986). Though the neurobiological mechanisms mediating this transmission have not been explored extensively, preliminary data suggest that the transmission of abusive phenotypes in rhesus monkey mothers is related to a decrease in the CSF circulating levels of serotonin. Females that receive abuse, and who become abusive, have lower circulating levels of a CSF serotonin metabolite than those females who receive abuse but do not become abusive (Maestripieri et al., 2006).

In rodents, pups exposed to reduced maternal behavior exhibit lower maternal care toward their offspring. Reducing the normal exposure of female mouse pups to maternal interactions through early weaning is associated with lower levels of LG and nursing toward their own pups (Kikusui, Isaka, & Mori, 2005). Female rat pups that are artificially separated from their mothers, either for short repeated periods (Lovic, Gonzalez, & Fleming, 2001) or for more prolonged periods (Gonzalez et al., 2001), exhibit impaired maternal care; they retrieve fewer pups during a retrieval test and exhibit reduced LG and crouching behaviors. Natural variations in maternal care are also transmitted across generations. The offspring of High LG rat dams exhibit high levels of maternal LG toward their own offspring whereas the offspring of Low LG dams are themselves low in LG (Champagne et al., 2003a; Fleming et al., 2002; Francis et al., 1999b). Moreover, cross-fostering female offspring between High and Low LG dams confirms the role of postnatal care in mediating this transmission.

The mechanisms through which the maternal care of one generation can influence the maternal behavior of subsequent generations may involve the sensitivity to hormones that normally serve to upregulate gene expression and promote both the physiological and behavioral aspects of maternal care. In rats, complete maternal deprivation in infancy is associated with reduced maternal behavior in response to estrogen and progesterone administration (Novakov & Fleming, 2005a). Offspring of Low LG dams exhibit decreased estrogen-mediated upregulation of oxytocin receptor binding and c-fos immunoreactivity in hypothalamic regions implicated in maternal care such as the medial preoptic area (MPOA) (Champagne,

Diorio, Sharma, & Meaney, 2001). This sensitivity may be mediated by decreased levels of estrogen receptor alpha mRNA in the MPOA that are found in offspring of Low compared to High LG dams (Champagne, Weaver, Diorio, Sharma, & Meaney, 2003b). Differential levels of ERα mRNA are observed in infancy and maintained into adulthood, suggesting a long-term suppression of gene expression in response to low levels of LG. Analysis of MPOA levels of DNA methylation within the ERα promoter indicates that low levels of maternal LG are associated with high levels of ERα methylation among female offspring whereas high levels of LG are associated with low levels of ERα methylation (Champagne et al., 2006). Thus LG is associated with epigenetic regulation of genes in female offspring that mediates maternal behavior and as such mediates the transmission of maternal care across generations.

Reversibility of Early Maternal Effects

The influence of the early environment can be extremely pervasive and the long-term effects of maternal care can be observed from infancy into adulthood. However, there is evidence that experiences at other periods of development reverse or reinforce the effects attributed to the quality of the mother–infant relationship. The question of reversibility has been addressed in the context of prenatal stress, maternal separation, and experience of low levels of postnatal maternal care in rodents. Offspring born to prenatally stressed females experience both the gestational and postnatal disruptions to maternal care. Offspring of prenatally stressed rat dams that are fostered to nonstressed dams experience fewer indices of increased HPA activity (Moore & Power, 1986). The adoption process itself has been found to stimulate postnatal maternal care in both stressed and nonstressed females and attenuate the stress response of adopted prenatally stressed offspring (Maccari et al., 1995). Postweaning exposure to environmental enrichment, consisting of enhanced levels of social and sensory stimulation, increases exploratory behavior, decreases stress responsivity, enhances performance on cognitive tasks, increases levels of hippocampal neurogenesis and dendritic branching, and increases serotonergic and dopaminergic activity (Leggio et al., 2005; van Praag, Kempermann, & Gage, 2000). These environmental conditions have been demonstrated to improve functioning of individuals exposed prenatally to gestational stress or alcohol (Hannigan, Berman, & Zajac, 1993; Laviola et al., 2004; Morley-Fletcher,

Rea, Maccari, & Laviola, 2003), attenuate the stress responsivity of maternally separated offspring (Francis, Diorio, Plotsky, & Meaney, 2002), and enhance the cognitive performance of offspring provided with low levels of postnatal maternal LG (Bredy, Humpartzoomian, Cain, & Meaney, 2003b). These studies also suggest that the effects of juvenile social experiences on phenotype may be mediated by different mechanisms that those associated with mother–infant interactions. Though environmental enrichment attenuates behavioral indices of stress responsivity, it does not alter the elevated CRF levels in the PVN and decreased levels of hippocampal GR mRNA found in maternally separated males (Francis et al., 2002). Likewise, though cognitive performance is enhanced in the offspring of Low LG dams exposed to pubertal enrichment levels of hippocampal N-methyl-D-aspartate (NMDA), receptor binding is not altered (Bredy et al., 2003b). Taken together, these studies suggest that though there are pervasive maternal influences on offspring phenotype, conditions beyond the period of mother–infant interaction can have a substantial influence on development.

Concluding Remarks

Variations in maternal care occur at preconceptional, prenatal, and postnatal periods of infant development and play an important role in modulating offspring neurobiology and behavior. In some instances, the early interactions between mother and infant are simply disruptive to development and lead to pathological outcomes. However, developmental plasticity in response to maternal care can also be an adaptive process enabling offspring to adjust their development so as to be better suited to their future infant, juvenile, and adult environments. This is demonstrated in the case of the "thrifty phenotype" in which maternal nutritional levels during pregnancy shift offspring into a metabolic phenotype more suited to nutrient-restricted environments (Barker, 2004; Gluckman et al., 2005). Prenatal stress, maternal deprivation, and reduced maternal care can likewise be viewed as signals to the quality of the environment. Offspring phenotype adjusts in response to these maternal cues in preparation to enter a stressful environment, leading to increased stress responsivity and reduced social behavior. Though we might view these outcomes as pathological, they may enhance survival under the conditions of environmental threat that are associated with disruptions of maternal care. Perhaps the pathology is not in the phenotype itself but rather in the mismatch between the environmental conditions of early development (which are critical to shaping phenotype) and adulthood. This mismatch has been implicated in metabolic disorders (Barker, 2004; Gluckman et al., 2005) but may be equally relevant to behavioral development. The plasticity in phenotype observed during the juvenile period in response to environmental enrichment may represent an adaptive strategy to prevent this mismatch, enabling offspring to adopt a phenotype that corresponds to environmental conditions that are more proximal to those of adulthood and thus the period of reproduction. However, under stable environmental conditions, maternal care itself can be transmitted across generations with implications for the gene expression and behavior of offspring within each generation (Champagne & Curley, 2005). Thus, through the influence of maternal care, infants can develop adaptive responses to the environmental conditions of a previous generation, providing evidence for the dynamic interplay between genes and environments in mediating the epigenetic inheritance of phenotype.

References

Ainsworth, M., Blehar, M., Waters, E., & Wall, S. (1978). *Patterns of attachment*. Hillsdale, MJ: Erlbaum.

Ainsworth, M., & Wittig, B. (1969). Attachment and exploratory behavior of one-year-olds in a strange situation. In B. Foss (Ed.), *Determinants of infant behavior* (Vol. 4, pp. 111–136). New York: Barnes & Noble.

Ammerman, R. T., Cassisi, J. E., Hersen, M., & van Hasselt, V. B. (1986). Consequences of physical abuse and neglect in children. *Clinical Psychology Reviews, 6*, 291–310.

Andrews, M. W., & Rosenblum, L. A. (1991). Attachment in monkey infants raised in variable- and low-demand environments. *Child Development, 62*, 686–693.

Andrews, M. W., & Rosenblum, L. A. (1994). The development of affiliative and agonistic social patterns in differentially reared monkeys. *Child Development, 65*, 1398–1404.

Anway, M. D., Cupp, A. S., Uzumcu, M., & Skinner, M. K. (2005). Epigenetic transgenerational actions of endocrine disruptors and male fertility. *Science, 308*, 1466–1469.

Arling, G. L., & Harlow, H. F. (1967). Effects of social deprivation on maternal behavior of rhesus monkeys. *Journal of Comparative and Physiological Psychology, 64*, 371–377.

Barbazanges, A., Piazza, P. V., Le Moal, M., & Maccari, S. (1996). Maternal glucocorticoid secretion mediates long-term effects of prenatal stress. *Journal of Neuroscience, 16*, 3943–3949.

Barker, D. J. (2004). The developmental origins of adult disease. *Journal of the American College of Nutrition, 23*, 588S–595S.

Benoit, D., & Parker, K. C. (1994). Stability and transmission of attachment across three generations. *Child Development, 65*, 1444–1456.

Berman, C. (1990). Intergenerational transmission of maternal rejection rates among free-ranging rhesus monkeys on Cayo Santiago. *Animal Behaviour, 44*, 247–258.

Bernstein, I. M., Mongeon, J. A., Badger, G. J., Solomon, L., Heil, S. H., & Higgins, S. T. (2005). Maternal smoking and its association with birth weight. *Obstetrics and Gynecology, 106*, 986–991.

Boccia, M. L., Razzoli, M., Vadlamudi, S. P., Trumbull, W., Caleffie, C., & Pedersen, C. A. (2006). Repeated long separations from pups produce depression-like behavior in rat mothers. *Psychoneuroendocrinology, 32*(1), 65–71.

Bowlby, J. (1988). *A secure base: Parent–child attachment and healthy human development*. New York: Basic Books.

Bredy, T. W., Grant, R. J., Champagne, D. L., & Meaney, M. J. (2003a). Maternal care influences neuronal survival in the hippocampus of the rat. *European Journal of Neuroscience, 18*, 2903–2909.

Bredy, T. W., Humpartzoomian, R. A., Cain, D. P., & Meaney, M. J. (2003b). Partial reversal of the effect of maternal care on cognitive function through environmental enrichment. *Neuroscience, 118*, 571–576.

Bukovsky, A., Caudle, M. R., Svetlikova, M., Wimalasena, J., Ayala, M. E., & Dominguez, R. (2005). Oogenesis in adult mammals, including humans: A review. *Endocrine, 26*, 301–316.

Caldji, C., Diorio, J., & Meaney, M. J. (2000). Variations in maternal care in infancy regulate the development of stress reactivity. *Biological Psychiatry, 48*, 1164–1174.

Caldji, C., Diorio, J., & Meaney, M. J. (2003). Variations in maternal care alter GABA(A) receptor subunit expression in brain regions associated with fear. *Neuropsychopharmacology, 28*, 1950–1959.

Carlson, E. A. (1998). A prospective longitudinal study of attachment disorganization/disorientation. *Child Development, 69*, 1107–1128.

Castle, J., Groothues, C., Bredenkamp, D., Beckett, C., O'Connor, T., & Rutter, M. (1999). Effects of qualities of early institutional care on cognitive attainment. E. R. A. Study Team. English and Romanian Adoptees. *American Journal of Orthopsychiatry, 69*, 424–437.

Catalano, R., Bruckner, T., Hartig, T., & Ong, M. (2005). Population stress and the Swedish sex ratio. *Paediatric and Perinatal Epidemiology, 19*, 413–420.

Champagne, F. A., Chretien, P., Stevenson, C. W., Zhang, T. Y., Gratton, A., & Meaney, M. J. (2004). Variations in nucleus accumbens dopamine associated with individual differences in maternal behavior in the rat. *Journal of Neuroscience, 24*, 4113–4123.

Champagne, F. A., & Curley, J. P. (2005). How social experiences influence the brain. *Current Opinion in Neurobiology, 15*, 704–709.

Champagne, F., Diorio, J., Sharma, S., & Meaney, M. J. (2001). Naturally occurring variations in maternal behavior in the rat are associated with differences in estrogen-inducible central oxytocin receptors. *Proceedings of the National Academy of Sciences, USA, 98*, 12736–12741.

Champagne, F. A., Francis, D. D., Mar, A., & Meaney, M. J. (2003a). Variations in maternal care in the rat as a mediating influence for the effects of environment on development. *Physiology & Behavior, 79*, 359–371.

Champagne, F. A., & Meaney, M. J. (2006). Stress during gestation alters postpartum maternal care and the development of the offspring in a rodent model. *Biological Psychiatry, 59*, 1227–1235.

Champagne, F. A., Weaver, I. C., Diorio, J., Dymov, S., Szyf, M., & Meaney, M. J. (2006). Maternal care associated with methylation of the estrogen receptor-alpha1b promoter and estrogen receptor-alpha expression in the medial preoptic area of female offspring. *Endocrinology, 147*, 2909–2915.

Champagne, F. A., Weaver, I. C., Diorio, J., Sharma, S., & Meaney, M. J. (2003b). Natural variations in maternal care are associated with estrogen receptor alpha expression and estrogen sensitivity in the medial preoptic area. *Endocrinology, 144*, 4720–4724.

Chapman, D., & Scott, K. (2001). The impact of maternal intergenerational risk factors on adverse developmental outcomes. *Developmental Review, 21*, 305–325.

Coplan, J. D., Altemus, M., Mathew, S. J., Smith, E. L., Sharf, B., Coplan, P. M., et al. (2005). Synchronized maternal–infant elevations of primate CSF CRF concentrations in response to variable foraging demand. *CNS Spectrums, 10*, 530–536.

Coplan, J. D., Smith, E. L., Altemus, M., Scharf, B. A., Owens, M. J., Nemeroff, C. B., et al. (2001). Variable foraging demand rearing: Sustained elevations in cisternal cerebrospinal fluid corticotropin-releasing factor concentrations in adult primates. *Biological Psychiatry, 50*, 200–204.

Coplan, J. D., Smith, E. L., Trost, R. C., Scharf, B. A., Altemus, M., Bjornson, L., et al. (2000). Growth hormone response to clonidine in adversely reared young adult primates: Relationship to serial cerebrospinal fluid corticotropin-releasing factor concentrations. *Psychiatry Research, 95*, 93–102.

Coplan, J. D., Trost, R. C., Owens, M. J., Cooper, T. B., Gorman, J. M., Nemeroff, C. B., et al. (1998). Cerebrospinal fluid concentrations of somatostatin and biogenic amines in grown primates reared by mothers exposed to manipulated foraging conditions. *Archives of General Psychiatry, 55*, 473–477.

Cox, B. J., Enns, M. W., & Clara, I. P. (2000). The Parental Bonding Instrument: Confirmatory evidence for a three-factor model in a psychiatric clinical sample and in the National Comorbidity Survey. *Social Psychiatry and Psychiatric Epidemiology, 35*, 353–357.

Cratty, M. S., Ward, H. E., Johnson, E. A., Azzaro, A. J., & Birkle, D. L. (1995). Prenatal stress increases corticotropin-releasing factor (CRF) content and release in rat amygdala minces. *Brain Research, 675*, 297–302.

De Sousa, P. A., Caveney, A., Westhusin, M. E., & Watson, A. J. (1998). Temporal patterns of embryonic gene expression and their dependence on oogenetic factors. *Theriogenology, 49*, 115–128.

Dowdney, L., Skuse, D., Rutter, M., Quinton, D., & Mrazek, D. (1985). The nature and qualities of parenting provided by women raised in institutions. *Journal of Child Psychology and Psychiatry and Allied Disciplines, 26*, 599–625.

Edwards, C. R., Benediktsson, R., Lindsay, R. S., & Seckl, J. R. (1996). 11-Beta-hydroxysteroid dehydrogenases: Key enzymes in determining tissue-specific glucocorticoid effects. *Steroids, 61*, 263–269.

Egeland, B., & Farber, E. A. (1984). Infant–mother attachment: Factors related to its development and changes over time. *Child Development, 55*, 753–771.

Egeland, B., Jacobvitz, D., & Papatola, K. (1987). *Child abuse and neglect: Biosocial dimensions*. New York: Aldine.

Egeland, B., & Sroufe, L. A. (1981). Attachment and early maltreatment. *Child Development, 52*, 44–52.

Eichenlaub-Ritter, U. (1998). Genetics of oocyte ageing. *Maturitas, 30*, 143–169.

Enns, M. W., Cox, B. J., & Clara, I. (2002). Parental bonding and adult psychopathology: Results from the US National Comorbidity Survey. *Psychological Medicine, 32*, 997–1008.

Fahlke, C., Lorenz, J. G., Long, J., Champoux, M., Suomi, S. J., & Higley, J. D. (2000). Rearing experiences and stress-induced plasma cortisol as early risk factors for excessive alcohol consumption in nonhuman primates. *Alcoholism, Clinical, and Experimental Research, 24*, 644–650.

Fairbanks, L. A. (1989). Early experience and cross-generational continuity of mother–infant contact in vervet monkeys. *Developmental Psychobiology, 22*, 669–681.

Fairbanks, L. A., & McGuire, M. T. (1988). Long-term effects of early mothering behavior on responsiveness to the environment in vervet monkeys. *Developmental Psychobiology, 21*, 711–724.

Feldman, S. S., & Ingham, M. E. (1975). Attachment behavior: A validation study in two age groups. *Child Development, 46*, 319–330.

Fisher, L. A., Ames, E. W., Chisholm, K., & Savoie, L. (1997). Problems reported by parents of romanian orphans adopted to British Columbia. *International Journal of Behavioral Development, 20*.

Fleming, A. S., Kraemer, G. W., Gonzalez, A., Lovic, V., Rees, S., & Melo, A. (2002). Mothering begets mothering: The transmission of behavior and its neurobiology across generations. *Pharmacology, Biochemistry and Behavior, 73*, 61–75.

Francis, D. D., Caldji, C., Champagne, F., Plotsky, P. M., & Meaney, M. J. (1999a). The role of corticotropin-releasing factor–norepinephrine systems in mediating the effects of early experience on the development of behavioral and endocrine responses to stress. *Biological Psychiatry, 46*, 1153–1166.

Francis, D., Diorio, J., Liu, D., & Meaney, M. J. (1999b). Nongenomic transmission across generations of maternal behavior and stress responses in the rat. *Science, 286*, 1155–1158.

Francis, D. D., Diorio, J., Plotsky, P. M., & Meaney, M. J. (2002). Environmental enrichment reverses the effects of maternal separation on stress reactivity. *Journal of Neuroscience, 22*, 7840–7843.

Francis, D. D., Szegda, K., Campbell, G., Martin, W. D., & Insel, T. R. (2003). Epigenetic sources of behavioral differences in mice. *Nature Neuroscience, 6*, 445–446.

Fulroth, R., Phillips, B., & Durand, D. J. (1989). Perinatal outcome of infants exposed to cocaine and/or heroin in utero. *American Journal of Diseases of Children, 143*, 905–910.

Gal, P., & Sharpless, M. K. (1984). Fetal drug exposure–behavioral teratogenesis. *Drug Intelligence and Clinical Pharmacy, 18*, 186–201.

Gavis, E. R., & Lehmann, R. (1992). Localization of nanos RNA controls embryonic polarity. *Cell, 71*, 301–313.

Gerra, G., Zaimovic, A., Garofano, L., Ciusa, F., Moi, G., Avanzini, P., et al. (2006). Perceived parenting behavior in the childhood of cocaine users: Relationship with genotype and personality traits. *American Journal of Medical Genetics. Part B, Neuropsychiatric Genetics, 144B*(1), 52–57.

Gluckman, P. D., Hanson, M. A., & Pinal, C. (2005). The developmental origins of adult disease. *Maternal & Child Nutrition, 1*, 130–141.

Goldfarb, W. (1943). Infant rearing and problem behavior. *American Journal of Orthopsychiatry, 13*, 249–265.

Gonzalez, A., & Fleming, A. S. (2002). Artificial rearing causes changes in maternal behavior and c-fos expression in juvenile female rats. *Behavioral Neuroscience, 116*, 999–1013.

Gonzalez, A., Lovic, V., Ward, G. R., Wainwright, P. E., & Fleming, A. S. (2001). Intergenerational effects of complete maternal deprivation and replacement stimulation on maternal behavior and emotionality in female rats. *Developmental Psychobiology, 38*, 11–32.

Grant, J. E., & Kim, S. W. (2002). Parental bonding in pathological gambling disorder. *Psychiatric Quarterly, 73*, 239–247.

Hall, W. G. (1975). Weaning and growth of artificially reared rats. *Science, 190*(4221), 1313–1315.

Hannigan, J. H., Berman, R. F., & Zajac, C. S. (1993). Environmental enrichment and the behavioral effects of prenatal exposure to alcohol in rats. *Neurotoxicology and Teratology, 15*, 261–266.

Harkness, K. L., Bruce, A. E., & Lumley, M. N. (2006). The role of childhood abuse and neglect in the sensitization to stressful life events in adolescent depression. *Journal of Abnormal Psychology, 115*, 730–741.

Harlow, H. F., & Suomi, S. J. (1971). Social recovery by isolation-reared monkeys. *Proceedings of the National Academy of Sciences, USA, 68*, 1534–1538.

Heider, D., Matschinger, H., Bernert, S., Alonso, J., & Angermeyer, M. C. (2006). Relationship between parental bonding and mood disorder in six European countries. *Psychiatry Research, 143*, 89–98.

Heider, D., Matschinger, H., Bernert, S., Vilagut, G., Martinez-Alonso, M., Dietrich, S., et al. (2005). Empirical evidence for an invariant three-factor structure of the Parental Bonding Instrument in six European countries. *Psychiatry Research, 135*, 237–247.

Hickie, I., Parker, G., Wilhelm, K., & Tennant, C. (1991). Perceived interpersonal risk factors of non-endogenous depression. *Psychological Medicine, 21*, 399–412.

Higgins, S. (2002). Smoking in pregnancy. *Current Opinion in Obstetrics and Gynecology, 14*, 145–151.

Hodges, J., & Tizard, B. (1989a). IQ and behavioural adjustment of ex-institutional adolescents. *Journal of Child Psychology and Psychiatry and Allied Disciplines, 30*, 53–75.

Hodges, J., & Tizard, B. (1989b). Social and family relationships of ex-institutional adolescents. *Journal of Child Psychology and Psychiatry and Allied Disciplines, 30*, 77–97.

Hook, E. B. (1981). Rates of chromosome abnormalities at different maternal ages. *Obstetrics and Gynecology, 58*, 282–285.

Hoyseth, K. S., & Jones, P. J. (1989). Ethanol induced teratogenesis: Characterization, mechanisms and diagnostic approaches. *Life Sciences, 44*, 643–649.

Ichise, M., Vines, D. C., Gura, T., Anderson, G. M., Suomi, S. J., Higley, J. D., et al. (2006). Effects of early life stress on [11C]DASB positron emission tomography imaging of serotonin transporters in adolescent peer- and mother-reared rhesus monkeys. *Journal of Neuroscience, 26*, 4638–4643.

Isabella, R. A. (1993). Origins of attachment: Maternal interactive behavior across the first year. *Child Development, 64*, 605–621.

Isabella, R. A., & Belsky, J. (1991). Interactional synchrony and the origins of infant–mother attachment: A replication study. *Child Development, 62*, 373–384.

Jacobvitz, D., Leon, K., & Hazen, N. (2006). Does expectant mothers' unresolved trauma predict frightened/frightening maternal behavior? Risk and protective factors. *Development and Psychopathology, 18*, 363–379.

Jaenisch, R., & Bird, A. (2003). Epigenetic regulation of gene expression: How the genome integrates intrinsic and environmental signals. *Nature Genetics, 33*(Suppl.), 245–254.

Janny, L., & Menezo, Y. J. (1996). Maternal age effect on early human embryonic development and blastocyst formation. *Molecular Reproduction and Development, 45*, 31–37.

Jans, J. E., & Woodside, B. C. (1990). Nest temperature: Effects on maternal behavior, pup development, and interactions with handling. *Developmental Psychobiology, 23*, 519–534.

Jones, P. A., & Taylor, S. M. (1980). Cellular differentiation, cytidine analogs and DNA methylation. *Cell, 20*, 85–93.

Kikusui, T., Isaka, Y., & Mori, Y. (2005). Early weaning deprives mouse pups of maternal care and decreases their maternal behavior in adulthood. *Behavioural Brain Research, 162*, 200–206.

Laviola, G., Rea, M., Morley-Fletcher, S., Di Carlo, S., Bacosi, A., De Simone, R., et al. (2004). Beneficial effects of enriched environment on adolescent rats from stressed pregnancies. *European Journal of Neuroscience, 20*, 1655–1664.

Lee, M., & Williams, D. (1974). Changes in licking behaviour of rat mother following handling of young. *Animal Behaviour, 22*, 679–681.

Lee, R. J., Gollan, J., Kasckow, J., Geracioti, T., & Coccaro, E. F. (2006). CSF corticotropin-releasing factor in personality disorder: Relationship with self-reported parental care. *Neuropsychopharmacology, 31*, 2289–2295.

Leggio, M. G., Mandolesi, L., Federico, F., Spirito, F., Ricci, B., Gelfo, F., et al. (2005). Environmental enrichment promotes improved spatial abilities and enhanced dendritic growth in the rat. *Behavioural Brain Research, 163*, 78–90.

Lehmann, J., Pryce, C. R., Bettschen, D., & Feldon, J. (1999). The maternal separation paradigm and adult emotionality and cognition in male and female Wistar rats. *Pharmacology, Biochemistry and Behavior, 64*, 705–715.

Lehmann, J., Pryce, C. R., Jongen-Relo, A. L., Stohr, T., Pothuizen, H. H., & Feldon, J. (2002a). Comparison of maternal separation and early handling in terms of their neurobehavioral effects in aged rats. *Neurobiology of Aging, 23*, 457–466.

Lehmann, J., Russig, H., Feldon, J., & Pryce, C. R. (2002b). Effect of a single maternal separation at different pup ages on the corticosterone stress response in adult and aged rats. *Pharmacology, Biochemistry and Behavior, 73*, 141–145.

Lesage, J., Blondeau, B., Grino, M., Breant, B., & Dupouy, J. P. (2001). Maternal undernutrition during late gestation induces fetal overexposure to glucocorticoids and intrauterine growth retardation, and disturbs the hypothalamo-pituitary adrenal axis in the newborn rat. *Endocrinology, 142*, 1692–1702.

Levine, S. (1957). Infantile experience and resistance to physiological stress. *Science, 126*, 405.

Liu, D., Caldji, C., Sharma, S., Plotsky, P. M., & Meaney, M. J. (2000). Influence of neonatal rearing conditions on stress-induced adrenocorticotropin responses and norepinephrine release in the hypothalamic paraventricular nucleus. *Journal of Neuroendocrinology, 12*, 5–12.

Liu, D., Diorio, J., Day, J. C., Francis, D. D., & Meaney, M. J. (2000). Maternal care, hippocampal synaptogenesis and cognitive development in rats. *Nature Neuroscience, 3*, 799–806.

Liu, D., Diorio, J., Tannenbaum, B., Caldji, C., Francis, D., Freedman, A., et al. (1997). Maternal care, hippocampal glucocorticoid receptors, and hypothalamic-pituitary-adrenal responses to stress. *Science, 277*, 1659–1662.

Lovic, V., & Fleming, A. S. (2004). Artificially-reared female rats show reduced prepulse inhibition and deficits in the attentional set shifting task—Reversal of effects with maternal-like licking stimulation. *Behavioural Brain Research, 148*, 209–219.

Lovic, V., Gonzalez, A., & Fleming, A. S. (2001). Maternally separated rats show deficits in maternal care in adulthood. *Developmental Psychobiology, 39*, 19–33.

Lyons-Ruth, K., Bronfman, E., & Parsons, E. (1999). Atypical attachment in infancy and early childhood among children at developmental risk. IV. Maternal frightened, frightening, or atypical behavior and disorganized infant attachment patterns. *Monographs of the Society for Research in Child Development, 64*, 67–96; discussion 213–220.

Maccari, S., Piazza, P. V., Kabbaj, M., Barbazanges, A., Simon, H., & Le Moal, M. (1995). Adoption reverses the long-term impairment in glucocorticoid feedback induced by prenatal stress. *Journal of Neuroscience, 15*, 110–116.

Mackinnon, A., Henderson, A. S., & Andrews, G. (1993). Parental 'affectionless control' as an antecedent to adult depression: A risk factor refined. *Psychological Medicine, 23*, 135–141.

Mackinnon, A. J., Henderson, A. S., Scott, R., & Duncan-Jones, P. (1989). The Parental Bonding Instrument (PBI): An epidemiological study in a general population sample. *Psychological Medicine, 19*, 1023–1034.

MacLean, K. (2003). The impact of institutionalization on child development. *Development and Psychopathology, 15*, 853–884.

Maestripieri, D. (1998). Parenting styles of abusive mothers in group-living rhesus macaques. *Animal Behaviour, 55*, 1–11.

Maestripieri, D. (1999). Fatal attraction: Interest in infants and infant abuse in rhesus macaques. *American Journal of Physical Anthropology, 110*, 17–25.

Maestripieri, D. (2005). Early experience affects the intergenerational transmission of infant abuse in rhesus monkeys. *Proceedings of the National Academy of Sciences, USA, 102*, 9726–9729.

Maestripieri, D., & Carroll, K. A. (1998). Child abuse and neglect: Usefulness of the animal data. *Psychological Bulletin, 123*, 211–223.

Maestripieri, D., Higley, J. D., Lindell, S. G., Newman, T. K., McCormack, K. M., & Sanchez, M. M. (2006). Early maternal rejection affects the development of monoaminergic systems and adult abusive parenting in rhesus macaques (*Macaca mulatta*). *Behavioral Neuroscience, 120*, 1017–1024.

Maestripieri, D., Lindell, S. G., Ayala, A., Gold, P. W., & Higley, J. D. (2005). Neurobiological characteristics of rhesus macaque abusive mothers and their relation to social and maternal behavior. *Neuroscience and Biobehavioral Reviews, 29*, 51–57.

Maestripieri, D., Tomaszycki, M., & Carroll, K. A. (1999). Consistency and change in the behavior of rhesus macaque abusive mothers with successive infants. *Developmental Psychobiology, 34*, 29–35.

Maestripieri, D., Wallen, K., & Carroll, K. A. (1997). Infant abuse runs in families of group-living pigtail macaques. *Child Abuse and Neglect, 21*, 465–471.

Main, M., & Hesse, E. (1990). Parents' unresolved traumatic experiences are related to infant disorganized attachment status: Is frightened and/or frightening parental behavior the linking mechanism? In M. Greenberg, D. Cicchetti, & E. Cummings (Eds.), *Attachment in the preschool years* (pp. 161–182). Chicago: University of Chicago Press.

McMillen, I. C., & Robinson, J. S. (2005). Developmental origins of the metabolic syndrome: Prediction, plasticity, and programming. *Physiological Reviews, 85*, 571–633.

Meaney, M. J. (2001). Maternal care, gene expression, and the transmission of individual differences in stress reactivity across generations. *Annual Review of Neuroscience, 24*, 1161–1192.

Meaney, M. J., Aitken, D. H., Bhatnagar, S., & Sapolsky, R. M. (1991). Postnatal handling attenuates certain neuroendocrine, anatomical, and cognitive dysfunctions associated with aging in female rats. *Neurobiology of Aging, 12*, 31–38.

Meaney, M. J., Aitken, D. H., Viau, V., Sharma, S., & Sarrieau, A. (1989). Neonatal handling alters adrenocortical negative feedback sensitivity and hippocampal type II glucocorticoid receptor binding in the rat. *Neuroendocrinology, 50*, 597–604.

Meaney, M. J., Diorio, J., Francis, D., Widdowson, J., LaPlante, P., Caldji, C., et al. (1996). Early environmental regulation of forebrain glucocorticoid receptor gene expression: Implications for adrenocortical responses to stress. *Developmental Neuroscience, 18*(1–2), 49–72.

Melo, A. I., Lovic, V., Gonzalez, A., Madden, M., Sinopoli, K., & Fleming, A. S. (2006). Maternal and littermate deprivation disrupts maternal behavior and social-learning of food preference in adulthood: Tactile stimulation, nest odor, and social rearing prevent these effects. *Developmental Psychobiology, 48*(3), 209–219.

Miller, L., Kramer, R., Warner, V., Wickramaratne, P., & Weissman, M. (1997). Intergenerational transmission of parental bonding among women. *Journal of the American Academy of Child and Adolescent Psychiatry, 36*, 1134–1139.

Moore, C. L., & Power, K. L. (1986). Prenatal stress affects mother–infant interaction in Norway rats. *Developmental Psychobiology, 19*, 235–245.

Morley-Fletcher, S., Rea, M., Maccari, S., & Laviola, G. (2003). Environmental enrichment during adolescence reverses the effects of prenatal stress on play behaviour and HPA axis reactivity in rats. *European Journal of Neuroscience, 18*, 3367–3374.

Murphy, E., Brewin, C. R., & Silka, L. (1997). The assessment of parenting using the parental bonding instrument: Two or three factors? *Psychological Medicine, 27*, 333–341.

Myers, M. M., Brunelli, S. A., Shair, H. N., Squire, J. M., & Hofer, M. A. (1989). Relationships between maternal behavior of SHR and WKY dams and adult blood pressures of cross-fostered F1 pups. *Developmental Psychobiology, 22*, 55–67.

Myers, M. M., Brunelli, S. A., Squire, J. M., Shindeldecker, R. D., & Hofer, M. A. (1989). Maternal behavior of SHR rats and its relationship to offspring blood pressures. *Developmental Psychobiology, 22*, 29–53.

Nothias, J. Y., Majumder, S., Kaneko, K. J., & DePamphilis, M. L. (1995). Regulation of gene expression at the beginning of mammalian development. *Journal of Biological Chemistry, 270*, 22077–22080.

Novakov, M., & Fleming, A. S. (2005a). The effects of early rearing environment on the hormonal induction of maternal behavior in virgin rats. *Hormones and Behavior, 48*, 528–536.

Novakov, M., & Fleming, A. S. (2005b). The effects of early rearing environment on the hormonal induction of maternal behavior in virgin rats. *Hormones and Behavior,, 48*(5), 528–536.

O'Connor, T. G., & Rutter, M. (2000). Attachment disorder behavior following early severe deprivation: Extension and longitudinal follow-up. English and Romanian Adoptees Study Team. *Journal of the American Academy of Child and Adolescent Psychiatry, 39*, 703–712.

Olegard, R., Sabel, K. G., Aronsson, M., Sandin, B., Johansson, P. R., Carlsson, C., et al. (1979). Effects on the child of alcohol abuse during pregnancy. Retrospective and prospective studies. *Acta Paediatrica Scandinavica Supplement, 275*, 112–121.

Painter, R. C., Roseboom, T. J., & Bleker, O. P. (2005). Prenatal exposure to the Dutch famine and disease in later life: An overview. *Reproductive Toxicology, 20*, 345–352.

Parker, G. (1981). Parental reports of depressives. An investigation of several explanations. *Journal of Affective Disorders, 3*, 131–140.

Parker, G. (1984). The measurement of pathogenic parental style and its relevance to psychiatric disorder. *Social Psychiatry, 19*, 75–81.

Parker, G. (1990). The Parental Bonding Instrument: A decade of research. *Social Psychiatry and Psychiatric Epidemiology, 25*, 281–282.

Parker, G. (1993). Parental rearing style: Examining for links with personality vulnerability factors for depression. *Social Psychiatry and Psychiatric Epidemiology, 28*, 97–100.

Parker, G., Hadzi-Pavlovic, D., Greenwald, S., & Weissman, M. (1995). Low parental care as a risk factor to lifetime depression in a community sample. *Journal of Affective Disorders, 33*, 173–180.

Parker, G., Kiloh, L., & Hayward, L. (1987). Parental representations of neurotic and endogenous depressives. *Journal of Affective Disorders, 13*, 75–82.

Parker, G., Tupling, H., & Brown, L. B. (1979). A parental bonding instrument. *British Journal of Medical Psychology, 52*, 1–10.

Patin, V., Lordi, B., Vincent, A., & Caston, J. (2005). Effects of prenatal stress on anxiety and social interactions in adult rats. *Brain Research. Developmental Brain Research, 160*, 265–274.

Pedersen, C. A., & Boccia, M. L. (2002). Oxytocin links mothering received, mothering bestowed and adult stress responses. *Stress, 5*, 259–267.

Pederson, D. R., Gleason, K. E., Moran, G., & Bento, S. (1998). Maternal attachment representations, maternal sensitivity, and the infant–mother attachment relationship. *Developmental Psychology, 34*, 925–933.

Pederson, D. R., & Moran, G. (1996). Expressions of the attachment relationship outside of the strange situation. *Child Development, 67*, 915–927.

Peters, D. A. (1982). Prenatal stress: Effects on brain biogenic amine and plasma corticosterone levels. *Pharmacology, Biochemistry and Behavior, 17*, 721–725.

Plotsky, P. M., & Meaney, M. J. (1993). Early, postnatal experience alters hypothalamic corticotropin-releasing factor (CRF) mRNA, median eminence CRF content and stress-induced release in adult rats. *Brain Research. Molecular Brain Research, 18*, 195–200.

Plotsky, P. M., Thrivikraman, K. V., Nemeroff, C. B., Caldji, C., Sharma, S., & Meaney, M. J. (2005). Long-term consequences of neonatal rearing on central corticotropin-releasing factor systems in adult male rat offspring. *Neuropsychopharmacology, 30*, 2192–2204.

Priebe, K., Romeo, R. D., Francis, D. D., Sisti, H. M., Mueller, A., McEwen, B. S., et al. (2005). Maternal influences on adult stress and anxiety-like behavior in C57BL/6J and BALB/cJ mice: A cross-fostering study. *Developmental Psychobiology, 47*, 398–407.

Pruessner, J. C., Champagne, F., Meaney, M. J., & Dagher, A. (2004). Dopamine release in response to a psychological stress in humans and its relationship to early life maternal care: A positron emission tomography study using [11C] raclopride. *Journal of Neuroscience, 24*, 2825–2831.

Quinton, D., Rutter, M., & Liddle, C. (1984). Institutional rearing, parenting difficulties and marital support. *Psychological Medicine, 14*, 107–124.

Radke-Yarrow, M., Cummings, E. M., Kuczynski, L., & Chapman, M. (1985). Patterns of attachment in two- and three-year-olds in normal families and families with parental depression. *Child Development, 56*, 884–893.

Razin, A. (1998). CpG methylation, chromatin structure and gene silencing—A three-way connection. *The EMBO Journal, 17*, 4905–4908.

Reti, I. M., Samuels, J. F., Eaton, W. W., Bienvenu, O. J., 3rd, Costa, P. T., Jr., & Nestadt, G. (2002a). Adult antisocial personality traits are associated with experiences of low parental care and maternal overprotection. *Acta Psychiatrica Scandinavica, 106*, 126–133.

Reti, I. M., Samuels, J. F., Eaton, W. W., Bienvenu, O. J., 3rd, Costa, P. T., Jr., & Nestadt, G. (2002b). Influences of parenting on normal personality traits. *Psychiatry Research, 111*, 55–64.

Rondo, P. H., Ferreira, R. F., Nogueira, F., Ribeiro, M. C., Lobert, H., & Artes, R. (2003). Maternal psychological stress and distress as predictors of low birth weight, prematurity and intrauterine growth retardation. *European Journal of Clinical Nutrition, 57*, 266–272.

Roseboom, T., de Rooij, S., & Painter, R. (2006). The Dutch famine and its long-term consequences for adult health. *Early Human Development, 82*, 485–491.

Roseboom, T. J., van der Meulen, J. H., Osmond, C., Barker, D. J., Ravelli, A. C., Schroeder-Tanka, J. M., et al. (2000). Coronary heart disease after prenatal exposure to the Dutch famine, 1944–45. *Heart, 84*, 595–598.

Rosenblum, L. A., Forger, C., Noland, S., Trost, R. C., & Coplan, J. D. (2001). Response of adolescent bonnet macaques to an acute fear stimulus as a function of early rearing conditions. *Developmental Psychobiology, 39*, 40–45.

Rosenblum, L. A., & Paully, G. S. (1984). The effects of varying environmental demands on maternal and infant behavior. *Child Development, 55*, 305–314.

Rosenfeld, P., Wetmore, J. B., & Levine, S. (1992). Effects of repeated maternal separations on the adrenocortical response to stress of preweanling rats. *Physiology & Behavior, 52*, 787–791.

Rutter, M. (2002). Maternal deprivation. In M. H. Bornstein (Ed.), *Handbook of parenting: Vol. 4, Social conditions and applied parenting* (2nd ed., pp. 181–202). Mahwah, NJ: Erlbaum Associates.

Saadat, M., & Ansari-Lari, M. (2004). Sex ratio of birth during wartime and psychological tensions. *Human Reproduction, 19*, 465.

Sato, T., Narita, T., Hirano, S., Kusunoki, K., Sakado, K., & Uehara, T. (1999). Confirmatory factor analysis of the Parental Bonding Instrument in a Japanese population. *Psychological Medicine, 29*, 127–133.

Sato, T., Sakado, K., Uehara, T., Narita, T., Hirano, S., Nishioka, K., et al. (1998). Dysfunctional parenting as a risk factor to lifetime depression in a sample of employed Japanese adults: Evidence for the 'affectionless control' hypothesis. *Psychological Medicine, 28*, 737–742.

Schuengel, C., Bakermans-Kranenburg, M. J., & Van, I. M. H. (1999). Frightening maternal behavior linking unresolved loss and disorganized infant attachment. *Journal of Consulting and Clinical Psychology, 67*, 54–63.

Scott, L. A. (2000). Oocyte and embryo polarity. *Seminars in Reproductive Medicine, 18*, 171–183.

Seay, B., Alexander, B. K., & Harlow, H. F. (1964). Maternal Behavior of Socially Deprived Rhesus Monkeys. *Journal of Abnormal Psychology, 69*, 345–354.

Seay, B., & Harlow, H. F. (1965). Maternal separation in the rhesus monkey. *Journal of Nervous and Mental Disease, 140*, 434–441.

Seckl, J. R., Nyirenda, M. J., Walker, B. R., & Chapman, K. E. (1999). Glucocorticoids and fetal programming. *Biochemical Society Transactions, 27*, 74–78.

Shannon, C., Champoux, M., & Suomi, S. J. (1998). Rearing condition and plasma cortisol in rhesus monkey infants. *American Journal of Primatology, 46*, 311–321.

Shannon, C., Schwandt, M. L., Champoux, M., Shoaf, S. E., Suomi, S. J., Linnoila, M., et al. (2005). Maternal absence and stability of individual differences in CSF 5-HIAA concentrations in rhesus monkey infants. *American Journal of Psychiatry, 162*, 1658–1664.

Shulman, S., Elicker, J., & Sroufe, L. A. (1994). Stages of friendship growth in preadolescence as related to attachment history. *Journal of Social and Personal Relationships, 11*, 341–361.

Sigal, J. J. (2004). Studies of Unwanted Babies. *American Psychologist, 59*, 183–184.

Sigal, J. J., Perry, J. C., Rossignol, M., & Ouimet, M. C. (2003). Unwanted infants: Psychological and physical consequences of inadequate orphanage care 50 years later. *American Journal of Orthopsychiatry, 73*, 3–12.

Sigal, J. J., Rossignol, M., & Perry, J. C. (1999). Some psychological and physical consequences in middle-aged adults of underfunded institutional care in childhood. *Journal of Nervous and Mental Disease, 187*, 57–59.

Silove, D., Parker, G., Hadzi-Pavlovic, D., Manicavasagar, V., & Blaszczynski, A. (1991). Parental representations of patients with panic disorder and generalised anxiety disorder. *British Journal of Psychiatry, 159*, 835–841.

Simpson, M., & Howe, S. (1986). Group and matriline differences in the behaviour of rhesus monkey infants. *Animal Behaviour, 34*, 444–459.

Sroufe, L. A. (2005). Attachment and development: A prospective, longitudinal study from birth to adulthood. *Attachment & Human Development, 7*, 349–367.

Sroufe, L. A., Egeland, B., Carlson, E., & Collins, W. (2005). *The development of the person: The Minnesota study of risk and adaptation from birth to adulthood.* New York: The Guildford Press.

Statistics, O. O. A. (2005). *Substance use during pregnancy: 2002 and 2003 update.* Rockville, MD: Substance Abuse and Mental Health Services Administration.

Steckler, T. K., Kalin, N. H., & Reul, J. M. H. M. (2005). *Handbook of stress and the brain. Part 1: The neurobiology of stress, 15, Part 1.* New York: Elsevier.

Stevenson-Hinde, J., & Shouldice, A. (1995). Maternal interactions and self-reports related to attachment classifications at 4.5 years. *Child Development, 66*, 583–596.

Stohr, T., Schulte Wermeling, D., Szuran, T., Pliska, V., Domeney, A., Welzl, H., et al. (1998). Differential effects of prenatal stress in two inbred strains of rats. *Pharmacology, Biochemistry and Behavior, 59*, 799–805.

Strathdee, G., & Brown, R. (2002). Aberrant DNA methylation in cancer: Potential clinical interventions. *Expert Reviews in Molecular Medicine, 2002*, 1–17.

Sullivan, R. M., Shokrai, N., & Leon, M. (1988). Physical stimulation reduces the body temperature of infant rats. *Developmental Psychobiology, 21*, 225–235.

Sullivan, R. M., Wilson, D. A., & Leon, M. (1988). Physical stimulation reduces the brain temperature of infant rats. *Developmental Psychobiology, 21*, 237–250.

Suomi, S. J., Harlow, H. F., & Kimball, S. D. (1971). Behavioral effects of prolonged partial social isolation in the rhesus monkey. *Psychological Reports, 29*, 1171–1177.

Symonds, M. E., Budge, H., Stephenson, T., & Gardner, D. S. (2005). Experimental evidence for long-term programming effects of early diet. *Advances in Experimental Medicine and Biology, 569*, 24–32.

Symonds, M. E., Budge, H., Stephenson, T., & McMillen, I. C. (2001). Fetal endocrinology and development—Manipulation and adaptation to long-term nutritional and environmental challenges. *Reproduction, 121*, 853–862.

Takahashi, L. K., Turner, J. G., & Kalin, N. H. (1992). Prenatal stress alters brain catecholaminergic activity and potentiates stress-induced behavior in adult rats. *Brain Research, 574*, 131–137.

Tambyrajia, R. L., & Mongelli, M. (2000). Sociobiological variables and pregnancy outcome. *International Journal of Gynaecology and Obstetrics, 70*, 105–112.

Tarin, J. J., Gomez-Piquer, V., Manzanedo, C., Minarro, J., Hermenegildo, C., & Cano, A. (2003). Long-term effects of delayed motherhood in mice on postnatal development and behavioural traits of offspring. *Human Reproduction, 18*, 1580–1587.

Taylor, S. M., & Jones, P. A. (1985). Cellular differentiation. *International Journal of Obesity, 9*(Suppl. 1), 15–21.

Torresani, S., Favaretto, E., & Zimmermann, C. (2000). Parental representations in drug-dependent patients and their parents. *Comprehensive Psychiatry, 41*, 123–129.

Trickett, P., & McBride-Chang, C. (1995). The developmental impact of different forms of child abuse and neglect. *Developmental Reviews, 15*, 11–37.

van Ijzendoorn, M. H. (1995). Adult attachment representations, parental responsiveness, and infant attachment: A meta-analysis on the predictive validity of the Adult Attachment Interview. *Psychological Bulletin, 117*, 387–403.

van Ijzendoorn, M. H., Schuengel, C., & Bakermans-Kranenburg, M. J. (1999). Disorganized attachment in early childhood: Meta-analysis of precursors, concomitants, and sequelae. *Development and Psychopathology, 11*, 225–249.

van Praag, H., Kempermann, G., & Gage, F. H. (2000). Neural consequences of environmental enrichment. *Nature Reviews. Neuroscience, 1*, 191–198.

Veijola, J., Maki, P., Joukamaa, M., Laara, E., Hakko, H., & Isohanni, M. (2004). Parental separation at birth and depression in adulthood: A long-term follow-up of the Finnish Christmas Seal Home Children. *Psychological Medicine, 34*, 357–362.

Vorria, P., Papaligoura, Z., Sarafidou, J., Kopakaki, M., Dunn, J., van, I. M. H., et al. (2006). The development of adopted children after institutional care: A follow-up study. *Journal of Child Psychology and Psychiatry and Allied Disciplines, 47*(12), 1246–1253.

Wagner, C. L., Katikaneni, L. D., Cox, T. H., & Ryan, R. M. (1998). The impact of prenatal drug exposure on the neonate. *Obstetrics and Gynecology Clinics of North America, 25*, 169–194.

Wassarman, P. M., & Kinloch, R. A. (1992). Gene expression during oogenesis in mice. *Mutation Research, 296*, 3–15.

Waterland, R. A. (2006). Assessing the effects of high methionine intake on DNA methylation. *Journal of Nutrition, 136*, 1706S–1710S.

Weaver, I. C., Cervoni, N., Champagne, F. A., D'Alessio, A. C., Sharma, S., Seckl, J. R., et al. (2004a). Epigenetic programming by maternal behavior. *Nature Neuroscience, 7*, 847–854.

Weaver, I. C., Champagne, F. A., Brown, S. E., Dymov, S., Sharma, S., Meaney, M. J., et al. (2005). Reversal of maternal programming of stress responses in adult offspring through methyl supplementation: Altering epigenetic marking later in life. *Journal of Neuroscience, 25*, 11045–11054.

Weaver, I. C., Diorio, J., Seckl, J. R., Szyf, M., & Meaney, M. J. (2004b). Early environmental regulation of hippocampal glucocorticoid receptor gene expression: Characterization of intracellular mediators and potential genomic target sites. *Annals of the New York Academy of Sciences, 1024*, 182–212.

Weaver, I. C., Grant, R. J., & Meaney, M. J. (2002). Maternal behavior regulates long-term hippocampal expression of BAX and apoptosis in the offspring. *Journal of Neurochemistry, 82*, 998–1002.

Weaver, I. C., Meaney, M. J., & Szyf, M. (2006). Maternal care effects on the hippocampal transcriptome and anxiety-mediated behaviors in the offspring that are reversible in adulthood. *Proceedings of the National Academy of Sciences, USA, 103*, 3480–3485.

Weinstock, M. (2005). The potential influence of maternal stress hormones on development and mental health of the offspring. *Brain, Behavior, and Immunity, 19*, 296–308.

Weinstock, M., Fride, E., & Hertzberg, R. (1988). Prenatal stress effects on functional development of the offspring. *Progress in Brain Research, 73*, 319–331.

Weissgerber, T. L., & Wolfe, L. A. (2006). Physiological adaptation in early human pregnancy: Adaptation to balance maternal-fetal demands. *Applied Physiology: Nutrition and Metabolism, 31*, 1–11.

Wilhelm, K., Niven, H., Parker, G., & Hadzi-Pavlovic, D. (2005). The stability of the Parental Bonding Instrument over a 20-year period. *Psychological Medicine, 35*, 387–393.

Wilhelm, K., & Parker, G. (1990). Reliability of the parental bonding instrument and intimate bond measure scales. *Australian and New Zealand Journal of Psychiatry, 24*, 199–202.

Winslow, J. T. (2005). Neuropeptides and non-human primate social deficits associated with pathogenic rearing experience. *International Journal of Developmental Neuroscience, 23*, 245–251.

Zhang, T. Y., Chretien, P., Meaney, M. J., & Gratton, A. (2005). Influence of naturally occurring variations in maternal care on prepulse inhibition of acoustic startle and the medial prefrontal cortical dopamine response to stress in adult rats. *Journal of Neuroscience, 25*, 1493–1502.

Zimmerberg, B., Brunelli, S. A., & Hofer, M. A. (1994). Reduction of rat pup ultrasonic vocalizations by the neuroactive steroid allopregnanolone. *Pharmacology, Biochemistry and Behavior, 47*, 735–738.

Zorn, B., Sucur, V., Stare, J., & Meden-Vrtovec, H. (2002). Decline in sex ratio at birth after 10-day war in Slovenia: Brief communication. *Human Reproduction, 17*, 3173–3177.

Mechanisms of Plasticity in the Development of Cortical Somatosensory Maps

Reha S. Erzurumlu

Abstract

The mouse barrel cortex is discussed in this chapter as a model system for the studies of cortical somatosensory map formation and developmental plasticity. The critical period plasticity in this system underscores the importance of sensory periphery in patterning of parietal cortical zone allocated to the representation of the somatosensory space. Findings from recent studies show that intrinsic cortical molecular mechanisms set up the positioning, location, and amount of space devoted to the somatosensory cortex, and neural activity involving glutamatergic and serotonergic systems pattern the somatosensory map. The molecular and cellular mechanisms that underlie the plasticity of the cortical somatosensory map are not fully understood. Signals transmitted from the sensory periphery or brain stem most likely set the parameters of cortical plasticity during development.

Keywords: cortical somatosensory, development plasticity, sensory periphery, parietal cortical zone, somatosensory space, glutamatergic systems, serotonergic systems

Introduction

Decades of research have unraveled much about how somatotopic maps are established in the neocortex of mammals, and the manifestations of cortical plasticity that follow sensory deprivation or deafferentation during development. Cortical plasticity of somatosensory maps in adults has been studied in a variety of species including humans, nonhuman primates, cats, ferrets, and rodents, using imaging and in vivo electrophysiological recording techniques. However, the vast majority of developmental studies aimed at uncovering the underlying molecular and cellular mechanisms have examined the somatosensory cortex of rodents, particularly that of mice. Patterned organization of the rodent somatosensory cortex is readily visible through investigation using common histological and histochemical staining methods. Moreover, with the widespread application of transgenic technologies in mice, they have become a useful species for loss-of-function and gain-of-function experiments at the molecular, morphological, physiological, and behavioral levels. In this chapter, I review recent progress in our understanding of developmental plasticity in the rodent somatosensory cortex.

The idea of somatotopic organization in the neocortex emerged from both the observations of John Hughlings Jackson (1835–1911), who worked with epileptic patients and from the experimental studies of Hitzig and Fritsch (1870), who applied electrical stimulations to the dog motor cortex (see Penfield & Rasmussen, 1950, for a detailed historical perspective). The notion that there is a topographic body map in the motor and sensory

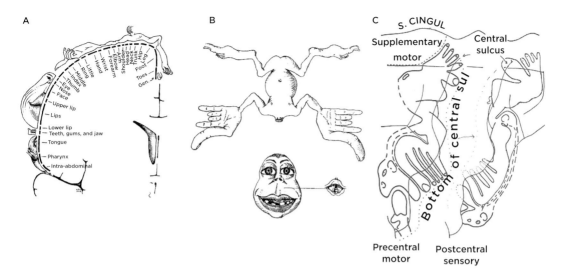

A

B

C

S. CINGUL

Supplementary motor

Central sulcus

Bottom of central sul

Precentral motor

Postcentral sensory

Figure 17.1 The original somatosensory (A) and motor (B) homunculus drawings of H. P. Cantlie (A from Penfield & RasMussen, 1950, and B from Penfield & Baldrey, 1937). (C) "Simiunculus" (sensory and motor representations) in the monkey cortex. (From Woolsey, 1964.)

cortices (pre- and postcentral gyri along the banks of the Rolandic fissure or central sulcus) originated at the Montreal Neurological Institute beginning in the 1930s with the systematic electrophysiological explorations of Wilder Penfield and his colleagues. In 1937, Penfield and Boldrey published their now classic article "Somatic and motor sensory representation in the cerebral cortex of man as studied by electrical stimulation." This article contains extensive illustrations of stimulation sites along the banks of the central sulcus and the somatosensory and motor responses evoked in locally anesthetized, awake patients. Figure 28 in that seminal article is a drawing by Mrs. H. P. Cantlie, which illustrates a distorted human figure reflecting the relative cortical space devoted to different body parts and their positioning within the motor and sensory neocortex. Cantlie's drawings and their variations have become known as the somatosensory or motor "homunculus" (Figure 17.1). They have been reproduced in the pages of numerous text books ever since.

The concept and the term "homunculus" (literally, little man) originated in philosophy and alchemy, subsequently finding its way into such diverse fields as literature, film, pop culture, games, and of course, neuroscience. Contemporaneous with Penfield and his colleagues, Clinton Woolsey, Wade Marshall, and Philip Bard were employing the newly devised evoked potential technique to map the cat and monkey somatosensory cortices

in detail at Johns Hopkins University (Marshall, Woolsey, & Bard, 1937, 1941; Woolsey, Marshall, & Bard, 1942). The pioneering studies of this group led to the description of "animalculi" in numerous mammalian species (Figure 17.2). In addition, the cortical mapping studies of the early 1940s were extended to other cortical areas, thereby revealing a general feature of the primary sensory cortex, namely, its "receptotopic" organization.

Peripheral receptor-related patterning of the somatosensory cortical map was discovered by Clinton Woolsey's son Thomas Woolsey and his mentor Hendrik Van der Loos at Johns Hopkins University (Woolsey & Van der Loos, 1970; for a detailed, first-hand account of this discovery, see Woolsey, 2005). In the face representation area of the primary somatosensory cortex of mice (and as noted subsequently in other rodent species), neurons in layer IV form cylindrical aggregates, replicating the patterned array of whiskers and sinus hairs on the contralateral snout. This region of the mouse neocortex had been studied earlier by Lorente de Nó using the Golgi impregnation technique. He referred to these cellular aggregates as "glomérulos" (Lorente de Nó, 1922). Woolsey and Van der Loos coined the term "barrels" to describe the morphological organization of mouse layer IV neuronal organization. When they performed neonatal whisker follicle lesions, they found that each barrel corresponds to a single whisker on the contralateral snout (Figure 17.3).

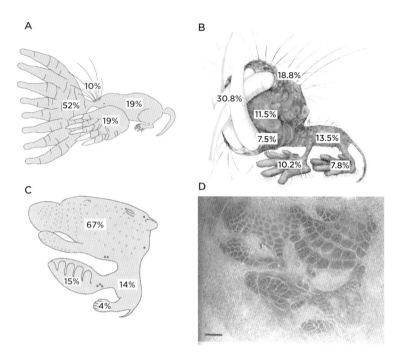

Figure 17.2 "Animalculi." Proportions of cortical area within the somatotopic map devoted to different body regions in (A) the star-nosed mole (from Catania & Kaas, 1997), (B) the naked mole rat (from Catania & Remple, 2002), and (C) the Sprague-Dawley rat (from Dawson & Killackey, 1986). (D) Histochemical staining of the rat somatosensory cortex in a tangential section illustrating the patterning (barrels) within different portions of the "rattunculus," the somatotopic body map. (From Dawson & Killackey, 1986.) Scale bar, 1 mm.

Barrel Cortex

In layer IV of the rodent primary somatosensory cortex, "barrels" are formed by discrete patches or "bouquets" of thalamocortical axon terminals, which arise from the ventroposteromedial (VPM) nucleus of the thalamus (Agmon, Yang, O'Dowd, & Jones, 1993; Erzurumlu & Jhaveri, 1990; Killackey, 1973; Killackey & Leshin, 1975; Rebsam, Seif, & Gaspar, 2002; Senft & Woolsey, 1991). These terminals are surrounded by layer IV spiny stellate neurons, which form the barrel "walls" and their dendrites embrace the thalamocortical axon terminals crowding the barrel "hollows" (Datwani, Iwasato, Itohara, & Erzurumlu, 2002a; Jeanmonod, Rice, & Van der Loos, 1981; Steffen & Van der Loos, 1980; Woolsey, Dierker, & Wann, 1975). Each barrel with its presynaptic (thalamocortical terminals) and postsynaptic (spiny stellate cells and their dendrites) elements receive and process information predominantly from a single whisker (Welker, 1971). Furthermore, in a plane through layer IV, parallel to the pial surface, the distribution of barrels replicates that of the whiskers and sinus hairs on the snout. A similar

but less distinct barrel-type patterning is present in cortical body map representing the lower jaw (with small hairs) as well as forepaw and hind paw areas, reflecting the receptor-dense pads of the paws (Belford & Killackey, 1978; Dawson & Killackey, 1987; Killackey, Rhoades, & Bennett-Clarke, 1995). The paw-related patterning is conveyed via the dorsal column lemniscal pathway to the ventroposterolateral (VPL) nucleus of the thalamus and to the paw representation regions of the primary somatosensory cortex (Figures 17.2 and 17.4). Such patterned cellular modules are called "barreloids" in the VPM–VPL nuclei and "barrelettes" in the brain stem (Ma & Woolsey, 1984; Van der Loos, 1976; Woolsey & Van der Loos, 1970).

The instructive role of the sensory periphery in sculpting central neural patterns has been demonstrated by lesion studies performed in perinatal rodents (Killackey et al., 1995; O'Leary, Schlaggar, & Tuttle, 1994; Welker & Van der Loos, 1986; Woolsey, 1990). Before the introduction of homologous recombination and gene targeting methods in mice, Van der Loos and his colleagues in Lausanne, Switzerland, selectively

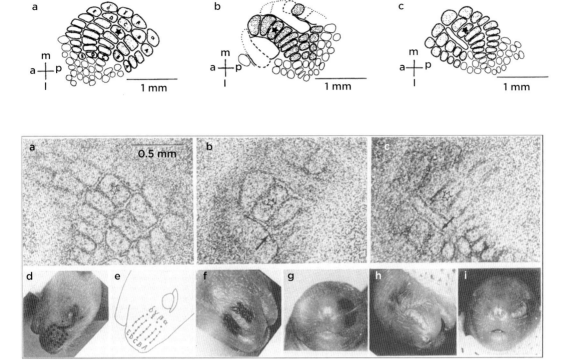

Figure 17.3 Original figure from Van der Loos and Woolsey (1970) showing the effects of neonatal whisker follicle lesions on the cytoarchitectonic organization of the barrel cortex. Top row: camera lucida drawings of normal and altered barrel fields following whisker row lesions. Bottom row: photomicrographs of Nissl-stained tangential sections through the barrel cortex of control and lesioned mice.

bred mice with aberrant numbers of whiskers. Beginning with an outbred population of mice, they inbred (by brother–sister matings) for bilaterally symmetric patterns of mystacial vibrissae characterized by the presence of supernumerary whiskers (Van der Loos, Dorfl, & Welker, 1984; Van der Loos, Welker, Dorfl, & Rumo, 1986; Welker & Van der Loos, 1986). They found that supernumerary barrels developed in the barrel cortex were corresponding to the supernumerary whiskers. The instructive role of sensory periphery in patterning of cortical maps was further corroborated by several lines of evidence, which indicated that somatosensory periphery-related neural maps and patterns are conveyed by the afferents to their target cells at each synaptic relay station (Erzurumlu & Jhaveri, 1990, 1992a, 1992b; Senft & Woolsey, 1991). However, the mechanisms by which thalamocortical afferent terminals develop patterns, and how they are detected by their postsynaptic partners, and further, how these cells orient their dendrites toward clusters of afferent terminals are poorly understood.

In the 1990s, simultaneous labeling of thalamocortical axons, postsynaptic cells, extracellular elements, and other pattern-forming elements revealed that in the developing rodent cortex, thalamocortical afferents are the first to form periphery-related patterns, which are then used as a template for patterning of cortical elements (Blue, Erzurumlu, & Jhaveri, 1991; Erzurumlu & Jhaveri, 1990, 1992b; Jhaveri, Erzurumlu, & Crossin, 1991). The clustering of thalamocortical terminals into whisker-related patterns emerges during the first 3 postnatal days (Agmon et al., 1993; Erzurumlu & Jhaveri, 1990; Rebsam et al., 2002; Senft & Woolsey, 1991). During this period, the cortical somatosensory map exhibits plasticity in response to changes induced by peripheral sensory nerve lesions (Belford & Killackey, 1980; Durham & Woolsey, 1984; Van der Loos & Woolsey, 1973).

Critical Period Plasticity in the Barrel Cortex

The sensory periphery provides a template for the formation of axonal and cellular patterns in

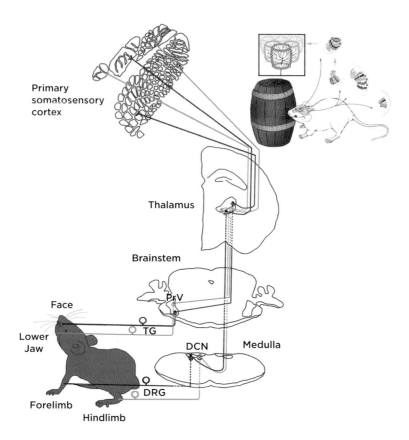

Figure 17.4 Schematic representations of the ascending somatosensory pathways from the periphery to the barrel cortex in mice (left) and patterned face maps (right) leading to the barrel cortex. Six rows of whiskers are first represented as neural modules (barrelettes) in the brain stem trigeminal nuclei, then in the thalamus as barreloids, and finally, in the cortex as barrels. The top left inset in the right cartoon illustrates the organization of Barrels with thalamocortical axon terminals filling in the barrel hollows and layer IV stellate cells forming the barrel walls. (From Lee & Erzurumlu, 2005; Erzurumlu & Kind, 2001.)

the barrel cortex during a critical period in development (see Jhaveri & Erzurumlu, 1992; Killackey et al., 1995; O'Leary et al., 1994; Woolsey, 1990, for reviews). On the rodent snout, whisker follicles are arranged into five curvilinear arrays (rows A–E). Whisker follicle cautery or lesions of the infraorbital branch of the trigeminal nerve (the sole afferent source to the whisker and sinus hair follicles on the snout) before postnatal day (P) 4 irreversibly alter the organization of central neural patterns. For example, when the middle row whiskers (row C) are cauterized before P4, cortical barrels corresponding to these whiskers form a narrow fused band, and the adjacent barrels representing the intact whiskers expand (Figure 17.3; Belford & Killackey, 1980; Jeanmonod et al., 1981; Woolsey & Wann, 1976). If the infraorbital nerve is transected, barrels do not form and the thalamocortical axons are distributed in an aberrant fashion (Bates & Killackey, 1985; Belford & Killackey, 1980; Jensen & Killackey,

1987). A similar defect in the projection zones of the dorsal column lemniscal pathway in the cortex has been noted following embryonic paw amputations (Dawson & Killackey, 1987; Killackey et al., 1995).

The mechanisms that underlie pattern formation and developmental plasticity are poorly understood. For example, how does the disruption of the sensory periphery, three synapses away from the cortex, alter thalamocortical afferent clustering and consequently, dendritic organization of barrel cells? How does sensory activity shape cortical neuronal connections and architecture early in development? Such observed plasticity events in the rodent trigeminal system have led several investigators suggest that there might be common mechanisms in the developmental plasticity of several sensory systems. This possibility has been most rigorously studied in the visual system (for reviews, see Cramer & Sur, 1995; Goodman & Shatz, 1993; Katz & Shatz, 1996).

In the 1960s, Hubel and Wiesel demonstrated the influence of visual experience on ocular dominance columns in the visual cortex (Hubel & Wiesel, 1964; Wiesel & Hubel, 1963), another distinct sensory cortical region with a receptotopic and patterned map. To manipulate early visual experience, investigators have typically reared newborns in the dark or prevented the entry of light into one or both eyes by suturing the eyelids shut. These studies, mostly done in cats and monkeys, revealed that there is a critical period for the establishment of ocular dominance columns. In the rodent somatosensory system, most studies have employed neonatal whisker follicle lesions or sensory nerve damage. Clearly, the two approaches utilized in the visual and somatosensory systems are different; in one, the experimental animal is deprived of sensory experience without damaging the sense organ, whereas the other entails sensory deprivation by damaging or deafferenting the sense organ. Thus, the generally used term "critical period" plasticity in the rodent somatosensory system actually refers more appropriately to a "sensitive period" during which the somatosensory pathway is vulnerable to the effects of peripheral receptor damage and subsequent sensory deprivation (Erzurumlu & Killackey, 1982).

The Role of Neural Activity in Patterning and Plasticity of the Barrel Cortex and its Molecular Basis

With technical advances in molecular genetics and in vivo imaging, the molecular mechanisms underlying developmental plasticity in the organization of cortical maps are now being elucidated (Cramer & Sur, 1995; Fox & Wong, 2005; Goodman & Shatz, 1993; Katz & Shatz, 1996; Sur & Rubenstein, 2005). For example, gradient expression of positional cues such as fibroblast growth factor 8 (FGF8), Wnts, bone morphogenetic proteins (BMPs), sonic hedgehog (SHH), and transcription factors Pax6, Emx2 in the developing telencephalic primordium help to shape the positioning of somatosensory maps before the arrival of thalamocortical afferents (for reviews, see Shimogori & Groove, 2006; Sur & Rubenstein, 2005).

Target-specific development of thalamocortical projections and their topographic alignment is directed by a variety of axon guidance cues. For example, ephrins and their Eph receptors have been implicated in the topographic alignment of thalamocortical axons in the barrel cortex (Vanderhaeghen & Polleux, 2004). Developing thalamocortical axons express high levels of the growth-associated phosphoprotein, GAP43 (Erzurumlu, Jhaveri, & Benowitz, 1990). In *GAP43* knockout (KO) mice, thalamocortical topography is severely disrupted, and thalamocortical terminals form aberrant patches (Maier et al., 1999). On the other hand, patterning of neural connections within "somatotopic" maps is controlled by neural activity-mediated mechanisms. It has long been known that neonatal infraorbital nerve injury leads to aberrant and broader arborization of thalamocortical axons (Jensen & Killackey, 1987), even when the above mentioned cortical positioning cues and thalamocortical axon guidance cues, three synapses away from the site of injury, are presumably unaffected.

In recent years, glutamatergic neural transmission, its regulation by serotonin (5-HT), and downstream signaling pathways have received considerable attention for their role in the developmental patterning of somatosensory maps. Targeted mutations in the genes encoding *N*-methyl-D-aspartate receptors (NMDARs), metabotropic glutamate receptors, 5-HT receptors, 5-HT transporters (5-HTTs), and altered levels of cortical 5-HT have led to mouse phenotypes with specific defects in pre- and/or postsynaptic patterning (or both) along the mouse trigeminal pathway (for reviews, see Erzurumlu & Iwasato, 2006; Erzurumlu & Kind, 2001). So far, no mutant phenotypes have been identified with the typical patterning of postsynaptic elements (i.e., barrels, barreloids, or barrelettes), without patterning of the presynaptic elements. In fact, if the patterns do not initially develop in the brain stem, pre- or postsynaptic patterning could not be observed upstream in the thalamus or somatosensory cortex (Iwasato et al., 2000; Lee & Erzurumlu, 2005). By contrast, a number of mutants display cortical defects with normal subcortical patterning. These observations further strengthen the conclusions drawn from the pioneering whisker lesion and selective breeding studies discussed above that the sensory periphery plays an instructive role in barrel cortex patterning and the patterns are relayed sequentially from the periphery to the brain stem, the thalamus, and the neocortex.

Most of the mouse lines with specific deficits in thalamocortical patterning involve various aspects of glutamatergic and serotonergic synaptic function (Cases et al., 1996; Hannan et al., 2001; Iwasato et al., 1997, 2000; Salichon et al., 2001; Vitalis et al., 1998) and related intracellular signaling pathways (Figure 17.5; Abdel-Majid

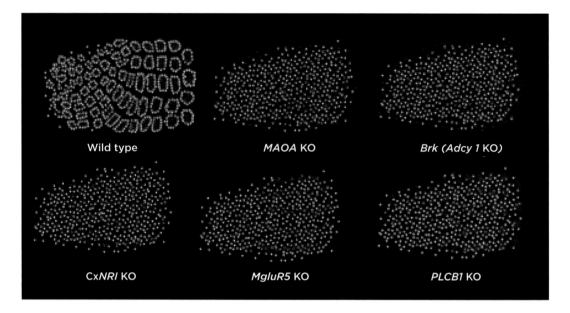

Figure 17.5 Pre- and postsynaptic pattern defects in genetically altered mice (from Erzurumlu & Kind, 2001). Barrel cells are depicted as blue spheres and thalamocortical axons as red arbors. In wild-type mice, thalamocortical axons form patches, which reflect the patterned distribution of whiskers and sinus hairs on the snout. Layer IV stellate cells organize around these presynaptic terminal patches forming the barrels. In various mouse mutants, thalamocortical axons either fail to form patches (consequently no postsynaptic patterns develop, as in *MAOA* KO and *brl* mice) or their patterning is impaired (as in Cx*NR1*, *mGluR5, and PLCβ1* KO mice) and barrels do not form.

et al., 1998; Hannan et al., 2001; Hannan, Kind, & Blakemore, 1998; Welker et al., 1996). The first line of gene targeted mice with whisker-specific patterning defects in the brain was *NR1* KO mice (Li, Erzurumlu, Chen, Jhaveri, & Tonegawa, 1994). NR1 is the obligatory subunit of NMDARs; without this subunit, NMDARs are not functional. Because of early postnatal lethality of the *NR1* KOs, defects in whisker-specific patterns could only be studied in the brain stem (where barrelette patterns can be seen at birth in normal mice), but not in the barrel cortex (Li et al., 1994). A couple of years after the generation of these *NR1* KOs, a spontaneous mutation was noted in the mouse colony in Van der Loos' laboratory in Lausanne. These mice had the normal pattern of whiskers, but barrels were absent in the somatosensory cortex; hence, these mice were classified as "barrelless" (Welker et al., 1996). The underlying mutation was later determined to be in the adenylyl cyclase type I gene (*Adcy1*) (Abdel-Majid et al., 1998). Adcy1 is one of nine adenylyl cyclases and is activated by increases in intracellular calcium (Ca^{2+}) in an NMDAR-dependent fashion (see Sheng & Kim, 2002). Activated Adcy1 catalyzes the formation of cAMP, a second messenger whose primary target is cAMP-dependent protein kinase A

(PKA) (Ferguson & Storm, 2004; Wang & Storm, 2003). In barrelless (*brl*) mice, thalamocortical axon arbors were broader than normal, suggesting a presynaptic role for Adcy1 in pattern formation (Gheorghita, Kraftsik, Dubois, & Welker, 2006; Welker et al., 1996). In the *brl* mice, the response of presumptive barrel cortex neurons to whisker stimulation was abnormal, and there was a prominent disruption of AMPA receptor surface expression, and long-term potentiation (LTP) and long-term depression (LTD) in layer IV neurons (Lu et al., 2003; Welker et al., 1996).

Generation of a cortex-specific KO of the *NR1* subunit (Cx*NR1*) presented a phenotype (Datwani et al., 2002a; Iwasato et al., 2000; Lee, Iwasato, Itohara, & Erzurumlu, 2005) somewhat similar to the *brl* mice described above. In Cx*NR1* KO mice, thalamocortical axons formed rudimentary patterns still faithfully replicating the patterned organization of whiskers on the snout. However, individual arbors had widespread territories. Furthermore, the organization of stellate cells into barrels and their skewed dendritic orientation toward the thalamocortical axon terminals was disrupted (Datwani et al., 2002a). The thalamocortical axon terminal phenotypes and absence of postsynaptic patterning in the barrel cortex of Cx*NR1* KO and *brl* mice indicate that activity-dependent mechanisms are at play in the patterning of the barrel cortex.

A similar barrel cortex defect has been observed in mice lacking one of the regulatory subunits of protein kinase A, PKARIIβ subunit, a signaling molecule downstream from Adcy1 (Inan, Lu, Albright, She, & Crair, 2006; Watson et al., 2006). These mice have defective barrels and lack LTP in layer IV; however, the thalamocortical axon patterning in these mice was better defined than those in CxNR1 KO mice. Because PKARIIβ is present only in layer IV neurons but not in thalamocortical axons (Inan et al., 2006; Watson et al., 2006), the observed pattern deficits further support the notion that postsynaptic components of the cortical barrels can be perturbed independent of afferent patterning. Similar barrel cortex defects have also been reported for mice with defects in other components of the glutamatergic pathway, such as metabotropic glutamate receptor 5 (mGluR5) and phospholipase C-β (PLCβ1) (Hannan et al., 2001).

Another aspect of neural activity at the developing thalamocortical synapse involves serotonin-mediated regulation of glutamatergic transmission. Thalamocortical axons transiently express 5-HT$_{1B}$ receptors (Bennett-Clarke, Leslie, Chiaia, & Rhoades, 1993) and the neurons of the primary sensory thalamic nuclei express the genes encoding the serotonin transporter (SERT) and the vesicular monoamine transporter (VMAT2) (Lebrand et al., 1996, 1998). Whereas thalamic neurons do not synthesize 5-HT, their terminals in the barrel cortex bind exogenous 5-HT via high-affinity 5-HT$_{1B}$ receptors. Mutant mice with increased 5-HT levels or abolished 5-HTT or 5-HT$_{1B}$ function also offer insights into mechanisms of pattern formation in the barrel cortex (Cases et al., 1996; Salichon et al., 2001; Vitalis et al., 1998). Normally, the monoamine neurotransmitters such as serotonin, norepinephrine, and epinephrine are broken down by monoamine oxidase A. Disruption of the monoamine oxidase A (MAOA) gene led to a seven- to ninefold increase in 5-HT levels and to a significant expansion of the thalamocortical axon terminal fields in the somatosensory cortex. Subsequent to disrupted segmentation of thalamocortical axons, barrels did not form (Cases et al., 1996). These cortical deficits were seen even though brain stem and thalamic somatosensory patterns were normal. Pharmacological inhibition of MAOA activity during the sensitive period for pattern formation in normal mice also mimicked the effects observed in transgenic mice (Cases et al., 1996; Vitalis et al., 1998).

As mentioned above, the deleterious effects of excess 5-HT are mediated via the 5-HT$_{1B}$ receptors. 5-HTT KO mice show partial patterning in the barrel cortex. In MAOA and 5-HTT double KO mice, 5-HT accumulates in extracellular spaces and severely disrupts patterning of thalamocortical axons. Deletion of the gene encoding 5-HT$_{1B}$ receptors in MAOA or 5-HTT KOs or in MAOA/5-HTT double KO mice restores barrel phenotypes. Namely, thalamocortical axons segregate and barrels form (Salichon et al., 2001). In vitro recordings from thalamocortical slices indicated that 5-HT has a strong presynaptic inhibitory effect on glutamatergic transmission between somatosensory thalamic axons and barrel cortex cells (Laurent et al., 2002; Rhoades, Bennett-Clarke, Shi, & Mooney, 1994), suggesting that thalamocortical axons autoregulate their glutamate release via uptake of 5-HT present in their target. It should be noted, however, that pharmacological depletion of serotonin in the barrel cortex does not affect barrel formation, but only delays formation for a couple of days. Moreover, such manipulations do not affect the duration of the sensitive period plasticity that follows neonatal whisker follicle damage (Blue et al., 1991; Turlejski, Djavadian, & Kossut, 1997).

Glutamatergic neural transmission, in particular, NMDAR activation has been implicated in patterning and refinement of retinotopic maps in the vertebrate visual system. For example, the NMDA antagonist, APV prevents eye-specific segregation of retinal inputs in three-eyed tadpoles (Cline, Debski, & Constantine-Paton, 1987), ocular dominance plasticity in the visual cortex of cats (Bear, Kleinschmidt, Gu, & Singer, 1990; Kleinschmidt, Bear, & Singer, 1987), segregation of sublaminar projections in the retinogeniculate pathway of ferrets (Hahm, Langdon, & Sur, 1991), and refinement of retinotectal projections in rats (Simon, Prusky, O'Leary, & Constantine-Paton, 1992). Early studies, which examined the role of activity during the sensitive period on the rodent somatosensory system, reported that pharmacological blockade of action potentials by localized applications of tetrodotoxin or NMDA receptor blockade by APV, either in the neocortex or in the infraorbital nerve, did not affect cortical patterning (Chiaia, Fish, Bauer, Bennett-Clarke, & Rhoades, 1992; Henderson, Woolsey, & Jacquin, 1992; Schlaggar, Fox, & O'Leary, 1993). Later pharmacological blockade experiments noted significant alterations in single whisker responsiveness of barrel neurons and functional organization of cortical columns (Fox, Schlaggar, Glazewski, & O'Leary, 1996) and in the morphological integrity of barrels (Mitrovic, Mohajeri, &Schachner, 1996).

One mutant mouse line (Cx*NR1* KO mice) has selective loss of the *NR1* gene in cortical excitatory neurons (Iwasato et al., 2000). In these region- and cell-specific NMDAR-deficient mice, the whiskers on the snout and all subcortical whisker-related patterns are similar to those seen in wild-type mice. But in these mice, barrels as cellular aggregations are missing, the dendritic field bias of layer IV spiny stellate cells (barrel cells) is lost, and the thalamocortical axons form exuberant terminal arbors within which there is some clustering, that is, rudimentary whisker-specific patterning (Datwani et al., 2002a; Iwasato et al., 2000; Lee et al., 2005). Despite these structural defects, the rudimentary patterning of thalamocortical axons exhibited "normal" levels of whisker lesion-induced plasticity and the window of plasticity (through P3) did not change (Figure 17.5). Since thalamocortical axon patterning is the first to appear in the barrel cortex (Erzurumlu & Jhaveri, 1990), and this pattern is subsequently used as a template by the layer IV barrel cells, it appears that postsynaptic NMDAR function in cortical excitatory neurons is not essential for thalamocortical axon plasticity. Thus, it is highly likely that sensitive period plasticity and its duration are set by the levels of afferent activity that start in the sensory periphery and propagate along the trigeminal neuraxis to the barrel cortex. Sensitive period plasticity responses of thalamocortical axons may simply reflect the extension of plasticity effects from subcortical trigeminal centers. Another possibility in explaining thalamocortical axon plasticity in the Cx*NR1* KO mice is the residual NMDAR function in GABAergic cells. Approximately 15%–20% of neurons in the barrel cortex are inhibitory, aspiny stellate cells that express GABA, and migrate to the cortex from the ganglionic eminence during embryonic development (Lavdas, Grigoriou, Pachnis, & Parnavelas, 1999; Metin, Baudoin, Rakic, & Parnavelas, 2006; Parnavelas Alifragis & Nadarajah, 2002). In the barrel cortex, GABAergic elements also show patterns and alterations after peripheral lesions during the critical period (Akhtar & Land, 1991; Kiser, Cooper, & Mower, 1998; Lin, Lu, & Schmechel, 1985). Thus, residual NMDAR function in the GABAergic barrel-field neurons might contribute to the thalamocortical axon plasticity observed in the Cx*NR1* KO mice.

Which molecular and cellular changes along the developing trigeminal pathway lead to the abrupt end of the sensitive period for structural plasticity around postnatal day 3? Is there a "molecular switch" that controls the timing of this period in the barrel cortex? Investigators have sought to discover a potential "molecular switch," which regulates the timing of the barrel cortex plasticity in neonatal rodents. In answering these questions, the NMDA receptor, mainly due to its coincidence detection properties and subunit composition (which regulates channel opening and closure times), has been a prime candidate. The possibility that developmentally regulated changes in the NMDAR subunit composition could act as a "plasticity switch" has been considered. NMDARs are heteromeric tetramers, which contain the essential NR1 subunits with a combination of NR2 or NR3 subunits (Wenthold, Prybylowski, Standley, Sans, & Petralia, 2003). In the barrel cortex, there is a gradual switch from slow NR2B-containing NMDAR and kainite receptor-mediated synaptic transmission to faster NR2A-containing NMDAR and AMPA receptor-mediated transmission after the end of the sensitive period for structural plasticity (Lu, Gonzalez, & Crair, 2001). Experimental evidence from the visual cortex suggests that a developmentally regulated increase in NR2A subunit expression is related to the end of the critical period for ocular dominance plasticity (Carmignoto & Vicini, 1992). Hypothetically, a shortening of the channel opening time for NMDARs with NR2A subunits would block sufficient Ca^{2+} entry for LTP induction. Sensory deprivation (in the form of dark rearing) also extends the period of predominant NR2B expression and light exposure results in a rapid increase in NR2A expression (Philpot, Sekhar, Shouval, & Bear, 2001; Quinlan, Olstein, & Bear, 1999a; Quinlan, Philpot, Huganir, & Bear, 1999b). A similar scenario has been envisioned for the barrel cortex. However, no change in the closure of the critical period plasticity could be detected in *NR2A* KO mice, even though the NMDAR subunit composition and current kinetics remained immature (Lu et al., 2001).

Several other molecular and cellular events known to play a role in synaptic plasticity, most notably in LTP and LTD, have been considered in the context of barrel cortex critical period plasticity. A variety of protein kinases important in synaptic plasticity have been implicated. Genetic invalidation of calcium/calmodulin-dependent kinase II (CaMKII), an enzyme necessary for LTP, blocks receptive field plasticity and NMDAR-dependent LTP in the barrel cortex (Glazewski, Chen, Silva, & Fox, 1996; Glazewski, Giese, Silva, & Fox, 2000; Hardingham et al., 2003); postsynaptic activation of protein kinase C (PKC) increases synaptic strength and is involved in LTP in the barrel cortex (Scott, Braud, Bannister, & Isaac, 2007). Despite the involvement of known players of hippocampal synaptic plasticity in the synaptic maturation of the barrel cortex, none of these molecules has been shown to be essential in governing the timing of the sensitive period for structural plasticity.

Is there a molecular switch for developmental critical period plasticity and its timing in neocortex or in subcortical structures? Clearly, genetic disruption of NMDARs in cortical excitatory cells did not alter the sensitive period plastic responses of thalamocortical axons and the developmental window during which plasticity events take place (Datwani, Iwasato, Itohara, & Erzurumlu, 2002b). In an attempt to distinguish between pattern formation and the effects of peripheral lesion-induced plasticity in the barrel cortex, investigators have focused on the effects of excess serotonin (Boylan, Kesterson, Bennett-Clarke, Chiaia, & Rhoades, 2001; Rebsam, Seif, & Gaspar, 2005). Administering the MAOA inhibitor clorgyline in neonatal rats (Boylan et al., 2001) delays barrel formation but has no apparent effects on the duration of the sensitive period. In *MAOA* KO mice with excess levels of 5-HT accumulation in the cortex, barrels do not form (Cases et al., 1996). When these mice are given daily injections of parachlorophenylalanine (PCPA), an inhibitor of tryptophan hydroxylase that significantly lowers 5-HT levels, barrel formation is delayed (up to P10). Even with this significant delay in barrel formation, whisker lesions after P3 did not have an effect, suggesting that the end of the sensitive period might be set subcortically (Rebsam et al., 2005) (Figure 17.6). Thus, the available evidence indicates that lesion-induced plasticity in the barrel cortex is not dependent on the time of emergence of thalamocortical axons and subsequent cellular patterning in the cerebral cortex. Thalamocortical axon segregation into barrel hollows can be significantly delayed, but the imprints of peripheral lesion-induced plastic changes are still enforced in the cortex.

When anterograde transport from the periphery is interrupted by vinblastine application (an agent that prevents microtubule assembly and thereby blocks axonal transport) to the infraorbital nerve in neonatal rats, the barrel cortex's structural organization resembles that of rats with damage to the infraorbital nerve (Chiaia et al., 1996). However, the nature of this peripheral signal mediating this effect is unknown. Neurotrophic factors produced in the whisker pad, such as brain-derived neurotrophic factor (BDNF) or neurotrophin 3 (Calia, Persico, Baldi, & Keller, 1998), have been implicated in this process, as application of neurotrophin into the lesioned whisker follicles appears to ameliorate structural cortical plasticity.

BDNF mRNA is also expressed in the barrel cortex, and a transient increase in mRNA levels has been detected following whisker stimulation (Rocamora, Welker, Pascual, & Soriano, 1996). Field potential recordings and optical imaging studies with voltage-sensitive dyes in *BDNF* KO mice demonstrate impaired thalamocortical synaptic communication similar to that observed in normal mice that have undergone whisker deprivation (Itami, Mizuno, Kohno, & Nakamura, 2000). *BDNF* KO mice also exhibit a higher proportion of silent synapses, which can be reversed by exogenous application of BDNF (Itami et al., 2003). Thus, BDNF may be one of the factors affecting synaptic plasticity in the barrel cortex, but it does not appear to play a major role in initial pattern formation and sensitive period plasticity.

Concluding Remarks

The molecular and cellular mechanisms that govern developmental plasticity of the cortical somatosensory map are not yet fully understood. Experimental clues lead us to search for these mechanisms in subcortical structures. Molecular signals transmitted from the sensory periphery or brain stem are most likely to set the parameters of cortical plasticity downstream. Thus, thalamocortical axon patterning in the cortex and the duration of the sensitive period for peripheral lesion–induced plasticity probably resides in the templates first formed in the brain stem, which are conveyed to the thalamus en route to the cerebral cortex. This prediction is in line with the conclusions reached by the pioneering studies that demonstrated how the sensory periphery plays an instructive role in shaping the patterning and plasticity of cortical maps.

Acknowledgments

The author's work is supported by NIH/NINDS (NS 039050 and NS 037070) and the University of Maryland School of Medicine Research Scholar Program. I thank Drs. J. Komins, H. Cinar, and Ms. C. Tosun for their help with manuscript preparation, Dr. T. Woolsey for discussions and providing

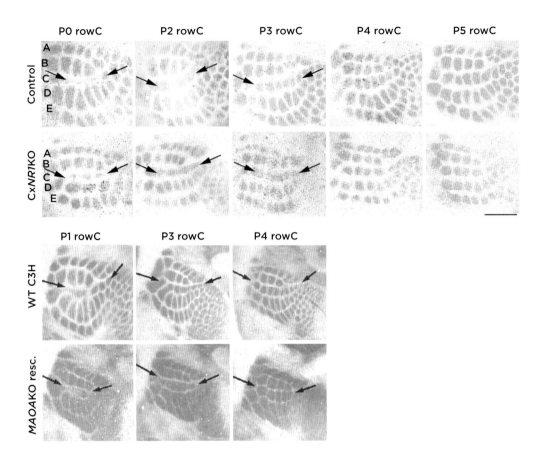

Figure 17.6 Unaltered critical period plasticity in Cx*NR1* KO mice (from Datwani et al., 2002b) and in *MAOA* KO mice with delayed barrel formation (from Rebsam et al., 2005). 5-HTT is used as a marker for thalamocortical axons. Row C whisker lesions at P0 result in shrinkage and fusion of the row C representation (arrows), and expansion of the neighboring thalamocortical patches in the cortex in both control and Cx*NR1* KO subjects. Lesions produced at later ages (i.e., P2 and P3) result in progressively less dramatic alterations. P4 or P5 lesions do not yield any plastic changes in either the control or Cx*NR1* KO mice, thus indicating that P3 denotes the end of the sensitive period for structural plasticity. Scale bar, 500 μm. Barrels can be restored in *MAOA* KO mice by daily injections of parachlorophenylalanine (PCPA), which lowers excess serotonin levels. In these mice, the duration of the row C lesion-induced sensitive period plasticity is also unaltered.

me with some of the original manuscripts of his father C. N. Woolsey, and Dr. M. Blumberg for reviewing and editing the manuscript.

References

Abdel-Majid, R. M., Leong, W. L., Schalkwyk, L. C., Smallman, D. S., Wong, S. T., Storm, D. R., et al. (1998). Loss of adenylyl cyclase I activity disrupts patterning of mouse somatosensory cortex. *Nature Genetics, 19,* 289–291.

Agmon, A., Yang, L. T., O'Dowd, D. K., & Jones, E. G. (1993). Organized growth of thalamocortical axons from the deep tier of terminations into layer IV of developing mouse barrel cortex. *The Journal of Neuroscience, 13,* 5365–5382.

Akhtar, N. D., & Land, P. W. (1991). Activity-dependent regulation of glutamic acid decarboxylase in the rat barrel cortex: Effects of neonatal versus adult sensory deprivation. *The Journal of Comparative Neurology, 307,* 200–213.

Bates, C. A., & Killackey, H. P. (1985). The organization of the neonatal rat's brainstem trigeminal complex and its role in the formation of central trigeminal patterns. *The Journal of Comparative Neurology, 240,* 265–287.

Bear, M. F., Kleinschmidt, A., Gu, Q. A., & Singer, W. (1990). Disruption of experience-dependent synaptic modifications in striate cortex by infusion of an NMDA receptor antagonist. *The Journal of Neuroscience, 10,* 909–925.

Belford, G. R., & Killackey, H. P. (1978). Anatomical correlates of the forelimb in the ventrobasal complex and the cuneate nucleus of the neonatal rat. *Brain Research, 158,* 450–455.

Belford, G. R., & Killackey, H. P. (1980). The sensitive period in the development of the trigeminal system of the neonatal rat. *The Journal of Comparative Neurology, 193,* 335–350.

Bennett-Clarke, C. A., Leslie, M. J., Chiaia, N. L., & Rhoades, R. W. (1993). Serotonin 1B receptors in the developing somatosensory and visual cortices are located on thalamocortical axons. *Proceedings of the National Academy of Sciences, USA, 90*, 153–157.

Blue, M. E., Erzurumlu, R. S., & Jhaveri, S. (1991). A comparison of pattern formation by thalamocortical and serotonergic afferents in the rat barrel field cortex. *Cerebral Cortex, 1*, 380–389.

Boylan, C. B., Kesterson, K. L., Bennett-Clarke, C. A., Chiaia, N. L., & Rhoades, R. W. (2001). Neither peripheral nerve input nor cortical NMDA receptor activity are necessary for recovery of a disrupted barrel pattern in rat somatosensory cortex. *Developmental Brain Research, 129*, 95–106.

Calia, E., Persico, A. M., Baldi, F., & Keller, F. (1998). BDNF and NT-3 applied in the whisker pad reverse cortical changes after peripheral deafferentation in neonatal rats. *The European Journal of Neuroscience, 10*, 3194–31200.

Carmignoto, G., & Vicini, S. (1992). Activity-dependent decrease in NMDA receptor responses during development of the visual cortex. *Science, 258*, 1007–1011.

Cases, O., Vitalis, T., Seif, I., De Maeyer, E., Sotelo, C., & Gaspar, P. (1996). Lack of barrels in the somatosensory cortex of monoamine oxidase A-deficient mice: Role of a serotonin excess during the critical period. *Neuron, 16*, 297–307.

Catania, K. C., & Kaas, J. H. (1997). Somatosensory fovea in the star-nosed mole: Behavioral use of the star in relation to innervation patterns and cortical representation. *The Journal of Comparative Neurology, 387*, 215–233.

Catania, K. C., & Remple, M. S. (2002). Somatosensory cortex dominated by the representation of teeth in the naked mole-rat brain. *Proceedings of the National Academy of Sciences, USA, 99*, 5692–5697.

Chiaia, N. L., Bennett-Clarke, C. A., Crissman, R. S., Zheng, L., Chen, M., & Rhoades, R. W. (1996). Effect of neonatal axoplasmic transport attenuation in the infraorbital nerve on vibrissae-related patterns in the rat's brainstem, thalamus and cortex. *The European Journal of Neuroscience, 8*, 1601–1612.

Chiaia, N. L., Fish, S. E., Bauer, W. R., Bennett-Clarke, C. A., & Rhoades, R. W. (1992). Postnatal blockade of cortical activity by tetrodotoxin does not disrupt the formation of vibrissa-related patterns in the rat's somatosensory cortex. *Developmental Brain Research, 66*, 244–250.

Cline, H. T., Debski, E. A., & Constantine-Paton, M. (1987). *N*-methyl-D-aspartate receptor antagonist desegregates eye-specific stripes. *Proceedings of the National Academy of Sciences USA, 84*, 4342–4345.

Cramer, K. S., & Sur, M. (1995). Activity-dependent remodeling of connections in the mammalian visual system. *Current Opinion in Neurobiology, 5*, 106–111.

Datwani, A., Iwasato, T., Itohara, S., & Erzurumlu, R. S. (2002a). NMDA receptor dependent pattern transfer from afferents to postsynaptic cells and dendritic differentiation in the barrel cortex. *Molecular and Cellular Neurosciences, 21*, 477–492.

Datwani, A., Iwasato, T., Itohara, S., & Erzurumlu, R. S. (2002b). Lesion-induced thalamocortical axonal plasticity in the S1 cortex is independent of NMDA receptor function in excitatory cortical neurons. *The Journal of Neuroscience, 22*, 9171–9175.

Dawson, D. R., & Killackey, H. P. (1987). The organization and mutability of the forepaw and hind paw representations in the somatosensory cortex of the neonatal rat. *The Journal of Comparative Neurology, 256*, 246–256.

Durham, D., & Woolsey, T. A. (1984). Effects of neonatal whisker lesions on mouse central trigeminal pathways. *The Journal of Comparative Neurology, 223*, 424–447.

Erzurumlu, R. S., & Iwasato, T. (2006). Patterning of the somatosensory maps with NMDA receptors. In R. Erzurumlu, W. Guido, & Z. Molnár (Eds.), *Development and plasticity in sensory thalamus and cortex* (pp. 158–182). New York: Springer.

Erzurumlu, R. S., & Jhaveri, S. (1990). Thalamic axons confer a blueprint of the sensory periphery onto the developing rat somatosensory cortex. *Developmental Brain Research, 56*, 229–34.

Erzurumlu, R. S., & Jhaveri, S. (1992a). Emergence of connectivity in the embryonic rat parietal cortex. *Cerebral Cortex, 2*, 336–352.

Erzurumlu, R. S., & Jhaveri, S. (1992b). Trigeminal ganglion cell processes are spatially ordered prior to the differentiation of the vibrissa pad. *The Journal of Neuroscience, 12*, 3946–3955.

Erzurumlu, R. S., Jhaveri, S., & Benowitz, L. I. (1990). Transient patterns of GAP-43 expression during the formation of barrels in the rat somatosensory cortex. *The Journal of Comparative Neurology, 292*, 443–456.

Erzurumlu, R. S., & Killackey, H. P. (1982). Critical and sensitive periods in neurobiology. *Current Topics in Developmental Biology, 17*(Pt. 3), 207–240.

Erzurumlu, R. S., & Kind, P. C. (2001). Neural activity: Sculptor of 'barrels' in the neocortex. *Trends in Neurosciences, 24*, 589–595.

Ferguson, G. D., & Storm, D. R. (2004). Why calcium-stimulated adenylyl cyclases? *Physiology, 19*, 271–276.

Fox, K., Schlaggar, B. L., Glazewski, S., & O'Leary, D. D. (1996). Glutamate receptor blockade at cortical synapses disrupts development of thalamocortical and columnar organization in somatosensory cortex. *Proceedings of the National Academy of Sciences, USA, 93*, 5584–5589.

Fox, K., & Wong, R. O. (2005). A comparison of experience-dependent plasticity in the visual and somatosensory systems. *Neuron, 48*, 465–477.

Gheorghita F., Kraftsik, R., Dubois, R., & Welker E. (2006). Structural basis for map formation in the thalamocortical pathway of the barrelless mouse. *The Journal of Neuroscience, 26*, 10057–10067.

Glazewski, S., Chen, C. M., Silva, A., & Fox, K. (1996). Requirement for alpha-CaMKII in experience-dependent plasticity of the barrel cortex. *Science, 272*, 421–423.

Glazewski, S., Giese, K. P., Silva, A., & Fox, K. (2000). The role of alpha-CaMKII autophosphorylation in neocortical experience-dependent plasticity. *Nature Neuroscience, 3*, 911–918.

Goodman, C. S., & Shatz, C. J. (1993). Developmental mechanisms that generate precise patterns of neuronal connectivity. *Cell, 72*(Suppl.), 77–98.

Hahm, J. O., Langdon, R. B., & Sur, M. (1991). Disruption of retinogeniculate afferent segregation by antagonists to NMDA receptors. *Nature, 351*, 568–570.

Hannan A. J., Blakemore, C., Katsnelson, A., Vitalis, T., Huber, K. M., Bear, M., et al. (2001). PLC-beta1, activated via mGluRs, mediates activity-dependent differentiation in cerebral cortex. *Nature Neuroscience, 4*, 282–288.

Hannan, A. J., Kind, P. C., & Blakemore, C. (1998). Phospholipase C-beta1 expression correlates with neuronal differentiation and synaptic plasticity in rat somatosensory cortex. *Neuropharmacology, 37*, 593–605.

Hardingham, N., Glazewski, S., Pakhotin, P., Mizuno, K., Chapman, P. F., Giese, K. P., et al. (2003). Neocortical long-term potentiation and experience-dependent synaptic plasticity require alpha-calcium/calmodulin-dependent protein kinase II autophosphorylation. *The Journal of Neuroscience, 23,* 4428–4436.

Henderson, T. A., Woolsey, T. A., & Jacquin, M. F. (1992). Infraorbital nerve blockade from birth does not disrupt central trigeminal pattern formation in the rat. *Developmental Brain Research, 66,* 146–152.

Hitzig, E., & Fritsch, G. T. (1870). Über die elektrische Erregbarkeit des Grosshirns. *Archives für Anatomische Physiologie und wissenschaftlich Medizin (Leipzig), 37,* 300–332.

Hubel, D. H., & Wiesel, T. N. (1964). Effects of monocular deprivation in kittens. *Naunyn-Schmiedebergs Archiv fuer Experimentelle Pathologie und Pharmakologie, 248,* 492–497.

Inan, M., Lu, H. C., Albright, M. J., She, W. C., & Crair, M. C. (2006). Barrel map development relies on protein kinase A regulatory subunit II beta-mediated cAMP signaling. *The Journal of Neuroscience, 26,* 4338–4349.

Itami, C., Kimura, F., Kohno, T., Matsuoka, M., Ichikawa, M., Tsumoto, T., et al. (2003). Brain-derived neurotrophic factor-dependent unmasking of "silent" synapses in the developing mouse barrel cortex. *Proceedings of the National Academy of Sciences, USA, 100,* 13069–13074.

Itami, C., Mizuno, K., Kohno, T., & Nakamura, S. (2000). Brain-derived neurotrophic factor requirement for activity-dependent maturation of glutamatergic synapse in developing mouse somatosensory cortex. *Brain Research, 857,* 141–150.

Iwasato, T., Datwani, A., Wolf, A. M., Nishiyama, H., Taguchi, Y., Tonegawa, S., et al. (2000). Cortex-restricted disruption of NMDAR1 impairs neuronal patterns in the barrel cortex. *Nature, 406,* 726–731.

Iwasato, T., Erzurumlu, R. S., Huerta, P. T., Chen, D. F., Sasaoka, T., Ulupinar, E., et al. (1997). NMDA receptor-dependent refinement of somatotopic maps. *Neuron, 19,* 1201–1210.

Jeanmonod, D., Rice, F. L., & Van der Loos, H. (1981). Mouse somatosensory cortex: Alterations in the barrel field following receptor injury at different early postnatal ages. *Neuroscience, 6,* 1503–1535.

Jensen, K. F., & Killackey, H. P. (1987). Terminal arbors of axons projecting to the somatosensory cortex of the adult rat. II. The altered morphology of thalamocortical afferents following neonatal infraorbital nerve cut. *The Journal of Neuroscience, 7,* 3544–3553.

Jhaveri, S., & Erzurumlu, R. S. (1992). Two phases of pattern formation in the developing rat trigeminal system. In S. C. Sharma & A. M. Goffinet (Eds.), *Development of the central nervous system in vertebrates* (pp. 167–178). New York: Plenum Press.

Jhaveri, S., Erzurumlu, R. S., & Crossin, K. (1991). Barrel construction in rodent neocortex: Role of thalamic afferents versus extracellular matrix molecules. *Proceedings of the National Academy of Sciences, USA, 88,* 4489–4493.

Katz, L. C., & Shatz, C. J. (1996). Synaptic activity and the construction of cortical circuits. *Science, 274,* 1133–1138.

Killackey, H. P. (1973). Anatomical evidence for cortical subdivisions based on vertically discrete thalamic projections from the ventral posterior nucleus to cortical barrels in the rat. *Brain Research, 51,* 326–331.

Killackey, H. P., & Leshin, S. (1975). The organization of specific thalamocortical projections to the posteromedial barrel subfield of the rat somatic sensory cortex. *Brain Research, 86,* 469–472.

Killackey, H. P., Rhoades, R. W., & Bennett-Clarke, C. A. (1995). The formation of a cortical somatotopic map. *Trends in Neurosciences, 18,* 402–407.

Kiser, P. J., Cooper, N. G., & Mower, G. D. (1998). Expression of two forms of glutamic acid decarboxylase (GAD67 and GAD65) during postnatal development of rat somatosensory barrel cortex. *The Journal of Comparative Neurology, 402,* 62–74.

Kleinschmidt, A., Bear, M. F., & Singer, W. (1987). Blockade of "NMDA" receptors disrupts experience-dependent plasticity of kitten striate cortex. *Science, 238,* 355–358.

Laurent, A., Goaillard, J. M., Cases, O., Lebrand, C., Gaspar, P., & Ropert, N. (2002). Activity-dependent presynaptic effect of serotonin 1B receptors on the somatosensory thalamocortical transmission in neonatal mice. *The Journal of Neuroscience, 22,* 886–900.

Lavdas, A. A., Grigoriou, M., Pachnis, V., & Parnavelas, J. G. (1999). The medial ganglionic eminence gives rise to a population of early neurons in the developing cerebral cortex. *The Journal of Neuroscience, 19,* 7881–7888.

Lebrand, C., Cases, O., Aldebrecht, C., Doye, A., Alvarez, C., El-Mestikawy, S., et al. (1996). Transient uptake and storage of serotonin in developing thalamic neurons. *Neuron, 17,* 823–835.

Lebrand, C., Cases, O., Wehrle, R., Blakely, R. D., Edwards, R. H., & Gaspar, P. (1998). Transient developmental expression of monoamine transporters in the rodent forebrain. *The Journal of Comparative Neurology, 401,* 506–524.

Lee, L. J., & Erzurumlu, R. S. (2005). Altered parcellation of neocortical somatosensory maps in *N*-methyl-D-aspartate receptor-deficient mice. *The Journal of Comparative Neurology, 485,* 57–63.

Lee, L. J., Iwasato, T., Itohara, S., & Erzurumlu, R. S. (2005). Exuberant thalamocortical axon arborization in cortex-specific NMDAR1 knockout mice. *The Journal of Comparative Neurology, 485,* 280–292.

Li, Y., Erzurumlu, R. S., Chen, C., Jhaveri, S., & Tonegawa, S. (1994). Whisker-related neuronal patterns fail to develop in the brainstem trigeminal nuclei of NMDAR1 knockout mice. *Cell, 76,* 427–437.

Lin, C. S., Lu, S. N., & Schmechel, D. E. (1985). Glutamic acid decarboxylase immunoreactivity in layer IV of barrel cortex of rat and mouse. *The Journal of Neuroscience, 5,* 1934–1939.

Lorente de Nó, R. (1922). La corteza cerebral del ratón. *Trabajos del Laboratorio de Investigaciones Biológicas (Madrid), 20,* 41–78.

Lu, H. C., Gonzalez, E., & Crair, M. C. (2001). Barrel cortex critical period plasticity is independent of changes in NMDA receptor subunit composition. *Neuron, 32,* 619–634.

Lu, H. C., She, W. C., Plas, D. T., Neumann, P. E., Janz, R., & Crair, M. C. (2003). Adenylyl cyclase I regulates AMPA receptor trafficking during mouse cortical 'barrel' map development. *Nature Neuroscience, 6,* 939–947.

Ma, P. M., & Woolsey, T. A. (1984). Cytoarchitectonic correlates of the vibrissae in the medullary trigeminal complex of the mouse. *Brain Research, 306,* 374–379.

Maier, D. L., Mani, S., Donovan, S. L., Soppet, D., Tessarollo, L., McCasland, J. S., et al. (1999). Disrupted cortical map and absence of cortical barrels in growth-associated protein (GAP)-43 knockout mice. *Proceedings of the National Academy of Sciences, USA, 96,* 9397–9402.

Marshall, W. H., Woolsey, C. N., & Bard, P. (1937). Cortical representation of tactile sensibility as indicated by cortical potentials. *Science, 85,* 388–390.

Marshall, W. H., Woolsey, C. N., & Bard, P. (1941). Observations on cortical somatic sensory mechanisms of cat and monkey. *Journal of Neurophysiology, 4,* 1–24.

Metin, C., Baudoin, J. P., Rakic, S., & Parnavelas, J. G. (2006). Cell and molecular mechanisms involved in the migration of cortical interneurons. *The European Journal of Neuroscience, 23,* 894–900.

Mitrovic, N., Mohajeri, H., & Schachner, M. (1996). Effects of NMDA receptor blockade in the developing rat somatosensory cortex on the expression of the glia-derived extracellular matrix glycoprotein tenascin-C. *The European Journal of Neuroscience, 8,* 1793–1802.

O'Leary, D. D., Schlaggar, B. L., & Tuttle, R. 1994. Specification of neocortical areas and thalamocortical connections. *Annual Review of Neuroscience, 17,* 419–439.

Parnavelas, J. G., Alifragis, P., & Nadarajah, B. (2002). The origin and migration of cortical neurons. *Progress in Brain Research, 136,* 73–80.

Penfield, W., & Boldrey, E. (1937). Somatic motor and sensory representation in the cerebral cortex of man as studied by electrical stimulation. *Brain, 60,* 389–443.

Penfield, W., & Rasmussen, T. (1950). *The cerebral cortex of man.* New York: Macmillan.

Philpot, B. D., Sekhar, A. K., Shouval, H. Z., & Bear, M. F. (2001). Visual experience and deprivation bidirectionally modify the composition and function of NMDA receptors in visual cortex. *Neuron, 29,* 157–169.

Quinlan, E. M., Olstein, D. H., & Bear, M. F. (1999a). Bidirectional, experience-dependent regulation of *N*-methyl-D-aspartate receptor subunit composition in the rat visual cortex during postnatal development. *Proceedings of the National Academy of Sciences, USA, 96,* 12876–12880.

Quinlan, E. M., Philpot, B. D., Huganir, R. L., & Bear, M. F. (1999b). Rapid, experience dependent expression of synaptic NMDA receptors in visual cortex in vivo. *Nature Neuroscience, 2,* 352–357.

Rebsam, A., Seif, I., & Gaspar, P. (2002). Refinement of thalamocortical arbors and emergence of barrel domains in the primary somatosensory cortex: A study of normal and monoamine oxidase a knock–out mice. *The Journal of Neuroscience, 22,* 8541–8552.

Rebsam, A., Seif, I., & Gaspar, P. (2005). Dissociating barrel development and lesion-induced plasticity in the mouse somatosensory cortex. *The Journal of Neuroscience, 25,* 706–710.

Rhoades, R. W., Bennett-Clarke, C. A., Shi, M. Y., & Mooney, R. D. (1994). Effects of 5-HT on thalamocortical synaptic transmission in the developing rat. *Journal of Neurophysiology, 72,* 2438–2450.

Rocamora, N., Welker, E., Pascual, M., & Soriano, E. (1996). Upregulation of BDNF mRNA expression in the barrel cortex of adult mice after sensory stimulation. *The Journal of Neuroscience, 16,* 4411–4419.

Salichon, N., Gaspar, P., Upton, A. L., Picaud, S., Hanoun, N., Hamon, M., et al. (2001). Excessive activation of serotonin (5-HT) 1B receptors disrupts the formation of sensory maps in monoamine oxidase A and 5-HT transporter knock-out mice. *The Journal of Neuroscience, 21,* 884–896.

Schlaggar, B. L., Fox, K., & O'Leary, D. D. (1993). Postsynaptic control of plasticity in developing somatosensory cortex. *Nature, 364,* 623–626.

Scott, H. L., Braud, S., Bannister, N. J., & Isaac, J. T. R. (2007). Synaptic strength at the thalamocortical input to layer IV neonatal barrel cortex is regulated by protein kinase C. *Neuropharmacology, 52,* 185–192.

Senft, S. L., & Woolsey, T. A. (1991). Growth of thalamic afferents into mouse barrel cortex. *Cerebral Cortex, 1,* 308–335.

Sheng, M., & Kim, M. J. (2002). Postsynaptic signaling and plasticity mechanisms. *Science, 298,* 776–780.

Shimogori, T., & Grove, E. A. (2006). Subcortical and neocortical guidance of area-specific thalamic innervation. In R. Erzurumlu, W. Guido, & Z. Molnár (Eds.), *Development and plasticity in sensory thalamus and cortex* (pp. 42–53). New York: Springer.

Simon, D. K., Prusky, G. T., O'Leary, D. D., & Constantine-Paton, M. (1992). *N*-methyl-D-aspartate receptor antagonists disrupt the formation of a mammalian neural map. *Proceedings of the National Academy of Sciences, USA, 89,* 10593–10597.

Steffen, H., & Van der Loos, H. (1980). Early lesions of mouse vibrissal follicles: Their influence on dendrite orientation in the cortical barrel field. *Experimental Brain Research, 40,* 419–431.

Sur, M., & Rubenstein, J. L. R. (2005). Patterning and plasticity of the cerebral cortex. *Science, 310,* 805–810.

Turlejski, K., Djavadian, R. L., & Kossut, M. (1997). Neonatal serotonin depletion modifies development but not plasticity in rat barrel cortex. *Neuroreport, 8,* 1823–1828.

Vanderhaeghen, P., & Polleux, F. (2004). Developmental mechanisms patterning thalamocortical projections: Intrinsic, extrinsic and in between. *Trends in Neurosciences, 27,* 384–391.

Van der Loos, H. (1976). Barreloids in mouse somatosensory thalamus. *Neuroscience Letters, 2,* 1–6.

Van der Loos, H., Dörfl, H., & Welker, E. (1984). Variation in pattern of mystacial vibrissae in mice. A quantitative study of ICR stock and several inbred strains. *Journal of Heredity, 75,* 326–336.

Van der Loos, H., Welker, E., Dörfl, J., & Rumo, G. (1986). Selective breeding for variations in patterns of mystacial vibrissae of mice. Bilaterally symmetrical strains derived from ICR stock. *Journal of Heredity, 77,* 66–82.

Van der Loos, H., & Woolsey, T. A. (1973). Somatosensory cortex: Structural alterations following early injury to sense organs. *Science, 179,* 395–398.

Vitalis, T., Cases, O., Callebert, J., Launay, J. M., Price, D. J., Seif, I., et al. (1998). Effects of monoamine oxidase A inhibition on barrel formation in the mouse somatosensory cortex: Determination of a sensitive developmental period. *The Journal of Comparative Neurology, 393,* 169–184.

Wang, H., & Storm, D. R. (2003). Calmodulin-regulated adenylyl cyclases: Cross-talk and plasticity in the central nervous system. *Molecular Pharmacology, 63,* 463–468.

Watson, R. F., Abdel-Majid, R. M., Barnett, M. W., Willis, B. S., Katsnelson, A., Gillingwater, T. H., et al. (2006).

Involvement of protein kinase A in patterning of the mouse somatosensory cortex. *The Journal of Neuroscience, 26*, 5393–5401.

Welker, C. (1971). Microelectrode delineation of fine grain somatotopic organization of (SmI) cerebral neocortex in albino rat. *Brain Research, 26*, 259–275.

Welker, E., Armstrong-James, M., Bronchti, G., Ourednik, W., Gheorghita-Baechler, F., Dubois, R., et al. (1996). Altered sensory processing in the somatosensory cortex of the mouse mutant barrelless. *Science, 271*, 1864–1867.

Welker, E., & Van der Loos, H. (1986). Quantitative correlation between barrel-field size and the sensory innervation of the whisker pad: A comparative study in six strains of mice bred for different patterns of mystacial vibrissae. *The Journal of Neuroscience, 6*, 3355–3373.

Wenthold, R. J., Prybylowski, K., Standley, S., Sans, N., & Petralia, R. S. (2003). Trafficking of NMDA receptors. *Annual Review of Pharmacology and Toxicology, 43*, 335–358.

Wiesel, T. N., & Hubel, D. H. (1963). Single-cell responses in striate cortex of kittens deprived of vision in one eye. *Journal of Neurophysiology, 26*, 1003–1017.

Woolsey, C. N. (1964). Cortical localization as defined by evoked potential and electrical stimulation studies. In G. Schaltenbrand & C. N. Woolsey (Eds.), *Cerebral localization and organization* (pp. 17–26). Madison and Milwaukee, WI: The University of Wisconsin Press.

Woolsey, C. N., Marshall, W. H., & Bard, P. (1942). Representation of cutaneous tactile sensibility in the cerebral cortex of the monkey as indicated by evoked potentials. *Bulletin of the Johns Hopkins Hospital, 70*, 399–441.

Woolsey, T. A. (1990). Peripheral alteration and somatosensory development. In E. J. Coleman (Ed.), *Development of sensory systems in mammals* (pp. 461–516). New York: Wiley.

Woolsey, T. A. (2005). Barrel Cortex. *IBRO Science Issues/ Neuro History*. Retrieved April 20, 2009, from http://www.ibro.org/Pub_Main_Display.asp?Main_ID=21

Woolsey, T. A., Dierker, M. L., & Wann, D. F. (1975). Mouse SmI cortex: Qualitative and quantitative classification of golgi-impregnated barrel neurons. *Proceedings of the National Academy of Sciences, USA, 72*, 2165–2169.

Woolsey, T. A., & Van der Loos, H. (1970). The structural organization of layer IV in the somatosensory region (SI) of mouse cerebral cortex. The description of a cortical field composed of discrete cytoarchitectonic units. *Brain Research, 17*, 205–242.

Woolsey, T. A., & Wann, J. R. (1976). Areal changes in mouse cortical barrels following vibrissal damage at different postnatal ages. *The Journal of Comparative Neurology, 170*, 53–66.

Cross-Modal Plasticity in the Mammalian Neocortex

Sarah J. Karlen, Deborah L. Hunt, *and* Leah Krubitzer

Abstract

Cross-modal plasticity refers to how the loss of sensory activity within one modality affects the development of the remaining modalities at cortical and subcortical levels. Two approaches are used to understand how this plasticity is generated. A comparative approach is used to determine how aspects of cortical organization are altered across species with natural enhancement of a sensory system, whereas a developmental approach is used to determine the factors that contribute to sensory domain allocation as well as the functional assignment of cortical fields. Together, comparative and developmental studies suggest that a cortical field is a combination of the sensory-driven input each sensory system receives during development and the genes that contribute to basic aspects of cortical field emergence including location, size, and connectivity.

Keywords: Sensory-driven activity, congenital sensory loss, development, multimodal plasticity, cortical fields, sensory domains, evolution

Introduction

The neocortex is a highly dynamic structure, particularly during development. In fact, recent studies in humans and other animals indicate that a substantial amount of the neocortex can be reorganized following the early loss of sensory inputs. Specifically, neurons in the deprived cortex become responsive to stimulation of the remaining sensory modalities. Even in adults, the functional organization of cortical areas can be significantly modified by sensory experiences (e.g., Merzenich & Kaas, 1982; Recanzone, Merzenich, Jenkins, Grajski, & Dinse, 1992). This remarkable plasticity throughout the life of an animal seems to be at odds with recent developmental studies, which demonstrate that highly conserved patterns of gene expression play a pivotal role in the emergence and development of cortical fields in mammals. Further, the precise nature of the spatial and temporal patterns of gene expression, as well as the developmental cascades upon which their expression depends, must constrain the types of changes that can be made to the developing and evolving neocortex. While a number of studies have demonstrated that sensory experience or sensory-driven activity can influence the development of cortical fields in terms of their connections and functional properties, most studies have only focused on limited portions of the nervous system and have not explored how sensory activity within one modality affects the other sensory systems (e.g., see Majewska & Sur, 2006; O'Leary & Nakagawa, 2002; Pallas, 2001, for review). This phenomenon, in which changes in one sensory system alter the development of the remaining sensory systems, is called cross-modal plasticity. In this chapter, we will discuss the cross-modal plasticity of the neocortex, particularly in terms of functional organization and connectivity.

The relative contributions of sensory experience and genetic factors to the development of cortical fields continue to be debated. For example, some believe that genetic factors play the leading role in establishing the location, size, and connectivity of cortical fields (e.g., Sur & Rubenstein, 2005; O'Leary, Chou, & Sahara, 2007). By contrast, others believe that sensory experience not only refines existing organization, but also plays an equal role with genetic factors in the development of cortical fields (e.g., Krubitzer & Kahn, 2003; Krubitzer, 2007). While one must concede that genes do control many processes, it is hard to isolate their exact role because genes do not work in a vacuum; there is an ongoing interaction between the expression of genes intrinsic to the cortex, intrinsic to the animal, and the environment that an animal inhabits. Nevertheless, there are aspects of the developmental process that seem to be invariant from one generation to the next regardless of alterations in the body or the environment. This indicates that certain developmental processes are intrinsically regulated by genes, whereas other processes are based on the sensory experience of the individual animal.

In some ways, it seems intuitive that the physical parameters of the environment should play a fundamental role in shaping the structure that will ultimately enable an animal to detect, perceive, and execute appropriate behaviors in their unique and dynamic environment. However, like genes, the physical stimuli that impinge on sensory receptor arrays, although variable in their distribution in time and space, are invariant in nature. For example, there are invariant forms of physical energy that obey fundamental, physical laws that control how energy moves, such as how photons travel, how sound waves propagate, and how molecules combine and interact with each other. Consequently, these fixed features of the world limit the way in which sensory receptors, such as photoreceptors, mechanoreceptors, and chemoreceptors, can be modified. These limitations have shaped the evolution of sensory transduction, which in turn constrains the patterns of sensory-driven activity that can be delivered to the developing brain. Thus, as with genes, the physical parameters of the environment constrain brain development and evolution (Krubitzer, 2009).

Given these genetic and environmental constraints, how is cross-modal plasticity generated in the neocortex? There are two general approaches to address this question. First, one can adopt a comparative approach and examine neocortical organization in species with naturally modified sensory receptor arrays and peripheral morphology, and determine if and how the neocortex was altered in different lineages that have evolved extreme modifications in their sensory periphery. Alternatively, one can adopt a developmental approach and examine the effect of altered sensory array activity on cortical field organization. In this chapter, we utilize a combined comparative and developmental approach. First, we begin by discussing the primary subdivisions of the neocortex and how aspects of cortical organization are altered across species. We then describe the development of the neocortex and factors that contribute to cortical field emergence and organization. Finally, we discuss the organizational changes to the neocortex that occur following congenital loss of sensory arrays or impairment of sensory-driven activity in human and nonhuman animals.

Sensory Neocortex in Mammals: Evolutionary Cross-Modal Plasticity

As noted above, one way to understand the role of sensory-driven activity on neocortical organization is to examine mammals with naturally modified sensory systems. This has been done for a variety of mammalian species, and a strong relationship has been observed between peripheral sensory morphology and the two major features of neocortical organization: cortical fields and sensory domains.

Cortical Fields

Traditionally, the neocortex is divided into cortical fields or areas, which are defined using a number of criteria including architectonic appearance, neuronal response properties, and cortical and subcortical connections (Kaas, 1982, 1983). While all mammals possess a basic plan of cortical organization that is composed of several cortical fields with specific patterns of connections, different species have different relative sizes of cortical areas, numbers of cortical fields, functional organization, and connectivity (Figure 18.1). This variability in cortical field organization is thought to generate the behavioral diversity exhibited by various mammals. Cortical areas common to all mammals include the primary visual area (V1; Rosa & Krubitzer, 1999), the primary somatosensory area (S1; Johnson, 1990; Kaas, 1983), and the primary auditory area (A1; Ehret, 1997; see Krubitzer & Kaas, 2005, for review).

Comparative studies indicate that in all mammals, V1 is always located caudally on the cortical

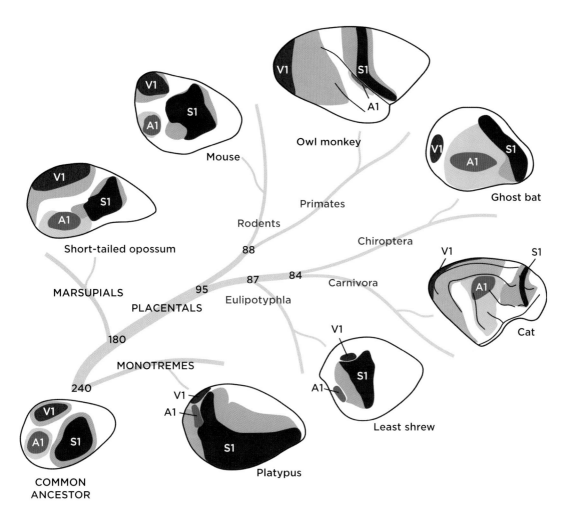

Figure 18.1 All mammals studied possess a primary visual area (V1; dark blue), a primary somatosensory area (S1, dark red), and a primary auditory area (A1, dark green). These primary areas contain a complete representation of the sensory epithelium that is coextensive with a unique architectonic appearance and pattern of connectivity. In addition, most animals possess other cortical fields devoted to processing information from a single sensory system. Combined, these larger subdivisions of the neocortex are termed sensory domains. Shown here is the visual domain depicted in light and dark blue, the somatosensory domain in light and dark red, and the auditory domain in light and dark green. While all mammals possess a basic plan of cortical organization, different species have different relative sizes of cortical areas and sensory domains, and this variability is thought to generate the behavioral diversity exhibited by various mammals. Short-tailed opossum (Huffman, Nelson, Clarey, & Krubitzer, 1999; Kahn, Huffman, & Krubitzer, 2000); mouse (Carvell & Simons, 1986; Woolsey, 1967); owl monkey (Kaas, 2004); ghost bat (Krubitzer, 1995); cat (Scannell, Blakemore, & Young, 1995); least shrew (Catania, Lyon, Mock, & Kaas, 1999); platypus (Krubitzer et al., 1995); phylogeny (Murphy, Pevzner, & O'Brien, 2004); timescale in millions of year ago. Medial (M) is up; rostral (R) is to the right.

sheet, S1 is always located rostral to V1, and A1 is always located lateral to V1 (Figure 18.1). Each of these primary areas contains a complete representation of the corresponding sensory epithelium that is coextensive with a unique architectonic appearance and pattern of connectivity. Regardless of the morphological and behavioral specializations of many mammals (e.g., Catania, 2000; Henry, Marasco, & Catania, 2005; Krubitzer, 1995), the conserved constellation of fields is always present, even in the

absence of apparent use. For example, the blind mole rat (*Spalax ehrenbergi*) still has a "visual" cortex even though this species is functionally blind (Bronchti et al., 2002; Cooper, Herbin, & Nevo, 1993; Heil, Bronchti, Wollberg, & Scheich, 1991). The ubiquity of these fields, their consistent patterns of corticocortical and thalamocortical connectivity, and their conserved geographic arrangement on the cortical sheet across all mammals indicate that the primary cortical fields were present in the common ancestor, cannot be eliminated under most or all circumstances, and reflect the genetic constraints imposed upon the evolving neocortex.

On the other hand, there are a number of alterations that have been made to this basic plan of cortical organization in different mammals, and to a large extent, these evolutionary changes reflect alterations in peripheral morphology, sensory receptor arrays (such as number and distribution of receptors), and patterns of behavior. For example, in the short-tailed opossum (*Monodelphis domestica*), an arboreal, highly visual marsupial, the size of V1 is large in relation to other primary sensory areas (Figure 18.1; Kahn, Huffman, & Krubitzer, 2000). By contrast, in the least shrew (*Cryptotis parva*), a small insectivore that lives in subterranean burrows, the size of S1 is large in relation to V1 and A1 (Figure 18.1; Catania, Lyon, Mock, & Kaas, 1999). This is consistent with the least shrew's reliance on its somatosensory system for exploring the environment and detecting prey. Finally, in the ghost bat (*Macroderma gigas*), which uses echolocation for navigating its environment and catching prey, the size of A1 is large in relation to other primary fields (Figure 18.1), similar to the organization observed in other echolocating bats (e.g., Suga, 1984, 1994).

In addition to these alterations in the overall size of primary cortical fields, some species have expanded representations within a cortical field of behaviorally important morphological structures. For instance, the duck-billed platypus (*Ornithorhynchus anatinus*) uses its bill for many activities including navigating in water, prey capture, predator avoidance, and mating, and approximately two-thirds of the cortex is involved in processing input from the bill (Krubitzer, Manger, Pettigrew, & Calford, 1995). Similarly, in the star-nosed mole (*Condylura cristata*), much of the cortical sheet is devoted to processing input from the 22 appendages that surround the nose and are used for navigating and foraging (Catania, 2000; Catania & Kaas, 1995). Finally, in the naked mole rat (*Heterocephalus glaber*), the representation of the upper and lower incisors, which are used for foraging, digging, and moving objects, occupy over 30% of S1 (Henry, Remple, O'Riain, & Catania, 2006). These examples serve to illustrate that species with highly specialized body morphology have expanded representations of these behaviorally relevant structures within a cortical field.

Although the size of primary fields can vary dramatically among species, the expansion (or contraction) of individual primary fields does not occur in isolation. Rather, cortical fields that increase their relative size seem to do so at the expense of other fields. This change in the size of cortical fields is directly related to peripheral morphology, the types and distribution of sensory receptor arrays, and the unique sensory-driven behaviors of an animal. We term these types of changes to the neocortex that occur in different mammalian lineages across time *evolutionary cross-modal plasticity*.

Sensory Domains

Recently, we have considered larger divisions of the cortex when making cross-species comparisons. These larger subdivisions of the neocortex are termed sensory domains and are defined as the amount of cortex allotted to each sensory system. As with cortical fields, some aspects of sensory domain allocation are similar across species. For example, the visual domain is located in the occipital lobe, the auditory domain in the temporal lobe, and the somatosensory domain in the parietal lobe. Further, as with cortical fields, the size of sensory domains can vary across species, and this variability is related to the sensory systems that are most behaviorally relevant to the animal. For instance, in the highly visual short-tailed opossum, a large proportion of the neocortex is devoted to the visual system (Figure 18.1), which includes several cortical fields such as V1, second visual area (V2), and caudotemporal area (CT). Similarly, mice (*Mus musculus*) and other rodents rely more on their vibrissae than on their visual system, and relatively more of the neocortex is devoted to processing information from this sensory system (Figure 18.1), which includes S1, second somatosensory area (S2), and parietal ventral area. Finally, chiroptera, such as ghost bats, are echolocating mammals that rely heavily on their auditory system and a large proportion of their neocortex is devoted to processing auditory information (Figure 18.1), which includes A1 and surrounding auditory fields.

We have purposely described extreme examples of sensory domain allocation to emphasize our point that cortical organization in mammals can vary dramatically and, moreover, that this organization reflects and supports peripheral morphology, receptor array distribution, and behavior. However, in most instances, animals do not depend exclusively on a single sensory system. For example, cats (*Felis catus*) rely on both vision and audition, which is reflected by the functional organization of their neocortex (Figure 18.1; Scannell, Blakemore, & Young, 1995). Similarly, prairie voles (*Microtus ochrogaster*) rely on both somatosensation and audition, and the neocortex in this species primarily processes information from these two modalities (Campi, Karlen, Bales, & Krubitzer, 2007). Finally, owl monkeys (*Aotus trivirgatus*) and other primates rely on both vision and somatosensation, and they have a large proportion of their neocortex devoted to processing input from both modalities (Figure 18.1; Kaas, 2004). Thus, the amount of the cortical sheet that is allocated to each sensory domain closely reflects the sensory systems that are most behaviorally relevant to the animal.

As with the organization of individual cortical fields, these studies demonstrate that sensory domain allocation also varies across lineages, and suggests that cross-modal plasticity within the neocortex is related to alterations in peripheral sensory morphology, sensory-driven activity, and use. However, the extent to which these cortical field and sensory domain differences between species are genetically mediated, and thus heritable, or are due to sensory-driven activity during development, and not directly heritable, is not known.

Development of the Neocortex

Traditionally, developmental mechanisms involved in parceling the neocortex into separate fields have been broken down into intrinsic and extrinsic factors. Intrinsic factors are defined here as features of development that occur solely within the neocortex, such as changes in cell division and cell death, shifts in the global patterns of gene expression, and variations in protein translation and posttranslational modifications. Extrinsic factors influence neocortical development but do not originate within the cortex, such as shifts in circulating hormonal levels, changes in thalamocortical connectivity, and variations in the pattern of activity received from the external environment and relayed through sensory receptors. Extrinsic factors, as defined here, refer to the more limited set of features, such as sensory-driven activity patterns that occur outside of the cortex entirely, but directly influence the developing neocortex. There is strong evidence that both intrinsic and extrinsic factors play a role in neocortical development and that both contribute to the differences observed across species, although extrinsic factors are likely to play a larger role in cross-modal plasticity within the lifetime of an individual.

Intrinsic Factors That Shape Cortical Field Development and Evolution

There is ample evidence indicating that intrinsic factors, such as genes expressed within the developing neocortex, play a significant role in specifying the gross geometric, anatomical relationships of the neocortex. Early in development, positional information is provided to the cortical primordium by signaling centers that produce secreted molecules, such as fibroblast growth factor (FGF) proteins that are involved with patterning of the anterior/posterior axis and other molecules that pattern the dorsal/ventral axis, such as bone morphogenetic proteins (BMPs) and Wingless-Int (Wnt) proteins (e.g., see Grove & Fukuchi-Shimogori, 2003; Monuki & Walsh, 2001; Rash & Grove, 2006; Sur & Rubenstein, 2005, for review). These patterning centers are highly conserved across lineages (see Barembaum & Bronner-Fraser, 2005, for review).

Secreted proteins, such as FGF, BMP, and Wnt, interact to generate graded expressions of transcription factors in the ventricular and subventricular zones of the neocortex, which in turn regulate different aspects of cortical development. For example, FGF8 has been shown to play a role in establishing the anterior–posterior axis of the neocortex (Fukuchi-Shimogori & Grove, 2001), and Wnt signaling has been shown to be involved in patterning the dorsal–ventral axis (Grove, Tole, Limon, Yip, & Ragsdale, 1998). Changes in FGF8 and Wnt signaling interact to regulate the expression of two transcription factors important for the regionalization of the neocortex, *Emx2* and *Pax6*, which are expressed in opposing gradients (see O'Leary & Nakagawa, 2002; Rash & Grove, 2006; O'Leary et al., 2007, for review). By changing the graded expression of these transcription factors, the size and location of cortical fields on the cortical sheet can be altered. For example, *Emx2* is expressed in a low-rostral/high-caudal and low-lateral/high-medial gradient, whereas *Pax6* is expressed in a low-caudal/high-rostral and low-medial/high-lateral gradient (Figure 18.2) (Bishop, Goudreau, & O'Leary, 2000). In *Emx2* knockout mice, rostral cortical areas, such as somatosensory cortex, expand while caudal areas, such as visual cortex, contract (Figure 18.2). *Pax6* mutants show shifts in cortical areas in the opposite direction from *Emx2* mutants, as predicted by their complementary expression patterns, with caudal areas showing expansion and rostral areas showing contraction (Bishop et al., 2000). In addition, when *Emx2* is overexpressed, using nestin-*Emx2* transgenic mice, an expansion of visual cortex is observed (Figure 18.2; Hamasaki, Leingartner, Ringstedt, & O'Leary, 2004).

These transcription factors regulate the region-specific expression of other genes that appear to be directly related to the emergence and further development of cortical fields into the adult phenotype, as well as in the development of thalamocortical and corticocortical connections. For example, *cadherin 6* (*Cad6*), *Cad8*, and *Cad11* are cell adhesion molecules that are regionally expressed in both the neocortex and thalamus; furthermore, there is a matching expression pattern between the primary sensory areas in cortex and their corresponding thalamic nuclei (Nakagawa, Johnson, & O'Leary, 1999; Suzuki, Inoue, Kimura, Tanaka, & Takeichi, 1997). Similarly, the Eph family of receptors, in conjunction with the ephrin ligands, act as axon guidance molecules for incoming thalamocortical axons in both the visual and somatosensory systems (e.g., see Bolz et al., 2004; O'Leary & Nakagawa, 2002; Vanderhaeghen & Polleux, 2004, for review).

Taken together, these studies in developing animals indicate that several of the ubiquitous features of cortical organization, such as the presence of primary sensory fields and their location are intrinsically regulated and predominantly under the influence (control) of genes. The size and connectivity of primary sensory areas can be intrinsically regulated as well, but they are also shaped by extrinsic influences as well (described below). What is not clear is how alterations in the features of cortical organization are accomplished during the life of an individual, given the control that genes have on the formation of cortical areas and patterns of connections during development.

Extrinsic Factors That Shape Cortical Field Development and Evolution

During development, genes do not function in isolation, but are influenced by a number of extrinsic factors present in the internal and external environment of the developing neocortex. For example, the physical properties of the environment are necessarily conveyed through sensory receptors, which transmit patterns of activity to the developing neocortex via thalamocortical afferents. Historically, studies have addressed the role of patterned activity in cortical field development within a single sensory system. For example, Wiesel and Hubel (1963, 1974; Hubel, Wiesel,

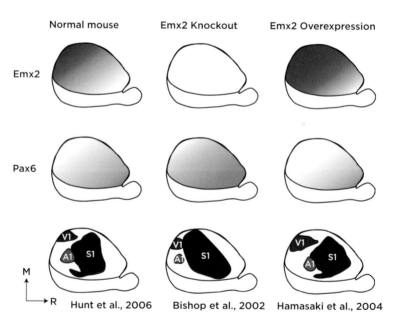

Figure 18.2 Genes intrinsic to the neocortex play a substantial role in determining cortical field size and location. By changing the graded expression of transcription factors, the size and location of cortical fields on the cortical sheet can be altered. Shown here is *Emx2* (purple) expressed in a low-rostral/high-caudal and low-lateral/high-medial gradient, while *Pax6* (orange) expressed in a low-caudal/high-rostral and low-medial/high-lateral gradient (Bishop et al., 2000). In *Emx2* knockout mice, rostral areas, such as S1 (red), expand while caudal areas, such as A1 (green) and V1 (blue), contract. Conversely, when *Emx2* is overexpressed, using nestin-*Emx2* transgenic mice, V1 expands more rostrally, and S1 and A1 are shifted forward (Hamasaki et al., 2004). Conventions as in previous figure; abbreviations defined in Table 18.1.

& LeVay, 1977) demonstrated that experience-dependent mechanisms were involved in normal ocular dominance column development in cats and monkeys. Specifically, they found that monocular deprivation led to a larger cortical representation of the nondeprived eye. Similarly, Rakic (1981) demonstrated that when rhesus monkeys (*Macaca mulatta*) were monocularly enucleated before birth, they failed to develop ocular dominance columns, which suggested that binocular competition is necessary for ocular dominance column formation. Further studies on ocular dominance columns have shown that both sensory-driven activity and spontaneously generated activity are critical for the normal development of visual cortex (e.g., see Katz & Shatz, 1996, for review; Shatz, 1990; Stryker & Harris, 1986). Similarly, Chapman and Stryker (1993) have demonstrated that visually driven activity is necessary for the maturation of orientation-selective responses in visual cortex (see Chapman, Godecke, & Bonhoeffer, 1999, for review).

In the somatosensory system, multiple studies in mice have demonstrated that lesions of vibrissae follicles early in development lead to the absence of the corresponding barrels in the adult neocortex (Rice & Van der Loos, 1977; Van der Loos & Woolsey, 1973) and in strains of mice with supernumerary vibrissae, the barrel field in S1 exhibits extra barrels that correspond to the location of the additional vibrissae (Van der Loos & Dorfl, 1978; Van der Loos, Dorfl, & Welker, 1984; Van der Loos, Welker, Dorfl, & Rumo, 1986). In the auditory system, Zhang and colleagues (2002) examined developmental plasticity by introducing white noise pulses during rat pup development (P9–P28) and found that in the adult rat the A1 tonotopic representation was disordered and frequency-response selectivity was degraded.

Together, these studies demonstrate the effects of extrinsic factors on the development of a single cortical field; however, the effect that a loss or enhancement of sensory-driven activity in one sensory system has on the organization, connections, and functions of the neocortex associated with the remaining sensory systems is less understood. As discussed below, recent studies in both humans and other animals have begun to address this issue of cross-modal plasticity within the life of an individual.

Cross-Modal Plasticity Resulting from Congenital Sensory Loss in Humans

Psychophysical studies have demonstrated cross-modal plasticity following early sensory loss in humans (see Bavelier & Neville, 2002, for review). For example, blind individuals exceed sighted individuals in monaural sound source localization (Doucet et al., 2005; Lessard, Pare, Lepore, & Lassonde, 1998), particularly in peripheral auditory space (Roder, Rosler, & Neville, 1999). Further, early blind subjects perform better than normal subjects on self-localization when auditory cues are used to define the space in which the subject is tested (Despres, Boudard, Candas, & Dufour, 2005). They also exceed sighted individuals in auditory memory for verbal encoding and retrieval tasks (Raz, Amedi, & Zohary, 2005; Roder, Rosler, & Neville, 2001), and auditory memory for environmental sounds (Roder & Rosler, 2003). Moreover, blind subjects have shorter reaction times for tactile and auditory spatial attention tasks (Collignon, Renier, Bruyer, Tranduy, & Veraart, 2006).

Similarly, psychophysical studies have shown that deaf subjects are significantly faster than hearing subjects at detecting a visual stimulus in the periphery, although the reaction time of deaf and hearing subjects is the same for stimuli presented in the central visual field (Loke & Song, 1991; Neville & Lawson, 1987). Further, deaf subjects experienced in American Sign Language show greater right visual field sensitivity for motion processing than hearing subjects (Bosworth & Dobkins, 2002). Finally, deaf subjects are more accurate than hearing subjects in detecting suprathreshold tactile changes, although frequency discrimination is not significantly different between the two groups (Levanen & Hamdorf, 2001). Thus, in humans with early visual or auditory loss, sensory-driven abilities mediated through the remaining sensory systems exceed those of normal individuals and the underlying source of these psychophysical differences appears to be due to functional changes in the neocortex.

Noninvasive functional imaging and electrophysiological studies in both early blind and deaf humans indicate that cortex normally activated by the lost sensory system becomes activated by the remaining sensory systems. For example, positron emission tomography (PET) studies in blind humans indicate that auditory localization tasks activate occipital cortex in regions normally involved in visual localization and motion detection (Weeks et al., 2000). Similarly, functional magnetic resonance imaging (fMRI) studies in blind individuals indicate that Braille reading activates occipital cortex (Burton et al., 2002; Gizewski, Gasser, de Greiff, Boehm, & Forsting,

2003; Sadato et al., 1996; Sadato, Okada, Honda, & Yonekura, 2002), and vibrotactile stimulation elicits activation throughout "visual" cortex (Burton, Sinclair, & McLaren, 2004). Even for high-level perceptual and cognitive tasks, such as language processing, fMRI and repetitive transcranial magnetic stimulation (rTMS) studies indicate that the occipital cortex is activated (Amedi, Floel, Knecht, Zohary, & Cohen, 2004; Burton, Snyder, Diamond, & Raichle, 2002).

Functional MRI studies have also shown that "visual" cortical areas, including V1, process auditory information (Kujala et al., 2005), although not all auditory stimuli have been found to elicit a response in the "visual" cortex. Similarly, event-related potential (ERP) studies demonstrate that for auditory stimulation, the N1 and P3 waves peak over occipital cortex (Leclerc, Saint-Amour, Lavoie, Lassonde, & Lepore, 2000). For higher-level processing, such as auditory memory, ERP and fMRI studies have shown that the occipital cortex is activated in blind individuals, as compared to normal controls (Raz et al., 2005; Roder, Rosler, & Neville, 2000). Finally, a desynchronization of the electroencephalogram (EEG) has been found over the occipital lobe in congenitally blind subjects, as compared to normal adults (Noebels, Roth, & Kopell, 1978). Together, these studies demonstrate that the regions of cortex, normally activated by visual stimulation, become responsive to auditory and tactile stimulation in congenitally blind individuals.

There are only a handful of studies that have examined the anatomical substrate for this cross-modal plasticity in humans. In one study, rTMS over S1 generated significantly higher levels of activity, as measured by PET, in area 17 of early blind individuals as compared to late blind individuals (Wittenberg, Werhahn, Wassermann, Herscovitch, & Cohen, 2004). This suggests that S1 provides input to "visual" cortex through corticocortical connections in early blind individuals. Similarly, a study by Shimony and colleagues (2006) found a decrease in geniculocortical projections in early blind individuals as compared to normally sighted individuals using diffusion tensor imaging (DTI) and diffusion tensor tractography (DTT). These results indicate that the observed functional reorganization is mediated by alterations in corticocortical connections, although no additional projections were detected in the blind individuals as compared to sighted individuals (Shimony et al., 2006).

Cross-modal cortical plasticity has also been demonstrated in congenitally deaf subjects. For instance, functional imaging studies indicate that "auditory" areas are active during a variety of visual tasks in congenitally deaf individuals (e.g., Catalan-Ahumada et al., 1993; Finney, Clementz, Hickok, & Dobkins, 2003; Finney, Fine, & Dobkins, 2001; Nishimura et al., 1999). Further, congenitally deaf individuals exhibit enhanced ERP N1 amplitudes, which are associated with the processing of visual motion (Armstrong, Neville, Hillyard, & Mitchell, 2002) when attending to the peripheral visual field (Neville & Lawson, 1987). Finally, using magnetoencephalographic (MEG) techniques, Levanen and colleagues (1998) found that vibrotactile stimuli applied to the palm and fingers activated "auditory" cortex in congenitally deaf subjects.

While the studies noted above in humans represent only a few of the many studies that demonstrate cross-modal plasticity with early sensory loss, the data clearly indicate that following the loss of one sensory modality, behaviors mediated by the remaining modalities are enhanced. This is likely due to an increase in the amount of cortex devoted to the remaining sensory systems (Bavelier & Neville, 2002; Shimony et al., 2006), alterations in the development of the attentional system (Bavelier, Dye, & Hauser, 2006; Forster, Eardley, & Eimer, 2007; Loke & Song, 1991; Poirier et al., 2006), as well as changes in connectivity along the entire neuroaxis. The details of the functional and anatomical changes that occur both in the neocortex and at subcortical levels following early sensory loss have been recently described in nonhuman animals.

Cross-Modal Plasticity Resulting from Early Sensory Loss in Other Mammals

Sensory compensation has been demonstrated behaviorally following early visual loss in a variety of nonhuman animals. For example, bilateral lid suture at birth in cats results in enhanced precision for sound localization, especially for lateral and rear positions, as compared to normal animals (Rauschecker & Kniepert, 1994). Further, ferrets that were deprived of early visual experience by binocular eyelid suture have enhanced sound localization as compared to normal animals when tested in the lateral field; however, there is no clear difference when they are tested at the midline (King & Parsons, 1999), a finding similar to the results of psychophysical studies in humans. Finally, in bilaterally enucleated hamsters, an unconditioned orienting reflex paradigm was used to examine the direction of orientation and habituation to an auditory stimulus (Izraeli et al., 2002). This study found that bilaterally enucleated hamsters performed like normal animals in terms of correctly orienting toward the stimulus, but they were slower to habituate to the stimulus than normal animals. Although there was no difference in sensory ability, the blind animals were more responsive to auditory stimuli. As in human studies, the cause of these behavioral differences can be traced to functional changes in the nervous system.

In the visual system, there are a number of studies in cats and ferrets that examine the functional and anatomical changes that occur with early visual deprivation via either binocular lid suture or dark rearing. In cats deprived of early visual experience, the majority of neurons in areas 17 and 18 show no orientation selectivity or directional selectivity (Blakemore & Price, 1987; Blakemore & Van Sluyters, 1975). Dark rearing in cats also decreases contrast sensitivity of neurons in area 17 (Gary-Bobo, Przybyslawski, & Saillour, 1995). In ferrets, dark rearing decreases direction selectivity (Li, Fitzpatrick, & White, 2006) and decreases or disrupts orientation selectivity (Chapman & Stryker, 1993; Coppola & White, 2004; White, Coppola, & Fitzpatrick, 2001). Early visual deprivation also decreases the volume, surface area, cortical thickness, and numerical density of neurons in area 17 (Takacs, Saillour, Imbert, Bogner, & Hamori, 1992). When responsiveness to other modalities was specifically investigated in these animals, it was found that 6% of cells in area 17 responded to auditory stimulation (Sanchez-Vives et al., 2006; Yaka, Yinon, & Wollberg, 1999). Further, when higher-order "visual" areas in the suprasylvian sulcus (areas, anterolateral lateral suprasylvian area [ALLS] and anteromedial lateral suprasylvian area [AMLS]) were examined in bilaterally enucleated or lid-sutured cats, most neurons were responsive to auditory stimulation (Yaka et al., 1999).

Similar findings have been reported in areas of the anterior ectosylvian region of early visually deprived cats. In cats with early binocular lid suture, neurons in the anterior ectosylvian "visual" area, which are normally only responsive to visual stimulation, contain neurons that respond predominantly to auditory stimulation (Rauschecker, 1996; Rauschecker & Korte, 1993). Finally, not only are visual areas affected by early loss of vision, but neural responses in nonvisual areas are also modified with early visual deprivation. For example, in cats with early binocular lid suture, a higher proportion of neurons in auditory fields, including the anterior auditory field (AAF) and the anterior ectosylvian auditory field (AEA), are spatially tuned to a particular direction and are more sharply tuned (Korte & Rauschecker, 1993; see Rauschecker, 1995, for review). These findings are similar to those seen in naturally blind animals, like the blind mole rat, in which neurons in "visual" cortex respond to auditory stimuli (Heil et al., 1991).

Since spontaneous visual activity still occurs in dark-reared animals and in those with eyelids bilaterally sutured, as well as in congenitally blind animals, like the blind mole rat, bilateral enucleation experiments have been used to prevent the effects of both spontaneous and sensory-driven activity on cortical field development. In bilaterally enucleated cats, Yaka and colleagues (1999) found that 6% of neurons in area 17 (Figure 18.3), as well as roughly 65% of neurons in extrastriate "visual" areas ALLS and AMLS, respond to auditory stimuli. Further, they found that substantially more cells were responsive to auditory stimulation in bilaterally enucleated cats than in bilaterally eyelid-sutured cats (Yaka et al., 1999). Similarly, about 63% of cells in "visual" cortex responded to auditory stimulation in bilaterally enucleated hamsters, whereas no auditory responsive cells were found in V1 in normal hamsters (Figure 18.3; Izraeli et al., 2002). In rats that were enucleated later in development, about one-third of the cells in "visual" cortex responded to auditory stimulation, although the tuning properties differed from auditory cells in the auditory cortex of normal and enucleated rats, and no tonotopic organization could be identified (Piche et al., 2007).

Finally, in our laboratory, we have found that bilaterally enucleated short-tailed opossums show functional reorganization of visual cortex such that neurons in area 17 as well as extrastriate cortex respond to auditory, somatosensory, or auditory and somatosensory stimulation (Figure 18.3; Kahn & Krubitzer, 2002; Karlen, Kahn, & Krubitzer, 2006). Which sensory system dominates the invaded area varies between animals and is most likely due to differences in strategies implemented by individual animals to explore their surroundings (see Karlen et al., 2006, for more detail).

The differences between these studies in the extent to which "visual" cortex is reorganized (see Figure 18.3) could be due to species differences, but are more likely due to the progressively later developmental ages at which the bilateral enucleations

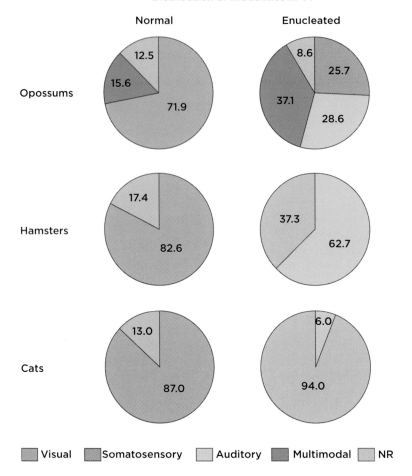

Figure 18.3 Bilateral enucleations early in development result in the functional reorganization of "visual" cortex. Shown here are the percentage of recording sites in architectonically defined V1, which contain neurons that respond to visual (light blue), somatosensory (light red), auditory (light green), and multimodal (teal) stimuli. Lack of response to stimuli from any modality is indicated in gray. The differences between these three studies could be due to species differences, but are more likely due to the progressively later developmental ages at which the bilateral enucleations took place. In enucleated short-tailed opossums, which were enucleated very early in development before retinal axons reach the diencephalon and well before thalamic axons reach the cortex, the majority of recording sites contain neurons that respond to auditory and somatosensory stimulation (Kahn & Krubitzer, 2002; Karlen et al., 2006). In enucleated hamsters, which were enucleated later in development when retinal axons had reached the LGd and thalamocortical axons had reached the subplate but before the formation of cortical layers, most of the cells responded to auditory responses (Izraeli et al., 2002). Finally, in enucleated cats, which were enucleated at the latest developmental timepoint after the retinal axons innervated the LGd and thalamocortical axons innervated layer IV of the cortex, very few of the cells responded to auditory responses (Yaka et al., 1999).

took place. Specifically, opossums were enucleated at an age before retinal axons reach the diencephalon and well before thalamic axons reach the cortex; hamsters were enucleated later in development when retinal axons had reached the dorsal lateral geniculate nucleus (LGd) and thalamocortical axons had reached the subplate but before the formation of cortical layers; and cats were enucleated only after the retinal axons innervated the LGd and thalmocorical axons innervated layer IV of

the cortex. Thus, future research in these and other species should consider the timing of sensory loss relative to other important developmental events.

The functional reorganization that occurs in the neocortex with the early loss of a sensory system (Figure 18.3) appears to be driven by dramatic changes in cortical and subcortical connectivity. For example, Asanuma and Stanfield (1990) showed that in both congenitally blind mice and those bilaterally enucleated at birth, ascending somatosensory projections from the dorsal column nuclei innervate the LGd. Further, in bilaterally enucleated hamsters (Izraeli et al., 2002; Piche, Robert, Miceli, & Bronchti, 2004) and in naturally blind animals, such as the blind mole rat (Doron & Wollberg, 1994), the inferior colliculus has been shown to be the major source of input to the LGd. Likewise, in bilaterally enucleated short-tailed opossums, area 17 receives input from thalamic nuclei associated with somatosensory (ventral posterior nucleus [VP]), auditory (medial geniculate nucleus [MG]), motor (ventrolateral nucleus [VL]), and limbic/hippocampal systems (anterior dorsal nucleus [AD], anterior ventral nucleus [AV]) (Karlen et al., 2006). Finally, there are alterations in corticocortical connections. The callosal pathway between areas 17 and 18 was significantly altered in bilaterally enucleated rats (Olavarria & Li, 1995) and cats (Berman, 1991; Innocenti & Frost, 1980), and in bilaterally enucleated macaque monkeys area 18 had significantly more callosal projections than in normal animals (Dehay, Horsburgh, Berland, Killackey, & Kennedy, 1989). Izraeli and colleagues (2002) did not find any changes in corticocortical connections in bilaterally enucleated hamsters; however, in short-tailed opossums that were bilaterally enucleated very early in development, we found substantial changes in the density of cortical projections as well as the cortical fields projecting to area 17 (Karlen et al., 2006). Specifically, bilaterally enucleated opossums exhibit projections to area 17 from S1, A1, and frontal cortex, in addition to normal cortical projections to V1 from V2, CT, multimodal area (MM), and entorhinal cortex.

There are only a few studies that have examined the functional organization of "auditory" cortex in congenitally deaf animals. In congenitally deaf cats, Kral and colleagues (2003) were unable to find any evidence of cross-modal plasticity in A1 (Figure 18.4). From these results, they concluded that only higher-order auditory areas undergo substantial reorganization following congenital sensory loss. This differs from our own work in congenitally deaf mice, where we have seen extensive cortical reorganization of A1 and the surrounding auditory cortex in adult animals (Figure 18.4; see Hunt, Yamoah, & Krubitzer, 2006, for more detail). Specifically, we found that cortex, which would normally contain neurons that respond to auditory stimulation, contained neurons that responded to somatosensory (36%), visual (15%), or somatosensory and visual (24%) stimulation. In addition to changes in A1, the other primary fields, V1 and S1,

were also functionally reorganized in congenitally deaf animals such that there were more bimodal responses. Further, V1 was significantly larger and A1 was significantly smaller in congenitally deaf mice compared to normal animals, as measured using myeloarchitecture (Hunt et al., 2006). The results of these studies indicate that cortical domain territories shift dramatically in congenitally deaf mice such that "auditory" cortex is taken over by the visual and somatosensory system.

The difference in the extent to which "auditory" cortex is reorganized (see Figure 18.4) between our findings and those of Kral and colleagues could be due to species differences, but are more likely due to methodological differences in the timing of sensory loss in the two studies. Specifically, in the deaf cat study, the organ of Corti progressively deteriorates postnatally (Heid, Hartmann, & Klinke, 1998), whereas in the congenitally deaf mouse study, there is never any sensory-driven activity from the cochlea (Delpire, Lu, England, Dull, & Thorne, 1999; Kozel et al., 1998). Despite this lack of patterned activity in the deaf cats, the brief exposure to spontaneous activity, which occurs normally during development and precedes the onset of hearing, could be sufficient to establish normal auditory connections and prevent the more substantial changes observed in the congenitally deaf mice.

Very few anatomical studies have examined the effect of early auditory loss on neocortical and subcortical development. However, the studies that have been done demonstrate that the loss of auditory stimulation also leads to changes in cross-modal connectivity. For example, in congenitally deaf mice, the loss of auditory activity results in aberrant projections of the retina into nonvisual auditory structures, such as the MG and the intermediate layers of the superior colliculus (Hunt et al., 2005).

Animal models of cross-modal plasticity following early sensory loss are consistent with the results described in humans in that the data clearly indicate that with the early loss of one sensory modality, behaviors mediated by the remaining modalities are improved. As in human studies, there seems to be a negative correlation between the age of sensory loss and the amount of cortical reorganization (Figures 18.3 and 18.4); however, the relationship between the age of sensory loss and the amount of cortical reorganization may not be straightforward. For example, in ferrets deafened as adults, 84% of neurons recorded in auditory cortex responded to

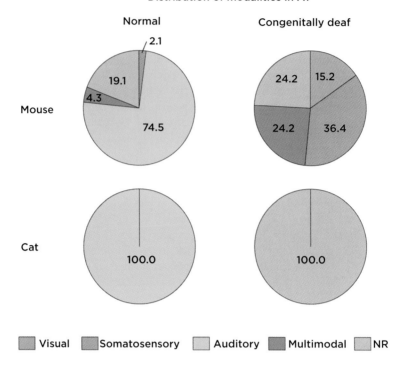

Figure 18.4 Congenital deafness early in development results in the functional reorganization of "auditory" cortex. In mice, congenital deafness results in the functional reorganization of "auditory" cortex. Shown here are the percentage of recording sites in architectonically defined A1 that contain neurons, which respond to visual (light blue), somatosensory (light red), auditory (light green), and multimodal (teal) stimuli. Gray indicates a lack of response to any stimulus. The differences between these two studies could be due to species differences, but are more likely due to the timing of auditory loss in the two experiments. In congenitally deaf mice, which never have any sensory-driven activity from the cochlea, the majority of recording sites in A1 contain neurons that responded to somatosensory and visual stimulation (Hunt et al., 2006). In congenitally deaf cats, Kral and colleagues (2003) were unable to find any evidence of cross-modal plasticity in A1 and concluded that only higher-order auditory areas undergo substantial reorganization following congenital sensory loss; however, in these animals, the organ of Corti progressively deteriorates postnatally, so the animals do have a brief exposure to spontaneous activity during early development.

somatosensory stimulation (Allman, Keniston, & Meredith, 2009). These changes in neuronal response properties did not seem to be due to unmasking or the formation of new cortical connections; instead the authors hypothesize that these changes may be due to subcortical alterations (Allman et al., 2009). Although the mechanisms generating cross-modal plasticity in the neocortex may differ between early development and adults, the data indicate that the loss of one sensory system can lead to changes in the remaining modalities. Further, these changes in functional organization likely result from alterations in cortical and/or subcortical connectivity.

How is Cross-Modal Plasticity Generated in the Neocortex?

Given the examples above, it is clear that the neocortex can be globally affected by changes in

sensory-driven activity during early development, regardless of which modality is deprived of activity. For example, both in bilaterally enucleated and congenitally deaf individuals, not only do we observe reorganization of the neocortical area directly affected by the lost modality, but substantial portions of the remaining cortical sheet also reorganize (Figure 18.5). In some ways, this is analogous to a pebble thrown in the water. The largest displacement (ripple) occurs at the point of entry, which in terms of the neocortex, would be the sensory modality directly affected by the loss. But, successive alterations in neocortical organization can occur a good deal away from the cortical area directly associated with the lost modality. Although the changes do not disperse in a uniform fashion, like ripples in a pond, changes in the affected modality induce alterations in the remaining,

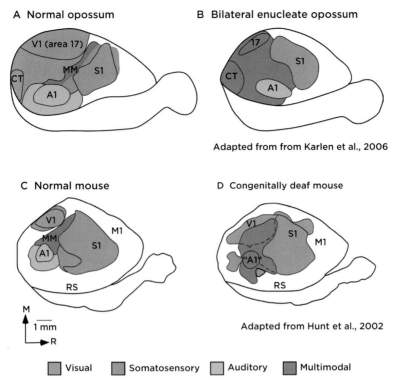

A Normal opossum

V1 (area 17)
MM
CT
S1
A1

B Bilateral enucleate opossum

17
CT
S1
A1

Adapted from from Karlen et al., 2006

C Normal mouse

V1
MM
A1
M1
S1
RS

D Congenitally deaf mouse

V1
S1
M1
"A1"
RS

Adapted from Hunt et al., 2002

M
1 mm
R

☐ Visual   ☐ Somatosensory   ☐ Auditory   ☐ Multimodal

Figure 18.5 In both bilaterally enucleated and congenitally deaf animals, not only is the cortical area that is directly affected by the lost modality reorganized, but substantial portions of the remaining cortical sheet also reorganize. The cortical fields (outlined) and sensory domains (colored) are illustrated for a normal opossum (A), bilaterally enucleated opossum (B), normal mouse (C), and congenitally deaf mouse (D). In the bilaterally enucleated opossum (B), the entire cortex, which would normally be devoted to visual processing, contains neurons responsive to somatic, auditory, or both somatic and auditory stimulation. In the congenitally deaf mouse (D), the entire cortex, which would normally be devoted to processing auditory inputs, contains neurons responsive to somatic, visual, or both somatic and visual stimulation. In both these examples, the cross-modal plasticity is substantial such that all of cortex that is deprived of normal inputs is responsive to new types of sensory stimulation. In opossums and mice, sensory-specific cortical areas can be identified architectonically, although in sensory-deprived animals (B,D), the fields are smaller. (Modified from Krubitzer & Hunt, 2006.) Conventions as in previous figures; abbreviations defined in Table 18.1.

intact sensory systems. In essence, what happens at one point in a fluid, highly dynamic structure like the neocortex affects the development of adjacent points.

The patterns of cortical and subcortical connections provide insight into the neuroanatomical substrates underlying the observed cross-modal plasticity. The fact that normal patterns of connections are intact in both experimental and naturally modified sensory systems suggests that these connections are inherently specified and not easily affected by changes in activity. Conversely, the presence of abnormal wiring, such that normally unimodal structures receive inputs from more than one sensory system, suggests that other connections are greatly affected by sensory-driven activity during development. Whether these are exuberant connections that fail to be pruned or new

connections that sprout during development is not known. Regardless, these activity-driven changes in connections most likely drive the changes in functional reorganization of the neocortex following early sensory loss, which in turn contributes to the observed behavioral changes.

Data from both comparative and developmental studies indicate that sensory systems do not develop or evolve in isolation. Instead, they develop in the presence of other sensory systems, each transmitting some form of patterned activity from a unique environment that governs the combinatorial patterns of activity across sensory systems. While genes appear to determine the global organization of the neocortex, the ultimate adult cortical phenotype (which includes sensory domain allocation and cortical field size, organization, and connectivity) can be altered significantly. Thus, despite the

Table 18.1 Abbreviations

A1	Primary auditory area
AAF	Anterior auditory field
AD	Anterior dorsal nucleus
AEA	Anterior ectosylvian auditory field
ALLS	Anterolateral lateral suprasylvian area
AMLS	Anteromedial lateral suprasylvian area
AV	Anterior ventral nucleus
BMP	Bone morphogenetic protein
Cad	Cadherin
CT	Caudotemporal area
DTI	Diffusion tensor imaging
DTT	Diffusion tensor tractography
EEG	Electroencephalogram
ERP	Event-related potential
FGF	Fibroblast growth factor
fMRI	Functional magnetic resonance imaging
LGd	Dorsal lateral geniculate nucleus
M	Medial
MEG	Magnetoencephalograph
MG	Medial geniculate nucleus
MM	Multimodal area
PET	Positron emission tomography
R	Rostral
rTMS	Repetitive transcranial magnetic stimulation
S1	Primary somatosensory area
S2	Second somatosensory area
V1	Primary visual area
V2	Second visual area
VL	Ventrolateral nucleus
VP	Ventral posterior nucleus
Wnt	Wingless-Int

formidable constraints imposed by genes and the invariant nature of physical energy on the development and evolution of the neocortex, the patterns of sensory activity set up across sensory systems allow for a wide range of cortical phenotypes within the lifetime of an individual and across evolutionary time.

Acknowledgment

This work was supported by a McDonnell Foundation grant and in part by an NINDS award (R01-NS35103) to L.K., and by a NRSA fellowship to S.K.

References

Amedi, A., Floel, A., Knecht, S., Zohary, E., & Cohen, L. G. (2004). Transcranial magnetic stimulation of the occipital pole interferes with verbal processing in blind subjects. *Nature Neuroscience*, *7*(11), 1266–1270.

Armstrong, B. A., Neville, H. J., Hillyard, S. A., & Mitchell, T. V. (2002). Auditory deprivation affects processing of motion, but not color. *Cognitive Brain Research*, *14*(3), 422–434.

Asanuma, C., & Stanfield, B. B. (1990). Induction of somatic sensory inputs to the lateral geniculate nucleus in congenitally blind mice and in phenotypically normal mice. *Neuroscience*, *39*(3), 533–545.

Barembaum, M., & Bronner-Fraser, M. (2005). Early steps in neural crest specification. *Seminars in Cell & Developmental Biology*, *16*(6), 642–646.

Bavelier, D., Dye, M. W., & Hauser, P. C. (2006). Do deaf individuals see better? *Trends in Cognitive Sciences*, *10*(11), 512–518.

Bavelier, D., & Neville, H. J. (2002). Cross-modal plasticity: Where and how? *Nature Reviews. Neuroscience*, *3*(6), 443–452.

Berman, N. E. (1991). Alterations of visual cortical connections in cats following early removal of retinal input. *Developmental Brain Research*, *63*(1–2), 163–180.

Bishop, K. M., Goudreau, G., & O'Leary, D. D. (2000). Regulation of area identity in the mammalian neocortex by *Emx2* and *Pax6*. *Science*, *288*(5464), 344–349.

Blakemore, C., & Price, D. J. (1987). Effects of dark-rearing on the development of area 18 of the cat's visual cortex. *The Journal of Physiology*, *384*, 293–309.

Blakemore, C., & Van Sluyters, R. C. (1975). Innate and environmental factors in the development of the kitten's visual cortex. *The Journal of Physiology*, *248*(3), 663–716.

Bolz, J., Uziel, D., Muhlfriedel, S., Gullmar, A., Peuckert, C., Zarbalis, K., et al. (2004). Multiple roles of ephrins during the formation of thalamocortical projections: Maps and more. *Journal of Neurobiology*, *59*(1), 82–94.

Bosworth, R. G., & Dobkins, K. R. (2002). The effects of spatial attention on motion processing in deaf signers, hearing signers, and hearing nonsigners. *Brain and Cognition*, *49*(1), 152–169.

Bronchti, G., Heil, P., Sadka, R., Hess, A., Scheich, H., & Wollberg, Z. (2002). Auditory activation of "visual" cortical areas in the blind mole rat (*Spalax ehrenbergi*). *The European Journal of Neuroscience*, *16*(2), 311–329.

Burton, H., Sinclair, R. J., & McLaren, D. G. (2004). Cortical activity to vibrotactile stimulation: An fMRI study in blind and sighted individuals. *Human Brain Mapping*, *23*(4), 210–228.

Burton, H., Snyder, A. Z., Conturo, T. E., Akbudak, E., Ollinger, J. M., & Raichle, M. E. (2002). Adaptive changes in early and late blind: A fMRI study of Braille reading. *Journal of Neurophysiology*, *87*(1), 589–607.

Burton, H., Snyder, A. Z., Diamond, J. B., & Raichle, M. E. (2002). Adaptive changes in early and late blind: A fMRI study of verb generation to heard nouns. *Journal of Neurophysiology*, *88*(6), 3359–3371.

Campi, K. L., Karlen, S. J., Bales, K. L., & Krubitzer, L. (2007). Organization of sensory neocortex in prairie voles (*Microtus ochrogaster*). *The Journal of Comparative Neurology*, *502*(3), 414–426.

Carvell, G. E., & Simons, D. J. (1986). Somatotopic organization of the second somatosensory area (SII) in the cerebral cortex of the mouse. *Somatosensory Research*, *3*(3), 213–237.

Catalan-Ahumada, M., Deggouj, N., De Volder, A., Melin, J., Michel, C., & Veraart, C. (1993). High metabolic activity demonstrated by positron emission tomography in human auditory cortex in case of deafness of early onset. *Brain Research*, *623*(2), 287–292.

Catania, K. C. (2000). Cortical organization in insectivora: The parallel evolution of the sensory periphery and the brain. *Brain Behavior and Evolution*, 55(6), 311–321.

Catania, K. C., & Kaas, J. H. (1995). Organization of the somatosensory cortex of the star-nosed mole. *The Journal of Comparative Neurology*, 351(4), 549–567.

Catania, K. C., Lyon, D. C., Mock, O. B., & Kaas, J. H. (1999). Cortical organization in shrews: Evidence from five species. *The Journal of Comparative Neurology*, 410(1), 55–72.

Chapman, B., Godecke, I., & Bonhoeffer, T. (1999). Development of orientation preference in the mammalian visual cortex. *Journal of Neurobiology*, 41(1), 18–24.

Chapman, B., & Stryker, M. P. (1993). Development of orientation selectivity in ferret visual cortex and effects of deprivation. *The Journal of Neuroscience*, 13(12), 5251–5262.

Collignon, O., Renier, L., Bruyer, R., Tranduy, D., & Veraart, C. (2006). Improved selective and divided spatial attention in early blind subjects. *Brain Research*, 1075(1), 175–182.

Cooper, H. M., Herbin, M., & Nevo, E. (1993). Visual system of a naturally microphthalmic mammal: The blind mole rat, *Spalax ehrenbergi*. *The Journal of Comparative Neurology*, 328(3), 313–350.

Coppola, D. M., & White, L. E. (2004). Visual experience promotes the isotropic representation of orientation preference. *Visual Neuroscience*, 21(1), 39–51.

Dehay, C., Horsburgh, G., Berland, M., Killackey, H., & Kennedy, H. (1989). Maturation and connectivity of the visual cortex in monkey is altered by prenatal removal of retinal input. *Nature*, 337(6204), 265–267.

Delpire, E., Lu, J., England, R., Dull, C., & Thorne, T. (1999). Deafness and imbalance associated with inactivation of the secretory Na-K-2Cl co-transporter. *Nature Genetics*, 22(2), 192–195.

Despres, O., Boudard, D., Candas, V., & Dufour, A. (2005). Enhanced self-localization by auditory cues in blind humans. *Disability and Rehabilitation*, 27(13), 753–759.

Doron, N., & Wollberg, Z. (1994). Cross-modal neuroplasticity in the blind mole rat *Spalax ehrenbergi*: A WGA-HRP tracing study. *Neuroreport*, 5(18), 2697–2701.

Doucet, M. E., Guillemot, J. P., Lassonde, M., Gagne, J. P., Leclerc, C., & Lepore, F. (2005). Blind subjects process auditory spectral cues more efficiently than sighted individuals. *Experimental Brain Research*, 160(2), 194–202.

Ehret, G. (1997). The auditory cortex. *The Journal of Comparative Physiology. A*, 181(6), 547–557.

Finney, E. M., Clementz, B. A., Hickok, G., & Dobkins, K. R. (2003). Visual stimuli activate auditory cortex in deaf subjects: Evidence from MEG. *Neuroreport*, 14(11), 1425–1427.

Finney, E. M., Fine, I., & Dobkins, K. R. (2001). Visual stimuli activate auditory cortex in the deaf. *Nature Neuroscience*, 4(12), 1171–1173.

Forster, B., Eardley, A. F., & Eimer, M. (2007). Altered tactile spatial attention in the early blind. *Brain Research*, 1131(1), 149–154.

Fukuchi-Shimogori, T., & Grove, E. A. (2001). Neocortex patterning by the secreted signaling molecule FGF8. *Science*, 294(5544), 1071–1074.

Gary-Bobo, E., Przybyslawski, J., & Saillour, P. (1995). Experience-dependent maturation of the spatial and temporal characteristics of the cell receptive fields in the kitten visual cortex. *Neuroscience Letters*, 189(3), 147–150.

Gizewski, E. R., Gasser, T., de Greiff, A., Boehm, A., & Forsting, M. (2003). Cross-modal plasticity for sensory and motor activation patterns in blind subjects. *Neuroimage*, 19(3), 968–975.

Grove, E. A., & Fukuchi-Shimogori, T. (2003). Generating the cerebral cortical area map. *Annual Review of Neuroscience*, 26, 355–380.

Grove, E. A., Tole, S., Limon, J., Yip, L., & Ragsdale, C. W. (1998). The hem of the embryonic cerebral cortex is defined by the expression of multiple Wnt genes and is compromised in Gli3-deficient mice. *Development*, 125(12), 2315–2325.

Hamasaki, T., Leingartner, A., Ringstedt, T., & O'Leary, D. D. (2004). *Emx2* regulates sizes and positioning of the primary sensory and motor areas in neocortex by direct specification of cortical progenitors. *Neuron*, 43(3), 359–372.

Heid, S., Hartmann, R., & Klinke, R. (1998). A model for prelingual deafness, the congenitally deaf white cat-population statistics and degenerative changes. *Hearing Research*, 115(1–2), 101–112.

Heil, P., Bronchti, G., Wollberg, Z., & Scheich, H. (1991). Invasion of visual cortex by the auditory system in the naturally blind mole rat. *Neuroreport*, 2(12), 735–738.

Henry, E. C., Marasco, P. D., & Catania, K. C. (2005). Plasticity of the cortical dentition representation after tooth extraction in naked mole-rats. *The Journal of Comparative Neurology*, 485(1), 64–74.

Henry, E. C., Remple, M. S., O'Riain, M. J., & Catania, K. C. (2006). Organization of somatosensory cortical areas in the naked mole-rat (*Heterocephalus glaber*). *The Journal of Comparative Neurology*, 495(4), 434–452.

Hubel, D. H., Wiesel, T. N., & LeVay, S. (1977). Plasticity of ocular dominance columns in monkey striate cortex. *Philosophical Transactions of the Royal Society of London. Series B, Biological Sciences*, 278(961), 377–409.

Huffman, K. J., Nelson, J., Clarey, J., & Krubitzer, L. (1999). Organization of somatosensory cortex in three species of marsupials, *Dasyurus hallucatus*, *Dactylopsila trivirgata*, and *Monodelphis domestica*: Neural correlates of morphological specializations. *The Journal of Comparative Neurology*, 403(1), 5–32.

Hunt, D. L., King, B., Kahn, D. M., Yamoah, E. N., Shull, G. E., & Krubitzer, L. (2005). Aberrant retinal projections in congenitally deaf mice: How are phenotypic characteristics specified in development and evolution? *The Anatomical Record. Part A, Discoveries in Molecular, Cellular, and Evolutionary Biology*, 287(1), 1051–1066.

Hunt, D. L., Yamoah, E. N., & Krubitzer, L. (2006). Multisensory plasticity in congenitally deaf mice: How are cortical areas functionally specified? *Neuroscience*, 139(4), 1507–1524.

Innocenti, G. M., & Frost, D. O. (1980). The postnatal development of visual callosal connections in the absence of visual experience or of the eyes. *Experimental Brain Research*, 39(4), 365–375.

Izraeli, R., Koay, G., Lamish, M., Heicklen-Klein, A. J., Heffner, H. E., Heffner, R. S., et al. (2002). Cross-modal neuroplasticity in neonatally enucleated hamsters: Structure, electrophysiology and behaviour. *The European Journal of Neuroscience*, 15(4), 693–712.

Johnson, J. I. (1990). Comparative development of somatic sensory cortex. In E. G. Jones & A. Peters (Eds.), *Cerebral cortex* (pp. 335–449). New York: Plenum.

Kaas, J. H. (1982). The segregation of function in the nervous system: Why do the sensory systems have so many subdivisions? *Contributions to Sensory Physiology, 7*, 201–240.

Kaas, J. H. (1983). What, if anything, is SI? Organization of first somatosensory area of cortex. *Physiological Reviews, 63*(1), 206–231.

Kaas, J. H. (2004). Early visual areas: V1, V2, V3, DM, DL, and MT. In J. H. Kaas & C. E. Collins (Eds.), *The primate visual system* (pp. 139–159). Boca Raton, FL: CRC Press.

Kahn, D. M., Huffman, K. J., & Krubitzer, L. (2000). Organization and connections of V1 in *Monodelphis domestica*. *The Journal of Comparative Neurology, 428*(2), 337–354.

Kahn, D. M., & Krubitzer, L. (2002). Massive cross-modal cortical plasticity and the emergence of a new cortical area in developmentally blind mammals. *Proceedings of the National Academy of Sciences, USA, 99*(17), 11429–11434.

Karlen, S. J., Kahn, D. M., & Krubitzer, L. (2006). Early blindness results in abnormal corticocortical and thalamocortical connections. *Neuroscience, 142*(3), 843–858.

Katz, L. C., & Shatz, C. J. (1996). Synaptic activity and the construction of cortical circuits. *Science, 274*(5290), 1133–1138.

King, A. J., & Parsons, C. H. (1999). Improved auditory spatial acuity in visually deprived ferrets. *The European Journal of Neuroscience, 11*(11), 3945–3956.

Korte, M., & Rauschecker, J. P. (1993). Auditory spatial tuning of cortical neurons is sharpened in cats with early blindness. *Journal of Neurophysiology, 70*(4), 1717–1721.

Kozel, P. J., Friedman, R. A., Erway, L. C., Yamoah, E. N., Liu, L. H., Riddle, T., et al. (1998). Balance and hearing deficits in mice with a null mutation in the gene encoding plasma membrane Ca2+-ATPase isoform 2. *Journal of Biological Chemistry, 273*(30), 18693–18696.

Kral, A., Schroder, J. H., Klinke, R., & Engel, A. K. (2003). Absence of cross-modal reorganization in the primary auditory cortex of congenitally deaf cats. *Experimental Brain Research, 153*(4), 605–613.

Krubitzer, L. (1995). The organization of neocortex in mammals: Are species differences really so different? *Trends in Neurosciences, 18*(9), 408–417.

Krubitzer, L. (2007). The magnificent compromise: Cortical field evolution in mammals. *Neuron, 56*(2), 201–208.

Krubitzer, L. (2009). In search of a unifying theory of complex brain evolution. *Annals of the New York Academy of Sciences, 1156*, 44–67.

Krubitzer, L., & Hunt, D. L. (2006). Captured in the net of space and time: Understanding cortical field evolution. In J. H. Kaas & L. Krubitzer (Eds.), *The evolution of nervous systems in mammals* (Vol. IV, pp. 49–72). Oxford: Academic Press.

Krubitzer, L., & Kaas, J. (2005). The evolution of the neocortex in mammals: How is phenotypic diversity generated? *Current Opinion in Neurobiology, 15*(4), 444–453.

Krubitzer, L., & Kahn, D. M. (2003). Nature versus nurture revisited: An old idea with a new twist. *Progress in Neurobiology, 70*(1), 33–52.

Krubitzer, L., Manger, P., Pettigrew, J., & Calford, M. (1995). Organization of somatosensory cortex in monotremes: In search of the prototypical plan. *The Journal of Comparative Neurology, 351*(2), 261–306.

Kujala, T., Palva, M. J., Salonen, O., Alku, P., Huotilainen, M., Jarvinen, A., et al. (2005). The role of blind humans' visual cortex in auditory change detection. *Neuroscience Letters, 379*(2), 127–131.

Leclerc, C., Saint-Amour, D., Lavoie, M. E., Lassonde, M., & Lepore, F. (2000). Brain functional reorganization in early blind humans revealed by auditory event-related potentials. *Neuroreport, 11*(3), 545–550.

Lessard, N., Pare, M., Lepore, F., & Lassonde, M. (1998). Early-blind human subjects localize sound sources better than sighted subjects. *Nature, 395*(6699), 278–280.

Levanen, S., & Hamdorf, D. (2001). Feeling vibrations: Enhanced tactile sensitivity in congenitally deaf humans. *Neuroscience Letters, 301*(1), 75–77.

Levanen, S., Jousmaki, V., & Hari, R. (1998). Vibration-induced auditory-cortex activation in a congenitally deaf adult. *Current Biology, 8*(15), 869–872.

Li, Y., Fitzpatrick, D., & White, L. E. (2006). The development of direction selectivity in ferret visual cortex requires early visual experience. *Nature Neuroscience, 9*(5), 676–681.

Loke, W. H., & Song, S. (1991). Central and peripheral visual processing in hearing and nonhearing individuals. *Bulletin of the Psychonomic Society, 29*(5), 437–440.

Majewska, A. K., & Sur, M. (2006). Plasticity and specificity of cortical processing networks. *Trends in Neurosciences, 29*(6), 323–329.

Merzenich, M. M., & Kaas, J. (1982). Reorganization of mammalian somatosensory cortex following peripheral nerve injury. *Trends in Neurosciences, 5*, 434–436.

Monuki, E. S., & Walsh, C. A. (2001). Mechanisms of cerebral cortical patterning in mice and humans. *Nature Neuroscience, 4*(Suppl.), 1199–1206.

Murphy, W. J., Pevzner, P. A., & O'Brien, S. J. (2004). Mammalian phylogenomics comes of age. *Trends in Genetics, 20*(12), 631–639.

Nakagawa, Y., Johnson, J. E., & O'Leary, D. D. (1999). Graded and areal expression patterns of regulatory genes and cadherins in embryonic neocortex independent of thalamocortical input. *The Journal of Neuroscience, 19*(24), 10877–10885.

Neville, H. J., & Lawson, D. (1987). Attention to central and peripheral visual space in a movement detection task: An event-related potential and behavioral study. II. Congenitally deaf adults. *Brain Research, 405*(2), 268–283.

Nishimura, H., Hashikawa, K., Doi, K., Iwaki, T., Watanabe, Y., Kusuoka, H., et al. (1999). Sign language 'heard' in the auditory cortex. *Nature, 397*(6715), 116.

Noebels, J. L., Roth, W. T., & Kopell, B. S. (1978). Cortical slow potentials and the occipital EEG in congenital blindness. *Journal of the Neurological Sciences, 37*(1–2), 51–58.

Olavarria, J. F., & Li, C. P. (1995). Effects of neonatal enucleation on the organization of callosal linkages in striate cortex of the rat. *The Journal of Comparative Neurology, 361*(1), 138–151.

O'Leary, D. D., & Nakagawa, Y. (2002). Patterning centers, regulatory genes and extrinsic mechanisms controlling arealization of the neocortex. *Current Opinion in Neurobiology, 12*(1), 14–25.

O'Leary, D. D., Chou, S. J., & Sahara, S. (2007). Area patterning of the mammalian cortex. *Neuron, 56*(2), 252–269.

Pallas, S. L. (2001). Intrinsic and extrinsic factors that shape neocortical specification. *Trends in Neurosciences, 24*(7), 417–423.

Piche, M., Chabot, N., Bronchti, G., Miceli, D., Lepore, F., & Guillemot, J. P. (2007). Auditory responses in the visual cortex of neonatally enucleated rats. *Neuroscience*, *145*(3), 1144–1156.

Piche, M., Robert, S., Miceli, D., & Bronchti, G. (2004). Environmental enrichment enhances auditory takeover of the occipital cortex in anophthalmic mice. *The European Journal of Neuroscience*, *20*(12), 3463–3472.

Poirier, C., Collignon, O., Scheiber, C., Renier, L., Vanlierde, A., Tranduy, D., et al. (2006). Auditory motion perception activates visual motion areas in early blind subjects. *Neuroimage*, *31*(1), 279–285.

Rakic, P. (1981). Development of visual centers in the primate brain depends on binocular competition before birth. *Science*, *214*(4523), 928–931.

Rash, B. G., & Grove, E. A. (2006). Area and layer patterning in the developing cerebral cortex. *Current Opinion in Neurobiology*, *16*(1), 25–34.

Rauschecker, J. P. (1995). Compensatory plasticity and sensory substitution in the cerebral cortex. *Trends in Neurosciences*, *18*(1), 36–43.

Rauschecker, J. P. (1996). Substitution of visual by auditory inputs in the cat's anterior ectosylvian cortex. *Progress in Brain Research*, *112*, 313–323.

Rauschecker, J. P., & Kniepert, U. (1994). Auditory localization behaviour in visually deprived cats. *The European Journal of Neuroscience*, *6*(1), 149–160.

Rauschecker, J. P., & Korte, M. (1993). Auditory compensation for early blindness in cat cerebral cortex. *The Journal of Neuroscience*, *13*(10), 4538–4548.

Raz, N., Amedi, A., & Zohary, E. (2005). V1 activation in congenitally blind humans is associated with episodic retrieval. *Cerebral Cortex*, *15*(9), 1459–1468.

Recanzone, G. H., Merzenich, M. M., Jenkins, W. M., Grajski, K. A., & Dinse, H. R. (1992). Topographic reorganization of the hand representation in cortical area 3b owl monkeys trained in a frequency-discrimination task. *Journal of Neurophysiology*, *67*(5), 1031–1056.

Rice, F. L., & Van der Loos, H. (1977). Development of the barrels and barrel field in the somatosensory cortex of the mouse. *The Journal of Comparative Neurology*, *171*(4), 545–560.

Roder, B., & Rosler, F. (2003). Memory for environmental sounds in sighted, congenitally blind and late blind adults: Evidence for cross-modal compensation. *International Journal of Psychophysiology*, *50*(1–2), 27–39.

Roder, B., Rosler, F., & Neville, H. J. (1999). Effects of interstimulus interval on auditory event-related potentials in congenitally blind and normally sighted humans. *Neuroscience Letters*, *264*(1–3), 53–56.

Roder, B., Rosler, F., & Neville, H. J. (2000). Event-related potentials during auditory language processing in congenitally blind and sighted people. *Neuropsychologia*, *38*(11), 1482–1502.

Roder, B., Rosler, F., & Neville, H. J. (2001). Auditory memory in congenitally blind adults: A behavioral-electrophysiological investigation. *Brain Research. Cognitive Brain Research*, *11*(2), 289–303.

Rosa, M. G., & Krubitzer, L. A. (1999). The evolution of visual cortex: Where is V2? *Trends in Neurosciences*, *22*(6), 242–248.

Sadato, N., Okada, T., Honda, M., & Yonekura, Y. (2002). Critical period for cross-modal plasticity in blind humans: A functional MRI study. *Neuroimage*, *16*(2), 389–400.

Sadato, N., Pascual-Leone, A., Grafman, J., Ibanez, V., Deiber, M. P., Dold, G., et al. (1996). Activation of the primary visual cortex by Braille reading in blind subjects. *Nature*, *380*(6574), 526–528.

Sanchez-Vives, M. V., Nowak, L. G., Descalzo, V. F., Garcia-Velasco, J. V., Gallego, R., & Berbel, P. (2006). Crossmodal audio-visual interactions in the primary visual cortex of the visually deprived cat: A physiological and anatomical study. *Progress in Brain Research*, *155*, 287–311.

Scannell, J. W., Blakemore, C., & Young, M. P. (1995). Analysis of connectivity in the cat cerebral cortex. *The Journal of Neuroscience*, *15*(2), 1463–1483.

Shatz, C. J. (1990). Impulse activity and the patterning of connections during CNS development. *Neuron*, *5*(6), 745–756.

Shimony, J. S., Burton, H., Epstein, A. A., McLaren, D. G., Sun, S. W., & Snyder, A. Z. (2006). Diffusion tensor imaging reveals white matter reorganization in early blind humans. *Cerebral Cortex*, *16*(11), 1653–1661.

Stryker, M. P., & Harris, W. A. (1986). Binocular impulse blockade prevents the formation of ocular dominance columns in cat visual cortex. *The Journal of Neuroscience*, *6*(8), 2117–2133.

Suga, N. (1984). The extent to which biosonar information is represented in the bat auditory cortex. In G. M. Edelman, W. E. Gall, & W. M. Cowan (Eds.), *Dynamic aspects of neocortical function* (pp. 315–373). New York: John Wiley & Sons.

Suga, N. (1994). Multi-function theory for cortical processing of auditory information: Implications of single-unit and lesion data for future research. *Journal of Comparative Physiology. A*, *175*(2), 135–144.

Sur, M., & Rubenstein, J. L. (2005). Patterning and plasticity of the cerebral cortex. *Science*, *310*(5749), 805–810.

Suzuki, S. C., Inoue, T., Kimura, Y., Tanaka, T., & Takeichi, M. (1997). Neuronal circuits are subdivided by differential expression of type-II classic cadherins in postnatal mouse brains. *Molecular and Cellular Neurosciences*, *9*(5–6), 433–447.

Takacs, J., Saillour, P., Imbert, M., Bogner, M., & Hamori, J. (1992). Effect of dark rearing on the volume of visual cortex (areas 17 and 18) and number of visual cortical cells in young kittens. *Journal of Neuroscience Research*, *32*(3), 449–459.

Van der Loos, H., & Dorfl, J. (1978). Does the skin tell the somatosensory cortex how to construct a map of the periphery? *Neuroscience Letters*, *7*, 23–30.

Van der Loos, H., Dorfl, J., & Welker, E. (1984). Variation in pattern of mystacial vibrissae in mice. A quantitative study of ICR stock and several inbred strains. *Journal of Heredity*, *75*(5), 326–336.

Van der Loos, H., Welker, E., Dorfl, J., & Rumo, G. (1986). Selective breeding for variations in patterns of mystacial vibrissae of mice. Bilaterally symmetrical strains derived from ICR stock. *Journal of Heredity*, *77*(2), 66–82.

Van der Loos, H., & Woolsey, T. A. (1973). Somatosensory cortex: Structural alterations following early injury to sense organs. *Science*, *179*(71), 395–398.

Vanderhaeghen, P., & Polleux, F. (2004). Developmental mechanisms patterning thalamocortical projections: Intrinsic, extrinsic and in between. *Trends in Neurosciences*, *27*(7), 384–391.

Weeks, R., Horwitz, B., Aziz-Sultan, A., Tian, B., Wessinger, C. M., Cohen, L. G., et al. (2000). A positron emission tomographic study of auditory localization in the congenitally blind. *The Journal of Neuroscience*, *20*(7), 2664–2672.

White, L. E., Coppola, D. M., & Fitzpatrick, D. (2001). The contribution of sensory experience to the maturation of orientation selectivity in ferret visual cortex. *Nature, 411*(6841), 1049–1052.

Wiesel, T. N., & Hubel, D. H. (1963). Single-cell responses in striate cortex of kittens deprived of vision in one eye. *Journal of Neurophysiology, 26,* 1003–1017.

Wiesel, T. N., & Hubel, D. H. (1974). Ordered arrangement of orientation columns in monkeys lacking visual experience. *The Journal of Comparative Neurology, 158*(3), 307–318.

Wittenberg, G. F., Werhahn, K. J., Wassermann, E. M., Herscovitch, P., & Cohen, L. G. (2004). Functional connectivity between somatosensory and visual cortex in early blind humans. *The European Journal of Neuroscience, 20*(7), 1923–1927.

Woolsey, T. A. (1967). Somatosensory, auditory and visual cortical areas of the mouse. *The Johns Hopkins Medical Journal, 121*(2), 91–112.

Yaka, R., Yinon, U., & Wollberg, Z. (1999). Auditory activation of cortical visual areas in cats after early visual deprivation. *The European Journal of Neuroscience, 11*(4), 1301–1312.

Zhang, L. I., Bao, S., & Merzenich, M. M. (2002). Disruption of primary auditory cortex by synchronous auditory inputs during a critical period. *Proceedings of the National Academy of Sciences, USA, 99*(4), 2309–2314.

Factors Influencing Neocortical Development in the Normal and Injured Brain

Bryan Kolb, Celeste Halliwell, *and* Robbin Gibb

Abstract

It has long been known that experience alters the organization of neural networks in the brain. It has only recently been shown, however, that although experiences during brain development alter cerebral organization and behavior, these effects vary exquisitely with both the precise age at experience (e.g., prenatal vs. postnatal vs. juvenile) and the type of experience (e.g., sensory stimulation vs. drug exposure). Thus, prenatal, early postnatal, and juvenile experience all act to modify developing neural networks but do so in qualitatively and quantitatively different ways that influence behavioral development. In addition, perinatal brain injury interacts with these experience-dependent neural changes to lead yet another unique set of neural networks that underlie behavioral recovery.

Keywords: experience, neural networks, prenatal, postnatal, sensory stimulation, drug exposure, behavioral recovery

The development of behavior is shaped not only by the emergence of brain structures but also by a wide range of experiences that shape the emerging brain. Brains exposed to different environmental events such as sensory stimuli, stress, drugs, or diet thus may develop in very different ways. The goal of the current chapter is to review the way in which the developing brain can be influenced by a variety of prenatal and postnatal factors and how these factors can modulate recovery from perinatal brain injury. We will begin by briefly reviewing some basic stages in brain development and then consider how the normal and injured brains are shaped differently by a wide range of prenatal and postnatal events. Because most of what we know about the changes in the normal and injured brain is based on studies of the rat brain, our discussion will focus on the rat. Further, because most of what we know about modulation of brain development

is based on studies of neocortical development, we will focus on neocortical development. It is our belief, however, that other brain regions, and especially other forebrain regions, will be found to change in a similar manner.

Brain Development
Stages of Brain Development

The cells that will form the nervous system begin as a lining of the neural tube. The generation of the cells that will eventually form the neocortex of the rat begins on about embryonic day 11 (E11) and continues until E22, the day before birth (see Figure 19.1; for a review, see Bayer & Altman, 1991). The first stage in this development goes from about E11 to E14, by which time there is a rudimentary band of cells, which surrounds the emerging ventricles, and that will form the cortical plate. The second stage is from E15 to E21 during which

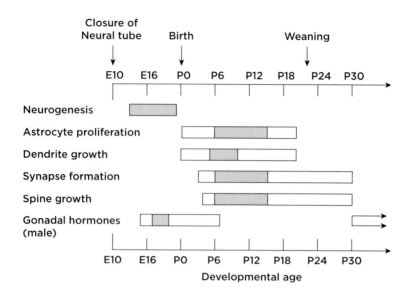

Figure 19.1 Main cellular events related to cortical plasticity. Bars mark the approximate beginning and ending of different processes. The shaded area illustrates the time of maximum activity.

time the neocortex increases in volume about 24 times. Cortical development is not uniform, however, as the ventrolateral and anterior regions develop faster than the dorsomedial and posterior regions. Distinct layers become visible by about E17 and continue to differentiate until birth. The deep layers (V and VI) are formed first, and are composed of pyramidal cells that project to subcortical targets. Layer IV, which is formed by local interneurons, forms next, followed by the pyramidal cells of layers II and III. Cells continue to travel to their final destinations throughout the first week of postnatal development with migration largely complete by about postnatal day 6 (P6). Once cells have reached their correct cortical region and layer, they begin to develop axons and dendrites, a process that is intense until about P20, after which it reduces to a much slower rate into adulthood. The dendritic and axonal growth is associated with the formation of synapses, the birth of glial cells, and the arborization of blood vessels. Because the pattern of connections of neurons is so complex, it would be impossible to have a genetic blueprint for them. Thus, the brain's solution is to overproduce neurons and synapses early in development, followed by a pruning of neurons, glia, and synapses in the juvenile period.

Brain development, therefore, is composed of a cascade of events beginning with mitosis and ending with selective cell and synaptic death. We shall see that a wide range of factors can influence cortical development and the effect of these factors varies with the precise embryological age. Furthermore, perturbations to the developing nervous system, such as injury or exposure to toxins, will have specific consequences depending upon the stage of brain development. We should not be surprised to find, for example, that experiences and/or perturbations during mitosis would have quite different effects than similar events during synaptogenesis. Events essentially are acting on a very different brain at different times.

Two features of brain development are especially important for understanding how experiences can modify cortical organization. First, the cells lining the ventricles in the subventricular zone are stem cells that remain active throughout life. These cells can produce progenitor cells that can divide to produce neurons and/or glia that can migrate away from the subependymal zone and may lie quiescently in the white or gray matter. While in these locations, they can be activated to produce neurons and/or glia. These cells likely form the basis of at least one form of postnatal neurogenesis, especially after injury (for useful reviews, see Becq, Jorquera, Ben-Ari, Weiss, & Represa, 2005; Gregg, Shingo, & Weiss, 2001). One challenge with activating quiescent progenitor cells is to find the "switch" to turn on controlled cell production when they are needed after an injury. There is now considerable evidence that the mammalian brain, including the primate brain, can generate neurons destined for the olfactory bulb, hippocampal formation, and possibly even the neocortex of the frontal and temporal lobes (e.g., Eriksson et al., 1998; Gould, Tanapat, Hastings, & Shors, 1999; Kempermann & Gage, 1999). The functional role of this generation is not clear at present, but the cell generation can be influenced by experience, hormones, drugs, and injury. Second, although it is difficult to quantify synapse numbers in the cortex, synapses do not form randomly on pyramidal neurons. Most excitatory inputs (up to 95%) synapse on spines, which are found on the dendrites, but rarely on or near the cell bodies (Figure 19.2). This means that it is possible to estimate excitatory synaptic numbers by estimating the number of spines, which is typically done by estimating both the length of dendritic material and the density of spines on the dendrites. Both dendrites and spines grow rapidly during development and show remarkable plasticity in response to experience and can form synapses in hours and possibly even minutes after some experiences (e.g., Greenough & Chang, 1989). This process is most rapid during development and is modified by changes in the developing brain, including experience and injury.

Experiential Control of Brain Development

The first and simplest way to manipulate experience across ages is to compare brain structure in animals living in standard laboratory caging to animals placed either in severely impoverished environments or so-called enriched environments, which we shall refer to as complex environments. Such studies have identified a large range of neural changes associated with complex housing. These include increases in brain size, cortical thickness, neuron size, dendritic branching, spine density, synapses per neuron, glial numbers and complexity, and vascular arborization (e.g., Greenough & Chang, 1988; Siervaag & Greenough, 1987). The magnitude of these changes should not be underestimated. For example, in our own studies of the effects of housing young rats for 60 days in enriched environments, we reliably observe changes in overall brain weight on the order of 7%–10% (e.g., Kolb, 1995). This increase in brain weight reflects increases in the number of glia and blood vessels, neuron soma size, dendritic elements, and synapses. It would be difficult to estimate the total number of increased synapses but it is probably on the order of 20% in the cortex, which is an extraordinary change. The magnitude of the effect is easily seen by examining the gross morphology of cortical

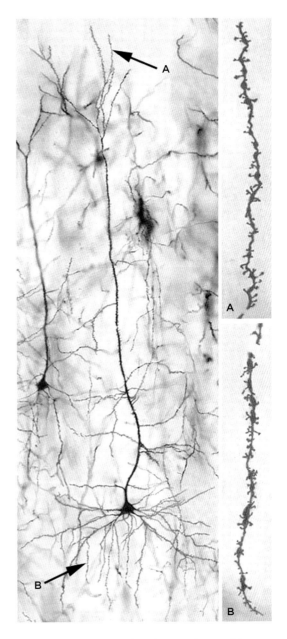

Figure 19.2 An example of a Golgi-stained pyramidal neuron. (A) A photomicrograph (200×) of the entire neuron. (B) A higher-power photo (1500×) of a terminal tip of an apical dendrite showing the spines. (C) A higher-power photo of a terminal tip of a basilar dendrite.

neurons using Golgi-type stains, as illustrated in Figure 19.2. The effects of restricted housing are not as well studied but the general trend is that there is a simplification of synaptic organization.

As we began to investigate the effects of complex housing at different times during development we anticipated that the general effects would be the same, but they would be enhanced if the experience of the offspring was manipulated earlier (i.e., in the juvenile period rather than postadolescence) (Table 19.1). This expectation turned out to be rather naïve. To investigate the effects of experience we placed rats in complex environments for 3 months beginning either at weaning or in young adulthood and measured dendritic length and spine density in the pyramidal cells in the parietal cortex at the end of the treatment. Our underlying assumption was that an increase in dendritic length and/or spine density would reflect an increase in the synapse number on the cells, which in turn would reflect an increase in the complexity of the computations by the cells (see Jacobs & Scheibel, 1993). We also presumed that increasing complexity of computations would be reflected in some type of behavioral advantage. For example, women have more complex dendritic organization in the posterior speech area than do men, and women have superior verbal abilities (Jacobs, Schall, & Scheibel, 1993).

Young adult rats showed a large increase in dendritic length in cortical neurons and an associated increase in spine density. By contrast, juvenile rats show a similar increase in dendritic length but a decrease in spine density. That is, the young animals show a qualitatively different change in the distribution of synapses on pyramidal neurons compared to older animals (Kolb, Gibb, & Gorny, 2003). Not only was the qualitative difference surprising but also was the fact that there was a decrease in spine density, which would imply a decrease in the complexity of the cells' computations. Given

the age-related difference, we wondered what earlier experience might do. To our surprise, we found yet a different outcome. Pregnant dams were placed in complex environments for 8 h a day prior to their pregnancy and then throughout the 3-week gestation. Analysis of the brains of their infants when they reached adulthood showed a decrease in dendritic length and an increase in spine density. We were surprised both that there was a large effect of prenatal experience and that it was qualitatively different from experience either in the juvenile period or in adulthood.

The question that immediately arises from these results is whether there is a behavioral advantage to the complex housing and whether the advantage is the same regardless of the age at experience. Our early results suggest that there is a small advantage in both cognitive and motor tasks and that it does not matter when the experience occurred. This makes it a real challenge to understand what is providing the advantage. A drop in dendritic length or spine density implies a drop in the number of synapses per neuron, which is a curious result because we might expect fewer synapses to be a functional disadvantage. Our new working hypothesis is that whenever we see a decrease in spine density in response to experience, it reflects a decrease in the number synapses per neuron but this is only going to be a behavioral disadvantage if the number of neurons remains constant. For example, if there were more neurons, either because there were more cells generated or less cell death during development, then having less dense synapses per neuron could still be associated with

Table 19.1 Modification of Cerebral Development by Experience

Treatment	Result	Basic Reference
Complex housing at weaning	Increased dendritic growth; decreased spine density	Kolb et al. (2003)
Complex housing in adulthood	Increased dendritic growth; increased spine density	Kolb et al. (2003)
Complex housing prenatally	Decreased dendritic length; increased spine density	Gibb et al. (2009)
Postnatal "handling"	Decreased dendritic length; spines unchanged	Gibb & Kolb (2005)
Postnatal tactile stimulation	Decreased dendritic length; decreased spine density	Gibb & Kolb (2009a)
Prenatal tactile stimulation	Decreased dendritic length; increased spine density	Gibb & Kolb (2009b)
Prenatal exercise	Decreased dendritic length; decreased spine density	Gibb et al. (2005)

an overall increase in synapse number if there was a large increase in neuron number. Furthermore, we can imagine that if the dendritic fields are large but the spines are spaced further apart, it might be easier to add spines (and their associated synapses) later. We must also point out that it is possible that there are increases in synaptic density in other regions of the brain that we did not measure and that these synaptic changes could compensate for the decreases that we observe in sensorimotor cortex.

A second way to manipulate early experience is to provide animals with specific sensory or motor experiences. To this end, we used four different procedures. In the first, which is referred to as "handling" in the stress literature (for a review of how this word is used, see Gibb & Kolb, 2005), rat pups were removed from their nest (and mother) for 15 min, 3 times per day for 10 days. In the second procedure, which was based on the one first used by Schanberg and Field (1987), infant rats were given tactile stimulation with a small brush for 15 min, 3 times per day for 10 days. In the third, we gave the pregnant dams the tactile stimulation beginning prior to their pregnancy and then until parturition. The logic was that if tactile stimulation of the skin increases some factor that influences the brain, it might be possible to influence prenatal brain development via induction of skin factors in the dam, which would cross the placental barrier. Finally, the female rats were allowed access to running wheels both before and throughout their pregnancy. We had seen this as a control for increased activity by the pregnant dams in the complex environments. All four procedures produced a drop in dendritic length but spine density varied with the specific experience: handling had no effect; postnatal tactile stimulation and prenatal exercise decreased the spine density; and, prenatal stimulation increased the spine density.

It is clear that the effects of experience on brain organization are far more complex than we ever imagined from previous studies of experience-dependent changes in adult rats. The challenge will be to determine the basis for the changes produced and how the changes relate to behavior. In adult studies of experience-dependent changes in cortical neurons there is a consistent relationship between function and dendritic change: longer dendrites and/or increased spine density is related to better function. All bets are off when the developing animal is given the same experiences, however.

Role of Other Developmental Factors

Our working hypothesis has been that factors that are normally fluctuating during development must play some role in cortical organization. There is a seemingly endless list of such possible factors and so our choice of those to study may appear somewhat arbitrary—and it is. We have focused on a single neurotrophic factor (fibroblast growth factor-2 [FGF-2]) and chose it because it plays an important developmental role in neurogenesis, synaptogenesis, cell death, and wound healing. We have looked at two different ages (P4–P11 vs. P11–P18) because FGF has a changing function from the first to the second week of development. We have looked at noradrenaline (NA) depletion because it had previously been found to influence cortical neural networks including the formation of barrel fields (Loeb, Chang, & Greenough, 1987), the response to complex housing (Brenner, Mirmiran, Uylings, & van der Gugten, 1983), and the development of ocular dominance columns (Kasamatsu, Pettigrew, & Ary, 1979). We therefore depleted forebrain NA in newborn rats, which can be accomplished with subdural doses of the neurotoxin 6-hydroxydopamine in the young animal. This method is effective because the forebrain blood–brain barrier is permeable to the toxin in the first few days of postnatal life and the noradrenergic terminals are destroyed selectively, leaving dopaminergic terminals and cells undisturbed. We modified diet because it has been shown that diet can influence gene expression during development (e.g., Afman & Muller, 2006; Stover & Garza, 2006) and changes in dendritic morphology must somehow be related to gene expression. We manipulated gonadal hormones because they are known to interact with the effects of complex housing (Juraska, 1990; Kolb et al., 2003) and, finally, we looked at the effect of prenatal stress because we had found it to influence cortical thickness, which normally is related to dendritic morphology (Stewart & Kolb, 1988). (We are currently investigating the effect of psychoactive drugs including nicotine, fluoxetine, and diazepam as we have found that all of these drugs affect dendritic morphology in adulthood.)

The results of our studies are summarized in Table 19.2, which shows that all of the factors have an impact upon synaptic organization, but again in a complex manner. Consider the effects of subcutaneous FGF-2 administration at different developmental times. The adult brains of rats that received FGF-2 from P4 to P11 showed a decrease in dendritic length, whereas those that received FGF-2

Table 19.2 Modification of Cerebral Development by Nonexperiential Factors

Treatment	Result	Basic Reference
Neurotrophic modification		
Postnatal FGF-2 (P3–P11)	Decreased dendritic length; spines unchanged	Gibb & Kolb (2009b)
Postnatal FGF-2 (P11–P18)	Increased dendritic length; spines NYA	Gibb & Kolb (20069b
Neuromodulatory modification		
NA depletion	Decreased dendritic length; increased spine density	Kolb et al. (1997)
Dietary modification		
High choline diet	Increased dendritic length; spines NYA	Halliwell et al. (2009)
Enhanced vitamins and minerals	Increased dendritic length; spines NYA	Halliwell & Kolb (unpublished)
Hormonal modification		
Neonatal GDX (male)	Decreased dendritic length; decreased spine density	Kolb & Stewart (1995)
Neonatal TP (female)	Increased dendritic length; decreased spine density	Kolb & Stewart (1995)
Prenatal stress	Dendritic length NA; increased spine density	Gibb, Gonzalez, & Kolb (2009)

Abbreviations: NYA, not yet available; GDX, castration on day of birth; TP, testosterone propionate; NA, noradrenaline.

from P11 to P18 showed just the opposite, namely, an increase in dendritic length. Curiously, the latter group was relatively impaired on tests of both cognitive and motor function, again suggesting that more is not necessarily better.

The hormonal results are perhaps more intuitive. There is a sex difference with males having more dendritic material in their cortical pyramidal neurons than females. Removal of testosterone in the developing male rat reduced the dendritic length, making the cells more "female-like," and adding testosterone to females increased dendritic length, making the cells similar to those of intact males. Curiously, although there is no endogenous difference in spine density, either eliminating testosterone in males or adding it to females reduced the density.

Summary

There are four important messages in these data. First, developmental events have profound effects on brain development and these effects vary exquisitely with the precise age and type of experience. It is daunting to realize that it would literally take an entire career to do a thorough study expanding our research to look at multiple cortical and subcortical regions. Nonetheless, such studies clearly will be needed if we are to provide a complete story as to how these perinatal factors alter cortical organization and behavior. Second, it is clear that prenatal experience can influence later brain development. The mechanism of this influence is likely different than that associated with the postnatal treatments because there are virtually no cortical synapses formed when the prenatal events are experienced, whereas when the postnatal (infant and juvenile) events occur, synapses are present and can be modified. Third, at this point, we have little understanding of how the morphological changes relate to function in the developing brain. Finally, it is clear that measuring only spine density or dendritic length can lead to very different conclusions. Future studies should measure both.

Brain Injury
Model of Early Brain Injury

It was generally assumed up until the 1970s that the earlier brain injury occurred during development, the better the outcome would be. This idea dates back to the late nineteenth century, when Broca and others noticed that children rarely had persistent aphasia after damage to the cortical language zones. Beginning in the 1930s, studies by Margaret Kennard supported this general notion of "earlier is better." She made unilateral motor cortex lesions in infant and adult monkeys. The behavioral impairments in the infant monkeys were milder than those in the adults, which led Kennard to hypothesize that there had been a change in cortical organization in the infants and these changes supported the behavioral recovery. In particular, she hypothesized that if some synapses were removed as a consequence of brain injury, "others would be formed in less usual combinations" and that "it is possible that factors, which facilitate cortical organization in the normal young are the same by which reorganization is accomplished in the imperfect cortex after injury" (Kennard, 1942, p. 239). In contrast with Kennard's findings, Donald Hebb's studies of children with early brain injury in the 1940s led to a different conclusion (Hebb, 1947, 1949). Hebb noticed that children with frontal lobe injuries often had worse outcomes than adults with similar injuries and proposed that the early injuries prevented a normal initial organization of the brain, thus making it difficult for the child to develop many behaviors, especially socioaffective behaviors. Thus, whereas Kennard hypothesized that recovery from early brain damage was associated with a novel reorganization of neural networks that supported functional recovery, Hebb postulated that the failure to recover was correlated with a failure of initial organization that prevented the normal development of many behaviors. Extensive studies of both cats and rats with cortical injuries have shown that both views are partially correct (e.g., Kolb, 1995; Schmanke & Villablanca, 2001; Villablanca, Hovda, Jackson, & Infante, 1993). It is the precise developmental age at injury that predicts the Kennard or Hebb outcome.

The critical relationship between age at injury and functional outcome can be illustrated in our studies looking at the effect of cortical injury at ages ranging from birth to adulthood. We have examined the behavior of adult rats that had injuries to the prefrontal, motor, posterior parietal, temporal, or posterior cingulate cortex at postnatal days 1, 4, 7, 10, or 90 (Table 19.3). The key finding is that regardless of the location of injury, the functional outcome is always best after injury during the second week of life. The best functional outcomes are seen after lesions of the prefrontal and posterior cingulate cortex, whereas the worst outcome is seen after lesions of the posterior parietal and occipital cortex. A similar pattern of results can be seen in parallel studies of the effects of cortical lesions in kittens by Villablanca and his colleagues (e.g.,

Table 19.3 Effects of Early Cortical Injury

Region	Basic References
Medial prefrontal cortex	Kolb & Whishaw 1981; Kolb (1987)
Orbital prefrontal cortex	Kolb, Gibb, & Gorny (2006); Kolb & Nonneman (1976)
Motor cortex	Kolb & Holmes (1983)
Posterior cingulate cortex	Gonzalez, Gibb, & Kolb (2002); Gonzalez, Whishaw, & Kolb (2003)
Posterior parietal cortex	Kolb, Holmes, & Whishaw (1987); Kolb & Cioe (1998)
Occipital cortex	Kolb, Ladowski, Gibb, & Gorny (1996)
Temporal cortex	Kolb & Cioe (2003)

Villablanca et al., 1993), although because the rat and cat develop at different rates the precise ages are different in the two species. Specifically, damage in the first few weeks after birth in the cat is equivalent to damage in the second postnatal week in the rat, and thus is associated with a relatively good outcome, whereas damage in the last few prenatal weeks in the cat is equivalent to damage in the first postnatal week in the rat and is associated with a very poor functional outcome. Thus, birth date is irrelevant—it is the stage of neural development that is important.

Given that prenatal factors can influence later brain development in the rat, we were interested in knowing how prenatal cortical injury would influence brain and behavioral development. We made prenatal lesions in putative frontal cortex and concluded that damage during the period of neurogenesis, which in the rat cortex is from about E12 to E20, appears to be associated with a good functional outcome on tests of spatial learning and skilled motor behavior (see also Hicks & D'Amato, 1961) provided there is no hydrocephalus (Kolb, Cioe, & Muirhead, 1998). We hasten to point out, however, that our injuries were focal and it is possible that more diffuse injuries, such as those that might be seen in head trauma, ischemia, or response to teratogens, could produce a different outcome.

Brain Development after Early Brain Injury

Regardless of the time of injury (prenatal or in the first 3 postnatal weeks), there is always a reduction in overall brain size relative to similar injuries later in life. Thus, given that we have seen that age at injury leads to very different outcomes, there must be some difference in the synaptic organization of the brain that is critical—rather than simply brain size because brain size does not predict the functional outcome.

Golgi analyses of cortical neurons in rats with perinatal lesions consistently show a general atrophy of dendritic arborization and a decrease in spine density across the cortical mantle (e.g., Kolb, Gibb, & van der Kooy, 1994). By contrast, rats with cortical lesions produced on P10 show an increase in dendritic arborization and an increase in spine density relative to control littermates. Thus, animals with the best functional outcome show the greatest synaptic increase, whereas animals with the worst functional outcome have a decrease in synapses relative to control animals.

We might expect that the changes in dendritic organization are related to obvious changes in cortical connectivity. Indeed, the elegant work of Payne and his colleagues on the effects of perinatal cortical lesions in the visual system of kittens (e.g., Payne & Cornwell, 1994; Payne & Lomber, 2001) have shown a major rewiring of thalamocortical and corticocortical connections of the visual system. Although there are certainly behavioral deficits in these animals, there is impressive sparing of visual system function. Parallel studies in rats and cats with unilateral motor cortex injuries have shown that there is a major expansion of the ipsilateral corticospinal pathway from the undamaged hemisphere, which is correlated with partial recovery of skilled forelimb use (e.g., Castro, 1990; Villablanca & Gomez-Pinella, 1987; Whishaw & Kolb, 1988). It appears, however, that the anomalous corticospinal projections sometimes may be formed at a significant cost. For example, when we compared the effects of motor cortex lesions on P4, P10, and P90, we found that although it was only the youngest animals that showed the enhanced ipsilateral connections, it was the P10 animals that showed the best functional outcome. Furthermore, animals with P4 lesions showed unexpected deficits on cognitive tasks (e.g., a spatial navigation task). It thus seems likely that the aberrant corticospinal pathway interfered with the normal functioning of cortical areas. This possibility has been termed "crowding" to reflect the idea that the normal functions of a cortical region can be crowded out by the development of abnormal connections (e.g., Teuber, 1975).

In sum, it would appear that the best way to look for anatomical correlates of functional outcomes after early brain injury is to look at patterns of synaptic organization. Although the Golgi-type analysis is an imperfect estimation of synaptic changes, it remains one of the most useful surrogate measures of synaptic change and we shall focus on these changes.

Modulation of the Effects of Early Brain Injury

The fact that age at injury shows such a consistent relationship with functional outcome after injury within so many different cortical regions provides us with a nice model to investigate the effects of a wide range of factors on brain development after injury. We have taken advantage of the poor outcome after injury in the first week of postnatal life in the rat to look for factors that would facilitate recovery. We then have contrasted facilitory effects in week 1 to the effect of factors that interfere with recovery after injury in the week 2. We hasten to point out that we are not simply talking about postinjury factors but also prenatal factors that can modulate the outcome of a brain injury that occurs postnatally. Because most of our studies on modulating factors have been using rats with medial frontal lesions, our discussion will focus on this preparation, with reference to other lesions where appropriate.

BEHAVIORAL THERAPY

Although it is generally assumed that behavioral therapies will improve recovery from cerebral injury in humans, there have been few direct studies of mechanism underlying the benefits, when the optimal time for therapy might be, or even whether it is actually effective (e.g., Kwakkel, Wagennar, Koelman, Lankhorst, & Doetsier, 1997). There have been surprisingly few studies using animals with perinatal cortical injuries and the few that are available have not reported any anatomical correlates. We thus began our studies by looking at the effects of the prenatal and postnatal experiential treatments (e.g., complex housing, tactile stimulation, exercise) that we had found to influence cortical development in intact animals and in each case we collected anatomical measures to see if they might provide insight into why the treatments did or did not work. There were two general results. First, nearly all treatments enhanced performance on measures of both cognitive and motor functions after P4 cortical injuries (Table 19.4). Second, there were morphological correlates of the enhanced recovery.

Curiously, however, the morphological changes in the intact and injured brain were different. Consider an example. Recall that tactile stimulation reduced spine density in intact animals and so did early cortical injury. But when brain-injured animals were given tactile stimulation there was an increase in spine density (Figure 19.3). It appears that the intact and injured brain respond differently to the same experiences, a finding that we certainly did not predict a priori. At any rate, the cortex appears to be capable of considerable environment-mediated modification after early injury, although the timing of the postinjury therapy appears to make some difference.

One treatment was ineffective, however. Complex housing that was delayed until adulthood did not facilitate recovery from P4 injury. Perhaps the synaptic organization of the remaining brain can be more easily remodeled if the reorganization occurs while the brain is still developing.

FGF-2

In the course of trying to determine how stimulating the skin might facilitate brain repair, we discovered that FGF-2 levels were increased in skin and brain after tactile stimulation in infant rats and that there was also an increase in FGF-2 receptor in brain. This led us to administer FGF-2 directly as a therapy. In our first series of studies, we gave animals with P4 medial frontal or posterior parietal lesions FGF-2 either prenatally, postinjury, or both (e.g., Comeau, Hastings, & Kolb, 2007, 2008, 2009; Gibb & Kolb, 2009b. All three treatment regimens proved to be beneficial, with the combined prenatal and postnatal treatments being the most advantageous. Although the anatomical studies are not completed, it appears that the FGF-2 treatment produces a unique set of

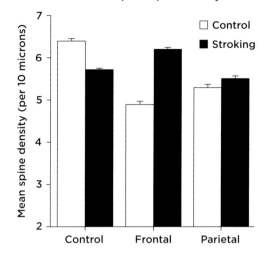

Par 1 Apical Spine Density

Figure 19.3 Terminal tip spine density in apical branches of layer III pyramidal cells in the parietal cortex of rats with or without tactile stimulation. Intact rats showed a chronic decrease in spine density, whereas lesion rats showed an increase in spine density relative to unstimulated animals.

morphological changes at each age. For example, prenatal FGF reversed the decrease in brain weight in the lesion rats, whereas postnatal FGF reversed the lesion-induced decrease in cortical thickness but did not affect brain weight. Combined pre- and postinjury treatment reversed the reductions in both brain weight and cortical thickness. Postinjury treatment also reversed the decrease in dendritic length and spine density normally seen after the early lesions—a result that is identical to the effects of tactile stimulation.

In a second series of experiments we administered FGF-2 to P10 rats with motor cortex lesions. We reasoned that although rats with P10 motor cortex lesions show partial recovery of function,

Table 19.4 Modification of the Effects of Early Frontal Cortical Injury by Experiential Treatments

Treatment	Result	Basic
Complex housing at weaning	Enhanced recovery after P1–7 injury	Kolb & Elliott (1987) Gibb et al. (2006)
Complex housing in adulthood	No functional recovery after P1–5 injury	Comeau et al. (2006)
Complex housing prenatally	Enhanced recovery after P4 injury	Gibb et al. (2009)
Postinjury tactile stimulation	Enhanced recovery after P4 injury	Gibb & Kolb (2009a)
Prenatal tactile stimulation	Enhanced recovery after P4 injury	Gibb & Kolb (2009b)
Postnatal handling; prenatal exercise	No effect on behavior; functional recovery blocked after P10 injury	Gibb & Kolb (2005) Gibb et al. (2009)

they are still impaired and the FGF might further enhance the recovery. To our surprise, the FGF-2 treatment not only improved motor recovery but recovery was correlated with a regeneration of the lost tissue (Monfils, Driscoll, Vavrek, Kolb, & Faoud, 2008; Monfils et al., 2005, 2006). This tissue does not have normal cortical lamination but the tissue does have connections with the spinal cord that are functional and the cells have fairly normal patterns of spontaneous discharge. Removing the regenerated tissue produces immediate loss of the recovered functions. It is not yet known whether there is a price to pay for this regeneration, such as crowding of other functions or a later change in experience-dependent plasticity.

OTHER BENEFICIAL TREATMENTS

Dietary manipulations (high choline and vitamin supplements) facilitated recovery after P4 frontal lesions (Figure 19.4). In the choline studies, animals received a high choline diet prenatally and postnatally via water that the pregnant dam drank and that the infants drank until weaning. When studied in adulthood, the lesioned animals showed improved spatial cognition, and motor functions were correlated with an increase in dendritic length in cortical pyramidal neurons (spine density was not measured) (Halliwell, Tees, & Kolb, 2009). In a follow-up study, dams and later their pups were given a diet enriched with vitamins and minerals using a formula that had been found to be beneficial in treating human bipolar patients (Kaplan et al., 2001; Kaplan, Fisher, Crawford, Field, & Kolb, 2004). Like the choline treatment, there was a facilitation of recovery correlated with dendritic growth in cortical pyramidal cells (C. Halliwell & B. Kolb, unpublished observations).

The final beneficial treatment was exposure to a low dose (0.3 mg/kg twice daily) of nicotine prenatally. Animals given P4 frontal lesions following prenatal nicotine exposure showed better recovery than animals without the treatment. Curiously, however, animals that were given nicotine but not the later lesions fared worse than saline controls (McKenna et al., 2000). Once again, it appears that experiential events can differentially affect intact and injured brains.

DETRIMENTAL TREATMENTS

Depletion of NA, manipulation of testosterone, exposure to prenatal stress, and prenatal exposure to fluoxetine (Prozac) all blocked

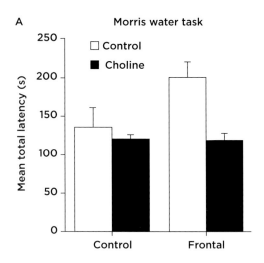

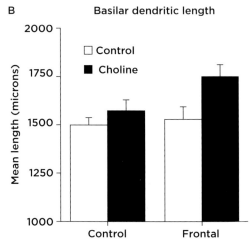

Figure 19.4 The effects of choline administration on recovery from perinatal frontal injury. (A) Day 4 frontal lesions produced a deficit in the acquisition of the Morris water task that was reversed by the addition of choline to the diet, beginning at conception and continuing until weaning. (B) The choline treatment increased dendritic length of layer III parietal pyramidal neurons in the lesion animals but not in the control animals.

recovery from lesions performed during the second postnatal week and all blocked the dendritic changes that are normally associated with recovery (Table 19.5). Consider an example. Rats were depleted of NA in the first few postnatal days and then received large frontal lesions at P7 and were later tested in spatial cognition tasks before undergoing a Golgi analysis of dendritic and spine morphology (Kolb & Sutherland, 1992; Kolb, Stewart, & Sutherland, 1997; Sutherland, Kolb, Whishaw, & Becker, 1982). The results showed that in the absence of NA there was no

Table 19.5 Modification of the Effects of Early Frontal Cortical Injury by Nonexperiential Treatments

Treatment	Result	Basic Reference
Neurotrophic modification		
Postinjury FGF-2	Functional recovery after P4 injury; dendritic growth	Comeau et al. (2007)
Prenatal FGF-2	Functional recovery after P4 injury	Comeau et al. (2008)
Postinjury FGF-2	Functional recovery after P10 injury; neurogenesis	Monfils et al. (2006)
Neuromodulatory modification		
NA depletion before day 7 lesion	Blocked recovery; dendritic atrophy; drop in spine density	Kolb & Sutherland (1992)
Diet modification		
High choline diet after P4 lesion	Stimulated recovery; enhanced dendritic growth	Halliwell et al. (2009)
Vitamin supplement	Stimulated recovery; enhanced dendritic growth	Halliwell & Kolb (unpublished)
Hormonal modification		
GDX before P7 lesion	Blocked recovery; reduced dendritic growth; reversed spine increase	Kolb & Stewart (1995)
TP in females before P7 lesion	Blocked recovery; decreased spine density	Kolb & Stewart (1995)
Prenatal drugs		
Fluoxetine	Blocks recovery after P10 injury; small brain	Day et al. (2003)
Nicotine	Facilitates recovery after P4 injury	McKenna et al. (2000)

Abbreviations: P4, P7, P10, postnatal day 4, 7, 10; P1–5, postnatal days 1–5; GDX, castration on day of birth; TP, testosterone propionate; NA, noradrenaline.

functional recovery. Analysis of the dendritic and spine changes showed that the NA depletion produced a drop in dendritic length and branch complexity in both sham control and lesion animals relative to saline-treated controls. The drop in dendritic length was greater in the lesion animals, as might be expected given that they essentially had two injuries—NA depletion and direct cortical injury. The sham NA-depleted animals, which had no obvious behavioral disturbance, apparently compensated for the dendritic loss with an increase in spine density. A similar increase was observed in the lesion animals as well but their overall loss of dendritic length was greater than the controls and the increase in spine density was unable to compensate effectively and the animals thus failed to show recovery.

Our finding that prenatal exposure to fluoxetine blocked later recovery from P10 frontal lesions was completely unexpected as we had anticipated that fluoxetine might actually enhance functional recovery from P4 lesions (it did not). This was a case, however, in which the intact and injured brain responded the same to

the treatment—both types of animals had severe functional impairments. Our anatomical analyses are in progress but our expectation is that both groups are likely to show reduced dendritic length and spine density.

Potential Mechanisms of Plasticity in the Normal and Injured Brain

Our demonstration of plastic changes in the normal and injured brain clearly show the remarkable capacity of the developing brain to form novel neural networks that can be inferred from changes in dendritic morphology. A key question, however, is how this happens. At this point, our understanding of the mechanisms underlying synaptic changes in either normal or injured brains is clearly in its infancy. It seems likely that there are genetic or epigenetic steps but exactly how changes in FGF-2, neuromodulators, stress hormones, and other factors might modify mRNA remains a mystery. We do have preliminary evidence that prenatal stress can decrease gene methylation in the cortex but we do not know how altered gene methylation might be related to changes in spine density. There might be some relatively direct link or there could be multiple steps, such as change in growth factor production or behavior that mediates the synaptic changes. This is clearly grist for future studies.

Acknowledgments

This research was supported by Natural Science and Engineering Research Council of Canada and Canadian Institute for Health Research grants to B.K. and R.G. The authors wish to thank the late G.G for her technical help in many of the experiments described here.

References

Afman, L., & Muller, M. (2006). Nutrigenomics: From molecular nutrition to prevention of disease. *Journal of the American Dietetic Association, 106,* 569–576.

Bayer, S. A., & Altman, J. (1991). *Neocortical development.* New York: Pergamon.

Becq, H., Jorquera, I., Ben-Ari, Y., Weiss, S., & Represa, A. (2005). Differential properties of dentate gyrus and CA1 neural precursors. *Journal of Neurobiology, 62,* 243–261.

Brenner, E., Mirmiran, M., Uylings, H. B., & van der Gugten, J. (1983). Impaired growth of the cerebral cortex of rats treated neonatally with 6-hydroxydopamine under different environmental conditions. *Neuroscience Letters, 42,* 13–17.

Castro, A. (1990). Plasticity in the motor system. In B. Kolb & R. Tees (Eds.), *Cerebral cortex of the rat* (pp. 563–588). Cambridge, MA: MIT Press.

Comeau, W. Gibb, R., Hastings, E., Cioe, J., & Kolb, B. (2008). Therapeutic effects of complex rearing or bFGF after perinatal frontal lesions. *Developmental Psychobiology, 50,* 134–146.

Comeau, W., Hastings, E., & Kolb, B. (2007). Differential effect of pre and postnatal FGF-2 following medial prefrontal cortical injury. *Behavioural Brain Research, 180,* 18–27.

Comeau, W., Hastings, E., & Kolb, B. (2009). *Pre and Post-injury FGF-2 act synergistically in enhancing functional outcome in rats with perinatal injury.* Manuscript submitted for publication.

Day, M., Gibb, R., & Kolb, B. (2003). Prenatal fluoxetine impairs functional recovery and neuroplasticity after perinatal frontal cortex lesions in rats [Abstract]. *Society for Neuroscience Abstracts, 29,* 459.10.

Eriksson, P. S., Perfilieva, E., Björk-Eriksson, T., Alborn, A. M., Nordborg, C., Peterson, D. A., et al. (1998). Neurogenesis in the adult human hippocampus. *Nature Medicine, 4,* 1313–1317.

Gibb, R., Gonzalez, C. L. R., & Kolb, B. (2009). *Complex environmental experience during pregnancy facilitates recovery from perinatal cortical injury in the offspring.* Manuscript submitted for publication.

Gibb, R., & Kolb, B. (2005). Neonatal handling alters brain organization but does not influence recovery from perinatal cortical injury. *Behavioral Neuroscience, 119,* 1375–1383.

Gibb, R., & Kolb, B. (2009a). *Prenatal tactile stimulation alters brain and behavioral development and facilitates recovery from perinatal brain injury.* Manuscript submitted for publication.

Gibb, R., & Kolb, B. (2009b). *Tactile-stimulation that facilitates functional recovery after perinatal cortical injury is mediated by FGF-2.* Manuscript submitted for publication.

Gonzalez, C. L. R., Gibb, R., & Kolb, B. (2002). Functional recovery and dendritic hypertrophy after posterior and complete cingulate lesions on postnatal day 10. *Developmental Psychobiology, 40*(2), 138–46.

Gonzalez, C. L. R., Whishaw, I. Q., & Kolb, B. (2003). Complete sparing of spatial learning following posterior and posterior plus anterior cingulate cortex lesions at 10 days of age in the rat. *Neuroscience, 122,* 563–571.

Gould, E., Tanapat, P., Hastings, N. B., & Shors, T. J. (1999). Neurogenesis in adulthood: a possible role in learning. *Trends in Cognitive Science, 3,* 186–192.

Greenough, W. T., & Chang, F. F. (1989). Plasticity of synapse structure and pattern in the cerebral cortex. In A. Peters & E. G. Jones (Eds.), *Cerebral cortex* (Vol. 7, pp. 391–440). New York: Plenum Press.

Gregg, C. T., Shingo, T., & Weiss, S. (2001). Neural stem cells of the mammalian forebrain. *Symposia of the Society for Experimental Biology, 53,* 1–19.

Halliwell, C., Tees, R., & Kolb, B. (2009). *Prenatal choline treatment enhances recovery from perinatal frontal injury in rats.* Manuscript submitted for publication.

Hebb, D. O. (1947). The effects of early experience on problem solving at maturity. *American Psychologist, 2,* 737–745.

Hebb, D. O. (1949). *The organization of behaviour.* New York: McGraw-Hill.

Hicks, S., & D'Amato, C. J. (1961). How to design and build abnormal brains using radiation during development. In W. S. Fields & M. M. Desmond (Eds.), *Disorders of the developing nervous system* (pp. 60–79). Springfield, IL: Thomas.

Jacobs, B., Schall, M., & Scheibel, A. B. (1993). A quantitative dendritic analysis of Wernicke's area in humans: II. Gender, hemispheric, and environmental factors. *The Journal of Comparative Neurology, 327,* 97–111.

Jacobs, B., & Scheibel, A. B. (1993). A quantitative dendritic analysis of Wernicke's area in humans: I. Lifespan changes. *The Journal of Comparative Neurology, 327,* 83–96.

Kaplan, B. J., Fisher, J. E., Crawford, S. G., Field, C. J., & Kolb, B. (2004). Improved mood and behavior during treatment with a mineral-vitamin supplement: An open-label case series of children. *Journal of Child and Adolescent Psychopharmacology, 14,* 115–122.

Kaplan, B. J., Simpson, J. S., Ferre, R. C., Gorman, C. P., McMullen, D. M., & Crawford, S. G. (2001). Effective mood stabilization with a chelated mineral supplement: An open-label trial in bipolar disorder. *The Journal of Clinical Psychiatry, 62,* 936–944.

Kasamatsu, T., Pettigrew, J. D., & Ary, M. (1979). Restoration of visual cortical plasticity by local microperfusion of norepinephrine. *The Journal of Comparative Neurology, 185,* 163–182.

Kennard, M. (1942). Cortical reorganization of motor function. *Archives of Neurology, 48,* 227–240.

Kempermann, G., & Gage, F. H. (1999). New nerve cells for the adult brain. *Scientific American, 280*(5), 48–53.

Kolb, B. (1987). Recovery from early cortical damage in rats. I. Differential behavioural and anatomical effects of frontal lesions at different ages of neural maturation. *Behavioural Brain Research, 25,* 205–220.

Kolb, B. (1995). *Brain plasticity and behavior.* Mahwah, NJ: Erlbaum.

Kolb, B., & Cioe, J. (1998). Absence of recovery or dendritic reorganization after neonatal posterior parietal lesions. *Psychobiology, 26*, 134–142.

Kolb, B., & Cioe, J. (2003). Recovery from early cortical damage in rats. IX. Differential behavioral and anatomical effects of temporal cortex lesions at different ages of neural maturation. *Behavioural Brain Research, 144*, 67–76.

Kolb, B., Cioe, J., & Muirhead, D. (1998). Cerebral morphology and functional sparing after prenatal frontal cortex lesions in rats. *Behavioural Brain Research, 91*, 143–155.

Kolb, B., & Elliott, W. (1987). Recovery from early cortical damage in rats. II. Effects of experience on anatomy and behavior following frontal lesions at 1 or 5 days of age. *Behavioural Brain Research, 26*, 47–56.

Kolb, B., & Gibb, R. (2009). *Tactile stimulation after posterior parietal cortical injury in infant rats stimulates functional recovery and altered cortical morphology.* Manuscript submitted for publication.

Kolb, B., Gibb, R., & Gorny, G. (2003). Experience-dependent changes in dendritic arbor and spine density in neocortex vary with age and sex. *Neurobiology of Learning and Memory, 79*, 1–10.

Kolb, B., Gibb, R., & Gorny, G. (2009). *Therapeutic effects of enriched rearing after frontal lesions in infancy vary with age and sex.* Manuscript submitted for publication.

Kolb, B., Gibb, R., & van der Kooy, D. (1994). Neonatal frontal cortical lesions in rats alter cortical structure and connectivity. *Brain Research, 645*, 85–97.

Kolb, B., & Holmes, C. (1983). Neonatal motor cortex lesions in the rat: Absence of sparing of motor behaviors and impaired spatial learning concurrent with abnormal cerebral morphogenesis. *Behavioral Neuroscience, 97*, 697–709.

Kolb, B., Holmes, C., & Whishaw, I. Q. (1987). Recovery from early cortical lesions in rats. III. Neonatal removal of posterior parietal cortex has greater behavioral and anatomical effects than similar removals in adulthood. *Behavioural Brain Research, 26*, 119–137.

Kolb, B., Ladowski, R., Gibb, R., & Gorny, G.. (1996). Does dendritic growth underlie recovery from neonatal occipital lesions in rats? *Behavioural Brain Research, 11*, 125–133.

Kolb, B., & Nonneman, A. J. (1976). Functional development of the prefrontal cortex in rats continues into adolescence. *Science, 193*, 335–336.

Kolb, B., & Stewart, J. (1995). Changes in neonatal gonadal hormonal environment prevent behavioral sparing and alter cortical morphogenesis after early frontal cortex lesions in male and female rats. *Behavioral Neuroscience, 109*, 285–294.

Kolb, B., Stewart, J., & Sutherland, R. J. (1997). Recovery of function is associated with increased spine density in cortical pyramidal cells after frontal lesions and/or noradrenaline depletion in neonatal rats. *Behavioural Brain Research, 89*, 61–70.

Kolb, B., & Sutherland, R. J. (1992). Noradrenaline depletion blocks behavioral sparing and alters cortical morphogenesis after neonatal frontal cortex damage in rats. *Journal of Neuroscience, 12*, 2221–2330.

Kolb, B., & Whishaw, I. Q. (1981). Neonatal frontal lesions in the rat: Sparing of learned but not species-typical behavior in the presence of reduced brain weight and cortical thickness. *Journal of Comparative and Physiological Psychology, 95*, 863–879.

Kwakkel, G., Wagennar, R. C., Koelman, T. W., Lankhorst, G. J., & Koetsier, J. (1997). Effects of intensity of rehabilitation after stroke: A research synthesis. *Stroke, 28*, 1550–1556.

Loeb, E. P., Chang, F. F., & Greenough, W. T. (1987). Effects of neonatal 6-hydroxydopamine treatment upon morphological organization of the posteromedial barrel subfield in mouse somatosensory cortex. *Brain Research, 403*, 113–120.

McKenna, J. E., Brown, R. W., Kolb, B., & Gibb, R. (2000). The effects of prenatal nicotine exposure on recovery from perinatal frontal cortex lesions [Abstract]. *Society for Neuroscience Abstracts, 26*, 653.17.

Monfils, M. H., Driscoll, I., Vandenberg, P. M., Thomas, N. J., Danka, D., Kleim, J. A., et al. (2005). Basic fibroblast growth factor stimulates functional recovery after neonatal lesions of motor cortex in rats. *Neuroscience, 131*, 1–8.

Monfils, M. H., Driscoll, I., Kamitakahara, H., Wilson, B., Flynn, C., Teskey, G. C., et al. (2006). FGF-2-induced cell proliferation stimulates anatomical, neurophysiological, and functional recovery from neonatal motor cortex injury. *The European Journal of Neuroscience, 24*, 739–749.

Monfils, M. H., Driscoll, I., Vavrek, R., Kolb, B., & Faoud, K. (2008). FGF-2 promotes restoration of functional corticospinal neurons after neonatal motor cortex injury. *Experimental Brain Research, 185*, 453–460.

Payne, B. R., & Cornwell, P. (1994). System-wide repercussions of damage of immature visual cortex. *Trends in Neurosciences, 17*, 126–130.

Payne, B. R., & Lomber, S. (2001). Reconstructing functional systems after lesions of the cerebral cortex. *Nature Reviews. Neuroscience, 2*, 911–919.

Schanberg, S. M., & Field, T. M. (1987). Sensory deprivation stress and supplemental stimulation in the rat pup and preterm human neonate. *Child Development, 58*, 1431–1447.

Schmanke, T. D., & Villablanca, J. R. (2001). A critical maturational period of reduced brain vulnerability to injury. A study of cerebral glucose metabolism in cats. *Developmental Brain Research, 26*, 127–141.

Sirevaag, A. M., & Greenough, W. T. (1987). A multivariate statistical summary of synaptic plasticity measures in rats exposed to complex, social and individual environments. *Brain Research, 441*, 386–392.

Stewart, J., & Kolb, B. (1988). The effects of neonatal gonadectomy and prenatal stress on cortical thickness and asymmetry in rats. *Behavioral and Neural Biology, 49*, 344–360.

Stover, P. J., & Garza, C. (2006). Nutrition and developmental biology—implications for public health. *Nutrition Reviews, 64*, S60–S71.

Sutherland, R. J., Kolb, B., Becker, J. B., & Whishaw, I. Q. (1982). Cortical noradrenaline depletion eliminates sparing of spatial learning after neonatal frontal cortex damage in the rat. *Neuroscience Letters, 32*, 125–130.

Teuber, H. L. (1975). Recovery of function after brain injury in man. *Outcome of severe damage to the nervous system.* Ciba Foundation Symposium 34. Amsterdam: Elsevier North Holland.

Villablanca, J. R., & Gomez-Pinilla, F. (1987). Novel crossed corticothalamic projections after neonatal cerebral hemispherectomy. A quantitative autoradiography study in cats. *Brain Research, 410*, 2119–231.

Villablanca, J. R., Hovda, D. A., Jackson, G. F., & Infante, C. (1993). Neurological and behavioral effects of a unilateral frontal cortical lesion in fetal kittens: II. Visual system tests, and proposing a 'critical period' for lesion effects. *Behavioural Brain Research, 57*, 79–92.

Whishaw, I. Q., & Kolb, B. (1988). Sparing of skilled forelimb reaching and corticospinal projections after neonatal motor cortex removal or hemidecortication in the rat: Support for the Kennard Doctrine. *Brain Research, 451*, 97–114.

PART 5

Regulatory Systems

The Form and Function of Infant Sleep: From Muscle to Neocortex

Mark S. Blumberg and Adele M. H. Seelke

Abstract

Despite the predominance of sleep during the perinatal period in mammals, most investigations of the mechanisms and functions of sleep continue to focus on adults. This chapter reviews recent progress in our understanding of infant sleep and its development, including developmental transitions in the temporal expression of ultradian and circadian rhythms, the developmental emergence of sleep components (e.g., cortical delta activity), the neural mechanisms of infant sleep, and the contributions of sleep processes to neural development. In addition, it is argued that a thorough understanding of the development of sleep can help us to understand the relations between normal and pathological states as well as the evolutionary modification of developmental mechanisms to shape species-specific features of sleep and wakefulness.

Keywords: sleep, infancy, REM, ultradian rhythms, circadian rhythms, neural development, wakefulness, evolution

Introduction

Everyday experience and decades of research inform us that the infants of many mammalian species, including humans, spend most of their days and nights asleep (Jouvet-Mounier, Astic, & Lacote, 1970; Kleitman & Engelmann, 1953; Roffwarg, Muzio, & Dement, 1966). Nonetheless, our understanding and appreciation of infant sleep have been impeded by a variety of obstacles. These obstacles reflect in part the technical and methodological challenges that small, fragile infants pose to the experimental scientist, as well as the challenges that arise when we attempt to interpret infant behavior using concepts that have emerged from research using adult subjects. Although these issues are very familiar to developmental psychobiologists (Alberts & Cramer, 1988; Hall & Oppenheim, 1987), they are—in

our experience—less familiar to the majority of sleep researchers.

In the 1990s, doubts were raised as to whether the state that we identify as sleep in infants is qualitatively similar to the sleep that we recognize in adults (Frank & Heller, 1997b, 2003). Specifically, it was suggested that infant sleep is initially best described as an amalgam of sleep states (called "presleep"). The fine details of the presleep hypothesis and the ensuing debate have been reviewed elsewhere (Blumberg, Karlsson, Seelke, & Mohns, 2005a; Frank & Heller, 2005). Instead, this chapter is devoted primarily to recent studies that have resolved this debate by advancing our understanding of the phenomenology of sleep during the early postnatal period. By way of introduction here, we focus first on several broad issues that are foundational to any attempt to understand infant sleep and its development.

First, it behooves us to appreciate the distinction between descriptions and explanations of sleep. To borrow the famous line from Supreme Court Justice Potter Stewart as he struggled to define pornography, we know sleep when we see it. But good science, like the good law, demands more precise definitions. Accordingly, sleep researchers in the 1960s produced *A Manual of Standardized Terminology, Techniques and Scoring System* to aid communication among laboratories and guide the work of future investigators (Rechtschaffen & Kales, 1968).

Although this manual provided the necessary criteria for describing (or "diagnosing") sleep in adult humans, it did little to explain the causal mechanisms controlling it. Nor did the manual provide a theory of sleep or even hypotheses concerning sleep's functions. Indeed, to their credit, the authors of the manual explicitly advised readers regarding its aims and limitations:

> Although there is considerable comparability of sleep stage manifestations among various species, the differences are sufficiently great to require a separate scoring system for most species. This proposal is designed for adult humans.... [I]t is well known that human infants show combinations of polygraphic features which defy classification by the criteria proposed here. A strict adherence to the proposed system *would not yield* an adequate description of infant sleep. (italics added)

Despite these caveats, the manual would have a pervasive influence on how we interpret sleep in other species and in infants. Perhaps most influential was the adoption of three electrographic measures—the electroencephalogram (EEG), electrooculogram (EOG), and electromyogram (EMG)—for categorizing the major states of sleep and wakefulness. Once these criteria were established, it became difficult to avoid analyzing sleep–wake states in nonhumans and nonadults without reference to them.

An alternative approach—one that grew out of the European ethological tradition—has relied predominantly on behavioral measures alone to categorize behavioral states (Gramsbergen, Schwartze, & Prechtl, 1970; Nijhuis, Martin, & Prechtl, 1984). This approach is particularly useful for investigations of subjects that are not amenable to more invasive approaches. For example, the body size of infant rats and the fragility of preterm human infants have impeded the use of the kinds of instrumentation procedures that are easily accomplished

in larger and more robust human and nonhuman animals. In infant rats, investigators were able to distinguish high-amplitude movements of limbs (e.g., stretching, kicking) as indicators of wakefulness and myoclonic twitches of the limbs and tail as indicators of active sleep (Gramsbergen et al., 1970). As we will see, however, such motor activity alone does not fully capture all aspects of behavioral state expression in perinates.

Regardless of whether one relies on behavioral or electrographic criteria (or both) for classifying behavioral states, there is little doubt that state assignments become more reliable (in the sense that interrater reliability increases) the more measures one has at one's disposal. But it is also true that the selection and interpretation of particular criteria reflect underlying assumptions that can critically influence our assessment of sleep.

For example, the traditional reliance on epochs to categorize behavioral states, a reliance codified in Rechtschaffen and Kale's manual, has the practical effect of filtering out events that occur at a temporal scale that is smaller than the epoch (in other words, the epoch technique functions as a low-pass filter). Similarly, although the neocortical EEG can provide valuable information when assessing sleep and wake states under many circumstances, we must be careful not to elevate this single measure to a status that it does not deserve. As we will see, overestimation of the value of the neocortical EEG, particularly delta activity, can be particularly confusing when we are examining animals that do not exhibit easily identifiable state-dependent neocortical activity.

The broader message is simple: Electrographic and behavioral measures are tools for categorizing states to animals, but we must exercise caution so as not to confuse these measures with the inferred state themselves. In effect, these measures are useful for *describing* a state, but for *explanation* we need formal, testable hypotheses that address the mechanistic links among the various measures and their functional significance.

One guiding theme of developmental psychobiology is that infants are adapted to the developmental niche in which they live as well as prepare for the likely niches that are to come. This notion of the "dual infant," connected as it is to the related concept of ontogenetic adaptation, helps us to appreciate the significance of the developmental period as more than a period of stasis and dependency (Alberts & Cramer, 1988). For example, if we wish to understand thermal homeostatic capabilities in infant rats, then we should not test them under ambient conditions appropriate to adults (Blumberg, 2001). Indeed, when thermal challenges are scaled to the size of the animal under study, infants reveal a regulatory capacity that is otherwise masked.

These lessons are equally important in the field of sleep research as we strive to develop criteria for measuring sleep and wakefulness that are not constrained by those criteria that apply most readily only later in life. Again, the fact that the EEG is useful for assigning behavioral states in adults does not imply that its absence in infants precludes effective descriptions of sleep and wakefulness. Rather than attempt to fit infants into slots custom-built for adults, we should strive to develop descriptive and explanatory tools and that are relevant for and appropriate to our infant subjects.

We note that the field of animal learning made its greatest strides as investigators turned to "simple" animal models of learning in invertebrates (e.g., *Aplysia*) (Kandel & Schwartz, 1982) and well-defined model systems in adult mammals (e.g., eyeblink conditioning) (Gormezano, Kehoe, & Marshall, 1983; Thompson, 1986). Accordingly, sleep researchers are considering the potential benefits of using "simple" animal models, including invertebrates (Hendricks, Sehgal, & Pack, 2000). We believe that the infants of altricial species (e.g., rats, mice), with their strong drive for sleep and their rapidly changing sleep patterns, also offer valuable opportunities for making progress in our understanding of the mechanisms and functions of sleep.

These and other related themes are explored in this chapter as we review recent research relating to the form and function of infant sleep. We first describe the various approaches that have been used to provide a modern description of behavioral states in infants, particularly infant rats. Then, we aim to show how, through developmental analysis, we can move beyond description to explanations of the mechanisms and functions of sleep across the lifespan.

The Phenomenology of Infant Sleep

A behavioral state is an outward manifestation of a stable but reversible and recurring pattern of internal conditions of an animal that exhibits two general features: first, a state must exhibit concordance or coherence among the components comprising it; second, it must exhibit persistence, that is, temporal stability (Nijhuis, 1995).

As characterized in adults—and even in older infants—behavioral states such as quiet sleep (QS, or nonrapid eye movement [NREM] or slow-wave sleep), active sleep (AS, or rapid eye movement [REM] or desynchronized sleep), and waking seem to be global phenomena comprising persistent and concordant components regulated by specific regions of the brain (Pace-Schott & Hobson, 2002; Siegel, 2005b). As for younger infants, however, it has been suggested that sleep states comprise relatively few components that are poorly integrated (Adrien & Lanfumey, 1984; Jouvet-Mounier et al., 1970; McGinty et al., 1977) and, further, that the brain does not modulate infant behavioral states (Frank & Heller, 1997b, 2003). Such claims present a challenge to the development of a comprehensive description of sleep across the lifespan.

This challenge becomes particularly acute when sleep is defined using an arbitrary number of privileged components or when it is asserted that a single, "essential" component must be present in order for sleep to be expressed. One response to the latter claim is to suggest alternative names to behavioral states that lack the essential component (Frank & Heller, 2003). Although such a classification strategy is appropriate and even useful in a clinical setting, no classification scheme alone is sufficient for revealing the mechanisms that produce and regulate sleep–wake states.

We suggest that any theory of sleep development must account for the addition and integration of individual sleep components, as well as changes in the persistence of sleep and wakefulness across ontogeny (Blumberg & Lucas, 1996; Corner, 1985; Dreyfus-Brisac, 1970). To that end, it is important that we recognize the role that behavioral assessment can play in providing a firm foundation for further explorations of the mechanisms underlying behavioral states. Thus, we begin with behavior.

The Foundation: Behavior

The earliest behavior of invertebrate and vertebrate animals is characterized by spontaneous movements of the head, limbs, and tail (Corner, 1977). In mammalian and avian embryos, this spontaneous motor activity (SMA) is a ubiquitous feature of behavioral expression and has been a major focus of investigation for behavioral embryologists (Hamburger, 1973; Narayanan, Fox, & Hamburger, 1971; Provine, 1973). In considering these various embryonic and infant movements, Corner (1977) proposed that they exhibit continuity across the life span. Indeed, he maintained that "sleep motility in its entirety... is nothing less than the continued postnatal expression of primordial nervous functional processes" (p. 292).

The SMA of fetal and infant rats exhibits organization in both spatial and temporal dimensions. One form of spatiotemporal organization that has received relatively little attention is movement synchrony, in which one limb moves in temporal proximity to another (Robinson & Smotherman, 1987). Although these synchronous movements occur predominantly at intermovement intervals of 0.5 s or less (Lane & Robinson, 1998), they are not simultaneous and do not resemble the whole-body startles[1] that have long been recognized (Gramsbergen et al., 1970; Hamburger & Oppenheim, 1967). Furthermore, movement synchrony reflects more than simply a temporal dependence among pairs of limbs; rather, patterns of movements among two or more limbs are organized into discrete bouts[2] (Fagen & Young, 1978). Using this bout-analytic approach (Robinson, Blumberg, Lane, & Kreber, 2000), similarities in bout structure between fetuses (embryonic day [E]17–E21) and infants (P1–P9) become readily apparent, thus providing additional empirical support for Corner's continuity hypothesis for SMA.

To further understand this organization, a computational model of SMA was developed that incorporated spontaneous activity of spinal motor neurons, intrasegmental and intersegmental interactions within the spinal cord, recurrent inhibition within the spinal cord, and descending influences from the brain; this model produced bouts with the same structure that we observed in perinatal rats (Robinson et al., 2000). Moreover, consistent with the model, bouts were not eliminated on embryonic day (E)20 after cervical spinal transection, suggesting that the brain is not necessary to produce bout organization in fetuses. Thus, the organization of limb movements into bouts appears to be a highly robust phenomenon that is consistently expressed by fetal and infant rats, and exhibits systematic changes during prenatal and postnatal development.

When an infant rat is placed in a humidified and thermoneutral environment—that is, an environment that allows for the minimal expenditure of energy[3]—it cycles rapidly between sleep and wakefulness. When awake, the pup often exhibits high-amplitude movements including locomotion, head-lifting, kicking, stretching, and yawning. When this activity ceases, there ensues a period of behavioral quiescence as muscles in the body relax.

After this period of QS, AS commences with the onset of myoclonic twitching of the fore and hind limbs, tail, and head. These periods of twitching wax and wane until the pup suddenly reawakens and resumes high-amplitude movements. A typical cycle of waking, QS, and AS exhibit this basic order of expression, with the duration of each bout of sleep and wakefulness varying significantly within and between individuals, as well as across age.

Careful analysis of the behavior of infant rats indicates that they conform to many of the standard criteria used by other researchers to assess the existence of sleep in a variety of vertebrate and invertebrate species (Campbell & Tobler, 1984; Hendricks et al., 2000). These criteria include (a) an absence of high-amplitude movements (often designated in the literature as voluntary, coordinated, or purposeful), (b) spontaneity, as indicated by transitions between behavioral states that occur in a protected environment and are therefore not triggered by exogenous stimuli, and (c) reversibility, a criterion that helps to distinguish sleep from irreversible pathological states (e.g., coma). Other criteria for defining sleep, including circadian rhythmicity, increased sensory and/or arousal thresholds, homeostatic regulation, and neural control are addressed later in this chapter.

We have used behavior alone to examine the effects of air temperature and endogenous heat production on the expression of sleep and wakefulness (Blumberg & Stolba, 1996; Sokoloff & Blumberg, 1998). In addition, as discussed above, behavioral analysis was used to assess the temporal structure of twitching in fetal and neonatal rats (Robinson et al., 2000), as well as the contributions of the spinal cord to twitching (Blumberg & Lucas, 1994) and the reliance of twitching upon mesopontine neural circuitry (Kreider, 2003). Nonetheless, there are limitations to complete reliance upon behavioral measures. For example, using this method, it is not possible to discern the transition between quiet wakefulness and QS, both of which are marked by behavioral quiescence (Gramsbergen et al., 1970). Thus, demonstrating a stable relationship between the expression of sleep–wake behaviors and a second component would provide an important step forward in our understanding of state organization in infants.

Beyond Behavior: Nuchal Muscle Activity

As we began our search for a second measure of sleep and wakefulness to complement behavior in our infant subjects, we turned to the "trio" of electrographic measures—EMG, EOG, and EEG—that had been codified in the manual of Rechtschaffen and Kales. Of these three, state-dependent EEG is not expressed in rats younger than P11 (Corner & Mirmiran, 1990; Frank & Heller, 1997b; Gramsbergen, 1976; Jouvet-Mounier et al., 1970; Seelke & Blumberg, 2008; Seelke, Karlsson, Gall, & Blumberg, 2005). Of the other two, we initially doubted our ability to measure the EOG, in part because we doubted that rapid eye movements occur early in infancy. So, we chose to measure EMG activity in the nuchal muscle, the primary elevator muscle of the head. To do this, we implanted fine-wire bipolar hook electrodes into the nuchal muscles of infant rats at P2, P5, and P8 (Karlsson & Blumberg, 2002) and recorded nuchal EMG activity and behavior, including twitches of the limbs and tail.

Figure 20.1A depicts a sleep–wake cycle in a 1-week-old rat, illustrating the progression from wakefulness to QS as indicated by the transition from high muscle tone to atonia. AS commences with the onset of twitching, as determined by behavioral analysis as well as the presence of twitch-related spikes in the nuchal EMG. Finally, with the onset of wakefulness, twitching is replaced by high-amplitude movements and nuchal atonia is replaced by high muscle tone, thus completing the cycle.

We noted that isolated spikes in the nuchal EMG occur only against a background of atonia and often result in noticeable twitch-like movements of the head. The relationship between these spikes and behaviorally scored twitches of the limbs and tail was examined, and we found a strong temporal relationship between them (Seelke & Blumberg, 2005). Specifically, during atonia periods, the onset of spikes in the nuchal EMG coincides with the onset of twitching in the limbs and tail (Figure 20.1B) and the two categories of twitching are highly correlated with each other (Figure 20.1C). Finally, bouts of twitching in the nuchal muscle and limbs are temporally linked across atonia periods, producing bouts of synchronized phasic activity interspersed with bouts of quiescence (Figure 20.1D) (Seelke & Blumberg, 2005; Seelke et al., 2005). Based on these and other observations, we can see that sleep and wakefulness in infant rats can be defined accurately using two measures—nuchal EMG and behavior—and, surprisingly, these measures are highly concordant at a very early age in this altricial species.

Using EMG and behavior, we were able to explore further whether the infant sleep state meets other standard criteria in the field (Hendricks et al., 2000). For example, to assess changes in sensory threshold during sleep, P8 rats were instrumented with nuchal EMG electrodes as well as electrodes for measuring respiration. Then, dimethyl disulfide, an olfactory stimulus, of various concentrations was presented to these subjects during periods of AS or wakefulness (Seelke & Blumberg, 2004). When awake, the threshold to exhibit polypnea (i.e., bursts of increased respiratory rate indicative of sniffing) was lower than when pups were in AS, suggesting a heightened sensory threshold during this sleep state.

Still another traditional criterion of sleep concerns the regulatory response to deprivation—commonly referred to as sleep homeostasis. Sleep homeostasis is typically assessed by depriving a subject of sleep and monitoring corrective responses (Bonnet, 2000; Rechtschaffen, Bergmann, Gilliland, & Bauer, 1999). Specifically, sleep deprivation is thought to evoke two compensatory responses: sleep pressure, which occurs during the period of deprivation and is indicated by an increase in the number of attempts to enter sleep (and a corresponding increase in the difficulty of producing and maintaining arousal), and sleep rebound, which occurs when sleep is permitted after a period of deprivation and is indicated by a compensatory increase in sleep.

To explore sleep regulation in early infancy, P5 rats were deprived of sleep for 30 min by delivering brief flank shocks whenever the nuchal muscle became atonic (Blumberg, Middlemis-Brown, & Johnson, 2004). Because it was increasingly difficult to maintain arousal over the period of sleep deprivation—as indicated by the need to increase the number of shocks and their intensity—we concluded that the procedure was inducing increased sleep pressure. In contrast to sleep pressure, sleep rebound was not detected at P5 in this study, consistent with an earlier study that suggested that rebound does not occur until after P14 (Frank, Morrissette, & Heller, 1998).

However, more recently (Todd & Blumberg, 2007), we developed an alternative method for depriving pups of sleep—one that allowed us to assess with greater confidence the effectiveness of the sleep deprivation procedure.[4] This method entailed the application of a cold stimulus to the snout, which possesses a high concentration of cold receptors (Dickenson, Hellon, & Taylor, 1979). Using this method in P2 and P8 rats, we again saw pronounced increases in sleep pressure. Moreover,

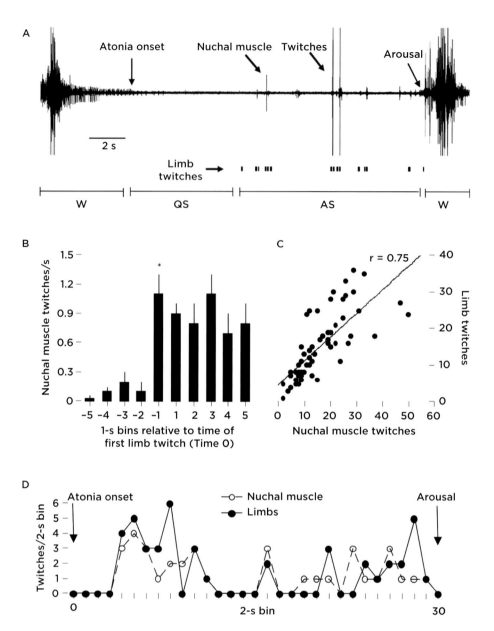

Figure 20.1 Relationship between myoclonic twitching as measured by visual observation of the limbs and activity in nuchal EMG. (A) Representative cycle of high nuchal muscle tone and atonia in a P8 rat tested at thermoneutrality (i.e., 35°C). Nuchal muscle twitches against a background of atonia are indicated, as are instances of visually scored limb twitches. This cycle has been divided into periods of wakefulness (W), quiet sleep (QS), and active sleep (AS). (B) Perievent histogram indicating increase in nuchal muscle twitching within 1 s of the first visually scored limb twitch of an atonia period. Data are from 10 atonia periods across 6 P8 rats . * Significant difference from previous time bin. (C) Regression relating the number of behaviorally scored limb twitches and the number of nuchal muscle twitches during periods of atonia. Data are from the same atonia periods as in (B). $N = 60$ data points. The best-fit line is shown. (D) Representative data from a single period of atonia in a P8 rat showing the number of twitches measured during successive 2-s bins. Behaviorally scored limb twitches (filled circles) and nuchal muscle twitches (open circles) are shown separately and indicate synchronized bursts of phasic activity during the atonia period. (From Seelke & Blumberg, 2005.)

when the deprivation period was over and the pups were allowed to sleep without disturbance, they exhibited pronounced increases in sleep duration, consistent with sleep rebound. Finally, when precollicular transections were performed at P2, sleep pressure increased significantly during the deprivation period, but sleep rebound was now prevented. This dissociation between pressure and rebound with precollicular transection has also been reported in adult cats (de Andres, Garzon, & Villablanca, 2003).

The studies just described are the first to address the effects of sleep deprivation before P12 in rats (Feng, Ma, & Vogel, 2001; Frank et al., 1998; Mirmiran et al., 1983; Mirmiran, Van De Poll, Corner, Van Oyen, & Bour, 1981). Clearly, important questions remain and more work in this area is needed.

Rapid Eye Movements and Extraocular Muscle Activity

During AS in adults, REMs occur along with other forms of phasic activity, such as myoclonic twitching. Jouvet-Mounier et al. (1970) reported that REMs occur as early as P6, but they did not mention whether REMs are present at earlier ages. Other researchers, including van Someren et al. (1990), reported the presence of REMs at P8 that exhibited an "adult-like appearance" by P15, that is, around the time of eye opening. These reports left several unanswered questions. First, do the eyes exhibit state-dependent movements, or indeed any activity, before P6? Second, what is the mechanism that generates the sleep-related rapid eye movements?

A novel perspective on the mechanisms of REM generation was proposed by Chase and Morales (1983, 1990). Specifically, in their 1983 paper examining the origin of myoclonic twitches, they asked whether the

> mechanisms responsible for the phasic contraction
> of the peripheral musculature during REM periods
> may reflect a general pattern that affects other
> somatomotor functions as well. For example, the
> striated muscles that move the orbits are active dur-
> ing REM periods.... It is possible that the central

neural areas that give rise to myoclonic activation of the limb muscles during REM periods also initiate a pattern of twitches and jerks that affect all striated muscles. REMs are an example.... (p. 1198)

This hypothesis—that the same mechanisms responsible for generating myoclonic twitches of the limbs could also be responsible for generating twitches of the eyes—provided us with a framework for examining the development of REMs in infant rats. We wondered: If REMs are indeed produced by twitches of the extraocular muscles, and if these extraocular muscle twitches are phenomenologically similar to the twitches produced by other striated muscles, then perhaps direct measurement of extraocular muscle activity would reveal ontogenetic precursors of REMs that had heretofore gone unnoticed.

Thus, we examined extraocular EMG activity in rats at P3, P8, and P14 (Seelke et al., 2005). EMG electrodes were implanted in the medial and lateral rectus muscle of each eye and the signals from the electrodes were filtered to allow for the examination of both gross eye movements and extraocular muscle activity. EMG electrodes were implanted in the nuchal muscle of each subject and, in P14 subjects, EEG activity was also measured.

As shown in Figure 20.2, each extraocular EMG record could be filtered in two ways to reveal two kinds of activity. First, filtering for high-frequency activity (i.e., 300–5000 Hz, top row of Figure 20.2) revealed spiking in the EMG record indicative of muscle twitching. At all three ages—P3, P8, and P14—distinct twitching was observed in the extraocular EMG. Second, filtering for low-frequency activity (i.e., 1–35 Hz, bottom row of Figure 20.2) revealed movements of the eyeball, similar to the information provided by the EOG. Sleep-related rapid eye movements were most easily identified

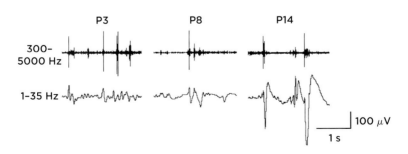

Figure 20.2 Representative extraocular EMG activity and eye movements at P3, P8, and P14. Top row: High-pass (300–5000 Hz) filtering to reveal myoclonic twitching. Bottom row: Low-pass (1–35 Hz) filtering to reveal eye movements. (From Seelke et al., 2005.)

at P14, but some evidence of such movements was found at P8 and even P3. Significantly, these REMs were typically accompanied by twitches of the extraocular muscles, thus providing direct support for the Chase and Morales hypothesis. Moreover, because twitching was easily identified as early as P3, an age when eye movements were not robust, it was apparent that twitching in the EMG record reveals features of early oculomotor activity that are not easily detectible using conventional EOG techniques.

Although REMs are often afforded privileged status by sleep researchers, our findings indicated that the eye muscles are, like those controlling any limb, prone to twitching during AS. One implication of this interpretation is that conventional assessments of the EMG and EOG may reveal tonic and phasic aspects of muscle activity, respectively, but a single record of skeletal muscle activity—when less restrictive filtering and sampling methods are used—can capture both tonic fluctuations in muscle tone as well as occurrences of phasic twitching (Seelke et al., 2005).

Having established that REMs are produced by twitches of the extraocular muscles, we next turned our attention to the relationship between these twitches and other forms of sleep-related phasic activity. As described above (see also Figure 20.1D), atonia periods begin with a bout of behavioral quiescence, soon followed by the onset of twitches as detected from the extraocular and nuchal EMGs as well as behavioral observations of the limbs and tail. Perhaps most striking, we found that as early as P3 (see Figure 20.3A), all of the phasic movements occur together to define a coherent period of AS. Moreover, when these movements are analyzed in greater detail, we see again that they are expressed as synchronized "waves" of phasic activity occurring in the extraocular muscles, nuchal muscle, and limbs. This highly organized structure of AS contrasts sharply with the perspective of infant sleep as diffuse, primitive, and dissociated (Adrien & Lanfumey, 1984; Frank & Heller, 1997b, 2003).

Completing the Trio: Neocortical EEG

As already mentioned, it is widely accepted that the neocortical EEG in rats does not exhibit state-dependent differentiation, especially delta (or slow-wave) activity, until approximately P11 (Frank & Heller, 1997b; Gramsbergen, 1976; Mirmiran & Corner, 1982). In other species, this milestone is reached at 115–120 days postconception in sheep (Clewlow, Dawes, Johnston, & Walker, 1983;

Szeto & Hinman, 1985), 50 days postconception in guinea pigs (Umans et al., 1985), and approximately 32 weeks postconception in preterm human infants (Dreyfus-Brisac, 1975). Despite the fact that neocortical activity is a noncausal correlate of sleep and wakefulness and not an integral component of the neural circuitry that modulates state, its inclusion as one of the critical criteria in the Rechtschaffen and Kales sleep manual elevated its status among sleep researchers (e.g., see Frank & Heller, 2003).

The absence of the EEG as a reliable measure of behavioral state in infants had forced earlier investigators to rely on other measures, including body movements, respiration, heart rate, and muscle tone (Gramsbergen et al., 1970; Nijhuis et al., 1984; Parmelee, Wenner, Akiyama, Schultz, & Stern, 1967). Perhaps inevitably, disagreement and confusion emerged as different investigators relied on different measures and adopted different criteria for categorizing sleep at these early ages (Dreyfus-Brisac, 1970; Prechtl, 1974). One of the aims of our research program was to avoid conceptual and semantic confusion through systematic and unbiased analysis of the components of sleep as they are elaborated through developmental time (Blumberg & Lucas, 1996). As detailed until this point, our research had indicated the presence of an ultradian rhythm comprising bouts of high and low muscle tone linked with other state-related phenomena (e.g., myoclonic twitches).

The relatively late postnatal emergence of delta activity in rats provides an opportunity to observe the real-time linking of a new sleep component with those that have already developed. We did this by examining the relationship between the neocortical EEG, nuchal and extraocular EMGs, and limb movements (Seelke et al., 2005). First, as shown for the P3 subject in Figure 20.3A, note once again how wakefulness is followed by a period of QS which, in turn, is followed by an AS period defined by the presence of phasic muscle activity. The question we addressed was whether delta activity, once it emerged, would occupy the "location" designated as QS in younger subjects. As shown for the P14 subject in Figure 20.3B, the period of nuchal atonia before the onset of twitching was accompanied by high-amplitude EEG activity; this EEG activity exhibited a dominant frequency of 2.5–4 Hz, characteristic of delta activity. Because the records at the two ages are, with the exception of EEG activity and timescale, nearly identical, we concluded that the states designated as QS and AS

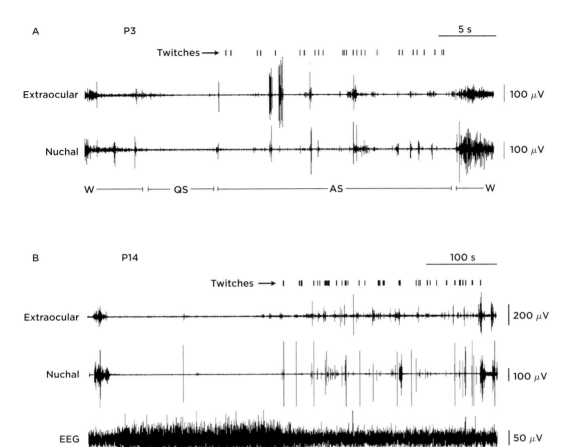

Figure 20.3 Phasic and tonic behavioral and electrographic events across a complete sleep–wake cycle in a P3 and P14 rat. (A) Behaviorally scored limb twitches and extraocular and nuchal EMGs for a P3 rat. Periods of wakefulness (W), quiet sleep (QS), and active sleep (AS) are indicated. (B) Same as (A) except the subject is a P14 rat and neocortical EEG is also recorded. The twitch occurring in the middle of the QS period is actualy due to a startle. Note the different timescales for (A) and (B). (From Seelke et al., 2005.)

before the emergence of delta activity are homologous with those that come later.

In subsequent work, we assessed the structure of sleep bouts in P9, P11, and P13 rats—that is, before, during, and after the emergence of delta activity (Seelke & Blumberg, 2008). At all three ages, using EMG and behavioral measures alone, we found that QS predominates during the first third of each sleep period. At P11 and P13, delta activity similarly predominates during the first third of each atonia period, declines during the second third, and is rare during the final third. When delta occurs during the final third of a sleep period, it occurs during those brief interludes between bursts of myoclonic twitching. Thus, with the developmental emergence of delta activity, we can positively identify multiple cycles

of QS and AS, as in adults (Zepelin, Siegel, & Tobler, 2005).

Based on previous studies, it is clear that QS dominates the first third of sleep periods in rats as early as P3 (Seelke et al., 2005) and that this pattern continues up until the emergence of delta activity at P11 (Seelke & Blumberg, 2008). These results seem inconsistent with the findings of Jouvet-Mounier et al., who reported that QS in infant rats is virtually nonexistent before P10 and increases explosively thereafter (Jouvet-Mounier et al., 1970). The discrepancy between these findings is likely due to the restrictive criteria used by those earlier investigators for defining QS. Specifically, in the Jouvet-Mounier et al. study, 30 s of behavioral quiescence were required before the designation of QS was applied. When we consider that the mean

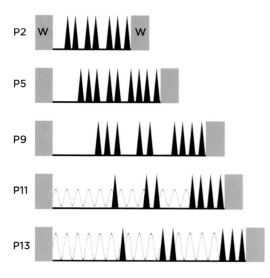

Figure 20.4 Schematic depiction of developmental changes in the temporal organization of sleep and wakefulness and the emergence of delta activity in infant rats. Gray rectangles represent periods of high muscle tone, indicative of wakefulness (W). Interposed periods of sleep are defined by nuchal atonia, depicted as black lines. Phasic bursts of myoclonic twitching, indicative of active sleep, are depicted as black triangles. At P9 and earlier, each sleep period comprises an initial bout of quiet sleep followed by bursts of phasic activity interrupted by brief bouts of behavioral quiescence. By P11, delta activity (depicted as sinusoidal waves) is detected during the first quiet sleep episode as well as during some of the subsequent periods of quiescence between bouts of twitching. By P13, delta power has increased and is more reliably expressed during periods of quiescence. Overall, with age, sleep durations increase and the intervals between bouts of twitching also increase, thus providing greater opportunity for the expression of delta activity during the final third of a sleep bout. (Adapted from Seelke & Blumberg, 2008.)

sleep bout duration during the first postnatal week ranges from 20 s at P3 to 45 s at P8 (Blumberg, Seelke, Lowen, & Karlsson, 2005b), and that mean QS duration only exceeds 30 s by P13 (Seelke & Blumberg, 2008), a 30-s criterion for the identification of QS effectively precluded its detection in that earlier study.

Thus, using the methods and criteria outlined above, within days after birth we can identify sleep periods comprising periods of quiescence interspersed with bursts of myoclonic twitching (see Figure 20.4). These bursts, comprising synchronized activity in multiple muscle groups throughout the body, begin shortly after the onset of atonia and continue throughout the duration of the sleep period. The periods of quiescence are initially very brief—during the first postnatal week they often last less than 2 s. The duration of these periods of

quiescence increases with age and, by P11, are often accompanied by delta activity.

We should stress that no classification scheme, including ours, provides perfect assessments across all spatial and temporal scales. Accordingly, it has long been appreciated that the inclusion of as many components as possible into a scheme helps to resolve uncertainties. However, given the fluidity of state development and the unavailability of certain state components at earlier ages, our goal should be to devise classification schemes that capture the full range of developmental phenomena in an unbiased fashion. Then, to move beyond classification toward explanation, we should seek to understand the neural mechanisms that produce the components as well as their functional relations.

State-dependent Neocortical Activity Revisited

The traditional reliance on surface EEG recordings and the focus on delta activity gave rise to the notion that the EEG is undifferentiated prior to the emergence of delta activity around P11 in rats. For a variety of reasons, however, this perspective is no longer accurate. First, the use of electrodes that can detect infraslow activity has revealed bursts of sleep-related "slow activity transients" in premature human infants during sleep that disappear around 40 postconceptional weeks (Vanhatalo et al., 2005; see Chapter 6).

Second, while recording from the primary sensory areas of newborn rats, Khazipov and colleagues detected brief oscillations that they call "spindle-bursts" (Khazipov et al., 2004; see Chapter 8). In somatosensory cortex, these bursts occur in response to spontaneous or evoked peripheral stimulation in a somatotopic manner. Subsequent work indicates that spindle-bursts within the forelimb region of primary somatosensory cortex are closely associated with the proprioceptive stimulation that accompanies twitching of the forelimb during AS (Marcano-Reik & Blumberg, 2008). Thus, already at P2–6, the infant neocortex exhibits somatotopic organization and a distinct neurophysiological response to discrete sensory stimulation. Because spindle-bursts occur in response to self-generated movements, they will occur predominantly during wakefulness or AS; in the nest, sensory stimulation from the dam and from other pups will also evoke them.

Spindle-bursts have also been detected in barrel and visual cortex after whisker stimulation and retinal waves, respectively (Hanganu, Ben-Ari, &

Khazipov, 2006; Hanganu, Staiger, Ben-Ari, & Khazipov, 2007; Minlebaev, Ben-Ari, & Khazipov, 2007). Thus, in conjunction with the previous findings in somatosensory cortex, it is clear that the neocortex of the altricial infant rat exhibits complex activity soon after birth. Some forms of this activity—as with spindle-bursts—are detected exclusively within primary sensory areas, whereas others may be found predominantly outside these areas. Regardless, it now appears that the infant neocortex exhibits state-dependent activity long before delta activity emerges. This early activity may play a critical role in the establishment and refinement of cortical connections, including those necessary for somatotopy (Khazipov et al., 2004; Seelke et al., 2005).

In P9, P11, and P13 rats (Seelke & Blumberg, 2008), we found evidence of very low-frequency cortical events that appear similar to the slow activity transients (SATs) described in premature human infants (Vanhatalo & Kaila, 2006; Vanhatalo et al., 2005). Also, as with SATs in humans, we found that SATs in infant rats are sleep-related. Specifically, we found that SATs predominate during the first third of the sleep period (Seelke & Blumberg, 2008), thus suggesting a close association with QS (although SATs also occur during wakefulness and in temporal proximity to AS-related twitching).

The developmental disappearance of SATs has been associated with the upregulation of the neuronal chloride extruder K+–Cl- cotransporter 2 (KCC2) and the associated emergence of the hyperpolarizing effects of GABA (Vanhatalo et al., 2005; see Chapter 6), which occurs during the second postnatal week in rats (Payne, Rivera, Voipio, & Kaila, 2003). Using calcium imaging, similar high-amplitude, low-frequency events have been observed in infant rat cortical tissue in vitro (Garaschuk, Linn, Eilers, & Konnerth, 2000) and neonatal mice in vivo (Adelsberger, Garaschuk, & Konnerth, 2005) and are referred to as "early network oscillations" (ENOs). As with SATs, the developmental disappearance of ENOs also appears to depend upon emerging GABAergic inhibition (Garaschuk et al., 2000). Thus, the disappearance of SATs/ENOs is mirrored by the appearance of delta activity, which may also depend upon GABAergic inhibition (Steriade, Curro Dossi, & Nunez, 1991; Terman, Bose, & Kopell, 1996).

Neural Substrates of Infant Sleep and Wakefulness

The successful integration of sleep research with neuroscience has contributed to the belief that sleep is "of the brain, by the brain, and for the brain" (Hobson, 2005). As a consequence, it is now expected that true sleep processes will be reflected in discernible neural activity, so much so that the identification of state-dependent neural activity has been mentioned as one criterion of sleep (Hendricks et al., 2000).

With regard to sleep in infant rats, technical obstacles have hampered the search for state-dependent neural activity. In only two early studies was it reported that the infant brain—specifically, the pontine and mesencephalic reticular formation—exhibits state-dependent activity (Corner & Bour, 1984; Tamásy, Korányi, & Lissák, 1980). Nonetheless, some had come to believe that the sleep–wake cycles of infant rats are not regulated by the brain, or at least are not controlled by the kinds of specific brain nuclei that have been identified in adults. Thus, in 1984, it was written that infant sleep comprises "a very primitive system of diffuse activation within the whole central nervous system" (Adrien & Lanfumey, 1984). More recently, Frank and Heller (2003) declared that infant sleep "is not controlled by executive sleep centers." In contrast with these views, we now review recent work documenting the contributions of central neural mechanisms to the modulation of infant sleep–wake states and the components that comprise them.

Spinal Cord

Myoclonic twitching has often been compared with other forms of SMA that are prevalent in vertebrate embryos, including birds and mammals (Corner, 1977; Narayanan et al., 1971; Robinson et al., 2000). Indeed, as already discussed, spontaneous activity in rats exhibits temporal structure that varies continuously across the prenatal-to-postnatal period (Robinson et al., 2000). Because this spontaneous activity provides useful information concerning the organization of behavioral states in early infancy, it is important to understand the neural mechanisms that produce it.

In order to investigate the mechanisms underlying the generation of myoclonic twitches, newborn rats received midthoracic spinal transections within several days after birth. When they were examined 1 week later, it was found that the hindlimbs (i.e., the limbs caudal to the transection) exhibited 50% fewer twitches than control pups (Blumberg & Lucas, 1994). Moreover, activity of the forelimbs (i.e., the limbs rostral to the transection) were unaffected by the spinal transection. It was concluded that spinal mechanisms alone can produce twitching, especially in fetuses and soon after birth in rats, but that there are increasing contributions with age from more rostral structures, including cervical spinal cord and brain.

Subsequent work demonstrated that the mesopontine region is a likely area of importance for the expression of twitching in rats within 1 week of birth. This was demonstrated by transecting the brain at various levels just caudal and rostral to the mesopontine region (Kreider & Blumberg, 2000). When the transections were placed anterior to the mesopontine region, twitching was no longer affected.

Therefore, both the brain and spinal cord contribute to the production of spontaneous activity, and specifically myoclonic twitching, soon after birth in rats. Furthermore, it appears that myoclonic twitching is initially produced independently by neural circuits within the spinal cord and that those circuits gradually come under the control of rostral brain structures (Stelzner, 1982).

Medulla

The demonstrated linkage between motor behavior (including myoclonic twitching) and nuchal EMG provided additional opportunities for exploring the neural bases of behavioral state organization in early infancy, provided that certain technical difficulties could be overcome. In particular, the soft, uncalcified skull of infant rats precludes many of the techniques that are readily used in larger and less fragile subjects. Over time, we developed a method for stimulating and recording from the brain of unanesthetized, head-fixed infants as nuchal EMG activity and behavior are also monitored.

The sleep-related nuchal atonia observed in infant rats could result from two distinct and mutually exclusive processes: the active inhibition of spinal motoneurons, as in adults (Chase & Morales, 1990), or from mere passive withdrawal of excitation to spinal motoneurons. If infant and adult atonia are produced by similar mechanisms, then the infant brain stem should contain neurons within the ventromedial medulla that produce atonia when stimulated (Hajnik, Lai, & Siegel, 2000) and exhibit atonia-related discharge properties (Sakai, 1988; Siegel et al., 1991); moreover, lesions of this area should produce a state reminiscent of "REM without atonia" (Schenkel & Siegel, 1989).

Using P7–10 rats, we found support for each of these predictions (Karlsson & Blumberg, 2005).

First, we used electrical stimulation to identify an inhibitory area within the medial medulla. As shown in Figure 20.5A, muscle tone inhibition was consistently found on or near the midline within the ventromedial medulla in an area that includes nucleus gigantocellularis, nucleus paramedianis, and raphe obscurus. Figures 20.5B and C depict the effect of electrical stimulation within this region on nuchal muscle tone in a representative subject. It is clear that each pulse of electrical stimulation produces a discrete and reversible inhibition of nuchal tone. To ensure that these observed effects were not due to stimulation of fibers of passage, we infused the glutamate agonist quisqualic acid into this same region and produced rapid inhibition of muscle tone (similar infusions of the cholinergic agonist carbachol or corticotropin-releasing factor had no effect).

Second, as shown in Figure 20.5D, extracellular recordings from this same area in the medulla revealed the presence of neurons exhibiting "atonia-on" profiles, that is, they became active during periods of nuchal atonia and went silent during period of high nuchal muscle tone (neurons with "EMG-on" profiles were also found during periods of high muscle tone, but at more lateral sites). Finally, chemical lesions within the inhibitory area resulted in significant reductions in atonia durations, as well as decoupling of atonia from myoclonic twitching; specifically, twitches occasionally occurred during periods of high muscle tone, a condition reminiscent of "REM without atonia" as described in adults (Morrison, 1988; Schenkel & Siegel, 1989).

Based on the results of this study employing three experimental approaches—stimulation, recording, and lesioning—we concluded that the brain of infant rats, like that of adults, contains a medullary inhibitory area (MIA) that must be activated in order to produce the atonia of sleep. These results were then used as a foundation for further investigations of the neural contributions to infant sleep and wakefulness at other levels of the neuraxis.

Mesopontine Region

Having established a foothold in the medulla with the identification of the MIA, we used a variety of experimental approaches to delineate the components of the neural circuit mediating behavioral state in 1-week-old rats (Karlsson, Gall, Mohns, Seelke, & Blumberg, 2005). First, to establish the presence of efferents to the MIA, we

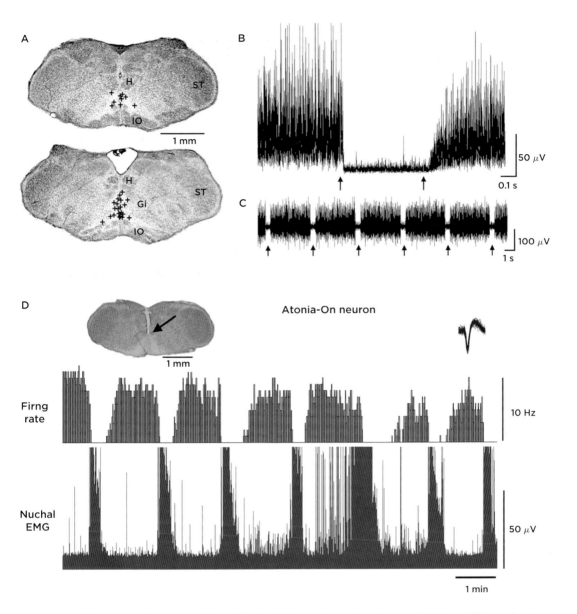

Figure 20.5 Inhibitory sites in the ventromedial medulla identified using electrical stimulation in P8–10 rats. (A) Coronal sections of the medullary inhibitory area. Each symbol (+) represents one inhibitory site from one pup (H, hypoglossal nucleus; ST, spinal trigeminal nucleus; Gi, nucleus gigantocellularis; IO, inferior olive). (B) Averaged nuchal EMG trace from 10 stimulus pulses applied to the inhibitory area of one pup; the arrows depict pulse onset and offset. (C) Representative sample of raw nuchal EMG responses to stimulation pulses; the arrows indicate periods of stimulation-induced atonia. (D) The discharge profile of a representative atonia-on unit in the ventromedial medulla (top) and its associated nuchal EMG trace (bottom). In the photomicrograph, the arrow indicates the tip of the electrode. The inset in the upper-right corner depicts 50 superimposed action potentials of the sorted unit. For purposes of illustration, the EMG trace is full-wave rectified. (From Karlsson & Blumberg, 2005.)

infused the fluorescent tracer DiI into that region and searched for the presence of cell bodies projecting to it. As expected, we found inputs to the MIA from medullary and mesopontine structures—including the nucleus subcoeruleus (SubLC), nucleus pontis caudalis (PC), and laterodorsal tegmental nucleus (LDT)—that are similar to those reported in adults (Cobos, Lima, Almeida, & Tavares, 2003; Malinowska & Kubin, 2004; Vertes, Martin, & Waltzer, 1986).

Using the tracing study as a guide, we next searched within the medulla and mesopontine region for sites that exhibited state-dependent activity. In particular, we were searching for neurons exhibiting firing patterns that mirrored sleep–wake states identified using the nuchal EMG, including atonia-on neurons (indicative of sleep, such as those identified in the MIA), EMG-on neurons (indicative of wakefulness), as well as other patterns that have been identified in adults. For example, as shown in Figure 20.6, atonia-on and EMG-on neurons, and even neurons associated particularly with AS ("AS-on"), were found within the SubLC and PC.

In contrast, the LDT contained many EMG-on neurons. Also, and perhaps most surprising was the identification of neurons within the LDT that exhibited a burst of activity in anticipation of myoclonic twitches; this finding is consistent with our earlier claim (Kreider & Blumberg, 2000; see discussion above) that neurons within the mesopontine region of 1-week-old rats contribute to twitching. All together, these findings demonstrate a remarkable diversity of state-dependent neural activity in neonatal rats.

Next, building on this neurophysiological evidence, we performed electrical and chemical lesions within the mesopontine region. Consistent with the recording data, we demonstrated that atonia durations are decreased after lesions of SubLC or nucleus pontis oralis (PO) and myoclonic twitching is reduced after lesions within the dorsolateral pontine tegmentum (DLPT), despite a dramatic increase in atonia duration. Moreover, lesions of SubLC and PO decoupled myoclonic twitching from nuchal atonia, producing a condition resembling "REM sleep without atonia" similar to that found after lesions within the MIA (Karlsson & Blumberg, 2005).

More recently, we tested the hypothesis that nuchal muscle tone is modulated, at least in part, by cholinergically mediated interactions between the DLPT and PO (Gall, Poremba, & Blumberg, 2007). Again using unanesthetized P8–10 rats, we found that chemical infusion of the cholinergic agonist carbachol within the DLPT activated high muscle tone. Next, chemical lesions of the PO were used to produce a chronic state of high nuchal muscle tone, at which time the cholinergic antagonist scopolamine was infused into the DLPT. Scopolamine effectively decreased nuchal muscle tone, suggesting that lesions of the PO increase muscle tone via cholinergic activation of the DLPT. Indeed, activation of the DLPT after PO lesions was effectively visualized using 2-deoxyglucose (2-DG) autoradiography. Finally,

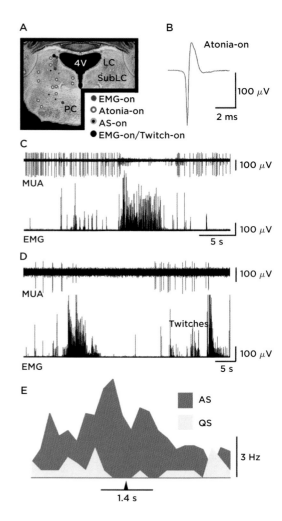

Figure 20.6 State-dependent neural activity within the mesopontine region. (A) Recording sites of state-dependent neurons reconstructed on a coronal section at the mesopontine level of a P8 rat. Note the predominance of atonia-on neurons. (B) Averaged waveform of a representative atonia-on neuron. (C) Upper trace: multiunit activity. Lower trace: concurrently recorded nuchal EMG. Spike sorting revealed 2 units that are easily distinguished by their amplitudes. The higher-amplitude unit is atonia-on; note its tonic discharge throughout the atonia period. (D) Upper trace: multiunit activity. Lower trace: concurrently recorded nuchal EMG. Spike sorting revealed 2 units that are easily distinguished by their amplitudes. The higher-amplitude unit is AS-on; note the absence of multiunit activity at the onset of the atonia period and then the increase in activity coinciding with the appearance of nuchal twitches. (E) Mean discharge rates of a representative AS-on neuron during bouts of AS and QS as defined, respectively, by the presence or absence of phasic nuchal twitches during periods of atonia. The arrowhead indicates the midpoint of the AS and QS bouts. 4V: fourth ventricle; LC: locus coeruleus; SubLC: subcoeruleus; PC: nucleus pontis caudalis. (From Karlsson et al., 2005.)

consistent with the hypothesis that PO inactivation produces high muscle tone, infusion of the sodium channel blocker lidocaine into the PO of unanesthetized pups produced a rapid increase in muscle tone. Thus, it appears that, even early in infancy, the DLPT is critically involved in the regulation of muscle tone and behavioral state and that its activity is modulated by a cholinergic mechanism that is directly or indirectly controlled by the PnO.

Forebrain

In light of recent doubts concerning medullary and mesopontine contributions to behavioral state organization in infant rats, the notion that the forebrain would make its own contributions would appear even more unlikely. In addressing this issue, an examination of the representative data presented in Figure 20.7A is particularly instructive. In noting the durations of sleep and wake bouts in that figure, it is apparent that the atonia periods depicted for the P2 subjects are substantially shorter in duration than that for the P8 subject; in contrast, the high-tone durations are similar at these two ages. When we quantified these durations across P2 and P8 subjects, as shown in Figure 20.7B, we found that mean atonia durations (i.e., sleep durations) increase from approximately 15 to 40 s between P2 and P8, whereas mean tone durations (i.e., wake durations) increase from approximately 5 to 15 s (Karlsson, Kreider, & Blumberg, 2004).

We hypothesized that the increasing durations of sleep and wake bouts across this early developmental period result, at least in part, from increasing modulatory effects of the forebrain on brainstem

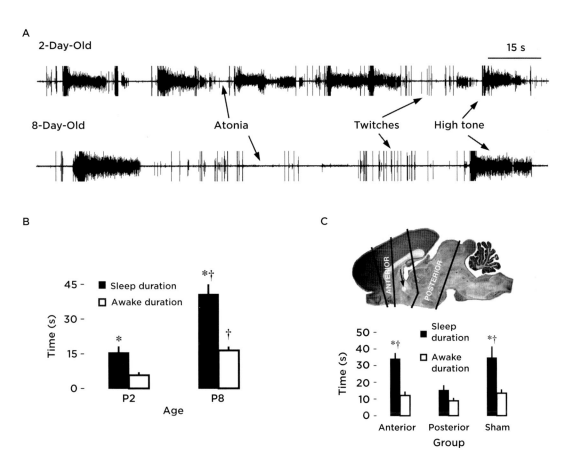

Figure 20.7 (A) Nuchal EMG data from representative P2 (top) and P8 (bottom) rats. Each segment is 2.4 min long. Atonia (i.e., sleep) and high-tone (i.e., awake) periods are indicated by arrows. The P2 rat cycles between the two EMG states more rapidly than the P8 rat. Instances of myoclonic twitching against a background of atonia are also indicated. (B) Mean sleep and wake bout durations for unrestrained P2 and P8 rats. * Significant difference from Awake Duration. † Significant difference from Sleep Duration. (C) Top: Mid-sagittal section in a P8 rat, with the rostral-caudal range of anterior and posterior transections depicted. Arrow indicates anterior commissure. Bottom: Mean sleep and wake bout durations for pups with anterior and posterior transections and for sham controls. * Significant difference from Awake Duration. † Significant difference from posterior transection group. (From Karlsson et al., 2004.)

structures. We initially tested this hypothesis by performing transections at two different levels of the neuraxis in P8 rats. As illustrated in Figure 20.7C, one set of "posterior" transections was placed ventrally within the caudal hypothalamus, and another set of "anterior" transection was placed rostral to the preoptic hypothalamus (POA). Figure 20.7C also presents the effects of these transections on mean sleep and wake bout durations. Whereas the anterior and sham transections exhibited similar bout durations, the posterior transections significantly decreased the sleep durations, resulting in pups that cycled very rapidly between sleep and wakefulness.

In a subsequent study (Mohns, Karlsson, & Blumberg, 2006), we identified the regions between the posterior and anterior transections that were responsible for the effects of transection on sleep and wake bouts. We focused on the ventrolateral preoptic area (VLPO) and basal forebrain because of their roles in adult sleep–wake regulation (Saper, Chou, & Scammell, 2001; Szymusiak, Steininger, Alam, & McGinty, 2001) and because these structures were spared by the most rostral posterior transections and the most caudal anterior transections in the earlier transection study. Electrolytic lesions placed selectively in the VLPO or basal forebrain produced discrete changes in sleep and wakefulness. Critically, however, only combined lesions of the two regions reproduced the reduced sleep and wake bouts produced by the posterior decerebrations in the earlier study.

Interestingly, the P8 subjects with posterior transections, described above, exhibited bout durations that resemble those of intact P2 subjects. Such a finding could suggest that sleep–wake regulation at P2 occurs without any contribution from forebrain structures. However, when similar transections were performed in P2 subjects, mean sleep durations were also significantly decreased (Mohns et al., 2006). Thus, it is not the case that the consolidation of sleep bouts across the first postnatal week arises entirely from the onset of a functional POA. Rather, it appears that both brainstem and forebrain mechanisms contribute.

In this same study, we also recorded extracellular neural activity within the preoptic area and basal forebrain of unanesthetized P9 subjects, the first such recordings in infant rats. Both sleep- and wake-on neural activity was found, consistent with a role for these forebrain areas in the modulation of sleep and wakefulness.

To investigate the possibility that the POA's modulatory effects on sleep and wakefulness change across early development, we administered the wake-promoting drug modafinil at P2 and P9. Although modafinil's wake-promoting (and sleep-inhibiting) mechanisms are not completely understood, this drug has been shown to potentiate the inhibition of GABAergic POA neurons in vitro (Gallopin, Luppi, Rambert, Frydman, & Fort, 2004). In our infant subjects, we found that modafinil had a strong wake-promoting effect at both P2 and P9, whereas the drug's ability to suppress sleep was significantly greater at P9 (perhaps resulting in part from the existence of longer sleep bout durations at P9). These results further support the hypothesis that the POA, through its modulation of more caudal regions, contributes to increasing sleep bout durations across the first postnatal week.

Summary

As reviewed here, and contrary to the predictions of the presleep hypothesis, the infant brainstem and forebrain are intimately involved in the generation of cyclic changes in muscle tone and the production of the phasic activity that defines AS. We still have much to learn about the neural circuit involved in infant sleep and how it changes across development. Nonetheless, it is notable that rapid progress in this area of research followed upon the development of the nuchal EMG as a measure of tonic and phasic changes in behavioral state. Used in its proper context, and divorced from expectations imported from work with adults, the nuchal EMG has proven a reliable indicator of sleep and wakefulness. Its usefulness has proven itself further as we developed new methods for acquiring neurophysiological data from unanesthetized infant subjects. Such methods have been, and are being developed in several laboratories (Karlsson et al., 2005; Khazipov et al., 2004; Lahtinen et al., 2001; Leinekugel et al., 2002; see Chapters 6 and 8). As these methods improve, they should provide an impetus to further investigations of the neural bases of infant behavior in general, and infant sleep in particular.

The Developing Temporal Structure of Sleep and Wakefulness

As discussed above, differing perspectives of the organization of infant behavioral states have largely concerned the brain and its role in that organization. The research reviewed above clarified this issue by showing that the brain plays a significant role in the organization of sleep and wakefulness in infants. But over the last several years, what has been most striking to us is not the presence or identity of the neural mechanisms involved in infant sleep, but the temporal structure of infant sleep and how it changes with age. For example, perhaps the most striking difference between the P3 and P14 records in Figure 20.3 concerns the timing of the sleep–wake cycles. Specifically, note how the time-scale bar for the P3 subject indicates 5 s, whereas the time scale bar for the P14 subject indicates 100 s. Similar differences in timing can be seen for the P2 and P8 subjects in Figure 20.7.

Such dramatic developmental shifts in the temporal structure of sleep and wakefulness are well known (Gramsbergen et al., 1970; Kleitman & Engelmann, 1953; Roffwarg et al., 1966). Recently, using analytical procedures that are relatively new to the field, we have sought to fully describe the statistical structure of sleep and wake bout durations across development. Such analyses have revealed previously unsuspected statistical structure in sleep and wake bouts and provide a foundation for future developmental, comparative, and neurophysiological investigations of sleep–wake organization.

Statistical Distributions of Sleep and Wake Bouts across Normal Development

Total amounts of sleep and wakefulness are accumulated in short bouts—produced by transitions between states—such as those depicted in Figure 20.8A for an infant rat. When such bouts are plotted to depict their distribution in real-time, as in Figure 20.8B for a P2 and P21 rat, we see highly variable distributions of sleep and wake bouts. Note also how this variability seems to change with age (and note the different timescales in the two plots). The issue to which we now turn concerns the statistical distributions that best describe this variability. A guiding assumption underlying this discussion is that a better understanding of the rules guiding transitions between behavioral states will provide valuable insight into the mechanisms that modulate sleep and wakefulness, including their development.

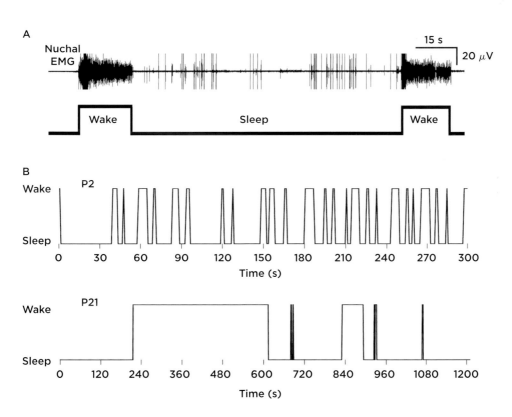

Figure 20.8 (A) A 2.4-min record in a P8 rat of nuchal EMG (upper trace) showing two brief periods of high muscle tone, indicative of wakefulness, separated by a longer period of muscle atonia, indicative of sleep. These dichotomous states are also depicted (lower trace). (B) Cycling between sleep and wakefulness in a P2 (upper trace) and P21 (lower trace) rat. Note the different time scales in the two traces. (From Blumberg et al., 2005.)

A. Raw Data: Bout durations

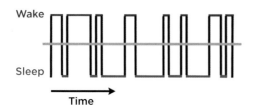

B. Frequency Distributions of durations

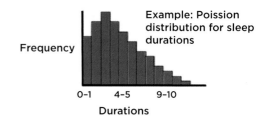

C. Survivor analysis

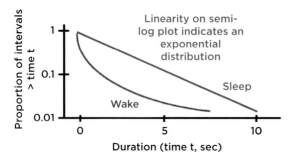

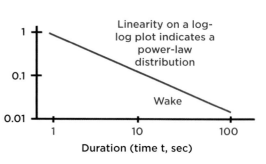

Figure 20.9 Illustration of method for converting raw nuchal EMG data to sleep–wake states in preparation for log-survivor analysis. (1) EMG amplitude is dichotomized into sleep (blue) and wake (red) states. (2) After bout durations are derived, frequency distributions can be produced. Illustrated here is the frequency distribution for sleep bouts for the case in which they follow a Poisson distribution. (3) Left: Plot of sleep and wake bouts on a semi-log plot. When sleep bouts follow a Poisson distribution (blue), they fall on a straight line on a semi-log plot. If wake bouts follow, for example, a power-law distribution, then they do not fall along a straight line on a semilog plot. Right: When power-law wake bouts are replotted on a log-log plot, they now fall along a straight line.

Figure 20.9 illustrates our approach to assessing these distributions. First, as in the previous figure, a continuous record of nuchal EMG is analyzed and dichotomized into sleep and wake bouts (Figure 20.9A). Second, without concern for the ordering of these bouts, frequency distributions are constructed (Figure 20.9B). Finally, the frequency distributions are converted to log-survivor plots. (Log-survivor analysis was originally devised for epidemiological assessment of medical treatments. Rather than assessing the survival of, for example, cancer patients, we are assessing the "survival" of sleep and wake bouts. That is, at each successive bout interval—i.e., 1 s, 2 s, etc.—we ask what percentage of the entire distribution "survived.") As shown in Figure 20.9C, an exponential distribution (such that the frequency distribution $f(t)$ of bout durations of duration t was proportional to $e^{(-t/\tau)}$, where τ is the characteristic timescale) falls along a straight line on a semilog plot. In contrast, a power-law distribution (such that $f(t) \sim t^{-\alpha}$, where α is a characteristic power-law exponent) falls along a straight line on a log–log plot.

Using this basic approach, Lo and colleagues analyzed the distributions of sleep and wake bouts in human adults (Lo et al., 2002). They found that sleep bouts exhibited an exponential distribution, whereas wake bouts exhibited a power-law distribution. In a subsequent report (Lo et al., 2004), similar findings were reported in adult rats, cats, and mice. In addition, these investigators found that the exponential timescale, τ, for sleep bout durations increases with body size, thus possibly implicating a constitutional variable (e.g., metabolic rate) in the regulation of sleep bouts. In contrast, the power-law exponent, α, for wake bout durations did not vary across species.

We suspected that data from developing animals could provide additional critical information for testing the generalizability of Lo et al.'s claims. Indeed, we had found earlier that both sleep and wake bout durations of P2 and P8 rats are better captured by exponential, not power-law, distributions (Karlsson et al., 2004). Because wake bout durations do not exhibit power-law behavior in early infancy, we inferred that this feature develops after P8. In addition, because the precise nature of these distributions critically shapes the models that we adopt to describe the temporal dynamics of sleep and wakefulness (Lo et al., 2002), we knew that establishing the statistical properties of these bout durations across development was important. Therefore, using archival and specially collected data from rats at P2, P8, P10, P14, and P21, we assessed the statistical behavior of sleep and wake bout durations (Blumberg et al., 2005b).

Survivor distributions for data at P2 and P21 are presented in Figure 20.10 for pooled data and for individual representative subjects. Again, survival data that follow an exponential distribution fall along a straight line on a semilog plot and those that follow a power-law distribution fall along a straight line on a log–log plot. For sleep durations, the data for both the P2 and P21 rats are best described by an exponential function, as they follow a straight line on the semilog plot. This is also true of the data for the wake durations at P2; in contrast, by P21, these data are now linearly distributed on a log–log plot, thus indicating a shift from an exponential distribution at P2 to a power-law distribution at P21.

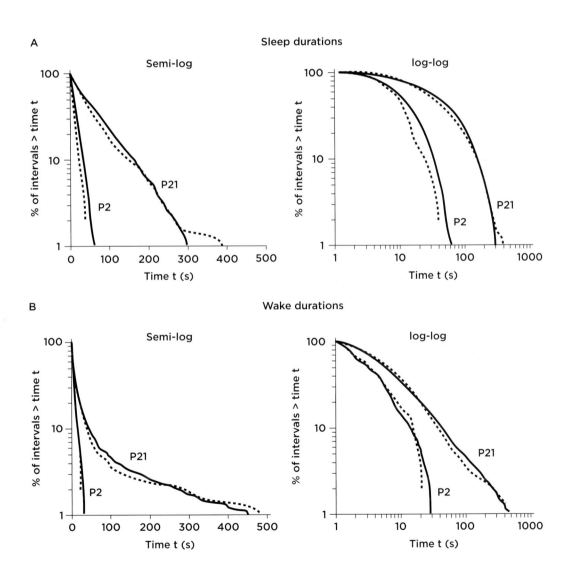

Figure 20.10 Survivor plots of sleep (A) and wake (B) bout durations for rats at P2 and P21. Each plot was constructed using pooled data at each age (solid lines) and data from one representative pup at each age (dotted line). The plots on the left were constructed using semi-log coordinates; straight lines on these plots indicate that the data follow an exponential distribution. The plots on the right were constructed using log-log coordinates; straight lines on these plots indicate that the data follow a power-law distribution. (From Blumberg et al., 2005.)

To determine whether the functions of the sleep and wake bout durations are best described as exponential or power-law distributions at each age, regression analyses were performed for each pup when data were plotted using semilog and log–log coordinates. Then, r^2 values were computed, averaged across subjects, and plotted across age. As shown in Figure 20.11A, sleep bout durations are best fit to an exponential distribution at all ages. In contrast, as shown in Figure 20.11B, wake bout

durations are best fit to an exponential distribution through P10 but to a power-law distribution thereafter.

Based on these and other analyses, we concluded that as infant rats cycle between sleep and wakefulness, there is no memory for the duration of previous intervals. For example, whether an infant rat exhibits a long or short sleep bout is completely uninfluenced by the length of its previous wake or sleep bouts. Accordingly, we concluded that transitions between sleep and wakefulness most closely resemble an alternating renewal process (Lowen & Teich, 1993a, 1993b); at the youngest ages tested, where both sleep and wake durations distribute exponentially, the sleep–wake state model further specializes to a two-state Markov process (a subset of alternating renewal processes). In other words, the system resets every time the animal wakes up or goes to sleep; no memory of the past persists beyond these events. However, some memory can exist *within* intervals, particularly for those that exhibit a power-law distribution. For example, a wake bout that has already persisted for a long time is likely to persist even longer, producing a relative lack of intermediate-duration wake times. Thus, as these older pups stay awake, they are more likely to stay awake longer. That this phenomenon occurs after P15 suggests a connection between the onset of sustained wakefulness and the initiation of weaning.

Development of Circadian Sleep–Wake Activity

During the early postnatal period in rats, several physiological and behavioral systems are known to exhibit circadian rhythmicity, including body temperature, metabolism, and pineal serotonin *N*-acetyltransferase (Ellison, Weller, & Klein, 1972; Kittrell & Satinoff, 1986; Nuesslein-Hildesheim, Imai-Matsumura, Döring, & Schmidt, 1995; Spiers, 1988). But in comparison to the vast literature detailing circadian rhythms of sleep and wakefulness in adults (Fuller, Gooley, & Saper, 2006), very little is known about these rhythms in infants. In one study, it was reported that nocturnal wakefulness is established in rats during the third postnatal week (Frank & Heller, 1997a).

As described already in this chapter, nuchal EMG has proven a very sensitive measure of sleep–wake cyclicity beginning soon after birth in rats. Thus, we wondered whether we could use this measure to reveal day–night differences in sleep–wake cyclicity and relate these differences to early suprachiasmatic nucleus (SCN) function. To explore

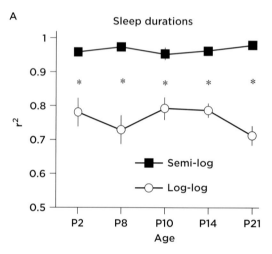

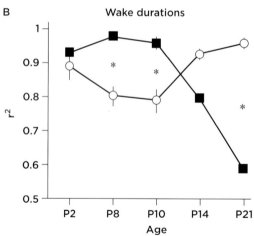

Figure 20.11 Values of r^2 produced using regression analysis of survivor data at five postnatal ages in infant rats. For each individual pup, the degree of fit of the data to power-law and exponential distributions was determined, yielding a value of r^2 that was then averaged across subjects at each age. (A) Values of r^2 for sleep bout durations showing that the data follow an exponential distribution. (B) Values of r^2 for wake bout durations showing that the data follow an exponential distribution at P8 and P10 and a power-law distribution at P21. * Significant within-age difference. Mean + S.E. (From Blumberg et al., 2005.)

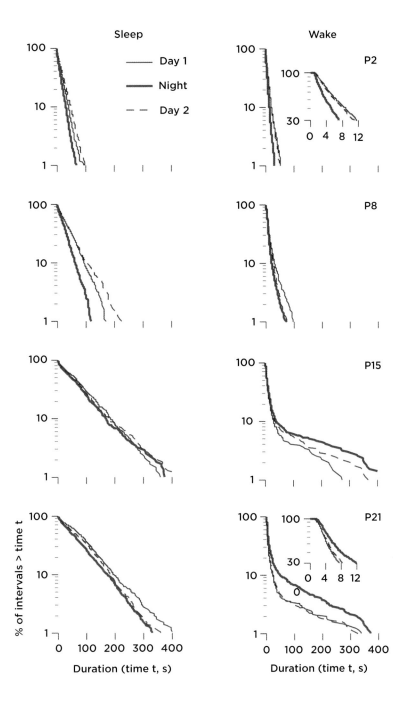

this possibility, we examined day–night differences in sleep–wake cyclicity in rats at P2, P8, P15, and P21 (Gall, Todd, Ray, Coleman, & Blumberg, 2008). At each age, data were collected from three littermates in succession about noon, midnight, and noon on the next day. Pups were always tested at thermoneutrality.

Figure 20.12 presents log-survivor data for the subjects in this study. Surprisingly, day–night differences in sleep–wake activity were detected as early as P2; specifically, pups at this age exhibited significantly more sleep–wake cycles at night than during the day (due to shorter bout durations of both sleep and wakefulness at night). By P15 and especially by P21, the wake bouts were now significantly longer at night, revealing the emergence of the nocturnal pattern of wakefulness that characterizes the adults of this species.

The SCN of the hypothalamus plays a major role in the regulation of circadian rhythms in mammals (Moore, 1983; Rusak & Zucker, 1979). In rats, nearly all neurons in the SCN are formed by embryonic day E18 (Ifft, 1972) and, by E19, the fetal SCN is more metabolically active during the day than during the night and is synchronized to the dam's SCN activity (Reppert & Schwartz, 1984; Reppert, Weaver, & Rivkees, 1988). The entraining effect of the dam on her pups continues through the first postnatal week, at which time light becomes the predominant entraining stimulus (Duncan, Banister, & Reppert, 1986; Ohta, Honma, Abe, & Honma, 2002; Takahashi & Deguchi, 1983). Thus, it is plausible that the pup's SCN circadian activity, entrained to that of the dam's, modulates the sleep–wake rhythmicity detected during the first postnatal week.

The transition from maternal to light entrainment parallels the development of the retinohypothalamic tract's (RHT) connections with the SCN (Felong, 1976; Speh & Moore, 1993). Within the retina, the RHT arises from intrinsically photosensitive ganglion cells that contain the photopigment, melanopsin (Berson, Dunn, & Takao, 2002; Hattar, Liao, Takao, Berson, & Yau, 2002). These melanopsin-containing cells respond to light passing through the eyelids, which in rats do not open until P15. It now appears that this nonimage-forming irradiance detection system is able to modulate SCN activity at birth (Hannibal & Fahrenkrug, 2002; Leard, Macdonald, Heller, & Kilduff, 1994; Sekaran et al., 2005; Sernagor, 2005). Thus, this system is poised to play an important role in the early development of circadian rhythms, including sleep–wake rhythms, and underlies the transition to light entrainment over the first postnatal week.

We hypothesized that eliminating RHT–SCN connectivity during the early postnatal period in rats—before and after SCN entrainment to light—would alter the later emergence of nighttime wakefulness in this nocturnal species. We investigated this possibility by enucleating pups at P3 or P11 and testing their subsequent sleep–wake patterns at P21 (Gall et al., 2008). Pups enucleated at P3 or P11 were similar to the extent that both exhibited power-law wake behavior at P21. In contrast, whereas enucleation at P11 did not prevent P21 rats from exhibiting the normal pattern of longer wake bout durations at night, enucleation at P3 resulted in subjects exhibiting longer wake bout durations during the day. To ensure that pups enucleated at P3 were not free-running and that the observed

daytime wakefulness was reliable, we repeated the study but tested weanlings at P28 and P35—with similar results.

This experiment suggests that enucleated infant rats differentially entrain to zeitgebers within the nest environment depending on when—in relation to the development of the RHT—the enucleation takes place. Specifically, it is possible that visual system stimulation—from light and/or spontaneous activity within the retina—transmitted through the RHT to the SCN, induces functional changes in SCN interactions with its downstream neural structures. Interestingly, in adults, the effect of light as a zeitgeber is to stimulate upregulation of growth factors (e.g., NGF1-A, BDNF) in the SCN and thereby entrain SCN activity (Allen & Earnest, 2005; Liang, Allen, & Earnest, 2000; Tanaka, Iijima, Amaya, Tamada, & Ibata, 1999). Such upregulation of gene activity—seen during everyday entrainment to light in adults—could also play an inductive, organizational role during a sensitive period when the RHT is forming functional connections with the SCN.

On the Similarly Fragmented Sleep–Wake Patterns of Infants and Narcoleptics

The development of sensitive indicators of infant sleep and wakefulness, as discussed above, may provide additional insights into the development and treatment of sleep disorders in infants and adult humans. For example, narcolepsy is a sleep disorder characterized in humans by excessive daytime sleepiness, the sudden loss of muscle tone (i.e., cataplexy), sleep-onset hallucinations, and paralysis at sleep transitions (Taheri, Zeitzer, & Mignot, 2002). Its prevalence has been reported to be 20–60 incidences per 100,000 persons, similar to multiple sclerosis and Parkinson's disease (Overeem, Mignot, Gert, van Dijk, & Lammers, 2001).

Narcolepsy has recently been recognized as a neurodegenerative disorder (Siegel, Moore, Thannickal, & Nienhuis, 2001; Taheri et al., 2002; van den Pol, 2000). Central to this reclassification has been the recent discovery of a neurotransmitter, orexin (or hypocretin) (de Lecea et al., 1998; Sakurai et al., 1998), which is produced by a distinct set of neurons within the caudal hypothalamus that project to the locus coeruleus and other nuclei implicated in the regulation of sleep and wakefulness (Peyron et al., 1998). Degeneration or deficient functioning of the orexinergic system has been linked to narcolepsy in humans (Peyron et al., 2000; Thannickal et al., 2000), dogs (Lin et al., 1999), and mice (Chemelli et al., 1999). Moreover, adult orexin knockout mice exhibit patterns of sleep and wakefulness that mirror those seen in narcoleptic humans (Chemelli et al., 1999; Mochizuki et al., 2004; Willie et al., 2003).

As with narcolepsy and as discussed above, the sleep and wake bouts of infant humans (Kleitman & Engelmann, 1953) and rats (Blumberg et al., 2005b; Gramsbergen et al., 1970) are highly fragmented, characterized by rapid transitions between short-duration states. We wondered whether the sleep–wake fragmentation observed in narcoleptics and infants result from a common neural mechanism. Specifically, we hypothesized that orexin knockout mice would retain the more fragmented sleep and wake bout durations that characterize normal infancy. Such an observation would indicate that narcolepsy in orexin knockout mice, though characterized in part by the novel expression of pathological symptoms such as cataplexy, is also characterized by retention of the infantile pattern of sleep–wake fragmentation. By extension, adult-onset narcolepsy in humans might entail reversion back toward that infantile pattern.

To test this hypothesis, we assessed sleep and wakefulness in orexin knockout and wild-type mice at P4, P12, and P21 (Blumberg, Coleman, Johnson, & Shaw, 2007). As shown in Figure 20.13, we found little difference between the two strains at P4 and P12, although both exhibited age-related consolidation of sleep and wake bouts. By P21, further consolidation occurred in both strains, along with the emergence of power-law wake behavior. But now, the knockouts were lagging behind their same-age wild-type counterparts, retaining the more fragmented bouts characteristic of earlier ages. Thus, it appears that the orexinergic system is not necessary for consolidation of sleep and wake bouts during the first 2 postnatal weeks, nor is it necessary for the developmental emergence of power-law wake behavior. Orexin does appear, however, to further consolidate bouts beyond the values attained in early infancy.

Thus, the infant's sleep–wake system operates, like a narcoleptic's, without a fully functioning orexinergic system and that the result—for both infant and narcoleptic—is fragmentation of sleep and wake bouts. Moreover, if the normally fragmented sleep of infants and the abnormally fragmented sleep of narcoleptic adults arise through the action of a common neural mechanism, then infants may provide a useful model for understanding the etiology of narcolepsy and for developing effective treatments.

Beyond narcolepsy, this analytical approach may provide useful information concerning normal and pathological human development. Because sleep disturbances are associated with many aspects of disease and psychopathology (Kryger, Roth, &

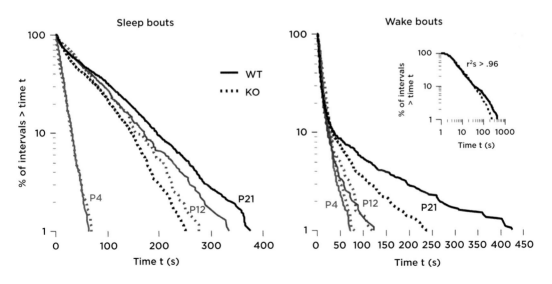

Figure 20.13 Survivor plots of sleep and wake bout durations for wild-type (WT; solid lines) and orexin knockout (KO; dashed lines) mice at P4 (blue), P12 (red), and P21 (black). Straight lines on these plots indicate that the data follow an exponential distribution. The inset is a replotting of the P21 wake data using log–log coordinates; straight lines on these plots indicate that the data follow a power-law distribution. Individual data points were pooled across all subjects. (From Blumberg et al., 2007.)

Dement, 2000; Nishino, Taheri, Black, Nofzinger, & Mignot, 2004), any method that provides greater sensitivity for tracking developmental milestones, detecting the onset of sleep disturbances, and assessing responses to treatment could be of use to clinicians. Accordingly, the analyses of sleep and wake bout durations described here may prove superior to gross measures of total sleep and wake time because they reveal more about the fine structure of sleep–wake organization and they more closely reflect the neural processes that govern transitions between states.

Functional Aspects of Infant Sleep

How we conceptualize the phenomenology of infant sleep and its relation to adult sleep can have a profound influence on the kinds of functional theories that will be entertained and tested. For example, if the "presleep hypothesis" had been correct, then we might understand the tendency among most sleep researchers to disregard infant sleep in the formulation of sleep function hypotheses. However, as reviewed in this chapter, that hypothesis is not supported by the available evidence, leading us to argue, once again (Blumberg & Lucas, 1996), that theories of sleep function should strive for applicability to infants as well as adults.

Although there is no dearth of theories of sleep function, emphasis continues to be placed on theories that posit a role in learning and memory, especially memory consolidation in humans (Stickgold, 2005). Some investigators are highly critical of such theories (Siegel, 2001; Vertes, 2004) and highlight instead the usefulness of comparative data as a source of valuable information concerning the phylogenetic history of sleep and, therefore, its functional importance (Siegel, 2005a).

Comparative analysis has long been used to test hypotheses concerning the evolution, function, and mechanistic control of sleep (Campbell & Tobler, 1984; Dave & Margoliash, 2000; Flanigan, 1973; Flanigan, Wilcox, & Rechtschaffen, 1973; Hendricks & Sehgal, 2004; Hendricks et al., 2000; Huntley & Cohen, 1980; Rattenborg, Amlaner, & Lima, 2000; Rattenborg et al., 2004; Siegel, 1999, 2005a; Siegel, Manger, Nienhuis, Fahringer, & Pettigrew, 1998; Tobler, 1995; Tobler & Deboer, 2001; Zepelin, 2000; Zepelin & Rechtschaffen, 1974). Relatively few studies, however, have combined comparative with developmental analysis. We believe, however, that systematic examination of the development of sleep and wakefulness in carefully chosen nontraditional species will help

to answer a variety of interesting and important questions.

As already discussed, a recent comparison of data from adult mice, rats, cats, and humans yielded useful insights into the temporal structure of sleep and wakefulness (Lo et al., 2004). A similar comparative analysis of sleep and wake development would be valuable. For example, Figure 20.14 compares the log-survivor plots of infant Norway rats (Blumberg et al., 2005b) and mice (Blumberg et al., 2007). The similar patterns exhibited by these two species are striking: sleep and wake bouts during the early postnatal period follow an exponential function, whereas wake bouts exhibit a power-law function several weeks later. This developmental correspondence attests to an underlying conservation of sleep processes in these two rodent species. But what can we really conclude from comparison of these two species alone? After all, rats and mice are both muroid rodents, both are nocturnal, both are omnivorous, and both are altricial. Therefore, to determine whether the developmental trajectories illustrated in Figure 20.14 represent a widely shared feature among mammals, it is necessary to examine additional species that differ from rats and mice on critical dimensions. Such comparisons may then inspire novel hypotheses concerning the mechanisms and functions of sleep.

Historically, the single most influential developmental hypothesis regarding the function of active sleep remains that of Roffwarg et al. (1966) who, noting the developmental relation between sleep and brain development in newborns, suggested that the two processes are related. Later, this hypothesis was elaborated further by considering all that we have learned in recent decades regarding the developmental significance of activity-dependent neural processes during fetal and postnatal development (Blumberg & Lucas, 1996). For example, we now know that spontaneous activity by retinal ganglion cells, even in the rat fetus, contributes significantly to the development of topographic relations in the visual system (Galli & Maffei, 1988; Shatz, 1990). Indeed, researchers continue to identify effects of sleep processes on neural plasticity in the developing brain, especially within the visual system (Frank, Issa, & Stryker, 2001; Shaffery, Sinton, Bissette, Roffwarg, & Marks, 2002). More broadly, recent evidence supports a role for myoclonic twitching in the developmental of somatotopic maps in the spinal cord (Petersson, Waldenström, Fåhraeus, & Schouenborg, 2003; Schouenborg, 2003; see Chapter 12).

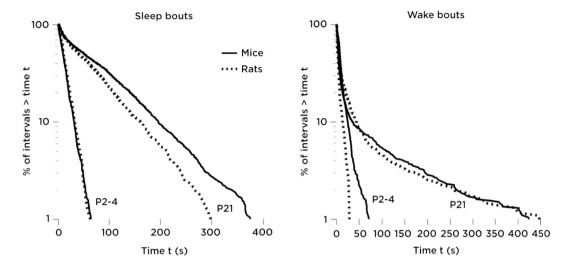

Figure 20.14 Log-survivor plots of sleep and wake bout durations for the P2–4 and P20–22 wild-type mice (solid lines) in Blumberg et al. (2007) and P2 and P21 Norway rats (dotted lines) from Blumberg et al. (2005). All plots were constructed using data pooled from multiple subjects. The gestation length of mice is 3 days shorter than that of rats. Regardless, the distributions are remarkably similar, including the development of wake-related power-law behavior by P21. (From Blumberg et al., 2007.)

Within the context of this chapter, we may move closer to an understanding of the functions of sleep through close examination of the temporal and spatial organization of the various sleep components. Consider Figure 20.15A, which depicts the traditional trio of electrographic measures of sleep in the form of a Venn diagram: nuchal EMG provides a measure of muscle tone; the EOG provides a measure of phasic extraocular muscle activity; and cortical EEG allows for the detection of delta waves. As we have seen, however, conventional methods for measuring EMG and EOG mask the redundant information provided by these two measures of muscle activity. Specifically, phasic activity can be detected in the nuchal EMG at appropriate filter settings and sampling frequencies; similarly, tonic activity can be detected from the eye muscles if their activity is measured directly (Seelke et al., 2005). Of course, as a practical matter, especially when recording in humans, these two measures are treated as separate entities. But as a conceptual matter, the underlying activity in all skeletal muscles provides similar information: oscillations between high and low tone and occasional bursts of phasic activity. Thus, the trio of electrographic measures in Figure 20.15A can be reduced to the two indicators depicted in Figure 20.15B.

Now we can assess the necessity of two electrographic measures. With regard to the EEG, it was recently shown in adult rats that the forebrain exhibits global EEG patterns that are sufficiently

distinct to discriminate between AS, QS, and wakefulness (Gervasoni et al., 2004). It was suggested that these EEG patterns provide the basis for the "classification of global states without reference to behavioral or electromyogram data" (p. 11141). Interestingly, the work reviewed in this chapter strongly suggests that the EMG alone is also sufficient for differentiating the behavioral states of infants and, presumably, adults as well. Indeed, EMG data are sufficient for revealing neural mechanisms that have been implicated in adult sleep–wake states using the conventional trio of electrographic measures (Karlsson & Blumberg, 2005; Karlsson et al., 2004, 2005; Seelke et al., 2005). Thus, the reduced Venn diagram in Figure 20.15B can be morphed into the qualitatively distinct arrangement of Figure 20.15C. In that figure, homologous behavioral states defined using EEG or EMG measures alone are linked by their association with common neural sources within the brainstem.

The perspective captured by Figure 20.15C indicates a mechanistic connection between the activational states of the forebrain (EEG) and skeletal muscle (EMG). And through this mechanistic connection it is possible to glimpse the basis for an approach to sleep that transcends description and diagnosis and moves toward explanation. Specifically, the conception depicted in Figure 20.15C presents sleep as a body-wide process that links muscle and brain into a single system that

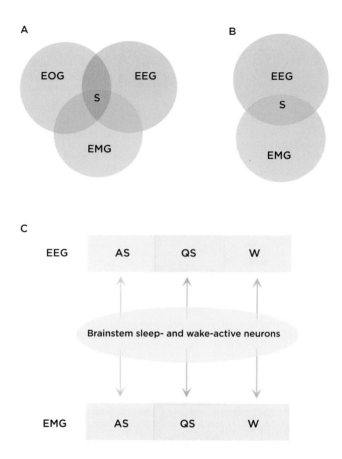

Figure 20.15 Conceptual representations of sleep. (A) Venn diagram depicting conventional diagnostic criteria for assessing sleep–wake states in adults using a trio of electrographic measures: EOG, EMG, and EEG. S denotes the behavioral state (i.e., active or quiet sleep, wakefulness) defined using these three parameters. (B) Reorganization of the Venn diagram in (A) based on the notion that the EOG and EMG provide redundant information. Specifically, REMs (detected from the EOG record) can be viewed as phasic events produced by twitches of the extraocular muscles; in addition, fluctuations in extraocular muscle tone are mirrored by fluctuations in nuchal muscle tone. Now, S denotes the behavioral state defined using only two parameters. (C) Alternative conceptualization that builds on the notion that either EEG (after P11) or EMG (as early as P2) is alone sufficient to define behavioral states in rats. According to this notion, homologous sleep–wake states (AS, QS, W) can be identified in the EEG and EMG records. This homology arises because EEG- and EMG-defined states are generated by common brainstem mechanisms. (From Seelke et al., 2005.)

must develop and maintain topographic relations for proper functioning to occur. The need for integrated relations between muscle and brain forms the basis for the suggestion that infant sleep states, including myoclonic twitching, contribute to neural and neuromuscular development (Blumberg & Lucas, 1996; Corner, van Pelt, Wolters, Baker, & Nuytinck, 2002; Mirmiran, 1995; Roffwarg et al., 1966). The discrete nature of a myoclonic twitch, especially when performed against a background of muscle atonia, provides, we suggest, an enhanced signal-to-noise ratio for accurately processing relationships between outgoing motor signals and sensory feedback. Such conditions may provide the basis by which twitch-related movements of

the limbs contribute to the self-organization of topographically organized maps and refinement of neural circuits in spinal cord (Petersson et al., 2003) and somatosensory cortex (Khazipov et al., 2004; Marcano-Reik & Blumberg, 2008), as well as hippocampus (Mohns & Blumberg, 2008).

Conclusions and Future Directions

Our aim in this chapter was to demonstrate how an accurate description of the phenomenology of sleep in early infancy helps us move toward a broader and deeper appreciation of its developmental and evolutionary origins. The work reviewed here builds upon a conceptual framework clearly enunciated by Michael Corner (Corner, 1977), which in turn was inspired by the embryological research of Viktor Hamburger and his colleagues (Hamburger & Oppenheim, 1967; Narayanan et al., 1971). Their ideas and research challenged subsequent investigators to extend the insights gained from behavioral embryology to later periods of development. Indeed, Corner himself performed important studies in this area, including examination of the development of the brain in relation to sleep (Corner, 1973, 1985).

In our work, focusing on the early postnatal period in altricial rodents, we have adopted the general approach encouraged by Corner and Hamburger while also keeping an eye on the methods and concepts of traditional sleep research—research performed largely in adults. Straddling these two traditions, we were convinced, would be essential to attaining our goal of building a durable bridge between them. In turn, such a bridge might help to convince clinically oriented sleep researchers that the proper study of development can offer useful insights into the mechanisms and functions of sleep.

Also central to our conceptual approach is a commitment to the epigenetic perspective championed by Gilbert Gottlieb and others (Blumberg, 2005; Gottlieb, 1997; Oyama, Griffiths, & Gray, 2001; see Chapters 2 and 3). Within the context of sleep, the epigenetic perspective places balanced emphasis on genetic and nongenetic factors in the development of ultradian and circadian rhythms. Our work, described earlier, on the possible inductive effects of photic stimulation on the development of the RHT–SCN system provides one example of how epigenetic factors can produce long-term organizational effects on sleep–wake behavior (Gall et al., 2008).

Our task now is to provide comprehensive accounts of the development and evolution of sleep across a diversity of species. As we engage this task, we will benefit from the lessons learned from investigations of sleep in rats and other altricial rodents. Perhaps the most seminal lesson concerns the need to incorporate multiple behavioral and electrographic measures of sleep in our assessments, but never fool ourselves into thinking that any one measure best captures the "essence" of sleep.

Thus, as has been shown many times, behavior alone provides a reliable estimate of wakefulness and sleep, including QS and AS (Corner, 1977; Gramsbergen et al., 1970; Kreider & Blumberg, 2000). With the addition of nuchal EMG (Dugovic & Turek, 2001; Karlsson & Blumberg,

2002), estimates become sharper as, for example, the transition from quiet wakefulness to quiet sleep is now discernible. In addition, the nuchal EMG—when filtered and sampled adequately—also provides a measure of phasic activity (i.e., myoclonic twitching) that complements behavioral assessments. Indeed, this is true of any measure of skeletal muscle activity, including that of the extraocular muscles (Seelke et al., 2005). Finally, the addition of cortical EEG is useful for detecting bouts of QS interposed between bouts of AS in rats older than P11 (Seelke & Blumberg, 2008).

Thus, during the early newborn period in altricial rodents, sleep and wakefulness are constructed developmentally upon a foundation that rests firmly on cyclic changes in skeletal muscle tone. This foundation rests, in turn, on medullary and mesopontine circuits that, with age, are increasingly modulated by forebrain mechanisms (Gall et al., 2007; Karlsson & Blumberg, 2005; Karlsson et al., 2004, 2005; Mohns et al., 2006). It is within the context of this developing circuit that the defining features of sleep, including homeostatic and circadian regulation, emerge. And it is within this context that we can see how sleep and wakefulness are body-wide processes that entail homologous activational states in muscle, spinal cord, brainstem, and forebrain. These homologous states, we believe, provide critical clues regarding the form and function of sleep across the lifespan.

Acknowledgments

We thank Kai Kaila and William Todd for helpful comments on an earlier draft of this manuscript. Preparation of this chapter was supported by a grant (MH50701) and a Research Scientist Award (MH66424) from the National Institute of Mental Health to M.S.B.

References

Adelsberger, H., Garaschuk, O., & Konnerth, A. (2005). Cortical calcium waves in resting newborn mice. *Nature Neuroscience, 8*, 988–990.

Adrien, J., & Lanfumey, L. (1984). Neuronal activity of the developing raphe dorsalis: Its relation with the states of vigilance. *Experimental Brain Research, Suppl. 8*, 67–78.

Alberts, J. R., & Cramer, C. P. (1988). Ecology and experience: Sources of means and meaning of developmental change. In E. M. Blass (Ed.), *Handbook of behavioral neurobiology* (Vol. 8, pp. 1–39). New York: Plenum Press.

Allen, G. C., & Earnest, D. J. (2005). Overlap in the distribution of TrkB immunoreactivity and retinohypothalamic tract innervation of the rat suprachiasmatic nucleus. *Neuroscience Letters, 376*, 200–204.

Berson, D. M., Dunn, F. A., & Takao, M. (2002). Phototransduction by retinal ganglion cells that set the circadian clock. *Science, 295*, 1070–1073.

Blumberg, M. S. (2001). The developmental context of thermal homeostasis. In E. M. Blass (Ed.), *Handbook of behavioral neurobiology* (Vol. 13, pp. 199–228). New York: Plenum Press.

Blumberg, M. S. (2005). *Basic instinct: The genesis of behavior*. New York: Thunder's Mouth Press.

Blumberg, M. S., Coleman, C., Johnson, E. D., & Shaw, C. S. (2007). Developmental divergence of sleep–wake patterns in orexin knockout and wild-type mice. *The European Journal of Neuroscience, 25*, 512–518.

Blumberg, M. S., Karlsson, K. Æ., Seelke, A. M. H., & Mohns, E. J. (2005a). The ontogeny of mammalian sleep: A response to Frank and Heller (2003). *Journal of Sleep Research, 14*, 91–101.

Blumberg, M. S., & Lucas, D. E. (1994). Dual mechanisms of twitching during sleep in neonatal rats. *Behavioral Neuroscience, 108*, 1196–1202.

Blumberg, M. S., & Lucas, D. E. (1996). A developmental and component analysis of active sleep. *Developmental Psychobiology, 29*, 1–22.

Blumberg, M. S., Middlemis-Brown, J. E., & Johnson, E. D. (2004). Sleep homeostasis in infant rats. *Behavioral Neuroscience, 118*, 1253–1261.

Blumberg, M. S., Seelke, A. M., Lowen, S. B., & Karlsson, K. A. (2005b). Dynamics of sleep–wake cyclicity in developing rats. *Proceedings of the National Academy of Sciences, USA, 102*, 14860–14864.

Blumberg, M. S., & Stolba, M. A. (1996). Thermogenesis, myoclonic twitching, and ultrasonic vocalization in neonatal rats during moderate and extreme cold exposure. *Behavioral Neuroscience, 110*, 305–314.

Bonnet, M. H. (2000). Sleep deprivation. In M. H. Kryger, T. Roth, & W. C. Dement (Eds.), *Principles and practice of sleep medicine* (pp. 53–71). Philadelphia: W. B. Saunders.

Campbell, S. S., & Tobler, I. (1984). Animal sleep: A review of sleep duration across phylogeny. *Neuroscience and Biobehavioral Reviews, 8*, 269–300.

Chase, M. H., & Morales, F. R. (1983). Subthreshold excitatory activity and motoneuron discharge during REM periods of active sleep. *Science, 221*, 1195–1198.

Chase, M. H., & Morales, F. R. (1990). The atonia and myoclonia of active (REM) sleep. *Annual Review of Psychology, 41*, 557–584.

Chemelli, R. M., Willie, J. T., Sinton, C. M., Elmquist, J. K., Scammell, T., Lee, C., et al. (1999). Narcolepsy in orexin knockout mice: Molecular genetics of sleep regulation. *Cell, 98*, 437–451.

Clewlow, F., Dawes, G. S., Johnston, B. M., & Walker, D. W. (1983). Changes in breathing, electrocortical and muscle activity in unanaesthetized fetal lambs with age. *The Journal of Physiology, 341*, 463–476.

Cobos, A., Lima, D., Almeida, A., & Tavares, I. (2003). Brain afferents to the lateral caudal ventrolateral medulla: A retrograde and anterograde tracing study in the rat. *Neuroscience, 120*, 485–498.

Corner, M. A. (1973). Sleep and wakefulness during early life in the domestic chicken, and their relationship to hatching and embryonic motility. In G. Gottlieb (Ed.), *Behavioral embryology* (Vol. 1, pp. 245–279). New York: Academic Press.

Corner, M. A. (1977). Sleep and the beginnings of behavior in the animal kingdom—Studies of ultradian motility cycles in early life. *Progress in Neurobiology, 8*, 279–295.

Corner, M. A. (1985). Ontogeny of brain sleep mechanisms. In D. J. McGinty (Ed.), *Brain mechanisms of sleep* (pp. 175–197). New York: Raven Press.

Corner, M. A., & Bour, H. L. (1984). Postnatal development of spontaneous neuronal discharges in the pontine reticular formation of free-moving rats during sleep and wakefulness. *Experimental Brain Research, 54*, 66–72.

Corner, M. A., & Mirmiran, M. (1990). Spontaneous neuronal firing patterns in the occipital cortex of developing rats. *International Journal of Developmental Neuroscience, 8*, 309–316.

Corner, M. A., van Pelt, J., Wolters, P. S., Baker, R. E., & Nuytinck, R. H. (2002). Physiological effects of sustained blockade of excitatory synaptic transmission on spontaneously active developing neuronal networks—an inquiry into the reciprocal linkage between intrinsic biorhythms and neuroplasticity in early ontogeny. *Neuroscience and Biobehavioral Reviews, 26*(2), 127–185.

Dave, A. S., & Margoliash, D. (2000). Song replay during sleep and computational rules for sensorimotor vocal learning. *Science, 290*, 812–816.

de Andres, I., Garzon, M., & Villablanca, J. R. (2003). The disconnected brain stem does not support rapid eye movement sleep rebound following selective deprivation. *Sleep, 26*, 419–425.

de Lecea, L., Kilduff, T. S., Peyron, C., Gao, X., Foye, P. E., Danielson, et al. (1998). The hypocretins: Hypothalamus-specific peptides with neuroexcitatory activity. *Proceedings of the National Academy of Sciences, USA, 95*, 322–327.

de Vries, J. I. P., Visser, G. H. A., & Prechtl, H. F. R. (1984). Fetal motility in the first half of pregnancy. In H. F. R. Prechtl (Ed.), *Continuity of neural functions from prenatal to postnatal life* (pp. 46–64). Oxford: Blackwell Scientific.

Dickenson, A. H., Hellon, R. F., & Taylor, C. M. (1979). Facial thermal input to the trigeminal spinal nucleus of rabbits and rats. *The Journal of Comparative Neurology, 185*, 203–210.

Dreyfus-Brisac, C. (1970). Ontogenesis of sleep in human prematures after 32 weeks of conceptional age. *Developmental Psychobiology, 3*, 91–121.

Dreyfus-Brisac, C. (1975). Neurophysiological studies in human premature and full-term newborns. *Biological Psychiatry, 10*, 485–496.

Dugovic, C., & Turek, F. W. (2001). Similar genetic mechanisms may underlie sleep–wake states in neonatal and adult rats. *Neuroreport, 12*, 3085–3089.

Duncan, M. J., Banister, M. J., & Reppert, S. M. (1986). Developmental appearance of light-dark entrainment in the rat. *Brain Research, 369*, 326–330.

Ellison, N., Weller, J. L., & Klein, D. C. (1972). Development of a circadian rhythm in the activity of pineal serotonin *N*-acetyltransferase. *Journal of Neurochemistry, 19*, 1335–1341.

Fagen, R. M., & Young, D. Y. (1978). Temporal patterns of behaviors: Durations, intervals, latencies and sequences. In P. W. Colgan (Ed.), *Quantitative ethology* (pp. 79–114). New York: Wiley.

Felong, M. (1976). Development of the retinohypothalamic projection in the rat. *Anatomical Record, 184*, 400–401.

Feng, P., Ma, Y., & Vogel, G. W. (2001). Ontogeny of REM rebound in postnatal rats. *Sleep, 24*, 645–653.

Flanigan, W. F. (1973). Sleep and wakefulness in iguanid lizards, Ctenosaura pectinata and Iguana iguana. *Brain, Behavior, and Evolution, 8*, 401–436.

Flanigan, W. F., Wilcox, R. H., & Rechtschaffen, A. (1973). The EEG and behavioral continuum of the crocodilian Caiman sclerops. *Electroencephalography and Clinical Neurophysiology, 34*, 521–538.

Frank, M. G., & Heller, H. C. (1997a). Development of diurnal organization of EEG slow-wave activity and slow-wave sleep in the rat. *The American Journal of Physiology, 273*, R472–R478.

Frank, M. G., & Heller, H. C. (1997b). Development of REM and slow wave sleep in the rat. *The American Journal of Physiology, 272*, R1792–R1799.

Frank, M. G., & Heller, H. C. (2003). The ontogeny of mammalian sleep: A reappraisal of alternative hypotheses. *Journal of Sleep Research, 12*, 25–34.

Frank, M. G., & Heller, H. C. (2005). Unresolved issues in sleep ontogeny: A response to Blumberg et al. *Journal of Sleep Research, 14*, 98–101.

Frank, M. G., Issa, N. P., & Stryker, M. P. (2001). Sleep enhances plasticity in the developing visual cortex. *Neuron, 30*, 275–287.

Frank, M. G., Morrissette, R., & Heller, H. C. (1998). Effects of sleep deprivation in neonatal rats. *The American Journal of Physiology, 44*, R148–R157.

Fuller, P. M., Gooley, J. J., & Saper, C. B. (2006). Neurobiology of the sleep–wake cycle: Sleep architecture, circadian regulation, and regulatory feedback. *Journal of Biological Rhythms, 21*, 482–493.

Gall, A. J., Poremba, A. L., & Blumberg, M. S. (2007). Brainstem cholinergic modulation of muscle tone in infant rats. *The European Journal of Neuroscience, 25*, 3367–3375.

Gall, A. J., Todd, W. D., Ray, B., Coleman, C. M., & Blumberg, M. S. (2008). The development of day-night differences in sleep and wakefulness in Norway rats and the effect of bilateral enucleation. *Journal of Biological Rhythms, 23*, 232–241.

Galli, L., & Maffei, L. (1988). Spontaneous impulse activity of rat retinal ganglion cells in prenatal life. *Science, 242*, 90–91.

Gallopin, T., Luppi, P. H., Rambert, F. A., Frydman, A., & Fort, P. (2004). Effect of the wake-promoting agent modafinil on sleep-promoting neurons from the ventrolateral preoptic nucleus: An in vitro pharmacologic study. *Sleep, 27*, 19–25.

Garaschuk, O., Linn, J., Eilers, J., & Konnerth, A. (2000). Large-scale oscillatory calcium waves in the immature cortex. *Nature Neuroscience, 3*, 452–459.

Gervasoni, D., Lin, S. C., Ribeiro, S., Soares, E. S., Pantoja, J., & Nicolelis, M. A. (2004). Global forebrain dynamics predict rat behavioral states and their transitions. *The Journal of Neuroscience, 24*, 11137–11147.

Gormezano, I., Kehoe, E. J., & Marshall, B. S. (1983). Twenty years of classical conditioning with the rabbit. *Progress in Psychobiology and Physiological Psychology, 10*, 197–275.

Gottlieb, G. (1997). *Synthesizing nature-nurture: Prenatal roots of instinctive behavior.* Mahway: Lawrence Erlbaum Associates.

Gramsbergen, A. (1976). The development of the EEG in the rat. *Developmental Psychobiology, 9*, 501–515.

Gramsbergen, A., Schwartze, P., & Prechtl, H. F. R. (1970). The postnatal development of behavioral states in the rat. *Developmental Psychobiology, 3*, 267–280.

Hajnik, T., Lai, Y. Y., & Siegel, J. M. (2000). Atonia-related regions in the rodent pons and medulla. *Journal of Neurophysiology, 84*, 1942–1948.

Hall, W. G., & Oppenheim, R. W. (1987). Developmental psychobiology: Prenatal, perinatal, and early postnatal aspects of behavioral development. *Annual Review of Psychology, 38*, 91–128.

Hamburger, V. (1973). Anatomical and physiological bases of embryonic motility in birds and mammals. In G. Gottlieb (Ed.), *Studies on the development of behavior and the nervous system, Behavioral embryology* (Vol. 1, pp. 51–76). New York: Academic Press.

Hamburger, V., & Oppenheim, R. (1967). Prehatching motility and hatching behavior in the chick. *Journal of Experimental Zoology, 166*, 171–204.

Hanganu, I. L., Ben-Ari, Y., & Khazipov, R. (2006). Retinal waves trigger spindle bursts in the neonatal rat visual cortex. *The Journal of Neuroscience, 26*, 6728–6736.

Hanganu, I. L., Staiger, J. F., Ben-Ari, Y., & Khazipov, R. (2007). Cholinergic modulation of spindle bursts in the neonatal rat visual cortex in vivo. *The Journal of Neuroscience, 27*, 5694–5705.

Hannibal, J., & Fahrenkrug, J. (2002). Melanopsin: A novel photopigment involved in the photoentrainment of the brain's biological clock? *Annals of Medicine, 34*, 401–407.

Hattar, S., Liao, H. W., Takao, M., Berson, D. M., & Yau, K. W. (2002). Melanopsin-containing retinal ganglion cells: Architecture, projections, and intrinsic photosensitivity. *Science, 295*, 1065–1070.

Hendricks, J. C., & Sehgal, A. (2004). Why a fly? Using *Drosophila* to understand the genetics of circadian rhythms and sleep. *Sleep, 27*, 334–342.

Hendricks, J. C., Sehgal, A., & Pack, A. (2000). The need for a simple animal model to understand sleep. *Progress in Neurobiology, 61*, 339–351.

Hobson, J. A. (2005). Sleep is of the brain, by the brain and for the brain. *Nature, 437*, 1254–1256.

Huntley, A. C., & Cohen, H. B. (1980). Further comments on "sleep" in the desert iguana, *Dipsosaurus dorsalis*. *Sleep Research, 9*, 11.

Ifft, J. D. (1972). An autoradiographic study of the time of final division of neurons in rat hypothalamic nuclei. *The Journal of Comparative Neurology, 144*, 193–204.

Jouvet-Mounier, D., Astic, L., & Lacote, D. (1970). Ontogenesis of the states of sleep in rat, cat, and guinea pig during the first postnatal month. *Developmental Psychobiology, 2*, 216–239.

Kandel, E. R., & Schwartz, J. H. (1982). Molecular biology of learning: Modulation of transmitter release. *Science, 218*, 433–443.

Karlsson, K. Æ., & Blumberg, M. S. (2002). The union of the state: Myoclonic twitching is coupled with nuchal muscle atonia in infant rats. *Behavioral Neuroscience, 116*, 912–917.

Karlsson, K. Æ., & Blumberg, M. S. (2005). Active medullary control of atonia in week-old rats. *Neuroscience, 130*, 275–283.

Karlsson, K. Æ., Gall, A. J., Mohns, E. J., Seelke, A. M. H., & Blumberg, M. S. (2005). The neural substrates of infant sleep in rats. *PLoS Biology, 3*, 891–901.

Karlsson, K. Æ., Kreider, J. C., & Blumberg, M. S. (2004). Hypothalamic contribution to sleep–wake cycle development. *Neuroscience, 123,* 575–582.

Karlsson, K. Æ., Mohns, E. J., Vianna di Prisco, G., & Blumberg, M. S. (2006). On the co-occurrence of startles and hippocampal sharp waves in newborn rats. *Hippocampus, 16,* 959–965.

Khazipov, R., Sirota, A., Leinekugel, X., Holmes, G. L., Ben-Ari, Y., & Buzsaki, G. (2004). Early motor activity drives spindle-bursts in the developing somatosensory cortex. *Nature, 432,* 758–761.

Kittrell, E. M. W., & Satinoff, E. (1986). Development of the circadian rhythm of body temperature in rats. *Physiology & Behavior, 38,* 99–104.

Kleitman, N., & Engelmann, T. G. (1953). Sleep characteristics of infants. *Journal of Applied Physiology, 6,* 269–282.

Kreider, J. C. (2003). *The neural substrates of active sleep in infant rats.* Unpublished doctoral dissertation, University of Iowa, Iowa City.

Kreider, J. C., & Blumberg, M. S. (2000). Mesopontine contribution to the expression of active 'twitch' sleep in decerebrate week-old rats. *Brain Research, 872,* 149–159.

Kryger, M. H., Roth, T., & Dement, W. C. (2000). *Principles and practice of sleep medicine.* Philadelphia: W. B. Saunders.

Lahtinen, H., Palva, J. M., Sumanen, S., Voipio, J., Kaila, K., & Taira, T. (2001). Postnatal development of rat hippocampal gamma rhythm in vivo. *Journal of Neurophysiology, 88,* 1469–1474.

Lane, M. S., & Robinson, S. R. (1998). Interlimb dependencies in the spontaneous motor activity of the rat fetus and neonate and preterm human infant. *Developmental Psychobiology, 33,* 376.

Leard, L. E., Macdonald, E. S., Heller, H. C., & Kilduff, T. S. (1994). Ontogeny of photic-induced c-fos mRNA expression in rat suprachiasmatic nuclei. *Neuroreport, 5,* 2683–2687.

Leinekugel, X., Khazipov, R., Cannon, R., Hirase, H., Ben-Ari, Y., & Buzsáki, G. (2002). Correlated bursts of activity in neonatal hippocampus in vivo. *Science, 296,* 2049–2052.

Liang, F. Q., Allen, G., & Earnest, D. (2000). Role of brain-derived neurotrophic factor in the circadian regulation of the suprachiasmatic pacemaker by light. *The Journal Neuroscience, 20,* 2978–2987.

Lin, L., Faraco, J., Li, R., Kadotani, H., Rogers, W., Lin, X., et al. (1999). The sleep disorder canine narcolepsy is caused by a mutation in the hypocretin (orexin) receptor 2 gene. *Cell, 98,* 365–376.

Lo, C. C., Amaral, L. A. N., Havlin, S., Ivanov, P. C., Penzel, T., Peter, J. H., et al. (2002). Dynamics of sleep–wake transitions during sleep. *Europhysics Letters, 57,* 625–631.

Lo, C. C., Chou, T., Penzel, T., Scammell, T. E., Strecker, R. E., Stanley, H. E., et al. (2004). Common scale-invariant patterns of sleep–wake transitions across mammalian species. *Proceedings of the National Academy of Sciences, USA, 101,* 17545–17548.

Lowen, S. B., & Teich, M. C. (1993a). Fractal renewal processes. *IEEE Transactions on Information Theory, 39,* 1669–1671.

Lowen, S. B., & Teich, M. C. (1993b). Fractal renewal processes generate 1/f noise. *Physical Review E, 47,* 992–1001.

Malinowska, M., & Kubin, L. (2004). Neurons of the dorsomedial pontine tegmentum make synaptic contacts with caudal pontomedullary neurons sending projections to the dorsomedial pons. *Sleep, 27,* A35.

Marcano-Reik, A. J., & Blumberg, M. S. (2008). The corpus callosum modulates spindle-burst activity within homotopic regions of somatosensory cortex in newborn rats. *The European Journal of Neuroscience, 28,* 1457–1466.

McGinty, D. J., Stevenson, M., Hoppenbrouwers, T., Harper, R. M., Sterman, M. B., & Hodgman, J. (1977). Polygraphic studies of kitten development: Sleep state patterns. *Developmental Psychobiology, 10,* 455–469.

Minlebaev, M., Ben-Ari, Y., & Khazipov, R. (2007). Network mechanisms of spindle-burst oscillations in the neonatal rat barrel cortex in vivo. *Journal of Neurophysiology, 97,* 692–700.

Mirmiran, M. (1995). The function of fetal/neonatal rapid eye movement sleep. *Behavioural Brain Research, 69,* 13–22.

Mirmiran, M., & Corner, M. (1982). Neuronal discharge patterns in the occipital cortex of developing rats during active and quiet sleep. *Brain Research, 255,* 37–48.

Mirmiran, M., Scholtens, J., van de Poll, N. E., Uylings, H. B. M., van der Gugten, J., & Boer, G. J. (1983). Effects of experimental suppression of active (REM) sleep during early development upon adult brain and behavior in the rat. *Developmental Brain Research, 7,* 277–286.

Mirmiran, M., Van De Poll, N. E., Corner, M. A., Van Oyen, H. G., & Bour, H. L. (1981). Suppression of active sleep by chronic treatment with chlorimipramine during early postnatal development: Effects upon adult sleep and behavior in the rat. *Brain Research, 204,* 129–146.

Mochizuki, T., Crocker, A., McCormack, S., Yanagisawa, M., Sakurai, T., & Scammell, T. E. (2004). Behavioral state instability in orexin knock-out mice. *The Journal of Neuroscience, 24,* 6291–6300.

Mohns, E. J., & Blumberg, M. S. (2008). Synchronous bursts of neuronal activity in the developing hippocampus: Modulation by active sleep and association with emerging gamma and theta rhythms. *The Journal of Neuroscience, 28,* 10134–10144.

Mohns, E. J., Karlsson, K. Æ., & Blumberg, M. S. (2006). The preoptic area and basal forebrain play opposing roles in the descending modulation of sleep and wakefulness in infant rats. *The European Journal of Neuroscience, 23,* 1301–1310.

Mohns, E. J., Karlsson, K. Æ., & Blumberg, M. S. (2007). Developmental emergence of transient and persistent hippocampal events and oscillations and their association with infant seizure susceptibility. *The European Journal of Neuroscience, 26,* 2719–2730.

Moore, R. Y. (1983). Organization and function of a central nervous system circadian oscillator: The suprachiasmatic hypothalamic nucleus. *Federation Proceedings, 42,* 2783–2789.

Morrison, A. R. (1988). Paradoxical sleep without atonia. *Archives Italiennes de Biologie, 126,* 275–289.

Narayanan, C. H., Fox, M. W., & Hamburger, V. (1971). Prenatal development of spontaneous and evoked activity in the rat (*Rattus norvegicus*). *Behaviour, 40,* 100–134.

Nijhuis, J. G. (1995). Physiological and clinical consequences in relation to the development of fetal behavior and fetal behavioral states. In J. P. Lecanuet, N. A. Krasnegor, W. P. Fifer, & W. P. Smotherman (Eds.), *Fetal development: A psychobiological perspective* (pp. 67–82). New York: Lawrence Erlbaum Associates.

Nijhuis, J. G., Martin, C. B., Jr., & Prechtl, H. F. R. (1984). Behavioural states of the human fetus. In H. F. R. Prechtl (Ed.), *Continuity of neural functions from prenatal to postnatal life* (pp. 65–92). Oxford: Blackwell Scientific.

Nishino, S., Taheri, S., Black, J., Nofzinger, E., & Mignot, E. (2004). The neurobiology of sleep in relation to mental illness. In D. S. Charney & E. J. Nestler (Eds.), *Neurobiology of mental illness* (pp. 1160–1179). Oxford: Oxford University Press.

Nuesslein-Hildesheim, B., Imai-Matsumura, K., Döring, H., & Schmidt, I. (1995). Pronounced juvenile circadian core temperature rhythms exist in several strains of rats but not in rabbits. *Journal of Comparative Physiology B, 165,* 13–17.

Ohta, H., Honma, S., Abe, H., & Honma, K. (2002). Effects of nursing mothers on rPer1 and rPer2 circadian expressions in the neonatal rat suprachiasmatic nuclei vary with developmental stage. *The European Journal of Neuroscience, 15,* 1953–1960.

Overeem, S., Mignot, E., Gert, E., van Dijk, J., & Lammers, G. J. (2001). Narcolepsy: Clinical features, new pathophysiologic insights, and future perspectives. *Journal of Clinical Neurophysiology, 18,* 78–105.

Oyama, S., Griffiths, P. E., & Gray, R. D. (Eds.). (2001). *Cycles of contingency: Developmental systems and evolution.* Cambridge, MA: MIT Press.

Pace-Schott, E. F., & Hobson, J. A. (2002). The neurobiology of sleep: Genetics, cellular physiology and subcortical networks. *Nature Reviews. Neuroscience, 3,* 591–605.

Parmelee, A. H., Jr., Wenner, W. H., Akiyama, Y., Schultz, M., & Stern, E. (1967). Sleep states in premature infants. *Developmental Medicine and Child Neurology, 9,* 70–77.

Payne, J. A., Rivera, C., Voipio, J., & Kaila, K. (2003). Cation-chloride co-transporters in neuronal communication, development and trauma. *Trends in Neurosciences, 26,* 199–206.

Petersson, P., Waldenström, A., Fåhraeus, C., & Schouenborg, J. (2003). Spontaneous muscle twitches during sleep guide spinal self-organization. *Nature, 424,* 72–75.

Peyron, C., Faraco, J., Rogers, W., Ripley, B., Overeem, S., Charnay, Y., et al. (2000). A mutation in a case of early onset narcolepsy and a generalized absence of hypocretin peptides in human narcoleptic brains. *Nature Medicine, 6,* 991–997.

Peyron, C., Tighe, D. K., van den Pol, A. N., de Lecea, L., Heller, H. C., Sutcliffe, J. G., et al. (1998). Neurons containing hypocretin (orexin) project to multiple neuronal systems. *The Journal of Neuroscience, 18,* 9996–10015.

Prechtl, H. F. R. (1974). The behavioural states of the newborn infant. *Brain Research, 76,* 185–212.

Provine, R. R. (1973). Neurophysiological aspects of behavior development in the chick embryo. In G. Gottlieb (Ed.), *Behavioral embryology* (Vol. 1, pp. 77–102). New York: Academic Press.

Rattenborg, N. C., Amlaner, C. J., & Lima, S. L. (2000). Behavioral, neurophysiological and evolutionary perspectives on unihemispheric sleep. *Neuroscience and Biobehavioral Reviews, 24,* 817–842.

Rattenborg, N. C., Mandt, B. H., Obermeyer, W. H., Winsauer, P. J., Huber, R., Wikelski, M., et al. (2004). Migratory sleeplessness in the white-crowned sparrow (*Zonotrichia leucophrys gambelii*). *PLoS Biology, 2,* E212.

Rechtschaffen, A., Bergmann, B. M., Gilliland, M. A., & Bauer, K. (1999). Effects of method, duration, and sleep stage on rebounds from sleep deprivation in the rat. *Sleep, 22,* 11–31.

Rechtschaffen, A., & Kales, A. (Eds.). (1968). *A manual of standardized terminology, techniques, and scoring system for sleep stages of human subjects.* Los Angeles: UCLA Brain Information Service/Brain Research Institute.

Reppert, S. M., & Schwartz, W. J. (1984). The suprachiasmatic nuclei of the fetal rat: Characterization of a functional circadian clock using 14C-labeled deoxyglucose. *The Journal of Neuroscience, 4,* 1677–1682.

Reppert, S. M., Weaver, D. R., & Rivkees, S. A. (1988). Maternal communication of circadian phase to the developing mammal. *Psychoneuroendocrinology, 13,* 63–78.

Robinson, S. R., Blumberg, M. S., Lane, M. S., & Kreber, L. A. (2000). Spontaneous motor activity in fetal and infant rats is organized into discrete multilimb bouts. *Behavioral Neuroscience, 14,* 328–336.

Robinson, S. R., & Smotherman, W. P. (1987). Environmental determinants of behaviour in the rat fetus. II. The emergence of synchronous movement. *Animal Behaviour, 35,* 1652–1662.

Roffwarg, H. P., Muzio, J. N., & Dement, W. C. (1966). Ontogenetic development of the human sleep-dream cycle. *Science, 152,* 604–619.

Rusak, B., & Zucker, I. (1979). Neural regulation of circadian rhythms. *Physiological Reviews, 59,* 449–526.

Sakai, K. (1988). Executive mechanisms of paradoxical sleep. *Archives Italiennes de Biologie, 126,* 239–257.

Sakurai, T., Amemiya, A., Ishii, M., Matsuzaki, I., Chemelli, R. M., Tanaka, H., et al. (1998). Orexins and orexin receptors: A family of hypothalamic neuropeptides and G protein-coupled receptors that regulate feeding behavior. *Cell, 92,* 573–585.

Saper, C. B., Chou, T. C., & Scammell, T. E. (2001). The sleep switch: Hypothalamic control of sleep and wakefulness. *Trends in Neurosciences, 24,* 726–731.

Schenkel, E., & Siegel, J. M. (1989). REM sleep without atonia after lesions of the medial medulla. *Neuroscience Letters, 98,* 159–165.

Schouenborg, J. (2003). Somatosensory imprinting in spinal reflex modules. *Journal of Rehabilitation Medicine, 35*(Suppl. 41), 73–80.

Seelke, A. M. H., & Blumberg, M. S. (2004). Sniffing in infant rats during sleep and wakefulness. *Behavioral Neuroscience, 118,* 267–273.

Seelke, A. M. H., & Blumberg, M. S. (2005). Thermal and nutritional modulation of sleep in infant rats. *Behavioral Neuroscience, 19,* 603–611.

Seelke, A. M. H., & Blumberg, M. S. (2008). The microstructure of active and quiet sleep in rats during the developmental emergence of delta activity. *Sleep, 31,* 691–699.

Seelke, A. M. H., Karlsson, K. Æ., Gall, A. J., & Blumberg, M. S. (2005). Extraocular muscle activity, rapid eye movements, and the development of active and quiet sleep. *The European Journal of Neuroscience, 22,* 911–920.

Sekaran, S., Lupi, D., Jones, S. L., Sheely, C. J., Hattar, S., Yau, K. W., et al. (2005). Melanopsin-dependent photoreception provides earliest light detection in the mammalian retina. *Current Biology, 15,* 1099–1107.

Sernagor, E. (2005). Retinal development: Second sight comes first. *Current Biology, 15,* R556–R559.

Shaffery, J. P., Sinton, C. M., Bissette, G., Roffwarg, H. P., & Marks, G. A. (2002). Rapid eye movement sleep deprivation modifies expression of long-term potentiation in visual cortex of immature rats. *Neuroscience, 110*, 431–443.

Shatz, C. J. (1990). Impulse activity and the patterning of connections during CNS development. *Neuron, 5*, 745–756.

Siegel, J. M. (1999). The evolution of REM sleep. In R. Lydic & H. A. Baghdoyan (Eds.), *Handbook of behavioral state control* (pp. 87–100). Boca Raton, FL: CRC Press.

Siegel, J. M. (2001). The REM sleep-memory consolidation hypothesis. *Science, 294*, 1058–1063.

Siegel, J. M. (2005a). Clues to the functions of mammalian sleep. *Nature, 437*, 1264–1271.

Siegel, J. M. (2005b). REM sleep. In M. H. Kryger, T. Roth, & W. C. Dement (Eds.), *Principles and practice of sleep medicine*. Philadelphia: W. B. Saunders.

Siegel, J. M., Manger, P. R., Nienhuis, R., Fahringer, H. M., & Pettigrew, J. D. (1998). Monotremes and the evolution of rapid eye movement sleep. *Philosophical Transactions of the Royal Society of London. Series B, Biological Sciences, 353*, 1147–1157.

Siegel, J. M., Moore, R., Thannickal, R., & Nienhuis, R. (2001). A brief history of hypocretin/orexin and narcolepsy. *Neuropsychopharmacology, 25*, S14–S20.

Siegel, J. M., Nienhuis, R., Fahringer, H. M., Paul, R., Shiromani, P., Dement, W. C., et al. (1991). Neuronal activity in narcolepsy: Identification of cataplexy-related cells in the medial medulla. *Science, 252*, 1315–1318.

Sokoloff, G., & Blumberg, M. S. (1998). Active sleep in cold-exposed infant Norway rats and Syrian golden hamsters: The role of brown adipose tissue thermogenesis. *Behavioral Neuroscience, 112*, 695–706.

Speh, J. C., & Moore, R. Y. (1993). Retinohypothalamic tract development in the hamster and rat. *Brain Research. Developmental Brain Research, 76*, 171–181.

Spiers, D. E. (1988). Nocturnal shifts in thermal and metabolic responses of the immature rat. *Journal of Applied Physiology, 64*, 2119–2124.

Stelzner, D. J. (1982). The role of descending systems in maintaining intrinsic spinal function: A developmental approach. In B. Sjölund & A. Björklund (Eds.), *Brain stem control of spinal mechanisms* (pp. 297–321). Amsterdam: Elsevier Biomedical Press.

Steriade, M., Curro Dossi, R., & Nunez, A. (1991). Network modulation of a slow intrinsic oscillation of cat thalamocortical neurons implicated in sleep delta waves: Cortically induced synchronization and brainstem cholinergic suppression. *The Journal of Neuroscience, 11*, 3200–3217.

Stickgold, R. (2005). Sleep-dependent memory consolidation. *Nature, 437*, 1272–1278.

Szeto, H. H., & Hinman, D. J. (1985). Prenatal development of sleep–wake patterns in sheep. *Sleep, 8*, 347–355.

Szymusiak, R., Steininger, T., Alam, N., & McGinty, D. (2001). Preoptic area sleep-regulating mechanisms. *Archives Italiennes de Biologie, 139*, 77–92.

Taheri, S., Zeitzer, J. M., & Mignot, E. (2002). The role of hypocretins (orexins) in sleep regulation and narcolepsy. *Annual Review of Neuroscience, 25*, 283–313.

Takahashi, K., & Deguchi, T. (1983). Entrainment of the circadian rhythms of blinded infant rats by nursing mothers. *Physiology & Behavior, 31*, 373–378.

Tamásy, V., Korányi, L., & Lissák, K. (1980). Early postnatal development of wakefulness-sleep cycle and neuronal responsiveness: A multiunit activity study on freely moving newborn rat. *Electroencephalography and Clinical Neurophysiology, 49*, 102–111.

Tanaka, M., Iijima, N., Amaya, F., Tamada, Y., & Ibata, Y. (1999). NGFI-A gene expression induced in the rat suprachiasmatic nucleus by photic stimulation: Spread into hypothalamic periventricular somatostatin neurons and GABA receptor involvement. *The European Journal of Neuroscience, 11*, 3178–3184.

Terman, D., Bose, A., & Kopell, N. (1996). Functional reorganization in thalamocortical networks: Transition between spindling and delta sleep rhythms. *Proceedings of the National Academy of Sciences, USA, 93*, 15417–15422.

Thannickal, T. C., Moore, R. Y., Nienhuis, R., Ramanathan, L., Gulyani, S., Aldrich, M., et al. (2000). Reduced number of hypocretin neurons in human narcolepsy. *Neuron, 27*, 469–474.

Thompson, R. F. (1986). The neurobiology of learning and memory. *Science, 233*, 941–947.

Tobler, I. (1995). Is sleep fundamentally different between mammalian species? *Behavioural Brain Research, 69*, 35–41.

Tobler, I., & Deboer, T. (2001). Sleep in the blind mole rat *Spalax ehrenbergi*. *Sleep, 24*, 147–154.

Todd, W. D., & Blumberg, M. S. (2007). Sleep regulation in neonatal rats: A reexamination. *Developmental Psychobiology, 49*, 742.

Umans, J. G., Cox, M. J., Hinman, D. J., Dogramajian, M. E., Senger, G., & Szeto, H. H. (1985). The development of electrocortical activity in the fetal and neonatal guinea pig. *American Journal of Obstetrics and Gynecology, 153*, 467–471.

van den Pol, A. N. (2000). Narcolepsy: A neurodegenerative disease of the hypocretin system? *Neuron, 27*, 415–418.

Vanhatalo, S., & Kaila, K. (2006). Development of neonatal EEG activity: From phenomenology to physiology. *Seminars in Fetal Neonatal Medicine, 11*, 471–478.

Vanhatalo, S., Palva, J. M., Andersson, S., Rivera, C., Voipio, J., & Kaila, K. (2005). Slow endogenous activity transients and developmental expression of K^+-Cl^- cotransporter 2 in the immature human cortex. *The European Journal of Neuroscience, 22*, 2799–2804.

Van Someren, E. J. W., Mirmiran, M., Bos, N. P. A., Lamur, A., Kumar, A., & Molenaar, P. C. M. (1990). Quantitative analysis of eye movements during REM-sleep in developing rats. *Developmental Psychobiology, 23*, 55–61.

Vertes, R. P. (2004). Memory consolidation in sleep, dream or reality. *Neuron, 44*, 135–148.

Vertes, R. P., Martin, G. F., & Waltzer, R. (1986). An autoradiographic analysis of ascending projections from the medullary reticular formation in the rat. *Neuroscience, 19*, 873–898.

Willie, J. T., Chemelli, R. M., Sinton, C. M., Tokita, S., Williams, S. C., Kisanuki, Y. Y., et al. (2003). Distinct narcolepsy syndromes in orexin receptor-2 and orexin null mice: Molecular genetic dissection of Non-REM and REM sleep regulatory processes. *Neuron, 38*, 715–730.

Zepelin, H. (2000). Mammalian sleep. In M. H. Kryger, T. Roth, & W. C. Dement (Eds.), *Principles and practice of sleep medicine* (pp. 82–92). Philadelphia: W. B. Saunders.

Zepelin, H., & Rechtschaffen, A. (1974). Mammalian sleep, longevity, and energy metabolism. *Brain, Behavior, and Evolution, 10*, 425–470.

Zepelin, H., Siegel, J. M., & Tobler, I. (2005). Mammalian sleep. In M. H. Kryger, T. Roth, & W. Dement (Eds.), *Principles and practice of sleep medicine* (4th ed., pp. 91–100). Philadelphia: Elsevier Saunders.

Notes

1 Startles are distinct from twitches in that they comprise sudden, spontaneous, and simultaneous contraction of multiple skeletal muscle groups, as described in human fetuses (de Vries, Visser, & Prechtl, 1984) and infant rats (Gramsbergen et al., 1970). Thus, although multiple limbs can exhibit myoclonic twitches in rapid succession, such multilimb bouts of twitching are distinct from the simultaneous activation that characterizes startles. In addition, startles exhibit a unique profile of associated hippocampal activity (Karlsson, Mohns, Vianna di Prisco, & Blumberg, 2006; Mohns, Karlsson, & Blumberg, 2007). Also, whereas sleep-related twitching continues into adulthood, startles decline and largely disappear across the postnatal period in rats (Gramsbergen et al., 1970).

2 A multilimb bout is defined as the set of limb movements in which the interval between successive movements does not exceed an established criterion value.

3 For example, in week-old rats, an environmental temperature of 35°C is within the thermoneutral range (Blumberg, 2001) and provides favorable conditions for sleep (Seelke & Blumberg, 2005).

4 The use of electric shock during the sleep deprivation period interfered with the reliable EMG measurement of nuchal muscle activity.

Perinatal Gonadal Hormone Influences on Neurobehavioral Development

Joseph S. Lonstein *and* Anthony P. Auger

Abstract

Generating distinctly male or female brains during early development is a monumental process that forever modifies behavior. Relatively straightforward theories involving perinatal exposure to gonadal hormones have historically been used to explain the generation of sex-typical traits. These tenets are of great heuristic value, but are unable to explain much of sexual differentiation. By examining events leading to sexual dimorphism of some well-studied neural structures (medial preoptic area, medial amygdala, ventromedial hypothalamus), and some social behaviors these structures mediate (play, maternal behavior, copulation), it is clear that sexual differentiation is anything but simple. Instead, it is an active process in both sexes, requires hormonal as well as nonhormonal events, extends beyond early development, and occurs differently across mammalian species.

Keywords: male brains, female brains, perinatal, gonadal hormones, sexual differentiation, sexual dimorphism, medial preoptic area, medial amygdala, ventromedial hypothalamus

Introduction to Sex Differences in Brain and Behavior

Many of the chapters in this book focus on developmental events modifying central nervous system circuits underlying behavior, and how these modifications lead to varied behavioral phenotypes later in life. In most cases, variations in behavioral phenotypes are examined within groups of males or females. Some of the most dramatic differences in brain and behavior, however, are observed when one compares *between* the sexes rather than within them. Molding the undifferentiated central nervous system into one with both subtle and immense sexual dimorphisms is truly an extraordinary developmental process.

The purpose of this chapter is to describe the developmental events leading to sex differences in

the brain and the resulting consequences on behavior. Our goal is not to exhaustively review this immense field, portions of which have been recently reviewed in great detail (Arnold, 2002; De Vries & Simerly, 2002; Forger, 2001; Wallen & Baum, 2002). Instead, we review the well-known, traditional views of how sexual differentiation of the brain and behavior occurs, but highlight particularly recent and salient exceptions to these tenets. It will hopefully be clear that generating sex differences in the brain and behavior is the result of several active processes occurring in both sexes, and that these events are not restricted to early development. We will then scrutinize the often tenuous association between neural structure and function. Lastly, we call attention to the great diversity in how sexual differentiation occurs, even within *Rodentia*.

The rich array of mechanisms involved in generating sex-typical brains and behavior, and the range of outcomes these mechanisms produce within and across species, provide a unique and exciting context in which to study neurobehavioral development.

Generation of Sex Differences in the Brain and Behavior
Traditional View of Sexual Differentiation

Recent reviews of this field have comprehensively detailed how perinatal hormones are thought to sexually differentiate the vertebrate brain and behavior. We will, therefore, provide only a brief overview sufficient to comprehend the present chapter. Laboratory rodents have been the best-studied model for this process, so they will be the focus of this review. In the section on "What Do Rats and Mice Tell Us about Sexual Differentiation of Other Species?" , however, we will note the potential pitfalls in this approach.

Most people are familiar with the concept that genotypic sex in mammals is determined by the complement of sex chromosomes contained in an individual's genome. The male genome contains an X and a Y chromosome, while the female genome contains two X chromosomes. It is generally accepted that during early development, the presence of the Y chromosome in males sets forth a cascade of events leading to differentiation of both peripheral and central nervous system tissues. While several genes are likely involved, the widely studied *Sry* gene (*Sex-determining Region of the Y* chromosome), causes the bipotential gonadal *anlagen* to differentiate into testes. Formation of the testes is one of the first essential steps toward sexually differentiating a developing organism. The traditional view then posits that the testes alter brain development primarily through surges of testosterone during early development, which in rats occur around embryonic day 18 and again within hours after birth (Pang, Caggiula, Gay, Goodman, & Pang, 1979; Rhoda, Corbier, & Roffi, 1984; Weisz & Ward, 1980). These exposures to testosterone are largely responsible for the normal *masculinization* (the process of increasing male-typical traits) and *defeminization* (the process of decreasing female-typical traits) of males. Importantly, once testosterone reaches the brain, it can be metabolized into two other ligands: dihydrotestosterone (DHT) by the 5α-reductase enzyme, and estradiol by the aromatase enzyme. This metabolism is important, as the masculinizing effects of testosterone on the developing nervous system in many rodents are mediated through its aromatization to estradiol, and subsequent activation of estrogen receptors (ERs; MacLusky & Naftolin, 1981). It is traditionally thought that DHT and its activation of androgen receptors (ARs) have only a small role in masculiniziation, at least in rodents, but may have a more important role in primates (Wallen, 2005). These surges of testicular hormones and activation of neural ERs during discrete perinatal critical periods are thought to permanently "organize" neural networks and lead to neurobehavioral masculinization and defeminization.

In contrast to males, the absence of a Y chromosome and the *Sry* gene in females prevents the gonadal *anlagen* from forming testes, and a pair of ovaries is instead produced. The perinatal ovary is relatively steroidogenically quiescent during perinatal life (Lamprecht, Kohen, Ausher, Zor, & Lindner, 1976; Weniger, Zeis, & Chouraqui, 1993), which maintains *feminization* (i.e., increased female-typical traits) of the female brain (Baum, Woutersen, & Slob, 1991; Pang & Tang, 1984; Slob, Ooms, & Vreeburg, 1980; Vomachka & Lisk, 1986; Weisz & Gunsalus, 1973; Weisz & Ward, 1980). Developing females are not completely shielded from hormone exposure, though. First, the perinatal ovary and/or adrenal glands do produce some estrogens (e.g., Montano, Welshons, & vom Saal, 1995; Smeaton, Arcondoulis, & Steele, 1975; Weisz & Ward, 1980). Second, estradiol may be produced de novo in the neonatal brain (Amateau, Alt, Stamps, & McCarthy, 2004). Third, steroid hormones readily diffuse across amniotic membranes, resulting in females being exposed to testosterone produced by their male siblings (vom Saal, 1989). Lastly, estrogens readily cross transplacentally from mothers to fetuses, and these hormones have the potential to alter brain development in females (Witcher & Clemens, 1987); however, females are mostly protected by the actions of the estrogen-sequestering protein, alpha fetoprotein, found in their bloodstream and brain during prenatal and early postnatal life (Germain, Campbell, & Anderson, 1978). Therefore, even if potentially masculinizing amounts of estrogens enter the perinatal female bloodstream, much of it is unable to bind to and activate neural estradiol receptors (Bakker et al., 2006; Raynaud, Mercier-Bodard, & Baulieu, 1971). It is important to note here that exposure to low levels of estradiol may actually be necessary to differentiate the female brain, as discussed in the section "Sexual Differentiation of Social Behaviors: Sexual Behavior."

Through these processes, brains are "organized" differently in males and females. In many cases, these "organized" neural circuits must later be transiently "activated" by gonadal hormones to permit the expression of sex-specific behaviors. That is, the neural circuitry may be primed to mediate sex-typical behaviors, but the behaviors cannot be displayed until the appropriate hormonal triggers are secreted during adulthood. Not all sex differences in brain and behavior, though, rely on previous perinatal organization. The neural substrates for a behavior can often develop similarly in males and females, with sex differences in steroid hormones produced during adulthood singularly responsible for sex differences in behavior. For example, treating female rats with testosterone can readily elicit male-typical sexual behaviors, and the opposite effect occurs in some male rats treated with ovarian hormones (Olster & Blaustein, 1988). Indeed, males of two different strain of rats (Sprague-Dawley and Wistar) can show high levels of female sexual behavior following pulsatile administration of estradiol (Olster & Blaustein, 1988; Södersten, Pettersson, & Eneroth, 1983). These data reinforce the fact that male and female brains are not inflexibly different, but rather have the capacity of showing components of both male and female behavior depending on the sensory, hormonal, or social context (e.g., Dulac & Kimchi, 2007).

Sexual Differentiation of Social Behaviors

It is often assumed that sexually dimorphic social behaviors are differentiated by perinatal gonadal hormones in the simple and straightforward manner described above. Below we offer three counterexamples to this notion.

Play

In rodents, social play is highly sexually dimorphic, with males engaging in more social play than females (Olioff & Stewart, 1978). The sexually dimorphic patterns of social play are organized by exposure to testosterone during the perinatal period. Indeed, castration of neonatal males prior to postnatal day 6 reduces the frequency of social play to female-typical levels (Beatty, Dodge, Traylor, & Meaney, 1981; Meaney & Stewart, 1981). On the other hand, early neonatal injections of testosterone (Thor & Holloway, 1986), or implants of testosterone directly into the amygdala (Meaney & McEwen, 1986; Tonjes, Docke, & Dorner, 1987), masculinize the social play behavior of females. Unlike what might be expected in the traditional

view, the effects of testosterone on the sexual differentiation of social play are not mediated by testosterone aromatization to estradiol and activation of neural estradiol receptors, but instead are mediated by activity of the AR. In support, peripheral treatment with testosterone or its androgenic metabolite, DHT, masculinizes social play behavior, but a low dose of estradiol benzoate (EB, 5 μg) has no effect (Meaney & Stewart, 1981).

Although it is interesting to consider that social play is not sexually differentiated through aromatization of testosterone to estradiol, it remains possible that the lack of effect of EB was due to the relatively low dose. In fact, recent data indicate that it takes 100 μg of peripherally injected EB to reach male-typical levels of estradiol in the brain (Amateau et al., 2004), leaving open the possibility that ER does influence the development of social play. Furthermore, while males rendered insensitive to androgens by the testicular feminization mutation (Tfm) showed decreased levels of play behavior (Meaney, Stewart, Poulin, & McEwen, 1983), Tfm males still tended to engage in play more frequently than females, providing support for the idea that ERs may play some role in differentiating this behavior. Additional support for ERs in modulating the development of play behavior comes from studies in primates. While it is well documented that androgen systems play the primary role in masculinizing juvenile social play behavior in non-human primates (Wallen, 2005), estrogens may also influence social play. Goy and Deputte found that prenatally exposing monkeys to the synthetic estrogen, diethylstilbestrol (DES), increased social play behavior during the juvenile period (Goy & Deputte, 1996). Therefore, it appears that *both* ARs and ERs probably influence the organization of social play.

As will be discussed in the section "Distribution and Function of Neural Steroid Hormone Receptors" below, nonsteroidal factors can activate steroid hormone receptors in a ligand-independent fashion, opening the possibility that neurotransmitters can contribute to sex differences in play in ways similar to steroid hormones themselves (Vanderschuren, Niesink, & Van Ree, 1997). Indeed, treating newborn female rats with a dopamine agonist masculinizes their juvenile play behavior (Gotz, Tonjes, Maywald, & Dorner, 1991; Tonjes, Gotz, Maywald, & Dorner, 1989). We have recently replicated these findings, and report that dopamine-induced organization of social play behavior occurs by ligand-independently activating

ERs in the developing brain (Olesen, Jessen, Auger, & Auger, 2005). Further support comes from studies examining sex differences in dopamine-producing neurons. Females have significantly more cells containing tyrosine hydroxylase (TH; the rate-limiting enzyme for dopamine synthesis) compared to males within the anteroventral periventricular nucleus (AVPv) of the preoptic area (POA), and that this difference is due to perinatal steroid hormone exposure (Simerly, 1989). In contrast to the AVPv, the number of TH-expressing neurons within the mediobasal hypothalamus appears to be higher (Balan et al., 2000), and these cells are present earlier in males (Balan et al., 1996), suggesting that dopamine concentrations within the mediobasal hypothalamus may be greater in developing males. Consistent with these findings, dopamine metabolism is higher in males than females during the first few hours after birth (Lesage, Bernet, Montel, & Dupouy, 1996), and in response to stimulation, male hypothalamic tissue releases more dopamine than that of females (Melnikova et al., 1999). Males also have greater dopamine levels within the cortex on postnatal day 3 (Connell, Karikari, & Hohmann, 2004). Lastly, hypothalamic dopamine turnover rates are increased in androgenized females (Reznikov & Nosenko, 1995), suggesting increased activity of the dopamine system during early brain development in response to testicular hormones. Because neonatal dopaminergic activity also affects sexual differentiation of copulatory behaviors in rats (Gonzales, Ortega, & Salazar, 2000; Gotz et al., 1991; Hull, Nishita, Bitran, & Dalterio, 1984; Tonjes et al., 1989), greater attention to how sexually dimorphic neurotransmitter systems arise and then contribute to sex differences in behavior is warranted.

Sexual Behavior

Copulatory behaviors in most mammals are extremely sexually dimorphic and are often thought to be an exemplar for traditional organizational–activational effects of hormones. Castration on the day of birth, or perinatal inhibition of hormone synthesis, does severely attenuate normal sexual development in many males. When neonatally castrated males are raised to adulthood, they exhibit decreased masculine sexual behavior and increased feminine sexual behavior when treated with the appropriate hormones (Gerall, Hendricks, Johnson, & Bounds, 1967; Hart, 1968). These effects are prevented if castrated males are given replacement testosterone neonatally (Grady, Phoenix, & Young, 1965; Hart,

1977). Aromatization of testosterone into estradiol, and subsequent ER activation, it a critical step in defeminizing sexual behavior in male rats (Davis, Chaptal, & McEwen, 1979; Dominguez-Salazar, Portillo, Baum, Bakker, & Paredes, 2002; Fadem & Barfield, 1981; McCarthy, Schlenker, & Pfaff, 1993b; McEwen, Lieberburg, Chaptal, & Krey, 1977; Sodersten, 1978; Vreeburg, Van der Vaart, & Van der Schoot, 1977; Whalen & Edwards, 1967; Whalen & Olsen, 1981). Neonatal treatment with the nonaromatizable androgen DHT does not defeminize sexual behavior (Booth, 1977; Whalen & Rezek, 1974), though, suggesting little contribution of the AR in this process. Behavioral masculinization, on the other hand, can be influenced by AR activation, and many studies have shown that masculinization can be disrupted by neonatal treatment with an AR antagonist or null mutation of the AR (Clemens, Gladue, & Coniglio, 1978; Dominguez-Salazar et al., 2002; Nadler, 1969; Neumann & Elger, 1966; Sato et al., 2004). Consistent with this, administration of aromatase inhibitors that block the conversion of testosterone to estradiol does not necessarily disrupt masculinization (Casto, Ward, & Bartke, 2003; Davis et al., 1979; Tonjes et al., 1987; Van der Schoot, 1980; Vreeburg et al., 1977; Whalen & Edwards, 1967; Whalen & Olsen, 1981), and females treated neonatally with DHT are masculinized (Hart, 1977; Tonjes et al., 1987; van der Schoot, 1980). This is also consistent with recent data supporting a role for AR in masculinization of brain morphology (Garcia-Falgueras et al., 2005; Morris, Jordan, Dugger, & Breedlove, 2005).

Taken together, these studies suggest that the mechanisms mediating masculinization and defeminization in laboratory rats can be independently influenced by interfering with different steroid receptors during development. However, as discussed in the section below "What Do Rats and Mice Tell Us about Sexual Differentiation of Other Species?," rodent species differ from each other in their need for early AR or ER for masculinization of sexual behaviors. It is also important to note that male sexual behavior is often reflected by a composite of latencies and frequency of mounts, intromissions, and ejaculations, and different steroid receptors might play different roles in modulating these different aspects of male sexual behavior. For example, neonatal treatment with an aromatase inhibitor or an ER antagonist can interfere with ejaculatory behavior, but has less effect on mounting or intromission behavior (Gladue & Clemens, 1980;

Sodersten, 1978). Complicating the issue is the fact that there are also significant differences between strains of laboratory rats in the degree that perinatal hormone manipulations alter behavioral masculinization and defeminization (Brand & Slob, 1991; Whalen, Gladue, & Olsen, 1986). It is also complicated by the findings that not only ER or AR contribute to masculinization and defeminization of copulatory behaviors in male rats, but that other steroid hormone receptors are also important (e.g., progestin receptors [PRs]; see Lonstein, Quadros, & Wagner, 2001; Van der Schoot & Baumgarten, 1990; Weinstein, Pleim, & Barfield, 1992).

In contrast to males, females normally undergo neurobehavioral demasculinization and feminization. It is often believed that these are passive processes that do not require steroid hormones, but these processes are actually much more complicated. Female rats are exposed to significantly lower levels of circulating testosterone during perinatal life compared to males, and treatment of neonatal females with large doses of testosterone does defeminize and masculinize many aspects of their brain and behavior (Gerall, 1957; Phoenix, Goy, Gerall, & Young, 1959). However, some ER activity is necessary for typical female brain development (Fitch & Denenberg, 1998). For example, newborn females given the estrogen antagonist tamoxifen show decreased adult female sexual behavior, but not increased male sexual behavior (Dohler et al., 1984a). Additionally, treating newborn females with an estrogen antagonist (Dohler et al., 1984a) or antisense oligonucleotides directed at ER mRNA (McCarthy et al., 1993b) further feminizes their sexually dimorphic nucleus of the preoptic area (SDN-POA). In contrast, injection of tamoxifen on postnatal day 4 or removal of the ovaries during the second postnatal week defeminizes the corpus callosum (Fitch & Denenberg, 1998) and perinatal aromatase inhibition can further feminize sexual behavior in female rats (Witcher & Clemens, 1987; but see Dominguez-Salazar et al., 2002). Together, these studies suggest that some level of ER activation is important for appropriate feminization of the female rat brain and behavior (Figure 21.1), and opens the possibility that activation of other steroid receptors is similarly necessary for demasculinization and feminization of female rodents and other mammals.

Parental Behavior

For the vast majority of mammalian species, there is a distinct sex difference in the display of

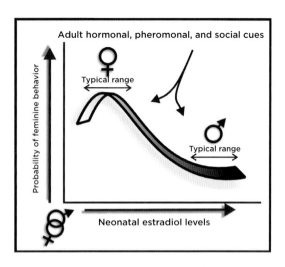

Figure 21.1 Simplified model of the role of estrogen on the development of adult female sexual behavior. The neonatal brain is relatively undifferentiated and differential exposure to steroid hormones organizes the later probability of showing male of female sexual behavior during adulthood. If perinatal exposure to estradiol is relatively high, the probability of exhibiting female sexual behavior in adulthood is decreased. Additionally, the capacity to show female sexual behavior in adulthood is modulated by the appropriate hormonal, pheromonal, and social cues.

parental behaviors, with females invariably taking the primary responsibility of caring for offspring. Laboratory rats are no exception, and males are rarely found in nests with lactating females and pups (Calhoun, 1962). Even as virgins, female rats have a higher propensity for maternal care compared to males when exposed to foster pups (see Lonstein & De Vries, 2000 for review). During this repeated exposure to pups, termed parental sensitization (Rosenblatt, 1967), virgin rats gradually become accustomed to neonates until they display parental behaviors that are similar in many ways to that of lactating females (Bridges, Zarrow, Gandelman, & Denenberg,1972; Fleming & Rosenblatt, 1974; Lonstein, Wagner, & De Vries, 1999). Most studies find that virgin females are more likely to be maternally sensitized, and are more consistently parental after sensitization, than males (Fleischer et al., 1981; Lonstein et al., 2001; Mayer, Freeman, & Rosenblatt, 1979; McCullough, Quandagno, & Goldman, 1974; Quadagno, McCullough, Ho, & Spevak, 1973; Rosenblatt, 1967; Samuels & Bridges, 1983).

One might expect that a behavior with such tremendous sexual dimorphism would have a correspondingly large literature examining how it is influenced by perinatal gonadal hormones. There are surprisingly few studies examining the effects of perinatal hormones on maternal responding, and the results are inconsistent. Injecting pregnant rats with testosterone, or injecting fetuses with it directly through the uterine wall, can reduce later maternal sensitization in the female offspring (Ichikawa & Fujii, 1982; Juarez, del Rio-Portilla, & Corsi-Cabrera, 1998). However, a lack of an effect of prenatal testosterone has also been reported (Quadagno, Briscoe, & Quadagno, 1977). Postnatal administration of testosterone generally does not reduce sensitization in virgin females (Bridges, Zarrow, & Denenberg, 1973; Ichikawa & Fujii, 1982; Leboucher, 1989; Quadagno, 1974; Quadagno et al., 1973; Rosenberg, Denenberg, Zarrow, Frank, 1971), but small reductions in maternal responsiveness in rats have been observed in some cases (Quadagno & Rockwell, 1972), particularly when the postnatal treatment is extensive and is followed by adult administration of testosterone (Rosenberg & Sherman, 1974, 1975).

In contrast to the relative inability of postnatal hormones to masculinize maternal responding in females, postnatal castration seems to readily feminize parental behavior in male rats. Castrated males are much more likely to resist infanticide and/or respond parentally if gonadectomy occurs during neonatal life, and even castration as late as postnatal day 60 or later has sometimes been seen to feminize their responses to pups (Leon, Numan, & Moltz, 1973; McCullough et al., 1974; Quadagno & Rockwell, 1972; Rosenberg, 1974; Rosenberg & Herrenkohl, 1976; Rosenberg et al., 1971; although see Rosenblatt, 1967). There has been virtually no examination of whether prenatal inhibition of gonadal hormone activity affects parental responding in male rats, other than one report showing that prenatal flutamide has no effect on the ability of later exogenous estrogen and progesterone to elicit rapid parental behavior (Tate-Ostroff & Bridges, 1988). It is unknown if flutamide would have an effect in a slow-onset sensitization paradigm that did not include exogenous hormones.

Not much is known about the neural basis underlying sex differences in parental behavior. The sexes differ in their sensitivity to gonadal hormones, as lower doses of exogenous gonadal hormones are required to compel virgin females to act parentally (Lubin, Numan, & Moltz, 1972). There are also sex differences in the sensitivity to pup-related cues (e.g., Stern, 1991). Thus, neural sites receiving and processing hormonal and sensory information

are obvious loci for generating sex differences in parental behaviors (Guillamon & Segovia, 1997).

In sum, the small literature on this topic suggests that early exposure to gonadal hormones can influence sex differences in the parental responding of rats. The critical period for parental responding seems to differ between the sexes. Females may be particularly sensitive to testosterone during gestation, if at all, whereas parental responding in males can apparently be suppressed by testicular hormones released not only soon after birth, but even through early adulthood. It is unknown if these are ER- or AR-mediated effects.

Distribution and Function of Neural Steroid Hormone Receptors

If gonadal hormones are to contribute to sexual differentiation of the brain and behavior, developmental expression of the appropriate receptors for these hormones is necessary. In the rat brain, gonadal steroid receptor-containing neurons are heterogeneously expressed (Pfaff & Keiner, 1973). Although steroid receptors are distributed throughout the brain, these regions are interconnected with each other to form a neural "network" (Cottingham & Pfaff, 1986; Newman, 1999), and that steroid hormones influence sexual differentiation and later complex behaviors by acting upon multiple components of this network. The distribution of steroid receptors in the developing and adult mammalian brain has been well documented and we highlight receptors for three major gonadal hormones involved in sexual differentiation—androgens, estrogens, progestins. Although these receptor systems are our focus, receptors for steroid hormones of extragonadal origin and those for nonsteroid hormones are also in the brain during early life, and also potentially contribute to sexual differentiation (Carter, 2003; McCormick, Smythe, Sharma, & Meaney, 1995; Reznikov, Nosenko, Tarasenko, 1999; Royster, Driscoll, Kelly, & Freemark, 1995; Snijdewint, Van Leeuwen, Boer, 1989).

ESTROGEN RECEPTORS

Relatively recent data suggest that there are at least two types of ERs—estrogen receptor α (ERα) and estrogen receptor β (ERβ). These isoforms have a high degree of sequence homology (Kuiper, Enmark, Peltohuikko, Nilsson, & Gustafsson, 1996), but their functions and transcriptional effects can differ greatly (Paech et al., 1997). It has long been known that neural ERs are present during development in the rat (e.g., Plapinger &

McEwen, 1973; White, Hall, & Lim, 1979). Before identification of multiple ER isoforms, early studies showed that ER mRNA, protein, or binding was found in many areas of the developing brain. ERs first appear in many sites of the fetal rat brain between mid- to late gestation and birth, with levels thereafter increasing and/or decreasing, depending on the neural site (DonCarlos, 1996; MacLusky, Chaptal, & McEwen, 1979a; MacLusky, Lieberburg, & McEwen, 1979b; Miranda & Toran-Allerand, 1992; O'Keefe & Handa, 1990; Pasterkamp et al., 1996). ERα expression is greater in neonatal females than males in some areas of the forebrain necessary for social and other complex motivated behaviors, including the cortex, hippocampus, POA, ventromedial nucleus of the hypothalamus (VMH), and bed nucleus of the stria terminalis (BST) (DonCarlos, 1996; DonCarlos & Handa, 1994; Kuhnemann, Brown, Hochberg, & MacLusky, 1994), and these differences exist on or soon after the day of birth (Hayashi, Hayashi, Ueda, & Papadopoulos, 2001; Ikeda & Nagai, 2006; Perez, Chen, & Mufson, 2003; Solum & Handa, 2001; Yokosuka, Okamura, & Hayashi, 1997; Zsarnovszky & Belcher, 2001; also see Belcher, 1999). There is little knowledge specifically about ERα expression in these sites throughout prenatal life, but ERα mRNA is present in the ventral midbrain and spinal cord during the last week of gestation (Burke et al., 2000; Raab, Karolczak, Reisert, & Beyer, 1999).

ERβ expression is found at birth or within the first few postnatal days in the rat cerebellum (Belcher, 1999), ventral midbrain (Raab et al., 1999; Ravizza, Galanopoulou, Veliskova, & Moshe, 2002), olfactory bulbs (Wong, Poon, Tsim, Wong, & Leung, 2000), cortex (Kritzer, 2006; Perez et al., 2003), amygdala, BST, paraventricular nucleus of the hypothalamus (PVN), and VMH (Ikeda, Nagai, Ikeda, & Hayashi, 2003; Perez et al., 2003). In addition, ERβ mRNA levels in the hypothalamus and POA are greater in neonatal male than female mice (Karolczak & Beyer, 1998), but ERβ protein immunoreactivity in the neonatal VMH is greater in female than male rats (Ikeda et al., 2003). Prenatal expression of ERβ has not been widely studied, but its mRNA is found in the hippocampus, hypothalamus, and POA of fetal mice (Ivanova & Beyer, 2000; Karolczak & Beyer, 1998). While sex differences in the perinatal expression of ERs may help contribute to sexual differentiation of the brain by amplifying the influence of estradiol in some sites, it seems intuitive that sex differences

in circulating testosterone and its ability to be aromatized (Lauber, Sarasin, & Lichtensteiger, 1997; MacLusky, Philip, Hurlburt, & Naftolin, 1985; Paden & Roselli, 1987; Tobet, Baum, Tang, Shim, & Canick, 1985) are primary contributors to subsequent sex differences in the brain.

Initial studies of mice with a selective mutation or deletion of the ERα or ERβ genes suggested that ERβ had little role in the development and mediation of sexually dimorphic behaviors (Ogawa et al., 1999). Mutation of all ERs eliminate copulatory behaviors in males (Ogawa et al., 2000), but males with only a disruption in ERβ still copulate normally (Ogawa et al., 1999), suggesting greater importance for ERα in the organization of male sexual behavior (Eddy et al., 1996; Rissman, Wersinger, Taylor, & Lubahna, 1997; Wersinger et al., 1997). It is impossible to determine if these effects reflect the lack of ER during development or adulthood, as ER mutation exists in these animals throughout their entire life span. Nonetheless, treating neonatal females with antisense oligodeoxynucleotides that disrupt ER mRNA synthesis does prevent the ability of exogenous testosterone to defeminize sexual behavior (McCarthy et al., 1993b), reinforcing the notion that the absence of ER expression during early life very likely contributes to the impairments in sexual behavior in mice without the ERα gene. Even so, more recent work demonstrates that ERβ does have important functions in copulatory behaviors in mice, with animals without ERβ showing delayed sexual development (Temple, Scordalakes, Bodo, Gustafsson, & Rissman, 2003). Male mice without functional ERβ are also less defeminized than controls, and more likely to show feminine sexual behavior when treated with ovarian hormones during adulthood (Kudwa, Bodo, Gustafsson, & Rissman, 2005). Further support of a role for ERβ in defeminization, neonatal treatment with an ERβ-specific agonist defeminizes sexual behavior, while neonatal treatment with an ERα-specific agonist has little effect (Kudwa, Michopoulos, Gatewood, & Rissman, 2006). These results suggest that ERα activity during development is necessary for behavioral masculinization of copulation and possibly other behaviors, while ERβ activity is necessary for behavioral defeminization.

Progestin receptors

PRs are expressed during the perinatal period in laboratory rats and occur in two forms, PR A and PR B (Conneely, Maxwell, Toft, Schrader,

& O'Malley, 1987). As PR A and B differ in the N-terminal sequence that conveys gene activation (Tora, Gronemeyer, Turcotte, Gaub, & Chambon, 1988), these isoforms can be functionally distinct (Mulac-Jericevic, Mullinax, Demayo, Lydon, Conneely, 2000). Indeed, data from PR isoform-specific gene disrupted mice suggest that PR A and B might influence different cellular pathways regulating adult female sexual behavior (Mani, Reyna, Chen, Mulac-Jericevic, & Conneely, 2006). PRs are present in the preoptic area of laboratory rats as early as gestational day 20, but not day 18, and notably, this PR expression is only found in males (Wagner, Nakayama, & De Vries, 1998; also see Kato, Onouchi, Okinaga, & Takamatsu, 1984). In adult rats, estradiol dramatically increases PR levels within the POA, ventromedial nucleus, and arcuate nucleus (Auger et al., 1996; MacLusky & McEwen, 1978; Moguilewsky & Raynaud, 1979), and to a small extent in the posterodorsal medial amygdala (Auger, Moffatt, & Blaustein, 1996). The same is true in developing rats, and the sex difference in PR is due to the males' naturally greater levels of estradiol, which is aromatized from testosterone and subsequently induces PR expression (Quadros, Pfau, Goldstein, De Vries, & Wagner, 2002a). Female rats begin to express PR on postnatal day 10, but levels remain significantly lower than that found in males until after weaning (Quadros, Goldstein, De Vries, & Wagner, 2002b). A much smaller sex difference is found in the developing VMH, with females having more PR than do males (Wagner et al., 1998). PRs are also present in the cerebral cortex during perinatal development (Hagihara, Hirata, Osada, Hirai, & Kato, 1992; Kato & Anouchi, 1981; Kato, Hirata, Nozawa, & Mouri, 1993; Sakamoto, Shikimi, Ukena, & Tsutsui, 2003), but appear not to be sexually dimorphic or affected by perinatal hormones (Jahagirdar, Quadros, & Wagner, 2005). The prenatal and early neonatal PR expression reflect high PR B synthesis, while PR expression after the first week of life includes more PR A synthesis (Kato et al., 1993); how this shift influences responsiveness to progesterone and its effects on development are unknown.

ANDROGEN RECEPTORS

ARs are widely expressed in the brain during development in both rodents and primates (Choate, Slayden, & Resko, 1998). In late-fetal and neonatal rats and mice, ARs are found in homogenized hypothalamic and preoptic tissue from both sexes, and levels increase rapidly through the preweanling period (Lieberburg, MacLusky, & McEwen, 1980; Meaney, Aitken, Jensen, McGinnis, & McEwen, 1985; Vito et al., 1979). In the first study to examine AR in specific brain sites, McAbee and DonCarlos (1998, 1999a, 1999b) found that AR mRNA could be found in a large number of areas in the neonatal brain. The strongest presence was in the POA and ventral premammillary nucleus, but AR mRNA could also be found in many areas of the hypothalamus (VMH, arcuate, PVN, supraoptic nucleus [SON]), limbic system (BST, LS, hippocampus, medial and central amygdala), and cortex. Other studies have since demonstrated AR mRNA or protein presence in the developing olfactory bulb (Wong et al., 2000), substantia nigra (Ravizza et al., 2002), and visual and cingulate cortices (Nunez, Huppenbauer, McAbee, Juraska, & DonCarlos, 2003). No sex differences in AR mRNA or protein are found in neonates, but by 10 days after birth, the male pBST, medial amygdala, and POA have higher levels of AR than do females. It is important to note that AR and other steroid hormone receptors in the developing central nervous system are not only present in neurons, but also in glia (e.g., Lorenz, Garcia-Segura, & DonCarlos, 2005; Platania et al., 2003), which themselves can be sexually dimorphic (Mong, Kurzweil, Davis, Rocca, & McCarthy, 1996), and whose morphology and potential function are sensitive to gonadal hormones (Amateau & McCarthy, 2002).

Actions of Steroid Receptors and Hormone Coactivators

Steroid hormones and their receptors in the brain are clearly present during development, and the intracellular mechanisms occurring after they join together have been well studied. Activation of a steroid receptor results in release of heat shock proteins and conformational change of the receptor. This conformational change is believed to enhance the ability of the steroid–receptor complex to bind to a hormone response element (HRE) on DNA (Jensen et al., 1968; Walters, 1985). Once bound to DNA, the receptor complex interacts with various combinations of coregulatory proteins to influence genomic transcription (Carson-Jurica, Schrader, & O'Malley, 1990; McKenna, Lanz, & O'Malley, 1999; Walters, 1985). These could include changes in second-messenger systems (Etgen & Petitti, 1986), inducible transcription factors (Auger & Blaustein, 1995; Herbison, King, Tan, & Dye, 1995; Insel, 1990), peptide receptors (De Kloet, Voorhuis,

Boschma, & Elands, 1986; De Kloet, Voorhuis, & Elands, 1985), factors involved in growth and synaptogenesis (Lustig, Hua, Wilson, & Federoff, 1993; Shughrue & Dorsa, 1994; Yanase, Honmura, Akaishi, & Sakuma, 1988; although see Sugiyama, Kanba, & Arita, 2003), and neurotransmitter synthesis and release (Etgen et al., 1992; McCarthy, Pfaff, & Schwartz-Giblin, 1993a). Many steroid hormone-induced effects contributing to sexual differentiation occur via such actions at the genome (Tobet, 2002). For example, sexual differentiation involves sex-specific rates of neurogenesis during perinatal life (e.g., Al-Shamma & De Vries, 1996; Jacobson & Gorski, 1981). On the other hand, steroid-hormone-dependent cell death (apoptosis) also contributes to sex differences in brain structure (Chung, Swaab, & De Vries, 2000; Davis, Popper, & Gorski, 1996). Other sex differences, including differences in neurochemical phenotype or neuroanatomical projections, are also examples of genomically mediated consequences of steroid hormones (see De Vries & Simerly, 2002).

While the binding of hormones to steroid receptors is an important step for regulating gene transcription and ultimately brain development, steroid receptors are also under the control of coregulatory proteins. These proteins, referred to as coactivators or corepressors, can either enhance or repress steroid receptor induced gene transcription, respectively. One of the first coactivators identified was steroid receptor coactivator-1 (SRC-1), which interacts with receptors for progesterone, estrogens, androgens, glucocorticoids, and thyroid hormone (Onate, Tsai, Tsai, & O'Malley, 1995). Since SRC-1 was first characterized, other coactivators have been identified, including TIF2 (SRC-2) and GRIP1, ARA70, Trip1, and RIP140. These coactivators, sometimes referred to as nuclear receptor coactivators, influence steroid-induced gene transcription via their intrinsic histone acetyltransferase activity (Shibata et al., 1997). That is, they are thought to act by acetylating histones, which allows DNA to be more accessible to transcription factors. Nuclear receptor coactivators also increase the transcriptional activity of steroid receptors by interacting with other histone acetyltransferase factors, such as p/CAF (p300/CBP associated factor) and general transcription factors, such as TBP and TIFIIB (McKenna et al., 1999).

Relevant to the present discussion, recent data indicate that some of these coactivators are involved sexual differentiation. Transiently reducing the expression of either SRC-1 or CREB-binding protein (CBP), which was originally identified as a coactivator of the cAMP response element binding protein (CREB; Chrivia et al., 1993; Kwok et al., 1994), during the first few days of life interferes with steroid-induced defeminization of sexual behavior (Auger et al., 2002; Auger, Tetel, & McCarthy, 2000). Interestingly, reducing either SRC-1 or CBP alone does not interfere with masculinization (Auger et al., 2000, 2002). Expression of coactivators is an additional way to modulate steroid receptor–induced differentiation of the brain, and their function further provides support for the idea that different pathways mediate masculinization and defeminization of the brain and behavior.

Ligand-Independent Activation of Steroid Receptors

The traditional view of sexual differentiation posits that steroid hormone receptors produce their effects only after being bound by steroid hormones. Steroid hormone receptors, however, may also be activated by pathways that do not require the presence of steroid hormones. Indeed, both ERs (Aronica & Katzenellenbogen, 1993) and PRs (Power, Mani, Codina, Conneely, & O'Malley, 1991) can be activated in vitro in the absence of their respective ligand (Denner, Weigel, Maxwell, Schrader, & O'Malley, 1990; Kazmi, Visconti, Plante, Ishaque, & Lau, 1993), and both can be activated by the neurotransmitter dopamine (Figure 21.2; Gangolli, Conneely, & O'Malley, 1997; Power et al., 1991). A functional role for ligand-independent activation of steroid receptor in the brain was first reported by Mani and colleagues (1994). They found that the dopamine (D_1)-receptor agonist SKF 38393 facilitates adult female sexual behavior in estradiol-primed rats by acting upon PRs in a ligand-independent manner. Since then, numerous factors have been found to activate PRs in a similar manner, including gonadotropin releasing hormone, prostaglandin E2, dibutyryl cAMP, nitric oxide, 8-bromo-cGMP and even cocaine (Beyer, Gonzalez-Flores, & Gonzalez-Mariscal, 1997; Chu, Morales, Etgen, 1999; Mani et al., 1994). As neurotransmitters are sensitive to social and environmental changes, it is likely that these pathways relay information from the changing environment and alter brain function by activating steroid receptors. For example, ligand-independent activation of PRs in females occurs following a mating interaction with a male (Auger et al., 1997) and may have a role in sexual differentiation of play behavior (see section on "Play" above).

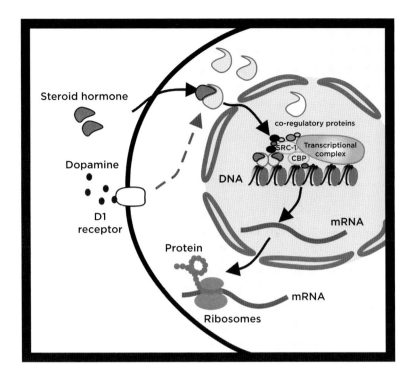

Figure 21.2 Conceptual model for ligand versus ligand-independent activation of steroid receptors. Steroid hormones diffuse into the cell and bind to their appropriate steroid receptor. Ligand-bound receptors then form dimer complexes on DNA and interact with a variety of coregulatory proteins, such as SRC-1 and CBP, which recruit additional proteins to the transcriptional complex to regulate gene transcription. While the mechanisms for ligand-independent activation of steroid receptors are currently unknown, dopamine can alter steroid receptor activity by acting upon membrane dopamine D1 receptors to elicit a cellular response that leads to increased transcriptional activity of steroid receptors.

Sexual Differentiation of Brains Areas Mediating Social Behaviors

It is often supposed that sex differences in behavior result from underlying sex differences in neural structure or function. This is likely to be true in some cases, and here we discuss perinatal steroid hormone effects on sexual differentiation of three neural structures often associated with the performance of sexually dimorphic social behaviors, including play, maternal, and/or sexual behaviors. To simplify these examples, we focus on sex differences in synaptic patterns and size of these structures, although sex differences in neurochemistry and other factors are also found in each region. The three brain areas used as examples are larger in males than females, but sex differences in volume also exist in the opposite direction (Davis et al., 1996; Garcia-Falqueras et al., 2005; Guillamon, de Blas, & Segovia, 1988; Simerly, Swanson, & Gorski, 1985; Sumida, Nishizuka, Kano, & Arai, 1993). Similar to some of the social behaviors discussed above, sexual differentiation of these neural

sites does not necessarily follow a particularly traditional path.

Preoptic Area

The POA was the first neural site reported to differ between males and females, and remains the most extensively studied model for how sexual differentiation occurs in the mammalian brain. In 1971, Raisman and Field reported that synapses of nonamygdaloid origin in the medial POA (mPOA) were sexually dimorphic, with synapses in males occurring almost exclusively upon dendritic shafts, and synapses in females more likely to be on dendritic spines. Neonatal castration could feminize this pattern in males, and conversely, early administration of TP masculinized it in females (Raisman & Field, 1973). Sex differences in electrophysiological function were also found, which could be reversed by manipulating perinatal hormones (Dyer, MacLeod, & Ellendorff, 1976). Although the greater functional significance was unknown, Raisman and Field (1971) proposed that sex differences in synaptic contacts within the mPOA were likely related to sex differences in gonadotropin release or sexual behavior. This was an insightful and reasonable proposition, but it is still unclear more than 35 years later if sex differences in the mPOA are necessary for sex differences in any reproductive behaviors.

The study of sex differences in ultrastructural and electrophysiological properties of the POA was quickly supplanted after a much more obvious sex difference was revealed. Gorski and colleagues (1978, 1980) found a gross morphological sex difference in the cell-dense medial preoptic nucleus (MPN), with male rats having five times as many cells, and larger cells, than females. They termed this the sexually dimorphic nucleus of the POA (SDN-POA), and an SDN-POA has since been found to exist in many laboratory mammals (e.g., Bleier, Byne, & Siggelkow, 1982; Commins & Yahr, 1985; Hines, Davis, Coquelin, Goy, & Gorski, 1985; Tobet, Zahniser, & Baum, 1986), nonmammalian species (Crews, Wade, & Wilczynski, 1990; Viglietti-Panzica et al., 1986), and in nonhuman and human primates (Byne, 1998; Swaab & Fliers, 1985). In rats, the sex difference in SDN-POA volume appears by postnatal day 5 (Hsu, Chen, & Peng, 1980) and is often thought to follow the traditional perinatal organization of the brain by gonadal hormones because early postnatal treatment with TP enlarges SDN-POA volume in females, while castrating males on the day of birth reduces its size (Gorski, Gordon, Shryne, & Southam, 1978). The critical sensitive period for hormone effects on the SDN-POA actually begins prenatally (around gestation day 18; Rhees, Shryne, & Gorski, 1990a) and the sex difference can be completely reversed if testosterone treatment of females extends from the prenatal period to the first few days after birth (Dohler et al., 1982; Rhees, Shryne, & Gorski, 1990b). Aromatization of testosterone to estradiol is necessary for the larger SDN-POA of males, with neonatal treatment with an aromatase inhibitor producing a female-like structure (Dohler et al., 1984a, 1984b), and estrogens as effective as TP in masculinizing SDN-POA volume in females (Dohler et al., 1984a, 1984b; Houtsmuller et al., 1994). There is apparently less of a role for perinatal AR activity for the sex difference in SDN-POA volume (Döhler et al., 1986; Morris et al., 2005; Rossi, Bestetti, Reymond, & Lemarchand-Beraud, 1991; although see Lund, Salyer, Fleming, & Lephart, 2000), but there may be some role for perinatal AR activity in the sex difference in SDN-POA soma size, because

it is smaller in male rats with a mutation of the AR gene (Morris et al., 2005).

One mechanism by which gonadal steroids sexually differentiate SDN-POA volume is differential birth of neurons during development, with neurogenesis greater on some gestational days in fetal male rats compared to females (Jacobson & Gorski, 1981; although see Bayer & Altman, 1987). Conversely, apoptosis is greater during the first postnatal week in females than in males (Chung et al., 2000; Davis et al., 1996; Yoshida, Yuri, Kizaki, Sawada, & Kawata, 2000). Testosterone is responsible for these effects, as neonatal castration increases apoptosis in males, while TP treatment prevents this increase in castrated males (Davis et al, 1996). Not surprisingly, aromatization of testosterone to estradiol is also necessary, as either testosterone or estradiol prevent perinatal apoptosis in the female rat SDN-POA (Arai, Sekine, & Murakami, 1996; Yang et al., 2004).

Although early work suggested a traditional perinatal sensitive period for steroid hormone-induced organization of the SDN-POA, the size of this structure can actually be modified by exposure to hormones later in life. Castrating males 29 days after birth still significantly reduces SDN-POA volume when measured around day 120 of age, although it is not as effective as a neonatal castration (23% vs. 48% decrease; Davis, Shryne, & Gorski, 1995). In contrast, castrating 82-day-old males does not significantly reduce SDN-POA volume when evaluated on day 120, but it is unknown if this lack of effect is due to the age at gonadectomy, or how long the animals were without gonads (Davis et al., 1995; also see Bloch & Gorski, 1988a, 1988b). Time since castration may be an important factor, as castrating males at 60 days of age decreases the size of SDN-POA somata when examined 4 weeks, but not 2 weeks, after surgery (Dugger, Morris, Jordan, & Breedlove, 2008; but see Bloch & Gorski, 1988b for lack of long-term castration effects). Another example of postperinatal effects of hormones on the SDN-POA is that ovarian hormones reduce SDN-POA volume by one-third in adult males (Bloch & Gorski, 1988a), but only if they are also castrated, suggesting that testicular hormones protect the male SDN-POA from feminizing effects of ovarian hormones through adulthood. There are clearly either multiple sensitive periods for development of this structure, or simply long-term persistence of steroid-mediated plasticity. Thus, the rat SDN-POA is not an exemplar for permanent, perinatally restricted organization of the nervous system. Rather, it demonstrates that steroid hormones can induce neural plasticity throughout the life span (Arnold & Breedlove, 1985).

Medial Amygdala

The medial amygdala is a critical part of the neural network processesing main and accessory olfactory cues (Price, 2003), and sex differences in the medial amygdala are likely related to sex differences in olfactory perception necessary for social behaviors in mammals, including parenting and sexual behaviors. Similar to the POA, the medial subnucleus of the amygdala (MeA) has sexually dimorphic synaptic patterns, with males having more synapses and dendritic spines than females (Nishizuka & Arai, 1982; Rasia-Fihlo, Fabian, Rigoti, & Achaval, 2004), and more excitatory synapses than females (Cooke & Wooley, 2005). In a traditional manner, neonatal testosterone masculinizes some synaptic patterns in females while neonatal castration feminizes them in males (Nishizuka & Arai, 1981). Volume differences are also found, with the posterodorsal medial amygdala (MeApd) up to twice as large in males as females (Cooke, Breedlove, & Jordan, 2003; Cooke, Tabibnia, Breedlove, 1999; Hines, Allen, & Gorski, 1992; Morris et al., 2005). Unlike the SDN-POA, which is sexually dimorphic by the time of birth, the sex difference in MeApd volume in rats emerges rather late, between postnatal days 11 and 21 (Mizukami, Nishizuka, & Arai, 1983). Other subnuclei of the amygdala are also sexually dimorphic, and males have a larger posteromedial cortical amygdala (PMCo) than females (Vinader-Caerols, Collado, Segovia, & Guillamon, 1998). The PMCo is particularly associated with the vomeronasal system, and as such, may also contribute to sex differences in pheromone-dependent behaviors. Volume of the PMCo can be feminized by neonatal castration, and "rescued" in neonatally males by neonatal injection of estradiol (Vinader-Caerols, Collado, Segovia, & Guillamon, 2000). Synaptic architecture in the PMco also differs between the sexes, which can be partially sex-reversed by giving testosterone to neonatal females (Akhmadeev & Kalimullina, 2005). The central nucleus of the amygdala is also larger in males, but appears to be organized by androgen exposure (Staudt & Dorner, 1976).

The existence of a developmental "window" when hormones can permanently influence sex differences in the medial amygdala is questionable. Mizukami and colleagues (1983) demonstrated that the volume of the medial amygdala could be greatly masculinized in females by prolonged postnatal estrogen treatment (postnatal days 1–30), suggesting organizational effects. In males, the reduction in size resulting from neonatal castration can be reversed with a single injection of testosterone on postnatal day 3, indicating that the window begins soon after birth at the latest (Staudt & Dorner, 1976). Nonetheless, hormones released during adulthood also affect the MeA, and equating circulating gonadal hormones in adult rats by gonadectomy, or gonadectomy followed by testosterone treatment of both sexes, virtually equates their MeApd volume and soma size (Cooke et al., 2003, 1999). Such MeApd plasticity also occurs naturally in response to fluctuations in circulating gonadal hormones across the estrous cycle (Rasia-Fihlo et al., 2004) and across seasons (Cooke, Hegstrom, Keen, & Breedlove, 2001). Unlike some sex differences in the brain, estrogenic and androgenic activity are both necessary to maintain a fully masculinized MeApd in rats (Cooke et al., 2003; Morris et al., 2005). Therefore, some sex differences in the MeApd appear to be due to activational—rather than organizational—effects of gonadal hormones.

Ventromedial Hypothalamus

Similar to the POA and MeA, the volume of the ventromedial nucleus of the hypothalamus (VMH) is larger in male than female laboratory rats (Chung et al., 2000; Madeira, Ferreira-Silva, & Paula-Barbosa, 2001; Matsumoto & Arai, 1983; although see Dorner & Staudt, 1969; Rossi et al., 1991), and differs between the sexes in its synaptic patterning and dendritic arborization (Madeira et al., 2001; Matsumoto & Arai, 1986b; Pozzo-Miller & Aoki, 1991; Segarra & McEwen, 1991). Castration during the first week after birth or anti-estrogenic treatment feminizes VMH synapses in males and TP treatment on postnatal day 5 masculinizes them in females (Matsumoto & Arai, 1983, 1986a, 1986b; Pozzo-Miller & Aoki, 1991). Unlike what is thought to be true for the SDN-POA, sex differences in VMH volume are apparently not due to differences in apoptosis, as apoptosis is not sexually dimorphic in the developing VMH (Chung et al., 2000). Neonatal castration reduces VMH volume in males, but testosterone injections beginning on postnatal day 5 cannot increase its size in females (Matsumoto & Arai, 1983). Thus, either the female VMH is insensitive to perinatal hormones, or the critical period for hormone effects on some sexually dimorphic qualities of the VMH differs between the sexes. Furthermore, similar to the POA and MeApd, VMH volume is *not* fully organized during perinatal life. Variations in circulating gonadal hormones during adulthood affect VMH volume, at least in female rats, with an increase during proestrus or during estrogen treatment (Carrer & Aoki, 1982; Madeira et al., 2001; although see Delville & Blaustein, 1989).

Relationship between Sex Differences in the Brain and Sex Differences in Behavior

Sex differences in the mammalian brain often exist in sites necessary for sexually dimorphic behaviors, often leading one to ascribe a relationship between neural structure and function. Nonetheless, as has been discussed previously (De Vries & Simerly, 2002), there are many examples where this hypothesis simply cannot be supported.

Consider parental behavior as an example. Neural activity in the medial POA is necessary for parental responding, whereas the VMH provides inhibitory control over this behavior (Numan & Insel, 2003). Both of these structures are larger in male rats, so any proposition of a positive correlation between size and function at a whole-brain level is immediately undermined. Even if one considers the converse relationship between size and function in some cases, such that a larger SDN-POA inhibits parental responding in male rats, then one might expect that SDN-POA destruction would facilitate the behavior in males. It does not, and similar to females, POA lesions impair parental behaviors in male rats (Rosenblatt, Hazelwood, & Poole, 1996). Further, the SDN-POA per se may not have a unique role in the performance of maternal behaviors at all, as maternal behavior is disrupted as much after small lesions specifically of the SDN-POA as it is after small lesions of the tissue surrounding it (Jacobson, Terkel, Gorski, & Sawyer, 1980). Another problem arises with the findings noted in sections " Distribution and Function of Neural Steroid Hormone Receptors" and "Sexual Differentiation of Brains Areas Mediating Social Behaviors" that postnatal injections of high doses of TP do not affect maternal responding in females, but such treatment readily masculinizes females' SDN-POA. Similar discordance is found in that castration up to 60 days of age increases positive responding to pups, but castration at these older ages does not reduce the size of their SDN-POA.

Any universal assumptions about size–function relationships are also undermined by the fact that some biparental rodents (e.g., Mongolian gerbils)

have sex differences in their POA as large as those found in uniparental rodents (Commins & Yahr, 1985), while the biparental prairie vole has no sex difference in POA volume (Shapiro, Leonard, Sessions, Dewsbury, & Insel, 1991). If the size of a neural structure was intimately related to its behavioral function, one might also expect it to change during periods of exceptional behavioral plasticity. Female rats are immediately maternal after experiencing pregnancy and parturition, while virgin females and males can require up to 1 week or more of exposure to pups before acting maternally. There is no evidence that the size of the SDN-POA changes in pregnant or parturient animals, which one might expect if its size was related to reproductive state or sex differences in its potential function. There is also no evidence that the rat SDN-POA changes over the course of maternal sensitization in either sex. Instead, changes in synaptogenesis, glial function, and neurochemistry—rather than gross morphological features—are probably responsible for behavioral differences between maternal and nonmaternal females (Numan & Insel, 2003). Remarkably, such gross morphological changes in POA volume may actually occur in California mice (*Peromyscus californicus*) when they become parents (Gubernick, Sengelaub, & Kurz, 1993). This is intriguing, but it is unknown if there is even a sex difference in parental responding before California mice mate and have pups. Virgin males are not parental (Gubernick & Nelson, 1989), but the behavior of virgin females to pups has apparently not been investigated.

Similar inconsistencies are found for the relationship between SDN-POA size and masculine copulatory behaviors in rats (Ito, Murakami, Yamanouchi, & Arai, 1986; Todd et al., 2005), and for VMH volume and feminine copulatory behaviors (Delville & Blaustein, 1989). One study in female rats reports no effects of prenatal TP on sexual behavior but a significant increase in SDN-POA volume (Ito et al., 1986). In another salient example, subjecting pregnant females to prolonged, daily stress greatly demasculinizes male offspring in numerous ways, including reducing SDN-POA volume (Anderson, Rhees, & Fleming, 1985; Herrenkohl, 1986; Ward, 1972). This gestational stress, however, does not always affect their latencies to mount stimulus females (Humm, Lambert, & Kinsley, 1995), and stressed males are still capable of copulating to ejaculation (Kerchner & Ward, 1992). Furthermore, prenatal exposure to alcohol reduces the size of the SDN-POA (Barron,

Tieman, & Riley, 1988) due to reduced perinatal testosterone secretion (McGivern, Handa, & Raum, 1998; McGivern, Handa, & Redei, 1993), but these males can sometimes still copulate normally (Barron et al., 1988; Ward, Bennett, Ward, Hendricks, & French, 1999). Because prenatal stress and alcohol also feminizes the behavior male rats (Ward, Ward, Winn, & Bielawski, 1994), it may be the case that instead of the size of SDN-POA being positively correlated to behavioral masculinization, it is positively correlated with the degree of behavioral defeminization (Todd et al., 2005). It also could be possible that the this sub-structure is really not related to copulatory behaviors at all; in support, lesions specifically of the SDN-POA do not eliminate copulation in sexually experienced rats (Arendash & Gorski, 1983). As pointed out by Ulibarri and Yahr (1996), sexual differentiation in most rodents occurs within a relatively narrow window, and correlations between structure and function probably often reflect a common response to the developmental hormone milieu, rather than suggesting a causal relationship.

A relatively new concept for understanding structure–function relationships proposed by DeVries and colleagues is to not assume that sex differences in the brain generate sex differences in behavior at all, but rather, that differences between male and female brains *prevent* overt behavioral and physiological differences between the sexes. That is, sex differences in the brain might exist to compensate for sex differences in circulating hormones, thereby avoiding sex differences in emotional, cognitive, or behavioral tasks (De Vries, 2004; De Vries & Boyle, 1998). Differences in neural structure, projections, or neurochemistry may allow the sexes to show similar behaviors without the need for similar hormonal profiles. This hypothesis is very intriguing, but choosing the appropriate neural sites and sexually monomorphic behaviors to test it could prove difficult.

What Do Rats and Mice Tell Us about Sexual Differentiation of Other Species?

The conflict between breadth and depth is a never-ending theme in neurobehavioral research. Does understanding the cellular and molecular basis of sexual differentiation primarily in rats and mice inform us about these developmental processes in other species? The answer is assuredly "yes," but it is also well accepted that sexual differentiation of the brain and behavior in many nonrodent species occurs via mechanisms quite different than those

for rats (Moore, Boyd, & Kelley, 2005; Wade & Arnold, 2004; Wallen & Baum, 2002). In fact, one does not have to look outside the order *Rodentia* to find such exceptions, as prairie voles (*Microtus ochrogaster*) and gerbils (*Meriones unguiculatus*) provide excellent examples.

Prairie voles have been valuable to examine the hormonal and neural control of social behaviors, because unlike most laboratory rodents, prairie voles display monogamous traits that include pair-bonding after copulation and biparental rearing of pups (Carter, DeVries, & Getz, 1995). Voles have not been a very widely studied model for sexual differentiation of brain and social behavior, probably because the earliest study of sexual differentiation in any *Microtus* species did not find anything unusual. Female prairie voles are induced ovulators, and require olfactory cues from the urine of unfamiliar males to initiate behavioral estrus (Hasler & Conaway, 1973). Smale, Nelson, and Zucker (1985) found that a single injection of TP within the first few days of life rendered female prairie voles unresponsive to the hormonal- and behavioral-estrus-inducing effects of either male urine or exogenous estradiol. Similarly, later work demonstrated that a single neonatal injection of TP defeminizes and masculinizes sexual behavior in the induced-ovulating and monogamous female pine vole (*Microtus pinetorum*) (Wekesa & Vandenbergh, 1996).

Nonetheless, recent work from our laboratory and the laboratories of others with prairie voles has revealed that they can be both typical and atypical models for sexual differentiation. Our typical model involves hypothalamic expression of tyrosine hydroxylase (TH), which we find is differentiated through a traditional route. Expression of tyrosine hydroxylase (TH) is sexually dimorphic in the AVPv of rats and mice, with females having three to four times more TH-expressing cells than males (Forger et al., 2004; Simerly, 1989; Simerly, Swanson, & Gorski, 1985). The same is also true for prairie voles, but subjects must first be gonadectomized, which results in a 50% decrease in TH-expressing cells in males (Lansing & Lonstein, 2006). Similar to rats, this sex difference in TH expression in the prairie vole AVPv is modified by perinatal gonadal hormones. Ovariectomized female prairie voles that had been treated neonatally with TP, EB, or DES are masculinized, such that they have fewer TH-expression cells than females that receive oil vehicle neonatally (Lansing & Lonstein, 2006). Conversely, neonatal males treated with the aromatase inhibitor ATD do not show the typically large loss of TH-expressing cells after castration (Northcutt & Lonstein, 2008). Remember that these effects are consistent with what is generally found for other laboratory rodents exposed to perinatal gonadal hormones or shielded from such exposure.

Another neural sex difference we have examined develops in a completely atypical manner. Similar to most other vertebrates (De Vries & Simerly, 2002), the number of cells and the density of projections in the extrahypothalamic arginine-vasopressin (AVP) system of prairie voles is greater in males than females (Bamshad, Novak, & De Vries, 1993; Wang, Smith, Major, & De Vries, 1994). Also similar to other rodents, we find that neonatal castration reduces male prairie voles' later AVP mRNA expression in the BST (where the cells of origin of this projection are found) and AVP-immunoreactive fiber content in the lateral septum (a major target of this projection) (Lonstein, Rood, & De Vries, 2005). The testicular hormones that masculinize this system in males require ER activity, as neonatal blockade of ERs with tamoxifen demasculinizes this AVP system (Lonstein et al., 2005). However, similarities between prairie voles and rats end there. Unlike female rats, perinatal TP simply cannot masculinize AVP expression in female prairie voles (Figure 21.3; Lonstein et al., 2005). Even more surprising, neonatal TP injections cannot even prevent demasculinization of the AVP system in neonatally castrated males (Lonstein et al., 2005). In sum, although testicular secretions are necessary for masculinization of parental behavior and extrahypothalamic AVP in male prairie voles, perinatal exposure to TP cannot substitute for the presence of testes to masculinize this system in either sex. We have found a similar situation for sex differences in parental responding in virgin prairie voles—males are feminized by neonatal castration, but females are not masculinized by perinatal TP (Lonstein, Rood, & De Vries, 2002). It may be that multiple hormones released from the testes during perinatal life act together to normally masculinize males' extrahypothalamic AVP and parental behavior. Our work does not support a multiple-hormone hypothesis, because postnatal injections of just the synthetic estrogen, DES, does masculinize AVP fiber content in the lateral septum of female prairie voles (Lonstein et al., 2005). It is clear that masculinization of the extrahypothalamic AVP system requires the presence of testes and ER activation. Strange as it may sound, this ER activation may not come from

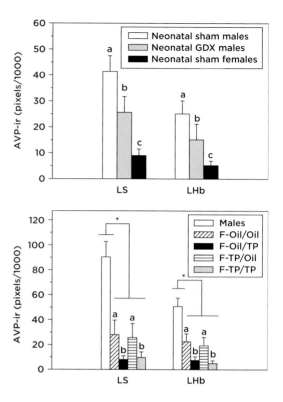

Figure 21.3 Arginine-vasopressin (AVP) immunoreactivity in the lateral septum (LS) and lateral habenula (LHb) of adult male or female prairie voles following (A) neonatal castration (GDX) or (B) prenatal and/or postnatal treatment with testosterone. Different letters above bars indicates significant differences between groups, * = sex difference within each site, $p < .05$. Experiments in the panels were performed at different times and involved different immunocytochemical runs, likely explaining differences in Y-axis range.

testicular testosterone's aromatization into estradiol. Instead, we conjecture that estradiol might be secreted directly from the testes in sufficient amounts to masculinize this neuropeptide system in male prairie voles.

The prairie vole brain has revealed yet a third mechanism for generating sex differences. We recently discovered that the principle bed nucleus of the stria terminalis (pBST) and posterodorsal medial amygdala (MeApd) contain a large number of TH-immunoreactive cells in male prairie voles, but not female prairie voles (Northcutt, Wang, & Lonstein, 2007). Unlike most sex differences in the rat brain, but similar to their MeApd volume (see section on "Medial Amygdala"), circulating gonadal hormones in adult prairie voles are largely responsible for this sex difference. Castrating adult males reduces the number of TH-immunoreactive cells in these sites almost to the level of females. Conversely, treating female prairie voles with testosterone increases the number of these cells to levels comparable to males (Figure 21.4; Northcutt et al., 2007). The sex difference is not completely reversed when gonadal hormone status is equated among the sexes, however, so there probably is still some role for developmental exposure to hormones on TH expression in these sites.

Mongolian gerbils provide another interesting exception to what rats and mice have told us about sexual differentiation because some aspects of gerbil sexual differentiation occur over an unusually prolonged period. Motor neurons in the spinal nucleus of the bulbocavernosus (SNB) innervate perineal muscles surrounding the phallus and are sexually dimorphic, and in rats this process is complete by postnatal day 10 (Nordeen, Nordeen, Sengelaub, & Arnold, 1985). In gerbils, these cells increase in number in males not only throughout postnatal development, but also through puberty (Fraley & Ulibarri, 2001). The gerbil analogue of the SDN-POA, the sexually dimorphic area pars compacta (SDApc), also has somewhat protracted development. Gerbils of both sexes have a similarly sized SDApc at birth, but over the next 2 weeks, this structure vanishes in females and enlarges in males (Ulibarri & Yahr, 1993). Similar to the SNB system, development of the male SDApc

continues through puberty (Holman, Collado, Rice, & Hutchison, 1995; Ulibarri & Yahr, 1993). Furthermore, unlike the SDN-POA of rats, which can be greatly modified in both sexes by neonatal gonadal hormones, the same is not true for the gerbil SDApc. Most females are masculinized by neonatal androgens or estrogens (Holman & Hutchison, 1991; Turner, 1975, Ulibarri & Yahr, 1988, 1996; Yahr, 1988), but it is unclear if neonatal castration has much effect on SDApc development (Holman & Hutchison, 1991; Ulibarri & Yahr, 1988, 1996). Although the SNB and SDApc of Mongolian gerbils may be "unusual," this is not universal in this particular species, because sexual differentiation of many other traits in gerbils occurs very traditionally (Clark, Santamaria, Robertson, & Galef, 1998; Forger, Galef, Clark, 1996; Holman, 1981; Holman et al., 1995, Holman, Collado, Skepper, & Rice, 1996; Sherry, Galef, & Clark, 1996; Turner, 1975; Ulibarri & Yahr, 1988, 1996).

In sum, understanding sexual differentiation in rats and mice does allow us to better understand and predict the course of sexual differentiation in other rodents. It is also true that unusual sexual differentiation can occur in species that also show completely usual sexual differentiation of other systems. Coming to terms with these "exceptions to the rules" would prevent us from being surprised or even skeptical about future examples of atypical sexual differentiation, and allow us to fully realize the rich diversity of mechanisms generating differences between the sexes even in common laboratory rodents.

Other Considerations about Sexual Differentiation
Direct Role of Sex Chromosome Genes on Sexual Differentiation

Differential exposure of the sexes to gonadal hormones is responsible for much of sexual differentiation, but because of some notable exceptions, it has been proposed that there must be other contributing factors. A recent review by Arnold (2004) describes how some sex differences in mammals arise prior to development of the gonads, so cannot be explained by sex differences in developmental exposure to gonadal hormones. For example, developing males are larger than females even before the gonads differentiate (Pedersen, 1980; Scott & Holson, 1977). Such examples are found both peripherally and centrally. Sexual differentiation of the external genitalia of the native Australian tammar wallaby begins prenatally, whereas differentiation of the gonads occurs *after* birth (Glickman,

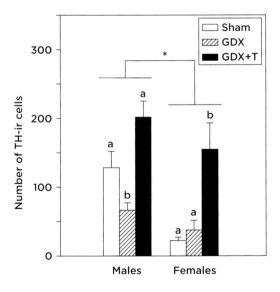

Figure 21.4 Tyrosine hydroxylase (TH) immunoreactivity in the pBST of adult male and female prairie voles that were gonadally intact (sham) or gonadectomized (GDX) and treated chronically with nothing or testosterone (T). * = Significant sex difference. Different letters above bars indicates significant differences between groups within each site, *p* < .05.

Short, & Renfree, 2005; Pask & Renfree, 2001). Centrally, there are sex differences in the number and size of catecholaminergic cells in the midbrain even when the cells are harvested before gonadal differentiation and thereafter maintained in vitro (Beyer, Pilgrim, & Reisert, 1991; Engele, Pilgrim, & Reisert, 1989). In a more general example, neural and behavioral sex differences often cannot be completely sex-reversed with perinatal hormone manipulations; this may be due to inappropriate doses or patterns of administration, but also suggests that additional, nonhormonal factors are probably involved.

There is experimental support for a direct contribution of sex chromosome genes to mammalian sexual differentiation, as opposed to the more indirect pathway by which the Y chromosome initiates testes development and subsequent hormone release. Using an ingenious paradigm where the testis-determining gene, *Sry*, is deleted from the Y-chromosome in male mice and inserted as a transgene into an autosome in both XX and XY genotypes, "males" and "females" with either XX or XY phenotype can be produced. In the former, mice with an XX or XY genotype have an *Sry* gene and develop testes, where in the latter case, mice with XX or XY genotypes do not have the *Sry* gene and develop ovaries. It was found that genetic sex does influence sexual differentiation, even when testes are present in both genetic males and genetic females. Indeed, genetic males with an *Sry* transgene have slightly, but significantly, more AVP immunoreactivity (5%–8%) in the lateral septum than genetic females with an *Sry* transgene (De Vries et al., 2002; also Gatewood et al., 2006). Behavior can also be affected by sex chromosome profile, as XY mice without an *Sry* gene (genetically male, but phenotypically female) are still more aggressive than XX mice (genetically female, but phenotypically female) (Gatewood et al., 2006). Parental behaviors are also influenced, and virgin XY mice that do not have an *Sry* gene (genetically male, but phenotypically female) are less parental on some measures than normal XX females (Gatewood et al., 2006). Other sex differences are unrelated to the presence or absence of the *Sry* gene (DeVries et al., 2002; Markham et al., 2003; Wagner et al., 2004), and are presumably due to differences in exposure to gonadal hormones. Transient manipulation of *Sry* directly in the brain are also effective, and reduction of *Sry* using antisense oligodeoxynucleotides disrupts masculization of nigral tyrosine hydroxylase expression (Dewing et al., 2006).

Puberty as a Critical Period for Sexual Differentiation

A plethora of research supports the view that early life is an important critical period for the permanently organizing effects of steroid hormones on sexual differentiation. Similar to the perinatal period, puberty is also a time of increased gonadal steroidogenesis and widespread neural maturation. Some have proposed that it is a second critical period when exposure to gonadal hormones permanently organizes the neural substrates underlying sexually differentiated behaviors (Scott, Stewart, & De Ghett, 1974; Schulz & Sisk, 2006; Sisk, Schulz, & Zehr, 2003). Work in hamsters reveals that copulatory behaviors and flank-marking (used to communicate identity and status) cannot be elicited by testosterone in prepubertal males, as is the case in postpubertal males (Sisk et al., 2003). If the brain was completely organized during perinatal life, one would expect testosterone to elicit these behaviors similarly at both ages. Therefore, events occurring after the perinatal period allow testosterone to activate the neural circuit necessary for copulation and flank marking. The presence and increased function of the gonads during puberty have been shown to be responsible for the different effects of testosterone on juvenile and adult behavior in hamsters, as castration just before puberty reduces testosterone's later ability to activate sexual and flank-marking behaviors (Sisk et al., 2003). Such effects can also be observed in rats, with prepubertal castration feminizing males' exploratory behavior in an open field (Brand & Slob, 1988) and their social interactions with other rats (Primus & Kellogg, 1990). Many areas of the brain probably undergo a second "organization" by gonadal hormones during puberty, including regions with well-established functions for social behavior—such as the amygdala, septum, POA, and BST (Romeo, Diedrich, & Sisk, 2000; Schulz, Menard, Smith, Albers, & Sisk, 2006; Zehr, Todd, Schulz, McCarthy, Sisk, 2006)—but also in other regions of the brain (Davis et al., 1995; Nunez, Sodhi, & Juraska, 2002; Pinos et al., 2001).

Maternal Contributions to Sexual Differentiation

For most sex-typical neural or behavioral characteristics there is often considerable variability within a sex. For examples, some females are more or less feminized than others, while some males are more or less masculinized than others. Some of this variability is due to variability in internal biological factors, such as higher or lower circulating testosterone during otherwise normal development (e.g., Hines et al., 2002; Udry, Morris, & Kovenock, 1995). However, some of this variability is instead due to postnatal environmental factors, including the type of maternal behavior that offspring receive from their mothers. As Champagne and Curley discuss in detail in this book, the amount of licking that mothers provide to their offspring greatly influences neurobehavioral development. This includes sexual differentiation of copulatory behaviors and the central nervous system structures that supports it.

Early research by Moore and colleagues revealed that mother rats interact differently with male and female neonates, licking the anogenital region of male offspring more often and for longer bouts than female offspring (Moore, 1982; Moore & Chadwick-Dias, 1986; Moore & Morelli, 1979). This differential licking is mediated by the preference of maternal, and even nonmaternal, female rats for testosterone-dependent olfactory cues emanating from male pup urine (Moore, 1982, 1985). The preferential licking given to males has functional consequences. When maternal licking of pups is reduced by impairing maternal olfaction, male offspring later require more sexual stimulation before ejaculating and take longer to resume copulating after ejaculating than do males raised by control mothers (Moore, 1984; also see Birke & Sadler, 1987). Possibly more interesting is that female offspring that received less licking from olfactory-impaired mothers showed normal feminine sexual behavior (Birke & Sadler, 1987), but were even more demasculinized than control females, and were less likely to mount other females and also slower to mate if they did respond (Moore, 1984). Some aspect of maternal licking, then, contributes to masculinization of copulatory responses in both males and female rats. In fact, perinatal insults that demasculinize offspring behavior may be partly due to maternal effects. As noted above, prenatal stress impairs later masculine copulatory behaviors in the offspring. It also reduces maternal licking of stressed pups, as mothers find the urine of prenatally stressed male offspring less attractive than that of nonstressed offspring (Moore & Power, 1986; Power & Moore 1986).

Instead of experimentally manipulating maternal olfaction to examine the effects of reduced maternal licking on offspring sexual differentiation, one can examine sexual differentiation in offspring reared by mothers who naturally lick more or less often. Male offspring of mothers who lick them more during the first week of life display more mounts to achieve the same number of ejaculation than males of low-licking mothers (Cameron, Fish, & Meaney, 2004). Females raised by low-licking mothers show more sexual proceptivity, are more receptive to males, receive intromissions faster, and have higher pregnancy rates than their counterparts that were licked more often during early life (Cameron et al., 2005). Virgin daughters of low-licking mothers also take almost twice as long to begin acting maternally in a maternal sensitization paradigm, indicating that not all behavioral end points are hyperfeminized by low licking (Champagne, Diorio, Sharma, & Meaney, 2001).

The neural basis for licking-induced differences in copulatory behaviors occurs at both spinal and supraspinal levels. The number of motor neurons of the SNB is slightly, but significantly, reduced in males and females that received less maternal licking (Moore, Dou, & Juraska, 1992). Such a reduction was not found in other motor neuron pools (Moore, Dou, & Juraska, 1996). How maternal licking affects these SNB motorneurons is unknown, but could be due to increased androgen release in frequently licked pups or a result of the increased afferent input to these cells or their target muscles (Moore et al., 1992). Within the brain, offspring of high- and low-licking mothers show differences in numerous neurochemical systems (e.g., Brake, Zhang, Diorio, Meaney, & Gratton, 2004; Caldji, Francis, Sharma, Plotsky, & Meaney, 2000; Champagne et al., 2001, 2006; Champagne, Weaver, Diorio, Sharma, & Meaney, 2003; Francis, Champagne, & Meaney, 2000; Zhang, Chrétien, Meaney, & Gratton, 2005) that could be substrates where maternal behavior affects sexual differentiation of copulatory and other behaviors.

Conclusions

Generating male-typical and female-typical brains and behaviors is essential for the propagation of almost all animal species. We have presented numerous concepts about how this can occur that are aimed at convincing readers that sexual differentiation of the brain and behavior does not depend only upon steroid hormones, is an active process in both females and males, does not only occur during very early development, and may not involve functional relationships between structure and function. Indeed, steroid receptors can be activated by nonsteroidal pathways and are influenced by coregulatory proteins. Active feminization and demasculinization in females is as critical as active defeminization and masculinization of males. The timing of these events is not confined to the end of gestation and first week after birth, but extends through puberty and beyond. Positive correlations between structure size and sexually dimorphic behaviors often do not exist, and sex differences may instead prevent sex differences in function.

It is important to understand that these issues are not purely esoteric. Humans cross-culturally show many reliable sex differences in brain function and behavior. Perhaps some of the most profound sex differences in humans are found in neurological and psychiatric disorders (Seeman, 1997; Zup & Forger, 2002). For example, women are more likely to suffer from depression, multiple sclerosis, and Alzheimer's disease. Boys and men are more susceptible to attention-deficit hyperactivity disorder, autism, and dyslexia. As most sex differences in the brain result from early steroid receptor action, it is possible that sex differences in some sexually dimorphic brain and behavioral disorders in humans are partly influenced by abnormal steroid receptor action during development, puberty, or adulthood. Therefore, understanding how steroid hormones and other factors shape brain development yields insight into how the human brain differentiates in a normal or abnormal manner.

References

Akhmadeev, A. V., & Kalimullina, L. B. (2005). Dendroarchitectonics of neurons in the posterior cortical nucleus of the amygdaloid body of the rat brain as influenced by gender and neonatal androgenization. *Neuroscience Behavior and Physiology, 35,* 393–397.

Al-Shamma, H. A., & De Vries, G. J. (1996). Neurogenesis of the sexually dimorphic vasopressin cells of the bed nucleus of the stria terminalis and amygdala of rats. *Journal of Neurobiology, 29,* 91–98.

Amateau, S. K., Alt, J. J., Stamps, C. L., & McCarthy, M. M. (2004). Brain estradiol content in newborn rats: sex differences, regional heterogeneity, and possible de novo synthesis by the female telencephalon. *Endocrinology 145,* 2906–2917.

Amateau, S. K., & McCarthy, M. M. (2002). Sexual differentiation of astrocyte morphology in the developing rat preoptic area. *Journal of Neuroendocrinology, 14,* 904–910.

Anderson, D. K., Rhees, R. W., & Fleming, D. E. (1985). Effects of prenatal stress on differentiation of the sexually dimorphic nucleus of the preoptic area (SDN-POA) of the rat brain. *Brain Research, 332,* 113–118.

Arai, Y., Sekine, Y., & Murakami, S. (1996). Estrogen and apoptosis in the developing sexually dimorphic preoptic area in female rats. *Neuroscience Research, 25,* 403–407.

Arendash, G. W., & Gorski, R. A. (1983). Effects of discrete lesions of the sexually dimorphic nucleus of the preoptic area or other medial preoptic regions on the sexual behavior of male rats. *Brain Research Bulletin, 10,* 147–154.

Arnold, A. P. (2002) Concepts of genetic and hormonal induction of vertebrate sexual differentiation in the twentieth century, with special reference to the brain. In D. W. Pfaff, A. P. Arnold, A. M. Etgen, S. E. Fahrbach, & R. T. Rubin (Eds.), *Hormones, brain and behavior* (Vol. IV, chap. 63 pp 105–135). New York: Academic Press.

Arnold, A. P., & Breedlove, S. M. (1985). Organizational and activational effects of sex steroids on brain and behavior: a reanalysis. *Hormones and Behavior, 19,* 469–498.

Aronica, S. M., & Katzenellenbogen, B. S. (1993) Stimulation of estrogen receptor-mediated transcription and alteration in the phosphorylation state of the rat uterine estrogen. *Molecular Endocrinology, 7,* 743–752.

Auger, A. P., & Blaustein, J. D. (1995). Progesterone enhances an estradiol-induced increase in Fos immunoreactivity in localized regions of female rat forebrain. *Journal of Neuroscience, 15,* 2272–2279.

Auger, A. P., Moffatt, C. A., & Blaustein, J. D. (1996). Reproductively-relevent stimuli induce Fos-immunoreactivity within progestin receptor-containing cells in localized regions of rat forebrain. *Journal of Neuroendocrinology 8,* 831–838.

Auger, A. P., Moffatt, C. A., & Blaustein, J. D. (1997). Progesterone-independent activation of rat brain progestin receptors by reproductive stimuli. *Endocrinology, 138,* 511–514.

Auger, A. P., Perrot-Sinal, T. S., Auger, C. J., Ekas, L. A., Tetel, M. J., & McCarthy, M. M. (2002). Expression of the nuclear receptor coactivator, cAMP response element-binding protein, is sexually dimorphic and modulates sexual differentiation of neonatal rat brain. *Endocrinology 143,* 3009–3016.

Auger, A. P., Tetel, M. J., & McCarthy, M. M. (2000). Steroid receptor coactivator-1 (SRC-1) mediates the development of sex-specific brain morphology and behavior. *Proceedings of the National Acadamy of Science, USA, 97,* 7551–7555.

Bakker, J., De Mees, C., Douhard, Q., Balthazart, J., Gabant, P., Szpirer, J., et al. (2006). Alpha-fetoprotein protects the developing female mouse brain from masculinization and defeminization by estrogens. *Nature Neuroscience, 9,* 220–226.

Balan, I. S., Ugrumov, M. V., Borisova, N. A., Calas, A., Pilgrim, C., Reisert, I., et al. (1996). Birthdates of the tyrosine hydroxylase immunoreactive neurons in the hypothalamus of male and female rats. *Neuroendocrinology, 64,* 405–411.

Balan, I. S., Ugrumov, M. V., Calas, A., Mailly, P., Krieger, M., & Thibault, J. (2000). Tyrosine hydroxylase-expressing and/or aromatic L-amino acid decarboxylase-expressing neurons in the mediobasal hypothalamus of perinatal rats: differentiation and sexual dimorphism. *Journal of Comparative Neurology, 425,* 167–176.

Bamshad, M., Novak, M. A., & De Vries, G. J. (1993). Sex and species differences in the vasopressin innervation of sexually naive and parental prairie voles, Microtus ochrogaster and meadow voles, *Microtus pennsylvanicus. Journal of Neuroendocrinology, 5,* 247–255.

Barron, S., Tieman, S. B., & Riley, E. P. (1988). Effects of prenatal alcohol exposure on the sexually dimorphic nucleus of the preoptic area of the hypothalamus in male and female rats. *Alcohol Clinical Experimental Research12,* 59–64.

Baum, M. J., Woutersen, P. J., & Slob, A. K. (1991). Sex difference in whole-body androgen content in rats on fetal days 18 and 19 without evidence that androgen passes from males to females. *Biology of Reproduction, 44,* 747–751.

Bayer, S. A., & Altman J. (1987). Development of the preoptic area: time and site of origin, migratory routes, and settling patterns of its neurons. *Journal of Comparative Neurology, 265,* 65–95.

Beatty, W. W., Dodge, A. M., Traylor, K. L., & Meaney, M. J. (1981). Temporal boundary of the sensitive period for hormonal organization of social play in juvenile rats. *Physiology and Behavior, 26,* 241–243.

Belcher, S. M. (1999). Regulated expression of estrogen receptor alpha and beta mRNA in granule cells during development of the rat cerebellum. *Developmental Brain Research, 115,* 57–69.

Beyer, C., Gonzalez-Flores, O., & Gonzalez-Mariscal, G. (1997). Progesterone receptor participates in the stimulatory effect of LHRH, prostaglandin E2, and cyclic AMP on lordosis and proceptive behaviors in rats. *Journal of Neuroendocrinology, 9,* 609–614.

Beyer, C., Pilgrim, C., & Reisert, I. (1991). Dopamine content and metabolism in mesencephalic and diencephalic cell cultures: sex differences and effects of sex steroids. *Journal of Neuroscience, 11,* 1325–1333.

Birke, L. I., & Sadler, D. (1987). Differences in maternal behavior of rats and the sociosexual development of the offspring. *Developmental Psychobiology, 20,* 85–99.

Bleier, R., Byne, W., & Siggelkow, I. (1982). Cytoarchitectonic sexual dimorphisms of the medial preoptic and anterior hypothalamic areas in guinea pig, rat, hamster, and mouse. *Journal of Comparative Neurology, 212,* 118–130.

Bloch, G. J., & Gorski, R. A. (1988a). Estrogen/progesterone treatment in adulthood affects the size of several components of the medial preoptic area in the male rat. *Journal of Comparative Neurology, 275,* 613–622.

Bloch, G. J., & Gorski, R. A. (1988b). Cytoarchitectonic analysis of the SDN-POA of the intact and gonadectomized rat. *Journal of Comparative Neurology, 275,* 604–612.

Booth, J. E. (1977). Sexual behaviour of neonatally castrated rats injected during infancy with oestrogen and dihydrotestosterone. *The Journal of Endocrinology, 72,* 135–141.

Brake, W. G., Zhang, T. Y., Diorio, J., Meaney, M. J., & Gratton, A. (2004). Influence of early postnatal rearing conditions on mesocorticolimbic dopamine and behavioural responses to psychostimulants and stressors in adult rats. *European Journal of Neuroscience, 19,* 1863–1874.

Brand, T., & Slob, A. K. (1988). Peripubertal castration of male rats, adult open field ambulation and partner preference behavior. *Behavioral Brain Research, 30,* 111–117.

Brand, T., & Slob, A. K. (1991). Perinatal flutamide and mounting and lordosis behavior in adult female Wistar and Sprague-Dawley rats. *Behavioral Brain Research, 44,* 43–51.

Bridges, R., Zarrow, M. X., & Denenberg, V. H. (1973). The role of neonatal androgen in the expression of hormonally induced maternal responsiveness in the rat. *Hormones and Behavior, 4,* 315–322.

Bridges, R., Zarrow, M. X., Gandelman, R., & Denenberg, V. H. (1972). Differences in maternal responsiveness between lactating and sensitized rats. *Developmental Psychobiology, 5,* 123–127.

Burke, K. A., Schroeder, D. M., Abel, R. A., Richardson, S. C., Bigsby, R. M., & Nephew, K. P. (2000). Immunohistochemical detection of estrogen receptor alpha in male rat spinal cord during development. *Journal of Neuroscience Research, 61,* 329–337.

Byne, W. (1998). The medial preoptic and anterior hypothalamic regions of the rhesus monkey: Cytoarchitectonic comparison with the human and evidence for sexual dimorphism. *Brain Research, 793,* 346–350.

Caldji, C., Francis, D., Sharma, S., Plotsky, P. M., & Meaney, M. J. (2000). The effects of early rearing environment on the development of GABA$_A$ and central benzodiazepine receptor levels and novelty-induced fearfulness in the rat. *Neuropsychopharmacology, 22,* 219–229.

Calhoun, J. (1962). *The ecology and sociology of the Norway rat.* Bethesda, MD: U.S. Department of Health, Education and Welfare.

Cameron, N. M., Champagne, F. A., Parent, C., Fish, E. W., Ozaki-Kuroda, K., & Meaney, M. J. (2005). The programming of individual differences in defensive responses and reproductive strategies in the rat through variations in maternal care. *Neuroscience and Biobehavioral Reviews, 29,* 843–865.

Cameron, N. M., Fish, E. W., & Meaney, M. J. (2004). Variations in maternal care influence mating preference of female rats. *Society for Neuroscience Abstracts, 212.3.*

Carrer, H. F., & Aoki, A. (1982). Ultrastructural changes in the hypothalamic ventromedial nucleus of ovariectomized rats after estrogen treatment. *Brain Research, 240,* 221–233.

Carson-Jurica, M. A., Schrader, W. T., & O'Malley, B. W. (1990). Steroid receptor family: Structure and functions. *Endocrine Reviews, 11,* 201–220.

Carter, C. S. (2003). Developmental consequences of oxytocin. *Physiology and Behavior, 79,* 383–397.

Carter, C. S., DeVries, A. C., & Getz, L. L. (1995). Physiological substrates of mammalian monogamy: the prairie vole model. *Neuroscience and Biobehavioral Reviews, 19,* 303–314.

Casto, J. M., Ward. O. B., & Bartke, A. (2003). Play, copulation, anatomy, and testosterone in gonadally intact male rats prenatally exposed to flutamide. *Physiology and Behavior, 79,* 633–641.

Champagne, F., Diorio, J., Sharma, S., & Meaney, M. J. (2001). Naturally occurring variations in maternal behavior in the rat are associated with differences in estrogen-inducible central oxytocin receptors. *Proceedings of the National Academy of Science, USA, 98,* 12736–12741.

Champagne, F. A., Weaver, I. C., Diorio, J., Dymov, S., Szyf, M., & Meaney, M. J. (2006). Maternal care associated with methylation of the estrogen receptor-alpha1b promoter and estrogen receptor-alpha expression in the medial preoptic area of female offspring. *Endocrinology, 147,* 2909–2915.

Champagne, F. A., Weaver, I. C., Diorio, J., Sharma, S., & Meaney, M. J. (2003). Natural variations in maternal care are associated with estrogen receptor alpha expression and estrogen sensitivity in the medial preoptic area. *Endocrinology, 144,* 4720–4724.

Choate, J. V., Slayden, O. D, & Resko, J. A. (1998). Immunocytochemical localization of androgen receptors in brains of developing and adult male rhesus monkeys. *Endocrine, 8,* 51–60.

Chrivia, J. C., Kwok, R. P., Lamb, N., Hagiwara, M., Montminy, M. R., & Goodman, R. H. (1993).

Phosphorylated CREB binds specifically to the nuclear protein CBP. *Nature, 365,* 855–859.

Chu, H. P., Morales, J. C., & Etgen, A. M. (1999) Cyclic GMP may potentiate lordosis behaviour by progesterone receptor activation. *Journal of Neuroendocrinology, 11,* 107–113.

Chung, W. C., Swaab, D. F., & De Vries, G. J. (2000). Apoptosis during sexual differentiation of the bed nucleus of the stria terminalis in the rat brain. *Journal of Neurobiology, 43,* 234–243.

Clark, M. M., Santamaria, B. T., Robertson, R. K., & Galef, B. G. (1998). Effects of gonadectomy in infancy and adulthood on handedness in male and female Mongolian gerbils. *Behavioral Neuroscience, 112,* 1026–1029.

Clemens, L. G., Gladue, B. A., & Coniglio, L. P. (1978). Prenatal endogenous androgenic influences on masculine sexual behavior and genital morphology in male and female rats. *Hormones and Behavior, 10,* 40–53.

Commins, D., & Yahr, P. (1985). Autoradiographic localization of estrogen and androgen receptors in the sexually dimorphic area and other regions of the gerbil brain. *Journal of Comparative Neurology, 231,* 473–489.

Conneely, O. M., Maxwell, B. L., Toft, D. O., Schrader, W. T., & O'Malley, B. W. (1987). The A and B forms of the chicken progesterone receptor arise by alternate initiation of translation of a unique mRNA. *Biochem Biophys Res Commun, 149,* 493–501.

Connell, S., Karikari, C., & Hohmann, C. F. (2004). Sex-specific development of cortical monoamine levels in mouse. *Developmental Brain Research, 151,* 187–191.

Cooke, B. M., Breedlove, S. M., & Jordan, C. L. (2003). Both estrogen receptors and androgen receptors contribute to testosterone-induced changes in the morphology of the medial amygdala and sexual arousal in male rats. *Hormones and Behavior, 43,* 336–346.

Cooke, B. M., Hegstrom, C. D., Keen, A., & Breedlove, S. M. (2001). Photoperiod and social cues influence the medial amygdala but not the bed nucleus of the stria terminalis in the Siberian hamster. *Neuroscience Letters, 312,* 9–12.

Cooke, B. M., Tabibnia, G., & Breedlove, S. M. (1999). A brain sexual dimorphism controlled by adult circulating androgens. *Proceedings of the National Academy of Sciences, USA, 96,* 7538–7540.

Cooke, B. M., & Woolley, C. S. (2005). Sexually dimorphic synaptic organization of the medial amygdala. *Journal of Neuroscience, 25,* 10759–10767.

Cottingham, S. L., & Pfaff, D. W. (1986). Interconnectedness of steroid hormone-binding neurons: Existence and implications. *Current Topics in Neuroendocrinology, 7,* 223–249.

Crews, D., Wade, J., & Wilczynski, W. (1990). Sexually dimorphic areas in the brain of whiptail lizards. *Brain Behavior and Evolution, 36,* 262–270.

Davis, P. G., Chaptal, C. V., & McEwen, B. S. (1979). Independence of the differentiation of masculine and feminine sexual behavior in rats. *Hormones and Behavior, 12,* 12–19.

Davis, E. C., Popper, P., & Gorski, R. A. (1996). The role of apoptosis in sexual differentiation of the rat sexually dimorphic nucleus of the preoptic area. *Brain Research, 734,* 10–18.

Davis, E. C., Shryne, J. E., & Gorski, R. A. (1995). A revised critical period for the sexual differentiation of the sexually dimorphic nucleus of the preoptic area in the rat. *Neuroendocrinology, 62,* 579–585.

De Kloet, E. R., Voorhuis, D. A., Boschma, Y., & Elands J. (1986). Estradiol modulates density of putative 'oxytocin receptors' in discrete rat brain regions. *Neuroendocrinology, 44,* 415–421.

De Kloet, E. R., Voorhuis, T. A., & Elands, J. (1985). Estradiol induces oxytocin binding sites in rat hypothalamic ventromedial nucleus. *European Journal of Pharmacology, 118,* 185–186.

Delville, Y., & Blaustein, J. D. (1989). Long-term ovariectomy and hormone-induced sexual behavior, progestin receptors, and hypothalamic morphology in female rats. *Hormones and Behavior, 23,* 269–278.

Denner, L. A., Weigel, N. L., Maxwell, B. L., Schrader, W. T., & O'Malley, B. W. (1990) Regulation of progesterone receptor-mediated transcription by phosphorylation. *Science, 250,* 1740–1743.

De Vries, G. J. (2004). Minireview: Sex differences in adult and developing brains: Compensation, compensation, compensation. *Endocrinology, 145,* 1063–1068.

De Vries, G. J., & Boyle, P. A. (1998). Double duty for sex differences in the brain. *Behavioral Brain Research, 92,* 205–213.

De Vries, G. J., Rissman, E. F., Simerly, R. B., Yang, L. Y., Scordalakes, E. M., Auger, C. J., et al. (2002). A model system for study of sex chromosome effects on sexually dimorphic neural and behavioral traits. *Journal of Neuroscience, 22,* 9005–9014.

De Vries, G. J., & Simerly, R. B. (2002). Anatomy, development, and function of sexually dimorphic neural circuits in the mammalian brain. In D. W. Pfaff, A. P. Arnold, A. M. Etgen, S. E. Fahrbach, R. L. Moss, & R. T, Rubin (Eds.), *Hormones, brain, and behavior, Vol. IV. Development of hormone-dependent neuronal systems* (pp. 137–191). New York: Elsevier.

Dewing, P., Chiang, C. W., Sinchak, K., Sim, H., Fernagut, P. O., Kelly, S., et al. (2006). Direct regulation of adult brain function by the male-specific factor SRY. *Current Biology, 16,* 415–420.

Dohler, K. D., Coquelin, A., Davis, F., Hines, M., Shryne, J. E., & Gorski, R. A. (1982). Differentiation of the sexually dimorphic nucleus in the preoptic area of the rat brain is determined by the perinatal hormone environment. *Neuroscience Letters, 33,* 295–298.

Döhler, K. D., Coquelin, A., Davis, F., Hines, M., Shryne, J. E., Sickmöller, P. M., et al. (1986). Pre- and postnatal influence of an estrogen antagonist and an androgen antagonist on differentiation of the sexually dimorphic nucleus of the preoptic area in male and female rats. *Neuroendocrinology, 42,* 443–448.

Dohler, K. D., Hancke, J. L., Srivastava, S. S., Hofmann, C., Shryne, .J. E., & Gorski, R. A. (1984a). Participation of estrogens in female sexual differentiation of the brain; neuroanatomical, neuroendocrine and behavioral evidence. *Progress in Brain Research, 61,* 99–117.

Dohler, K. D., Srivastava, S. S., Shryne, J. E., Jarzab, B., Sipos, A., & Gorski, R. A. (1984b). Differentiation of the sexually dimorphic nucleus in the preoptic area of the rat brain is inhibited by postnatal treatment with an estrogen antagonist. *Neuroendocrinology, 38,* 297–301.

Dominguez-Salazar, E., Portillo, W., Baum, M. J., Bakker, J., & Paredes, R. G. (2002). Effect of prenatal androgen receptor antagonist or aromatase inhibitor on sexual behavior, partner preference and neuronal Fos responses to estrous female odors in the rat accessory olfactory system. *Physiology and Behavior 75*, 337–346.

DonCarlos, L. L. (1996). Developmental profile and regulation of estrogen receptor (ER) mRNA expression in the preoptic area of prenatal rats. *Developmental Brain Research, 94*, 224–233.

DonCarlos, L. L., & Handa, R. J. (1994). Developmental profile of estrogen receptor mRNA in the preoptic area of male and female neonatal rats. *Developmental Brain Research, 79*, 283–289.

Dorner, G., & Staudt, J. (1969). Structural changes in the hypothalamic ventromedial nucleus of the male rat, following neonatal castration and androgen treatment. *Neuroendocrinology, 4*, 278–281.

Dugger, B. N., Morris, J. A., Jordan, C. L., & Breedlove, S. M. (2008). Gonadal steroids regulate neural plasticity in the sexually dimorphic nucleus of the preoptic area of adult male and female rats. *Neuroendocrinology, 88*(1), 17–24.

Dulac, C., & Kimchi, T. (2007). Neural mechanisms underlying sex-specific behaviors in vertebrates. *Current Opinion in Neurobiology, 17*, 675–683.

Dyer, R. G., MacLeod, N. K., & Ellendorff, F. (1976). Electrophysiological evidence for sexual dimorphism and synaptic convergence in the preoptic and anterior hypothalamic areas of the rat. *Proceedings of the Royal Society of London B: Biological Sciences, 193*, 421–440.

Eddy, E. M., Washburn, T. F., Bunch, D. O., Goulding, E. H., Gladen, B. C., Lubahn, D. B., et al. (1996). Targeted disruption of the estrogen receptor gene in male mice causes alteration of spermatogenesis and infertility. *Endocrinology, 137*, 4796–4805.

Engele, J., Pilgrim, C., & Reisert, I. (1989). Sexual differentiation of mesencephalic neurons in vitro: effects of sex and gonadal hormones. *International Journal of Developmental Neuroscience, 7*, 603–611.

Etgen, A. M., & Petitti, N. (1986). Norepinephrine-stimulated cyclic AMP accumulation in rat hypothalamic slices: effects of estrous cycle and ovarian steroids. *Brain Research, 375*, 385–390.

Fadem, B. H., & Barfield, R. J. (1981). Neonatal hormonal influences on the development of proceptive and receptive feminine sexual behavior in rats. *Hormones and Behavior, 15*, 282–288.

Fitch, R. H., & Denenberg, V. H. (1998). A role for ovarian hormones in sexual differentiation of the brain. *Behavioral Brain Science, 21*, 311–327.

Fleischer, S., Kordower, J. H., Kaplan, B., Dicker, R., Smerling, R., & Ilgner, J. (1981). Olfactory bulbectomy and gender differences in maternal behaviors of rats. P*hysiology and Behavior, 26*, 957–959.

Fleming, A. S., & Rosenblatt, J. S. (1974). Maternal behavior in the virgin and lactating rat. *Journal of Comparative and Physiological Psychology, 86*, 957–972.

Forger, N. G. (2001) The development of sex differences in the nervous system. In Blass, E. (ed.), *The handbook of behavioral neurobiology, Vol. 13: Developmental psychobiology* (pp. 153–208). New York: Plenum, New York.

Forger, N. G., Galef, B. G., & Clark, M. M. (1996). Intrauterine position affects motoneuron number and muscle size in a sexually dimorphic neuromuscular system. *Brain Research, 735*, 119–124.

Forger, N. G., Rosen, G. J., Waters, E. M., Jacob, D., Simerly, R. B., & de Vries, G. J. (2004). Deletion of Bax eliminates sex differences in the mouse forebrain. *Proceedings of the National Academy of Sciences, USA, 101*, 13666–13671.

Fraley, G. S., & Ulibarri, C. (2001). Sexual dimorphism in the number and size of SNB motoneurons: Delayed development during normal ontogeny. *Developmental Brain Research, 126*, 57–64.

Francis, D. D., Champagne, F. C., & Meaney, M. J. (2000). Variations in maternal behaviour are associated with differences in oxytocin receptor levels in the rat. *Journal of Neuroendocrinology, 12*, 1145–1148.

Gangolli, E. A., Conneely, O. M., & O'Malley, B. W. (1997). Neurotransmitters activate the human estrogen receptor in a neuroblastoma cell line. *Journal of Steroid Biochemistry and Molecular Biology, 61*, 1–9.

Garcia-Falgueras, A., Pinos, H., Collado, P., Pasaro, E., Fernandez, R., Jordan, C.L., et al. (2005). The role of the androgen receptor in CNS masculinization. *Brain Research, 1035*, 13–23.

Gatewood, J. D., Wills, A., Shetty, S., Xu, J., Arnold, A. P., Burgoyne, P.S., et al. (2006). Sex chromosome complement and gonadal sex influence aggressive and parental behaviors in mice. *Journal of Neuroscience, 26*, 2335–2342.

Gerall, A. A. (1957). Effects of early postnatal androgen and estrogen injections on the estrous activity cycles and mating behavior of rats. *Anatomical Record, 157*, 97–104.

Gerall, A. A., Hendricks, S. E., Johnson, L. L., & Bounds, T. W. (1967). Effects of early castration in male rats adult sexual behavior. *Journal of Comparative and Physiological Psychology, 64*, 206–212.

Germain, B. J, Campbell, P. S., & Anderson, J. N. (1978). Role of the serum estrogen-binding protein in the control of tissue estradiol levels during postnatal development of the female rat. *Endocrinology, 103*, 1401–1410.

Gladue, B. A., & Clemens, L. G. (1980). Flutamide inhibits testosterone–induced masculine sexual behavior in male and female rats. *Endocrinology, 106*, 1917–1922.

Glickman, S. E., Short, R. V., & Renfree, M. B. (2005). Sexual differentiation in three unconventional mammals: spotted hyenas, elephants and tammar wallabies. *Hormones and Behavior, 48*, 403–417.

Gonzales, F. G., Ortega, J. G., & Salazar, M. (2000) Effect of neonatal administration of an antidopaminergic drug (metoclopramide) on sexual behavior of male rats. *Archives of Andrology, 45*, 137–142.

Gorski, R. A., Gordon, J. H., Shryne, J. E., & Southam, A. M. (1978). Evidence for a morphological sex difference within the medial preoptic area of the rat brain. *Brain Research, 148*, 333–346.

Gorski, R. A., Harlan, R. E., Jacobson, C. D., Shryne, J. E., & Southam, A. M. (1980). Evidence for the existence of a sexually dimorphic nucleus in the preoptic area of the rat. *Journal of Comparative Neurology, 193*, 529–539.

Gotz, F., Tonjes, R., Maywald, J., & Dorner, G. (1991) Short- and long-term effects of a dopamine agonist (lisuride) on sex- specific behavioural patterns in rats. *Experimental and Clinical Endocrinology, 98*, 111–121.

Goy, R. W., & Deputte, B. L. (1996) The effects of diethylstilbestrol (DES) before birth on the development of masculine behavior in juvenile female rhesus monkeys. *Hormones and Behavior, 30*, 379–386.

Grady, K. L., Phoenix, C. H., & Young, W. C. (1965). Role of the developing rat testis in differentiation of the neural tissues mediating mating behavior. *Journal of Comparative and Physiological Psychology, 59*, 176–182.

Gubernick, D. J., & Nelson, R. J. (1989). Prolactin and paternal behavior in the biparental California mouse, *Peromyscus californicus. Hormones and Behavior, 23*, 203–210.

Gubernick, D. J., Sengelaub, D. R., & Kurz, E. M. (1993). A neuroanatomical correlate of paternal and maternal behavior in the biparental California mouse (*Peromyscus californicus*). *Behavioral Neuroscience, 107*, 194–201.

Guillamon, A., de Blas, M. R., & Segovia, S. (1988). Effects of sex steroids on the development of the locus coeruleus in the rat. *Brain Research, 468*, 306–310.

Guillamon, A., & Segovia, S. (1997). Sex differences in the vomeronasal system. *Brain Research Bulletin, 44*, 77–82.

Hagihara, K., Hirata, S., Osada, T., Hirai, M., & Kato, J. (1992). Expression of progesterone receptor in the neonatal rat brain cortex: detection of its mRNA using reverse transcription-polymerase chain reaction. *Journal of Steroid Biochemistry and Molecular Biology, 41*, 637–640.

Hart, B. L. (1968). Neonatal castration: Influence on neural organization of sexual reflexes in male rats. *Science, 160*, 1135–1136.

Hart, B. L. (1977). Neonatal dihydrotestosterone and estrogen stimulation: Effects on sexual behavior of male rats. *Hormones and Behavior, 8*, 193–200.

Hasler, M. J., & Conaway, C. H. (1973). The effect of males on the reproductive state of female *Microtus ochrogaster. Biology of Reproduction, 9*, 426–36.

Hayashi, S., Hayashi, H., Ueda, H., & Papadopoulos, G. C. (2001). Analysis of transient expression of estrogen receptor-alpha in newborn rat primary auditory cortex. *Hormones and Behavior, 40*, 191–195.

Herbison, A. E., King, I. S., Tan, K. K. C. & Dye, S. (1995). Increased fos expression in preoptic calcitonin gene-related peptide (CGRP) neurones following mating but not the luteinizing hormone surge in female rats, *Journal of Neuroendocrinology, 7*, 377–385.

Herrenkohl, L. R. (1986). Prenatal stress disrupts reproductive behavior and physiology in offspring. *Annals of the New York Academy of Sciences, 474*, 120–128.

Hines, M., Allen, L. S., & Gorski, R. A. (1992). Sex differences in subregions of the medial nucleus of the amygdala and the bed nucleus of the stria terminalis of the rat. *Brain Research, 579*, 321–326.

Hines, M., Davis, F. C., Coquelin, A., Goy, R. W., & Gorski, R. A. (1985). Sexually dimorphic regions in the medial preoptic area and the bed nucleus of the stria terminalis of the guinea pig brain: A description and an investigation of their relationship to gonadal steroids in adulthood. *Journal of Neuroscience, 5*, 40–47.

Hines, M., Golombok, S., Rust, J., Johnston, K. J., Golding, J., & Avon. Longitudinal Study of Parents and Children Study Team. (2002). Testosterone during pregnancy and gender role behavior of preschool children: a longitudinal, population study. *Child Development, 73*, 1678–1687.

Holman, S. D. (1981). Neonatal androgenic influences on masculine ultrasonic vocalizations of Mongolian gerbils. *Physiology and Behavior, 26*, 583–586.

Holman, S. D., & Hutchison, J. B. (1991). Differential effects of neonatal castration on the development of sexually dimorphic brain areas in the gerbil. *Developmental Brain Research, 61*, 147–150.

Holman, S. D., Collado, P., Rice, A., & Hutchison, J. B. (1995). Stereological estimates of postnatal structural differentiation in a sexually dimorphic hypothalamic nucleus involved in vocal control. *Brain Research, 694*, 167–176.

Holman, S. D., Collado, P., Skepper, J. N., & Rice, A. (1996). Postnatal development of a sexually dimorphic, hypothalamic nucleus in gerbils: a stereological study of neuronal number and apoptosis. *Journal of Comparative Neurology, 376*, 315–325.

Houtsmuller, E. J., Brand, T., de Jonge, F. H., Joosten, R. N., van de Poll, N. E., & Slob, A. K. (1994). SDN–POA volume, sexual behavior, and partner preference of male rats affected by perinatal treatment with ATD. *Physiology and Behavior, 56*, 535–541.

Hsu, H. K., Chen, F. N., & Peng, M. T. (1980). Some characteristics of the darkly stained area of the medial preoptic area of rats. *Neuroendocrinology, 31*, 327–330.

Hull, E. M., Nishita, J. K., Bitran, D., & Dalterio, S. (1984) Perinatal dopamine-related drugs demasculinize rats. *Science, 224*, 1011–1013.

Humm, J. L., Lambert, K. G., & Kinsley, C. H. (1995). Paucity of c-fos expression in the medial preoptic area of prenatally stressed male rats following exposure to sexually receptive females. *Brain Research Bulletin, 37*, 363–368.

Ichikawa, S., & Fujii, Y. (1982). Effect of prenatal androgen treatment on maternal behavior in the female rat. *Hormones and Behavior, 16*, 224–233.

Ikeda, Y., & Nagai, A. (2006). Differential expression of the estrogen receptors alpha and beta during postnatal development of the rat cerebellum. *Brain Research, 1083*, 39–49.

Ikeda, Y., Nagai, A., Ikeda, M. A., & Hayashi, S. (2003) Sexually dimorphic and estrogen-dependent expression of estrogen receptor beta in the ventromedial hypothalamus during rat postnatal development. *Endocrinology, 144*, 5098–5104.

Ito, S., Murakami, S., Yamanouchi, K., & Arai, Y. (1986). Prenatal androgen exposure, preoptic area and reproductive functions in the female rat. *Brain Development 8*, 463–468.

Ivanova, T., & Beyer, C. (2000). Ontogenetic expression and sex differences of aromatase and estrogen receptor-alpha/beta mRNA in the mouse hippocampus. *Cell and Tissue Research, 300*, 231–237.

Jacobson, C. D., & Gorski, R. A. (1981). Neurogenesis of the sexually dimorphic nucleus of the preoptic area in the rat. *Journal of Comparative Neurology, 196*, 519–529.

Jacobson, C. D., Terkel, J., Gorski, R. A., & Sawyer, C. H. (1980). Effects of small medial preoptic area lesions on maternal behavior: Retrieving and nest building in the rat. *Brain Research, 194*, 471–478.

Jahagirdar, V., Quadros, P. S., & Wagner, C. K. (2005). Transient expression of progesterone receptors in the subplate of developing rat cortex. *Society for Neuroscience Abstracts, 406.3.*

Jensen, E. V., Suzuki, T., Kawashima, T., Stumpf, W. E., Jungblut, P. W., & DeSombre, E. R. (1968). A two-step mechanism for the interaction of estradiol with rat uterus. *Proceedings of the National Academy of Science, USA 59*, 632–638.

Juarez, J., del Rio-Portilla, I., & Corsi-Cabrera, M. (1998). Effects of prenatal testosterone on sex and age differences in behavior elicited by stimulus pups in the rat. *Developmental Psychobiology, 32*, 121–129.

Karolczak, M., & Beyer, C. (1998). Developmental sex differences in estrogen receptor-beta mRNA expression in the mouse hypothalamus/preoptic region. *Neuroendocrinology, 68*, 229–234.

Kato, J., Hirata, S., Nozawa, A., & Mouri, N. (1993) The ontogeny of gene expression of progestin receptors in the female rat brain. *Journal of Steroid Biochemistry and Molecular Biology, 47*, 173–182.

Kato, J., & Onouchi, T. (1981). Progesterone receptors in the cerebral cortex of neonatal female rats. *Developmental Neuroscience, 4*, 427–432.

Kato, J., Onouchi, T., Okinaga, S., & Takamatsu, M. (1984). The ontogeny of cytosol and nuclear progestin receptors in male rat brain and its male-female differences. *Journal of Steroid Biochemistry, 20*, 147–152.

Kazmi, S. M. I., Visconti, V., Plante, R. K., Ishaque, A., & Lau, C. (1993) Differential regulation of human progesterone receptor-A and receptor-B form-mediated trans-activation by phosphorylation. *Endocrinology, 133*, 1230–1238.

Kerchner, M., & Ward, I. L. (1992). SDN-MPOA volume in male rats is decreased by prenatal stress, but is not related to ejaculatory behavior. *Brain Research, 581*, 244–251.

Kritzer, M. F. (2006). Regional, laminar and cellular distribution of immunoreactivity for ERbeta in the cerebral cortex of hormonally intact, postnatally developing male and female rats. *Cerebral Cortex, 16*, 1181–92.

Kudwa, A. E., Bodo, C., Gustafsson, J. A., & Rissman, E. F. (2005). A previously uncharacterized role for estrogen receptor beta: defeminization of male brain and behavior. *Proceedings of the National Academy of Science, USA 102*, 4608–4612.

Kudwa, A. E., Michopoulos, V., Gatewood, J. D., & Rissman, E. F. (2006). Roles of estrogen receptors alpha and beta in differentiation of mouse sexual behavior. *Neuroscience, 138*, 921–928.

Kuhnemann, S., Brown, T. J., Hochberg, R. B., & MacLusky, N. J. (1994). Sex differences in the development of estrogen receptors in the rat brain. *Hormones and Behavior, 28*, 483–491.

Kuiper, G. G. J. M., Enmark, E., Peltohuikko, M., Nilsson, S., & Gustafsson, J. A. (1996). Cloning of a novel estrogen receptor expressed in rat prostate and ovary. *Proceedings of the National Academy of Science, USA, 93*, 5925–5930.

Kwok, R. P., Lundblad, J. R., Chrivia, J. C., Richards, J. P., Bachinger, H. P., Brennan, R. G., et al. (1994). Nuclear protein CBP is a coactivator for the transcription factor CREB. *Nature, 370*, 223–226.

Lamprecht, S. A., Kohen, F., Ausher, J., Zor, U., & Lindner, H. R. (1976). Hormonal stimulation of oestradiol-17 beta release from the rat ovary during early postnatal development. *Journal of Endocrinology, 68*, 343–344.

Lansing, S. W., & Lonstein, J. S. (2006). Tyrosine hydroxylase-synthesizing cells in the hypothalamus of prairie voles (*Microtus ochrogaster*): sex differences in the anteroventral periventricular preoptic area and effects of adult gonadectomy or neonatal gonadal hormones. *Journal of Neurobiology, 66*, 197–204.

Lauber, M. E., Sarasin, A., & Lichtensteiger, W. (1997). Transient sex differences of aromatase (CYP19) mRNA expression in the developing rat brain. *Neuroendocrinology, 66*, 173–180.

Leboucher, G. (1989). Maternal behavior in normal and androgenized female rats: Effect of age and experience. *Physiology and Behavior, 45*, 313–319.

Leon, M., Numan, M., & Moltz, H. (1973). Maternal behavior in the rat: facilitation through gonadectomy. *Science, 179*, 1018–1019.

Lesage, J., Bernet, F., Montel, V., & Dupouy, J.P. (1996). Hypothalamic metabolism of neurotransmitters (serotonin, norepinephrine, dopamine) and NPY, and gonadal and adrenal activities, during the early postnatal period in the rat. *Neurochemistry Research, 21*, 87–96.

Lieberburg, I., MacLusky, N. J., & McEwen, B. S. (1980). Androgen receptors in the perinatal rat brain. *Brain Research, 196*, 125–138.

Lonstein, J. S., & De Vries, G. J. (2000). Sex differences in the parental behavior of rodents. *Neuroscience and Biobehavioral Reviews, 24*, 669–686.

Lonstein, J. S., Quadros, P. S., & Wagner, C. K. (2001). Effects of neonatal RU486 on adult sexual, parental, and fearful behaviors in rats. *Behavioral Neuroscience, 115*, 58–70.

Lonstein, J. S., Rood, B. D., & De Vries, G. J. (2002). Parental responsiveness is feminized after neonatal castration in virgin male prairie voles, but is not masculinized by perinatal testosterone in virgin females. *Hormones and Behavior, 41*, 80–87.

Lonstein, J. S., Rood, B. D., & De Vries, G. J. (2005). Unexpected effects of perinatal gonadal hormone manipulations on sexual differentiation of the extrahypothalamic arginine–vasopressin system in prairie voles. *Endocrinology, 146*, 1559–1567.

Lonstein, J. S., Wagner, C. K., & De Vries, G. J. (1999). Comparison of the "nursing" and other parental behaviors of nulliparous and lactating female rats. *Hormones and Behavior, 36*, 242–251.

Lorenz, B., Garcia-Segura, L. M., & DonCarlos, L. L. (2005). Cellular phenotype of androgen receptor-immunoreactive nuclei in the developing and adult rat brain. *Journal of Comparative Neurology, 492*, 456–468.

Lubin, M., Leon, M., Moltz, H., & Numan, M. (1972). Hormones and maternal behavior in the male rat. *Hormones and Behavior, 3*, 369–374.

Lund, T. D., Salyer, D. L., Fleming, D. E., & Lephart, E. D. (2000). Pre- or postnatal testosterone and flutamide effects on sexually dimorphic nuclei of the rat hypothalamus. *Developmental Brain Research, 120*, 261–266.

Lustig, R. H., Hua, P., Wilson, M. C., & Federoff, H. J. (1993). Ontogeny, sex dimorphism, and neonatal sex hormone determination of synapse-associated messenger RNAs in rat brain. *Molecular Brain Research, 20*, 101–110.

MacLusky, N. J., Chaptal, C., & McEwen, B. S. (1979a). The development of estrogen receptor systems in the rat brain and pituitary: postnatal development. *Brain Research, 178*, 143–160.

MacLusky, N. J., Lieberburg, I., & McEwen, B. S. (1979b). The development of estrogen receptor systems in the rat brain: perinatal development. *Brain Research, 178*, 129–142.

MacLusky, N. J., & McEwen, B. S. (1978). Oestrogen modulates progestin receptor concentrations in some rat brain regions but not in others. *Nature 274*, 276–278.

MacLusky, N. J., & Naftolin, F. (1981). Sexual differentiation of the central nervous system. *Science, 211*, 1294–302.

MacLusky, N. J., Philip, A., Hurlburt, C., & Naftolin. F. (1985). Estrogen formation in the developing rat brain: sex differences in aromatase activity during early post-natal life. *Sychoneuroendocrinology, 10*, 355–361.

Madeira, M. D., Ferreira-Silva, L., & Paula-Barbosa, M. M. (2001). Influence of sex and estrus cycle on the sexual dimorphisms of the hypothalamic ventromedial nucleus: stereological evaluation and Golgi study. *Journal of Comparative Neurology, 432,* 329–345.

Mani, S. K., Allen, J. M. C., Rettori, V., Mccann, S. M., O'Malley, B. W., & Clark, J. H. (1994). Nitric oxide mediates sexual behavior in female rats. *Proceedings of the National Academy of Science, USA, 91,* 6468–6472.

Mani, S. K., Reyna, A. M., Chen, J. Z., Mulac-Jericevic, B., & Conneely, O. M. (2006) Differential response of progesterone receptor isoforms in hormone-dependent and -independent facilitation of female sexual receptivity. *Molecular Endocrinology, 20,* 1322–1332.

Markham, J. A., Jurgens, H. A., Auger, C. J., De Vries, G. J., Arnold, A. P., & Juraska, J. M. (2003). Sex differences in mouse cortical thickness are independent of the complement of sex chromosomes. *Neuroscience, 116,* 71–75.

Matsumoto, A., & Arai, Y. (1983). Sex difference in volume of the ventromedial nucleus of the hypothalamus in the rat. *Endocrinology Japan, 30,* 277–280.

Matsumoto, A., & Arai, Y. (1986a). Male-female difference in synaptic organization of the ventromedial nucleus of the hypothalamus in the rat. *Neuroendocrinology, 42,* 232–236.

Matsumoto, A., & Arai, Y. (1986b). Development of sexual dimorphism in synaptic organization in the ventromedial nucleus of the hypothalamus in rats. *Neuroscience Letters, 68,* 165–8.

Mayer, A. D., Freeman, N. C., & Rosenblatt, J. S. (1979). Ontogeny of maternal behavior in the laboratory rat: factors underlying changes in responsiveness from 30 to 90 days. *Developmental Psychobiology, 12,* 425–439.

McAbee, M. D., & DonCarlos, L. L. (1998). Ontogeny of region-specific sex differences in androgen receptor messenger ribonucleic acid expression in the rat forebrain. *Endocrinology, 139,* 1738–1745.

McAbee, M. D., & DonCarlos, L. L. (1999a). Estrogen, but not androgens, regulates androgen receptor messenger ribonucleic acid expression in the developing male rat forebrain. *Endocrinology, 140,* 3674–3681.

McAbee, M. D., & DonCarlos, L. L. (1999b). Regulation of androgen receptor messenger ribonucleic acid expression in the developing rat forebrain. *Endocrinology, 140,* 1807–1814.

McCarthy, M. M., Pfaff, D. W., & Schwartz-Giblin, S. (1993a). The role of steroid modulation of amino acid transmitters in the regulation of female reproduction. *American Zoologist, 33,* 275–284.

McCarthy, M. M., Schlenker, E. H., & Pfaff D. W. (1993b). Enduring consequences of neonatal treatment with antisense oligodeoxynucleotides to estrogen receptor messenger ribonucleic acid on sexual differentiation of rat brain. *Endocrinology, 133,* 433–439.

McCormick, C. M., Smythe, J. W., Sharma, S., & Meaney, M. J. (1995). Sex-specific effects of prenatal stress on hypothalamic-pituitary-adrenal responses to stress and brain glucocorticoid receptor density in adult rats. *Developmental Brain Research, 84,* 55–61.

McCullough, J., Quandagno, D. M., & Goldman, B. D. (1974). Neonatal gonadal hormones: effect on maternal and sexual behavior in the male rat. *Physiology and Behavior, 12,* 183–188.

McEwen, B. S., Lieberburg, I., Chaptal, C., & Krey, L. C. (1977). Aromatization: important for sexual differentiation of the neonatal rat brain. *Hormones and Behavior, 9,* 249–263.

McGivern, R. F., Handa, R. J., & Raum, W. J. (1998). Ethanol exposure during the last week of gestation in the rat: inhibition of the prenatal testosterone surge in males without long-term alterations in sex behavior. *Neurotoxicology and Teratology, 20,* 483–490.

McGivern, R. F., Handa, R. J., & Redei, E. (1993). Decreased postnatal testosterone surge in male rats exposed to ethanol during the last week of gestation. *Alcohol Clinical and Experimental Research, 17,* 1215–1222.

McKenna, N. J., Lanz, R. B., & O'Malley, B. W. (1999). Nuclear receptor coregulators: cellular and molecular biology. *Endocrine Reviews, 20,* 321–344.

Meaney, M. J., Aitken, D. H., Jensen, L. K., McGinnis, M. Y., & McEwen, B. S. (1985). Nuclear and cytosolic androgen receptor levels in the limbic brain of neonatal male and female rats. *Brain Research, 355,* 179–185.

Meaney, M. J., & McEwen, B. S. (1986) Testosterone implants into the amygdala during the neonatal period masculinize the social play of juvenile female rats. *Brain Research, 398,* 324–328.

Meaney, M. J., & Stewart, J. (1981) Neonatal-androgens influence the social play of prepubescent rats. *Hormones and Behavior, 15,* 197–213.

Meaney, M. J., Stewart, J., Poulin, P., & McEwen, B. S. (1983). Sexual differentiation of social play in rat pups is mediated by the neonatal androgen-receptor system. *Neuroendocrinology, 37,* 85–90.

Melnikova, V., Orosco, M., Calas, A., Sapronova, A., Gainetdinov, R., Delhaye-Bouchaud, N., et al. (1999). Dopamine turnover in the mediobasal hypothalamus in rat fetuses. *Neuroscience, 89,* 235–241.

Miranda, R. C., & Toran-Allerand, C. D. (1992). Developmental expression of estrogen receptor mRNA in the rat cerebral cortex: a nonisotopic in situ hybridization histochemistry study. *Cerebral Cortex, 2,* 1–15.

Mizukami, S., Nishizuka, M., & Arai, Y. (1983). Sexual difference in nuclear volume and its ontogeny in the rat amygdala. *Experimental Neurology, 79,* 569–75.

Moguilewsky, M., & Raynaud, J. P. (1979). Estrogen-sensitive progestin-binding sites in the female rat brain and pituitary. *Brain Research, 164,* 165–175.

Mong, J. A., Kurzweil, R. L., Davis, A. M., Rocca, M. S., & McCarthy, M. M. (1996). Evidence for sexual differentiation of glia in rat brain. *Hormones and Behavior, 30,* 553–562.

Montano, M. M., Welshons, W. V., & vom Saal, F. S. (1995). Free estradiol in serum and brain uptake of estradiol during fetal and neonatal sexual differentiation in female rats. *Biology of Reproduction, 53,* 1198–1207.

Moore, C. L. (1982). Maternal behavior of rats is affected by hormonal condition of pups. *Journal of Comparative and Physiological Psychology, 96,* 123–129.

Moore, C. L. (1984). Maternal contributions to the development of masculine sexual behavior in laboratory rats. *Developmental Psychobiology, 17,* 347–356.

Moore, C. L. (1985). Sex differences in urinary odors produced by young laboratory rats (*Rattus norvegicus*). *Journal of Comparative Psychology, 99,* 336–41.

Moore, C. L., & Chadwick-Dias, A. M. (1986). Behavioral responses of infant rats to maternal licking: variations with age and sex. *Developmental Psychobiology, 19,* 427–438.

Moore, C. L., Dou, H., & Juraska, J. M. (1992). Maternal stimulation affects the number of motor neurons in a sexually dimorphic nucleus of the lumbar spinal cord. *Brain Research, 572,* 52–56.

Moore, C. L., Dou, H., & Juraska, J. M. (1996). Number, size, and regional distribution of motor neurons in the dorsolateral and retrodorsolateral nuclei as a function of sex and neonatal stimulation. *Developmental Psychobiology, 29,* 303–313.

Moore, C. L., & Morelli, G. A. (1979). Mother rats interact differently with male and female offspring. *Journal of Comparative and Physiological Psychology, 93,* 677–684.

Moore, C. L., & Power, K. L. (1986). Prenatal stress affects mother–infant interaction in Norway rats. *Developmental Psychobiology, 19,* 235–245.

Moore, F. L., Boyd, S. K., & Kelley, D. B. (2005). Historical perspective: Hormonal regulation of behaviors in amphibians. *Hormones and Behavior, 48,* 373–383.

Morris, J. A., Jordan, C. L., Dugger, B. N., & Breedlove, S. M. (2005). Partial demasculinization of several brain regions in adult male (XY) rats with a dysfunctional androgen receptor gene. *Journal of Comparative Neurology, 487,* 217–226.

Mulac-Jericevic, B., Mullinax, R. A., Demayo, F. J., Lydon, J. P., Conneely, O. M. (2000). Subgroup of reproductive functions of progesterone mediated by progesterone receptor-B isoform. *Science, 289,* 1751–1754.

Nadler, R. D. (1969). Differentiation of the capacity for male sexual behavior in the rat. *Hormones and Behavior, 1,* 53–63.

Neumann, F., & Elger, W. (1966). Permanent changes in gonadal function and sexual behavior as a result of early feminization of male rats by treatment with an antiandrogenic steroid. *Endokrinologie, 50,* 209–14.

Newman, S. W. (1999). The medial extended amygdala in male reproductive behavior. A node in the mammalian social behavior network. *Annals of the New York Academy of Science, 877,* 242–257.

Nishizuka, M., & Arai, Y. (1981). Sexual dimorphism in synaptic organization in the amygdala and its dependence on neonatal hormone environment. *Brain Research, 212,* 31–38.

Nishizuka, M., & Arai, Y. (1982). Synapse formation in response to estrogen in the medial amygdala developing in the eye. *Proceedings of the National Academy of Science, USA, 79,* 7024–7026.

Nordeen, E. J., Nordeen, K. W., Sengelaub, D. R., & Arnold, A. P. (1985). Androgens prevent normally occurring cell death in a sexually dimorphic spinal nucleus. *Science, 229,* 671–673.

Northcutt, K. V., & Lonstein, J. S. (2008). Sex differences and effects of neonatal aromatase inhibition on masculine and feminine copulatory potentials in prairie voles. *Hormones and Behavior, 54*(1), 160–169.

Northcutt, K. V, Wang, Z. & Lonstein, J. S. (2007). Sex and species differences in tyrosine hydroxylase-synthesizing cells of the rodent extended amygdala. *Journal of Comparative Neurology, 500,* 103–115.

Numan, M. J., & Insel, T. R. (2003). *The neurobiology of parental behavior,* 3rd ed. New York: Springer.

Nunez, J. L., Huppenbauer, C. B., McAbee, M. D., Juraska, J. M., & DonCarlos, L. L. (2003). Androgen receptor expression in the developing male and female rat visual and prefrontal cortex. *Journal of Neurobiology, 56,* 293–302.

Nunez, J. L., Sodhi, J., & Juraska, J. M. (2002). Ovarian hormones after postnatal day 20 reduce neuron number in the rat primary visual cortex. *Journal of Neurobiology, 52,* 312–321.

Ogawa, S., Chan, J., Chester, A. E., Gustafsson, J., Korach, K. S., & Pfaff, D. W. (1999). Survival of reproductive behaviors in estrogen receptor beta gene- deficient (betaERKO) male and female mice. *Proceedings of the National Academy of Science, USA, 96,* 12887–12892.

Ogawa, S., Chester, A. E., Hewitt, S. C., Walker, V. R., Gustafsson, J. A., Smithies, O., et al. (2000). Abolition of male sexual behaviors in mice lacking estrogen receptors alpha and beta (alpha beta ERKO). *Proceedings of the National Academy of Science, USA, 97,* 14737–14741.

O'Keefe, J. A., & Handa, R. J. (1990). Transient elevation of estrogen receptors in the neonatal rat hippocampus. *Developmental Brain Research, 57,* 119–127.

Olesen, K. M., Jessen, H. M., Auger, C. J., & Auger, A. P. (2005) Dopaminergic activation of estrogen receptors in neonatal brain alters progestin receptor expression and juvenile social play behavior. *Endocrinology, 146,* 3705–3712.

Olioff, M., & Stewart, J. (1978) Sex differences in the play behavior of prepubescent rats. *Physiology and Behavior, 20,* 113–115.

Olster, D. H., & Blaustein, J. D. (1988). Progesterone facilitation of lordosis in male and female Sprague-Dawley rats following priming with estradiol pulses. *Hormones and Behavior, 22,* 294–304.

Onate, S. A., Tsai, S. Y., Tsai, M. J., & O'Malley, B. W. (1995). Sequence and characterization of a coactivator for the steroid hormone receptor superfamily. *Science, 270,* 1354–1357.

Paden, C. M., & Roselli, C. E. (1987). Modulation of aromatase activity by testosterone in transplants of fetal rat hypothalamus-preoptic area. *Brain Research, 430,* 127–133.

Paech, K., Webb, P., Kuiper, G. G., Nilsson, S., Gustafsson, J., Kushner, P. J., et al. (1997). Differential ligand activation of estrogen receptors ER-alpha and ER-beta at AP1 sites. *Science, 277,* 1508–1510.

Pang, S. F., Caggiula, A. R., Gay, V. L., Goodman, R. L., & Pang, C. S. (1979). Serum concentrations of testosterone, oestrogens, luteinizing hormone and follicle-stimulating hormone in male and female rats during the critical period of neural sexual differentiation. *Journal of Endocrinology, 80,* 103–110.

Pang, S. F., & Tang, F. (1984). Sex differences in the serum concentrations of testosterone in mice and hamsters during their critical periods of neural sexual differentiation. *Journal of Endocrinology, 100,* 7–11.

Pask, A., & Renfree, M. B. (2001). Sex determining genes and sexual *differentiation* in a marsupial. *Journal of Experimental Zoology, 290,* 586–596.

Pasterkamp, R. J., Yuri, K., Visser, D. T., Hayashi, S., & Kawata M. (1996). The perinatal ontogeny of estrogen receptor-immunoreactivity in the developing male and female rat hypothalamus. *Developmental Brain Research, 91,* 300–303.

Pedersen, J. F. (1980). Ultrasound evidence of sexual difference in fetal size in first trimester. *British Medical Journal, 281,* 1253.

Perez, S. E., Chen, E. Y., & Mufson, E. J. (2003). Distribution of estrogen receptor alpha and beta immunoreactive profiles in the postnatal rat brain. *Developmental Brain Research,* *145,* 117–1139.

Pfaff, D., & Keiner, M. (1973). Atlas of estradiol-concentrating cells in the central nervous system of the female rat. *Journal of Comparative Neurology, 151,* 121–158.

Phoenix, C. H., Goy, R. W., Gerall, A. A., & Young, W. C. (1959). Organizing action of prenatally administered testosterone propionate on the tissues mediating mating behavior in the female guinea pig. *Endocrinology, 65,* 369–382.

Pinos, H., Collado, P., Rodriguez-Zafra, M., Rodriguez, C., Segovia, S., & Guillamon, A. (2001). The development of sex differences in the locus coeruleus of the rat. *Brain Research Bulletin, 56,* 73–78.

Plapinger, L., & McEwen, B. S. (1973). Ontogeny of estradiol-binding sites in rat brain. I. Appearance of presumptive adult receptors in cytosol and nuclei. *Endocrinology, 93,* 1119–1128.

Platania, P., Laureanti, F., Bellomo, M,. Giuffrida, R., Giuffrida-Stella, A. M., Catania, M. V., et al. (2003). Differential expression of estrogen receptors alpha and beta in the spinal cord during postnatal development: localization in glial cells. *Neuroendocrinology, 77,* 334–40.

Power, K. L., & Moore, C. L. (1986). Prenatal stress eliminates differential maternal attention to male offspring in Norway rats. *Physiology and Behavior, 38,* 667–671.

Power, R. F., Mani, S. K., Codina, J., Conneely, O. M., & O'Malley, B. W. (1991). Dopaminergic and ligand-independent activation of steroid hormone receptors. *Science, 254,* 1636–1639.

Pozzo Miller, L. D., & Aoki, A. (1991). Stereological analysis of the hypothalamic ventromedial nucleus. II. Hormone-induced changes in the synaptogenic pattern. *Developmental Brain Research, 61,* 189–196.

Price, J. L. (2003). Comparative aspects of amygdala connectivity. *Annals of the New York Academy of Science, 985,* 50–58.

Primus, R. J., & Kellogg, C. K. (1990). Gonadal hormones during puberty organize environment-related social interaction in the male rat. *Hormones and Behavior, 24,* 311–323.

Quadagno, D. M. (1974). Maternal behavior in the rat: aspects of concaveation and neonatal androgen treatment. *Physiology and Behavior, 12,* 1071–4.

Quadagno, D. M., Briscoe, R., & Quadagno, J. S. (1977). Effect of perinatal gonadal hormones on selected nonsexual behavior patterns: a critical assessment of the nonhuman and human literature. *Psychological Bulletin, 84,* 62–80.

Quadagno, D. M., McCullough, J., Ho, G. K., & Spevak, A. M. (1973). Neonatal gonadal hormones: effect on maternal and sexual behavior in the female rat. *Physiology and Behavior, 11,* 251–4.

Quadagno, D. M., & Rockwell, J. (1972). The effect of gonadal hormones in infancy on maternal behavior in the adult rat. *Hormones and Behavior, 3,* 55–62.

Quadros, P. S., Goldstein, A. Y., De Vries, G. J., & Wagner, C. K. (2002b). Regulation of sex differences in progesterone receptor expression in the medial preoptic nucleus of postnatal rats. *Journal of Neuroendocrinology, 14,* 761–767.

Quadros, P. S., Pfau, J. L., Goldstein, A. Y., De Vries, G. J., & Wagner, C. K. (2002a). Sex differences in progesterone receptor expression: A potential mechanism for estradiol-mediated sexual differentiation. *Endocrinology, 143,* 3727–3739.

Raab, H., Karolczak, M., Reisert, I., & Beyer, C. (1999). Ontogenetic expression and splicing of estrogen receptor-

alpha and beta mRNA in the rat midbrain. *Neuroscience Letters, 275,* 21–24.

Raisman, G., & Field, P. M. (1971). Sexual dimorphism in the preoptic area of the rat. *Science, 173,* 731–733.

Raisman, G., & Field, P .M. (1973). Sexual dimorphism in the neuropil of the preoptic area of the rat and its dependence on neonatal androgen. *Brain Research, 54,* 1–29.

Rasia-Filho, A. A., Fabian, C., Rigoti, K. M., & Achaval, M. (2004). Influence of sex, estrous cycle and motherhood on dendritic spine density in the rat medial amygdala revealed by the Golgi method. *Neuroscience, 126,* 839–847.

Ravizza, T., Galanopoulou, A. S., Veliskova, J., & Moshe, S. L. (2002). Sex differences in androgen and estrogen receptor expression in rat substantia nigra during development: An immunohistochemical study. *Neuroscience, 115,* 685–696.

Raynaud, J. P., Mercier-Bodard, C., & Baulieu, E. E. (1971). Rat estradiol binding plasma protein (EBP). *Steroids, 18,* 767–788.

Reznikov, A. G., & Nosenko, N. D. (1995). Catecholamines in steroid-dependent brain development. *Journal of Steroid Biochemistry and Molecular Biology, 53,* 349–353.

Reznikov, A. G., Nosenko, N. D., & Tarasenko, L. V. (1999). Prenatal stress and glucocorticoid effects on the developing gender-related brain. *Journal of Steroid Biochemistry and Molecular Biology, 69,* 109–115.

Rhees, R. W., Shryne, J. E., & Gorski, R. A. (1990a). Onset of the hormone-sensitive perinatal period for sexual differentiation of the sexually dimorphic nucleus of the preoptic area in female rats. *Journal of Neurobiology, 21,* 781–786.

Rhees, R. W., Shryne, J. E., & Gorski, R. A. (1990b). Termination of the hormone-sensitive period for differentiation of the sexually dimorphic nucleus of the preoptic area in male and female rats. *Developmental Brain Research, 52,* 17–23.

Rhoda, J., Corbier, P., & Roffi, J. (1984). Gonadal steroid concentrations in serum and hypothalamus of the rat at birth: aromatization of testosterone to 17 beta-estradiol. *Endocrinology, 114,* 1754–1760.

Rissman, E. F., Wersinger, S. R., Taylor, J. A., & Lubahn, D. B. (1997). Estrogen receptor function as revealed by knockout studies: neuroendocrine and behavioral aspects. *Hormones and Behavior, 31,* 232–243.

Romeo, R. D., Diedrich, S. L., & Sisk, C. L. (2000). Effects of gonadal steroids during pubertal development on androgen and estrogen receptor-alpha immunoreactivity in the hypothalamus and amygdala. *Journal of Neurobiology, 44,* 361–368.

Rosenberg, K. M. (1974). Effects of pre- and postpubertal castration and testosterone on pup-killing behavior in the male rat. *Physiology & Behavior, 13*(1), 159–161.

Rosenberg, K. M., Denenberg, V. H., Zarrow, M. X., & Frank, B. L. (1971). Effects of neonatal castration and testosterone on the rat's pup-killing behavior and activity. *Physiology and Behavior, 7,* 363–368.

Rosenberg, K. M., & Sherman, G. F. (1974). Testosterone induced pup-killing behavior in the ovariectomized female rat. *Physiology and Behavior, 13,* 697–699.

Rosenberg, K. M., & Sherman, G. F. (1975). Influence of testosterone on pup killing in the rat is modified by prior experience. *Physiology and Behavior, 15,* 669–672.

Rosenberg, P. A., & Herrenkohl, L. R. (1976). Maternal behavior in male rats: critical times for the suppressive action of androgens. *Physiology and Behavior, 16,* 293–297.

Rosenblatt, J. S. (1967). Nonhormonal basis of maternal behavior in the rat. *Science, 156*, 1512–1514.

Rosenblatt, J. S., Hazelwood, S., & Poole, J. (1996). Maternal behavior in male rats: Effects of medial preoptic area lesions and presence of maternal aggression. *Hormones and Behavior, 30*, 201–215.

Rossi, G. L., Bestetti, G. E., Reymond, M. J., & Lemarchand-Beraud, T. (1991). Morphofunctional study of the effects of fetal exposure to cyproterone acetate on the hypothalamo-pituitary-gonadal axis of adult rats. *Experimental Brain Research, 83*, 349–356.

Royster, M., Driscoll, P., Kelly, P. A., & Freemark, M. (1995). The prolactin receptor in the fetal rat: Cellular localization of messenger ribonucleic acid, immunoreactive protein, and ligand-binding activity and induction of expression in late gestation. *Endocrinology, 136*, 3892–3900.

Sakamoto, H., Shikimi, H., Ukena, K., & Tsutsui, K. (2003). Neonatal expression of progesterone receptor isoforms in the cerebellar Purkinje cell in rats. *Neuroscience Letters, 343*, 163–166.

Samuels, M. H., & Bridges, R. S. (1983). Plasma prolactin concentrations in parental male and female rats: Effects of exposure to rat young. *Endocrinology, 113*, 1647–1654.

Sato, T., Matsumoto, T., Kawano, H., Watanabe, T., Uematsu, Y., Sekine, K., et al. (2004) Brain masculinization requires androgen receptor function. *Proceedings of the National Academy of Science, USA, 101*, 1673–1678.

Schulz, K. M., Menard, T. A., Smith, D. A., Albers, H. E., & Sisk, C. L. (2006). Testicular hormone exposure during adolescence organizes flank-marking behavior and vasopressin receptor binding in the lateral septum. *Hormones and Behavior, 50*, 477–483.

Schulz, K. M., & Sisk, C. L. (2006). Pubertal hormones, the adolescent brain, and the maturation of social behaviors: Lessons from the Syrian hamster. *Molecular and Cellular Endocrinology, 254–255*, 120–126.

Scott, J. P., Stewart, J. M., & De Ghett, V. J. (1974). Critical periods in the organization of systems. *Developmental Psychobiology, 7*, 489–513.

Scott, W. J., & Holson, J. F. (1977). Weight differences in rat embryos prior to sexual differentiation. *Journal of Embryology and Experimental Morphology, 40*, 259–263.

Seeman, M. V. (1997). Psychopathology in women and men: focus on female hormones. *American Journal of Psychiatry, 154*, 1641–1647.

Segarra, A. C., & McEwen, B. S. (1991). Estrogen increases spine density in ventromedial hypothalamic neurons of peripubertal rats. *Neuroendocrinology, 54*, 365–372.

Shapiro, L. E., Leonard, C. M., Sessions, C. E., Dewsbury, D. A., & Insel, T. R. (1991). Comparative neuroanatomy of the sexually dimorphic hypothalamus in monogamous and polygamous voles. *Brain Research, 541*, 232–240.

Sherry, D. F., Galef, B. G., & Clark, M. M. (1996). Sex and intrauterine position influence the size of the gerbil hippocampus. *Physiology and Behavior, 60*, 1491–1494.

Shibata, H., Spencer, T. E., Onate, S. A., Jenster, G., Tsai, S. Y., Tsai, M. J., et al. (1997). Role of co-activators and co-repressors in the mechanism of steroid/thyroid receptor action. *Recent Progress in Hormones Research, 52*, 141–164.

Shughrue, P. J., & Dorsa, D. M. (1994). Estrogen and androgen differentially modulate the growth-associated protein GAP-43 (neuromodulin) messenger ribonucleic acid in postnatal rat brain. *Endocrinology, 134*, 1321–1328.

Simerly, R. B. (1989). Hormonal control of the development and regulation of tyrosine hydroxylase expression within a sexually dimorphic population of dopaminergic cells in the hypothalamus. *Molecular Brain Research, 6*, 297–310.

Simerly, R. B., Swanson, L. W., & Gorski, R. A. (1985). The distribution of monoaminergic cells and fibers in a periventricular preoptic nucleus involved in the control of gonadotropin release: Immunohistochemical evidence for a dopaminergic sexual dimorphism. *Brain Research, 330*, 55–64.

Sisk, C. L., Schulz, K. M., & Zehr, J. L. (2003). Puberty: A finishing school for male social behavior. *Annals of the New York Academy of Science, 1007*, 189–198.

Slob, A. K., Ooms, M. P., & Vreeburg, J. T. (1980). Prenatal and early postnatal sex differences in plasma and gonadal testosterone and plasma luteinizing hormone in female and male rats. *Journal of Endocrinology, 87*, 81–87.

Smale, L., Nelson, R. J., & Zucker, I. (1985). Neuroendocrine responsiveness to oestradiol and male urine in neonatally androgenized prairie voles (*Microtus ochrogaster*). *Journal of Reproduction and Fertility, 74*, 491–496.

Smeaton, T. C., Arcondoulis, D. E., & Steele, P. A. (1975). The synthesis of testosterone and estradiol-17beta by the gonads of neonatal rats in vitro. *Steroids, 261*, 181–192.

Snijdewint, F. G., Van Leeuwen, F. W., Boer, G. J. (1989). Ontogeny of vasopressin and oxytocin binding sites in the brain of Wistar and Brattleboro rats as demonstrated by light microscopical autoradiography. *Journal of Chemical Neuroanatomy, 2*, 3–17.

Sodersten, P. (1978). Effects of anti-oestrogen treatment of neonatal male rats on lordosis behaviour and mounting behaviour in the adult. *Journal of Endocrinology, 76*, 241–249.

Södersten, P., Pettersson, A., & Eneroth, P. (1983). Pulse administration of estradiol-17 beta cancels sex difference in behavioral estrogen sensitivity. *Endocrinology, 112*, 1883–1885.

Solum, D. T., & Handa, R. J. (2001). Localization of estrogen receptor alpha (ER alpha) in pyramidal neurons of the developing rat hippocampus. *Developmental Brain Research, 128*, 165–175.

Staudt, J., & Dorner, G. (1976). Structural changes in the medial and central amygdala of the male rat, following neonatal castration and androgen treatment. *Endokrinologie, 67*, 296–300.

Stern, J. M. (1991). Nursing posture is elicited rapidly in maternally naive, haloperidol-treated female and male rats in response to ventral trunk stimulation from active pups. *Hormones and Behavior, 25*, 504–517.

Sugiyama, N., Kanba, S., & Arita, J. (2003). Temporal changes in the expression of brain-derived neurotrophic factor mRNA in the ventromedial nucleus of the hypothalamus of the developing rat brain. *Molecular Brain Research, 115*, 69–77.

Sumida, H., Nishizuka, M., Kano, Y., & Arai, Y. (1993). Sex differences in the anteroventral periventricular nucleus of the preoptic area and in the related effects of androgen in prenatal rats. *Neuroscience Letters, 151*, 41–44.

Swaab, D. F., & Fliers, E. (1985). A sexually dimorphic nucleus in the human brain. *Science, 228*, 1112–1115.

Tate-Ostroff, B. A., & Bridges, R. S. (1988). Nipple development and pup-induced prolactin release in male rats treated prenatally with the antiandrogen flutamide. *Psychoneuroendocrinology, 13*, 309–316.

Temple, J. L., Scordalakes, E. M., Bodo, C., Gustafsson, J.A., & Rissman, E. F. (2003). Lack of functional estrogen receptor beta gene disrupts pubertal male sexual behavior. *Hormones and Behavior, 44,* 427–434.

Thor, D. H., & Holloway, W. R. (1986). Social play soliciting by male and female juvenile rats: Effects of neonatal androgenization and sex of cagemates. *Behavioral Neuroscience, 100,* 275–279.

Tobet, S.A. (2002). Genes controlling hypothalamic development and sexual differentiation. *European Journal of Neuroscience, 16,* 373–376.

Tobet, S. A., Baum, M. J., Tang, H. B., Shim, J. H., & Canick, J. A. (1985). Aromatase activity in the perinatal rat forebrain: effects of age, sex and intrauterine position. *Brain Research, 355,* 171–178.

Tobet, S. A., Zahniser, D. J., & Baum, M. J. (1986). Differentiation in male ferrets of a sexually dimorphic nucleus of the preoptic/anterior hypothalamic area requires prenatal estrogen. *Neuroendocrinology, 44,* 299–308.

Todd, B. J., Schwarz, J. M., & McCarthy, M. M. (2005). Prostaglandin-E2: A point of divergence in estradiol-mediated sexual differentiation. *Hormones and Behavior, 48,* 512–521.

Tonjes, R., Docke, F., & Dorner, G. (1987). Effects of neonatal intracerebral implantation of sex steroids on sexual behaviour, social play behaviour and gonadotrophin secretion. *Experimental and Clinical Endocrinology, 90,* 257–263.

Tonjes, R., Gotz, F., Maywald, J., & Dorner, G. (1989). Influence of a dopamine agonist (lisuride) on sex-specific behavioural patterns in rats. II. Long-term effects. *Experimental and Clinical Endocrinology, 94,* 48–54.

Tora, L., Gronemeyer, H., Turcotte, B., Gaub, M-P., & Chambon, P. (1988). The N-terminal region of the chicken progesterone receptor specifies target gene activation. *Nature, 333,* 185–188.

Turner, J. W. (1975). Influence of neonatal androgen on the display of territorial marking behavior in the gerbil. *Physiology and Behavior, 15,* 265–270.

Udry, J. R., Morris, N. M., & Kovenock, J. (1995). Androgen effects on women's gendered behaviour. *Journal of Biosocial Science, 27,* 359–368.

Ulibarri, C., & Yahr, P. (1988). Role of neonatal androgens in sexual differentiation of brain structure, scent marking, and gonadotropin secretion in gerbils. *Behavioral and Neural Biology, 49,* 27–44.

Ulibarri, C. M., & Yahr, P. (1993). Ontogeny of the sexually dimorphic area of the gerbil hypothalamus. *Developmental Brain Research, 74,* 14–24.

Ulibarri, C., & Yahr, P. (1996). Effects of androgens and estrogens on sexual differentiation of sex behavior, scent marking, and the sexually dimorphic area of the gerbil hypothalamus. *Hormones and Behavior, 30,* 107–130.

Van der Schoot, P. (1980). Effects of dihydrotestosterone and oestradiol on sexual differentiation in male rats. *Journal of Endocrinology, 84,* 397–407.

Van der Schoot, P., & Baumgarten, R. (1990). Effects of treatment of male and female rats in infancy with mifepristone on reproductive function in adulthood. *Journal of Reproduction and Fertility, 90,* 255–66.

Vanderschuren, L. J., Niesink, R. J., & Van Ree, J. M. (1997). The neurobiology of social play behavior in rats. *Neuroscience and Biobehavioral Reviews, 21,* 309–326.

Viglietti-Panzica, C., Panzica, G. C., Fiori, M. G., Calcagni, M., Anselmetti. G. C., & Balthazart, J. A. (1986). Sexually dimorphic nucleus in the quail preoptic area. *Neuroscience Letters, 64,* 129–134.

Vinader-Caerols, C., Collado, P., Segovia, S., & Guillamon, A. (1998). Sex differences in the posteromedial cortical nucleus of the amygdala in the rat. *Neuroreport, 9,* 2653–2656.

Vinader-Caerols, C., Collado, P., Segovia, S., & Guillamon, A. (2000). Estradiol masculinizes the posteromedial cortical nucleus of the amygdala in the rat. *Brain Research Bulletin, 53,* 269–73.

Vito, C. C., Wieland, S. J., & Fox, T.O. (1979). Androgen receptors exist throughout the "critical period" of brain sexual differentiation. *Nature, 282,* 308–310.

Vomachka, A. J., & Lisk, R. D. (1986). Androgen and estradiol levels in plasma and amniotic fluid of late gestational male and female hamsters: uterine position effects. *Hormones and Behavior, 20,* 181–193.

Vom Saal, F. S. (1989). Sexual differentiation in litter-bearing mammals: influence of sex of adjacent fetuses in utero. *Journal of Animal Science, 67,* 1824–40.

Vreeburg, J. T., Van der Vaart, P. D., & Van der Schoot, P. (1977). Prevention of central defeminization but not masculinization in male rats by inhibition neonatally of oestrogen biosynthesis. *Journal of Endocrinology, 74,* 375–382.

Wade, J., & Arnold, A. P. (2004). Sexual differentiation of the zebra finch song system. *Annals of the New York Academy of Science, 1016,* 540–559.

Wagner, C. K., Nakayama, A. Y., & De Vries, G. J. (1998). Potential role of maternal progesterone in the sexual differentiation of the brain. *Endocrinology, 139,* 3658–3661.

Wagner, C. K., Xu, J., Pfau, J. L., Quadros, P. S., De Vries, G. J.,& Arnold, A. P. (2004). Neonatal mice possessing an *Sry* transgene show a masculinized pattern of progesterone receptor expression in the brain independent of sex chromosome status. *Endocrinology, 145,* 1046–1049.

Wallen, K. (2005). Hormonal influences on sexually differentiated behavior in nonhuman primates. *Frontiers in Neuroendocrinology, 26,* 7–26.

Wallen, K., & Baum, M. J. (2002). Masculinization and defeminization in altricial and precocial mammals: Comparative aspects of steroid hormone action. In: D. W. Pfaff, A. P. Arnold, A. M. Etgen, S. E. Fahrbach, & R. T. Rubin (Eds.), *Hormones, brain and behavior* (Vol. IV, chap. 63, pp. 385–423). New York: Academic Press.

Walters, M. R. (1985). Steroid hormone receptors and the nucleus. *Endocrine Reviews, 6,* 512–543.

Wang, Z., Smith ,W., Major, D. E., & De Vries, G. J. (1994). Sex and species differences in the effects of cohabitation on vasopressin messenger RNA expression in the bed nucleus of the stria terminalis in prairie voles (*Microtus ochrogaster*) and meadow voles (*Microtus pennsylvanicus*). *Brain Research, 650,* 212–218.

Ward, I. L. (1972). Prenatal stress feminizes and demasculinizes the behavior of males. *Science, 175,* 82–84.

Ward, I. L., Bennett, A. L., Ward, O. B., Hendricks, S. E., & French, J. A. (1999). Androgen threshold to activate copulation differs in male rats prenatally exposed to alcohol, stress, or both factors. *Hormones and Behavior, 36,* 129–140.

Ward, I. L., Ward, O. B., Winn, R. J., & Bielawski, D. (1994). Male and female sexual behavior potential of male rats prenatally exposed to the influence of alcohol, stress, or both factors. *Behavioral Neuroscience, 108,* 1188–1195.

Weinstein, M. A., Pleim, E. T., & Barfield, R. J. (1992). Effects of neonatal exposure to the antiprogestin mifepristone, RU 486, on the sexual development of the rat. *Pharmacology Biochemistry and Behavior, 41,* 69–74.

Weisz, J., & Gunsalus, P. (1973). Estrogen levels in immature female rats: true or spurious—ovarian or adrenal? *Endocrinology, 93,* 1057–65.

Weisz, J., & Ward, I. L. (1980). Plasma testosterone and progesterone titers of pregnant rats, their male and female fetuses, and neonatal offspring. *Endocrinology, 106,* 306–316.

Wekesa, K. S., & Vandenbergh, J. G. (1996). Androgen exposure and reproductive behavior of an induced ovulator, the pine vole (*Microtus pinetorum*). *Hormones and Behavior, 30,* 416–423.

Weniger, J. P., Zeis, A., & Chouraqui, J. (1993). Estrogen production by fetal and infantile rat ovaries. *Reproduction Nutrition and Development, 33,* 129–136.

Wersinger, S. R., Sannen, K., Villalba, C., Lubahn, D. B., Rissman, E. F., & De Vries, G. J. (1997). Masculine sexual behavior is disrupted in male and female mice lacking a functional estrogen receptor alpha gene. *Hormones and Behavior, 32,* 176–183.

Whalen, R. E., & Edwards, D. A. (1967). Hormonal determinants of the development of masculine and feminine behavior in male and female rats. *Anatomical Record, 157,* 173–180.

Whalen, R. E, Gladue, B. A., & Olsen, K. L. (1986). Lordotic behavior in male rats: Genetic and hormonal regulation of sexual differentiation. *Hormones and Behavior, 20,* 73–82.

Whalen, R. E., & Olsen, K. L. (1981). Role of aromatization in sexual differentiation: Effects of prenatal ATD treatment and neonatal castration. *Hormones and Behavior, 15,* 107–122.

Whalen, R. E., & Rezek, D. L. (1974). Inhibition of lordosis in female rats by subcutaneous implants of testosterone, androstenedione or dihydrotestosterone in infancy. *Hormones and Behaviour, 5,* 125–128.

White, J. O., Hall, C., & Lim, L. (1979). Developmental changes in the content of oestrogen receptors in the hypothalamus of the female rat. *Biochemical Journal, 184,* 465–468.

Witcher, J. A., & Clemens, L. G. (1987). A prenatal source for defeminization of female rats is the maternal ovary. *Hormones and Behavior, 21,* 36–43.

Wong, C. C., Poon, W. H., Tsim, T. Y., Wong, E. Y., & Leung, M. S. (2000). Gene expressions during the development and sexual differentiation of the olfactory bulb in rats. *Developmental Brain Research, 119,* 187–194.

Yahr, P. (1988). Pars compacta of the sexually dimorphic area of the gerbil hypothalamus: Postnatal ages at which development responds to testosterone. *Behavioral and Neural Biology, 49,* 118–124.

Yanase, M., Honmura, A., Akaishi, T., & Sakuma, Y. (1988). Nerve growth factor-mediated sexual differentiation of the rat hypothalamus. *Neuroscience Research, 6,* 181–185.

Yang, S. L., Chen, Y. Y., Hsieh, Y. L., Jin, S. H., Hsu, H. K., & Hsu, C. (2004). Perinatal androgenization prevents age-related neuron loss in the sexually dimorphic nucleus of the preoptic area in female rats. *Developmental Neuroscience, 26,* 54–60.

Yokosuka, M., Okamura, H., & Hayashi, S. (1997). Postnatal development and sex difference in neurons containing estrogen receptor-alpha immunoreactivity in the preoptic brain, the diencephalon, and the amygdala in the rat. *Journal of Comparative Neurology, 389,* 81–93.

Yoshida, M., Yuri, K., Kizaki, Z., Sawada, T., & Kawata, M. (2000). The distributions of apoptotic cells in the medial preoptic areas of male and female neonatal rats. *Neuroscience Research, 36,* 1–7.

Zhang, T. Y., Chrétien, P., Meaney, M. J., & Gratton, A. (2005). Influence of naturally occurring variations in maternal care on prepulse inhibition of acoustic startle and the medial prefrontal cortical dopamine response to stress in adult rats. *The Journal of Neuroscience, 25,* 1493–1502.

Zehr, J. L., Todd, B. J., Schulz, K. M., McCarthy, M. M., & Sisk, C. L. (2006). Dendritic pruning of the medial amygdala during pubertal development of the male Syrian hamster. *Journal of Neurobiology, 66,* 578–590.

Zsarnovszky, A., & Belcher, S. M. (2001). Identification of a developmental gradient of estrogen receptor expression and cellular localization in the developing and adult female rat primary somatosensory cortex. *Developmental Brain Research, 129,* 39–46.

Zup, S. L., & Forger, N. G. (2002). Hormones and sexual differentiation. In V. S. Ramachandran (Ed.), *Encyclopedia of the human brain* (pp. 323–341). New York: Academic Press.

Development of Ingestive Behavior: The Influence of Context and Experience on Sensory Signals Modulating Intake

Susan E. Swithers

Abstract

The meaning of sensory signals related to ingestive behavior is shaped during development by ongoing behavior and by previous experience. For example, orosensory signals that accrue during the act of ingestion may influence meal size and may determine the impact of other sensory signals (such as hormone release or stomach fill). In addition, pre- and postnatal exposure to sensory cues related to food and to the relationship between these sensory cues and their postingestive consequences may alter food preferences and the regulation of food intake and body weight into adulthood. Determining how sensory signals modulate ingestion thus requires attention to the environmental, experiential, and ontogenetic contexts in which they operate.

Keywords: ingestive behavior, orosensory signals, meal size, hormone release, stomach fill, food

Experience and Context in the Development of Ingestive Behavior

The control of food intake depends on sensory signals that come from multiple sources, including those related to aspects of the food itself (e.g., taste, smell, texture) and those related to the consequences of eating that food (e.g., stomach fill, hormone release). In addition, the meaning of one sensory signal (such as taste) can be influenced both by simultaneous presence of other sensory signals (such as stomach fill), and by the animal's previous experience with such signals. The goal of the present chapter is to highlight how a developmental approach to the study of ingestion can provide critical information on how experience with sensory signals, and the behavioral context in which these signals are experienced, can shape ongoing behavior, and how experiences during one developmental stage can influence behavior at later stages. In particular, I consider how orosensory signals that

accrue during the act of ingestion may both contribute to the control of meal size and determine the consequences of other sensory signals, demonstrating a role of behavioral context in the meaning of sensory signals. Further, the chapter considers how sensory signals that are experienced both before birth and during the early postnatal period can shape ingestion by (1) altering food choices and (2) modifying associations between the sensory properties of a diet and its consequences (hedonic and/ or caloric). These effects can occur even when such experiences occur outside of the behavioral context that characterizes adult ingestion. In addition, the function of different behavioral contexts is illustrated by consideration of signals that appear to modulate intake during the early postnatal period, but whose consequences are subsequently modified by additional developmental events. Finally, while examining the development of food intake is one approach that informs us about influences on intake in adult animals, examining the development of food intake in young animals is also important because we cannot understand how young animals regulate food intake and body weight, without examining them. Young animals are not simply miniature adult animals; behavioral, physiological, neural, and experiential differences at different developmental ages or stages significantly affect how ingestion is modulated. Appreciation of these differences is fundamental when circumstances require intervention in early development. As the prevalence of energy dysregulation in humans continues to increase at an alarming rate, particularly in children, an understanding of the factors that control development of ingestive behavior may provide the best hope for ameliorating or reversing the negative health consequences associated with overweight and obesity.

Tinbergen argued forcefully that a full explanation of behavior demands investigations at multiple levels of analysis, including consideration of both proximate and ultimate causes (Tinbergen, 1963). Proximate causes entail the immediate physiological, environmental, and neural mechanisms that contribute to behavioral outcomes, as well as factors that are directly related to the age and previous experience of an individual. Proximate explanations must themselves be considered in light of ultimate considerations: for example, how has the present behavior been shaped by evolutionary pressures and what previous and present adaptive and functional purposes might it serve? Thus, a broad approach that considers each of these "four causes" (mechanism, evolution, development, and function) is necessary to fully appreciate and articulate the forces that shape behavior. Ingestive behaviors—that is, behaviors that contribute to the acquisition and consumption of foods and fluids—are no exception to this rule.

Infant Rats: A Simple System for Studying Ingestion?

One of the guiding premises of the research reviewed here is that neonatal rats provide a convenient and relatively simple system for exploring the mechanisms that control ingestion. As altricial mammals, rats are born in an immature state—physically, physiologically, neurologically, and behaviorally. At birth, they are blind and furless, exhibit limited mobility, and have sealed ears. They display few complex behaviors, but are competent to locate and attach to the dam's nipples (Hall, Cramer, & Blass, 1975). Outside of the laboratory,

suckling, the signature mammalian ingestive behavior, is the sole mechanism by which rats obtain food and fluid for the first 2 weeks of postnatal life (Blass, Hall, & Teicher, 1979). By the start of the third postnatal week, rats begin to sample solid food and water, although suckling remains the preeminent ingestive behavior (Babicky, Ostadalova, Parizek, Kolar, & Bibr, 1973a; Babicky, Parizek, Ostadalova, & Kolar, 1973b). The frequency of suckling begins to decrease during the fourth and fifth postnatal weeks and by postnatal day (P) 30, suckling behavior has been replaced entirely by the independent ingestion of food and water.

These rapid transitions in ingestive behavior during the first several postnatal weeks provide an opportunity to relate emerging behavioral capacities to the development of physiological and neural systems. In early studies of suckling, the utility of such a developmental approach appeared to be borne out, as it appeared that neonatal rat pups possessed rudimentary controls over suckling behavior that became increasingly sophisticated and complex over time (e.g., Blass & Teicher, 1980). To study the development of controls of suckling, techniques that isolated the pup's capabilities and behaviors during suckling from those contributed by the dam were employed (e.g., Hall et al., 1975; Hall, Cramer, & Blass, 1977). Typically, dams were anesthetized and both attachment to the dam's nipples and extraction of milk by pups were assessed.

This work suggested that during the first postnatal week, attachment to the dam's nipples was a highly potent behavior, which occurred rapidly and was relatively independent of physiological state. For example, neonatal rats deprived of the opportunity to suckle (which deprives them of food, fluid, and sensory stimulation) attached to the nipple no more rapidly than did nondeprived pups. In addition, during the first 2 postnatal weeks, maintenance of suckling behavior once pups were attached was demonstrated to be independent of the rate of milk delivery. Very young pups (e.g., P5) remained attached to nipples for hours even when milk was not delivered (Hall et al., 1977), and P10 or younger pups did not stop suckling, even if they were virtually drowned by an artificially inflated volume of milk delivery (Hall & Rosenblatt, 1977, 1978). These results suggested that during the first postnatal week, controls of suckling are minimal; pups attach to the dam's nipple and remain attached independent of sensory or physiological signals. During the second postnatal week, controls of suckling become more sophisticated. For example, when deprived of the opportunity to suckle during the second postnatal week, the latency to attach was significantly faster in deprived compared to non-deprived pups. This effect was principally due to removal of sensory stimulation related to suckling rather than physiological or nutritional deprivation, since pups that attached to the nipples of nonlactating females during deprivation (which provided the tactile, thermal, and other sensory properties of the dam, but not hydration or nutrition) eliminated the differences in the latency to attach. Not until after P20 do internal physiological signals related to nutritional deprivation appear to influence the latency to attach (e.g., Hall et al., 1977; Henning, Chang, & Gisel, 1979; Lorenz, Ellis, & Epstein, 1982). These data suggested that for neonatal rats, physiological signals that typically play a role in modulating ingestion in adults (e.g., food deprivation, stomach fill) have little impact on ingestion in the context of suckling. Thus, rats appear to be born with relatively simple controls of intake and these controls develop further over the first several postnatal weeks.

However, assessing the development of these controls is complicated, as suckling (like other motivated behaviors) does not represent a single unitary behavior, but instead requires the performance of a sequence of both appetitive and consummatory responses (Craig, 1913). In the case of suckling, these appetitive behaviors include locating, identifying, approaching, and attaching to the dam's nipples. Consummatory responses are behaviors that consummate the appetitive sequence; in the case of suckling and other ingestive behaviors, these consummatory responses also result in consumption of a commodity (i.e., milk). Thus, when considering suckling, and other ingestive behaviors, it is critical to appreciate the particular behavioral components under examination. Sensory signals that influence appetitive responses may differ from those that influence consummatory response. In fact, the results described above indicate that internal physiological signals (including nutritional deprivation and gastric fill) have little impact on appetitive aspects of suckling behavior (including the latency to initiate suckling and the maintenance of nipple attachment) until as late as the third postnatal week (e.g., Blass, 1990; Brake, Shair, & Hofer, 1988; Friedman, 1975; Houpt & Epstein, 1973; Houpt & Houpt, 1975; see Table 22.1). In contrast, several studies from multiple laboratories have demonstrated that physiological signals can

Table 22.1 Effects of Selected Stimuli on Appetitive and Consummatory Responses Related to Suckling and Independent Ingestion

Stimulus	Age	Context	Outcome
Deprivation (food, fluids, sensory signals)	<10 days	Suckling	No effect on appetitive behavior (latency to attach, maintenance of attachment)
Olfactory and tactile deprivation	10+ days	Suckling	Increased appetitive behavior (decreased latency to attach)
Deprivation (food, fluids)	Birth	Independent ingestion	Increased appetitive and consummatory behavior (decreased latency to initiate intake, amount consumed)
	< 20 days	Suckling	No effect on appetitive behavior (latency to attach)
	20+ days	Suckling	Increased appetitive behavior (decreased latency to attach)
CCK	1+ days	Exogenous administration—independent ingestion	Decreased consummatory behavior (amount consumed)
	2+ days	Receptor deletion—independent ingestion	Increased appetitive behavior (decreased latency) and consummatory behavior (amount consumed)
	<15 days	Exogenous administration—suckling	No effect on appetitive or consummatory behavior
	15+ days	Exogenous administration—suckling	No effect on appetitive behavior; decreased consummatory behavior (rate and vigor of suckling activity, amount consumed)

CCK, cholecystokinin.

modulate consummatory behaviors. For example, when allowed to suckle after a period of deprivation, deprived pups consume larger volumes of milk from the nipple than do nondeprived pups (Houpt & Epstein, 1973). In addition, young pups modulate intake at the nipple in response to gastric preloads, with both the volume and the composition of the preload influencing the amount of milk consumed (Houpt & Epstein, 1973; Houpt & Houpt, 1975).

Subsequent work suggested that regulation of intake at the nipple is accomplished by alterations in both the rate and vigor of suckling behavior. To demonstrate this, techniques were developed to record electomyographic activity from the digastric muscle (which controls jaw opening and tongue support) and intraoral pressure within the pup's mouth during suckling. Using this method, several distinct patterns of suckling activity were identified (Brake et al., 1988; Brake, Sager, Sullivan, & Hofer, 1982). These patterns were termed rapid rhythmic suckling (RRS), slow rhythmic suckling (SRS), and arrhythmic suckling (ARS). Each of these patterns appears to have a distinct relationship to milk availability. In rats, milk is not continuously released during suckling, but instead is let down in brief 10-s bursts separated by varying intervals of 5–20 min (Wakerley & Drewett, 1975; Wakerly & Lincoln, 1971). Thus, although young rats spend most of their time (i.e., 70%–80%; Plaut, 1974) attached to the nipples and suckling, for much of this time no milk is available and, during these periods, ARS is observed exclusively. In contrast, RRS is observed most frequently during milk delivery and when pups first attach to nipples, and SRS is displayed during the intervals between milk deliveries. Thus, changes in RRS may result in alterations in amount of milk consumed, whereas alterations in SRS may contribute to changes in maternal stimulation that influence milk letdown.

A variety of experiments suggested that pups regulate milk intake from the nipple by altering the proportion of time spent in RS (both RRS and SRS; see Brake et al., 1988, for review). For example, increasing deprivation produced increased amounts of SRS and RRS. In addition, deprived pups given a gastric preload prior to a suckling test show significantly lower levels of SRS for shorter durations compared to deprived pups that are not given preloads. Thus, from very young ages, rat pups appear to be able to adjust consummatory suckling behaviors to modulate intake in response to physiological challenges such as deprivation and stomach fill, whereas appetitive responses are unaffected by such physiological signals.

The precise mechanisms that influence intake during suckling remain unknown, but a number of candidate mechanisms have been examined. For example, the gut peptide, cholecystokinin (CCK), is released during food consumption, and a role for CCK in the modulation of food intake in adult rats is now well accepted: administration of exogenous CCK reduces food intake, stimulation of endogenous CCK release suppresses food intake, and administration of CCK antagonists increases food intake (e.g., Smith & Gibbs, 1975, 1985; Smith et al., 1981). Further, a spontaneous CCK-receptor deletion results in animals (OLETF rats) that are bigger, fatter, and consume larger meals than rats from the background control strain (LETO; e.g., Moran & Bi, 2006a).

Similarly, a large body of work on CCK suggests that early in development in rats, release of CCK provides a signal that can lead to the termination of food intake, an effect that is at least partly due to CCK's effects on gastric emptying (reviewed in Weller, 2006). In addition, developmental work indicates that OLETF pups are larger than LETO pups and the lack of CCK receptors may contribute to their greater milk intake during suckling (e.g., Blumberg, Haba, Schroeder, Smith, & Weller, 2006; Moran & Bi, 2006b; Schroeder et al., 2007; Schroeder, Zagoory-Sharon, Lavi-Avnon, Moran, & Weller, 2006). Despite this evidence, administration of exogenous CCK has not been demonstrated to modulate consummatory behavior in the context of suckling until at least 15 days of age (Blass, Beardsley, & Hall, 1979). This dissociation between the consequences of endogenous release of CCK and exogenous administration provides an illustration of an additional critical aspect of understanding the control of ingestive behavior. Signals, such as those produced by CCK, do not operate in isolation, but are interpreted in the context of ongoing ingestive behavior. For example, in adult rats, exogenous administration of CCK is more effective at reducing food intake if it is given while animals are actually eating (i.e., contingent with oral stimulation) compared with administration that occurs prior to the initiation of food intake (e.g., Forsyth, Weingarten, & Collins, 1985; Shillabeer & Davison, 1987; West et al., 1987). Thus, because milk letdowns during suckling are not continuous, it is likely that the failure of exogenous administration of CCK to affect suckling intake may reflect the temporal dissociation between the administration of the drug and the availability of milk during suckling. The ongoing consummatory responses may be necessary for the physiological signals produced by CCK to influence behavior.

Is Suckling Feeding?

The developing control of ingestive behavior in pups can be described as the emergence of an increasingly sophisticated system to modulate both appetitive and consummatory responses to physiological signals. However, such a notion must be tempered by questions that pertain to all developmental approaches: To what extent is the pup's behavior continuous with the similar behavior that is displayed in adults? With regard to the current topic, although suckling represents the method by which infant rats typically acquire food and fluids, does it in fact represent the developmental precursor to adult ingestion? Does understanding how rats modulate appetitive and consummatory aspects of suckling behavior inform us about how the controls of food and fluid intake function in adults?

Questions about developmental continuity in ingestive behaviors have been underscored by work that identified an alternative method for eliciting intake that is independent of the dam and the suckling situation even in neonatal rats. In these studies, neonatal animals that were separated from the dam and were provided with liquid diets would readily consume them. This behavior has been referred to as "independent ingestion" because it occurs independent of the dam and the context of suckling. Further, based on differences in response topography, external and internal controls, neural substrates, and experiential determinants, it has been argued, and generally accepted, that it is independent ingestion, rather than suckling, that represents the developmental precursor to adult intake (for review, see Hall & Williams, 1983; Smith, 2006).

Suckling, then, is an example of a behavior that is an "ontogenetic adaptation," that is, a behavior that is specialized and adapted to the capacities and demands of a particular developmental stage (e.g., Oppenheim, 1981; West, King, & Arberg, 1988). For example, the pup's challenge is to maximize the amount of milk obtained to support rapid and maximal growth. The pup accomplishes this by demonstrating a prepotent tendency to remain attached to the nipple even in the face of overwhelming quantities of milk, and to increase the rate and vigor with which it suckles in response to periods of deprivation. At the same time, there is little threat of overconsumption—and therefore little need for inhibitory mechanisms—as the amount of milk available is strongly limited by the dam's resources. In fact, the critical role of the dam's milk availability in modulating the pup's growth is clearly demonstrated by the profound acceleration of growth in pups reared in small compared to large litters (e.g., Babicky et al., 1973b). And, even in small litters, inhibitory mechanisms appear unnecessary as the increase in the supply of milk is not limitless, but remains constrained by the dam at higher levels.

The goal of suckling, then, may be to permit pups to maximize growth within a context that also provides thermal and social interactions with the dam and littermates. The mechanisms that have evolved to promote this goal need not be continuous with those that subsequently modulate ingestion independent of the dam. Note that these mechanisms need not be discontinuous either; some signals may modulate intake in multiple contexts. For example, gastric fill suppresses consummatory behavior both during suckling and independent ingestion from very early ages (Houpt & Epstein, 1973; Phifer, Sikes, & Hall, 1986). Thus, while some signals may differentially modulate suckling intake and independent ingestion, others may produce similar outcomes in both contexts.

Ongoing Experience and Ingestive Control

A principal advantage of studying independent ingestion in young rats is that it provides an opportunity to examine adult-like ingestive behavior in animals in which the physiological and neural systems that underlie its control may be simpler, and more easily identified and understood. Further, because young rats have relatively limited experience with the sensory properties of foods and their consequences, examining food intake in young rats has been considered an approach in determining how physiological signals operate in the absence of significant effects of previous experience (although see below for an alternative perspective). A variety of work, including work from our laboratory, examining the development of controls of independent ingestion has documented physiological signals (such as gastric fill) that can modulate appetitive and consummatory responses in young rats, and has described how signals that have little effect at early ages become functionally significant during the first several weeks of postnatal life (reviewed in Smith, 2006).

Among the conclusions that can be drawn from such work is that even in neonatal rats, the sensory signals that arise from ongoing ingestive behavior have a significant influence on the meaning of physiological signals. To illustrate, in adult animals, it has long been known that increasing the variety of foods available within a meal results in increased intake. While this phenomenon has been termed sensory-specific satiety in the clinical literature, work in young rats has suggested that one mechanism that may underlie this variety effect is habituation to the orosensory properties of a diet, such as its taste, smell, and/or texture (e.g., Swithers & Hall, 1994). Young rats given oral infusions of flavored diets in which the postingestive consequences (such as calories and stomach fill) were minimized showed significant decreases in ingestive responses to the specific flavored diet over the course of a testing session. Ingestive responsiveness could be restored by switching the flavor of the diet offered. More importantly, no decreases in ingestive responding were observed when the same infusions were delivered directly into the stomach; rats needed to experience the flavors orally for their behavior to be affected. In addition, when infusions into the stomach were combined with infusions in the mouth, greater effects were seen compared to infusions made into the mouth or stomach alone (Swithers-Mulvey & Hall, 1993). Thus, the consequences of both oral experience with a diet and the gastric fill that occurs as diets are consumed appear to interact. Stomach fill alone does not suppress intake (although the amount of stomach fill was designed to be minimal), oral experience alone does result in decreased intake, but oral experience combined with gastric fill results in significantly greater reductions in ingestive behavior.

Thus, ongoing oral experience may be a component necessary for appropriate modulation of intake, either by providing a context in which physiological signals can be interpreted or by stimulating subsequent physiological responses that interact to regulate ingestion (e.g., cephalic phase response, see below). The role of such interaction between ongoing ingestion and postingestive consequences mirrors the enhanced effects of CCK on intake when CCK administration is contingent with oral stimulation described above (e.g., Forsyth et al., 1985; Shillabeer & Davison, 1987; West et al., 1987). Finally, there is some evidence that when the stomach is filled in the absence of oral stimulation, intake may be artificially suppressed. For example, one mechanism for filling the stomach in the absence of oral stimulation is by delivering liquid diets through a gavage tube placed into the stomach. Using such methods, rat pups have been demonstrated to show decreased independent ingestion in response to stomach fill from very young ages (Phifer et al., 1986). An alternative method is to use an oral cannula to infuse a diet directly into the back of a pup's mouth. Using this procedure, the pup receives stimulation of the oral cavity (e.g., taste, smell, and texture), but reflexively swallows the diet ensuring that similar amounts of gastric fill are produced. Under these circumstances, gastric fill was demonstrated to have limited influence on intake even in pups at P15 (Davis, Doerflinger, McCurley, & Swithers, 2003). Taken together, these data argue that the consequences of physiological signals, like stomach fill or release of hormones, depends on the animal's current, ongoing behavior; a stomach that fills during a meal has greater consequences for intake than a stomach that fills when no eating has occurred.

Long-Term Consequences of Experience on Ingestive Controls

Identifying development of particular physiological and neural substrates that underlie the modulation of ongoing appetitive and consummatory responses during a meal (either suckling or independent ingestion) is one approach that may contribute to understanding the modulation of appetitive and consummatory responses during adult ingestion. However, equally important is understanding the impact of experiences that occur during the suckling period, and in fact, even during prenatal life, on adult ingestion and body weight regulation; the influence of such experience is considered here.

Tastes, Flavors, Experiences, and Preferences

Beginning at birth, humans and rats exposed to a variety of tastants exhibit "preference" or "acceptance" responses to sweet tastants and "rejection" responses to bitter, sour, salty, and other unfamiliar tastants (Desor, Maller, & Andrews, 1975; Ganchrow, Steiner, & Canetto, 1986; Hall & Bryan, 1981; Maller & Desor, 1973; Nowlis & Kessen, 1976; Petrov, Varlinskaya, & Spear, 2001; Rosenstein & Oster, 1988). Because of the early expression of these seemingly "innate" responses, a significant role for genetic influences has been inferred.

To the extent that "innate" is used to imply "present at birth" and, therefore, "independent of previous experience," such terminology is misleading. Indeed, a variety of direct and indirect evidence supports a significant influence of in utero experiences on neonatal ingestive responses. First, during the prenatal period, amniotic fluid bathes the oral cavity, and humans and other animals show evidence of active swallowing of amniotic fluid in utero (e.g., Brace, 1997; Ross & Nijland, 1997, 1998). Second, it is well established that the ability to detect and respond to changes in the sensory (olfactory and/or tastant) qualities of amniotic fluid develops prenatally; for example, in prenatal sheep, in utero infusions of sucrose solutions result in significant increases in swallowing behavior (El-Haddad, Ismail, Guerra, Day, & Ross, 2002). Third, it is also clear that the chemical composition of amniotic fluid is influenced by maternal diet, thus the sensory properties of the amniotic fluid reflect the sensory properties of the maternal diet (Friesen & Innis, 2006; Gurekian & Koski, 2005); alterations of the maternal diet may lead to altered flavor experiences in utero. Thus, it is clear that animals experience flavors in utero, and that these flavors vary based on maternal diet, thereby providing a potential source of information about odors, tastes, and their consequences before their first encounters with foods after birth.

That these prenatal experiences do actually influence ingestive responses postnatally has also been demonstrated. For example, in utero exposure of rats to flavors such as alcohol, cineole, apple, garlic, or onion result in either increases in positive orosensory reactivity or decreases in negative reactivity (e.g., Abate, Varlinskaya, Cheslock, Spear, & Molina, 2002; Chotro, Arias, & Laviola, 2007; Dominguez, Lopez, & Molina, 1998; Hepper, 1988; Schaal & Orgeur, 1992; Smotherman, 1982; Wuensch, 1978). Similarly, work in humans has documented increased preference responses for flavor cues experienced only in utero, including preferences for the odor of amniotic fluid or breast milk over the odor of formula in formula-fed infants (Marlier & Schaal, 2005; Marlier, Schaal, & Soussignan, 1998) and increased preference for carrot-flavored foods in infants whose mothers had consumed carrot juice prenatally (Mennella, Jagnow, & Beauchamp, 2001). Prenatal sensory experiences have the capacity to shape ingestive preferences exhibited during the early postnatal period. Note that these preferences need not be expressed in terms of intake during suckling, but instead may result in altered reactivity to diets offered in the context of independent ingestion. That is, prenatal exposures can have influences on ingestion that may not manifest themselves until

well after the experiences have occurred. As a result, simply examining food preferences in adult animals can ignore significant sources of influence. Understanding food preference and food choice demands a developmental approach.

Further, prenatal flavor exposures are likely reinforced by postnatal experience in both rats and breast-fed humans, since there is ample evidence that sensory cues from the maternal diet are readily transferred through maternal milk (Mennella, 1995; Mennella & Beauchamp, 2005; Mennella, Griffin, & Beauchamp, 2004). Such postnatal dietary cues also influence subsequent dietary preferences, with both rats and humans typically demonstrating increased preference and/or intake of diets containing flavors similar to those in the maternal diet (Galef & Henderson, 1972; Galef & Sherry, 1973; Mennella, 1995; Mennella et al., 2004). In addition, in formula-fed infants, flavor preferences are altered by the composition of the formula; human infants that consume hydrolysate or soy-based formulas (which are characterized by increased sourness and bitterness relative to milk-based formulas) subsequently show enhanced preference for sour and bitter tastes and altered acceptance of solid foods with different flavor profiles (e.g., Mennella & Beauchamp, 2005; Mennella, Kennedy, & Beauchamp, 2006).

These findings indicate that one mechanism by which flavors experienced in the context of the uterine environment or suckling may influence subsequent ingestive behavior is by altering dietary preferences (see above, Table 22.2). That is, increased preference or acceptance of flavors experienced prenatally or postnatally may contribute to increased propensity to consume such diets during the early postnatal period. But the consequences of these early dietary experiences can be influenced by the context in which they are encountered. For example, human infants whose mothers consume alcohol during times of stress actually show an aversion to the odor of alcohol, whereas the odor of alcohol is neutral or preferred in infants when maternal consumption is not associated with stress (Mennella & Garcia, 2000). Thus, flavor exposure does not necessarily mean enhanced flavor acceptance.

Tastes, Experience, and the Modulation of Food Intake and Body Weight

As described above, rats and humans respond to sweet-tasting fluids, and show pronounced preferences for those fluids from very early in life. In

Table 22.2 Examples of Experiential and Context-dependent Effects during Development on Flavor Preference, Acceptance, and Caloric Compensation

Sensory Stimulus	Species	Experience	Context	Outcome
Garlic Cineole Citral Alcohol Carrot Apple	Rat and human	Prenatal exposure	Amniotic fluid	Increased positive orosensory reponses, decreased negative orosensory responses, increased preference/ acceptance
Garlic Hydrolysate formulas Breast milk odor Soy formulas	Rat and human	Postnatal exposure	Breast milk/Formula	Increased preference and/or acceptance
Alcohol	Rat	Prenatal intoxication	Amniotic fluid	Increased preference and/or acceptance
	Human	Postnatal exposure	Associated with maternal stress	Aversion response
		Postnatal exposure	Not associated with maternal stress	Preference or neutral responses
Sweet	Rat, sheep, human	Prenatal exposure	Amniotic fluid	Preference?
		Prenatal association with calories/energy?	Amniotic fluid	Preference? Conditioning of cephalic phase responses?
	Rat, human	Postnatal exposure	Breast milk/Formula	Preference?
		Postnatal association with calories/energy?	Breast milk/Formula	Preference? Conditioning of cephalic phase responses
Low viscosity	Rat, human	Prenatal association with low calories/energy?	Amniotic fluid	Reduced compensation for low-viscosity calories?
		Postnatal association with low calories	Breast milk/Formula	Reduced compensation for low-viscosity calories?
Low viscosity	Rat	Postweaning exposure	Long-term exposure viscosity/calorie contingencies	Persistent increases in adiposity when consuming low-viscosity calories
High viscosity	Rat, human	Postnatal association with high calories (relative to milk and/or amniotic fluid)	Weaning diets	Reduced compensation for low-viscosity calories?

?: Postulated effects not yet experimentally tested.

addition, rats show strong preferences for diets that deliver calories, independent of their sensory properties (e.g., Capaldi, 1996; Sclafani, 2004). In the normal course of neonatal experience, animals typically experience sweet-tasting diets (milk) in association with the delivery of calories. Recent work from my laboratory has suggested that experiences such as this in which the sensory properties of a diet predict the consequences of that diet may have effects that go beyond altering food preferences and actually modulate food consumption and body weight regulation (Davidson & Swithers, 2004).

If animals do use predictive relationships between the sensory properties of a food (such as sweet taste) and its caloric consequences as a mechanism for modulating caloric intake, then experiences that disrupt this predictive relationship should disrupt the ability to regulate intake. And in fact, weanling-aged rats (25 days of age) given experience with diets where a sweet taste was always associated with calories of food intake showed a better ability to compensate for the calories provided in a novel, sweet-tasting meal compared to rats given experience with diets where a sweet taste was sometimes associated with calories and sometimes provided no calories (Figure 22.1; Davidson & Swithers, 2004). Subsequent experiments have supported the role of such associations in adult rats. Both the ability to compensate for the calories in a novel, sweet-tasting diet and the ability to regulate body weight and adiposity were impaired in animals given experience with diets in which a sweet taste did not predict the delivery of calories (Figure 22.2; Swithers & Davidson, 2008). Thus, in both weanling aged and adult rats, experiences with diets in which sweet tastes are not associated with increased calories results in impairments in control of ingestive behavior. While the mechanisms that produce these disruptions are not yet known, Pavlov first reported that how the sensory properties of food and stimuli that are associated with food (e.g., the sound of a metronome) that predict the delivery of nutrients can acquire the capacity to evoke what are termed "cephalic phase" responses (Pavlov, 1927). Cephalic phase responses are physiological reflexes that are evoked preabsorptively by stimuli related to food (Giduck, Threatte, & Kare, 1987; Mattes, 1997; Powley & Berthoud, 1985). These responses are usually transient, fractional components of larger physiological changes that occur when food actually enters the gastrointestinal tract. It has been argued that energy regulation may be critically dependent on Pavlovian conditioning of cephalic phase reflexes, as even small, consistent changes in energy intake or utilization could lead to significant long-term weight gain (Powley & Berthoud, 1985; Woods & Ramsay, 2000). Not only could such Pavlovian conditioning occur much earlier in development than is typically considered (e.g., potentially during the prenatal period), but the consequences of disrupting such taste–calorie conditioning could be profound.

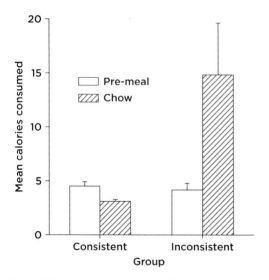

Figure 22.1 Mean calories consumed of a sweet, chocolate-flavored premeal (open bars) and of a subsequent laboratory chow test meal (cross-hatched bars) for rats that were given prior training with different sweet tastes that were consistently paired with calories (Group Consistent) and for rats that were trained with sweet tastes that were inconsistently paired with calories (Group Inconsistent). Inconsistent animals consumed significantly more chow than consistent animals. (Adapted from Davidson & Swithers, 2004.)

Diet Viscosity, Experience, and Regulation of Food Intake and Body Weight

Taste is not the only sensory property of food that may be associated with calories. In fact, the

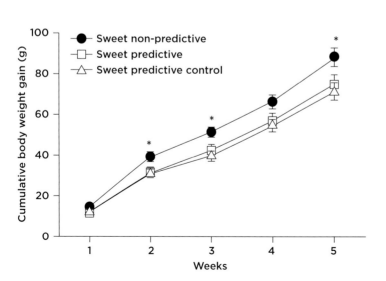

Figure 22.2 Adult male rats gained more weight (A) and had higher adiposity (B) when consuming yogurt diets in which sweet taste did not predict calories (Sweet Nonpredictive) compared to those yogurt diets in which sweet taste did predict increased calories (Sweet Predictive). (Adapted from Swithers & Davidson, 2008.) *$P < .05$ compared to Sweet Predictive.

consequences of prenatal and/or postnatal exposure to another sensory property of food, its viscosity, may influence food intake and body weight regulation. For example, during the suckling period, the only source of calories for these animals is provided in liquid form. The caloric composition of this liquid, milk, is not static but changes in concert with the demands of the neonate (e.g., Davis, Fiorotto, & Reeds, 1993; Del Prado, Delgado, & Villalpando, 1997; Hartmann, 1973; Keen, Lonnerdal, Clegg, & Hurley, 1981; Mitoulas, Sherriff, & Hartmann, 2000; Picciano, 1998). These changes can occur over multiple time frames, both within a suckling episode and across the duration of the preweaning period. Early milk (both within a single feeding episode and relative to the preweaning period) tends to be low in calories, with later milk becoming more calorically dense due to increases in the protein, carbohydrate, and fat content of the milk. These changes in caloric density may be associated with increases in the viscosity of the milk, providing mammalian neonates with the opportunity to learn that more calories are contained in more viscous diets compared to less viscous diets. Such information may be used to modulate intake during the suckling period. In addition, weaning foods are typically more calorically dense than milk, and the physical properties change in a manner consistent with increased caloric density: weaning diets are more viscous than milk. Thus, if neonatal mammals are responsive to differences in the viscosity of diets, food viscosity may be used to regulate intake during suckling, weaning, and into adulthood. Moreover, early experience with the natural contingency where high viscosity predicts high calories and low viscosity predicts low calories could play a role in producing overeating when high calories are provided in low-viscosity form.

Do calories provided in low-viscosity form lead to overeating and/or body weight gain compared to calories contained in high-viscosity foods? If so, then when calories are kept constant, food intake should be higher when viscosity is low compared to when viscosity is high. In fact, in adult rats, food intake was significantly higher following a low-viscosity, liquid, premeal compared to intake following an equicaloric, high-viscosity (pudding-like) meal (Figure 22.3; Davidson & Swithers, 2005). Further, when adult male rats were given a daily supplement of 15 g of Chocolate Ensure Plus® in addition to ad lib laboratory chow and water for 9 weeks, weight gain was significantly greater for rats receiving either the low-viscosity, liquid, chocolate

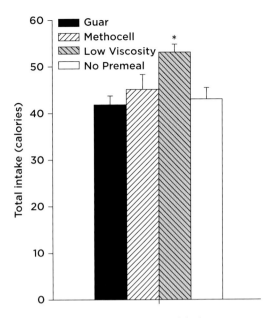

Figure 22.3 Effects of low-viscosity meal, high-viscosity meal (guar and Methocel), or no premeal on subsequent chow intake. (Adapted from Davidson & Swithers, 2005.) *$P < .05$ compared to guar, Methocel, or no premeal.

supplement compared to both a group that received the same chocolate supplement in a high-viscosity pudding or a control group that received no supplement at all (Figure 22.4; Davidson & Swithers, 2005; Swithers & Davidson, 2005b). Thus, in adult rats, short- and long-term exposure to diets that were low in viscosity and high in calories, overeating and increased weight gain were observed relative to the same diets delivered in a thicker form.

The impaired ability to control food intake after consuming liquid calories is not easily modified by postweaning experience, at least in rats. In several studies, as much as 9 weeks experience, starting as young as 35 days of age, in which low viscosity was explicitly paired with high calories failed to influence the rat's ability to reduce their food intake after consuming liquid, low-viscosity calories (Swithers & Davidson, 2005a). In addition, consumption of a low-viscosity diet beginning at 35–42 days of age led to increased adiposity that persisted for at least 3 months after the diet was discontinued (Figure 22.5; Swithers & Davidson, 2005a). These data support the idea that an animal's experience with the viscosity of a diet and its caloric content (e.g., low-viscosity diets such as milk have fewer calories than higher viscosity diets, like chow) influences its subsequent inability to

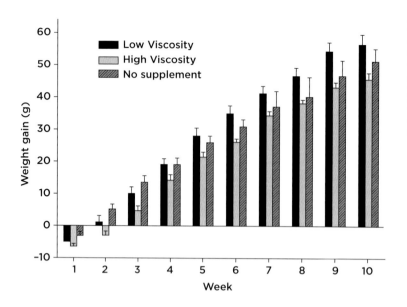

Figure 22.4 Body weight gain in adult male rats receiving daily exposure to 15 g of low- or high-viscosity versions of the same dietary supplement (Chocolate Ensure Plus). (Adapted from Davidson & Swithers, 2005.) *P < .05 compared to high viscosity or no supplement.

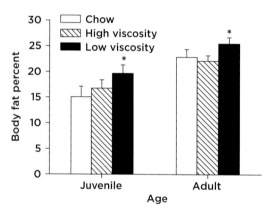

Figure 22.5 Adiposity (as assessed by dual-energy X-ray absorptiometry [DEXA]) in rats immediately following (Juvenile) 9 weeks exposure to high- or low-viscosity dietary supplements or chow alone or 3 months after discontinuation of the supplements (Adult). (Adapted from Swithers & Davidson, 2005a.) *P < .05 compared to high viscosity or chow groups.

overweight, and obesity (Bray, Nielsen, & Popkin, 2004; DiMeglio & Mattes, 2000; Malik, Schulze, & Hu, 2006; Mattes & Rothacker, 2001; Tam et al., 2006).

Taken together, these data support the idea that both adult and juvenile rats do a poor job of accounting for calories that come in liquid form. One factor that may contribute to this deficit is a developmental or evolutionary history of early experiences of liquid diets representing lower calorie foods compared to chow and other diets consumed after the onset of weaning. Because these types of experiences occur during a period of rapid growth, if animals possess an inherent bias toward acquisition of as many calories as are available, then young animals would be predisposed to overeat after getting liquid calories rather undereating to take account for them. Further, outside of the context of the suckling period, rats and humans (in an evolutionary sense) would have been unlikely to encounter calories in the form of liquids. After the suckling period, the principal role of liquids would have been to meet hydrational, not caloric needs. Thus, there may have been little pressure to make associations between liquids and calories. The role of associations between the sensory properties of foods and beverages and their postingestive consequences (such as calories or hydration) requires additional consideration. However, there is some evidence that experience with water and solid food is necessary for the modulation of appetitive responses with respect to energy or water deficits. For example, there is evidence that only rats

regulate calories that are delivered in liquid form. The long-term consequences of consuming calories delivered in low-viscosity, liquid form may therefore be significant and persistent, and likely extend beyond those demonstrated in our work in rats. For example, there is evidence from the clinical literature that humans overeat following consumption of calories in liquid form, and it has been argued that consumption of calories in low-viscosity, beverage form (such as soft drinks and juices) may be contributing to a major current public health issue, that have previously consumed water while dehydrated show enhanced water-seeking behavior following dehydration and rats that have previously eaten food while food deprived show food-seeking behavior following food deprivation (Table 22.3; Changizi, McGehee, & Hall, 2002; Hall, Arnold, & Myers, 2000; Myers & Hall, 2001). These data suggest that by the age of weaning, rat pups are capable of associating physiological state cues (like those produced by food and water deprivation) with the consequences of eating and drinking, and that these associations influence appetitive and consummatory responses related to food and water intake.

From Suckling to Feeding: Weaning as an Ontogenetic Niche

At weaning, pups must abandon the dam as a sole source of food and water and achieve independent ingestion. Rats have provided a convenient model system for examining the transition to independent ingestion, because the maturation of neural, physiological, and behavioral systems that may underlie this capacity occurs during the first 2 weeks of life. These systems result in increased locomotor, thermoregulatory, and sensory capacities,

all of which may be necessary for successful initiation of intake independent of the dam. In rats, this initiation typically begins during the third week of postnatal life. In a typical nesting situation, rat pups are observed consuming solid diets at approximately 15–18 days of age (Babicky et al., 1973a, 1973b). Previous work has documented that the timing of this process is influenced by a variety of environmental manipulations including environmental temperature and the number of animals in the litter (Babicky et al., 1973a; Gerrish & Alberts, 1996; Gerrish, Onischak, & Alberts, 1998; Thiels & Alberts, 1985). The mechanisms that promote this transition can be influenced by experience, including early exposures to flavors that modify food choices along with experiences related to the consequences of consuming novel substances under different physiological states.

The specific mechanisms that lead individual animals to initiate independent ingestion of food are unknown, but independent food intake typically occurs at a time when the pups' growth rate has slowed, likely due to an inability of the dam to meet the increasing needs of her pups. Work from our laboratory has suggested that the timing of independent ingestion may rely on pups' newly

Table 22.3 Developmental, Experiential, and Contextual Influences on Appetitive and Consummatory Response to Physiological Signals during Independent Ingestion

	Birth	P12–P15	P18	P21	P25	Adult
Food deprivation	Decreased latency to initiate food intake $\longrightarrow$					
	Increased food intake					
			Decreased latency to seek food $\longrightarrow$			
Dehydration	Increased water intake $\longrightarrow$					
	Increased milk intake $\longrightarrow$		Decreased latency to seek water $\longrightarrow$			
			Dehydration anorexia $\longrightarrow$			
Changes in fatty acid oxidation		Decreased latency to initiate milk intake	No effect $\longrightarrow$		Decreased latency to initiate chow intake	
		Increased milk intake	No effect $\longrightarrow$		Increased chow intake	
					No effect on food intake (intact females)	
Changes in glucose utilization				Decreased latency to initiate chow intake $\longrightarrow$		
					Increased chow intake	

*Previous experience with food deprivation/dehydration and food/water consumption necessary.

developed capacities to detect signals related to the energy deficit produced by the dam's inability to match output to the need. This hypothesis is supported by work from our laboratory and others that suggest that signals related to energy deficit are unable to modulate independent ingestion prior to P12–P15, instead the principal physiological signal that stimulates independent ingestion in very young rats appears to be hydrational (Hall, 1990; Phifer, Ladd, & Hall, 1991). In young rats, dehydration (cellular or extracellular) results in increased intake and preventing dehydration during overnight deprivation is as successful at modulating independent ingestion as preventing both dehydration and caloric privation in 6-day-old rats (Phifer et al., 1991). Not until pups are approximately P12–P15 do signals related to energy deficits influence the initiation of intake, a developmental time schedule that is coincident with the typical initiation of independent ingestion (see Table 22.3). A 15-day-old rat that is hydrated during overnight food deprivation consumes as much as a 15-day-old that is not hydrated, and much more than a 15-day-old given both fluids and calories (Phifer et al., 1991). Thus, by 15 days of age, the rats have developed the capacity to respond to a signal related to caloric deprivation.

Attempts to identify this signal focused first on glucose availability or utilization. In adult rats, glucose is the principal fuel for neurons, and injection of drugs such as insulin or 2-deoxyglucose reliably elicit food intake in adults. However, in rat pups, several studies have documented a failure of alterations in glucose availability or utilization to stimulate independent ingestion until well after the weaning period has begun (25–30 days of age; Gisel & Henning, 1980; Houpt & Epstein, 1973; Leshem, Flynn, & Epstein, 1990; Lytle, Moorcroft, & Campbell, 1971; Swithers, 2000).

A logical alternative was that changes in the availability or utilization of fat contributed to increased independent ingestion following deprivation. In neonatal rats, metabolism is biased toward fat utilization and the dam's milk is high in fat; a shift toward increased dietary carbohydrate and glucose metabolism occurs by the end of the weaning period (Bailey & Lockwood, 1971; Fernando-Warnakulasuriya, Staggers, Frost, & Wells, 1981; Lockwood & Bailey, 1970; Wells, 1985; Yeh & Sheehan, 1985; Yeung & Oliver, 1967). Consistent with these shifts are changes in the physiological consequences of mild to moderate food deprivation in young rats of different ages. In pups aged 9 to 18 days, circulating levels of both free fatty acids (FFA; the source of energy for fatty acid oxidation) and ketone bodies (a product of fatty acid oxidation) in animals that are not food deprived are high, and FFA levels increase with increasing food deprivation, suggesting that fatty acids are mobilized as a source of energy during food deprivation in rats at this age (e.g., Leshem et al., 1990). As a result, it is possible that a signal or signals related to the changes in fat availability or utilization play a role in the emergence of energy-related modulation of independent ingestion in pups between 6 and 15 days of age. If so, then interfering with the pup's ability to utilize fat would be expected to produce changes in ingestive behavior.

In fact, several studies have demonstrated that the capacity to respond to changes related to fat oxidation with the initiation of independent ingestion first appears to emerge between 12 and 15 days of age. These studies examined the effects of administration of drugs, such as 2-mercaptoacetate (MA) and methyl palmoxirate (MP), which interfere with one or more enzymes required for mitochondrial oxidation of fatty acids. In adult rats, administration of these drugs had been demonstrated to result in increased intake, with the effects more pronounced in animals maintained on diets that were high in fat (Friedman & Tordoff, 1986; Friedman, Tordoff, & Ramirez, 1986; Langhans & Scharrer, 1987a, 1987b; Scharrer & Langhans, 1986). However, while work in both very young pups (4 days) and older pups (14 and 20 days of age) had documented a failure of MA or MP to alter intake in the context of suckling (Leshem et al., 1990), the consequences of administration of these drugs for modulation of independent ingestion had not been examined. Thus, in our initial studies, we examined the effects of administration of MA on independent ingestion of milk from the floor of test containers in 6-, 9-, 12-, and 15-day-old rats, a task that required pups to perform both appetitive and consummatory aspects of ingestion. The results demonstrated that although intake was not affected by administration of MA in 6- or 9-day-old pups, it significantly increased milk intake in 12- and 15-day-old rats (Figure 22.6; Swithers, 1997).

The age-related differences in ingestive behavior were not directly due to differences in age-related physiological responses to administration of the drug. The magnitude of changes in ketone bodies and FFAs after administration of MA was similar in the younger pups that did not show a change in behavior as in the older pups that did show an

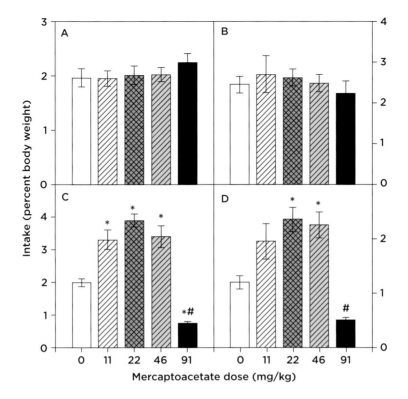

Figure 22.6 Intake (expressed as %pup's body wt.) of a commercial half-and-half diet during a 30-min intake test from the floor of test containers 1 h after administration of 2-mercaptoacetate (MA). (A) 6-day-old rats; (B) 9-day-old rats; (C) 12-day-old rats; and (D) 15-day-old rats. Note that scales are different for pups at different ages. *$P < .05$ compared with saline control; #, $P < .05$ compared with 11, 22, and 46 mg/kg MA. (Adapted from Swithers, 1997.)

increase in intake (Swithers, 1997). Based on these data, our hypothesis was that by 12 days of age, the rats had developed the capacity to respond to changes in the availability of fat as an energy source, by increasing their food intake independent of the dam, and that changes in the availability or utilization of fats, rather than glucose, as an energy source were the first energy-related signal to emerge developmentally.

Subsequent work, however, revealed a more complex pattern. As described above, previous work had documented a failure of administration of MA to stimulate intake in the context of suckling in animals at an age (14 days) when it did stimulate independent ingestion from the floor of a test container (Leshem et al., 1990; Swithers, 1997). Thus, the meaning of the signal generated by blocking fatty acid oxidation appeared to depend on the context in which it was tested. One possible explanation for this difference is that MA was influencing the *initiation of intake* (i.e., appetitive behavior) rather than *intake itself* (i.e., consummatory behavior). Additional work in pups of varying

ages has supported this notion by demonstrating that MA appeared to selectively decrease the latency with which food intake was initiated. First, we examined the consequences of administering MA to animals older than 15 days of age. Our hypothesis was that because MA stimulated intake in pups at 12 and 15 days of age, older pups would also increase intake after receiving MA. However, not only did MA fail to stimulate intake of milk in 18-, 21-, 25-, or 30-day-olds, but also milk intake in these older animals was often suppressed by the highest doses of MA employed (Swithers & McCurley, 2002; Swithers, McCurley, Scheibler, & Doerflinger, 2005). Subsequent work revealed that intake of the milk diet was typically initiated with very short latencies (within 20–25 s) in control animals aged either 9 or 21 days (Figure 22.7; Swithers, 2003). By contrast, the latency to initiate milk intake independent of the dam in 15-day-old control rats was significantly longer (approximately 300 s); administration of MA produced a significant reduction in this latency in 15-day-old rats (Swithers, 2003). These results suggested that MA

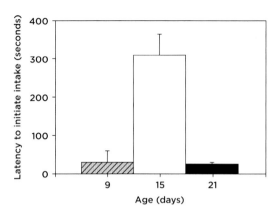

Figure 22.7 Latency to initiate independent ingestion of milk from the floor of a test container in nondeprived rats at 9, 15, and 21 days of age. (Adapted from Swithers, 2003.)

might not stimulate consummatory behavior, but instead, appetitive behavior.

Further evidence that MA was affecting the appetitive components of intake was based on studies in which we removed the pup's ability to control the initiation of intake by infusing diets directly into their mouths. In these studies, MA did not stimulate intake in P12 rats, even though intake was stimulated when the same diet was offered on the floor of the test container (Swithers, Peters, & Shin, 1999). Taken together, these data support the idea that when pups receive a signal that fatty acid oxidation has been reduced, they initiate food intake more rapidly at ages (P12 and P15) that anticipate the onset of weaning. This timing coincides with the age at which signals produced during food deprivation first come to stimulate food intake. In contrast, signals related to changes in glucose availability or utilization do not significantly affect food intake until at least P21 (decreased latency; Gisel & Henning, 1980) or P30 (increased intake; Leshem et al., 1990). Signals related to changes in the availability or utilization of fatty acids may represent an early emerging signal related to energy status that modulates ingestive behavior. The developmental of the ability to initiate food intake in response to changes in a fat-related energy signal may represent one stimulus that contributes to the timing of start of the weaning process. After weaning has been initiated, the meaning of such a signal may be altered by changes in the composition of the diet and/or the development of additional behavioral capacities, such as the ability to respond to changes in glucose availability. Increased appetitive behavior in preweanling pups in response to changes in fatty acid oxidation

may therefore represent an additional example of an ontogenetic niche. This signal is experienced by a young rat prior to the onset of weaning, but may have different consequences in adult animals.

After Weaning: The Consequences of Puberty

After weaning has been initiated, do signals related to changes in fatty acid oxidation continue to play a role in modulating food intake? To some extent, they do play a role. For example, as described above, in adult male rats, administration of MA or MP does stimulate food intake and these effects are amplified in animals maintained on diets high in fat (Friedman et al., 1986; Langhans & Scharrer, 1987b). In addition, in rats tested at P30, increases in food intake are displayed following administration of MA. One conclusion, therefore, might be that by P30, the physiological and neural systems that underlie a rat's ability to modulate intake in response to signals regarding energy status have matured completely, and there is developmental continuity in the ontogeny of the capacity to increase food intake in the face of signals related to energy deficits. However, more recent work suggests that such a conclusion is incorrect. Instead, developmental events that occur after P30 modulate subsequent behavioral responses to changes in oxidation of fatty acids. In particular, work in our laboratory has suggested that in female rats, exposure to estrogen during puberty appears to eliminate increases in food intake produced by administration of MA.

We had previously demonstrated that administration of MA resulted in increased intake of a standard low-fat chow diet in both male and female rats on P30 (Swithers et al., 2005). In adult animals, work examining the effects of MA on food intake had been done almost exclusively in adult males. However, in one recent report, administration of MA was demonstrated to have no effect on food intake in adult female rats (Shahab et al., 2006). While the authors attributed this outcome to the low-fat diet on which the animals were maintained, more recent data from our laboratory indicate that differences in ingestive responding in adult male and female rats do not stem the maintenance diet. Instead, they reflect fundamental developmental changes in behavioral responses to administration that occur in female rats. To demonstrate this, we first examined the effects of administration of MA to adult female rats that maintained high-fat and standard, low-fat chow diets. MA did not stimulate intake in either group of adult females (Swithers,

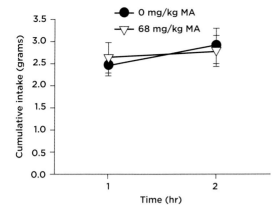

Figure 22.8 Chow intake following administration of MA in female rats that were OVX as adults. Rats were maintained and tested on a high-fat chow diet.

2006). Thus, unlike adult male rats, adult female rats do not appear to show increased food intake after administration of MA. One potential source of this sex difference was ovarian hormones. In adult female rats, food intake has been demonstrated to be sensitive circulating ovarian hormones; increased levels of estrogen (exogenous or endogenous) are associated with lower levels of food intake (Asarian & Geary, 2006; Wade & Zucker, 1970). Thus, it was possible that in intact female rats, circulating estrogen might be interacting with the signals generated by administration of MA. If so, then removing the source of estrogen through ovariectomy (OVX) in adult females should result in increased food intake after administration of MA. However, several experiments in adult female rats following OVX consistently indicated that administration of MA did not stimulate intake (Figure 22.8; Swithers, 2006). Taken together, these results indicated that

the failure of administration of MA to stimulate intake in adult females was not a result of either the fat composition of their maintenance diet or levels of ovarian hormone levels in adulthood.

In contrast to the results in adult females, previous work with juvenile rats had demonstrated that at P30, female rats do show an increase in food intake after MA. These results suggested that changes that occur during the pubertal period might reorganize behavioral responses to signals related to energy utilization in female rats. To test this, female rats were ovariectomized (OVX) between P23 and P27. When these females were then tested in adulthood, MA did stimulate food intake in OVX females, but not in control, sham OVX, females (Figure 22.9; Swithers, 2006). Further, when females OVX before P30 were given injections of estrogen between P35 and P65, their responses to MA in adulthood were similar to intact adult females; no increases in intake after administration of MA were observed, even though the estrogen administration had been discontinued at least 3 months prior to administration of MA (Figure 22.10; Swithers, 2006). These results suggest that in female rats, the behavioral response to a signal related to changes in fatty acid oxidation is permanently altered by exposure to estrogen during the time of puberty.

Unlike male rats, female rats no longer increase food intake in response to this signal related to changes in fat utilization. However, administration of MA may have other effects on behavior in adult females. For example, it has long been known that in rats, along with other species, ovulation, sexual behavior, and pulsatile release of gonadotropic hormones, such as GnRH and LH can be suppressed by changes in energy status, such as those produced by food deprivation or by the administration of

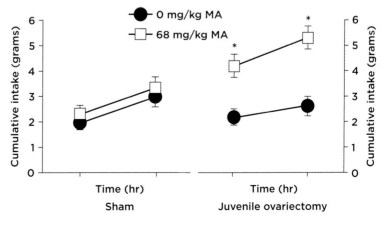

Figure 22.9 Chow intake following administration of MA in adult female rats following sham (left) or real (right) OVX at 23–27 days of age. Rats were maintained and tested on a high-fat chow diet. *P < .05 compared to 0 mg/kg MA.

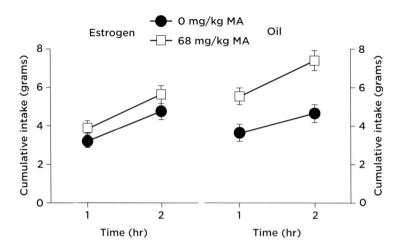

Figure 22.10 Chow intake after administration of MA in adult female rats following OVX at 23–27 days of age. Rats were maintained and tested on a high-fat chow diet and received 7 cycles (once every 4 days) of estrogen (left) or the oil vehicle (right). *$P<.05$ compared to 0 mg/kg MA.

drugs like MA and 2-deoxyglucose, which interferes with glucose utilization (Schneider, 2004, 2006; Shahab et al., 2006; Wade, Schneider, & Li, 1996). For a female animal that has gone through puberty, then, the behavioral response to signals that related to decreased energy availability is not to get additional energy by eating, but instead reduce reproductive behavior. Because both reproductive physiology and sexual behavior are impaired, the high energy demands associated with reproduction in the female are avoided (Schneider, 2006). Such a strategy may be unnecessary in male rats, or prepubertal female rats, and as a result, the predominant behavioral response to the same signal is to acquire additional energy by increasing food intake.

Taken as a whole, these data indicate that behavioral responses to signals related to changes in energy status depend on a variety of developmental factors. For example, in young rats prior to the onset of weaning (P12–P15), signals related to glucose utilization are not effective at increasing ingestive behavior, whereas signals related to changes in fat availability or utilization lead pups to initiate food intake independent of the dam. The early development of behavioral responses to fat-related signals may reflect the high-fat content of the diet (dam's milk) consumed by preweanling pups, and may represent one mechanism by which pups initiate the process of weaning. This behavioral response appears transient as only a few days later (P18–P21), pups fail to increase food intake when given MA, perhaps due to a change in dietary fat content that results from the initiation of chow intake. Alternatively, as seen with behavioral responses to food deprivation, pups may require experience with consumption of chow diets in

the context of an energy deficit in order to display enhanced intake. Such experience may naturally occur by P25–P30, since at this time, changes in either fatty acid oxidation or glucose utilization do stimulate chow intake. In male rats, significant developmental shifts do not appear to occur subsequent to this age, but dietary context continues to modulate the consequences of signals related to energy utilization. Adult males maintained on a high-fat diet show enhanced responses to altered fat utilization relative to males maintained on a low-fat diet. In female rats, an additional developmental shift does occur. Exposure to estrogen appears to produce a significant change in the behavioral response from a stimulation of food intake to a suppression of sexual behavior. This behavioral shift persists even if ovarian hormones are subsequently removed. While the role of estrogen in this shift seems clear, it is presently uncertain whether the timing of such estrogen exposure matters. For example, the long-term consequences of exposure to estrogen on ingestive behavior in females may depend on estrogen exposure occurring during puberty when significant neural organization is occurring (e.g., Sisk & Zehr, 2005), with estrogen exposure outside this time window producing less profound effects.

It seems clear that a variety of experiences can influence the development of controls of food intake in rats. These experiences include exposure to the sensory properties of foods and their caloric consequences, familiarity with the influence of signals related to food and water deprivation on the consequences of eating and drinking, and the integration of postingestive consequences of eating, such as stomach fill, with the ongoing sensory experiences that accumulate when a meal is being consumed. In addition, the meaning of such experiences can be modulated by the developmental context. Sensory signals may have different meanings in the context of suckling versus independent ingestion, and may result in differential behavioral outcomes in female rats before and after exposure to ovarian hormones during puberty. Together, the work argues that understanding the proximate factors that control food intake requires attention to past and present experience. And, as the prevalence of obesity and its attendant negative health consequences continues to rise drastically worldwide, identifying the signals that modulate intake, and determining how to reverse these trends becomes increasingly urgent. An important consideration in accomplishing such a goal will be to determine the physiological, genetic, and neural signals that modulate ingestion within the environmental, experiential, and ontogenetic contexts in which those signals operate.

References

Abate, P., Varlinskaya, E. I., Cheslock, S. J., Spear, N. E., & Molina, J. C. (2002). Neonatal activation of alcohol-related prenatal memories: Impact on the first suckling response. *Alcoholism, Clinical and Experimental Research*, *26*, 1512–1522.

Asarian, L., & Geary, N. (2006). Modulation of appetite by gonadal steroid hormones. *Philosophical Transactions of the Royal Society of London. Series B, Biological Sciences*, *361*, 1251–1263.

Babicky, A., Ostadalova, I., Parizek, J., Kolar, J., & Bibr, B. (1973a). Onset and duration of the physiological weaning period for infant rats reared in nests of different sizes. *Physiologia Bohemoslovaca*, *22*, 449–456.

Babicky, A., Parizek, J., Ostadalova, I., & Kolar, J. (1973b). Initial solid food intake and growth of young rats in nests of different sizes. *Physiologia Bohemoslovaca*, *22*, 557–566.

Bailey, E., & Lockwood, E. A. (1971). Formation and utilization of ketone bodies during development of the male rat. *Biochemical Journal*, *124*, 7P–8P.

Blass, E. M. (1990). Suckling: Determinants, changes, mechanisms, and lasting impressions. *Developmental Psychology*, *26*, 520–533.

Blass, E. M., Beardsley, W., & Hall, W. G. (1979). Age-dependent inhibition of suckling by cholecystokinin. *The American Journal of Physiology*, *236*, E567–E570.

Blass, E. M., Hall, W. G., & Teicher, M. H. (1979). The ontogeny of suckling and ingestive behaviors. *Progress in Psychobiology and Physiological Psychology*, *8*, 243–299.

Blass, E. M., & Teicher, M. H. (1980). Suckling. *Science*, *210*, 15–22.

Blumberg, S., Haba, D., Schroeder, M., Smith, G. P., & Weller, A. (2006). Independent ingestion and microstructure of feeding patterns in infant rats lacking CCK-1 receptors. *The American Journal of Physiology*, *290*, R208–R218.

Brace, R. A. (1997). Physiology of amniotic fluid volume regulation. *Clinical Obstetrics and Gynecology*, *40*, 280–289.

Brake, S. C., Sager, D. J., Sullivan, R., & Hofer, M. (1982). The role of intraoral and gastrointestinal cues in the control of sucking and milk consumption in rat pups. *Developmental Psychobiology*, *15*, 529–541.

Brake, S. C., Shair, H., & Hofer, M. (1988). Exploiting the nursing niche: The infant's suckling and feeding in the context of the mother-infant interaction. In E. M. Blass (Ed.), *Handbook of behavioral neurobiology:Vol. 9. Developmental psychobiology and behavioral ecology* (pp. 347–388). New York: Plenum Press.

Bray, G. A., Nielsen, S. J., & Popkin, B. M. (2004). Consumption of high-fructose corn syrup in beverages may play a role in the epidemic of obesity. *The American Journal of Clinical Nutrition*, *79*, 537–543.

Capaldi, E. D. (1996). Conditioned food preferences. In E. D. Capaldi (Ed.), *Why we eat what we eat: The psychology of eating* (pp. 53–80). Washington, D.C.: American Psychological Association.

Changizi, M. A., McGehee, R. M., & Hall, W. G. (2002). Evidence that appetitive responses for dehydration and food-deprivation are learned. *Physiology and Behavior*, *75*, 295–304.

Chotro, M. G., Arias, C., & Laviola, G. (2007). Increased ethanol intake after prenatal ethanol exposure: Studies with animals. *Neuroscience and Biobehavioral Reviews*, *31*, 181–191.

Craig, W. (1913). Appetites and aversions as consituents of instinct. *Biological Bulletin*, *34*, 91–107.

Davidson, T. L., & Swithers, S. E. (2004). A Pavlovian approach to the problem of obesity. *International Journal of Obesity and Related Metabolic Disorders*, *28*, 933–935.

Davidson, T. L., & Swithers, S. E. (2005). Food viscosity influences caloric intake compensation and body weight in rats. *Obesity Research*, *13*, 537–544.

Davis, R. J., Doerflinger, A., McCurley, M., & Swithers, S. E. (2003). Gastric emptying and control of ingestion in preweanling rat pups. *Nutritional Neuroscience*, *6*, 71–78.

Davis, T. A., Fiorotto, M. L., & Reeds, P. J. (1993). Amino acid compositions of body and milk protein change during the suckling period in rats. *The Journal of Nutrition*, *123*, 947–956.

Del Prado, M., Delgado, G., & Villalpando, S. (1997). Maternal lipid intake during pregnancy and lactation alters milk composition and production and litter growth in rats. *The Journal of Nutrition*, *127*, 458–462.

Desor, J. A., Maller, O., & Andrews, K. (1975). Ingestive responses of human newborns to salty, sour, and bitter stimuli. *Journal of Comparative and Physiological Psychology*, *89*, 966–970.

DiMeglio, D. P., & Mattes, R. D. (2000). Liquid versus solid carbohydrate: Effects on food intake and body weight. *International Journal of Obesity and Related Metabolic Disorders*, *24*, 794–800.

Dominguez, H. D., Lopez, M. F., & Molina, J. C. (1998). Neonatal responsiveness to alcohol odor and infant alcohol intake as a function of alcohol experience during late gestation. *Alcohol*, *16*, 109–117.

El-Haddad, M. A., Ismail, Y., Guerra, C., Day, L., & Ross, M. G. (2002). Effect of oral sucrose on ingestive behavior in the near-term ovine fetus. *American Journal of Obstetrics and Gynecology*, *187*, 898–901.

Fernando-Warnakulasuriya, G. J., Staggers, J. E., Frost, S. C., & Wells, M. A. (1981). Studies on fat digestion, absorption, and transport in the suckling rat. I. Fatty acid composition and concentrations of major lipid components. *Journal of Lipid Research, 22*, 668–674.

Forsyth, P. A., Weingarten, H. P., & Collins, S. M. (1985). Role of oropharyngeal stimulation in cholecystokinin-induced satiety in the sham feeding rat. *Physiology and Behavior, 35*, 539–543.

Friedman, M. I. (1975). Some determinants of milk ingestion in suckling rats. *Journal of Comparative and Physiological Psychology, 89*, 636–647.

Friedman, M. I., & Tordoff, M. G. (1986). Fatty acid oxidation and glucose utilization interact to control food intake in rats. *The American Journal of Physiology, 251*, R840–R845.

Friedman, M. I., Tordoff, M. G., & Ramirez, I. (1986). Integrated metabolic control of food intake. *Brain Research Bulletin, 17*, 855–859.

Friesen, R., & Innis, S. M. (2006). Maternal dietary fat alters amniotic fluid and fetal intestinal membrane essential n-6 and n-3 fatty acids in the rat. *The American Journal of Physiology, 290*, G505–G510.

Galef, B. G., Jr., & Henderson, P. W. (1972). Mother's milk: A determinant of the feeding preferences of weaning rat pups. *Journal of Comparative and Physiological Psychology, 78*, 213–219.

Galef, B. G., Jr., & Sherry, D. F. (1973). Mother's milk: A medium for transmission of cues reflecting the flavor of mother's diet. *Journal of Comparative and Physiological Psychology, 83*, 374–378.

Ganchrow, J. R., Steiner, J. E., & Canetto, S. (1986). Behavioral displays to gustatory stimuli in newborn rat pups. *Developmental Psychobiology, 19*, 163–174.

Gerrish, C. J., & Alberts, J. R. (1996). Environmental temperature modulates onset of independent feeding: Warmer is sooner. *Developmental Psychobiology, 29*, 483–495.

Gerrish, C. J., Onischak, C. M., & Alberts, J. R. (1998). Acute, early thermal experience alters weaning onset in rats. *Physiology and Behavior, 64*, 463–474.

Giduck, S. A., Threatte, R. M., & Kare, M. R. (1987). Cephalic reflexes: Their role in digestion and possible roles in absorption and metabolism. *The Journal of Nutrition, 117*, 1191–1196.

Gisel, E. G., & Henning, S. J. (1980). Appearance of glucoprivic control of feeding behavior in the developing rat. *Physiology and Behavior, 24*, 313–318.

Gurekian, C. N., & Koski, K. G. (2005). Amniotic fluid amino acid concentrations are modified by maternal dietary glucose, gestational age, and fetal growth in rats. *The Journal of Nutrition, 135*, 2219–2224.

Hall, W. G. (1990). The ontogeny of ingestive behavior: Changing control of components in the feeding sequence. In E. M. Stricker (Ed.), *Neurobiology of food and fluid intake. Handbook of behavioral neurobiology* (Vol. 10, pp. 77–123). New York: Plenum Press.

Hall, W. G., Arnold, H. M., & Myers, K. P. (2000). The acquisition of an appetite. *Psychological Science, 11*, 101–105.

Hall, W. G., & Bryan, T. E. (1981). The ontogeny of feeding in rats: IV. Taste development as measured by intake and behavioral responses to oral infusions of sucrose and quinine. *Journal of Comparative and Physiological Psychology, 95*, 240–251.

Hall, W. G., Cramer, C. P., & Blass, E. M. (1975). Developmental changes in suckling of rat pups. *Nature, 258*, 318–320.

Hall, W. G., Cramer, C. P., & Blass, E. M. (1977). The ontogeny of suckling in rats: Transitions toward adult ingestion. *Journal of Comparative and Physiological Psychology, 91*, 1141–1155.

Hall, W. G., & Rosenblatt, J. S. (1977). Suckling behavior and intake control in the developing rat pup. *Journal of Comparative and Physiological Psychology, 91*, 1232–1247.

Hall, W. G., & Rosenblatt, J. S. (1978). Development of nutritional control of food intake in suckling rat pups. *Behavioral Biology, 24*, 413–427.

Hall, W. G., & Williams, C. L. (1983). Suckling isn't feeding, or is it? A search for developmental continuities. *Advances in the Study of Behavior, 13*, 219–254.

Hartmann, P. E. (1973). Changes in the composition and yield of the mammary secretion of cows during the initiation of lactation. *Journal of Endocrinology, 59*, 231–247.

Henning, S. J., Chang, S. S., & Gisel, E. G. (1979). Ontogeny of feeding controls in suckling and weaning rats. *The American Journal of Physiology, 237*, R187–R191.

Hepper, P. (1988). Adaptive fetal learning: Prenatal exposure to garlic affects postnatal preference. *Animal Behaviour, 36*, 935–936.

Houpt, K. A., & Epstein, A. N. (1973). Ontogeny of controls of food intake in the rat: GI fill and glucoprivation. *The American Journal of Physiology, 225*, 58–66.

Houpt, K. A., & Houpt, T. R. (1975). Effects of gastric loads and food deprivation on subsequent food intake in suckling rats. *Journal of Comparative and Physiological Psychology, 88*, 764–772.

Keen, C. L., Lonnerdal, B., Clegg, M., & Hurley, L. S. (1981). Developmental changes in composition of rat milk: Trace elements, minerals, protein, carbohydrate and fat. *The Journal of Nutrition, 111*, 226–236.

Langhans, W., & Scharrer, E. (1987a). Evidence for a vagally mediated satiety signal derived from hepatic fatty acid oxidation. *Journal of the Autonomic Nervous System, 18*, 13–18.

Langhans, W., & Scharrer, E. (1987b). Role of fatty acid oxidation in control of meal pattern. *Behavioral and Neural Biology, 47*, 7–16.

Leshem, M., Flynn, F. W., & Epstein, A. N. (1990). Brain glucoprivation and ketoprivation do not promote ingestion in the suckling rat pup. *The American Journal of Physiology, 258*, R365–R375.

Lockwood, E. A., & Bailey, E. (1970). Fatty acid utilization during development of the rat. *Biochemical Journal, 120*, 49–54.

Lorenz, D. N., Ellis, S. B., & Epstein, A. N. (1982). Differential effects of upper gastrointestinal fill on milk ingestion and nipple attachment in the suckling rat. *Developmental Psychobiology, 15*, 309–330.

Lytle, L. D., Moorcroft, W. H., & Campbell, B. A. (1971). Ontogeny of amphetamine anorexia and insulin hyperphagia in the rat. *Journal of Comparative and Physiological Psychology, 77*, 388–393.

Malik, V. S., Schulze, M. B., & Hu, F. B. (2006). Intake of sugar-sweetened beverages and weight gain: A systematic review. *The American Journal of Clinical Nutrition, 84*, 274–288.

Maller, O., & Desor, J. A. (1973). Effect of taste on ingestion by human newborns. *Symposium on Oral Sensation and Perception, 4*, 279–291.

Marlier, L., & Schaal, B. (2005). Human newborns prefer human milk: Conspecific milk odor is attractive without postnatal exposure. *Child Development, 76,* 155–168.

Marlier, L., Schaal, B., & Soussignan, R. (1998). Bottle-fed neonates prefer an odor experienced in utero to an odor experienced postnatally in the feeding context. *Developmental Psychobiology, 33,* 133–145.

Mattes, R. D. (1997). Physiologic responses to sensory stimulation by food: Nutritional implications. *Journal of the American Dietetic Association, 97,* 406–413.

Mattes, R. D., & Rothacker, D. (2001). Beverage viscosity is inversely related to postprandial hunger in humans. *Physiology and Behavior, 74,* 551–557.

Mennella, J. A. (1995). Mother's milk: A medium for early flavor experiences. *Journal of Human Lactation, 11,* 39–45.

Mennella, J. A., & Beauchamp, G. K. (2005). Understanding the origin of flavor preferences. *Chemical Senses, 30*(Suppl. 1), i242–i243.

Mennella, J. A., & Garcia, P. L. (2000). Children's hedonic response to the smell of alcohol: Effects of parental drinking habits. *Alcoholism, Clinical and Experimental Research, 24,* 1167–1171.

Mennella, J. A., Griffin, C. E., & Beauchamp, G. K. (2004). Flavor programming during infancy. *Pediatrics, 113,* 840–845.

Mennella, J. A., Jagnow, C. P., & Beauchamp, G. K. (2001). Prenatal and postnatal flavor learning by human infants. *Pediatrics, 107,* E88.

Mennella, J. A., Kennedy, J. M., & Beauchamp, G. K. (2006). Vegetable acceptance by infants: Effects of formula flavors. *Early Human Development, 82,* 463–468.

Mitoulas, L. R., Sherriff, J. L., & Hartmann, P. E. (2000). Short-and long term variation in the production, content, and composition of human milk fat. *Advances in Experimental Medicine and Biology, 478,* 401–402.

Moran, T. H., & Bi, S. (2006a). Hyperphagia and obesity in OLETF rats lacking CCK-1 receptors. *Philosophical Transactions of the Royal Society of London. Series B, Biological Sciences, 361,* 1211–1218.

Moran, T. H., & Bi, S. (2006b). Hyperphagia and obesity of OLETF rats lacking CCK1 receptors: Developmental aspects. *Developmental Psychobiology, 48,* 360–367.

Myers, K. P., & Hall, W. G. (2001). Effects of prior experience with dehydration and water on the time course of dehydration-induced drinking in weanling rats. *Developmental Psychobiology, 38,* 145–153.

Nowlis, G. H., & Kessen, W. (1976). Human newborns differentiate differing concentrations of sucrose and glucose. *Science, 191,* 865–866.

Oppenheim, R. W. (1981). Ontogenetic adaptations and retrogressive processes in the development of the nervous system and behaviour: A neuroembryological perspective. In K. J. Connolly & H. F. R. Prechtl (Eds.), *Maturation and development: Biological and psychological perspectives* (pp. 73–109). Philadelphia, PA: Lippincott.

Pavlov, I. P. (1927). *Conditioned reflexes.* Oxford: Oxford University Press.

Petrov, E. S., Varlinskaya, E. I., & Spear, N. E. (2001). Self-administration of ethanol and saccharin in newborn rats: Effects on suckling plasticity. *Behavioral Neuroscience, 115,* 1318–1331.

Phifer, C. B., Ladd, M. D., & Hall, W. G. (1991). Effects of hydrational state on ingestion in infant rats: Is dehydration the only ingestive stimulus? *Physiology and Behavior, 49,* 695–699.

Phifer, C. B., Sikes, C. R., & Hall, W. G. (1986). Control of ingestion in 6-day-old rat pups: Termination of intake by gastric fill alone? *The American Journal of Physiology, 250,* R807–R814.

Picciano, M. F. (1998). Human milk: Nutritional aspects of a dynamic food. *Biology of the Neonate, 74,* 84–93.

Plaut, S. M. (1974). Adult-litter relations in rats reared in single and dual-chambered cages. *Developmental Psychobiology, 7,* 111–120.

Powley, T. L., & Berthoud, H. R. (1985). Diet and cephalic phase insulin responses. *The American Journal of Clinical Nutrition, 42,* 991–1002.

Rosenstein, D., & Oster, H. (1988). Differential facial responses to four basic tastes in newborns. *Child Development, 59,* 1555–1568.

Ross, M. G., & Nijland, M. J. (1997). Fetal swallowing: Relation to amniotic fluid regulation. *Clinical Obstetrics and Gynecology, 40,* 352–365.

Ross, M. G., & Nijland, M. J. (1998). Development of ingestive behavior. *The American Journal of Physiology, 274,* R879–R893.

Schaal, B., & Orgeur, P. (1992). Olfaction in utero: Can the rodent model be generalized? *The Quarterly Journal of Experimental Psychology. B, 44,* 245–278.

Scharrer, E., & Langhans, W. (1986). Control of food intake by fatty acid oxidation. *The American Journal of Physiology, 250,* R1003–R1006.

Schneider, J. E. (2004). Energy balance and reproduction. *Physiology and Behavior, 81,* 289–317.

Schneider, J. E. (2006). Metabolic and hormonal control of the desire for food and sex: Implications for obesity and eating disorders. *Hormones and Behavior, 50,* 562–571.

Schroeder, M., Lavi-Avnon, Y., Dagan, M., Zagoory-Sharon, O., Weller, A., & Moran, T. H. (2007). Diurnal and nocturnal nursing behavior in the OLETF rat. *Developmental Psychobiology, 49,* 323–333.

Schroeder, M., Zagoory-Sharon, O., Lavi-Avnon, Y., Moran, T. H., & Weller, A. (2006). Weight gain and maternal behavior in CCK1 deficient rats. *Physiology and Behavior, 89,* 402–409.

Sclafani, A. (2004). Oral and postoral determinants of food reward. *Physiology and Behavior, 81,* 773–779.

Shahab, M., Sajapitak, S., Tsukamura, H., Kinoshita, M., Matsuyama, S., Ohkura, S., et al. (2006). Acute lipoprivation suppresses pulsatile luteinizing hormone secretion without affecting food intake in female rats. *Journal of Reproductive Development, 52,* 763–772.

Shillabeer, G., & Davison, J. S. (1987). Endogenous and exogenous cholecystokinin may reduce food intake by different mechanisms. *The American Journal of Physiology, 253,* R379–R382.

Sisk, C. L., & Zehr, J. L. (2005). Pubertal hormones organize the adolescent brain and behavior. *Frontiers in Neuroendocrinology, 26,* 163–174.

Smith, G. P. (2006). Ontogeny of ingestive behavior. *Developmental Psychobiology, 48,* 345–359.

Smith, G. P., & Gibbs, J. (1975). Cholecystokinin: A putative satiety signal. *Pharmacology, Biochemistry, and Behavior, 3,* 135–138.

Smith, G. P., & Gibbs, J. (1985). The satiety effect of cholecystokinin. Recent progress and current problems. *Annals of the New York Academy of Sciences, 448,* 417–423.

Smith, G. P., Gibbs, J., Jerome, C., Pi-Sunyer, F. X., Kissileff, H. R., & Thornton, J. (1981). The satiety effect of cholecystokinin: A progress report. *Peptides*, *2*, 57–59.

Smotherman, W. P. (1982). In utero chemosensory experience alters taste preferences and corticosterone responsiveness. *Behavioral and Neural Biology*, *36*, 61–68.

Swithers, S. E. (1997). Development of independent ingestive responding to blockade of fatty acid oxidation in rats. *The American Journal of Physiology*, *273*, R1649–R1656.

Swithers, S. E. (2000). Effects of metabolic inhibitors on ingestive behavior and physiology in preweanling rat pups. *Appetite*, *35*, 9–25.

Swithers, S. E. (2003). Do metabolic signals stimulate intake in rat pups? *Physiology and Behavior*, *79*, 71–78.

Swithers, S. E. (2006). Ovarian hormones influence development of ingestive responding to alterations in fatty acid oxidation. *Developmental Psychobiology*, *48*, 627.

Swithers, S. E., & Davidson, T. L. (2005a). Influence of early dietary experience on energy regulation in rats. *Physiology and Behavior*, *86*, 669–680.

Swithers, S. E., & Davidson, T. L. (2005b). Obesity: Outwitting the wisdom of the body? *Current Neurology Neuroscience Reports*, *5*, 159–162.

Swithers, S. E., & Davidson, T. L. (2008). A role for sweet taste-calorie predictive relations in energy regulation by rats. *Behavioral Neuroscience,. 122*, 161–173.

Swithers, S. E., & Hall, W. G. (1994). Does oral experience terminate ingestion? *Appetite*, *23*, 113–138.

Swithers, S. E., & McCurley, M. (2002). Effects of 2-mercaptoacetate on ingestive behavior in 18- and 21-day-old rats. *Behavioural Brain Research*, *136*, 511–520.

Swithers, S. E., McCurley, M., Scheibler, A., & Doerflinger, A. (2005). Differential effects of lipoprivation and food deprivation on chow and milk intake in 25- and 30-day-old rats. *Appetite*, *45*, 86–93.

Swithers, S. E., Peters, R. L., & Shin, H. S. (1999). Behavioral specificity of effects of 2-mercaptoacetate on independent ingestion in developing rats. *Developmental Psychobiology*, *34*, 101–107.

Swithers-Mulvey, S. E., & Hall, W. G. (1993). Integration of oral habituation and gastric signals in decerebrate pups. *The American Journal of Physiology*, *265*, R216–R219.

Tam, C. S., Garnett, S. P., Cowell, C. T., Campbell, K., Cabrera, G., & Baur, L. A. (2006). Soft drink consumption and excess weight gain in Australian school students: Results from the Nepean study. *International Journal of Obesity and Related Metabolic Disorders*, *30*, 1091–1093.

Thiels, E., & Alberts, J. R. (1985). Milk availability modulates weaning in the Norway rat (*Rattus norvegicus*). *Journal of Comparative Psychology*, *99*, 447–456.

Tinbergen, N. (1963). On aims and methods of ethology. *Zeitschrift für Tierpsychologie*, *20*, 410–433.

Wade, G. N., Schneider, J. E., & Li, H. Y. (1996). Control of fertility by metabolic cues. *The American Journal of Physiology*, *270*, E1–E19.

Wade, G. N., & Zucker, I. (1970). Development of hormonal control over food intake and body weight in female rats. *Journal of Comparative and Physiological Psychology*, *70*, 213–220.

Wakerley, J. B., & Drewett, R. F. (1975). Pattern of sucking in the infant rat during spontaneous milk ejection. *Physiology and Behavior*, *15*, 277–281.

Wakerly, J. B., & Lincoln, D. W. (1971). Milk ejection in the rat: Recordings of intramammary pressure during suckling. *Journal of Endocrinology*, *51*, 13–14.

Weller, A. (2006). The ontogeny of postingestive inhibitory stimuli: Examining the role of CCK. *Developmental Psychobiology*, *48*, 368–379.

Wells, M. A. (1985). Fatty acid metabolism and ketone formation in the suckling rat. *Federation Proceedings*, *44*, 2365–2368.

West, D. B., Greenwood, M. R., Sullivan, A. C., Prescod, L., Marzullo, L. R., & Triscari, J. (1987). Infusion of cholecystokinin between meals into free-feeding rats fails to prolong the intermeal interval. *Physiology and Behavior*, *39*, 111–115.

West, M. J., King, A. P., & Arberg, A. A. (1988). The inheritance of niches: The role of ecological legacies in ontogeny. In E. M. Blass (Ed.), *Handbook of behavioral neurobiology: Developmental psychobiology and behavioral ecology* (Vol. 9, pp. 41–62). New York: Plenum Press.

Woods, S. C., & Ramsay, D. S. (2000). Pavlovian influences over food and drug intake. *Behavioural Brain Research*, *110*, 175–182.

Wuensch, K. L. (1978). Exposure to onion taste in mother's milk leads to enhanced preference for onion diet among weanling rats. *Journal of General Psychology*, *99*, 163–167.

Yeh, Y. Y., & Sheehan, P. M. (1985). Preferential utilization of ketone bodies in the brain and lung of newborn rats. *Federation Proceedings*, *44*, 2352–2358.

Yeung, D., & Oliver, I. T. (1967). Gluconeogenesis from amino acids in neonatal rat liver. *Biochemical Journal*, *103*, 744–748.

Multilevel Development: The Ontogeny of Individual and Group Behavior

Jeffrey R. Alberts *and* Jeffrey C. Schank

Abstract

The aim of this chapter is to bring back into focus the primacy of behavioral analysis both for its own sake and for integrating and understanding the discoveries made at genetic and neural levels of organization. This chapter argues that this integrative aspect of behavior requires tools and techniques that match the sophistication of those used by research focused more directly on genetic and neural levels. The chapter surveys the behavioral ontogeny of laboratory rats using a dialectic process that interweaves the study of individual and group behavior. The chapter ends with a preview of the directions technology and integration may take in the study of the behavioral development of individual and of groups.

Keywords: behavioral development, emergent, ontogeny, rats, individual behavior, group behavior, integrative, group selection

Behavioral neuroscience is a young field that has rapidly generated a large body of knowledge. The growth rate on one side of this body, however, its behavioral side, has been slower than on its now larger, "neuro" side. We think that the behavioral side can—and will—grow dramatically and change in important ways that will benefit the entire field.

In this chapter, we are particularly concerned with multiple levels of analysis and organization. Whether a behavioral neuroscientist emphasizes an organism's behavior, or a neural system, or some region of the genome that is affected by brain-mediated experience, the subject matter is that of a complex, dynamic system and there arise common conceptual barriers that have been difficult to penetrate (Alberts, 2002).

Reductionism is one traditional approach to such complex phenomena. Typically, one begins at the level of the individual organism and proceeds to look down to lower levels of organization (e.g.,

neural or endocrine systems, genomic systems, or even proteomic events). Such reductionistic studies involve stripping away the organism and most of its parts or from the parts with which it interacts (i.e., other organisms). This is a powerful strategy for revealing lower-level mechanisms but too often organismal behavior is lost and cannot be retrieved from the reductionistic levels.

Researchers have also been looking up. While remaining anchored at the level of the individual organism, these investigators cross to "higher" levels, usually involving one or more other organisms. In studies of mammalian development, the mother–infant relations can constitute a functional, integrated unit. In species that give birth to multiple offspring, the aggregate of offspring may itself constitute a group.

The nonreductionist strategy has paid good dividends. As we will see, the rewards include discoveries of how mechanisms on a lower level of organization (the individual) create, sometimes additively and at other times multiplicatively, a separable and higher level of organization (the group). We are learning how the two levels, the level of the individual and the emergent level of the group, interact and affect one another. This amounts to an advance in multilevel integration, important to all of behavioral neuroscience. After all, our ultimate goal is not simply to reduce behavior to the expression of genes or the firing of neurons, but rather to understand how lower-level entities such as genes and neurons interact to play a generative role in the emergence of individual and group behavior.

We think that behavioral studies will contribute importantly to expanding and refining our ability to conceptualize how multiple levels of organization operate and, especially, how they develop. Understanding dynamic, living systems must include understanding how they are formed and maintained at multiple levels of organization.

The ascendance of behavioral studies will occur largely in response to the challenge of linking genes, brain, and behavior. Behavior is paramount: It is bodies and interacting bodies that behave, not brains or genes. To discover the links, it is essential to cross levels of organization and to forge interdisciplinary connections. Indeed, multilevel integration is central to behavioral neurobiology itself. The present chapter was written in part to explore some of the ways in which behavioral studies within neurobiology can lead the way toward multilevel understanding and facilitate new and powerful integrative perspectives. It was also written to explore ways in which behavioral methods and approaches can be used as powerful tools for integrating lower-levels of organization with higher, behavioral levels.

Current directions in neurobiology and genetics have been driven by the development of new technologies that have enabled the exploration of previously unexplorable problems. We will argue that analogous technological developments are occurring for behavior that are allowing behavioral studies to take a new and leading role in behavioral neurobiology, largely because new methods have opened up new ways of seeing behavior and, importantly, of handling the massive sets of data that are characteristic of complex systems, such as living organisms and groups of organisms. Thus, we will begin with an overview of some of the technological innovations for the study of behavior.

By themselves, they can do little to solve the integrative problem we pose. With guiding precepts, however, we believe that these behavioral tools (and others yet to be developed) can provide a conceptual framework for the integration of individual and group behavior across multiple levels and through development.

Studies of the Norway rat (*Rattus norvegicus*) have probably contributed the most to our knowledge pertinent to understanding multilevel development and behavior. The present chapter will reflect the generous contributions of this species, which has long been appreciated for its adaptability to various laboratory conditions, its rapid and dramatic postnatal development, and its rich behavioral repertoire. *Mus musculus*, of course, is now growing in popularity due to rich knowledge of its genome, but *R. norvegicus* best helps us tell the story that comprises the present chapter. Indeed, both species typify the gap in levels of analysis this chapter aims to bridge conceptually and methodologically.

The dialectic of this review begins with an overview of new tools that enable new views of individuals and groups. We then turn to precepts to guide our investigative journey from individual to group and group to individual. By reviewing episodes in the study of ontogenies, we will discover how powerful the dialectic process of moving from part to whole, individual to group, and group to individual can be. We then return to some of the new tools and illustrate how they yield new insights and facilitate our integrative aims.

New Tools Enable New Views

New technologies have changed the study of behavior. So profound are these technology-enabled changes that they have engendered new conceptualizations of behavior and of causality, especially in relation to behavioral development. The advent of new views can be found on many levels of analysis, but is especially evident in the study of groups. Behavior in the context of groups is complicated, but new technological tools have made such complex observations increasingly possible and precise. Here we note a few of the more influential technological advances that have altered the ways we view behavior.

Video: Capturing Behavior and Making Time Elastic

The advent of video imaging and video recording, both analog and digital, has steadily transformed the study of behavior. Video enables images to be captured (i.e., recorded and stored), replayed, reanalyzed, duplicated, and shared. Infrared capabilities enable imaging in the dark. Video equipment has become increasingly miniaturized and remarkably inexpensive, replacing the older, celluloid film-based technologies that were bulky, slow, and expensive.

Video technologies also enable us to capture behavior in "elastic time." Standard, commercial formats provide about 30 frame-like shots per second. Time-lapse video, in contrast, samples at a specified, reduced rate, perhaps only 5 times per second. When playback is at the standard rate, the images from each second move at an accelerated pace. Observers can record without direct presence, perhaps continuously for 24 h or more, and then compress time during playback and see the behavior without interruption in a viewing session of 1 or 2 h. With these methods, we see more, we collect more, and come to understand a lot more.

Another way of appreciating the power of a time-lapse view is to contrast it with another, time-sampled view of behavior. "Time-sampling" is accomplished by observing an animal or group of animals at intervals, usually predetermined, fixed intervals. Time-sampled observations are usually recorded "live" with a keyboard or, perhaps voice recording, so they are limited to behaviors that can be discerned reliably in real time. In the same 15 min devoted to time-sampling one target, the time-lapse user can sample portions of each second and accumulate six hours of such data! These time-lapse records can be reexamined (frame by frame, if necessary), duplicated, and shared.

Video can also *expand time* by slowing down the stream of behavior. Such approaches are helpful when the behavior of interest occurs very rapidly or consists of small rapidly expressed components. Even after more than 20 years of observing cowbirds courting, it was not until West and King (1988) used high-speed video to expand time and examine the microstructure of the birds' behavior, could they discern the female's brief "wingstroke" that serves as a reinforcing signal, indicating an effective song from the male.

Other high-speed and high-throughput methods, beyond the scope of the present chapter, have been employed productively. These include kinematic methods enabled by video and other digitized tracking technologies, which provide two- and three-dimensional tracking of limb and joint positions. These data, which rapidly become voluminous during most applications, yield quantitative descriptions of movement-in-time that are used to analyze behavioral form and plasticity.

Appearing on the market now are a variety of video-/computer-based systems featuring software designed to recognize and categorize an animal's behavior. These systems not only can track movement and thus measure activity, but with pattern recognition capabilities, they can reliably categorize activities such as rearing and grooming. Such systems have great promise in replicating the tasks undertaken by some human observers, but more work is needed.

Computerization: Do More, Store More, See More

There are two correct views on the contribution of computerization to the study of behavior. The first, commonly held view, is that computers help us collect more data, store it, and analyze it. Such computerization greatly facilitates what we already do. We can do more per unit time, and so we do. Unbelievably, computer speed has evolved at the awesome pace prescribed by Moore's law, which states that computational speed will double every 18 months and may continue to do so for another 250 years (Lloyd, 2000). Computers have become really fast and will likely continue doing so.

Linked to blazing computational speed has been a corresponding evolution of affordable storage space. Memory got cheap and it continues to get cheaper. So, we can do more and store more. Because analytic speed has increased, we can collect and store digital video, handle vast data sets for three-dimensional, kinematic analyses, or on-line pattern recognition.

The second and more recent correct view is that computerization has evolved to a level that it now enables to see things in ways we could not have imagined before. Speed and storage boundaries now allow us to collect so much more data that there have been raised new questions about the organization and analysis of such data sets. For example, we have collected precise measures of position, orientation, and activity on each of eight rat pups, as they interact in a huddle. From the formidable data set generated by the group, we could for the first time, describe the dynamic behavior of the group as a whole, by "seeing" for the first time, the flow of aggregon formation—the 22 different combinations of bodies in contact that can be (and are) displayed by eight rat pups in a huddle. Later in this chapter, we examine and discuss the behavior of groups.

Perhaps it is time to start developing a new field called *psychobioinformatics*. We construe psychobioinformatics to include any technology, technique, or method that allows us to extract, organize, integrate, and analyze behavioral and biological data at multiple levels of organization and timescales. These new tools include not only the imaging technologies just mentioned but also a variety of new algorithms that allow us to use computers in new ways to study behavior. For example, progress is being made in computer-automated tracking and identification of behavior for specific applications (Delcourt et al., 2006; Noldus, Spink, & Tegelenbosch, 2001; Tsibidis & Tavernarakis, 2007), but much more remains to be done (Schank & Koehnle, 2007).

Robotics and Computer Simulation: Hypothesis Testing by Construction

We believe that thorough analysis of behavior and the integration of behavioral processes at different levels require more than traditional hypothesis testing. Empirical methods are necessary but probably insufficient to manage the complexities of behavioral problems. Additional approaches are needed. Whereas traditional empirical approaches accomplish hypothesis testing by *falsification*, in robotics hypothesis testing is by *construction*. This approach embodies the methodological precept that if you understand how something works, you should be able to build something like it to test your understanding.

Robotic and simulation-based approaches to hypothesis testing are just beginning to emerge, so it is premature to review and evaluate them. Instead, we can best describe an example and consider its contributions to knowledge of behavior and development. In short, this approach is based on demonstration of the possible, with reliance on elements that resemble biological realities.

Some of robotics' most powerful manifestations grow out of computational modeling. Central processor unit (CPU) technology is at the heart of both approaches. With the increasing power of CPUs and their miniaturization, we not only can construct multilevel simulation of robots and agents, but it is also possible to construct physical models (i.e., robots). Such robotic applications require the construction of predictive and explanatory models that connect multiple levels of organization. By building both virtual and physical models, we can test by construction (and not merely falsification) the theories and mechanisms we propose as explanations of multilevel development. That is, we can build model systems that behave like we think natural systems behave and then compare the behavior of our artificial systems to natural systems.

The Precepts

In this section, we present some general and basic formulations—precepts—that will help clarify themes that prevail throughout the research described in the remainder of the chapter. These precepts arise from findings propelled by research tools such as those discussed in our early remarks and analyses guided by innovative developmental perspectives. Although our discussions will focus on developmental and behavioral aspects of behavioral neurobiology, we think that the precepts are broadly applicable to the field, especially in the quest for improvements in multilevel integration.

Precept 1: Ontogeny Is a Collective Noun

Ontogeny is not a single process; rather, ontogeny comprises a number of interacting processes at different levels of organization. Thus, the term *ontogeny* is actually a collective noun referring to interacting ontogenies within ontogenies. That development proceeds on multiple levels is obvious when we begin to enumerate things that develop: neurons, neural systems, functional capabilities, individual behavior, and group behavior.

Such a multitude of levels presents patterns of activities. Obviously, there are interactions among units or "agents" on each level (e.g., neurons, systems, individuals). Less obvious but no less important, however, is that each of these levels can affect others. Behaviors and phenomena are emergent from lower-level interactions and therefore cannot be adequately understood without understanding the dynamic interactions of lower-level components. Interactions across levels are also apparent.

The perspective we will take in this chapter is that development is multilevel and emergent. Our focus will be on two special levels and their interactions: individual and group behavior. We will show that studying individual and group behavior is important as subject and as paradigm not only for understanding development but also for other integrative efforts. The behaving individual is analyzed at a fundamental level and such analysis is strategically positioned for reduction to other familiar, lower levels. Conveniently, the level of the individual is also below another important level, that of the group.

Nevertheless, focusing on just these two levels does not make our task simple. An ontogeny at any level contains ontogenies within it. Our task will not only be to describe these ontogenies and their mechanisms, but also how they interact across and within levels. Because our perspective is one of emergence, it seems untenable to consider ontogenies as programmed in genomes. Rather, they emerge from interacting parts and from ontogenies at numerous levels of organization including the genome. How ontogenies emerge from these interactions is heavily constrained by context.

Precept 2: Development Occurs in Context

Contextual features constrain and generate patterns of behavior. These contextual features include all kinds of environmental elements, such as temperature, gravity, light, sound, and chemical stimuli. Some less obvious, but influential features include other organisms, the geometry of the physical context, body size and shape, as well as the placement and orientation of receptors. Thus, context, as we define it, is always present and behavior is never context-free.

Development is sustained and constrained by context. The mammalian uterus is a context, as is the amniotic sac. Alberts and Cramer (1988) traced the rats' early postnatal development as a series of adaptations to series of contextual changes that comprised a series of "ontogenetic niches." These were, in sequence, the uterus, the exterior of the mother's body, the clump of siblings in the nest, and finally, the social coterie outside of the nest, first experienced by weanlings.

There have been a variety of essays that have explored the interrelations of development, adaptation, and context. Interestingly and importantly, in mammalian development, the study of behavior development is often best investigated in the context of social groups. This implies that mechanisms such as gene expression and regulation are also embedded in social contexts. Gene expression and regulation in a developing animal influences and is influenced by context. In this view, phenotypic expression during development is not merely gene expression in developmental context but it better characterized as a web of interactions within and between levels and contexts. What genes are expressed and how they are expressed are downwardly influenced and regulated by social context (Schank, 2001).

Precept 3: Groups Are Functional Entities

Conspecifics located together at the same time constitute a group. But there are different *kinds of groups*. For purposes of the present discussion, we will recognize two kinds: groups that are (a) the sum of their parts (i.e., aggregations independent of their interactions) and (b) groups that are *more* than the sum of their parts (i.e., aggregations emergent from their interactions, some of which can be adapted groups).

In the present framework, the most basic, minimally organized group structure emerges when individuals act or interact in a manner that merely results in physical association with one another. In such instances, we find each individual capable of autonomous behavior. Individuals respond to others, or perhaps they respond to a common cue in the environment, and thus enter into association with others through simple movements and/or sensory interactions (Fraenkel & Gunn, 1940). When such actions and interactions result in a group and the organization and characteristics of the aggregate are the basic, linear sum of the individuals, we have a simple group.

In contrast, emergent and adapted groups are attained when the aggregate displays functional characteristics or capabilities that are different or beyond those of the individuals comprising it. We say that the "group is more than the sum of its parts" and that it is an *adapted group*. Such groups define themselves in terms of the integration of their activities or the specialized, emergent, functional characteristics of the group. Specialized "functional characteristics" are demonstrable during interactions between levels, especially when one level alters or regulates the other. To use a distinction introduced by evolutionary biologist, Williams (1966), who discussed such properties of aggregations of insects, we will primarily focus on the distinction between *a group of adapted pups* and *an adapted group of pups*.

It should be kept in mind, however, that patterns of organization can emerge for which there is no obvious adaptive function. This can occur anytime context is changed, since changes in context affect emergent organization. Nevertheless, our proposed dichotomy of kinds of groups (i.e., *group of adapted pups* versus *an adapted group of pups*) is useful, for it helps us to discriminate between different forms of interaction and see their functional consequences. When we recognize such differences, we can better ask how they arise. Much of this chapter consists of different approaches to recognizing and analyzing groups and their organization.

Precept 4: Development Is Emergent

We identify *emergence* as a cause of development. To be sure, we are again invoking emergence, but previously, in Precept 3, we identified emergence as instances in which a new level of organization arises. The developmental emergence that we recognize here arises on the same level of organization as the interactions that induce the new form or function. This is a framework in which behavior can cause or invent new forms of behavior. This is a framework in which development is emergent.

Development emerges when tissues interact in ways that "induce" new elements (Saunders, 1982). Development emerges when tissue accumulates to produce changes in size and shape. It is often the case that the activity of such growing forms constitutes interaction among cells or systems and these interactions comprise information that alters form and function (Goodwin, 1994). The development of sensory systems provides a wealth of such examples (Gottlieb, 1976). Similarly, exercising nerves, muscles, and bones constitutes interactions and information across the body from which emerge stronger, more efficient, and adaptive movements (Thelen, 1988; Thelen, Kelso, & Fogel, 1987). Development also emerges from interactions across levels, just as was recognized earlier in Precept 3.

Both uses of emergent—as a cause of invention on another level of organization (Precept 3) and as a cause of development (Precept 4)—are valid. In fact, these two forms of emergence typically occur simultaneously. With the development of new capabilities on levels below that of the organism, new ontogenies emerge on higher levels of organization, i.e., on the level of the individual. As developing individuals interact, individual ontogenies create new interactions and thus developmental change is made more likely on the level of the group. Similarly, interactions on the level of the group can create new conditions within which there arises new behavior by the group. And, as we shall see, new developments on the level of the group can also exert downward influences to the level of the individual.

Together, the interactions on multiple levels constitute development. As proffered by Precept 1, there are ontogenies within ontogeny and the interactions that comprise these levels are developmental information. These elements of information comprise the nonprogrammed emergent instructions that determine development.

Behavioral Development on the Levels of the Individual and the Group: Episodes of Discovery

In the next two sections, we review research from our laboratories, from our collaborations, and from the laboratories of others in a manner that we think can help illustrate and illuminate dialectic processes of ontogenesis on the level of the individual and the group. In addition, we hope to demonstrate that there is much that can help us conceptualize and think about multilevel development by "looking up" from the level of the individual to the level of the group. When this upward view is combined with the more traditional downward, reductionistic perspective, we see new integrative possibilities.

We first examine some of the more traditional, descriptive accounts of development on the level of the individual. Even simple description of individual development is not that simple. For example, whether individuals are viewed in their normal context (*in situ*) or in some approximation of the normal context, or contrastingly, out of [normal] context—in isolation (*ex situ*)—assumes importance.

Behavior and Development on the Level of the Individual
DESCRIPTIVE ACCOUNTS OF RAT DEVELOPMENT

Williard Small's (1899) diary-like report was probably the first systematic description of the development of the domesticated rat. His account is based both on direct observations of pups in a nest box and of individuals removed from the nest for inspection, sometimes with quasiexperimental probes to test whether, for instance, a pup can detect a particular odorant. Presented as a description of "psychic development of the young white rat," Small included discussion of dimensions of behavior that are purely constructs, such as curiosity, fearfulness, greed, and the like. Small did not attempt to operationalize such constructs, so this aspect of his work is almost fanciful by today's standards. Small made a lasting contribution, however, and many of his observations of early sensory function have lasted as reliable accounts. His narrative remains a valuable read. It is filled with thoughtful percepts and integrative overviews of development.

Bolles and Woods (1964) conducted an informal type of time-sample study with 13 caged dams and litters. They observed and took notes on entire litters of pups by watching all of the individuals, documenting the ages at which different behaviors were displayed. Featured in this now classic report were "reflex figures" such as body flexions and sniffing, "functional activities" including eating, drinking, grooming, and climbing, as well as a few "social behaviors." The study provides an overview of "onsets" in pups, such as the onset of walking, running, and grooming behaviors. They also observed the behavior of single, "focal" pups in an additional six litters. Again, the data were mostly qualitative and focused on behavioral categories.

Alberts' (1984, 2005) reviews of sensory development and general development in rat exemplify another type of descriptive account. The approach used in such accounts is based on assembling and synthesizing findings from many different investigations, from different laboratories, conducted at different times and with a variety of different techniques. From such diversity, the goal is to create an idealized, unified overview of an "average" pup moving through a series of developmental transitions.

Altman and Sudarshan (1975) provided a kind of overview of motor development by testing pups of different ages with a battery of tests and measures. Some were largely observational and others were motoric challenges, such as balancing on narrow supports or hanging onto a wire. Their developmental description is designed to define a set of developmental milestones to characterize ontogenetic change and achievement.

MECHANISTIC REACTIONS THAT CREATE COMPLEX BEHAVIOR, *EX SITU*

Early in the twentieth century, research groups dedicated to a behavior-based, mechanistic perspective were motivated by a grand view of an evolutionary phylogeny of plant and animal behavior. In this framework, streams of complex behavior are composed of simple responses to stimuli in the immediate environment. A variety of basic reactions to stimuli were identified, including tropisms, taxes, and kineses (Frankel & Gunn, 1940).

Nevertheless, there is power in such mechanistic approaches. Recently, we tested individual, 10-day-old rat pups' behavior on a uniform, temperature-controlled surface that was tilted at a very modest angle (8° or less). Pups were observed to move downhill (Alberts, Motz, & Schank, 2004). In other words, we saw *positive geotaxis* on substrates tilted at 4° and 8°. Figure 23.1 illustrates the phenomenon of positive geotaxis on modest inclines.

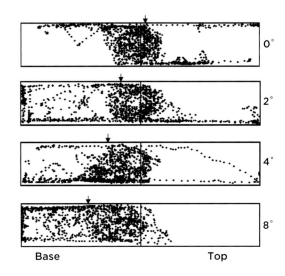

Figure 23.1 Locations of 10-day-old rats on a 91 × 20 cm surface that was either completely level (0°, uppermost rectangle) or tilted to an incline of 2°, 4°, or 8° (shown in series, below). Each dot represents the location of a rat pup's nose as recorded at 5-s intervals during a 15-min test. Trials began when pups were allowed to move freely from the central region of the temperature-controlled test surface. On a level surface, they remain predominantly in the middle. With increasing angles of inclination the distribution of locations shifts downward. Frame-by-frame analyses revealed a combination of taxis- and kinesis-like responses to tilt and to wall surfaces that account for the directional shift (Alberts et al., 2004). The arrows indicate average position.

With increasing slopes, pups increasingly orient and move downhill. This finding contrasts sharply with the "classic" result reported extensively by Crozier and his colleagues (e.g., Crozier & Pincus, 1926, 1936). It now appears that in their zeal, Crozier and his associates rushed to conclusions that were confounded methodologically and colored by preconceptions (cf., Krieder & Blumberg, 1999; Motz & Alberts, 2005).

Using an automatic frame-grabbing technique and software that helped measure, store, and analyze the *x–y* coordinates of the pup's snout, shoulders, and rump, we were able to examine position, angular changes in position, orientation, contact with walls, and velocity. We found that pups initially displayed nondirected activities, the frequency and velocity of which were independent of inclination. The size and configuration of the testing arena made it likely that the pups' initial movements would lead to contact with a wall, usually within 30 s. Once in contact with a wall, pups on an incline were likely to orient downhill, as illustrated in Figure 23.1. The probability and extent of positive geotaxis on an inclined, walled surface increased as a function of angle of inclination. Pups maintained contact and thus maintained downhill orientation. Average movement velocities during the 8 s following wall contact were significantly greater than during a comparable time sample for pups that had not yet encountered a wall. The contact-induced increase in speed, coupled with their orientation, accounts for the characteristic "positive geotaxis."

A coordinated, complex response (orientation and movement downhill) can result from an assembly of simpler, separable reactions to proximal cues. It was possible to diagnose and study this form of behavioral organization only by the careful control of numerous other factors such as temperature, texture, lighting, and the vibrations of nearby equipment that influenced the pups' responses. Clearly, the behavior of an individual involves multiple inputs, simultaneously at play. There is power and parsimony in analyses that focus on the proximal cues in an individual's immediate context that evoke or shape its behavior.

DEVELOPMENT OF BEHAVIORAL AROUSAL AND ACTIVITY

Campbell and associates miniaturized some of the classic stabilimeters for monitoring general locomotor activity of single animals and collected systematic, quantitative data under controlled conditions.

As an animal traverses the floor of a stabilimeter cage, it tips the floor and activates a microswitch and counter. It was not especially surprising that the pups' activity increased after postnatal day (P) 5, when locomotor competence improved dramatically, but it was remarkable that activity surged 10-fold on P15, as can be seen in Figure 23.2. Particularly unexpected was the dramatic decline in activity after P15 (see upper line in Figure 23.2). The P15 peak and subsequent diminution in activity became the focus of subsequent studies of the ontogeny of forebrain inhibition (Campbell, Lytle, & Fibiger, 1969; Campbell & Mabry, 1973; Moorcroft, Lytle, & Campbell, 1971).

Campbell and associates used pharmacological manipulations as well as lesions of forebrain structures to test the hypothesis that the decrease in activity after P15 reflected the development of descending inhibition on brainstem structures that produced the arousal reflected in locomotor activity. Sure enough, when cholinergic forebrain activity was disrupted, the age-related decrease in activity was disrupted, and activity was potentiated. The overall concept was that a variety of stimuli and agents can nonselectively increase arousal in the young pup, and therefore its general activity level. Then, beginning around P15, coincident with the maturation of neural structures such as descending inhibitory projections to the brain stem, behavioral modulation begins (e.g., Fibiger, Lytle, & Campbell, 1970).

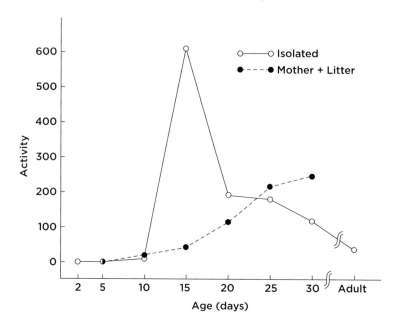

Figure 23.2 Locomotor activity of rats of different ages (infancy through adulthood) when tested alone (open circles) or in a social setting (mother and littermates present). The classic, 15-day-old's peak in activity is a reliable and robust (often 10-fold) potentiation of activity, as measured in a stabilimeter apparatus or via line crossings from video images. When activity is measured in situ—in the presence of the mother and/or littermates—a different picture of age-related activity emerges. The graph shown here is a composite of findings from several reports. (Campbell et al., 1969; Campbell & Mabry, 1973; Campbell & Randall, 1976.)

This picture of an early phase of unrestrained activity followed by reduced levels of activity appeared to be highly robust and reliable until Randall and Campbell (1976) examined the same developmental phenomenon in social settings, *viz.*, in the presence of the mother or littermates or both. Fifteen-day-old pups presented an entirely different picture. Behavioral activity of rat pups tested in either of the two social setting did not show the distinctive P15 peak seen reliably in studies of isolated pups. Instead, when the development of behavioral arousal was measured in a social context, pup activity increased gradually and steadily from day 5 to day 30, as shown by the filled points (broken line) in Figure 23.2. This shocking finding, from the same laboratory that had faithfully promoted a purely central nervous system (CNS)-based explanation for the development of behavioral arousal, was followed by a study examining "the role of environmental stimuli" in the ontogeny of behavioral arousal (Campbell & Raskin, 1978). Once again, it was found that a variety of contextual stimuli, including the presence of bedding material or nest odors, contributed to the modulation of activity in the isolated rat pup.

It was concluded from this long and rigorous line of research that the ontogeny of behavioral arousal is neither a purely brain maturation phenomenon nor a simple product of arousal-inducing external cues. Instead, the frequency, intensity, and duration of activities displayed by rat pups depend on a confluence of identifiable factors in the pup's brain, body, history, as well as its momentary state. This panoply of variables is best combined into a view of *situated behavior,* in which behavioral expression emerges from continuous interactions of organism-in-environment.

DEVELOPMENT OF INGESTIVE BEHAVIOR

In this section, rather than review, we select a set of findings that characterize development of ingestion when it is studied in the individual rat pup in and out of its social context. We will parse suckling into components, showing that the expression of these complex, adaptive behaviors can be understood as a system containing relatively simple and localized responses. Nonsuckling ingestion will also be examined. Once again, we see behaviors that are based on context-dependent, locally organized reactions.

The development of ingestion actually comprises two, separable ontogenies. One is the development and dissolution of suckling. The second is the onset and development of independent ingestion (i.e., feeding and drinking). The two processes are remarkably independent, in terms of the sensory controls, physiological cues, neural systems, and responses to pharmacological manipulations (see Hall & Williams, 1983; Chapter 22).

NIPPLE ATTACHMENT

Before an infant can suckle, it must locate and then attach to a nipple. Olfactory cues are key. Infant rats rendered anosmic do not suckle (cf., Alberts, 1976). Intact rat pups do not attach to the nipples of a dam if her ventrum has been thoroughly washed (Teicher & Blass, 1976). Applying to the clean maternal ventrum, the distillate of the original wash reinstates suckling, indicating that a key olfactory cue has been removed and replaced. Without the correct olfactory input, even a deprived infant will simply rest near a lactating dam and not display any form of searching or dam-directed behavior.

Amniotic fluid is or contains the necessary olfactory cues for the newborn rat's suckling sequence (Teicher & Blass, 1976; Blass & Teicher, 1980). It is instructive to note that during parturition, amniotic fluid is abundant and spread on the dam's body and around the natal environment. Odors that have become familiar *in utero* may be recognized in the new and dramatically different *ex utero* world and thus serve a crucial role in bridging the two environments.

The formative mechanism that prepares a newborn rat to respond to suckling involves *learning*. Amniotic olfactants—whether natural or inserted by an experimenter's injection—are learned by the fetus. If a lemon scent (citral) is added to each amniotic sac on embryonic day (E)17 and the pups are delivered at term, on E22, citral proves to be the necessary cue for nipple attachment. For the citral-conditioned pups, even natural amniotic fluid stimulus is not sufficient to activate the suckling sequence (Pedersen & Blass, 1983).

It is easy to conclude (albeit prematurely and incorrectly) that because olfactory input is necessary for nipple attachment and suckling, and because suckling from a washed dam can be reinstated by painting her nipples with an odor known to the pup, that nipple odor elicits apprehension of a teat. However, the critical and oft unappreciated finding is that a conditioned perinatal odor (i.e., one that was experienced in utero and during parturition) merely in the atmosphere is sufficient to facilitate nipple attachment to a washed dam (Pedersen & Blass, 1981; Pedersen, Williams, &

Blass, 1982). Under such conditions, there was no gradient to follow and no odor source emanating from the dam's body. Activation was the key.

CONDITIONED ACTIVATION

Behavioral activation, initially general and undirected, facilitates nipple attachment because odor cues potentiate movements that bring pups to the dam's body. The pups' head movements and probing brings the infants' perioral area in contact with a nipple, at which point perioral reflexes produce oral grasping of the teat. Thus, general activation of behavior, embodied in a pup with age-related sensory and motor characteristics, situated in a niche composed of a mother's ventrum, leads directly to topographically distinct behavior and a functional, adaptive outcome.

THE AUTOMATIC INFANT

In situ ingestion is reflexive and nonregulated. Friedman (1975) found that the limiting factor of suckling intake for P10 rats is the availability of mother's milk. In the "normal" context of suckling from the dam, intake stops when the mother's milk supply is depleted. When P10 rats were given access to a series of milk-laden dams (10 days postpartum), they continued to suckle and to gain weight.

Hall and Rosenblatt (1977) installed a cannula through which they could deliver milk into a pup's mouth, under its tongue. These cannulated pups moved freely attached to the nipples of an anesthetized dam. The experimenters then delivered milk through the cannula in long pulses (0.10 mL/15 s). Milk was delivered until the pups ceased ingesting it. The most stunning result was that the youngest pups showed no satiety. Even after consuming such large quantities of milk that breathing was difficult, the engorged 5-day-olds struggled back to a nipple.

P10 rats with full stomachs showed an average increase in latency to attach; 15- and 20-day-olds would abandon the nipple after reaching satiety. Hall and Rosenblatt (1977) describe the gradual diminution of the stretch response. Even "nipple shifting" (i.e., releasing a suckled nipple and switching to another one) only appears after P10, which seems to be another sign that internal cues are beginning to exert behavioral control along with the external, olfactory and perioral stimuli (Hall & Rosenblatt, 1977).

PRECOCIOUS FEEDING—*EX SITU*

For this discussion, feeding consists of nutrient ingestion from a source other than the mother's mammary glands. There are several dazzling demonstrations that infant rats are capable of independent, regulated ingestion. This discovery emphasizes how the infant rat can express independent, regulated ingestion, even though such behavior is never expressed under normal conditions during early postnatal life.

Hall (1979b) provided some of the founding demonstrations of precocious feeding in rats. Here he used the same cannula system described earlier, except the pup was in a warm incubator with no mother present and had been deprived for 0.5, 7, or 22 h. Testing involved a series of slow infusions. Pups consumed the diet, and intake increased with deprivation, up to about 78% of the infusate or 2% of their body weight.

The drawings in Figure 23.3 depict some of the movements evoked by the oral infusions. Hall noted that such activities included mouthing,

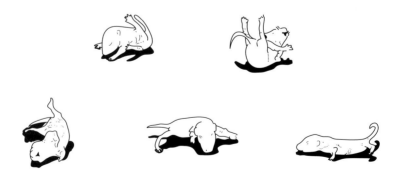

Figure 23.3 Rat pups activated by oral infusions of milk. These drawings (adapted from Hall, 1979b) show examples of 3-day-old pups that have received an infusion of milk into their mouth via an oral cannula (not shown). These pups became highly aroused and moved vigorously, often probing and mouthing the substrate, as well as exhibiting movements and postures rarely seen when with the mother and littermates. (See also Hall, 1979a.)

tongue protrusions, and probing "the surface in front of them." These postures are rarely seen when pups are with the dam and littermates. That setting, though highly variable, nevertheless contains a basic set of olfactory, tactile, contour, and thermal cues that engage the pups' movements and shape an entirely different topography of response. With a dam present, for example, the pups in Figure 23.3 would be observed to stretch and tread in response to the oral infusion and, if detached from the nipple, its aroused behavior would be directed at the dam. The pup would paddle and squirm into contact, and then push and probe into the dam's ventrum until a nipple was encountered. It would be grasped and sucking would resume.

A common feature in every successful demonstration of precocious ingestion is that infant is tested alone, away from the mother. In other words, regulatory competence is masked in the presence of the mother and litter. This is a stunning reminder of the potency of context. Pups can regulate their ingestion, if an appropriate niche (albeit an unusual one) is created.

Behavior and Development on the Level of the Group

By recognizing suckling and feeding as separable processes, we also see two examples of how the presence of social stimuli—the mother in some cases and littermates in others—creates a new order in each individual. This "new order" is evidence for the emergence of a new, functional level of organization, as evidenced by *downward regulation*, from higher-to-lower levels. In this case, we see litter → individual, and mother → offspring, forms of downward regulation. We will survey a few examples of such processes on the level of the group.

DOWNWARD REGULATION OF SUCKLING INTAKE EXERTED BY LITTER COHORT

The amount of milk obtained by pups begins to decrease between P15 and P20, although the amount of milk produced by the mother does not. Indeed, when pups begin to ingest solid food, there is milk available from the dam's mammary ducts (Thiels, Cramer, & Alberts, 1988). The dissolution of suckling comes from a combination of the pups' interactions with one another and the dynamics of the mother–litter relations (Thiels & Alberts, 1991).

Thiels et al. (1988) revealed the power of social setting when two 20-day-old rats were integrated into a litter of six 15-day-olds. Under this arrangement, the 20-day-olds consumed as much milk or more than their new littermates and significantly more than pups in homogenous, 20-day-old litters. Thiels et al. (1988) considered several aspects of the dam's behavior that could affect milk availability, but these did not account for the observed differences.

Also significant is that 20-day-old rats embedded in a litter of 15-day-olds exhibited nonsuckling behavior that also resembled that of the younger pups. For instance, 20-day-olds placed among 15-day-olds were more docile and oriented toward the dam more than did 20-day-olds with same-age littermates.

Observations of the behavior of 15- and 20-day-old litters placed nearby an anesthetized dam provided additional insight into the way the groups acted and interacted as a function of age. The proportion of pups attaching to the dams' nipples was higher and the latency to the first attachment was shorter in 15-day-olds compared to 20-day-olds. It appears that the presence of 15-day-old littermates acts as a form of social facilitation for suckling in the 20-day-olds. In contrast, milk consumption by 15-day-olds was relatively unaffected by the presence of 20-day-old of companion pups (Thiels et al., 1988).

Perhaps the most dramatic, if not most bizarre, demonstration of potent social influences was the demonstration that social stimulation from younger pups can override the diminishing tendency of older pups to attach to the nipple. Individual postweaning-age pups, housed with a series of preweaning-age mothers and their 16- to 21-day-old litters, continue to suckle until they are as old as 70 days of age, well beyond the time of normal weaning (Pfister, Cramer, & Blass, 1986). It is noteworthy that older pups never attach to a nipple when none or fewer than half of the younger pups are attached.

WEANING AT THE LEVEL OF THE GROUP

All mammalian offspring wean, i.e., they cease suckling and commence independent feeding. We have seen that the physical and physiological bases of suckling and feeding develop within each individual. Synchronized and coordinated with these individual ontogenies are transitions in maternal physiology and behavior (Alberts & Gubernick, 1983; Rosenblatt & Lehrman, 1963). In addition, there are also ontogenies on the level of the group. Thus, the diminution of suckling and the transition to feeding occurs within complex and dynamic social niches.

A rat pup's initial egressions from the nest are pivotal events in the weaning process because food is encountered remotely—in other areas of a burrow or in the outside world. The age at which pups leave the nest and begin to sample solid food varies, depending on many contextual factors, but weaning is often underway around P20. What factors account for the pups leaving the nest?

POSTSUCKLING ACTIVATION

Video observations of rats in a variety of laboratory-based habitats have provided much information on the weaning process (Alberts & Leimbach, 1980; Cramer, Thiels, & Alberts, 1990; Galef & Clark, 1971; Gerrish & Alberts, 1996, 1997; Thiels, Alberts, & Cramer, 1990). In the course of observing weanling rats' initial egressions from a nest box into an adjacent open field, we noticed that their forays from the nest often occurred during periods of heightened general activity. More careful, empirical examination revealed a pattern of postsuckling activation.

Shortly after a mother rat completes a nursing bout and leaves the nest, there is often a gradual increase in activity among the litter that can build into an explosion of activity, termed postsuckling behavioral arousal (Gerrish & Alberts, 1997). The aroused litter often displays tumultuous activity, dramatically obvious in a time-lapse videograph. The litter seethes and roils. With increasing turbulence within the nest, individual pups may be seen climbing over and revolving around the group. During this accelerated activity, individuals may zoom out of their orbital path, leaving the group and heading away. We studied this phenomenon in 20-day-old litters in a nest that was attached, via a couple of short tunnels, to an outside field where food and water were located. This postsuckling behavioral arousal was typically the prelude to leaving the nest and entering the field (Gerrish & Alberts, 1997).

The phenomenon can be produced by presenting P20 rats with an anesthetized dam, and then separating each one from a nipple by a tug to its tail. (A nondislodging tail tug was used as a control.) Loss of orally grasped nipple predicts the onset of activation. Figure 23.4 summarizes some experiments that specified the stimulus conditions for the phenomenon of postsuckling behavioral arousal. The behavioral effect was profound and led directly to food sampling (Gerrish & Alberts, 1997; see also Alberts & Leimbach, 1980).

SOCIAL CONTEXTS DETERMINE DIET SELECTION

Ingesting safe, nutritious food and avoiding toxic substances (especially the poisons intended for unwanted commensals) is a primary challenge in the life of wild *R. norvegicus* (Barnett, 2001). Galef and Clark (1971) showed that rat pups completely avoid eating a food that is avoided by the adult members of their colony and prefer foods preferred by adults in the colony. In one of their elegant experiments, rat pups emerged from nest boxes and approached adults that were feeding from a bowl containing a distinct, nutritious Diet A and avoiding another bowl containing a distinct, nutritious, Diet B, which the adults had previously experienced as toxic. (When pups were present, Diet B lacked toxic content.) Pups fed on Diet A hundreds of times and never sampled Diet B, even when a full bowl of this safe, palatable food was located as little as 3 in. from Diet A!

The adults never prevented the pups from sampling Diet B nor did they "mark" the food or its bowl with a chemical deterrent. In fact, Galef and Clark (1971) showed that pups did not learn an aversion to Diet B; they simply learned eating what the adults ate (Diet A).

Such powerful and reliable specificity proved to be formed by remarkably simple and nonspecific mechanisms. Basically, when weanlings approach other rats, this simply brings them into the vicinity of food. Pups choose to eat the same food that others are eating. Preexposure to cues that they can recognize from mother's milk may bias their choice (Galef & Henderson, 1972) as can an association of food odors with carbon disulfide, a constituent of rat breath (Galef, Mason, Petri, & Bean, 1988). Together, these findings suggest that social factors are the predominant guiding force for diet selection and much of the rats' feeding behavior. These factors are influential only because the pups are so exquisitely sensitive and responsive to them.

ONTOGENY OF HUDDLING

For *R. norvegicus*, huddling, or contact behavior, is a life-long behavior. Huddling among littermates begins immediately after birth; huddling with the dam also begins at about this time, as the mother broods and nurses her litter of propagules. Pups remain huddled together in the nest during maternal excursions until around P15 when the coherence of the group lessens, but does not fade. Under normal, group-living, colonial conditions, adult *R.*

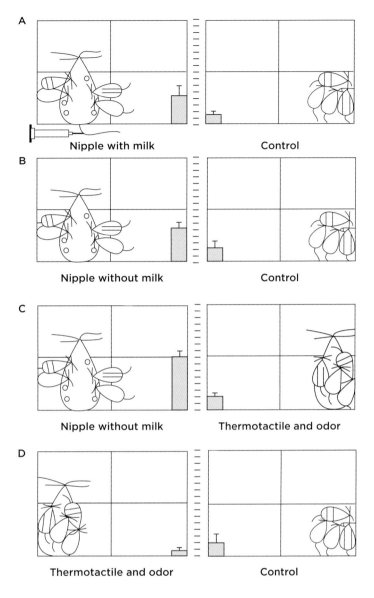

Figure 23.4 Summary of experimental manipulations and outcomes of studies of postsuckling behavioral arousal. Each row depicts a test condition and its control group. For instance, the top row (A) shows a condition in which a litter containing two "focal pups" (striped) can suckle on an anesthetized dam injected with oxytocin so that she provides milk. Their postsuckling activity, shown by the histogram in the lower right of panel, is greater than that of control pups that did not suckle but were handled similarly. The comparison in row B indicates that milk transfer is not necessary for the postsuckling phenomenon. We concluded that nipple attachment (and detachment) is the key stimulus for this form of behavioral arousal. (Gerrish & Alberts, 1997.)

norvegicus continue to engage in a variety of behaviors that involve cutaneous contact. These habits have earned *R. norvegicus* the label of "contact species" (Barnett, 1963).

A naturally occurring clump of pups is not a just a heap of bodies. There is usually activity somewhere within the group. Time-lapse views are especially revealing, for they enable a human observer to see the rhythms and flow of individual behavior within the group. In one observational study, groups of littermates were placed in a bowl-shaped nest for observation. Focal pups within each litter were marked for individual identification and the groups were observed with time-lapse videography

at a record:playback ratio of 12:1. Under these conditions, the huddle is a nearly continuously seething mass. Figure 23.5 depicts the amount of time a focal pup was observed on the surface of the group. Data in panels A and C, and B and D depict individual pups in the same clump so, by mentally sliding the paired panels together, it is possible to envision the alternations and in-phase movements of these individuals.

One answer, derived from studies of 10-day-old rats, is that pup flow can be understood as a group manifestation of individual regulations of exposed body surface shown in Figure 23.5. Litters were placed in nests that were either cool (24°C)

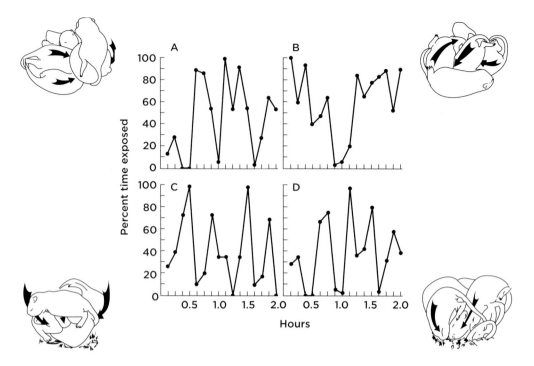

Figure 23.5 Pup flow in a huddle. The movements of individual pups within a huddle were quantified by measuring those times when marked individuals were visible on the huddle surface. These observations were of litters in a bowl-shaped nest. Data are shown as the percent of each 7.5-min interval of a 2-h observation session that a marked individual was visible. (Alberts, 1978.)

or warm (36°C). There were two focal pups, one experimental and the other the control. The experimental animal was injected with an anesthetic before the test and its littermate control was given a saline injection. Both were placed on the surface of their huddle for time-lapse video recording. The time that each focal pup was exposed on the huddle surface was quantified.

It is unusual to run a behavioral study in which the subject is anesthetized, but the point here was the fate of the anesthetized, nonparticipating pup. This pup provided a telling diagnostic. In the room-temperature nest, the unanesthetized pups actively burrowed down into the depths of the litter, thereby pushing the anesthetized pup to the surface of the huddle where it remained almost continuously. Thus, under these conditions, the anesthetized pup was a "floater." In contrast, its active littermate control periodically appeared and disappeared at the surface, as is characteristic of normal pup flow.

That this is a thermally determined, regulatory activity was further demonstrated by the fate of the anesthetized pup in the warm nest (right-hand panel, Figure 23.6). Now, as unanesthetized pups emerged at the surface of the nest to lose heat, the anesthetized pup becomes a "sinker," disappearing into the depths of the group. Thus, we see here a reversal of the direction of pup flow caused by a change in thermal conditions.

This group regulatory behavior can be explained in terms of individual adjustments. Developmental analyses of this phenomenon could prove informative (e.g., Sokoloff & Blumberg, 2001), because there are dramatic developments of individual behavioral thermoregulation in rats (Farrell & Alberts, 2007; Hoffman, Flory, & Alberts, 1999a, 1999b; Pfister, 1990).

We have been discussing the behavior of individual rat pups, sometimes seeing them as an individual within a complex family setting, often in contexts that were specially designed to isolate the rat pup from many of the myriad stimuli that can simultaneously affect pup behavior. Now we turn to the group, especially the group of littermates that comprise the huddle, the pup's first social setting.

By identifying the aggregation of littermates as a "huddle," we immediately invoke a term associated with defense against cold. The connotation is appropriate. Infant rats, often considered ectothermic, thus lacking self-produced body heat, were shown to be warmer and to have lower metabolic rates as a function of group size. Energy conservation by huddling was impressive in scale (Alberts, 1978).

How is this group effect on metabolic heat production achieved? We now know that even newborn rats can activate endogenous deposits of brown adipose tissue, a thermogenic organ, and thereby generate body heat (cf., Blumberg, 2001). But, due in part to the pups' lack of insulative fur and meager subcutaneous fat, they are susceptible to rapid loss of body heat. The pup's large body surface in relation to its small body volume or mass is the prime factor for such heat loss (Alberts, 1978). By huddling, a pup can greatly reduce its exposed surface area, thus reducing the surface:mass ratio, which governs heat transfer.

It is important to ask whether the metabolic benefits of huddling have functional significance. Small huddles of four littermates were placed in a temperature-regulated compartment. By changing the pups' ambient temperature from 20°C to 40°C and back to 20°C over the course of 2 h and measuring the exposed surface area of the group every 10 min, we obtain a picture of the group surface dynamics. Figure 23.7 summarizes the results. At each age, the group surface area was regulated behaviorally to increase and decrease with ambient temperature. These results show that rat pups behave in a manner that produces a form of *group regulatory behavior*. In this instance, the phenomenon is evidenced as the systematic control of the group's physical properties that control heat loss and heat gain.

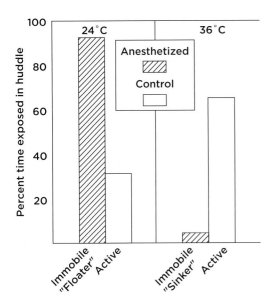

Figure 23.6 Time exposed on the surface of a huddle as a function of whether the focal pup is active or inactive (anesthetized) and temperature of the nest. The fate of an inactive pup reveals the temperature-dependent direction of pup flow. A non-participating pup becomes a "floater" in cool nests as the active pups flow down into the warm depths of the group. In a warm nest, however, pup flow reverses and the inactive littermate is a "sinker" and tends to disappear. (Alberts, 1978.)

GROUP REGULATORY BEHAVIOR

We have characterized this form of group regulatory behavior as an example of niche construction (Alberts, 2007; Alberts & Schank, 2006) whereby huddles of pups create a microenvironment in which the average surface:mass ratio of each individual is reduced. This effectively reduces the magnitude of the environmental challenge, and makes

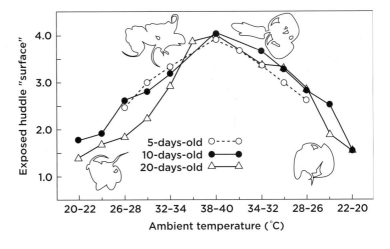

Figure 23.7 Group regulatory behavior in litters of 5-, 10-, and 20-day-old rats. The total exposed body surface area of the huddles increased and decreased as a direct function of ambient temperature. These groups exhibited behavioral and physiological regulations that are superior to those typically seen in isolated individuals. (Alberts, 1978.)

the pup's limited thermogenic abilities more effective (see also Blumberg, 2001; Sokoloff, Blumberg, & Adams, 2000). Therefore, in this niche of bodies, each pup benefits and can express its capabilities with greater efficacy. In this way, the group becomes each individual's niche, and in this niche, their physiological size and capabilities combine to make them more competent than they are as single individuals.

Reconstructing Individual and Group Development: New Tools and Techniques

We can begin to synthesize the diverse body of knowledge about rat pups by constructing models of group and individual behavior. Constructing even relatively simple models of interacting infant rats leads to detailed and unexpected issues. Here we provide a glimpse of what may be possible with these new tools and techniques.

In a typical study, which simplifies many contextual variables, litters of eight rat pups are placed in the stalls of a starting corral (Figure 23.8) centered in an arena (8 × 12 in.) that is a well-controlled, warm environment (e.g., 34°C floor; 34°C air). When the corral is removed, the pups can move freely and aggregate. Video images of pups' movements and aggregations provide a surfeit of information, from which we sample to make comparisons

with virtual or physical models. We have found that image sampling every 5 s is sufficient to collect meaningful data concerning individual and group behavior (May et al., 2006; Schank, 2008; Schank & Alberts, 1997, 2000; Schank, May, Tran, & Joshi, 2004).

Data on locomotion are obtained by recording pup positions as x–y coordinates in images; these data allow for analysis of activity, pup contact, wall contact, and aggregation (Schank & Koehnle, 2007). For example, how pups aggregate into patterns of contact with other pups can be measured as aggregon patterns (i.e., the distribution of individuals in contact groups formed on the surface of an arena) or as subgroups (i.e., the number of contact groups that form, which can range from 1 to the number of individuals in the group; Schank, 2008; Schank & Alberts, 1997, 2000). There are 22 possible aggregons combinations of 8 pups, as shown in the aggregon index of Figure 23.9 and eight possible subgroups, each consisting of subsets of aggregon combinations (Schank, 2008; Schank & Alberts, 2000). The dynamics of aggregon and subgroup frequencies provide detailed and diagnostic descriptions of group behavior (Schank, 2008).

To understand how blind and deaf pups could form the aggregon patterns, we built an agent-based model (Schank, 2008; Schank & Alberts,

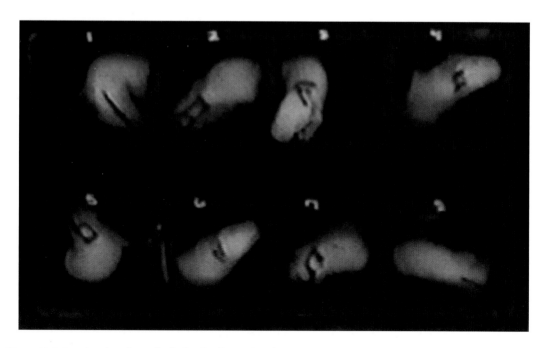

Figure 23.8 Pups (numbered) in individual stalls of a corral used to standardize starting positions for a trial of aggregation. The barrier separating pups is lifted and the trial begins with the free interactions of the pups.

Figure 23.9 Index of 22 possible aggregons created by 8 pups. The upper photo illustrates aggregon #1, with all pups separated. The middle photo shows them aggregated as 4, 2, 1 and 1 (#12). In the lower photo, all 8 pups are in contact (aggregon #22). Group organization changes constantly, and aggregon distribution/time is used to capture the dynamics of the group. When models are tested, the positions of the agent-pups are scored every 5 seconds and the aggregon distributions are compared to huddles of real pups.

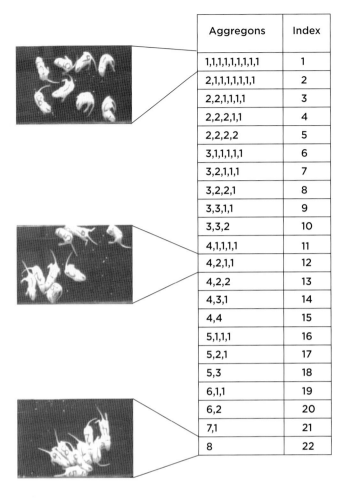

Aggregons	Index
1,1,1,1,1,1,1,1	1
2,1,1,1,1,1,1	2
2,2,1,1,1,1	3
2,2,2,1,1	4
2,2,2,2	5
3,1,1,1,1,1	6
3,2,1,1,1	7
3,2,2,1	8
3,3,1,1	9
3,3,2	10
4,1,1,1,1	11
4,2,1,1	12
4,2,2	13
4,3,1	14
4,4	15
5,1,1,1	16
5,2,1	17
5,3	18
6,1,1	19
6,2	20
7,1	21
8	22

1997, 2000). Pup *movement* was simplified: With each time-step, a pup could move to one of eight adjacent locations in the virtual arena. The rules of behavior were simple: (1) if one or more pups are located in front or on the side of a pup's head, then there is an increased probability that the pup moves towards that location. Similarly, we assumed that (2) pups moved toward the walls of the arena directly in front of them. The two other rules governed *activity*: (3) A pup remains active as a function of the number of active and inactive pups it contacts and (4) becomes inactive again as a function of the number of active and inactive pups contacted. These rules are conceptually simple. Where a pup moves and whether it is active is situation-dependent.

To find a model that behaves like real pups involves determining specific values for the probabilities of moving toward pups or toward wall and for the activity rules described in the previous paragraph. This can be accomplished by systematically simulating the parameter values, or in more complex cases, using optimization techniques such as simulated annealing or genetic algorithms (Schank, 2008; Schank & Alberts, 2000). We thereby fit movement and activity parameters to the aggregative patterns of groups of pups. As illustrated in Figure 23.10, the best fit model generates aggregon frequency distributions that mimic those of the real 7-day-old rat huddles using only the movement and activity rules previously described. We explored the landscape of results derived from changing parameters of the model and have shown that this is a robust phenomenon (Schank & Alberts, 1997).

It is important to emphasize that the model contains no rules of group behavior, but only rules for individual movement and activity. Nonetheless, in the absence of group instructions, pups aggregate and age-specific patterns of aggregation emerge (Schank, 2008; Schank & Alberts, 2000).

Perhaps the most interesting result of this model was the identification of social context-dependent activity during early development. Seven-day-olds exhibited the same probabilities of staying active or becoming active independent of the number or the activity state of pups contacted. Ten-day-olds, however, showed a clear and systematic activity relationship to the number and the activity state of pups contacted. We believe that the coupling of activity states characteristic of the 10-day-olds reflects the *onset of sociality* and reveals a fundamental development from the complete autonomy exhibited by the 7-day-olds in this context.

Converging on our interpretation of a developmental transition into sociality are the results of a separate study in which we infused either oxytocin (OT) or an OT antagonist (Vasotocin) intracisternally in 7- and 10-day-old pups that were tested under group conditions (Alberts, 2007; Odya, Sokoloff, & Alberts, 2002). We used OT because it is widely associated with modulating social behavior in a variety of species and behavioral contexts (e.g., Ferguson, Young, & Insel, 2002; Goodson, 2005; Insel & Fernald, 2004; Lim & Young, 2006), though there have been few developmental studies (cf., Carter, 2003). In this preliminary study, we measured group "size" (i.e., total area subtended by the aggregons) and found that in 10-day-olds OT treatment promoted proximity and group coherence whereas the antagonist decreased group coherence below levels seen in the control groups. Figure 23.11 illustrates these results. Thus, we believe that this research with rats (a) defines and validates emergent group behavior, (b) reveals an ontogeny of group behavior, and (c) provides quantitative and qualitative methods for isolating and synthesizing the rules and mechanisms for the patterns of aggregation we have observed.

Hypothesis Testing by Construction

Hypothesis testing in behavioral neuroscience has traditionally been accomplished by falsification. There is art to this kind of science: Beautiful experiments are devised to falsify, and thereby reject, well-articulated null hypotheses. Most often, we seek precise and specific hypotheses, which can be thoroughly tested and rejected. As noted early in this chapter, however, integrative problems as complex as understanding development of behavior on

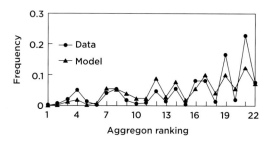

Figure 23.10 Frequency of aggregons during 15-min test exhibited by 7-day-old rat pups (data) and agent-based computational pups (model). Aggregon index is shown on the abscissa. The observed fit of Model and Data was lost when 10-day-old pups were run. By adding a rule that changes each pup's activity as a function of the activity of the other pup(s) with which it is in contact, the model again matches the real pups.

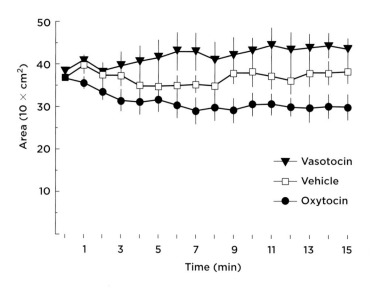

Figure 23.11 Total area created by 10-day-old rat aggregons following intracisternal infusion of either oxytocin, vasotocin (an oxytocin antagonist), or vehicle. Vertical axis shows total circumference of group (10× cm²). Whereas oxytocin increased huddle cohesion; vasotocin decreased it.

multiple levels needs more than a series of tests of specific hypotheses because the problem of integrating multiple levels is too complex. At this point, we need to synthesize the available information. We need to construct a system analog or model that we can test and analyze. We think that modeling is a valuable and important approach that can be used rigorously, and can contribute in special ways to a fuller understanding of complex processes. As mentioned above, one goal of constructing models is to integrate levels by creating models that behave like the natural systems. When we successfully construct models that behave like a natural living system, using biologically valid elements, we demonstrate a sufficiency or completeness of knowledge regarding a complex reality in relation to its simpler components. Such models become a source of testable hypotheses.

Models come in a variety of forms and compositions, ranging from pure mathematical entities to computation or even physical models (Koehnle & Schank, 2003). Robotic models pose a special challenge in this regard but offer special rewards. One reason for building physical robotic models of animals—in addition to building only virtual models—is to emulate physical interactions of bodies with their environment. Ideally, such interactions can be modeled virtually (Bish, Joshi, Schank, &Wexler, 2007) but in practice, the virtual models remain only approximations for physical properties, which may therefore miss important physical interactions. Moreover, physical robots also allow for the gradual evolution of increasingly complex robotic models of animals by adding components and then testing the new phenotype.

We see special value in using robots to learn about multilevel development using individual and group behavior as the prime phenomenological levels. Rat development is beautifully suited to this strategy. The infant's limited sensory and motor repertoires direct the modeler to begin with simple robots. Then, to account for the increased sensorimotor complexity that emerges in subsequent developmental states (e.g., the development of visual and auditory function), the modeler can reengineer the robots to include such sensory systems. Each stage requires testing and reengineering based on results and new data.

To build robots that behave like infant rats required us to model pup morphology and physical contact. These preliminary requirements proved instructive and provided lessons not readily learned from the virtual models alone.

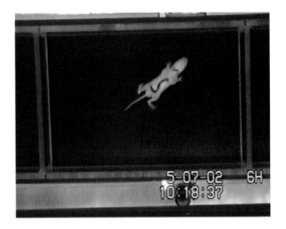

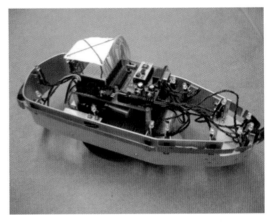

Figure 23.12 Ten-day-old rat pup in an arena (top) and one of our robots (bottom).

We learned that the *shape* of a robot's body (Figure 23.12) is important because it determines how the robot interacts with corners, walls, and other robots in an arena (see Figure 23.12, top), and thus whether a robot can behave like a pup. A 10-day-old rat pup measures about 7.6 × 2.5 cm, which is too small to model with available mechanical and electrical hardware. Thus, we built robots scaled to a rat pup's length-to-width ratio (3:1). The overall dimensions for the robots were 32.4 × 10.8 cm. We built a total of eight robots (May et al., 2006). Rat pups, up to 10 days old, primarily use their back legs for forward locomotion (Altman & Sudarshan, 1975). Robots with rear-driven wheels and differential drive on the chassis create forces on the body that resemble those of young rat pups (May et al., 2006; Schank et al., 2004).

We believe that the flexibility of pups' bodies and the rigidity of robots' bodies resulted in different patterns of motion. For example, rat pups often leave corners in an arena by flexing their body in an arc rather than backing up. Because flexing to turn is not possible for our robots, we simulated this maneuver by allowing a robot to back up slightly and then turn. We achieved different circular arc motions by shifting the center of motion along the lateral axis of the robot, which affected the overall turning trajectory. This center could be adjusted to accommodate data for pups at different ages. Because our strategy is to start with the "simple" and work to the complex on a developmental timescale, our robots modeled only an infant rat's dominant sensory modality during the first 12 days after birth, namely its tactile sense. To model tactile sensitivity, we mounted microswitch bump sensors around the skirt to mimic tactile sensory fields of rats (Figure 23.12, bottom). Because the majority of infant rat interactions occur rostrally, we mounted a number of adjustable sensors near the front of the robot. A total of 14 sensors were installed, with half located on the head and half along the body. To increase the range of each sensor, we mounted brass metal strips on them, which allowed sensing at all points along the robot's body.

The central processor of a robot implements sensorimotor rules that simulate the brain of an animal. There are many levels of abstraction for modeling a brain, ranging from a simple reactive architecture that deterministically relates peripheral sensory input and motor output to neural networks models with increasingly realistic representation of neural anatomy and physiology. Thus, a simple and natural starting point for modeling contact and aggregation in infant rats with robotic modes is to implement a reactive-control architecture that is responsive to contact alone. This approach—which is a simplified implementation of a brain—resembles the contextual simplification and control that we used when we began the testing of (real) rat pups in a warm, flat, evenly illuminated arena (Schank & Alberts, 1997; 2000).

A typical robot run, using this thigmotaxic-reactive architecture, produced patterns of movement that were highly stereotyped. Robots repeatedly followed walls, circling the arena over and over again, resembling the "stereotypies" often observed in animals in zoos. It was clear that a purely deterministic, thigmotaxic-reactive architecture could not explain the behavior of pups in an arena. There were, however, runs in which the robots' behavior did not appear so stereotypical. A robot's behavior can be influenced indeterminately when, for example, dust on the substrate causes wheels to slip

slightly, or if there are small differences in the servo motors that run each wheel. This suggested to us that randomness may be an important factor in generating behavior.

We then decided to test robots that moved completely randomly with no influence on their behavior from their tactile sensors. To produce a random control robot, a robot at each time step t (the interval between time steps was set to 2 s) randomly chooses one of 10 locomotor behaviors produced by modulating the two servo motors running the wheels: (1) forward; (2) 45° left; (3) 90° left; (4) 135° left; (5) 45° right; (6) 90° right; (7) 135° right; (8) backup left; (9) backup right; and (10) do nothing. To our great surprise, results from both individual and multiple robot experiments revealed that a simple random architecture with no contingency relationships between sensory inputs and motor outputs coupled with body-environment constraints accounted for a large proportion of the behavioral patterns observed in both individuals and groups. Individual random robots followed walls, got stuck in corners, escaped them, and visited a variable number of corners in each run. Individuals in groups produced the same movements and even aggregated in similar ways as illustrated in Figure 23.13 (see Table 23.1 for comparisons among all metrics).

It is striking that a randomly moving robot with a body shape similar to a pup placed in an arena is so constrained by arena geometry and body shape that its behavior alone and in a group is very similar to rat pups. But real infant rats have sensory systems that respond to tactile input. Surely their behavior cannot be purely random? Probably the best interpretation of these results is that body morphology and its interactions with the environment can generate emergent patterns of aggregation even though the robots are using no rules at all to move about! We are currently simulating various ways in which these robots can have flexible bodies because having rigid bodies greatly constrains movement and is unrealistic as a model of flexible bodied rat pups. Our initial results are that flexibility does make a difference and that flexible bodied robots, which move randomly, do not match pup behavior nearly as well though body morphology still contributes substantially to the patterns of aggregation we observe (May, 2007). We are now at the stage where we can begin to model the contribution of simple sensorimotor rules with an understanding of how morphology and the physical structure of the environment constrain behavior.

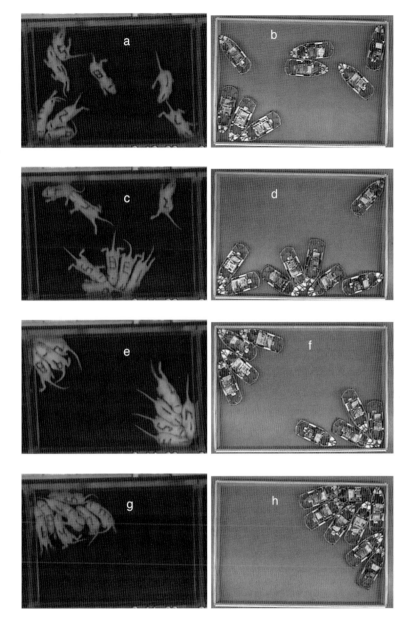

Figure 23.13 Examples of aggregation patterns of P10 pups (left column) and robots (right column) in the arenas. Pups (A) and robots (B) shortly after they are released. Pups (C) and robots (D) forming a subgroup that is not in a corner. Pups (E) and robots (F) forming two subgroups in opposite corners. Pups (G) and robots (H) aggregating in a single corner.

Final Overview: Individuals and Groups during Natural Selection

Recognition of groups as coherent, functional units has a long history in biology. By 1872 and with each edition of the *Origin of the Species*, Darwin increasingly recognized the importance of natural selection operating at the level of the group. Yet, in the 1960s, adaptation at the level of the group was strongly challenged—so strongly in fact, that the idea was essentially rejected outright and considered an anathema if raised for discussion

(Darlington, 1980). The demise of group selection can be attributed, at least in part, to overemphasis on the idea that the interests of the individual are sacrificed or subordinated to those of the group. After group selection was narrowed and isolated this way, there was room to popularize mutually exclusive viewpoints. Proponents of the view that natural selection is limited to the level of the individual scored big with inclusive fitness theory (Hamilton, 1964, 1975) and selfish gene theory (Dawkins, 1976; Williams, 1966).

Table 23.1 Comparison of Robots to 7-Day and 10-Day Rats on All Metrics

Measure	Pup Age vs. Robots Pup Age
Individual wall contact	7 days = Robots = 10 days
Individual corner contact	7 days < Robots = 10 days
Individual center contact	7 days > Robots > 10 days
Individual distance moved	7 days < Robots = 10 days
Individual aim	7 days > Robots = 10 days
Group wall contact	7 days < Robots = 10 days
Group corner contact	7 days < Robots > 10 days
Group center contact	7 days > Robots < 10 days
Group aggregation	7 days < Robots < 10 days

Robots either statistically match 10-day-old pups or are intermediate between 7- and 10-day-old pups, except for Group corner contact and Group center contact.

There is now, however, a growing revival of interest in group selection as an important force in evolution (e.g., Wade, 1976; Wilson, 1975, 1983), even among some previous detractors (Wilson & Wilson, 2007). We see the precepts and much of the research discussed in this chapter as amenable with the more modern ideas about selection and adaptation at the level of the group.

In contemporary treatments of the topic, efforts are made to recognize that selection occurs simultaneously on the levels of individual and group: "... anything that is good for the group must be good for one or more of the individuals in it" (Darlington, 1980, p. 140). As we have found, the key to understanding group function lies in detailed attention to individuals in it. The basic argument is that when group advantages are achieved, the advantages are experienced by individuals in the group, not just by the group itself. And, if more than one such group exists, then the relative advantages (improved fitness of individuals) of one over the other can contribute to the selection of those individuals and hence, an adaptive advantage to the groups comprising those individuals. When group selection operates positively at both individual and group levels, evolution can be rapid (e.g., Wilson & Wilson, 2007).

Group adaptation and group selection is multileveled and context-dependent, much like the individual and group processes outlined in the present chapter. We see great potential in a coherent, multilevel and multi-timescale view of developmental and evolutionary thinking. Behavioral analyses can forge new paths into this terrain.

References

Alberts, J. R. (1976). Olfactory contributions to behavioral development in rodents. In R.L. Doty (Ed.), *Mammalian olfaction, reproductive processes, and behavior* (pp. 67–93). New York: Academic Press.

Alberts, J. R. (1978). Huddling by rat pups: Group behavioral mechanisms of temperature regulation and energy conservation. *Journal of Comparative and Physiological Psychology, 92*, 231–245.

Alberts, J. R. (1984). Sensory-perceptual development in the Norway rat: A view toward comparative studies. In: R. Kail & N. Spear (Eds.), *Comparative perspectives on memory development* (pp. 65–101). New York: Plenum

Alberts, J. R. (1985). Ontogeny of social recognition: An essay on metaphor and mechanism in behavioral development. In: E.S. Gollin (Ed.), *Comparative development of adaptive skills: Evolutionary implications* (pp. 65–101). Hillsdale, NJ: Erlbaum,.

Alberts, J. R. (2002). Simply complex: Essentialism trumps reductionism. *Current Neurology and Neurosciences Reports, 2*, 379–381.

Alberts, J. R. (2005). Infancy. In I.Q. Whishaw & B. Kolb (Eds.), *The behavior of the laboratory rat: A handbook with tests* (pp. 266–277). New York: Oxford University Press.

Alberts, J. R. (2007). Huddling by rat pups: Ontogeny of individual and group behavior. *Developmental Psychobiology, 49*, 22–32.

Alberts, J. R., & Cramer, C. P. (1988). Ecology and experience; Sources of means and meaning of developmental change. In: E.M. Blass (Ed.), *Handbook of behavioral neurobiology, Vol. 9: Behavioral ecology and developmental psychobiology* (pp. 1–39). New York: Plenum Press.

Alberts, J. R., & Gubernick, D. J. (1983). Reciprocity and resource exchange: A symbiotic model of parent–offspring relations. In: L.A. Rosenblum & H. Moltz (Eds.), *Symbiosis in parent–offspring relations* (pp. 7–44). New York: Plenum Press.

Alberts, J. R., & Leimbach, M. P. (1980). The first foray: Maternal influences on nest egression in the weanling rat. *Developmental Psychobiology, 13*, 417–430.

Alberts, J. R., & May, B. (1984). Non-nutritive, thermotactile induction of olfactory preferences for huddling in rat pups. *Developmental Psychobiology, 17*, 161–181.

Alberts, J. R., Motz, B. A., & Schank, J. C. (2004). Positive geotaxis in rats: A natural behavior and a historical correction. *Journal of Comparative Psychology, 118*, 123–132.

Alberts, J. R., & Schank, J. C. (2006). Constructing ontogenetic niches. AlifeX Conference. Bloomington, IN.

Altman, J., & Sudarshan, K. (1975). Postnatal development of locomotion in the laboratory rat. *Animal Behaviour, 23*, 896–920.

Barnett, S. A. (1963). *The rat: A study in behaviour*. London: The Camelot Press Ltd.

Barnett, S. A. (2001). *The story of rats: Their impact on us, our impact on them*, Crows Nest, Australia: Allen and Unwen.

Bish, R., Joshi, S., Schank, J., & Wexler, J. (2007). Mathematical modeling and computer simulation of a robotic rat pup. *Mathematical and Computer Modeling, 54*, 981–1000.

Blass, E. M., & Teicher, M. H. (1980). Suckling. *Science, 210*, 15–22.

Blumberg, M. S. (2001). The developmental context of thermal homeostasis. In E. M. Blass (Ed.), *The Handbook of behavioral neurobiology. Volume 13: Developmental* psychobiology, developmental neurobiology and behavioral ecology: Mechanisms and early principles (pp. 199–228). New York: Plenum Press.

Bolles, R. C., & Woods, P. J. (1964). The ontogeny of behavior in the albino rat. Animal Behaviour, 12, 427–441.

Campbell, B. A., & Mabry, P. D. (1973). The role of catecholamines in behavioral arousal during ontogenesis. Psychopharmacolgia, 31, 253–264.

Campbell, B. A., Lytle, L. D., & Fibiger, H. C. (1969). Ontogeny of adrenergic arousal and cholinergic inhibitory mechanisms in the rat. Science, 166, 637–638.

Campbell, B. A., & Randall, P. K. (1976). Ontogeny of behavioral arousal in rats: Effect of maternal and sibling presence. Journal of Comparative and Physiological Psychology, 90, 453–459.

Campbell, B. A., & Raskin, L. A. (1978). Ontogeny of behavioral arousal: The role of environmental stimuli. Journal of Comparative and Physiological Psychology, 92, 176–184.

Carter, C. S. (2003). Developmental consequences of oxytocin. Physiology & Behavior, 79, 383–397.

Cramer, C. P., Thiels, E., & Alberts, J. R. (1990). Weaning in Norway Rats: I. Maternal Behavior patterns. Developmental Psychobiology, 23, 479–494.

Crozier, W. J., & Pincus, G. (1926). The geotropic conduct of young rats. Journal of General Physiology, 10, 257–269.

Crozier, W. J., & Pincus, G. (1936). Analysis of the geotropic orientation of young rats. X. Journal of General Physiology, 20, 111–124.

Darlington, P.J., Jr. (1980). Evolution for naturalists: The simple principles and complex realities. New York: John Wiley & Sons.

Darwin, C. R. (1872). The origin of species by means of natural selection, or the preservation of favoured races in the struggle for life (6th ed.). London: John Murray.

Dawkins, R. (1976). The selfish gene. Oxford: Oxford University Press.

Delcourt, J., Becco, C., Ylieff, M. Y., Caps, H., Vandewalle N., & Poncin P. (2006). Comparing the EthoVision 2.3 system and a new computerized multitracking prototype system to measure the swimming behavior in fry fish. Behavior Research Methods, 38, 704–710.

Farrell, W. J., & Alberts J. R. (2007). Rat behavioral thermoregulation integrates with nonshivering thermogenesis during postnatal development. Behavioral Neuroscience, 121, 1333–1341.

Ferguson, J. N., Young, L. J., & Insel, T. R. (2002). The neuroendocrine basis of social recognition. Frontiers in neuroendocrinology, 23, 200–224.

Fibiger, H. C., Lytle, L. D., & Campbell, B. A. (1970). Cholinergic modulation of adrenergic arousal in the developing rat, Journal of Comparative and Physiological Psychology, 72, 384–389.

Fraenkel, G. S., & Gunn, D. L. (1940). The orientation of animals. London: Oxford University Press.

Friedman, M. I. (1975). Some determinants of milk ingestion in suckling rats. Journal of Comparative and Physiological Psychology, 89, 636–647.

Galef, B. G., Jr., & Clark, M. M. (1971). Social factors in the poison avoidance and feeding behavior of wild and domesticated rat pups. Journal of Comparative and Physiological Psychology, 75, 341–357.

Galef, B.G., Jr., & Henderson, P. W. (1972). Mother's milk: A determinant of the feeding preferences of weaning rat pups. Journal of Comparative and Physiological Psychology, 78, 213–219.

Galef, B. G., Jr., Mason, J. R., Preti, G., & Bean, N. J. (1988). Carbon disulfide: A semiochemical mediating socially-induced diet choice in rats. Physiology and Behavior, 42, 119–124.

Gerrish, C., & Alberts, J. R. (1996). Environmental temperature modulates onset of independent feeding: Warmer is sooner. Developmental Psychobiology, 29, 483–495.

Gerrish, C., & Alberts, J. R. (1997). Post-suckling behavioral arousal contributes to weaning in Norway rats (Rattus norvegicus). Journal of Comparative Psychology, 111, 37–49.

Goodson, J. L. (2005). The vertebrate social behavior network: Evolutionary themes and variations. Hormones and Behavior, 48, 11–22.

Goodwin, B. (1994). How the leopard changed its spots. New York: Scribner.

Gottlieb, G. (1976). The roles of experience in the development of behavior and the nervous system. In G. Gottlieb (Ed.), Studies in the development of behavior and the nervous system (Vol. 3, pp. 25–54). New York: Academic Press.

Hall, W. G. (1979a). Feeding and behavioral activation in infant rats. Science, 205, 206–209.

Hall, W. G. (1979b). The ontogeny of feeding in rats: I. Ingestive and and behavioral responses to oral infusions. Journal of Comparative and Physiological Psychology, 93, 977–1000.

Hall, W. G., & Rosenblatt, J. S. (1977). Suckling behaior and intake control in the developing rat. Journal of Comparative and Physiological Psychology, 91, 1232–1237.

Hall, W. G., & Williams, C. L. (1983). Suckling isn't feeding, or is it? Advances in the Study of Behavior, 13, 219–254.

Hamilton, W. D. (1964). The genetical evolution of social behavior: I and II. Journal of Theoretical Biology, 7, 1–52.

Hamilton, W. D. (1975). Innate social aptitudes in man: An approach from evolutionary genetics. In R. Fox (Ed.), Biosocial anthropology (pp. 133–153), London: Malaby Press.

Hoffman, C. M., Flory, S. G., & Alberts, J. R. (1999a). Neonatal thermotaxis improves reversal of a thermally-reinforced instrumental response. Developmental Psychobiology, 34, 87–99.

Hoffman, C. M, Flory, S. G., & Alberts, J. R. (1999b). Ontogenetic adaptation and learning: A developmental constraint in learning for a thermal reinforcer. Developmental Psychobiology, 34, 73–86.

Insel, T. R., & Fernald, R. D. (2004). How the brain processes social information: Searching for the social brain. Annual Review of Neuroscience, 27, 697–722.

Koehnle, T. J., & Schank, J. C. (2003). Power tools needed for the dynamical toolbox. Adaptive Behavior, 11, 291–295.

Krieder, J. C., & Blumberg, M. S. (1999). Geotaxis in 2-week-old Norway rats (Rattus norvegicus). Developmental Psychobiology, 35, 35–42.

Lim, M. M., & Young, L. J. (2006). Neuropeptidergic regulation of affiliative behavior and social bonding in animals. Hormones and Behavior, 50, 506–517.

Lloyd, S. (2000). Ultimate physical limits to computation. Nature, 406, 1047–1054.

May, C. J. (2007). Modeling the behavior of infant Norway rats (Rattus norvegicus). Unpublished doctoral dissertation, University of California, Davis.

May, C. J., Schank, J. C., Joshi, S., Tran, J., Taylor, R. J., & Scott, I. (2006). Rat pups and random robots generate similar self-organized and intentional behavior. *Complexity,* *12* (1), 53–66.

Moorcroft, W. H., Lytle, L. D., & Campbell, B. A. (1971). Ontogeny of starvation-induced behavioral arousal in the rat. *Journal of Comparative and Physiological Psychology, 75,* 59–67.

Motz, B. A., & Alberts, J. R. (2005). The validity and utility of geotaxis in young rodents. *Neurotoxicology and Teratology, 27,* 543–544.

Noldus, L. P., Spink, A. J., & Tegelenbosch, R. A. (2001). EthoVision: A versatile video tracking system for automation of behavioral experiments. *Behavioral Research Methods, Instrumentation and Computation, 33,* 398–414.

Odya, E. C., Sokoloff, G., & Alberts, J. R. (2002). *The effects of oxytocin on the aggregation of infant rats.* Orlando, FL: Society for Neuroscience.

Pedersen, P., & Blass, E. M. (1981). Olfactory control over suckling in albino rats. In R. N. Aslin, J. R. Alberts, & M. R. Petersen (Eds.), *The development of perception: Psychobiological perspectives* (pp. 359–381). New York: Academic Press.

Pedersen, P., & Blass, E. M. (1983). Prenatal and postnatal determinants of the 1ˢᵗ suckling episode in albino rats. *Developmental Psychobiology, 15,* 349–355.

Pedersen, P. E., Williams, C. L., & Blass, E. M. (1982). Activation and odor conditioning of suckling behavior in 3-day-ole albino rats. *Journal of Experimental Psychology: Animal Behavior Processes, 8,* 329–341.

Pfister, J. F. (1990). *The development of responses to hot and cold challenges in the Norway rat: Preferences, regulation, and learning.* Unpublished doctoral dissertation, Indiana University, Bloomington, IN.

Pfister, J. P., Cramer, C. P., & Blass, E. M. (1986). Suckling in rats extended by continuous living with dams and their preweaning litters. *Animal Behaviour, 34,* 415–420.

Randall, P. K., & Campbell, B. A. (1976). Ontogeny of behavioral arousal in rats: Effect of maternal and sibling presence. *Journal of Comparative and Physiological Psychology, 90,* 453–459.

Rosenblatt, J. S., & Lehrman, D. S. (1963). Maternal behavior in the laboratory rat. In H. L. Rheingold (Ed.), *Maternal behavior in mammals* (pp. 8–57). New York: Wiley.

Saunders, J. W. (1982). *Developmental biology. Patterns, problems, principles.* New York: Macmillan.

Schank, J. C. (2001). Beyond reductionism: Refocusing on the individual with individual-based modeling. *Complexity. 6,* 33–40.

Schank, J. C. (2008). The development of locomotor kinematics in neonatal rats: An agent-based modeling analysis in group and individual contexts. *Journal of Theoretical Biology, 254,* 826–842.

Schank, J. C., & Alberts, J. R. (1997). Self-organized huddles of rat pups modeled by simple rules of individual behavior. *Journal of Theoretical Biology, 189,* 11–25.

Schank, J. C., & Alberts, J. R. (2000). The developmental emergence of coupled activity as cooperative aggregation in rat pups. *Proceedings of the Royal Society of London, 267,* 2307–2345.

Schank J. C., & Koehnle T. J. (2007). Modeling complex biobehavioral systems. In: Laubichler, M.D., & Muller G.B, (Eds.), *Modeling biology: Structures, behaviors, evolution* (pp. 219–240). Cambridge, MA: MIT Press.

Schank, J. C., May, C. J., Tran, J. T., & Joshi, S. S. (2004). A biorobotic investigation of Norway rat pups (*Rattus norvegicus*) in an arena. *Adaptive Behavior, 12,* 161–173.

Small, W. S. (1899). Notes on the psychic development of the young white rat. *American Journal of Psychology. 11,* 80–100.

Sokoloff, G., & Blumberg, M.S. (2001). Competition and cooperation among huddling infant rats. *Developmental Psychobiology, 39,* 65–75.

Sokoloff, G., Blumberg, M. S., & Adams, M. M. (2000). A comparative analysis of huddling in infant Norway rats and Syrian hamsters: Does endothermy modulate behavior? *Behavioral Neuroscience, 114,* 585–583.

Teicher, M. H., & Blass, E. M. (1976). Suckling in newborn rats: Eliminated by nipple lavage, reinstated by pup saliva. *Science, 193,* 422–425.

Thelen, E. (1988). Dynamical approaches to the development of behavior. In: J. A. S. Kelso, A. Mandell, & M. F. Schlesinger (Eds.), *Dynamical patterns in complex systems* (pp. 348–369). Singapore: World Scientific.

Thelen, E., Kelso, J. A. S., & Fogel, A. (1987). Self-organizing systems and infant motor development. *Developmental Review, 7,* 39–65.

Thiels, E., & Alberts, J. R. (1991). Weaning in the Norway rat: Relation between suckling and milk, and suckling and independent ingestions. *Developmental Psychobiology, 24,* 19–38.

Thiels, E., Alberts, J. R., & Cramer, C. P. (1990). Weaning in Norway rats: II. Pup behavior patterns. *Developmental Psychobiology, 23,* 495–510.

Thiels, E., Cramer, C. P., & Alberts, J. R. (1988). Behavioral interactions rather than milk availability determine decline in milk intake of weaning rats. *Physiology and Behavior, 42,* 507–515.

Tsibidis G. D. & Tavernarakis, N. (2007). Nemo: A computational tool for analyzing nematode locomotion. *BMC Neuroscience,* 8(1), 86–92.

Wade, M. J. (1976). Group selection among laboratory populations of tribolium. *Proceedings of the National Academy of Sciences, 73,* 4604–4607.

West, M. J., & King, A. P. (1988). Female visual displays alter the development of male song in the cowbird, *Nature, 334,* 244–246.

Williams, G. C. (1966). *Adaptation and natural selection.* Princeton, NJ: Princeton University Press.

Wilson, D. S. (1975). A theory of group selection. *Proceedings of the National Academy of Sciences. 72,* 143–146.

Wilson, D. S. (1983). The group selection controversy: History and current status. *Annual Review of Ecology and Systematics, 14,* 159–187.

Wilson, D. S., & Wilson, E. O. (2007). Rethinking the theoretical foundations of sociobiology, *Quarterly Review of Biology, 82,* 327–348.

PART 6

Learning and Memory

Ontogeny of Multiple Memory Systems: Eyeblink Conditioning in Rodents and Humans

Mark E. Stanton, Dragana Ivkovich Claflin, *and* Jane Herbert

Abstract

This chapter reviews developmental studies of eyeblink conditioning in rodents and humans that have been pursued from a multiple memory systems perspective. It extends previous summaries of the ontogeny of eyeblink conditioning in humans and in rodents, including previous rodent research on multiple memory systems. Past and current views of multiple memory systems, including developmental views, are reviewed and how studies of eyeblink conditioning can advance research in this area is shown. Research in developing rodents and humans is then described and some general conclusions are presented.

Keywords: eyeblink conditioning, ontogeny of eyeblink, humans, rodents, multiple memory systems, developmental views

Introduction

The purpose of this chapter is to review developmental studies of eyeblink conditioning in rodents and humans that have been pursued from a multiple memory systems perspective (Stanton, 2000). It extends previous summaries of the ontogeny of eyeblink conditioning in humans (Ivkovich, Eckerman, Krasnegor, & Stanton, 2000b) and rodents (Freeman & Nicholson, 2004; Stanton & Freeman, 2000), including previous rodent research on multiple memory systems (Stanton, 2000). In this introductory section, we briefly review past and current views of multiple memory systems, including developmental views, and then indicate how studies of eyeblink conditioning can advance research in this area. We then describe our research in developing rodents and humans, and present some general conclusions.

Multiple Memory Systems

The idea that there is more than one kind of memory is now generally accepted. It has "arrived," after a 200-year journey across the disciplines of "…philosophy, then psychology, and now biology" (Squire, 2004, p. 175; Figure 24.1). Squire (2004) describes the origination of the idea in nineteenth-century philosophy (James, 1890; Maine de Biran, 1804/1929), its appearance most often as a dichotomy by the mid-twentieth century in psychology (Bruner, 1969; Ryle, 1949; Tolman, 1948; Winograd, 1975), its extension to neurology beginning in the 1950s (Milner, 1962), and its subsequent rapid transformation by the burgeoning field of behavioral neuroscience into its present taxonomic form today (Figure 24.1). This taxonomy illustrates some important points concerning how the term "multiple memory systems" is used in this chapter. One use of the term focuses on *two categories of memory*, a category that depends on the medial temporal lobe and diencephalon and another category that does not ("declarative vs. nondeclarative memory," second row in Figure 24.1). Another use of the term focuses on individual brain memory systems (bottom row in Figure 24.1) and recognizes them as distinct and distinctly important, regardless of which of the two broad categories of memory they may belong to (e.g., Stanton, 2000; other contributions to this volume). By this view, there are a least six "memory systems," not just two.

The contrast in these perspectives is a natural consequence of historical trends in the biological study of multiple memory systems so cogently reviewed by Squire (2004). Early progress centered on characterizing memory functions that depend on the hippocampus and related structures, and how these functions differ *psychologically* from those that do not depend on the temporal lobe (Milner, 1962; Mishkin, Malamut, & Bachevalier, 1984; O'Keefe & Nadel, 1978; Olton, 1983; Schacter, 1984; Squire, 1987; Sutherland & Rudy, 1989). Only later did progress in the neurobiology of learning provide us with the rich and detailed descriptions of how the striatum (Packard, Hirsh, & White, 1989), amygdala (Davis, 1992; Fanselow, 1994; LeDoux, 1992), and cerebellum (Thompson, 1986, 2005) serve memory functions that do not depend on the hippocampus and related temporal cortical structures. As Squire (2004) notes, this progress has probably done more to reinforce the distinction between declarative versus nondeclarative memory than has progress in understanding the neural basis of declarative memory itself. However, the proliferation of brain memory systems that fall in the nondeclarative category also raises questions about the utility of a dichotomous view of memory. Why talk about two memory systems when, as far as the nervous system is concerned, there are many more than that? At the neural level, is the distinction between memory functions of, for example, the amygdala versus the cerebellum not just as important as the distinction between their functions and those of the medial temporal lobe? The dichotomous view of memory is also likely to be further transformed by another important recent trend in the neurobiology of learning—the growing appreciation that brain memory systems *interact* to produce different forms of memory at the psychological level (Columbo & Gold, 2004). Declarative memory is now seen to depend on *interactions* between the hippocampus and temporal cortical structures—the "hippocampal system"—rather than the hippocampal formation itself (Squire& Zola-Morgan, 1991), and the specialized roles and relative importance of the components of the hippocampal system are still being clarified (Baxter & Murray, 2001; Murray & Wise, 2004; Zola & Squire, 2001). More importantly, although the memory systems summarized in Figure 24.1 are accepted as distinct and dissociable, it is also becoming increasingly recognized that these systems may also compete or cooperate during a given memory task to alter

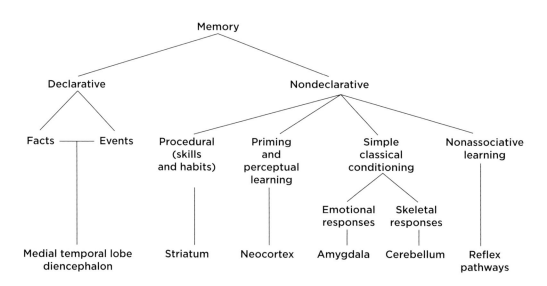

Figure 24.1 A taxonomy of memory indicating types of memory and underlying brain structures. (From Squire, 2004.)

how experience is represented and/or how behavior is controlled (Columbo & Gold, 2004; Kesner & Rogers, 2004; Squire, 2004; Stanton, 2000). We elaborate on this point in the case of eyeblink conditioning below.

So, what does this mean for our use of the term "multiple memory systems" in this chapter? First, this chapter is concerned more with the cerebellum and the hippocampus than it is with declarative versus nondeclarative memory. We review developmental studies of eyeblink conditioning phenomena, which depend on the cerebellum either with or without the additional involvement of the hippocampus. Second, by "hippocampus" we really mean the "hippocampal system." Distinguishing the contribution of the hippocampal formation proper versus related cortical structures is beyond the scope of what we have done thus far, if not indeed what *anyone* studying the role of the hippocampus in the ontogeny of memory in rodent models or humans has done thus far (see below). This is an important avenue for future research. Third, we do no take a position concerning what psychological theory best captures the role of the hippocampus in learning and memory. This is also a consequence of our methods and findings and does not mean that we believe the issue is unimportant. The model systems tradition in the neurobiology of learning, of which eyeblink conditioning is a prominent example, is a strongly empirical tradition. The role of the hippocampus in conditioning has been determined empirically by lesion, inactivation, neural recording, and stimulation studies, without much regard for memory theories. Psychological theories of hippocampal function can be tested with eyeblink conditioning but they are not required. For example, it has been shown that human temporal lobe amnesics are impaired on trace but not delay eyeblink conditioning because the former task requires "awareness" of conditioned stimulus–unconditioned stimulus (CS–US) relationships whereas the latter does not (Clark & Squire, 1998; Weiskrantz & Warrington, 1979). This supports the role of the temporal lobe and of declarative memory in human trace eyeblink conditioning. However, the role of the hippocampal system in trace eyeblink conditioning was first demonstrated in rabbits many years earlier, as an empirical extension of unit recording studies (Solomon, Vander Schaaf, Thompson, & Weisz, 1986). Thus far, our developmental experiments implicate the hippocampal system in the ontogeny of some eyeblink conditioning tasks but our experiments are largely silent concerning psychological theories of hippocampal function. This is also a potentially important avenue for further research.

In summary, we consider "multiple memory systems" in both senses in which the term has been widely used: to distinguish memory that depends on the hippocampal system from memory that does not and to exploit advances that have been made in identifying numerous brain memory systems, particularly the cerebellum (see also Chapter 26).

Ontogeny of Multiple Memory Systems

In this section, we provide a brief history of research directed at the role of the hippocampal system in the ontogeny of memory. The first reviews of this issue focused on rats and were not concerned with memory dichotomies. Rather, they focused on learning tasks that were commonly used during that period in hippocampal aspiration lesion studies involving adult rats, and for which there was behavioral data involving developing rats (Altman, Brunner, & Bayer, 1973; Amsel & Stanton, 1980; Douglas, 1975). Extensive neuroanatomical work on hippocampal development in the rat also provided an important context (Altman & Bayer, 1975). Altman et al. (1973) noted that performance of hippocampus-dependent tasks such as passive avoidance is poor prior to weaning, and emerges around 21–25 days of age. They noted that the ontogenetic profile of performance on these tasks parallels maturation of the hippocampus. Altman et al. (1973) also noted that neonatal irradiation of dentate granule cells impairs adult performance of runway extinction and single alternation learning (Brunner, Hagbloom, & Gazzara, 1974). Douglas (1975) argued that the normative development of spontaneous alternation, combined with his adult lesion work involving this task, suggests that the role of the hippocampus in memory emerges around 25 days of age in the rat. Amsel and Stanton (1980) noted that their studies of the normative development of a wide range of appetitive runway learning, extinction, and contrast effects in 12- to 25-day-old rats also supported a role of the hippocampus in the ontogeny of learning. However, they differed from earlier researchers by suggesting that this role emerges developmentally as early as 14–16 days of age. This was subsequently confirmed empirically in studies of runway learning in 16-day-old rats that had undergone hippocampal lesions (Lobaugh, Bootin, & Amsel, 1985) or x-irradiation of dentate granule cells (Diaz-Granadas, Greene, & Amsel, 1992).

Beginning in the 1980s, attention turned to memory dichotomies, to the idea that memory systems can be dissociated developmentally as well as neuroanatomically, and to cross-species comparisons involving rats, monkeys, and humans (Bachevalier & Mishkin, 1984; Diamond, 1990a; Freeman & Stanton, 1991; Green & Stanton, 1989; Nadel & Zola-Morgan, 1984; Rovee-Collier, Hayne, & Columbo, 2001; Rudy, 1992). By this time, the role of the hippocampal system in memory was being studied by comparing two tasks that engage common sensory, motor, and motivational processes but that engage different memory processes, one involving the hippocampal system and the other not involving this system. A common finding with these task dissociations was that performance of the hippocampus-dependent task emerges *later* in ontogeny than performance on the other memory task (Bachevalier & Mishkin, 1984; Diamond, 1990b; Freeman & Stanton, 1991; Green & Stanton, 1989).

This is illustrated in a developmental study of spatial-delayed alternation versus position habit learning in the rat (Green & Stanton, 1989; Figure 24.2; Freeman & Stanton, 1991; Figure 24.3). Delayed alternation is a hippocampus-dependent spatial working memory task in which rats are subjected to trials consisting of a rewarded "forced-run" to one of the arms of a T-maze followed after a short delay by a "choice-run" in which both arms are available and reward is contingent on choosing the alternate arm that was just visited on the forced run. After an intertrial interval, the trial is repeated with the direction of forced runs varying quasirandomly across the trial series. This task has also been called delayed-nonmatching-to-position. The position habit task, in contrast, consists of a series of trials, each involving only a single choice-run with one of the arms (left or right) always rewarded and the other always nonrewarded. Green and Stanton (1989) compared the performance of 15-, 21-, and 27-day-old rats on these two tasks (Figure 24.2, "Expmnt," filled symbols) relative to versions of these tasks ("Control," open symbols) in which reward was delivered regardless of which arm was chosen on the choice run (noncontingently rewarded control). Delayed alternation developed between 15 and 21 days of age whereas position habit was present at all three ages (Figure 24.2).

Freeman and Stanton (1991) subsequently showed that neonatal fornix transactions, which disrupt hippocampal system function by removing its subcortical afferent and efferent connections,

selectively disrupt the ontogeny of delayed alternation (Figure 24.3, Shift, filled symbols) without altering the performance of noncontingently rewarded control groups (SNC, open symbols). Freeman and Stanton (1991) also showed that neonatal fornix cuts did not disrupt the ontogeny of position habit learning (data not shown). These rat studies support the view that memory processes that depend on the hippocampal system emerge later in ontogeny than memory processes that do not depend on this system but otherwise engage similar sensory, motor, and motivational processes. Similar developmental findings were obtained with delayed-nonmatching-to-sample (DNMS) for objects versus simple object discrimination in developing monkeys (Bachevalier, 1990) and humans (Diamond, 1990b; Overman, 1990). Rudy's (1992) large body of behavioral research in developing rats, much of it based on Pavlovian conditioning techniques, together with some studies of preschool children, also supported the view that an "elemental associative system," which does not depend on the hippocampus, emerges earlier in ontogeny than a "configural association system," which critically depends on the hippocampus and related structures (Sutherland & Rudy, 1989). Thus, research on memory development seemed to join neuropsychological research in support of the notion that there are "two kinds of memory" (Diamond, 1990a; Squire, 1987, 2004). This view that explicit memory (hippocampal system–dependent) necessarily develops later than implicit memory (nonhippocampal) was subsequently challenged (Rovee-Collier, 1997; Rovee-Collier, Hayne, & Columbo, 2001). We return to this issue in the concluding section of this chapter.

It is one thing to determine that, within a given experimental preparation, task variants that depend on the hippocampal system develop later than those that do not. It is quite another thing to identify absolute ages at which the hippocampal system is or is not playing a causal role in a broader range of behaviors (Stanton, 2000). As noted previously, researchers working with rats have historically considered 21–25 days of age to be *the* period in development when the hippocampus "comes online," behaviorally speaking (Altman et al., 1973; Douglas, 1975; Nadel & Zola-Morgan, 1984; Rudy, 1992). The idea that it is important to identify such a period has also been considered by researchers working with monkeys or humans (Diamond, 1990a). The idea has appeal because of its parsimony. If such a period could be identified,

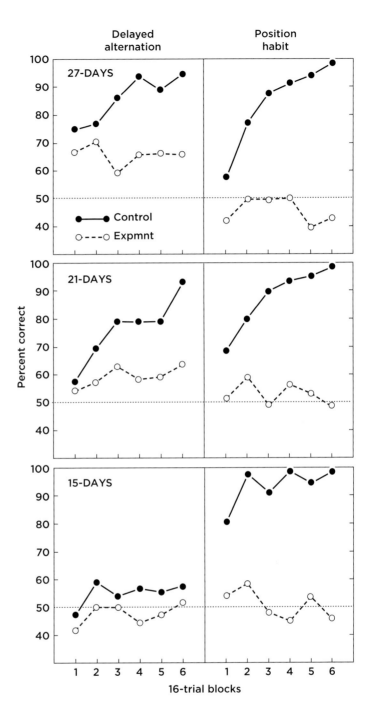

Figure 24.2 Performance of 15-, 21-, and 27-day-old rats on two appetitive T-maze tasks, spatial delayed alternation (left panels) and position discrimination (position habit, right panels). Experimental rats (EXPMNT) were rewarded contingent on correct choice. Control rats (CONTROL) were rewarded regardless of choice. Dashed horizontal line at 50% indicates chance performance. Note the ontogenetic increase in spontaneous alternation in Control rats tested on delayed alternation. (Adapted from Green and Stanton, 1989.)

then simple and specific predictions could be made concerning when a broad range of hippocampus-dependent behaviors will develop, the specific neural and molecular mechanisms underlying this development would be easier to identify, and clinical disorders involving early injury or aberrant maturation of the hippocampal system would be far easier to study and manage. Unfortunately,

the idea that all behavioral functions of the hippocampus emerge during a narrow developmental period is clearly wrong. When one looks across a broad range of behavioral tasks for converging evidence concerning the onset of hippocampal function in the rat, one finds enormous variation across development (Stanton, 2000; Table 24.1). In general, the role of the hippocampal system in

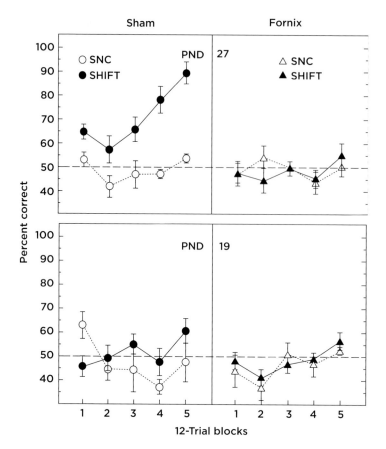

Figure 24.3 Performance of rats on spatial delayed alternation (Shift) or noncontingently rewarded control task (SNC) on Postnatal Day (PND) 19 or 27 as a function of fimbria-fornix transections (Fornix, right panels) or sham lesions (Sham, left panels) performed on PND10. Delayed alternation emerged across age in Sham but not Fornix rats. (From Freeman and Stanton, 1991.)

visuospatial memory tasks develops much later than its role in nonspatial memory tasks, tasks which are impaired by hippocampal injury at 16 days of age (Diaz-Granadas et al., 1992; Lobaugh et al., 1985), an age when intact rats are generally unable to perform conventional spatial memory tasks (Stanton, 2000; Table 24.1). Part of this variation likely reflects quantitative differences in the extent to which different behavioral phenomena engage the hippocampal system, with greater engagement associated with later ontogenetic emergence (e.g., Daly, 1991), but most of this variation occurs because different hippocampus-dependent phenomena engage different "behavioral systems" (Timberlake & Fanselow, 1994) and the developmental emergence of hippocampal system function "…depends as much on the developmental status of [these] other behavioral systems that both drive and express this function as it does on the developmental status of the hippocampus itself" (Stanton, 2000, p. 29). It is worth noting that this principle is not unique to the rat but seems to apply to human and nonhuman primates as well. Visual-paired

comparison (e.g., Overman, Bachevalier, Sewell, & Drew, 1993), DNMS (Diamond, 1990b; Overman, 1990), transverse patterning (Rudy, 1992), and spatial navigation (Overman, Pate, Moore, & Peuster, 1996), tasks that are all thought to depend on the hippocampus and/or related temporal lobe structures in these species, emerge in that order over an ontogenetic period that spans several years. Thus, the key to understanding memory development requires that we shift our attention away from the hippocampal system alone and, rather focus on the *interactions* of this system with other behavioral or memory systems, particularly systems that are themselves amenable to developmental and neurobiological analysis (Stanton, 2000). We next describe how the eyeblink conditioning paradigm can be used for this purpose.

Using Eyeblink Conditioning to Study the Ontogeny of Multiple Memory Systems

Eyeblink conditioning is a simple form of Pavlovian reflex learning that was first demonstrated in humans about 77 years ago (Hilgard,

Table 24.1 Approximate Age of Developmental Onset (in days) of Learning and Memory Phenomena Involving the Hippocampal System in the Rat (from Stanton, 2000)

Behavioral Task	Age	Reference
Patterned alternation (runway)	11	Stanton, Dailey, & Amsel, 1980
		Dias-Granadas et al., 1992
Partial reinforcement extinction effect (runway)	12–14	Letz, Burdette, Gregg, Kittrell, & Amsel, 1978
		Lobaugh et al., 1985
Olfactory reversal	18	Saperstein, Kucharski, Stanton, & Hall, 1989
Glucocorticoid conditioning	20	Jacobs, Stanton, & Levine, 1986
		Smotherman et al., 1981
Magnitude of reward extinction effect (runway)	18–19	Amsel & Chen, 1976
Spatial delayed alternation	18–21	Green & Stanton, 1989
		Freeman & Stanton, 1991
Auditory trace fear conditioning	21	Moye & Rudy, 1987
Passive avoidance	21	Riccio & Schulenburg, 1969
Spatial navigation	21–23	Rudy, Stadler-Morris, & Alberts, 1987
		Altemus & Almli, 1997
Contextual fear conditioning	23	Pugh & Rudy, 1996
Exploratory habituation	21–25	Fiegley, Parsons, Hamilton, & Spear, 1972
Spontaneous alternation	25	Douglas, 1975
Successive negative contrast (runway)	25	Chen, Gross, & Amsel, 1980
Visual trace fear conditioning	30	Moye & Rudy, 1987
Latent inhibition	21–32	Nicolle, Barry, Veronesi, & Stanton, 1989
		Rudy, 1994
Spatial delayed alternation (long delay)	31–40	Castro, Paylor, & Rudy, 1987

1931). At an operational level, it is a nonverbal associative learning task in which a conditioned stimulus (CS), usually a pure tone, precedes and coterminates with an unconditioned stimulus (US), usually a mild airpuff to the eye, which elicits the reflexive eyeblink unconditioned response (UR). Initially, the tone fails to elicit eyeblink responses reliably. However, with repeated pairings of the tone and airpuff, the tone CS comes to elicit eyeblink responses on a large percentage of trials. Over the past half century, a massive amount of behavioral and neuroscientific research has transformed eyeblink conditioning into a powerful paradigm for the interdisciplinary study of brain and behavior, as summarized in several books and proceedings (Baudry, Davis, & Berger, 2001; Gormezano, Prokasy, & Thompson, 1987; Steinmetz, Gluck, & Solomon, 2001; Woodruff-Pak & Steinmetz, 2000a, 2000b). This interdisciplinary power arises from the operational simplicity and minimal sensory, motor, and motivational demands of the procedure, which have made its behavioral and neurobiological mechanisms more tractable to study than other forms of learning that involve more complex patterns of instrumental behavior. This simplicity has also made the preparation applicable with little or no modification, across a range of animal species–rodents, ferrets, rabbits, cats, dogs, monkeys, humans–and across the life span, beginning in early infancy (Ivkovich et al., 2000b; Little, Lipsitt, & Rovee-Collier, 1984; Stanton & Freeman, 1994, 2000; Woodruff-Pak & Thompson, 1988). Being a form of Pavlovian conditioning, the preparation can be used to examine cognitive processes by contrasting "higher order" conditioning phenomena with simple delay conditioning (see below). Studies in both animals and humans indicate that simple associative learning is mediated by well-characterized brain stem–cerebellar circuitry (Thompson, 1986, 2005), whereas more complex, "higher order" conditioning phenomena appear to depend on interactions of this circuitry with forebrain structures (see below). Applying advances in the neurobiology of eyeblink conditioning to developing animals has yielded important new insights concerning brain development and the emergence of associative learning (Chapter 26; Freeman & Nicholson, 2004) and has made the paradigm useful for developmental studies of learning and cognition from a "multiple memory systems" perspective.

Figure 24.4 illustrates three brain memory systems that are known to be engaged during eyeblink conditioning (Stanton, 2000). These systems were encountered previously in Squire's taxonomy, which emphasizes that they are dissociable neuroanatomically (Squire, 2004; Figure 24.1). They are also dissociable developmentally (Stanton, 2000; see below). However, these memory systems are also known to *interact* (Fanselow, 1994; Schmajuk & DiCarlo, 1991; Thompson et al., 1987; Wagner & Brandon, 1989) and that is how they are represented here (Figure 24.4). During a conditioning episode, associative learning takes place simultaneously in all three systems. These systems encode different aspects of the conditioning episode, have different operating characteristics, and are expressed in different ways at the behavioral level (Stanton, 2000). The cerebellar system is responsible for conditioning of the discrete eyeblink reflex (Chapter 26; Thompson, 1986, 2005). The amygdala mediates learned "fear" (Davis, 1992; Fanselow, 1994; LeDoux, 1992) that is established during eyeblink conditioning (Wagner & Brandon, 1989). The cognitive system encodes a mental representation that includes the spatial and episodic (temporal) context in which the CS and US are embedded. This representation is multidimensional and "flexible" in that it can be accessed and updated by a broader range of inputs and is expressed behaviorally via multiple outputs, which tend to be indirect and conditional on the operation of other brain systems. Simple associative learning (delay conditioning) engages the hippocampal system, which encodes the episode and receives an "efferent copy" from other systems, but is not critically dependent on it. The cerebellum and amygdala are sufficient for simple delay conditioning of the eyeblink reflex

or fear states, respectively, regardless of whether the hippocampal system is intact, but "higher-order" conditioning phenomena such as trace conditioning, discrimination reversal, configural conditioning, and contextual conditioning depend critically on the cognitive system and its interaction with the other two systems, which derive their cognitive properties from the cognitive system (Clark & Squire, 1998; Fanselow, 1994; Moyer, Deyo, & Disterhoft, 1990; Solomon et al., 1986). The interaction between the cerebellum and hippocampus has been reviewed and summarized with a neural network model (Schmajuk & DiCarlo, 1991). The interaction between hippocampus and amygdala is captured in Fanselow's (1994) model of contextual versus cued fear conditioning and by demonstrations that trace fear conditioning depends on both the hippocampus and amygdala whereas delay fear conditioning depends only on the amygdala (McEchron, Bouwmeester, Tseng, Weiss, & Disterhoft, 1998). Finally, the interaction between the amygdala and cerebellum is consistent with the well-known theoretical distinction between conditioning of preparatory versus consummatory responses (Konorski, 1967; Wagner & Brandon, 1989) and is supported by developmental and neurobiological studies of eyeblink conditioning (Blankenship, Huckfeldt, Steinmetz, & Steinmetz, 2005; Freeman, Barone, & Stanton, 1995; Lee & Kim, 2004; Stanton, 2000; Thompson et al., 1987; Weisz, Harde, & Xiang, 1992).

Developmental studies of eyeblink conditioning indicate that these three memory systems can be dissociated ontogenetically. Cued-fear conditioning emerges earlier in development (P16–18) than the conditioned eyeblink reflex (P20–24) or contextual-fear conditioning (P23, Stanton, 2000). Disrupting

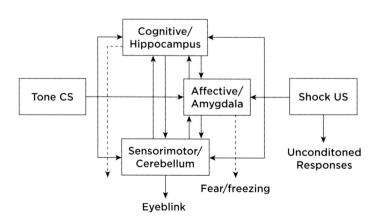

Figure 24.4 A schematic diagram of the associative components of eyeblink conditioning and the neural systems which subserve them. See text for further explanation. (From Stanton, 2000.)

cerebellar development impairs the ontogeny of eyeblink conditioning but not cued-fear conditioning or spatial-delayed alternation (Freeman, Barone, & Stanton, 1995). While these developmental dissociations are relatively easy to demonstrate, gathering evidence of ontogenetic changes in memory system *interactions* is more challenging. The ontogeny of amygdala–cerebellar interactions during eyeblink conditioning has not been studied directly at either the behavioral or neurobiological levels (Stanton, 2000). However, "arousal states" can modulate rate of eyeblink conditioning as early as P17 (Stanton, Freeman, & Skelton, 1992; Experiment 3) and the early development of fear conditioning makes it likely that preparatory fear states could alter the eyeblink conditioned response (CR) as soon as it emerges in ontogeny. Stanton, Fox, and Carter (1998) speculated that fear established during eyeblink conditioning on P17 subsequently accelerates conditioning of the eyeblink reflex on P20 (relative to groups receiving unpaired training or no training on P17), but there are other plausible interpretations of this effect. Stanton (2000) reviewed indirect behavioral evidence that interactions of the hippocampal system with the amygdala emerge earlier in ontogeny than its interactions with the cerebellum. The phenomenon of latent inhibition, in which CS preexposure retards subsequent conditioning, has been attributed to a process of decremental attention involving the septohippocampal system, which acts to reduce the CS input to the cerebellum at the level of the pons (Schmajuk & Dicarlo, 1991). Latent inhibition of eyeblink conditioning is not seen until P24 whereas latent inhibition of fear established during eyeblink conditioning is seen at P20, an age at which CS-preexposure enhances rather than attenuates acquisition of the eyeblink CR (Stanton, 2000). Thus, the eyeblink conditioning paradigm makes it possible to study developmental variation in when hippocampal system function "comes online" (Table 24.1) in relation to known memory-system interactions, all in the context of a single experimental preparation (Stanton, 2000).

The remainder of this chapter describes studies that further examine the role of the hippocampal system in the ontogeny of eyeblink conditioning. We extend our analysis to include other conditioning tasks, such as learned irrelevance and trace versus delay conditioning. We also describe rodent studies of the effects of early hippocampal injury on trace versus delay conditioning. We also extend this analysis in a comparative direction by studying eyeblink conditioning in human infancy using some of the same task dissociations that we have studied in developing rodents (see "Human Studies").

Rodent Studies

Rush, Robinette, and Stanton (2001) performed a study of learned irrelevance (LIr) in developing rats. In this phenomenon, random or unpaired preexposure to a CS and US retards subsequent paired conditioning involving these stimuli (Mackintosh, 1974). Learning that two events occur reliably together is a relatively simple associative process compared to learning that two events reliably do *not* occur together, which is thought to involve higher-order learning. LIr has been attributed to cognitive processes such as priming of stimulus representations in short-term memory (Wagner, 1981), attention (Mackintosh, 1975), explicit learning that events are unrelated (Bennett, Maldonado, & Mackintosh, 1995; Mackintosh, 1974), and, in the case of unpaired preexposure, to conditioned inhibition (Rescorla, 1973). The effect was first demonstrated in (adult) rabbit eyeblink conditioning by Siegel and Domjan (1971). We encountered clues that this effect may not exist in preweanling rats when we incidentally found—in a study directed at a different issue (acquisition vs. expression of conditioning)—that unpaired US/CS preexposure on PND17 *facilitated* rather than retarded subsequent paired conditioning relative to naïve controls on PND20 (Stanton, Fox, & Carter, 1998). The effect is relevant to multiple memory systems because of evidence that temporal cortical damage (entorhinal cortex) eliminates LIr of eyeblink conditioning in adult rabbits (Allen, Chelius, & Gluck, 2002). Because entorhinal cortex continues to mature past the periweanling period in the rat (Loy, Lynch, & Cotman, 1977; Ulfig, 1993), we hypothesized that the effect may emerge after this period in the rat. Unpaired or random US/CS preexposure impairs subsequent conditioning more than CS-preexposure does, indicating that LIr is generally a stronger preexposure effect than latent inhibition (Mackintosh, 1974). We therefore also thought it would be of interest to determine if LIr would emerge earlier in ontogeny than latent inhibition.

The main developmental finding appears in Figure 24.5 (Rush et al., 2001; Experiment 3). Rats aged PND20, 25, and 30 on the day of training received three 100-trial sessions about 5 h apart in a single day. During the first session, animals received

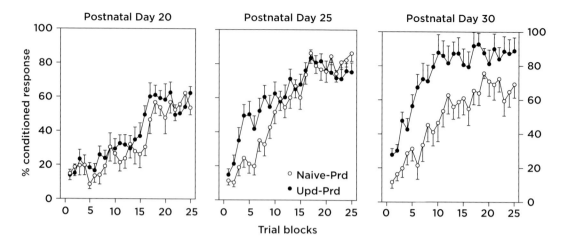

Figure 24.5 Acquisition of delay eyeblink conditioning in rats at different postnatal ages in groups that either received prior unpaired exposure to conditioned and unconditioned stimuli (Upd-Prd) or exposure only to the conditioning chamber (Naïve-Prd). Impairment of conditioning by unpaired preexposure was not found at the youngest age but this effect emerged at the older ages. (From Rush, Robinette. and Stanton, 2001.)

either 50 unpaired presentations of US and CS (Group Upd-Prd) or 50 "blank trials" (no stimulus presentations, Group Naïve-Prd), followed immediately by 50 paired trials (Prd). During the next two sessions, all animals received paired training. In this study, LIr would appear as slower learning in Group Upd-Pd versus Naïve-Prd across the twenty-five 10-trial blocks of paired training (Figure 24.5). LIr was absent on PND20, was weak on PND25, and was robust on PND30. At the youngest age, performance of the two groups never differed and both reached conditioning asymptote of about 60% CRs (Rush et al., 2001). At the intermediate age, Group Upd-Prd performed significantly more poorly that its control group early in training but both groups reached the same conditioning asymptote. At the oldest age, Group Upd-Prd differed from its control group throughout training and failed to reach the same asymptote within the 250-trial limit of this experiment. CS-alone and US-alone groups were added to the experimental design in a separate study of PND30 rats (Rush et al., 2001; Experiment 2). This experiment confirmed that impairment of conditioning was produced by unpaired preexposure to US and CS rather than preexposure to either stimulus alone, an important control in studies of LIr (e.g., Siegel & Domjan, 1971).

Although these findings are consistent with the idea that higher-order processes involving temporal cortex develop later in ontogeny than simple cerebellar-dependent eyeblink conditioning, the rate and asymptote of conditioning continued to change during the same developmental period in which LIr was emerging, particularly from PND20 to 25. Further studies are needed to determine the precise psychological mechanism of this LIr effect, whether its ontogenetic emergence is causally related to the ontogeny of simple associative learning, or indeed whether it depends on maturation of temporal cortical structures (Rush et al., 2001).

To gather additional evidence with a different eyeblink conditioning task, we undertook a developmental study of trace eyeblink conditioning (Ivkovich, Paczkowski, & Stanton, 2000a) and followed this with a study of the effects of neonatal aspiration lesions of the hippocampus on trace conditioning (Ivkovich & Stanton, 2001). As noted previously, trace eyeblink conditioning is impaired in human temporal lobe amnesia (Clark & Squire, 1998) and trace (fear) conditioning is a task that has been related to the emergence of hippocampal function in rats (Table 24.1; Moye & Rudy, 1987). The primary questions of interest were how the ontogeny of trace eyeblink conditioning would compare with that of other hippocampal-dependent learning tasks in the rat (Table 24.1) and with other higher-order eyeblink conditioning tasks such as latent inhibition (Stanton, 2000) and LIr (Rush et al., 2001).

ONTOGENY OF TRACE VERSUS DELAY EYEBLINK CONDITIONING

As operational procedures, the defining difference between delay and trace conditioning is that, in the former, the CS overlaps temporally with the US, whereas in the latter, the CS is temporally separated from the US by a stimulus-free interval, termed the "trace interval." To examine the effect of these two types of procedures on conditioning requires a three-group design (Figure 24.6). This design involves two delay-conditioning groups, a short-delay group that matches the trace group for CS duration and a long-delay group that matches the trace group for interstimulus interval (ISI). In our developmental studies of trace conditioning, our "standard" delay conditioning procedure ("Delay 280," D280) involves a 380-ms tone CS, which overlaps and coterminates with a 100-ms periocular-shock US, yielding an ISI of 280 ms (the delay interval). Our trace conditioning procedure ("Trace 500," T500) uses the same duration tone but adds a 500 ms "trace interval" between CS offset and US onset, resulting in an ISI of 880 ms. Our "long-delay" procedure ("Delay 880," D880) uses the same 880-ms ISI as the trace procedure. However, the CS overlaps and coterminates with

the US. Comparison of the trace conditioning group with the delay and long-delay groups reveals the effect of development on the three factors that are necessarily involved in any trace versus delay comparison: CS–US overlap, CS-duration, and ISI. For example, if overlap were the key factor, performance of the trace group would develop differently (e.g., later) than that of the two delay groups (which would themselves not differ). Without this three-group design, interpretation of an experimental outcome would be confounded by two factors (e.g., overlap and ISI).

Ivkovich et al. (2000a; Experiment 1) applied this design in studies of weanling-juvenile rats and found clear acquisition of eyeblink CRs on all three of these tasks (Figure 24.7). Conditioned responding increased across sessions during paired but not unpaired training in all groups. However, acquisition of CRs during standard delay conditioning (D280) was more rapid and reached a higher asymptote across six training sessions than acquisition of CRs during trace and long-delay conditioning

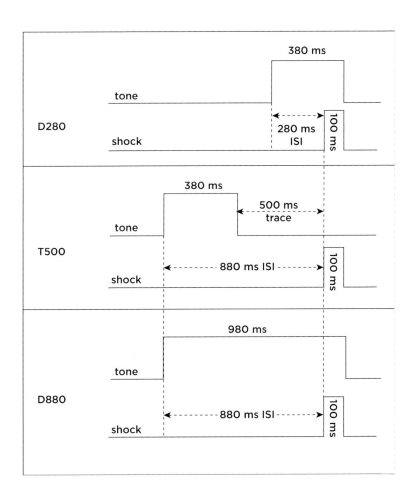

Figure 24.6 Schematic diagram of standard-delay (D280), trace (T500) and long-delay (D880) eyeblink conditioning procedures used in developing rats. See text for further explanation. (From Ivkovich, Paczkowski, and Stanton, 2000a.)

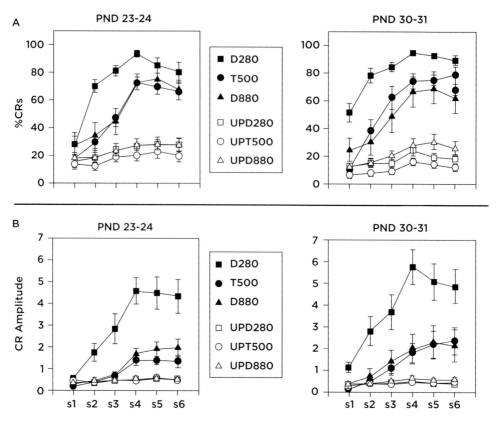

Figure 24.7 Mean eyeblink CR percentage (upper panels) or amplitude (lower panels) in postnatal day (PND) 23–24 or 30–31 rats trained with the three conditioning paradigms shown in Figure 24.6, relative to corresponding unpaired (UP) control groups. See text for further explanation. (From Ivkovich et al., 2000a.)

(T500 and D880). Importantly, the latter two groups acquired CRs at the same rate, indicating that ISI rather than overlap of CS–US is the factor that accounts for the superior performance of the standard delay group during this period of development. Across a broader age range, delay conditioning develops earlier than trace and long-delay conditioning. The latter two tasks show identical ontogenetic profiles, at least during this developmental period (Claflin, Garrett, & Buffington, 2005; Ivkovich et al., 2000a; Experiment 2, Figure 24.8).

These findings underscore the importance of using the three-group design in biological studies of trace conditioning. Inclusion of the long-delay group is particularly important because it provides a comparison of trace versus delay conditioning under conditions in which CR acquisition rates are similar and task difficulty is matched across delay versus trace conditioning procedures.

Effects of Early Damage to the Hippocampal System on Delay versus Trace Conditioning

Ivkovich and Stanton (2001) examined the effect of neonatal lesions of the hippocampus on delay, trace, and long-delay eyeblink conditioning in weanling rats. PND25–27 rats were tested with the same behavioral procedures as in the previous study (Ivkovich et al, 2000a; except the 6 sessions were distributed 2/day across 3 days rather than 3/day across 2 days). On PND10, rats received aspiration lesions of hippocampus plus overlying neocortex, control lesions of neocortex, or no treatment (Figure 24.9). The effects of neonatal lesions on acquisition of trace conditioning were examined in Experiment 1 whereas effects on standard versus long-delay conditioning were examined in Experiment 2.

Experiment 1 found that the hippocampal lesion group (HIPP) was dramatically impaired on trace conditioning relative to the control

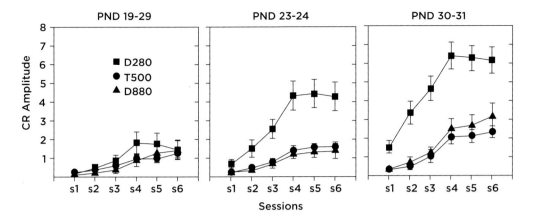

Figure 24.8 Mean CR amplitude in rats aged PND19–20 (left panel), PND23–24 (middle panel) or PND30–31 (right panel) trained with standard delay (D280), trace (T500) and long-delay (D880) procedures. (From Ivkovich et al., 2000a.)

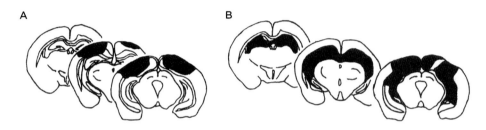

Figure 24.9 Reconstructions of typical cortical control (A) and hippocampal (B) aspiration lesions performed on PND10 and assessed following eyeblink conditioning on PND25–27. (From Ivkovich and Stanton, 2001.)

groups—cortical (CTX) and normal unoperated control (NORM) —which did not differ (Figure 24.10). There were no lesion effects on unlearned responses to the US (UR amplitude) or CS (startle or "alpha" responses), confirming that the lesions disrupted learning processes rather than sensory or motor processes involved in performance (Ivkovich & Stanton, 2001). These findings indicate that trace conditioning in weanling rats depends on the hippocampal system and that neonatal damage to the hippocampus impairs trace conditioning at the point in ontogeny when it is first emerging. The findings resemble the effect of adult hippocampal damage on trace conditioning (Moyer et al., 1990; Solomon et al., 1986; Weiss, Bouwmeester, Power, & Disterhoft, 1999). This agrees with the general principle, indicated previously (Table 24.1), that the effects of early damage on the emergence of hippocampal-dependent memory are qualitatively similar to the effects of adult damage on adult memory.

In Experiment 2, delay and long-delay conditioning were also impaired by the early aspiration lesion but to a much lesser extent than was observed for trace conditioning. All groups showed a significant increase in CR percentage across sessions, but CR percentage was reduced about 10% by the lesion in both delay conditioning groups, relative to their normal counterparts (cortical-lesion controls were omitted from Experiment 2 because they failed to differ from normal controls in Experiment 1). This suggests that the lesion effect in developing rats is less selective across trace versus delay conditioning than is the case for adults (see Ivkovich & Stanton, 2001, for discussion of possible explanations for this effect). To more directly examine the lesion effect across tasks, performance of long-delay versus trace conditioning was compared as a function of lesion group. This comparison was chosen because ISI and task difficulty were matched across these groups. This analysis revealed that hippocampal lesions produced a significantly

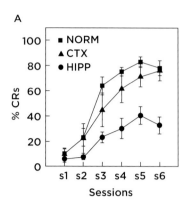

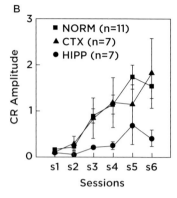

Figure 24.10 Mean CR percentage (A) and CR amplitude (B) in separate groups of PND25–27 rats trained on trace conditioning that underwent different surgical treatments on PND10 (HIPP, hippocampal aspiration; CTX, cortical control aspiration; NORM, normal rearing without surgery). (From Ivkovich and Stanton, 2001.)

greater impairment of trace conditioning (T500) relative to long-delay conditioning (D880, Figure 24.11). While normal rats did not differ across tasks (compare D880-N with T500-N), lesioned animals performed much more poorly on trace conditioning than long-delay conditioning (compare T500-H vs. D880-H).

This result is important for two reasons. First, it indicates that the dissociation of the effects of hippocampal injury on trace versus delay conditioning that is found in adulthood is also found during development (at least qualitatively). Second, it indicates that, in the case of this injury, trace interval rather than ISI is the critical factor determining the differential sensitivity of these tasks.

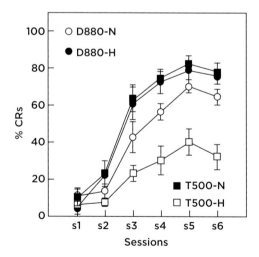

Figure 24.11 CR percentage in PND25–27 rats trained on long-delay (D880) or trace (T500) eyeblink conditioning following hippocampal aspiration on PND10 (H) or normal rearing (N). (From Ivkovich and Stanton, 2001.)

Thus, even though ISI is the factor that governs the normative development of trace versus long-delay conditioning (Claflin et al., 2005; Ivkovich et al., 2000a), the hippocampal system nevertheless appears to play a special role in learning procedures that involve a trace interval. This suggests that maturation of brain systems governing learning at long ISIs is "rate limiting" for the ontogeny of these tasks. This maturation apparently shows more protracted development than the hippocampal contribution to trace conditioning, which is normally "masked" by ISI effects but can be revealed by early hippocampal damage (Ivkovich & Stanton, 2001). There is evidence that cerebellar cortex plays a special role in ISI functions in eyeblink conditioning, particularly in learning at long ISIs (Mauk & Donegan, 1997; Perrett, Ruiz, & Mauk, 1993). Therefore one plausible interpretation of our developmental studies is that "the hippocampus is more important to the development of trace eyeblink conditioning than to that of long-delay eyeblink conditioning [but]…the hippocampus is functionally mature before cerebellar development is able to support learning over long ISIs" (Ivkovich & Stanton, 2001).

Taken together, these findings suggest that the hippocampal system plays a role in the ontogeny of higher-order eyeblink conditioning phenomenon but that this role does not necessarily cause these phenomena to emerge later in ontogeny than simple delay conditioning effects that are less dependent on the hippocampus. It is possible that the late development of the cerebellum makes the ontogenetic emergence of hippocampal versus nonhippocampal conditioning phenomenon more synchronous than occurs in other learning paradigms (see "Introduction"). We return to this point in the final section of this chapter.

Human Studies

In this section, we describe studies in human infants that examine some of the same conditioning phenomena that we have just described in developing rodents. The goal of such a comparative analysis is to develop and test hypotheses about the ontogeny of memory development in humans that is informed by recent progress in neural and behavioral studies of eyeblink conditioning in rodents.

Our methods for studying eyeblink conditioning in human infants have been described in great detail elsewhere (Ivkovich, Collins, Eckerman, Krasnegor, & Stanton, 1999; Ivkovich et al., 2000b; Figure 24.12). Participants were 4- and 5-month-old infants (±10 days) that sat on their parent's lap facing a visual display of objects that functioned as an infant version of the mild entertainment (silent movies) used in studies of eyeblink conditioning in adult humans. The tone CS (1 kHz, 80 dB) was delivered via two small speakers, positioned on each side of the infant's head. A soft head band supported the tubing for delivering the airpuff US (approximately 1/20 psi, measured at the eye) and gel pad electrodes for recording electromyographic activity in the vicinity of the eye. Infant's eyeblink responses were also scored frame by frame by two independent observers off video recordings

(Ivkovich et al., 2000b). Presentation of stimuli and recording of electromyogram (EMG) records was accomplished by the same custom-built system and software (JSA Designs, Raleigh, NC) that is used in our rodent conditioning studies (Stanton & Freeman, 2000). Sessions consisted of 50 trials and lasted about 15–20 min. Paired training trials consisted of a 750-ms tone that overlapped and coterminated with the 100 ms air puff. Unpaired training sessions consisted of the same number of CS and US presentations but the stimuli were presented 4–8 s apart so as to match the stimulus density of the paired condition.

Learned Irrelevance

In a study that was originally directed at the issue of acquisition versus expression of eyeblink conditioning between 4 and 5 months of age (Ivkovich et al., 2000b), we encountered evidence that LIr fails to appear in 5-month-old infants (Figure 24.13; Ivkovich et al., 1999). Three groups of infants were brought to the laboratory for 2 training sessions, spaced 6–8 days apart. All the infants received paired training during the second session but they differed in what they experienced during the first training session. During this session, one group received paired training

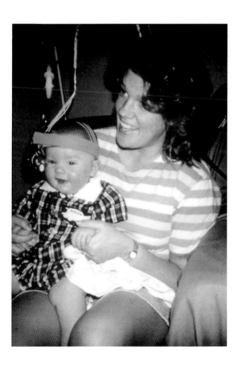

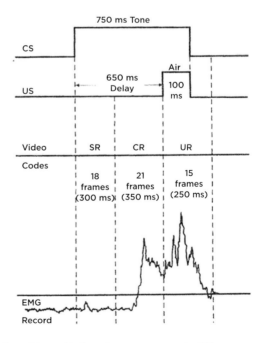

Figure 24.12 Illustration of the experimental preparation for studying delay eyeblink conditioning in 5-month-old human infants. See text for further explanation. (From Ivkovich et al., 2000b.)

(Paired group), one received unpaired training (CS/US-exposure group), and one was exposed only to the training situation without any stimulus presentations (Context-exposure group). The question was how these different experiences during the first session would influence eyeblink conditioning when all these groups received paired training during the second session. Paired training marginally elevated CR percentage during Session 1, relative to the other two groups (Figure 24.13) and resulted in robust conditioning with further paired training during Session 2 that exceeded that of the other two groups (Figure 24.13, Paired). Of most interest for the LIr effect was the contrast in performance between the unpaired CS/US-exposure versus Context-exposure groups. CR performance of these two groups did not differ significantly during Session 2, although the trend was for unpaired preexposure to *facilitate* rather than impair eyeblink conditioning (Figure 24.13). We have seen this facilitation effect of unpaired preexposure in rats initially trained on PND17 and retested on PND20 (Stanton et al., 1998) and in human infants initially trained at 4 months of age and retested at 5 months of age (Ivkovich et al., 2000b). Although further studies involving older age groups

and different amounts of unpaired stimulus preexposure are needed, these findings corroborate our rodent studies by suggesting that there are early stages of infancy when the LIr effect is not present. This is consistent with the idea that temporal lobe structures are involved in learning that events are unrelated and that this learning does not interfere with associative learning involving the developing cerebellum at this stage of human infancy.

Delay, Trace, and Long-Delay Eyeblink Conditioning

Herbert, Eckerman, and Stanton (2003) performed a study of delay, trace, and long-delay eyeblink conditioning in human infants and adults that, like our developmental rodent study (Ivkovich et al., 2000a), sought to examine developmental differences in trace versus delay conditioning with a design that addressed the roles of CS duration, ISI, and trace interval. Delay conditioning was examined in Experiment 1 whereas long-delay and trace conditioning were compared in Experiment 2.

Experiment 1 compared 5-month-old infants and young adults (college students) with the "standard delay" conditioning procedure described previously (Ivkovich et al., 1999, 2000b). Two 50-trial sessions were conducted 6–8 days apart. Infants sat on their parent's lap and were entertained by the visual display described previously (Ivkovich et al., 2000b). Adults sat in the same chair as the infant's parents but were entertained by a silent video (*Milo and Otis*) presented on a TV screen. In all other respects, the two age groups underwent the same training procedure.

The results of this 2 (infant vs. adult) × 2 (Delay 650 vs. Unpaired 650) × 2 (session) × 6 (blocks) mixed factorial design appear in Figure 24.14. At both ages, percentage CRs increased across blocks and sessions in the paired but not the unpaired groups, yielding a large pairing effect by the end of training. Performance of unpaired groups did not differ across age. Infants receiving paired training learned somewhat more slowly than their adult counterparts during Session 1 but reached the same asymptote of conditioning in Session 2.

UR latencies and durations (a measure of US efficacy) and alpha-responses (blinks during the first 300 ms of the trial epoch, a measure of CS orienting/processing) were analyzed to determine the possible contribution of differences in stimulus processing across age, or training group, to this outcome (Herbert et al., 2003). There were no training-group effects on any of these measures,

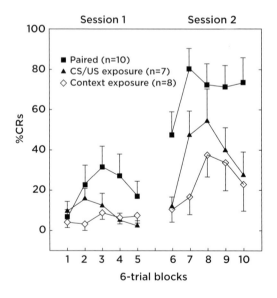

Figure 24.13 Percentage CR in groups of 5-month-old human infants that received different training experiences during Session 1 (Paired, CS-US pairings; CS/.US exposure, unpaired training; Context exposure, similar experience but with no stimulus exposure) and then all underwent paired training during Session 2. See text for further explanation. (From Ivkovich et al., 1999.)

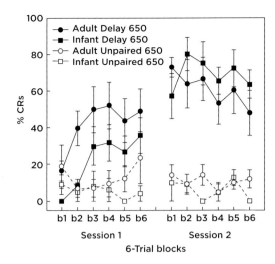

Figure 24.14 Mean CR percentage in 5-month-old human infants or adults receiving delay eyeblink conditioning with a 650-ms CS–US interval (Delay 650) or unpaired control training. See text for further explanation. (From Herbert, Eckerman, and Stanton, 2003.)

confirming that conditioning was not confounded with sensory or performance factors in this study. However, infants showed significantly longer UR latencies (~137 ms vs. 68 ms for adults, collapsed across training groups) and UR durations (~69 ms vs. 43.5 ms for adults, onset-to-peak). The differences in these UR measures suggest a possible age difference in US efficacy or motor performance. However, the fact that there were no age differences in the asymptotic level of CRs in the paired groups or in baseline responding in unpaired groups suggests that these measured differences in US efficacy were not enough to translate into different levels of CR performance (particularly since asymptotic CRs were not at "ceiling"). We have also found that UR amplitude is not predictive of learning in 4- to 5-month-old infants (Ivkovich et al., 1999). Studies manipulating airpuff intensity are needed to fully clarify this issue. Analysis of alpha responses also yielded a potentially important age difference. These responses were absent in infants but were robust in adults (Herbert et al., 2003). In adults, alpha responses occurred at comparable levels in both paired and unpaired groups, confirming that they are nonassociative "orienting" responses. The infants given paired training showed learning despite the absence of alpha responses, suggesting that orienting responses are not crucial for conditioning on the Delay 650 task. However, the absence of these responses may reflect a reduction in CS salience or attention that contributed to the

slower acquisition rates observed in infants compared with adults. Again, parametric studies of CS intensity, like those performed in developing rats (Stanton & Freeman, 2000), are needed to fully characterize the contribution of developmental changes in orienting responses to the ontogeny of human eyeblink conditioning.

In Experiment 2, a trace conditioning procedure ("Trace 500") was used in which the same 750-ms tone used in Experiment 1 was followed by a 500-ms stimulus-free "trace period" prior to the 100-ms airpuff. Because CS and US did not overlap, this yielded a 1250-ms ISI. In the long-delay procedure, a 1350-ms tone CS preceded and coterminated with the 100-ms airpuff, also yielding a 1250-ms delay between CS and US onset ("Delay 1250"). Each conditioning procedure was compared with an unpaired counterpart as a control for nonassociative effects. The procedure was otherwise the same as in Experiment 1. Thus, the experiment was a 2 (infant vs. adult) × 2 (paired vs. unpaired) × 2 (long delay vs. trace) × 2 (session) × 6 (blocks) mixed factorial design. Because infant performance was so poor on these tasks, many were invited back for an additional session. The effect of this training was analyzed in a separate 2 (paired vs. unpaired) × 2 (long delay vs. trace) × 3 (session) × 6 (blocks) mixed factorial design involving only these infants.

The main results appear in Figure 24.15. Infants exhibited no evidence of conditioning, relative to unpaired controls in either the long-delay or trace procedure during Session 1, and marginal (statistically nonsignificant) conditioning during Session 2. Infants were greatly and equivalently impaired on both tasks, relative to their performance in the Delay 650 condition in the previous experiment. In contrast, adults showed conditioning in the long-delay and trace tasks across two sessions that was comparable to their learning in the Delay 650 condition in Experiment 1, with clear differences between paired versus unpaired groups emerging in Session 1 and growing larger as asymptote was reached during Session 2. As in Experiment 1, unpaired controls performed comparably across age. In striking contrast to Experiment 1, infants in the paired groups failed entirely during the first two sessions to reach conditioning asymptotes that were reached by their adult counterparts. Even after a third training session, infants showed lower CR percentages than adults did after two sessions (Figure 24.15), although infant paired groups came to differ significantly from unpaired controls during the third training session.

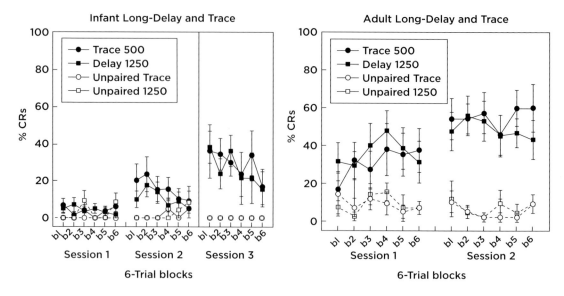

Figure 24.15 Mean CR percentage in 5-month-old human infants or adults receiving long-delay eyeblink conditioning with a 1250-ms CS–US interval (Delay 650), trace conditioning involving a 500-ms trace interval but matched for CS–US interval (Trace 500) or unpaired control training. See text for further explanation. (From Herbert et al., 2003.)

As in Experiment 1, UR onset latencies and durations did not explain differences between paired versus unpaired groups but were somewhat greater in infants versus adults. Alpha responses were also (again) generally not evident in infants but were striking in adults, regardless of task and (again) pairing condition. Infants in the paired groups also showed striking differences in CR timing, with CR onset appearing much earlier in the trial epoch than adults (see next section, "CR Timing").

The findings of Herbert et al. (2003) revealed some differences but several general parallels with studies of developing rodents (e.g., Ivkovich et al., 2000a; Ivkovich & Stanton, 2001). Notable differences were the developmental change in alpha responding and UR latency in humans but not in rodents. Nevertheless, the parallels across species in conditioned responding were striking. CR performance was stronger and developmental differences were attenuated under optimal (short) delay conditions. In contrast, performance of long-delay and trace conditioning was clearly impaired and developmental differences were enhanced. Most importantly, ISI rather than trace interval determined the effectiveness of conditioning, suggesting that in both humans and rats, the normative development of trace conditioning is determined largely by the difficulty of forming associations over long CS–US intervals rather than by short-

term memory processes engaged by the trace interval. As reviewed above (Figure 24.11), early damage to the hippocampal system in rats impairs trace conditioning more than long-delay conditioning, suggesting a greater hippocampal role in the short-term memory component than the ISI component (Ivkovich & Stanton, 2001). It remains to be determined whether early injury to the temporal lobe would have a similar disproportionate impact on trace conditioning in human infants, as has been demonstrated following temporal lobe injury in human adults (Clark & Squire, 1998). Further work is also needed to address the hypothesis, arising from our developmental rodent studies (see above), that learning in infant humans at long ISIs places greater demands on immature cerebellar circuitry that may "mask" hippocampal-system involvement in trace conditioning (see next section "CR Timing" for further discussion).

The study of Herbert et al. (2003) is the first to examine the ontogeny of trace conditioning in humans with a design that controls both for CS duration and ISI. The findings in adult subjects that delay, long-delay, and trace conditioning procedures yield comparable acquisition rates is consistent with other reports (e.g., Hansche & Grant, 1960; Kimble, 1947; Reynolds, 1945; Ross & Ross, 1971). However, the findings in infant subjects contrast with the outcome of a previous study of trace versus delay conditioning in human infants

(Little, 1973). In this study, delay and trace conditioning were matched for ISI (1500 ms) but trace conditioning involved a 100-ms CS followed by a 1400-ms trace interval. Infants aged 1.5 to 2.5 months received six daily 50-trial training sessions and reached an asymptote of 80% CRs on delay conditioning but failed entirely to learn trace conditioning. Although there are many variables that distinguish Little's (1973) study from ours, other studies (Claflin et al., 2002, see below; Little et al., 1984) suggests that trace conditioning was not observed by Little (1973) because the CS was too short. Because delay conditioning fails to occur in 5-month-olds with a 350 ms CS (ISI of 250 ms; Claflin et al., 2002) or in 1.5-month-olds at an ISI of 500 ms (Little et al., 1984), it is no surprise that infants cannot show trace conditioning to a 100-ms CS. Our findings show that when CS duration, ISI, and trace interval are controlled, ISI is the most important variable during development (Herbert et al., 2003).

CR Timing in Infant Eyeblink Conditioning

Recent advances in behavioral neuroscience have increased attention to CR timing as a property of eyeblink conditioning that has potentially important neurological implications. Neuropharmacological and neural recording studies of cerebellar circuitry suggest a distinction between CR expression and timing (Garcia & Mauk, 1998; Mauk & Ruiz, 1992; Ohyama & Mauk, 2001). In adult rabbits, the anterior interpositus nucleus is critically involved in the production of CRs, whereas the ipsilateral cerebellar cortex influences the amplitude and timing of responding (Garcia, Steele, & Mauk, 1999; McCormick & Thompson, 1984; Ohyama & Mauk, 2001). Disrupting modulation of interpositus activity by cerebellar cortex in rabbits produces CRs that are prematurely timed relative to normal rabbits, particularly during long-delay conditioning (e.g., Perrett, Ruiz, & Mauk, 1993). There is also evidence that damage to temporal lobe structures can result in premature CRs in both rabbits (Moyer et al., 1990) and humans (McGlinchey-Berroth, Brawn, & Disterhoft, 1999). This led us to examine CR timing during infant eyeblink conditioning (Claflin et al., 2002; Herbert et al., 2003). We found that human infants do indeed show premature CRs. As in our rodent studies, we followed established conventions in the field of using "adaptive CRs"—those that occurred at the end of the trial epoch (the last 350 ms before

US onset in our case)—as the primary measure of conditioning. This convention equates the duration of the sampling period across different ISIs and yields a conservative CR measure that does not include early responses that, in adult humans, are not classically conditioned (e.g., "voluntary responses," Spence & Ross, 1959). Figure 24.16 shows the distribution of responses during Delay 1250 conditioning in 5-month-old infants. The CR sampling period was divided into 25 successive 50-ms bins and CR onset in each bin of the CS period were averaged across each training session (Claflin et al., 2002). Infants trained on long-delay conditioning showed few responses during the first 300 ms (alpha responses) or during the final 350 ms (adaptive CRs). Rather, their CR onsets occurred early in the CR period and increased between Sessions 1 and 2. This increase was associative because their unpaired counterparts did not show CRs (Claflin et al., 2002) and bin counts in unpaired controls ranged between 0 and 0.5 in an evenly distributed manner across the trial epoch (Herbert et al., 2003). During standard delay conditioning (Delay 650), infant CR onsets occurred primarily during the adaptive period but they nevertheless "spiked" earlier than CR onsets in comparably trained adults (Herbert et al., 2003). The early-onset CRs of infants trained on long-delay

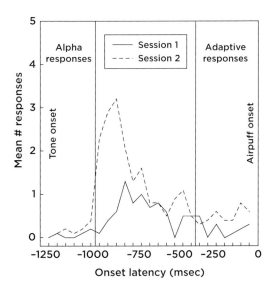

Figure 24.16 Mean number of CRs in 5-month-old infants trained on long-delay eyeblink conditioning (Delay 1250) as function of latency from CS-onset (Onset latency) and training session. (From Claflin, Stanton, Herbert, Greer, and Eckerman, 2002.)

conditioning were seen also during trace condition-ing, and differed dramatically from the temporal pattern of CR onsets shown by adults trained on these tasks, which generally showed a monotonic increase that was highest in the latter half of the adaptive period (Herbert et al., 2003).

To determine the impact of CR timing as opposed to CR generation on infant eyeblink conditioning, Claflin et al. (2002) performed an analysis of trials to criterion (TTC, see Ivkovich et al., 2000b) using either the adaptive CR measure, which counted responses occurring only during the 350 ms period preceding US onset, or a more inclu-sive "total CR" measure that counted all responses occurring between the end of the alpha period and US onset (Figure 24.17). The study examined ISI functions in infant delay conditioning by compar-ing groups trained with delay intervals of 250, 650, or 1250 ms (the latter two groups were also used by Herbert et al., 2003). In the case of the adaptive CR measure (Figure 24.17, left panel), 5-month-olds trained at the 650-ms delay interval reached crite-rion in about 43.2 trials whereas their counterparts trained with the 250- and 1250-ms delay intervals failed to reach criterion within 2 training sessions. When the Total CR measure was used (Figure 24.17, right panel), both the 650- and 1250-ms delay groups reached criterion within about 43–46 trials, although the 250-ms delay group still failed

to learn (even with an extended CR sampling period, Claflin et al., 2002). This result indicates that the failure to learn long- but not short-delay conditioning reflects a deficit in CR timing (rather than CR generation per se) that appears under long-ISI conditions in these infants.

It is unclear if premature CR timing has been found in other developmental studies of human eyeblink conditioning, or if the use of our adaptive versus total CR measures would alter the outcome of these studies. Little et al. (1984) used a more stringent adaptive-CR measure (last 170 ms prior to US onset) than ours whereas other researchers (Hoffman, Cohen, & DeVido, 1985; Ohlrich & Ross, 1968) used the equivalent of our total CR measure. The many procedural differences across studies, particularly age of testing, further compli-cate the issue. Hoffman et al. (1985) used a delay interval of 500 ms in 8-month-old infants, condi-tions that our data suggest would minimally influ-ence (or be influenced by) CR timing. Little et al. (1984) studied much younger infants (newborn to about 6 weeks old) and found better conditioning at long ISIs (1500 ms) than shorter ones (500 ms). Our findings do not suggest that using a total CR measure would have changed the outcome of their study. Our finding that 5-month-old infants do not condition at the shorter 250-ms ISI, a delay interval that supports strong conditioning in adult humans

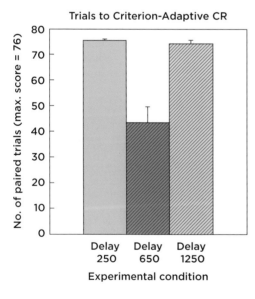
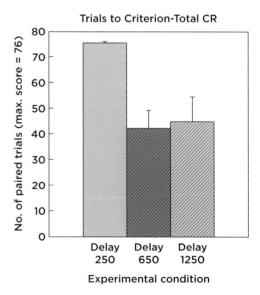

Figure 24.17 Trials-to-criterion in 5-month-old human infants trained on delay eyeblink conditioning with 250-, 650-, and 1250-ms CS–US intervals as function of whether Adaptive versus Total CRs were counted. See text for further explanation. (From Claflin, Stanton, Herbert, Greer, and Eckerman, 2002.)

(Kimble, 1947) supports a general principle of Little et al. (1984). Both studies show that infants cannot learn at shorter delays that support conditioning in adults. Taken together, they also suggest that the optimal ISI may shift downward between the neonatal period and 5 months of age.

The markedly premature CRs demonstrated in our studies of human infants trained with long-delay and trace conditioning procedures have not been seen in our studies of developing rodents. Premature CRs can occur but adaptive CRs generally predominate during trace and long-delay conditioning in developing rats (Ivkovich & Stanton, unpublished observations). However, studies using more complex CR-timing tasks in developing rodents indicate that accurate timing of adaptive CRs continues do undergo ontogenetic development beyond the weanling period under long-delay but not short-delay conditions. This has been shown with both temporal uncertainty (Freeman, Nicholson, Muckler, Rabinak, & DiPietro, 2003) and ISI discrimination tasks (Brown, Pagani, & Stanton, 2006). Thus, the general principle that timing of eyeblink CRs improves across ontogenetic development shows some generality across species. Advances in our understanding of the cerebellar and forebrain mechanisms underlying CR timing, particularly in humans, will have a potentially large impact on how studies in infant humans are designed and interpreted.

Summary and Conclusions

The studies reviewed in this chapter extend previous developmental studies of eyeblink conditioning in the rodent (Chapter 26; Freeman & Nicholson, 2004; Stanton, 2000; Stanton & Freeman, 2000) and in humans (Ivkovich et al., 2000b) by adding LIr and trace conditioning to the range of phenomena that have been examined (Claflin et al., 2002; Ivkovich et al., 2000a; Ivkovich & Stanton, 2001; Herbert et al., 2003; Rush et al., 2001). The main goal has been to gather converging evidence across behavioral tasks concerning the point in ontogeny when memory functions of the hippocampal system are expressed in eyeblink conditioning. The findings reveal both commonalities and contrasts across tasks and across species. Both LIr and trace conditioning appear to show more protracted development than standard delay conditioning. This is a common feature of both tasks in both species. Trace conditioning contrasts with LIr, however, in that ISI rather than trace interval is the factor that is responsible for the later emergence of trace

conditioning relative to standard delay conditioning. When ISI is held constant across trace- and long-delay conditioning, ontogenetic profiles across tasks are the same in both rodents (Figures 24.8) and humans (Figures 24.14 and 24.15). ISI is not the factor that causes hippocampal system damage to impair trace conditioning, neither in developing rats (Figure 24.11) nor in adult humans (Clark & Squire, 1998). This damage impairs trace conditioning with little or no effect on long delay conditioning that is matched for ISI. Whether early hippocampal system damage would impair trace conditioning more than long-delay conditioning in infant humans is not known. We can therefore not say whether the late development of long-delay conditioning in human infants "masks" the role of hippocampal development in trace conditioning the way it appears to do in developing rats. An advantage of the converging evidence approach is that one task can probe the ontogeny of neurological function in a manner that overcomes limitations of the other task. Thus, the LIr task assesses hippocampal system involvement in eyeblink conditioning without the interpretive problems arising from ontogenetic changes in optimal ISI functions or task difficulty that we have encountered with the trace conditioning task. It is tempting to invoke the principle of parsimony and conclude that the weanling period in rats and the first 6 months of life in humans represent developmental windows in which hippocampal involvement in eyeblink conditioning is still emerging. However, as noted previously, our work with LIr in human infants does not benefit from the extensive parametric studies that are needed to draw stronger conclusions about the ontogeny of this effect. Our work with rats suffers less in this regard but much more work remains to be done concerning the behavioral and neural determinants of this effect in developing rats (Rush et al., 2001).

An important species contrast in the work reviewed here is the large role that differences in CS orienting (alpha responses) and CR timing appear to play in infant versus adult eyeblink conditioning (Claflin et al., 2002; Herbert et al., 2003). These factors do not seem to play as much of a role (if any) in our rodent studies that involve the same tasks. Our rodent work is based on extensive analysis of the role of conditioning parameters in the ontogeny of eyeblink conditioning (Stanton & Freeman, 2000). Such parametric studies need to be performed in human infants in order to provide a clearer picture concerning which factors do or do not contribute importantly to the ontogeny of eyeblink conditioning in humans and how this picture compares with what is known in developing rodents. This is an important area for future research.

In the first section of this chapter (Introduction), we noted the historical emergence of a dichotomous view of memory (Squire, 2004). This view contrasts declarative (or explicit) memory that depends on the hippocampal system with nondeclarative (or implicit) memory that depends on other brain systems. We also noted how this view of memory stimulated developmental research that seemed to show that nondeclarative memory emerges earlier in ontogeny than declarative memory (e.g., Diamond, 1990a; Freeman & Stanton, 1991; Rudy, 1992). We also noted the historical tendency for researchers to attach absolute age ranges to the emergence of hippocampal system–dependent memory. This view of the development of two forms of memory has been challenged on the grounds that memory performance of infants in the conjugate mobile paradigm shows many properties of "explicit memory, which should not be present if this memory depends on hippocampal system function that does not mature until after the first year of life (Rovee-Collier, 1997; Rovee-Collier et al., 2001). Although it is not known whether memory performance on this paradigm depends on the hippocampal system because infants with hippocampal damage have not yet been tested on this paradigm, nor are there data from adult humans or a developmental animal model that might address this issue, we concur that the attempt to identify specific developmental periods when explicit, declarative, or hippocampal-dependent memory is *absent* is a misguided view of memory development. We also "…realize the risk inherent in proclaiming that infants cannot do this or that "(Rovee-Collier, Hayne, & Colombo, 2001, p. ix). We have instead emphasized that the emergence of hippocampal-dependent memory is better conceived from a perspective that is relative rather than absolute, that incorporate a "behavioral systems" view, and that emphasizes interactions rather than dissociations among memory systems (Table 24.1 and Figure 24.4; Stanton, 2000). From this perspective, the developmental order in which implicit or explicit memory appears depends on which behavioral system is engaged by a particular task and whether interactions between this system and the hippocampal system are present. In the rat, some forms of hippocampal system–dependent memory (runway patterned alternation, Diaz-Granadas et al., 1992, Table 24.1) emerge

earlier than other forms of nonhippocampal memory (eyeblink conditioning, Stanton, Freeman, & Skelton, 1992). Because the conjugate mobile paradigm takes advantage of behavioral predispositions that are strongly but transiently expressed only during infancy in humans, the neural basis of performance on this task can only be studied in human infants with early brain injuries. However, the developmental perspective concerning multiple memory systems presented in this chapter does not exclude a possible role for the hippocampal system in conjugate mobile performance.

At a methodological level, our studies of eyeblink conditioning permit the ontogeny of multiple memory systems to be examined with a behavioral paradigm that is probably better understood neurobiologically and developmentally, and is more directly comparable across species and developmental stages, than many of the other behavioral paradigms that have been directed at this issue in either humans or animal models. These advantages have not, however, yielded a simpler picture concerning the order in which different memory systems appear during ontogeny. Perhaps the best test of how implicit versus explicit memory develops in our paradigm is the comparison of trace versus long-delay conditioning. This is the best test because task demands and difficulty are so closely matched, something that often is not true of task-dissociations in the infant memory literature (Rovee-Collier et al., 2001). Our results with this comparison suggest that the two forms of memory develop in parallel. Our work with latent inhibition (Stanton, 2000) and LIr (Rush et al., 2001) in developing rats also falls far short of clearly showing that (nondeclarative) memory functions of the cerebellum emerge earlier in ontogeny than (declarative) memory functions arising from hippocampal–cerebellar interactions. Latent inhibition is seen in development as soon as delay eyeblink conditioning is strong enough to reveal it (Stanton, 2000). LIr emerges during a developmental period when delay conditioning is continuing to strengthen (Figure 24.5; Rush et al., 2001). Our experience with eyeblink conditioning suggests that the ontogeny of multiple memory systems is likely to be better understood by studying specific brain memory systems using empirical approaches from behavioral neuroscience—when and how these systems develop will be revealed by the empirical data. Studying memory system development from the perspective of broad psychological theories that predict various properties of memory will generalize across several experimental paradigms is less likely to be fruitful. Our experience also underscores the importance of considering memory-system interactions rather than memory dichotomies. Understanding these interactions is also best approached with empirical neuroscience methods. This is consistent with historical trends that have influenced multiple memory systems research (Squire, 2004). These trends place greater importance on gathering information concerning the neural basis of memory in human infants. Studies of developmental neurological disorders and infant brain imaging will become increasingly important, not just to advance clinical practice, but to advance our understanding of the ontogeny of multiple memory systems.

References

Allen, M. T., Chelius, L., & Gluck, M. A. (2002). Selective entorhinal and nonselective cortical-hippocampal region lesions, but not selective hippocampal lesions, disrupt learned irrelevance in rabbit eyeblink conditioning. *Cognitive, Affective & Behavioral Neuroscience, 2*, 214–226.

Altemus, K. L., & Almli, C. R. (1997). Neonatal hippocampal damage in rats: Long-term spatial memory deficits and associations with magnitude of hippocampal damage. *Hippocampus, 7*, 403–415 .

Altman, J., & Bayer, S. (1975). Postnatal development of the hippocampal dentate gyrus under normal and experimental conditions. In R. L. Isaacson & K. H. Pribram (Eds.), *The hippocampus: Structure and development* (Vol. 1, pp. 95–122). New York: Plenum.

Altman, J., Brunner, R. L., & Bayer, S. A. (1973). The hippocampus and behavioral maturation. *Behavioral Biology, 8*, 557–596.

Amsel, A., & Chen, J. (1976). Ontogeny of persistence: immediate and long-term persistence in rats varying in training age between 17 and 65 days. *Journal of Comparative and Physiological Psychology, 90*, 808–820.

Amsel, A., & Stanton, M. (1980). Ontogeny and phylogeny of paradoxical reward effects. In J. S. Rosenblatt, R. A. Hinde, C. Beer, & M. Busnel (Eds.), *Advances in the study of behavior* (pp. 227–274). New York: Academic Press.

Bachevalier, J. (1990). Ontogenetic development of habit and memory formation in primates, In A. Diamond (Ed.), *The development and neural basis of higher cognitive functions* (pp. 457–477). New York: New York Academy of Sciences Press.

Bachevalier, J., & Mishkin, M. (1984). An early and late developing system for learning and retention in infant monkeys. *Behavioral Neuroscience, 98*, 770–778.

Baudry, M., Davis, J. L., & Berger, T. W. (2001). A celebration of the scientific contributions of Richard F. Thompson. *Neurobiology of Learning and Memory, 76*(3), 225–461.

Baxter, M. G., & Murray, E. A. (2001). Effects of hippocampal lesions on delayed nonmatching-to-sample in monkeys: A reply to Zola and Squire (2001). *Hippocampus, 11*, 201–203.

Bennett, C. H., Maldonado, A., & Mackintosh, N. J. (1995). Learned irrelevance is not the sum of exposure to CS and US. *Quarterly Journal of Experimental Psychology, 48B*, 117–128.

Blankenship, M. R., Huckfeldt, R., Steinmetz, J. J., & Steinmetz, J. E. (2005). The effects of amygdala lesions on hippocampal activity and classical eyeblink conditioning in rats. *Brain Research, 1035*, 120–130.

Brown K. L., Pagani J. P., & Stanton, M. E. (2006). The ontogeny of interstimulus interval (ISI) discrimination of the conditioned eyeblink response in rats. *Behavioral Neuroscience, 120*, 1057–1070.

Bruner, J. S. (1969). Modalities of memory. In G. A. Talland & N. C. Waugh (Eds.), *The pathology of memory* (pp. 253–259). New York: Academic Press.

Brunner, R. L., Haggbloom, S. J., & Gazzara, R. A. (1974). Effects of hippocampal x-irradiation-produced granule-cell agenesis on instrumental runway performance in rats. *Physiology & Behavior, 13*, 485–494.

Castro, C. A., Paylor, R., & Rudy, J. W. (1987). A developmental analysis of the learning and short-term-memory processes mediating performance in conditional-spatial discrimination problems. *Psychobiology, 15*, 308–316.

Chen, J., Gross, K., & Amsel, A. (1980). Ontogeny of successive negative contrast and its dissociation from other paradoxical reward effects in preweanling rats. *Journal of Comparative and Physiological Psychology, 95*, 146–159.

Claflin, D.I., Garrett, T., & Buffington, M.L. (2005) A developmental comparison of trace and delay eyeblink conditioning in rats using matching interstimulus intervals. *Developmental Psychobiology, 47*, 77–88.

Claflin, D., Stanton, M. E., Herbert, J., Greer, J., & Eckerman, C. O. (2002). Effect of delay-interval on classical eyeblink conditioning in 5-month-old human infants. *Developmental Psychobiology, 41*, 329–340.

Clark, R. E., & Squire, L. R. (1998). Classical conditioning and brain systems: The role of awareness. *Science, 280*, 77–81.

Columbo, P. J., & Gold, P. E. (2004). Multiple memory systems (Editor's note for special issue). *Neurobiology of Learning and Memory, 82*, 169–170.

Daly, H. B. (1991). Changes in learning about aversive nonreward accounts for ontogeny of paradoxical appetitive reward effects in the rat pup: A mathematical model (DMOD) integrates results. *Psychological Bulletin, 109*, 325–339.

Davis, M. (1992). The role of the amygdala in conditioned fear. In J. P. Aggleton (Ed.) *The amygdala: Neurobiological aspects of emotion, memory, and mental dysfunction* (pp. 255–305). New York: Wiley-Liss.

Diamond, A. (1990a). *The development and neural basis of higher cognitive functions* (Vol. 608). New York: Annual New York Academy of Sciences.

Diamond, A. (1990b). Infant's and young children's peformance on delayed non-match-to-sample (direct and indirect) and visual paired comparison. In A. Diamond (Ed.), *The development and neural basis of higher cognitive functions* (pp. 394–426). New York: New York Academy of Sciences Press.

Diaz-Granados, J. L., Greene, P. L., & Amsel, A. (1992). Memory-based learning in preweanling and adult rats after infantile x-irradiation-induced hippocampal granule cell hypoplasia. *Behavioral Neuroscience, 106*, 940–946.

Douglas, R. (1975). The development of hippocampal function: Implications for theory and therapy. In R. Isaacson & K. H. Pribram (Eds.), *The hippocampus* (Part 1, pp. 327–361). New York: Plenum Press.

Fanselow, M. S. (1994). Neural organization of the defensive behavior system responsible for fear. *Psychonomic Bulletin & Review, 1*, 429–438.

Feigley, D. A., Parsons, P. J., Hamilton, L. W., & Spear, N. E. (1972). Development of habituation to novel environments in the rat. *Journal of Comparative and Physiological Psychology, 79*, 443–452.

Freeman, J. H., Jr., Barone, S., Jr., & Stanton, M. E. (1995). Disruption of cerebellar maturation by an antimitotic agent impairs the ontogeny of eyeblink conditioning in rats. *Journal of Neuroscience, 15*, 7301–7314.

Freeman, J. H., & Nicholson, D. A. (2004). Developmental changes in the neural mechanisms of eyeblink conditioning. *Behavioral and Cognitive Neuroscience Reviews, 3*, 3–13.

Freeman, J. H., Nicholson, D. A., Muckler, A. S., Rabinak, C. A., & DiPietro, N. T. (2003). Ontogeny of eyeblink conditioned response timing in rats. *Behavioral Neuroscience, 117*, 283–291.

Freeman, J. H., Jr., & Stanton, M. E. (1991). Fimbria-fornix transections disrupt the ontogeny of delayed alternation but not position discrimination in the rat. *Behavioral Neuroscience, 105*, 386–395.

Garcia, K. S., & Mauk, M. D. (1998). Pharmacological analysis of cerebellar contributions to the timing and expression of conditioned eyelid responses. *Neuropharmacology, 37*, 471–480.

Garcia, K. S., Steele, P. M., & Mauk, M. D. (1999). Cerebellar cortex lesions prevent acquisition of conditioned eyelid responses. *Journal of Neuroscience, 19*, 10940–10947.

Gormezano, I., Prokasy, W. F., & Thompson, R. F. (Eds.). (1987). *Classical conditioning* (3rd ed.). Hillsdale NJ: Erlbaum.

Green, R. J., & Stanton, M. E. (1989). Differential ontogeny of working and reference memory in the rat. *Behavioral Neuroscience, 103*, 98–105.

Hansche, W. J., & Grant, D. A. (1960). Onset versus termination of a stimulus as the CS in eyelid conditioning. *Journal of Experimental Psychology, 59*, 19–26.

Herbert, J. S., Eckerman, C. O., & Stanton, M. E. (2003). The ontogeny of human learning in delay, long-delay, and trace eyeblink conditioning. *Behavioral Neuroscience, 117*, 1196–1210.

Hilgard, E. R. (1931). Conditioned eyelid reactions to a light stimulus based on the reflex wink to sound. *Psychological Monographs, 41*, 184.

Hoffman, H. S., Cohen, M. E., & DeVido, C. J. (1985). A comparison of classical eyelid conditioning in adults and infants. *Infant Behavior and Development, 8*, 247–254.

Ivkovich, D., & Stanton, M. E. (2001). Effects of early hippocampal lesions on trace, delay, and long-delay eyeblink conditioning in developing rats. *Neurobiology of Learning and Memory, 76*, 426–446.

Ivkovich, D., Collins, K. L., Eckerman, C. O., Krasnegor, N. A., & Stanton, M. E. (1999). Classical delay eyeblink conditioning in 4- and 5-month-old human infants. *Psychological Science, 10*, 4–8.

Ivkovich, D., Eckerman, C. O., Krasnegor, N. A., & Stanton, M. E. (2000b). Using eyeblink conditioning to assess neurocognitive development in human infants. In D. S. Woodruff-Pak & J. E. Steinmetz (Eds.), *Eyeblink classical conditioning: Vol. I. Applications in humans* (pp. 119–142). Amsterdam: Kluwer Academic.

Ivkovich, D., Paczkowski, C. M., & Stanton, M. E. (2000a). Ontogeny of delay versus trace eyeblink conditioning in the rat. *Developmental Psychobiology, 36*, 148–160.

Jacobs, E., Stanton, M. E., & Levine, S. (1986). *Differential ontogeny of behavioral and endocrine conditioned responses in the rat*. International Society for Developmental Psychobiology, Annapolis, November.

James, W. (1890). *Principles of psychology*. New York: Holt.

Kesner, R.P., & Rogers, J. (2004). An analysis of independence and interactions of brain substrates that subserve multiple attributes, memory systems, and underlying processes. *Neurobiology of Learning and Memory, 82*, 199–215.

Kimble, G. A. (1947). Conditioning as a function of the time between conditioned and unconditioned stimuli. *Journal of Experimental Psychology, 37*, 1–15.

Konorski, J. (1967) *Integrative activity of the brain*. Chicago: University of Chicago Press.

LeDoux, J. E. (1992). Emotion and the amygdala. In J. P. Aggleton (Ed.), *The amygdala: Neurobiological aspects of emotion, memory, and mental dysfunction* (pp. 339–351). New York: Wiley-Liss.

Lee T., & Kim, J. J. (2004). Differential effects of cerebellar, amygdalar, and hippocampal lesions on classical eyeblink conditioning in rats. *Journal of Neuroscience, 24*, 3242–3250.

Letz, R., Burdette, D. R., Gregg, B., Kittrell, M. E., & Amsel, A. (1978). Evidence for a transitional period for the development of persistence in infant rats. *Journal of Comparative and Physiological Psychology, 92*, 856–866.

Little, A. H. (1973). *A comparative study of trace and delay conditioning in the human infants*. Unpublished doctoral dissertation, Brown University.

Little, A. H., Lipsitt, L. P., & Rovee-Collier, C. (1984). Classical conditioning and retention of the infant's eyelid response: Effects of age and interstimulus interval. *Journal of Experimental Child Psychology, 37*, 512–524.

Lobaugh, N. J., Bootin, M., & Amsel, A. (1985). Sparing of patterned alternation but not partial reinforcement effect after infant and adult hippocampal lesions in the rat. *Behavioral Neuroscience, 99*, 46–59.

Loy, R., Lynch, G., & Cotman, C. W. (1977). Development of afferent lamination in the fasica dentata of the rat. *Brain Research, 121*, 229–243.

Mackintosh, N. J. (1974). *The psychology of animal learning*. London: Academic Press.

Mackintosh, N. J. (1975). A theory of attention: Variations in the associability of stimuli with reinforcement. *Psychological Review, 82*, 276–298.

Maine de Biran, F. P. G. (1929). *The influence of habit on the faculty of thinking*. Baltimore, MD: Williams & Wilkins [first published in 1804].

Mauk, M. D., & Donegan, N. H. (1997). A model of Pavlovian eyelid conditioning based on the synaptic organization of the cerebellum. *Learning and Memory, 3*, 130–158.

Mauk, M. D., & Ruiz, B. P. (1992). Learning-dependent timing of Pavlovian eyelid responses: Differential conditioning using multiple interstimulus intervals. *Behavioral Neuroscience, 106*, 666–681.

McCormick, D. A., & Thompson, R. F. (1984) Cerebellum: Essential involvement in the classically conditioned eyelid response. *Science, 223*, 296–299.

McEchron, M. D., Bouwmeester, H., Tseng, W., Weiss, C., & Disterhoft, J. F. (1998). Hippocampectomy disrupts auditory trace fear conditioning and contextual fear conditioning in the rat. *Hippocampus, 8,* 638–646.

McGlinchey-Berroth, R., Brawn, C., & Disterhoft, J. F. (1999). Temporal discrimination learning in severe amnesic patients reveals an alteration in the timing of eyeblink conditioned responses. *Behavioral Neuroscience, 113,* 10–18.

Milner, B. (1962). Les troubles de la me′moire accompagnant des le′sions hippocampiques bilate′rales. In *Physiologie de l_hippocampe* (pp. 257–272). Paris: Centre National de la Recherche Scientifique. English translation: B. Milner and S. Glickman (Eds.), Princeton: Van Nostrand, 1965 (pp. 97–111).

Mishkin, M., Malamut, B., & Bachevalier, J. (1984). Memory and habits: Two neural systems. In G. Lynch, J. L. McGaugh, & N. M. Weinberger (Eds.), *Neurobiology of learning and memory* (pp. 66–77). New York: Guilford Press.

Moye, T. B., & Rudy, J. W. (1987). Ontogenesis of trace conditioning in young rats: Dissociation of associative versus memory processes. *Developmental Psychobiology, 20,* 405–414.

Moyer, J. F., Deyo, R. A., & Disterhoft, J. F. (1990). Hippocampectomy disrupts trace eye-blink conditioning in rabbits. *Behavioral Neuroscience, 104,* 243–252.

Murray, E. A., & Wise, S. P. (2004). What, if anything, is the medial temporal lobe, and how can the amygdala be part of it if there is no such thing? *Neurobiology of Learning and Memory, 82,* 178–198.

Nadel, L. & Zola-Morgan, S. (1984). Infantile amnesia: A neurobiological perspective. In M. Moscovitch (Ed.), *Infant memory* (pp. 145–172). New York: Plenum.

Nicolle, M. M., Barry, C. C., Veronesi, B., & Stanton, M. E. (1989). Fornix transections disrupt the ontogeny of latent inhibition in the rat. *Psychobiology, 17,* 349–357.

Ohlrich, E. S., & Ross, L. E. (1968). Acquisition and differential conditioning of the eyelid response in normal and retarded children. *Journal of Child Psychology, 6,* 181–193.

Ohyama, T., & Mauk, M. D. (2001). Latent acquisition of timed responses in cerebellar cortex. *Journal of Neuroscience, 21,* 682–690.

O'Keefe, J., & Nadel, L. (1978). *The hippocampus as a cognitive map.* London: Oxford University Press.

Olton, D. S. (1983). Memory functions and the hippocampus. In W. Seifert (Ed.), *Neurobiology of the hippocampus* (pp. 335–373). San Diego, CA: Academic Press.

Overman, W. H. (1990). Performance on traditional match-to-sample, non-match-to-sample, and object discrimination tasks by 12 to 32 month old children: A developmental progression. In Diamond, A. (Ed.), *The development and neural basis of higher cognitive functions* (pp. 365–385). New York: New York Academy of Sciences Press.

Overman, W. H., Bachevalier, J., Sewell, F., & Drew, J. (1993). A comparison of children's performance on two recognition memory tasks: Delayed nonmatch-to-sample versus visual paired-comparison. *Developmental Psychobiology, 26,* 345–357.

Overman, W., H., Pate, B. J., Moore, K., & Peuster, A. (1996). Ontogeny of place learning in children as measured in the radial arm maze, Morris search task, and open field task. *Behavioral Neuroscience. 110,* 1205–1228.

Packard, M. G., Hirsh, R., & White, N. M. (1989). Differential effects of fornix and caudate nucleus lesions on two radial maze tasks: Evidence for multiple memory systems. *Journal of Neuroscience, 9,* 1465–1472.

Perrett, S. P., Ruiz, B. P., & Mauk, M. D. (1993). Cerebellar cortex lesions disrupt learning-dependent timing of conditioned eyelid responses. *Journal of Neuroscience, 13,* 1708–1718.

Pugh, C. R., & Rudy, J. W. (1996). A developmental analysis of contextual fear conditioning. *Developmental Psychobiology, 29,* 87–100.

Rescorla, R. A. (1973). Informational variables in Pavlovian conditioning. In G. H. Bower (Ed.), *The psychology of learning and motivation* (Vol. 6, pp. 1–46). Orlando, FL: Academic Press.

Reynolds, B. (1945). The acquisition of a trace conditioned response as a function of the magnitude of the stimulus trace. *Journal of Experimental Psychology, 35,* 15–30.

Riccio, D. C., & Schulenburg, C. J. (1969). Age-related deficits in acquisition of a passive avoidance response. *Canadian Journal of Psychology, 23,* 429–437 .

Ross, S. M., & Ross, L. E. (1971). Comparison of trace and delay classical eyelid conditioning as a function of interstimulus interval. *Journal of Experimental Psychology, 91,* 165–167.

Rovee-Collier, C. (1997). Dissociations in infant memory: Rethinking the development of implicit and explicit memory. *Psychological Review, 104,* 467–498.

Rovee-Collier, C., Hayne, H., & Colombo, M. (2001). *The development of implicit and explicit memory.* Philadelphia: John Benjamins Publishing Company.

Rudy, J. W. (1992). Development of learning: From elemental to configural associative networks. In C. Rovee-Collier & L.P. Lipsit (Eds.), *Advances in infancy research* (pp. 247–289). New Jersey: ABLEX Publishing Corporation.

Rudy, J. W. (1994). Ontogeny of content-specific latent inhibition of conditioned fear: Implications for configural associations theory and hippocampal formation development *Developmental Psychobiology, 27,* 367–379.

Rudy, J. W., Stadler-Morris, S., & Albert, P. (1987). Ontogeny of spatial navigation behaviors in the rat: dissociation of "proximal"- and "distal"-cue based behaviors. *Behavioral Neuroscience, 101,* 62–73.

Rush, A. N., Robinette, B. L., & Stanton, M. E. (2001). Ontogenetic differences in the effects of unpaired stimulus preexposure on eyeblink conditioning in the rat. *Developmental Psychobiology, 39,* 8–18.

Ryle, G. (1949). *The concept of mind.* San Francisco, CA: Hutchinson.

Saperstein, L. A., Kucharski, D., Stanton, M. E., & Hall, W. G. (1989). Developmental change in reversal learning of an olfactory discrimination. *Psychobiology, 17,* 293–299.

Schacter, D. L. (1984) Toward the multidisciplinary study of memory: Ontogeny, phylogeny, and pathology of memory systems. In L. R. Squire and N. Butters (Eds.), *Neuropsychology of memory* (pp. 13–24). New York: Guilford Press.

Schmajuk, N. A., & DiCarlo, J. J. (1991). A neural network approach to hippocampal function in classical conditioning. *Behavioral Neuroscience, 105,* 82–105.

Siegel, S., & Domjan, M. (1971). Backward conditioning as an inhibitory procedure. *Learning and Motivation, 2,* 1–11.

Smotherman, W. P., Burt, G., Kimble, D. P., Strickrod, G., BreMiller, R., & Levine, S. (1981). Behavioral and corticosterone effects in conditioned taste aversion following hippocampal lesions. *Physiology & Behavior, 27,* 569–574 .

Solomon, P. R., Vander Schaaf, E. R., Thompson, R. F., & Weisz, D. J. (1986). Hippocampus and trace conditioning of the rabbit's classically conditioned nictitating membrane response. *Behavioral Neuroscience, 100,* 729–744.

Spence, K. W., & Ross, L. E. (1959). A methodological study of the form and latency of eyelid responses in conditioning. *Journal of Experimental Psychology, 58,* 376–381.

Squire, L. R. (1987). *Memory and brain.* New York: Oxford University Press.

Squire, L. R., & Zola-Morgan, S. (1991). The medial temporal lobe memory system. *Science, 253,* 1380–1386.

Squire, L. W. (2004). Memory systems of the brain: A brief history and current perspective. *Neurobiology of Learning and Memory, 82,* 171–177.

Stanton, M. E. (2000). Multiple memory systems, development and conditioning. *Behavioral Brain Research, 110,* 25–37.

Stanton, M. E., & Freeman, J. H., Jr. (1994). Eyeblink conditioning in the developing rat: An animal model of learning in developmental neurotoxicology. *Environmental Health Perspectives, 102,* 131–139.

Stanton, M. E., & Freeman, J. H. (2000). Developmental studies of eyeblink conditioning in the rat. In D. S. Woodruff-Pak & J. E. Steinmetz (Eds.), *Eyeblink classical conditioning, Vol. 2, Animal models* (pp 17–49). Boston: Kluwer Academic Publishers.

Stanton, M. E., Fox, G. D., & Carter, C. S. (1998). Ontogeny of the conditioned eyeblink response in rats: Acquisition or expression? *Neuropsychopharmacology, 37,* 623–632.

Stanton, M., Dailey, W., & Amsel, A. (1980). Patterned (single) alternation in 11- and 14-day-old rats under various reward conditions. *Journal of Comparative and Physiological Psychology, 94,* 459–471.

Stanton, M. E., Freeman, J. H., Jr., & Skelton, R. W. (1992). Eyeblink conditioning in the developing rat. *Behavioral Neuroscience, 106,* 657–665.

Steinmetz, J., Gluck, M., & Solomon, P. (2001). *Model systems and the neurobiology of associative learning: A Festshrift for Richard F. Thompson.* Mahwah, NJ: Lawrence Erlbaum Associates.

Sutherland, R. J., & Rudy, J. W. (1989). Configural association theory: The role of the hippocampal formation in learning, memory, and amnesia. *Psychobiology, 17,* 129–144.

Thompson, R. F. (1986). The neurobiology of learning and memory. *Science, 233,* 941–947.

Thompson, R.F. (2005). In search of memory traces. *Annual Review of Psychology, 56,* 1–23.

Thompson, R. F., Donegan, N. H., Clark, G. A., Lavond, D. G., Lincoln, J. S., Madden, J., et al. (1987). Neuronal substrates of discrete, defensive conditioned reflexes, conditioned fear states, and their interactions in the rabbit. In I. Gormezano, W.F. Prokasy, & R.F. Thompson (Eds.), *Classical conditioning* (3rd ed., pp. 371–399). Hillsdale, NJ: Erlbaum.

Timberlake, W., & Fanselow, M.S. (1994). Symposium on behavior systems, learning, neurophysiology, and development: Introduction. *Psychomic Bulletin and Review, 1,* 403–404.

Tolman, E. C. (1948). Cognitive maps in rats and man. *Psychological Review, 55,* 189–208.

Ulfig, N. (1993). Ontogeny of the entorhinal cortex. *Hippocampus, 3,* 27–32.

Wagner, A. R. (1981). SOP: A model of automatic memory processing in animal behavior. In N. E. Spear & R. R. Miller (Eds.), *Information processing in animals: Memory mechanisms* (pp. 5–47). Hillsdale, NJ: Erlbaum.

Wagner, A. R., & Brandon, S.E. (1989). Evolution of a structured connectionist model of Pavlovian conditioning (AESOP). In S. B. Klein & R. R. Mowrer (Eds.), *Contemporary learning theories: Pavlovian conditioning and the status of traditional learning theory* (pp.149–90). Hillsdale, NJ: Erlbaum.

Weiskrantz, L., & Warrington, E. K. (1979). Conditioning in amnesic patients. *Neuropsychologia, 17,* 187–194.

Weiss, C., Bouwmeester, H., Power, J. M., & Disterhoft, J. F. (1999). Hippocampal lesions prevent trace eyeblink conditioning in the freely moving rat. *Behavioural Brain Research, 99,* 123–132.

Weisz, D. J., Harde, D. G., & Xiang, Z. (1992). Effects of amygdala lesions on reflex facilitation and conditioned response acquisition during nictitating membrane response conditioning in rabbit. *Behavioral Neuroscience, 106,* 262–273.

Winograd, T. (1975). Frame representations and the declarative procedural controversy. In D. Bobrow & A. Collins (Eds.), *Representation and understanding: Studies in cognitive science* (pp. 185–210). New York: Academic Press.

Woodruff-Pak, D. S., & Steinmetz, J. E. (2000a). *Eyeblink classical conditioning, Volume 1: Applications in humans.* Boston: Kluwer Academic Publishers.

Woodruff-Pak, D. S., & Steinmetz, J. E. (2000b). *Eyeblink classical conditioning, Volume 2: Animal models.* Boston: Kluwer Academic Publishers.

Woodruff-Pak, D. S., & Thompson, R. F. (1988). Cerebellar correlates of classical conditioning across the life span. In P. B. Baltes, D. M. Featherman, & R. M. Lerner (Eds.), *Life-span development and behavior* (pp. 1–37). Hillsdale NJ: Erlbaum.

Zola, S. M., & Squire, L. R. (2001). Relationship between magnitude of damage to the hippocampus and impaired recognition memory in monkeys. *Hippocampus, 11,* 92–98.

Ontogeny of Fear Conditioning

Rick Richardson *and* Pamela S. Hunt

Abstract

This chapter describes research that measured a variety of fear responses (e.g., freezing, changes in heart rate, and fear-potentiated startle) to conditioned stimuli of different sensory modalities (olfactory, auditory, and visual) in rats of different ages in order to characterize the developmental emergence of fear responding. The major finding from this research is an invariant progression in the way in which fear is expressed ontogenetically, which cannot be explained entirely by maturation of neural systems. This research has direct implications not only for theoretical models of memory development, but also for current conceptualizations of the neural mechanisms of learned fear.

Keywords: fear responses, freezing, heart rate, fear-potentiated startle, memory development, neural mechanisms

For a number of years, we have studied associative learning during development. In this research, we have focused on fear conditioning in rats. We have used the rat as our subject because of the pronounced developmental changes it undergoes in the first few weeks after birth. Maturational changes that take years in humans can take only days or weeks in the rat. We have focused on fear conditioning for several reasons. First, fear is rapidly established using Pavlovian conditioning procedures. Given the rapid development of the rat, it is not feasible to study potential developmental differences using a procedure that may take several days or even weeks to train. Second, motivational levels across age can be equated in fear conditioning studies where electric shock is used (Campbell, 1967). In contrast, with appetitive tasks, it is nearly impossible to equate level of motivation using food or water deprivation in different age groups. Another reason we have chosen to focus on fear

conditioning is because there is a long and widely held belief that early adverse experiences can have a profound impact on later behavior (Mineka & Zinbarg, 2006). Jacobs and Nadel (1985, 1999), for example, suggested that fear acquired early in development forms the basis of anxiety disorders that emerge much later in life. However, there is surprisingly little known about the establishment of fear early in development, and there is even less known about how early-acquired fear memories are expressed at later ages. If we are to understand the processes (behavioral, cognitive, biological) through which early traumatic experiences can affect adult behavior, then we need much more research in this area, especially in regard to how early memories are retained and possibly modified across development. A final reason for our focus on fear conditioning is because there is a great deal known about the neural basis of learned fear (Davis, 1992; Fendt & Fanselow, 1999; LeDoux, 2000). Most of this evidence comes from experiments using adult animals with lesions to specific regions of the brain. Because of the considerable neural development in the rat in the first few weeks after birth, a developmental analysis of learning and memory offers a unique model preparation for testing hypotheses derived from research with lesioned rats. Indeed, it has been suggested that the developing rat might, in certain circumstances, be viewed as a "natural lesion" preparation (Fanselow & Rudy, 1998).

The general perspective taken in this chapter is that the developing animal is not only an interesting subject in itself, but it can also be used as a tool to ask questions about associative learning in general, and about the neurobiological substrates of such learning in novel and unique ways. Further, we believe that the study of the ways in which learning and memory changes developmentally can contribute to a broader understanding of how the brain changes during ontogeny. Information about known brain developmental processes can be tied to the ontogeny of more and more sophisticated learning processes. As described in greater detail below, our work in this area has resulted in quite novel findings that have substantial implications for contemporary models of the neural bases of learned fear as well as to conceptualizations of memory from infancy to adulthood.

This chapter is divided into three sections, each focusing on one of three related issues. In the first section, we describe some of our research that has focused on the manner in which animals of different ages express conditioned fear. There are a number of commonly used measures of learned fear in the rat and our research shows that these various learned fear responses emerge at different ages. This work then provides the foundation for the research described in the second section. By taking advantage of the sequential emergence of learned fear reactions, we examined whether memories acquired early in development are later expressed via response systems that matured after the learning experience. The conclusion drawn from this research has consistently been that early memories are expressed only through response systems that were mature at the time of encoding; these memories are not expressed through response systems that matured after the learning experience. Finally, in the third section of the chapter, we show that early-acquired fear memories *can* be expressed in a manner appropriate to the rat's age at the time of test, but only if the memory was activated and re-encoded at a later age. Taken together, this research

not only illustrates several interesting features of how memory develops, but also offers unique insights into the neural basis of learned fear and into some of the fundamental assumptions inherent in contemporary models of associative learning.

What Is Conditioned Fear?

Before proceeding further, we first provide a brief overview of fear conditioning. It is important to review some of the current conceptualizations and assumptions regarding fear and its acquisition because much of the empirical data that we will present leads us to question some of these assumptions and conceptualizations.

Fear is typically viewed as an emotional state that has evolved to increase survival. From this perspective, fear taps into an existing antipredator defensive system (Bolles, 1970; Fanselow, 1991). Stimuli that predict aversive events can come to activate this defense system. In the laboratory, fear can easily be established via a process of Pavlovian conditioning, in which an initially neutral stimulus (conditioned stimulus, CS) such as an odor or a light is paired with a biologically relevant, aversive stimulus (unconditioned stimulus, US) such as an electric shock. Following these pairings, the CS comes to elicit a conditioned fear response (CR). Fear is rapidly acquired, being asymptotic after only a few CS–US pairings. Fear can engage multiple response systems, and several behavioral and physiological manifestations of fear have been measured in the laboratory. These fear responses have been referred to as species-specific defense reactions (SSDRs; Bolles, 1970), and include changes in autonomic function, vocalizations, somatomotor behavior, hormonal release, and the modulation of skeletal reflexes.

Common Assumptions About Conditioned Fear

Results from many studies using intact adult rats have led to a number of widely accepted principles regarding learned fear. First, it is generally assumed that following CS–US pairings, the CR elicited by subsequent presentation of the CS is a central emotional state (fear) as opposed to a specific behavioral or physiological response (McAllister & McAllister, 1971). According to this S–S view of Pavlovian conditioning, the rat forms an association between two stimuli (the CS and the US), not between a stimulus and a response. From this perspective, subsequent presentation of the CS elicits an expectation of US occurrence, and if that US is an aversive stimulus (e.g., shock), then the emotional state of fear is elicited. The animal then responds to this state of fear with any available SSDR. This S–S view of Pavlovian conditioning has substantial theoretical support (e.g., Rescorla & Wagner, 1972; Wagner, 1981). A corollary to the notion of the CR being a diffuse emotional state is that the various possible fear responses will usually co-vary, given that they are reflections of this central state of fear. A consequence of this assumption is that the choice of which response to actually measure in any particular study is relatively arbitrary, and is mostly determined out of convenience to the experimenter or a specific interest in the response system itself. We have previously referred to this as the assumption of response equivalence (Hunt & Campbell, 1997). In other words, a fear response is a fear response. Finally, it is assumed that neural plasticity occurring within the amygdala is not only necessary, but is also sufficient, for the acquisition of fear. Expression of this learning then involves projections from the amygdala to brain stem and midbrain structures that mediate a specific SSDR. Importantly, these downstream structures are not thought to be sites of neural plasticity underlying fear acquisition. Rather, the structures that are efferent to the amygdala are thought to only be necessary for response production.

Our research with the developing rat has raised serious questions about each of these fundamental assumptions. Our data suggest that not all SSDRs are equivalent reflections of a fear state in young animals (cf., Collier & Bolles, 1980), that Pavlovian fear conditioning is probably not exclusively S–S in nature, and that neural plasticity involving areas of the fear circuit other than the amygdala is very likely necessary for the acquisition and expression of conditioned fear. In the next three sections of this chapter, we present some of the work that has led us to draw these conclusions.

The Ontogeny of Learned Fear

A number of years ago, we began to study developmental changes in the rat's ability to learn and remember. In our initial experiments, we simply recorded multiple measures of fear in order to test the assumption of response equivalence. The results of these experiments revealed some interesting developmental dissociations in the emergence of specific behavioral expressions of learned fear during the first several weeks of life. In this part of our research, we focused on three response measures that are commonly used by neuroscientists and learning theorists to index learned fear: freezing, changes in heart rate, and fear-potentiated startle.

Freezing is defined as the absence of observable movement (Bouton & Bolles, 1980; Fanselow, 1980) and is probably the most commonly used measure of learned fear. It has been shown to be highly correlated, in adult rats, with other measures of learned fear such as suppression of an ongoing operant behavior (e.g., bar-press or lick suppression; Bevins & Ayres, 1992; Bouton & Bolles, 1980), changes in heart rate (Black & de Toledo, 1972; Carrive, 2000; McEchron, Cheng, & Gilmartin, 2004), and fear-potentiated startle (Leaton & Borszcz, 1985; Leaton & Cranney, 1990). These observations, of course, offer support for the assumption of response equivalence. We also measured changes in autonomic activity in some experiments. Although there are a number of possible ways of assessing changes in the autonomic nervous system to index fear, we chose to focus on *changes in heart rate* as it is easy to record at all stages of development. Interestingly, the direction of heart rate change (increase or decrease) is not consistent across studies of learned fear. That is, some studies have reported decreases in heart rate to a CS that had previously been paired with a shock US (Campbell & Ampuero, 1985; Powell & Kazis, 1976) while others have reported increases in heart rate to such a CS (Iwata, LeDoux, & Reis, 1986; Supple & Leaton, 1990). The reasons for these differences have not been determined, and are not particularly important for the issues considered in this chapter. The interested reader is referred to discussions of this issue in other published works (Hunt, 1997; Hunt & Campbell, 1997; Iwata & LeDoux, 1988; Martin & Fitzgerald, 1980). The third measure that we recorded in our studies of learned fear in the developing rat was *fear-potentiated startle* (FPS). To assess FPS in the rat, a reflexive startle response is elicited by presentation of a loud, unexpected noise. This noise elicits a whole body jerk referred to as the startle reflex (Eaton, 1984). When the startle-eliciting noise is preceded by a cue that elicits fear, such as a light CS previously paired with a shock US, the startle response is greater in magnitude than when the startle-eliciting stimulus is presented alone. This enhancement in the startle response is referred to as fear-potentiated startle (Brown, Kalish, & Farber, 1951; Davis, Falls, Campeau, & Kim, 1993).

Using these three measures, we have shown that learned fear emerges developmentally in a response-specific sequence. Specifically, when the assessment of learning occurs during CS–US pairings, or immediately after conditioning, freezing is observed at a younger age than are changes in heart rate, and changes in heart rate occur at a younger age than does fear-potentiated startle (for review, see Hunt & Campbell, 1997). This sequential emergence of fear responses does not support the response equivalence notion of learned fear, but instead suggests that the selection of which fear response to measure may be a critical factor, at least when studying learned fear in the developing rat. We have observed a similar, but not identical, pattern of results when rats are tested 24 h after training. In this case, freezing and heart rate responses can be observed at roughly the same age, and both are evident at a younger age than is the potentiated startle response. Some representative findings from these latter studies, in which rats have been tested 24 h after conditioning, are described below.

Freezing versus Changes in Heart Rate

In several studies, we have reported a correspondence between freezing and decreases in heart rate. A representative experiment is described here. Hunt, Hess, and Campbell (1997a) trained rats that were 16 or 75 days of age. Some subjects were given trials in which a 10-s flashing light CS terminated with a footshock US (paired groups) while others were given the same number of light CSs and shock USs, but in an explicitly unpaired manner (unpaired groups). Twenty-four hours later, heart rate recording electrodes were implanted. After a brief (15 min) period of adaptation to a novel test context, subjects were given several nonreinforced CS presentations. Heart rate was measured throughout the test, and the session was videotaped for later

scoring of freezing. Thus, the responses of interest, freezing and changes in heart rate, were obtained simultaneously from each subject in this study.

The freezing data are shown in Figure 25.1. Baseline levels of freezing were low in all groups. A marked increase in freezing was elicited by the CS in rats of both ages that were in the paired condition but not in rats in the unpaired condition. This pattern of results shows that CS-elicited freezing was associatively mediated. A similar pattern of results was observed when we measured CS-elicited changes in heart rate (Figure 25.2); that is, rats in the paired condition exhibited a monophasic decrease in heart rate (bradycardia) during the CS, and the magnitude of this response was similar in preweanling and adult subjects.

We have observed very similar patterns of freezing and heart rate decreases to an olfactory CS that had been paired with a shock US. Hunt (1997), for example, demonstrated the co-occurrence of freezing and bradycardia in 16-day-old rats trained with a 30-s olfactory CS (amyl acetate) paired with a shock US. CS-elicited freezing and changes in heart rate were simultaneously recorded during a test session given 24 h after training. Taken together, these and other data (Hunt, Hess, & Campbell, 1997b, 1998; Hunt, Richardson, Hess, & Campbell, 1997c) illustrate that freezing and decreases in heart rate are exhibited to a CS previously paired with an aversive US, and additionally that both responses emerge at roughly the same age during ontogeny if testing occurs 24 h after training.

Freezing versus Fear-Potentiated Startle

A very different ontogenetic pattern is observed when one compares the emergence of freezing

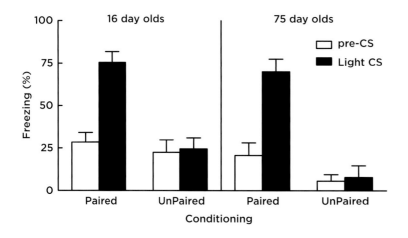

Figure 25.1 Percentage of intervals scored as freezing for 16- and 75-day-old rats during a test given 24 h after training. For training, subjects were given Paired or Unpaired presentations of a 10-s visual CS and 1-s shock US. For test, freezing was scored for a 10-s period prior to CS onset (pre-CS) and for the 10 s of the CS, averaged across nonreinforced test trials. (From Hunt, Hess, & Campbell, 1997a.)

and FPS. In contrast to the similar developmental emergence of freezing and heart rate response expression to a fear-eliciting CS that is described above, fear-potentiated startle is not observed until considerably later in development. Illustrative data are provided from an unpublished study by Hunt, Barnet, Rima, and Murdoch (2004). Subjects in that study were given paired or unpaired presentations of a light CS and a shock US at either 18 or 24 days of age. Half of the subjects at each age were tested, 24 h later, for CS-elicited freezing and the other half were tested for FPS. As can be seen in the left panel of Figure 25.3, subjects of both ages in the paired condition showed a substantial increase in freezing in response to CS presentation. The CS elicited virtually no freezing in the rats that had received unpaired light and shock presentations.

In contrast, there was a marked developmental difference in the expression of learned fear when potentiated startle was measured (see the right panel of Figure 25.3). The 24-day-old rats in the paired condition exhibited robust FPS compared to rats in the unpaired condition. However, the 18-day-old rats in the paired condition failed to exhibit FPS. The performance of the 18-day-old rats tested with the freezing procedure clearly indicates that rats of this age were able to acquire the CS–US association and retain it across the 24-h interval; however, rats of this age did not express this learning when tested in the potentiated startle procedure (see also Hunt, Richardson, & Campbell, 1994).

These findings replicate and extend previous results reported by Richardson, Paxinos, and Lee (2000) with an olfactory CS. In that study, odor

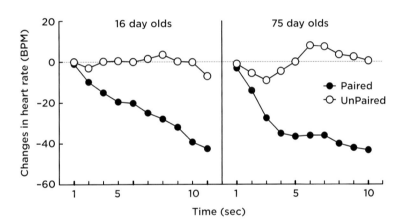

Figure 25.2 Mean beat-per-minute (BPM) changes in heart rate recorded for 16- and 75-day-old rats tested 24 h following Paired or Unpaired light CS and shock US. The dotted line represents baseline heart rate. The figure depicts the changes in heart rate on a second-by-second basis averaged across nonreinforced test trials. (From Hunt et al., 1997a.)

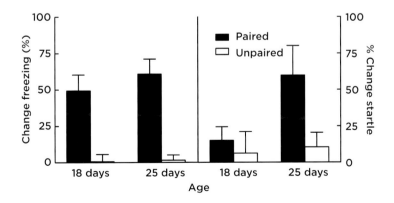

Figure 25.3 The left panel presents freezing data for 18 and 25 do rats previously trained with light CS and shock US presentations. The percentage of intervals scored as freezing during a pre-CS period was subtracted from the percentage during the CS period to yield a change score (CS-elicited freezing). The right panel presents the fear-potentiated startle data, expressed as a percentage change in startle. (From Hunt, Barnet, Rima, & Murdoch, 2004.) Percent change was calculated as (CS + N)/N * 100, where CS = startle amplitude on trials in which the startle-eliciting stimulus was presented at the end of the CS and N = startle amplitude on trials in which the startle-eliciting stimulus was presented alone.

avoidance, rather than freezing, was measured. Rats given odor–shock pairings at 16 days of age exhibited a pronounced avoidance of the odor CS but no FPS in the presence of the odor. In contrast, rats trained at 23 days of age, and tested the next day, exhibited both odor avoidance and FPS in the presence of the odor CS. While that study employed a between-groups design (i.e., separate groups were tested in the two procedures), the findings were subsequently replicated using a within-subjects design by Richardson and Fan (2002). The latter study is a particularly powerful illustration of the dissociation between these behavioral measures of learned fear in that an individual animal exhibited fear via one response system (avoidance) but not via another (FPS).

Taken together, these data highlight that the age at which fear "learning" first emerges is critically dependent on the response measured. As described above, 16- to 18-day-old rats can associate olfactory and visual CSs with a shock US, as inferred by changes in behavior (freezing, avoidance) and heart rate. However, when the FPS procedure is used, it appears as though learning did not occur at these ages. Evidence of learning usually is not observed with the FPS procedure until the rats are at least 23 days of age. These findings show that although the various fear-related responses (e.g., changes in heart rate and blood pressure, freezing, FPS) typically co-occur in the adult rat, they do not always do so in the immature rat. These findings are problematic for the notion of response equivalence. Clearly, these measures are not equally effective for inferring the presence of a fear state in young rats.

In addition to raising questions for the widely held assumption of response equivalence, the results described above also question the nature of the relationship between freezing and FPS. As noted previously, these two measures are often highly correlated, although it is unclear whether this relation is causal. For example, Wecker and Ison (1986) reported that general levels of motor activity affected the magnitude of the startle response in adult rats (see also Plappert, Pilz, & Schnitzler, 1993). Specifically, the startle response was smaller on trials in which the rats were naturally active, especially when they were grooming, compared with trials in which they were inactive. Similarly, Leaton and Borszcz (1985) reported a strong, positive correlation between CS-elicited freezing and FPS in adult rats. That is, there was a larger startle response on trials where the rat was also freezing. However, our work with the developing rat demonstrates that an aversive CS can elicit pronounced freezing responses while at the same time failing to result in an increase in startle magnitude (see Hunt et al., 1994, for our initial demonstration of this developmental dissociation, and Yap, Stapinski, & Richardson, 2005, for a replication using a within-subjects design). These latter findings indicate that the relation between freezing and FPS is not causal. Additional evidence, with adult rats, that FPS is not simply a consequence of reduced activity levels during the CS is provided by McNish, Gewirtz, and Davis (1997).

Exploring the Late Emergence of FPS

We have consistently found that FPS emerges much later in development than other expressions of learned fear, including freezing, avoidance, and changes in heart rate. Typically we do not observe potentiated startle in subjects trained prior to 22–23 days of age (Barnet & Hunt, 2006; Hunt et al., 1994; Richardson et al., 2000). Further, this finding seems to be general as it extends beyond situations that measure CS-evoked FPS. For example, Richardson and Vishney (2000) failed to observe shock sensitization of startle in rats younger than 23 days of age. In the shock sensitization procedure, the startle response to a series of loud noises is first measured. Then, some rats are given several unsignaled shocks. Responding to a subsequent series of loud noises shows that shocked rats exhibit a much larger magnitude startle response after the shock series than before. Nonshocked control rats do not show this increase. Davis (1989) first reported this effect, and suggested that it might be a reflection of unlearned fear. However, subsequent studies showed that this effect was actually due to context conditioning (Richardson & Elsayed, 1998). That is, fear conditioned to the contextual cues was responsible for the potentiated startle response observed in the shocked rats. So, conditioned FPS, whether it is to an olfactory CS, a visual CS, or more diffuse contextual cues, does not appear to occur in rats prior to about 23 days of age. Given the consistent finding that FPS emerges relatively late in development, compared with freezing, avoidance, and changes in heart rate, the question next becomes "Why?"

One of the great appeals of the FPS procedure is that the behavior is mediated by two relatively simple circuits—the primary startle circuit that underlies the actual startle response and a secondary circuit that can modulate (i.e., enhance) the magnitude of the startle response when it is activated by fear. The late emergence of conditioned FPS would have to be due to the delayed maturation of one or both of these circuits. Therefore, we set out to try to explore the functional maturation of these two circuits.

PRIMARY STARTLE CIRCUIT

The primary startle circuit basically consists of the cochlear root neurons, the caudal pontine nucleus (PnC) in the brain stem, and spinal motoneurons (Walker & Davis, 2002). Previous studies had shown that rats as young as 13–14 days of age exhibit a reliable startle response to a broadband white noise (approximately 110 dB; Parisi & Ison, 1979, 1981). But perhaps activity within the startle circuit cannot be modulated until later in development.

Although we have consistently found that fear does not potentiate the startle response in animals trained before 22–23 days of age, other research has shown that the response can be inhibited. For example, Parisi and Ison (1979) reported prepulse inhibition of startle in rats as young as 14 days of age. Prepulse inhibition is a reduction in startle amplitude produced by presentation of a low-intensity stimulus just prior to the loud noise. While that work shows that the primary circuit can be inhibited in young rats, it remains possible that activity within the circuit cannot be enhanced. Some of our work, however, has revealed that the response can be augmented in rats younger than 23 days of age. Specifically, Weber and Richardson (2001) demonstrated that the acoustic startle response could be potentiated in rats as young as 16 days of age as a result of systemic injection of strychnine, which increases activity in the spinal cord (Kehne & Davis, 1984), or by icv infusion of corticotropin-releasing hormone (CRH), which is thought to increase activity in the PnC (see Weber & Richardson, 2001). Both of these manipulations markedly enhanced the magnitude of the startle response in 16-day-old rats. These data suggest that activity in the primary startle pathway can be increased in young rats, leading to an increase in startle response magnitude. Other research has shown that presentation of a continuous, low-level background noise (Sheets, Dean, & Reiter, 1988) or constant high illumination levels (Weber, Watts, & Richardson, 2003) sensitizes the startle response in 16- to 18-day-old rats. Clearly, increased activity in the primary startle circuit can occur and can lead to a potentiated startle response in rats much younger than 23 days of age. Therefore, our consistent failure to observe potentiation of the startle response by a fear-eliciting stimulus, a stimulus that concurrently elicits freezing, behavioral avoidance, and changes in heart rate, cannot be due to general immaturity in the structures that comprise the primary startle circuit.

SECONDARY FEAR CIRCUIT

There is a great deal of evidence that the amygdala is critically involved in learned fear (e.g., Davis, 1992; LeDoux, 2000). Sensory neurons that convey CS and US information converge on cells within the basolateral amygdala (BLA) and cause a change in activity of these cells in an LTP-like manner. This associative information is then conveyed to the central nucleus of the amygdala (CeA), which is typically viewed as the primary output nucleus of the amygdala. Thus, "learning," in the form of synaptic plasticity, occurs in the BLA, and response production begins in the CeA (but see Goosens & Maren, 2003; Wilensky, Schafe, Kristensen, & LeDoux, 2006). The CeA projects to several brain stem regions that mediate the production of the specific components of the defense reaction. For example, a projection from the CeA to the PnC allows for the expression of FPS. Initially, this was thought to involve a direct projection from the amygdala to the PnC (e.g., Davis et al., 1993). However, subsequent research has shown that there are additional projections from the amygdala to the PnC that are relayed through other areas, such as the periaqueductal gray (PAG), which are also critically involved in the expression of FPS (Fendt, Koch, & Schnitzler, 1996: Walker & Davis, 1997; Zhao & Davis, 2004). The CeA also sends projections to the dorsal motor nucleus of the vagus/nucleus ambiguous, which regulates parasympathetically mediated decreases in heart rate (Kapp, Whalen, Supple, & Pascoe, 1992; McCabe et al., 1992), and to the ventral PAG, which is implicated in behavioral suppression (i.e., freezing; Fanselow, 1991; Fanselow, DeCola, De Oca, & Landeira-Fernandez, 1995). Each of these CeA efferents is separable and functions, for the most part, independently of the others. Lesions of the ventral PAG, for example, abolish the conditioned freezing response but have no effect on the expression of cardiovascular changes to the fear-eliciting CS (Iwata et al., 1986; LeDoux, Iwata, Cicchetti, & Reis, 1998). Thus, damage to a CeA efferent will eliminate a specific fear response, whereas damage to the CeA itself abolishes all expressions of learned fear.

Given the multiple, independent projections from the amygdala, it is perhaps not surprising that some fear responses emerge at older ages than do others. The emergence of FPS after freezing and heart rate could quite easily be explained by a later maturation of structures that are uniquely involved in FPS expression. If one was to take this anatomical approach to explaining the late development of conditioned FPS, then there are three distinct areas where functional maturity could possibly be delayed ontogenetically: (1) the CeA, (2) the PnC, or (3) one or more of the identified projections from the CeA to the PnC. We can immediately rule out the CeA as a candidate because animals that are much younger than 23 days of age quite readily show learned freezing and heart rate responses. If the CeA did not mature until about 23 days of age, then we should not observe any fear reactions in rats that are appreciably younger. We can similarly rule out the PnC as a candidate structure for the late emergence of conditioned FPS because of the evidence, reviewed above, that startle responses can be potentiated in rats as young as 16 days of age by various pharmacological and behavioral manipulations. The elimination of these first two possibilities leaves us with the third as the putative explanation. That is, the delayed development of FPS as a measure of learned fear is due to protracted maturation of projections from the CeA to the PnC. Rats younger than 23 days of age can certainly undergo the necessary neural plasticity within the amygdala to acquire fear to the CS, and also can exhibit the increased neural activity within the PnC that would result in an augmented startle response. But, it would seem that these animals fail to exhibit FPS because the projections between the CeA and the PnC are not yet sufficiently mature to support FPS. That is, both the fear system (amygdala) and the startle response system (primary startle circuit) are functional by about 2 weeks of age, but the two systems are not connected, or integrated with each

other, until at least 1 week later. We have referred to this proposal as the *neural maturation hypothesis* (Hunt & Campbell, 1997; Hunt et al., 1994), and have attempted to test this hypothesis indirectly in the series of experiments described in the next section.

Translation of Early-Acquired Memories across Stages of Development

The neural maturation hypothesis attributes the absence of FPS in rats younger than 23 days of age to neural immaturity, specifically immaturity somewhere along the CeA–PnC pathway (see Figure 25.4). A prediction that can be derived from the neural maturation hypothesis is that rats trained prior to this age will express their learned fear of the CS in term of FPS if testing is delayed until they are at least 23 days of age, i.e., an age at which the entire CeA–PnC pathway can support FPS expression.

At the time that we began this inquiry, there had been very few empirical studies that directly addressed the issue of whether early memories are expressed through response systems that become functionally mature after training. One early report by Johanson and Hall (1984) involved a Pavlovian appetitive conditioning procedure. Six- and 9-day-old rats were given pairings of a novel odor CS with intraoral infusions of milk (US). The CR recorded at both ages consisted of a range of overt behaviors, including general increases in activity, probing, and mouthing responses. However, the precise response profile was different between the two age groups. The CS elicited increases in general activity in the 6-day-olds, but not much probing or mouthing. In contrast, the CS elicited much less general activity in the 9-day-olds, but much more probing and mouthing. In other words, it appeared that the CS elicited a less precise CR in the 6-day-old rats than it did in the 9-day-old rats. Of particular relevance to the present discussion, Johanson and Hall

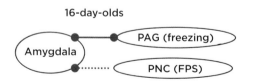

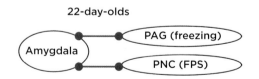

Figure 25.4 A schematic illustrating the neural maturation hypothesis, in regard to the late ontogenetic emergence of FPS relative to freezing. The dashed line in the figure on the left reflects the hypothesized immaturity of the projection from the amygdala to the PNC in preweanling (e.g., 16 days) subjects. Based on our FPS data this projection is functionally mature by 22 days of age, as depicted in the figure on the right.

determined the CR profile in rats that were trained at 6 days of age but not tested until 9 days of age. Basically, they examined whether the response pattern exhibited by these animals more closely resembled that of 6-day-olds (the age at which they were trained) or that of 9-day-olds (the age at which they were tested). Johanson and Hall found that subjects trained at 6 days of age but not tested until 9 days of age responded in a manner similar to rats that had been trained and tested at 9 days of age—the CR consisted primarily of probing and mouthing responses. Johanson and Hall concluded "the response profile changed because the same CS that elicited one response pattern at a younger age somehow gained access to the now more mature response system at a later age" (p. 152). This result is what is predicted by the neural maturation hypothesis and is what we expected to observe in our study on learned fear and potentiated startle.

Our initial attempts at evaluating this question consisted of training subjects at 16 days of age but delaying the test until they were 23 days of age. Inherent in the neural maturation hypothesis is the idea that as long as the animal is given CS–US pairings at an age at which their sensory systems are capable of detecting these two stimuli, and they have an associative system that can bind these stimuli together, then the CS will acquire the ability to later evoke an emotional state of fear. The rat should then express this fear via any response that is part of its current behavioral repertoire for fear. This should be true regardless of whether or not that response system was available at the time of fear conditioning. Therefore, rats trained at 16 days of age, but not tested until 23 days of age, should express the previously acquired fear to the CS via any of the defensive responses that we have examined to date, including FPS. The only caveat to this prediction is that care must be taken to ensure that the young rats actually remember the CS–US association across the retention interval. While learned fear associations are famously retained in adult rats (Gale et al., 2004), young rats typically forget much more rapidly (e.g., Campbell & Campbell, 1962). Therefore, in these experiments we included independent assessments of retention.

Our first effort at evaluating this idea was reported in Richardson et al. (2000; Experiment 4). Subjects in that experiment were 16-day-old rats that were given paired or unpaired presentations of an odor CS and a shock US. All rats were tested 7 days later, when 23 days of age. Half of the rats in each condition were tested for odor

avoidance while the other half was tested for FPS in the presence of the odor CS. As described above, rats trained with an odor CS at 16 days of age can express their learned fear in a number of ways (e.g., changes in heart rate, CS-elicited freezing, avoidance) although not via FPS. In contrast, rats trained at 23 days of age can express their learned fear via all of these responses. The question here was whether the responses exhibited at test in the animals trained at 16 days and tested at 23 days would more closely resemble those appropriate to the age of training (16 days) or the age of test (23 days). The outcome of this experiment was quite surprising—none of the subjects exhibited FPS. Performance on the FPS test by paired subjects was virtually the same as that in the unpaired group. These results are obviously in stark contrast to what we had predicted. This failure to observe FPS to the odor CS in these rats was not due to their forgetting of the CS–US association over the 7-day retention interval because rats in the paired condition exhibited a robust avoidance of the odor compared with those in the unpaired condition. The level of odor avoidance observed in this test was essentially the same as that measured in rats tested 1 day after training, implying good retention of the odor–shock association over the 1 week interval. Even though the rats clearly retained the odor–shock association, they did not express this learned fear via FPS, a response system that matured during the training-to-test interval. These results contrast with those reported by Johanson and Hall (1984) and they do not provide support for the neural maturation hypothesis (Hunt & Campbell, 1997). We have replicated these findings with olfactory CSs in a number of other experiments (e.g., Richardson, Fan, & Parnas, 2003; Yap et al., 2005), including one that used a within-subjects design (Richardson & Fan, 2002).

An analogous series of experiments were recently reported by Barnet and Hunt (2006). Slightly different age groups were used, and a visual stimulus served as the CS instead of an olfactory cue. Aside from these differences, however, the experiment was similar to those described above. Specifically, Barnet and Hunt (2006) gave rats either paired or unpaired presentations of a light CS with a shock US. The subjects were divided into three groups based on their age at the time of training and their age at the time of test. One group (18–19) was trained on day 18 and tested on day 19. A second group (24–25) was trained on day 24 and tested on day 25. The third group (18–25) was trained on day 18 but not tested until 1 week later, at 25 days of age. Half of the subjects in each group were tested for CS-elicited freezing and the other half were tested for FPS. As with the data described above, the results were not what were predicted by the neural maturation hypothesis. The only group to show significant FPS was the paired group that was trained at 24 days of age (group 24–25). Results of the freezing test, however, indicated that all subjects that had been given light–shock pairings showed marked increases in freezing during the CS, relative to those recorded during a pre-CS baseline period (Figure 25.5). The fact that subjects in group 18–25 showed robust freezing indicates retention of the light–shock association across the 1-week interval. Despite retaining the CS–US association, these rats failed to express fear to the visual CS via FPS. Additional support for this finding comes from several groups that were not included in the Barnet and Hunt (2006) paper. Specifically, rats in these groups were trained on day 24 and tested 1 week later. Half of the subjects were given paired presentations of the light CS with shock US and the other half were given unpaired stimulus presentations. Rats in the paired condition exhibited both CS-elicited freezing (%CS freezing–%pre-CS freezing; Paired 51.3%; Unpaired –9.4%) and FPS (Paired 52.2%; Unpaired –0.43%). These groups show that FPS can be expressed to the light CS by young rats tested 1 week after training—as long as the system mediating FPS was functionally mature at the time of training.

Perhaps even more impressive still are some data from Richardson's laboratory showing a lack of savings in acquisition of FPS in animals given odor–shock pairings when 16 days of age and then re-trained with the same odor CS when 22 days of age. As shown in Figure 25.6, the rats in this condition showed absolutely no benefit of the prior training in terms of the number of trials needed to "acquire" FPS compared to naive rats (Richardson & Fan, 2002; Experiment 3). These same animals showed clear retention when measured by odor avoidance. It is quite puzzling, especially when considering the prominent view that the CS elicits a central state of fear, how an individual animal can exhibit robust odor avoidance and yet, at the same time, fail to acquire and express FPS to that odor in fewer training trials than subjects that were completely naive when trained on day 22.

Collectively, the data reviewed in this section are at odds with the findings reported by Johanson and Hall (1984) that subjects tested following a retention interval exhibit responses appropriate for their age at test. From that perspective, memories are updated to include new responses that mature during the retention interval. That is not what we have found. While the difference between their findings and ours might be due to their use of an appetitive conditioning procedure and our use of a fear conditioning procedure, we believe that there is a more likely explanation for the difference—an explanation originally provided by Johanson and Hall. Specifically, the various CRs that were measured in their experiments were observed in both age groups, but in different proportions. The 6-day-old subjects exhibited primarily increases in general activity although they also displayed some, albeit minimal, mouthing and probing. In contrast, in our experimental situation, the target response

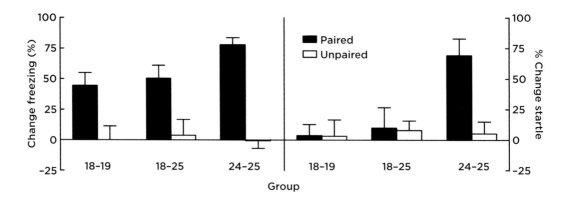

Figure 25.5 The left panel presents CS-elicited freezing obtained from subjects given paired or unpaired light CS and shock US presentations at 18 days of age and tested either one day later (group 18–19) or 1 week later (group 18–25), or trained on day 24 and tested one day later (group 24–25). The right panel presents the percentage change in startle of these same groups. (From Barnet & Hunt, 2006.)

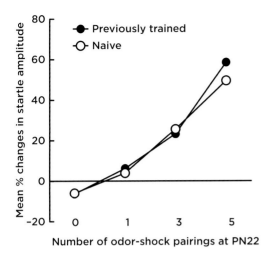

Figure 25.6 Mean percentage change in startle of 23-day-old animals during a test for fear-potentiated startle. Some subjects had been trained with pairings of the odor and shock on day 16 (Previously Trained group) and other subjects were experimentally naive (Naive group). On day 22, animals were given 0, 1, 3, or 5 odor–shock pairings, and subjects were tested for FPS the following day. The data show no savings in fear-potentiated startle of subjects given prior odor–shock training. (From Richardson & Fan, 2002.)

(FPS) was not observed at all in the younger age group. This latter circumstance, as Johanson and Hall noted, provides for a much more convincing test of whether or not early-acquired memories can gain access to later developing response systems. In considering the data we have presented, it is clear that this is not the case; early-acquired memories *do not* gain access to later developing response systems.

Our data also provide no support for the neural maturation hypothesis, at least as it was originally presented (Hunt & Campbell, 1997; Hunt, et al., 1994). Subjects do not express fear via all response systems that are functionally mature at the time of test. If a response system was not available at the time of training, then the memory of that experience is not expressed via that response system later in life. In other words, response systems that mature during the retention interval are apparently not integrated with previous learning, and therefore are not engaged to express an earlier acquired fear memory. Not only does this finding fail to support the neural maturation hypothesis but, considered more broadly, it also seriously challenges some of the principal assumptions regarding the underlying structure of Pavlovian fear conditioning.

It has long been held that a CS that is paired with an aversive US elicits a central state of fear

that, in turn, activates a defensive system comprised of several responses (SSDRs) that function to protect the individual from predation or other harm. This view of Pavlovian conditioning asserts an S–S associative structure and implies that the responses themselves are not integral to learning. However, our data challenge this fundamental concept of a Pavlovian conditioned emotional response because, even though the neural and motor systems that support FPS are unquestionably mature by 23 days of age, FPS is not expressed to a CS that was trained prior to this age. These findings appear to challenge the prevailing view of Pavlovian conditioning as exclusively involving associations between the CS and US. Although stimulus–response (S–R) learning has occasionally been suggested to play a role in Pavlovian conditioning under certain circumstances (e.g., Donahoe & Vegas, 2004; Gormezano & Kehoe, 1981; Holland & Rescorla, 1975), this approach to associative learning has not received broad support. Nonetheless, our data provide unique corroboration of the presence of S–R associations in Pavlovian conditioning by showing that only responses that can be engaged at the time of learning become part of the animal's repertoire of SSDRs to the CS.

One might suggest that our findings are a uniquely developmental phenomenon and are therefore not applicable to considerations of general models of Pavlovian conditioning. However, the basic result that we have repeatedly observed with the developing rat (i.e., memories are not expressed via response systems that were not functional at the time of training) does not appear to be unique to the developing animal. A very similar pattern of results has been observed in adult rats. Weber and Richardson (2004) reported a series of experiments in which the PnC of adult rats was temporarily inactivated during fear conditioning. The basic idea here was that temporarily inactivating this structure—which mediates FPS—would functionally turn the adult rat into a 16-day-old rat. In both cases, the basic circuitry for acquiring fear (i.e., the amygdala) would be functional, but the part of the circuit necessary for expressing that fear via FPS (i.e., the PnC) would be inactive at the time of training. Weber and Richardson tested the animals 24 h later, at a time when the chemical inactivation had worn off. In the first set of experiments, rats had an odor CS paired with a shock US. Subjects were tested for both odor-elicited freezing and FPS. The results showed that inactivating the PnC during CS–US pairings had absolutely no

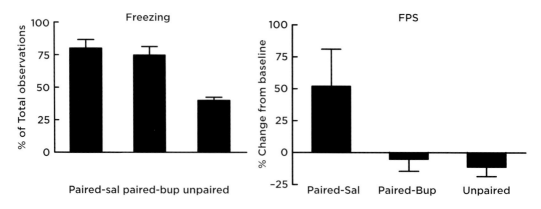

Figure 25.7 The left panel presents the percentage freezing data from adult rats that had been given Paired or Unpaired presentations of an odor CS with shock US. Some of the subjects were trained under temporary inactivation of the PNC (Bup) or were administered intra-PNC saline (Sal). The right panel shows the percentage change in startle to the odor CS in the same subjects. (From Weber & Richardson, 2004.)

effect on subsequent odor-elicited freezing (Figure 25.7, left panel), but completely abolished subsequent expression of FPS in the presence of this odor (Figure 25.7, right panel). As in Richardson and Fan's (2002) study with the developing rat, the same subjects were expressing fear to the CS via one response (freezing) but not via another response (FPS). Clearly, the neural circuitry necessary for both associative learning and for FPS expression are functional in the intact adult rat. However, when the part of this circuit that is necessary for FPS is inactivated during CS–US pairings, then that particular fear response is not expressed in a subsequent test of learned fear. Further, just like the developmental findings reported by Richardson and Fan (2002), the adult rats that were given odor–shock pairings while the PnC was inactivated exhibited no savings in terms of the number of trials needed to express FPS when they were later re-trained with the same odor CS. So, just like in the developing rat, it appears that if a response output system is not engaged in adult rats during CS–US pairings, then that particular response will not be expressed as a component of the fear reaction on a subsequent test.

However, it is important to note the results of another experiment reported by Weber and Richardson (2004). That study was essentially the same as the one described above except that a light CS was used rather than an odor CS. No differences were expected with this change in CS modality, especially given the developmental findings described earlier by Barnet and Hunt (2006) with a light CS. Nonetheless, in contrast to the results described above with an odor CS, temporary inactivation of the PnC had no effect on subsequent FPS (or freezing) to the light CS. This result is contrary to what was found with the olfactory CS, and to the findings that we consistently report in the developing rat. Clearly, there is a need for additional research in this area in order to more fully understand these modality differences.

Despite the very small, and admittedly inconsistent, literature on whether memories in adult rats are expressed via response systems that were functionally inactive at the time of training, our developmental data clearly show that early-acquired fear memories are not expressed via response systems that become functionally mature *after* the memory has been acquired. These latter data have significant implications for our understanding of memory development. Based on these data, one would have to conclude that early-acquired fear memories are not translated across stages of development, at least in terms of the response systems by which they can be expressed.

We have complementary demonstrations that memories are not translated across stages of development using other experimental procedures. For example, in a recent series of experiments, we examined latent inhibition and extinction in rats of different ages. Latent inhibition is the reduction in the observed CR produced by nonreinforced exposures to the CS prior to CS–US pairings (Lubow & Moore, 1959) while extinction is the reduction in the observed CR produced by nonreinforced exposures to the CS after CS–US pairings. Both of these phenomena have been shown to be contextually mediated in adult rats (see Bouton, 2004; Bouton & Bolles, 1979; Channel & Hall, 1983), with contextual cues serving to disambiguate which CS–US contingency (i.e., CS–US or CS–no US) is currently in effect. Because young rats have been shown to be impaired in learning about context (Rudy, 1993), we wondered whether latent inhibition and extinction would be contextually modulated in preweanling rats.

Our results showed that both latent inhibition and extinction were context-dependent in rats 23 days of age or older, but were context-independent in younger rats (Kim & Richardson, 2007; Yap & Richardson, 2005, 2007). We also examined whether the contextual dependence of these two phenomena would be appropriate to the rat's age at the time of "training" or their age at test. In each of these experiments, the rats were at least 23 days of age at test, an age for which both latent inhibition and extinction show context dependence. "Training" in these experiments was determined by the rat's age when their memory for the CS became ambiguous; that is, when CS–US pairings occurred in the latent inhibition procedure (after initial CS preexposures) and when CS-alone presentations were given in the extinction procedure (after initial CS–US pairings). The results of these experiments showed that the rat's age when the memory became ambiguous, not its age at the time of test, determined whether latent inhibition and extinction was contextually modulated. Specifically, rats that were 23 days of age at test exhibited context-dependent latent inhibition and extinction if the CS memory became ambiguous around this age. In contrast, if the CS memory became ambiguous when the rats were younger, at about 18 days of age, then both latent inhibition and extinction were context-independent. These findings extend our previous findings that early-acquired memories are expressed only via responses that were available at the time of training. Here, this general idea is shown to also apply to higher-order contextual modulation of ambiguous CS representations—whether an animal uses context to regulate their response to an ambiguous CS depends on their age when the CS became ambiguous rather than their age at test.

As mentioned in various instances in our discussion above, our results do not fit with current theoretical models of associative learning (which emphasize S–S learning; Rescorla & Wagner, 1972), models of the neural bases of learned fear (which emphasizes the role of the amygdala, but give little

consideration to plasticity involving downstream structures; LeDoux, 2000), or conceptualizations of memory development that emphasize the importance of early memories in guiding later behavior (Jacobs & Nadel, 1999). However, in regard to the latter issue, we are not suggesting that early memories are *never* translated across stages of development. Rather, we suggest that this translation of memory does not spontaneously occur, but rather only happens under special circumstances. In the next section we describe one such circumstance.

The Updating of Early Memories

The evidence presented in the previous section overwhelmingly implies that only those response systems that are functional at the time of learning are incorporated into an early-acquired fear memory. Moreover, response systems that mature after that learning has taken place are not later integrated into this memory; that is, these later-maturing response systems cannot be used to index that prior learning. From this, we infer that in order for a specific behavioral response to accurately reflect the central state of fear elicited by a CS previously paired with an aversive US, the specific neural systems responsible for that particular response must be active at the same time as the systems that are responsible for associative learning are active. A strong version of this inference would be that early-acquired fear memories can never be expressed via later-maturing response systems. As mentioned earlier, we do not hold this strong view. Rather, we suggest that early-acquired memories can be expressed via response systems that matured after the learning event, but only if the original memory is somehow "updated" to include these new responses. For example, if the original memory is somehow reactivated at a later age, then later-maturing response systems might be integrated into the reconsolidated memory (see Nader, 2003, for discussion of the process of memory reconsolidation in adult rats). This would allow for memories of recurrent aversive events to be translated across stages of development while highly infrequent aversive experiences would not be.

The idea that a response system must be functionally active at the time of training in order to be a part of the memory for that experience was captured by Barnet and Hunt (2006) in their *collateral activation hypothesis*. This hypothesis stipulates that the mechanisms required for response generation and those necessary for associative encoding must be activated concurrently in order for the response to become integrated with the CS–US memory. Put into neuroanatomical terms as they might relate to fear conditioning, we suspect that the amygdala, the PnC, and the projections connecting the two must all be activated during a training session in order for FPS to become one of the fear responses elicited by the CS. When preweaning rats (16–18 days of age) are given CS–US pairings, the amygdala is activated, but the PnC is not, due to anatomical immaturity. When subjects are later tested for responding to the fear-eliciting CS, FPS is not expressed because the "encoding" (e.g., amygdala) and "response" (PnC) systems had not been concurrently engaged and therefore had not been integrated. This hypothesis predicts that collateral activation of CS–US encoding mechanisms together with the FPS response pathway will allow for the integration of learning and response systems and therefore will allow the memory of acquired fear to the previously trained CS to be "updated" with the later developing response system. Note that, from this perspective, the effects of this concurrent activation are stimulus-independent; once the systems are integrated, they should afford activation by any CS. So, if rats are given CS–US pairings at an age prior to the functional maturation of the FPS circuit, but then are given a second training experience at a time when the FPS circuit is mature, then FPS should be evident to the original CS.

TESTING THE COLLATERAL ACTIVATION HYPOTHESIS

Yap et al. (2005; Experiment 1) gave 16-day-old rats pairings of an odor CS with a shock US. Some rats were also given pairings of a second odor CS with shock at 22 days of age. All subjects were tested for both FPS and freezing to both odor CSs (all tests occurred at 23 and 24 days of age). The results showed that an odor CS trained at 22 days of age (referred to as odor 2) elicited both FPS and freezing at test. Further, an odor CS trained at 16 days of age (referred to as odor 1) elicited freezing but not FPS. Finally, the most interesting results of that study were provided by a group of rats that had been trained with odor 1 at 16 days of age and then with odor 2 at 22 days of age. Rats in this group not only exhibited freezing and FPS to odor 2, they also expressed their fear of odor 1 via both of these responses. That is, the memory of the first CS had been updated and was now expressed via a response system that had matured during the training-to-test interval. This result offers support for the collateral activation hypothesis.

Further support for the collateral activation hypothesis was provided by Barnet and Hunt (2006). In that study, 18-day-old rats were assigned to one of three groups. One group was given paired presentations of a light CS and a shock US (group L+), a second group was given unpaired presentations of the light CS and shock US (group L/+), and a third group received no treatment (NT). All subjects were tested for FPS 1 week later. Recall that rats given CS–US pairings at 18 days of age do not ordinarily exhibit FPS to the CS, regardless of how old they are at test (as shown in Figure 25.5). In this experiment, however, all subjects were given pairings of an auditory CS (an 80 dB 1600 Hz pure tone) with shock 24 h prior to test. This additional training was intended to concurrently activate the learning and response systems that support FPS (i.e., the amygdala and PnC) at a time when the two could potentially be integrated. All rats were subsequently tested for FPS to both the light and tone CS, in a counterbalanced order. The question of interest was whether the nontarget training occurring on postnatal day 24 would promote the expression of FPS to the previously trained light CS. The data obtained from this experiment fully supported our prediction. First, FPS to the tone was evident, as expected. Second, and of most interest, fear conditioning to the tone CS promoted the expression of FPS to the light CS that had been trained 1 week earlier (Figure 25.8). This result was

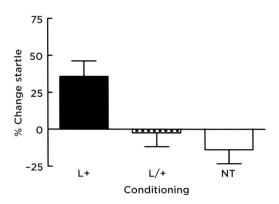

Figure 25.8 Percentage change in startle of subjects tested with a light CS. Subjects were trained at 18 days of age and were tested at 25–26 days for FPS to the light CS. On day 18, animals were given paired presentations of the light with shock (L+), unpaired presentations of the light and shock (L/+) or were given no treatment (NT). On day 24, one day prior to the FPS test, all animals were given pairings of a tone with the same shock US that was used for day 18 training. (From Barnet & Hunt, 2006.)

observed regardless of test sequence (i.e., tone CS first or light CS first). The design of this experiment also allowed us to rule out the possibility that FPS to the light CS was the result of simple stimulus generalization. Specifically, the other two groups of rats that had been given tone–shock pairings on day 24 did not express FPS to the light CS (groups L/+ and NT). Expression of FPS to the light required prior associative learning to that CS.

From the findings described above, it appears that providing subjects with a second training experience can promote the expression of FPS to an earlier-trained CS. A second training experience does not, however, always lead to the updating of the memory for the first CS. For example, the memory updating effect appears to be dependent on associative learning, as unpaired presentations of the second, nontarget CS and shock (Hunt & Barnet, unpublished data) or shock only (Yap et al., 2005) fail to result in observable FPS to the earlier-trained CS. Moreover, not all CS1–CS2 combinations are successful in producing the effect. Specifically, Yap et al. (2005) found that training with a visual CS2 at 23 days of age did not lead to FPS to an olfactory CS1 that had been trained at 16 days of age. Barnet and Hunt (2006) reported an identical result but used the opposite combination of stimuli; that is, an olfactory CS2 trained at 24 days did not promote FPS to a visual CS1 that had been trained at 18 days of age. The reasons for the modality dependence of this memory updating effect is not clear at present, but might reflect non-overlapping neural systems that convey auditory-visual versus olfactory stimulus information within and/or from the amygdala (Schwob & Price, 1984; Shi & Davis, 2001). In any case, this updating process can clearly serve as an effective means of allowing for repeated or recurrent experiences to be translated across stages of development.

Summary

In this chapter, we have highlighted some of our recent research on the ontogeny of fear conditioning. This research has yielded a number of extremely surprising results. These data not only contribute to a fuller understanding of the complexities underlying the ontogeny of learning and memory processes, but also raise serious questions about current theoretical models of (1) Pavlovian conditioning and (2) the neural bases of learned fear.

The first general issue examined in this chapter was the sequential emergence of learned fear responses, and we described research demonstrating that the manner in which learned fear is expressed changes dramatically during the first few weeks of life. Rats that are 16–18 days of age are quite capable of associating visual and olfactory CSs with an aversive US, and they reliably express their memory of this association by freezing and/or changing their heart rate when the CS is presented subsequently. However, rats at these ages do not express this fear memory via the FPS response; it is not until the rat is about 23 days of age that it can express learned fear via FPS. These findings argue against the central assumption of response equivalence in fear conditioning. When working with preweanling rats, the choice of which response to measure is certainly not arbitrary.

Another robust developmental dissociation reported in Pavlovian conditioning is that between freezing and eyeblink CRs. Stanton (2000), for example, has shown that preweanling rats given pairings of a brief auditory CS with periorbital shock display robust freezing to the CS but do not exhibit anticipatory eyeblink CRs. Eyeblink CRs are not consistently observed until about 24 days of age (Stanton, Freeman, & Skelton, 1992). It is interesting that the two response systems that emerge relatively late in development (i.e., FPS and eyeblink) both involve CS modulation of a skeletal reflex. The interested reader is directed to the chapters in this volume by John Freeman and Mark Stanton for a comprehensive discussion of the ontogeny of eyeblink conditioning (Chapters 24 and 26).

The second general issue examined in this chapter was whether early-acquired memories are translated across stages of development, and our research convincingly shows that memory is expressed in a manner appropriate to the rats' age at the time of training rather than their age at test. Specifically, rats given CS–US pairings at 16–18 days of age but not tested until they reach at least 23 days of age express fear to the CS by freezing but fail to express this fear in terms of potentiated startle. This finding causes considerable difficulty for contemporary models of fear conditioning that (1) rely on the assumption that the CS evokes a central emotional state and (2) embrace the notion that the structure of this learning is restricted to S–S associations.

A report by Simcock and Hayne (2002) with humans provides converging support for our findings on memory expression across development in rats. Briefly, in that study children ranging in age from 27 to 39 months interacted with a novel toy—the incredible "shrinking machine." At the time of this experience, children's productive vocabulary was measured. The children were tested for retention 6 months or 1 year later, and vocabulary was again assessed at the time of test. Children showed considerable retention of this unique experience, even after 1 year, as measured by picture recognition and behavioral reenactment. The most interesting data in that study, at least for the present purposes, were the number of words and phrases that the children used to describe the event at test. Remarkably, there was not a *single* instance of a child using a word to describe the event that had not been part of his or her productive vocabulary at the time the event was experienced, even though assessments of productive vocabulary at the time of test revealed that new words (relevant to a description of the event) had been acquired during the retention interval. So, just as we have observed that the developing rat normally only expresses an early-acquired memory via responses (fear responses) that were available at the time of training, Simcock and Hayne observed that children only express their verbal memory of an experience that happened 6 or 12 months previously via words that were in their productive vocabulary at the time of the experience. As noted by Simcock and Hayne, it appears that early-acquired memories are *frozen in time*, at least in terms of how they are behaviorally expressed.

The third general issue examined in this chapter concerned the possibility that early-acquired memories could be updated across stages of development. We described research illustrating that early-acquired memories can gain access to newly emerging response systems if the mechanisms of memory encoding are subsequently activated concurrently with those of response expression. Specifically, rats trained at 16–18 days of age were able to express their fear of the CS via the FPS procedure when tested 1 week later, *if and only if* they had been trained with a second CS the day prior to test. As described, there are constraints on this effect, primarily in terms of the modality of the two CSs. These modality effects certainly need to be explored more fully if we are to gain a more comprehensive understanding of the processes through which memory updating can and does occur.

Taken together, this research has a number of implications for current conceptualizations of the neural systems mediating the acquisition of fear. Our data with the developing rats suggest that current models of the neural bases of learned fear are incomplete. These models focus on the basolateral amygdala as a brain region that is not only necessary, but typically sufficient, for fear acquisition. Our developmental results are inconsistent with this general framework. While there is no doubt that the amygdala is critically involved in fear conditioning, synaptic plasticity in the BLA is not by itself sufficient for later expression of learned fear via FPS (cf., Wilensky et al., 2006). Rather, it may be the case that plasticity occurring at all levels of the circuit, including the BLA, the CeA, and the various downstream structures that mediate specific behavioral expressions of fear, is necessary for fear conditioning. Previous distinctions between those neural structures involved in "learning" (i.e., the BLA) versus those involved in "expression" (e.g., the PnC) may have led to research questions that limited our ability to develop a full understanding of the neural networks governing conditioned fear. It is certainly the case that our research with the developing rat suggests that fear conditioning requires plasticity at multiple levels of the fear circuit.

Finally, assumptions about the mechanisms underlying fear conditioning, including the prevailing view that Pavlovian conditioning is entirely governed by S–S processes, have guided the analysis of the neural systems involved. The possibility that Pavlovian conditioning may additionally involve S–R learning processes will open new avenues for future research into the neural bases of learned fear. Major questions regarding the nature of what is encoded during Pavlovian conditioning trials, and how memory for these events is governed by complex and interacting neural networks, should be at the forefront of current research into the neurobiological basis of associative learning. A developmental approach to this issue has not only uncovered this point, but will continue to provide what are likely to be unique insights into these and other areas of neuroscience and behavioral research.

Acknowledgment
The authors thank Marianne Weber for her assistance with the figures.

References
Barnet, R. C., & Hunt, P. S. (2006). The expression of fear-potentiated startle during development: Integration of learning and response systems. *Behavioral Neuroscience, 120*, 861–872.

Bevins, R. A., & Ayres, J. J. B. (1992). Rats' location during conditioned suppression training. *Animal Learning and Behavior, 20*, 8–16.

Black, A. H., & de Toledo, L. (1972). The relationship among classically conditioned responses: Heart rate and skeletal behavior. In A. H. Black & W. F. Prokasy (Eds.), *Classical conditioning II: Current research and theory* (pp. 290–311). New York: Appleton-Century-Crofts.

Bolles, R. C. (1970). Species-specific defense reactions and avoidance learning. *Psychological Review, 77*, 32–48.

Bouton, M. E. (2004). Context and behavioral processes in extinction. *Learning & Memory, 11*, 485–494.

Bouton, M. E., & Bolles, R. C. (1979). Contextual control of the extinction of conditioned fear. *Learning and Motivation, 10*, 455–466.

Bouton, M. E., & Bolles, R. C. (1980). Conditioned fear assessed by freezing and by the suppression of three different baselines. *Animal Learning and Behavior, 8*, 429–434.

Brown, J. S., Kalish, H. I., & Farber, I. E. (1951). Conditioned fear as revealed by magnitude of startle response to an auditory stimulus. *Journal of Experimental Psychology, 41*, 317–328.

Campbell, B. A. (1967). Developmental studies of learning and motivation in infra-primate mammals. In H. W. Stevenson, E. H. Hess, & H. L. Rheingold (Eds.), *Early behavior: Comparative and developmental approaches* (pp. 43–71). New York: Wiley.

Campbell, B. A., & Ampuero, M. X. (1985). Conditioned orienting and defensive responses in the developing rat. *Infant Behavior and Development, 8*, 425–434.

Campbell, B. A., & Campbell, E. H. (1962). Retention and extinction of learned fear in infant and adult rats. *Journal of Comparative and Physiological Psychology, 55*, 1–8.

Carrive, P. (2000). Conditioned fear to environmental context: Cardiovascular and behavioral components in the rat. *Brain Research, 858*, 440–445.

Channell, S., & Hall, G. (1983). Contextual effects in latent inhibition with an appetitive conditioning procedure. *Animal Learning and Behavior, 11*, 67–74.

Collier, A. C., & Bolles, R. C. (1980). The ontogenesis of defense reactions to shock in preweanling rats. *Developmental Psychobiology, 13*, 141–150.

Davis, M. (1989). Sensitization of the acoustic startle reflex by footshock. *Behavioral Neuroscience, 103*, 495–503.

Davis, M. (1992). The role of the amygdala in fear and anxiety. *Annual Review of Neuroscience, 15*, 353–375.

Davis, M., Falls, W.A., Campeau, S., & Kim, M. (1993). Fear-potentiated startle: A neural and pharmacological analysis. *Behavioural Brain Research, 58*, 175–198.

Donahoe, J. W., & Vegas, R. (2004). Pavlovian conditioning: The CS–UR relation. *Journal of Experimental Psychology: Animal Behavior Processes, 30*, 17–33.

Eaton, R. C. (Ed.). (1984). *Neural mechanisms of startle behavior.* New York: Plenum.

Fanselow, M. S. (1980). Conditional and unconditional components of postshock freezing. *Pavlovian Journal of Biological Sciences, 15*, 177–182.

Fanselow, M. S. (1991). The midbrain periaqueductal gray as a coordinator of action in response to fear and anxiety. In A. Depaulis & R. Bandler (Eds.), *The midbrain periaqueductal gray matter: Functional, anatomical, and neurochemical organization* (pp. 151–173). New York: Plenum.

Fanselow, M. S., DeCola, J. P., De Oca, B. M., & Landeira-Fernandez, J. (1995). Ventral and dorsolateral regions of the midbrain periaqueductal gray (PAG) control different stages of defensive behavior: Dorsolateral PAG lesions enhance the defensive freezing produced by massed and immediate shock. *Aggressive Behavior, 21*, 63–77.

Fanselow, M. S., & Rudy, J. W. (1998). Convergence of experimental and developmental approaches to animal learning and memory processes. In T. J. Carew, R. Menzel, & C. J. Shatz (Eds.), *Mechanistic relationships between development and learning* (pp. 15–28). New York: Wiley.

Fendt, M., & Fanselow, M. S. (1999). The neuroanatomical and neurochemical basis of conditioned fear. *Neuroscience and Biobehavioral Reviews, 23*,743–760.

Fendt, M., Koch, M., & Schnitzler, H.-U. (1996). Lesions of the central gray block conditioned fear as measured with the potentiated startle paradigm. *Behavioral Brain Research, 74*, 127–134.

Gale, G. D., Anagnostaras, S. G., Godsil, B. P., Mitchell S., Nozawa T., Sage J. R., et al. (2004). Role of the basolateral amygdala in the storage of fear memories across the adult lifetime of rats. *Journal of Neuroscience. 24,* 3810–3815.

Goosens, K. A.. & Maren, S. (2003). Pretraining NMDA receptor blockade in the basolateral complex, but not the central nucleus, of the amygdala prevents savings of conditional fear. *Behavioral Neuroscience, 117*, 738–750.

Gormezano, I., & Kehoe, E. J. (1981). Classical conditioning and the law of contiguity. In P. Harzem & M. D. Zeiler (Eds.), *Predictability, correlation, and contiguity* (pp. 1–45). New York: Wiley.

Holland, P. C., & Rescorla, R. A. (1975). Second-order conditioning with food unconditioned stimulus. *Journal of Comparative and Physiological Psychology, 88*, 459–467.

Hunt, P. S. (1997). Retention of conditioned autonomic and behavioral responses in preweanling rats: Forgetting and reinstatement. *Animal Learning and Behavior, 25*, 301–311.

Hunt, P. S., Barnet, R. C., Rima, B., & Murdoch, D. (2004). Dissociation of freezing and potentiated startle in the Sprague–Dawley rat. Unpublished data.

Hunt, P., & Campbell, B. A. (1997). Developmental dissociation of the components of conditioned fear. In M. E. Bouton & M. S. Fanselow (Eds.), *Learning, motivation and cognition: The functional behaviorism of Robert C. Bolles* (pp. 53–74). Washington, DC: American Psychological Association.

Hunt, P. S., Hess, M. F., & Campbell, B. A. (1997a). The effects of context novelty on defense behavior in rats. Paper presented at meetings of the International Society for Developmental Psychobiology, New Orleans, LA.

Hunt, P. S., Hess, M. F., & Campbell, B. A. (1997b). Conditioned cardiac and behavioral response topography to an olfactory CS dissociates with age. *Animal Learning and Behavior, 25*, 53–61.

Hunt, P. S., Hess, M. F., & Campbell, B. A. (1998). Inhibition of the expression of conditioned cardiac responses in the developing rat. *Developmental Psychobiology, 33*, 221–233.

Hunt, P. S., Richardson, R., & Campbell, B. A. (1994). Delayed development of fear-potentiated startle. *Behavioral Neuroscience, 108*, 69–80.

Hunt, P. S., Richardson, R., Hess, M. F., & Campbell, B. A. (1997c). Emergence of conditioned cardiac responses to an olfactory CS paired with an acoustic startle UCS during development: Form and autonomic origins. *Developmental Psychobiology, 30*, 151–163.

Iwata, J., & LeDoux, J. E. (1988). Dissociation of associative and nonassociative concomitants of classical fear conditioning in the freely behaving rat. *Behavioral Neuroscience, 102*, 66–76.

Iwata, J., LeDoux, J. E., & Reis, D. J. (1986). Destruction of intrinsic neurons in the lateral hypothalamus disrupts the classical conditioning of autonomic but not behavioral emotional responses in the rat. *Brain Research, 368*, 161–166.

Jacobs, W. J., & Nadel, L. (1985). Stress-induced recovery of fears and phobias. *Psychological Review, 92*, 512–531.

Jacobs, W. J., & Nadel, L. (1999). The first panic attack: A neurobiological theory. *Canadian Journal of Experimental Psychology, 53*, 92–107.

Johanson, I. B., & Hall, W. G. (1984). Ontogeny of appetitive learning: Independent ingestion as a model motivational system. In R. Kail & N. E. Spear (Eds.), *Comparative perspectives on the development of memory* (pp. 135–157). Hillsdale, NJ: Erlbaum.

Kapp, B. S., Whalen, P. J., Supple, W. F., & Pascoe, J. P. (1992). Amygdaloid contributions to conditioned arousal and sensory information processing. In J. P. Aggleton (Ed.), *The amygdala: Neurobiological aspects of emotion, memory, and mental dysfunction* (pp. 289–254). New York: Wiley-Liss.

Kehne, J. H., & Davis, M. (1984). Strychnine increases acoustic startle amplitude but does not alter short-term or long-term habituation. *Behavioral Neuroscience, 98*, 955–968.

Kim, J. H., & Richardson R. (2007). A developmental dissociation of context and GABA effects on extinguished fear in rats. *Behavioral Neuroscience, 121*, 131–139.

Leaton, R. N., & Borszcz, G. S. (1985). Potentiated startle: Its relation to freezing and shock intensity in rats. *Journal of Experimental Psychology: Animal Behavior Processes, 11*, 421–428.

Leaton, R. N., & Cranney, J. (1990). Potentiation of the acoustic startle response by a conditioned stimulus paired with acoustic startle stimulus in rats. *Journal of Experimental Psychology: Animal Behavior Processes, 16*, 279–287.

LeDoux, J. E. (2000). Emotion circuits in the brain. *Annual Review of Neuroscience, 23*, 155–184.

LeDoux, J. E., Iwata, J., Cicchetti, P., & Reis, D. J. (1988). Different projections of the central amygdaloid nucleus mediate autonomic and behavioral correlates of conditioned fear. *Journal of Neuroscience, 8*, 2517–2529.

Lubow, R. E., & Moore, A.U. (1959). Latent inhibition: The effects of nonreinforced pre-exposure to the conditional stimulus. *Journal of Comparative and Physiological Psychology, 52*, 415–419.

Martin, G. K., & Fitzgerald, R. D. (1980). Heart rate and somatomotor activity in rats during signaled escape and yoked classical conditioning. *Physiology and Behavior, 25*, 519–526.

McAllister, W. R., & McAllister, D. E. (1971). Behavioral measurement of conditioned fear. In F. R. Brush (Ed.), *Aversive conditioning and learning* (pp. 105–179). New York: Academic Press.

McCabe, P. M., Schneiderman, N., Jarrell, T. W., Gentile, C. G., Teich, A. H., Winters, R. W., et al. (1992). Central pathways involved in classical differential conditioning of heart rate responses in rabbits. In I. Gormezano & E. A. Wasserman (Eds.), *Learning and memory: The behavioral and biological substrates* (pp. 321–346). Hillsdale, NJ: Erlbaum.

McEchron, M. D., Cheng, A. Y., & Gilmartin, M. R. (2004). Trace fear conditioning is reduced in the aging rat. *Neurobiology of Learning and Memory, 82*, 71–76.

McNish, K. A., Gewirtz, J. C., & Davis, M. (1997). Evidence of contextual fear after lesions of the hippocampus:

A disruption of freezing but not fear potentiated startle. *Journal of Neuroscience, 17*, 9353–9360.

Mineka, S., & Zinbarg, R. (2006). A contemporary learning theory perspective on the etiology of anxiety disorders. *American Psychologist, 61*, 10–26.

Nader, K. (2003). Memory traces unbound. *Trends in Neurosciences, 26*, 65–72.

Parisi, T., & Ison, J. R. (1979). Development of the acoustic startle response in the rat: Ontogenetic changes in the magnitude of inhibition by prepulse stimulation. *Developmental Psychobiology, 12*, 219–230.

Parisi, T., & Ison, J, R. (1981). Ontogeny of control over the acoustic startle reflex by visual prestimulation in the rat. *Developmental Psychobiology. 14*, 31, 1–6.

Plappert, C. F., Pilz, P. K. D., & Schnitzler, H.-U. (1993). Acoustic startle response and habituation in freezing and nonfreezing rats. *Behavioral Neuroscience, 107*, 981–987.

Powell, D. A., & Kazis, E. (1976). Blood pressure and heart rate changes accompanying classical eyeblink conditioning in the rabbit (*Oryctolagus cuniculus*). *Psychophysiology, 13*, 441–447.

Rescorla, R. A., & Wagner, A. R. (1972). A theory of Pavlovian conditioning: Variations in the effectiveness of reinforcement and nonreinforcement. In A. H. Black & W. F. Prokasy (Eds.), *Classical conditioning II: Current research and theory* (pp. 64–99). New York: Appleton-Century-Crofts.

Richardson, R., & Elsayed, H. (1998). Shock-sensitization of startle: The role of contextual conditioning. *Behavioral Neuroscience, 112*, 1136–1141.

Richardson, R., & Fan, M. (2002). Behavioral expression of learned fear in rats is appropriate to their age at training, not their age at testing. *Animal Learning and Behavior, 30*, 394–404.

Richardson, R., Fan, M., & Parnas, S. (2003). Latent inhibition of conditioned odor potentiation of startle: A developmental analysis. *Developmental Psychobiology, 42*, 261–268.

Richardson, R., Paxinos, G., & Lee, J. (2000). The ontogeny of conditioned odor potentiation of startle. *Behavioral Neuroscience, 114*, 1167–1173.

Richardson, R., & Vishney, A. (2000). Shock sensitization of startle in the developing rat. *Developmental Psychobiology, 36*, 282–291.

Rudy, J. W. (1993). Contextual conditioning and auditory cue conditioning dissociate during development. *Behavioral Neuroscience, 197*, 887–891.

Schwob, J. E., & Price, J. L. (1984). The development of axonal connections in the central olfactory system of rats. *Journal of Comparative Neurology, 223*, 177–202.

Sheets, L. P., Dean, K. F., & Reiter, L. W. (1988). Ontogeny of the acoustic startle response and sensitization to background noise in the rat. *Behavioral Neuroscience, 102*, 706–713.

Shi, C., & Davis, M. (2001). Visual pathways involved in fear conditioning measured with fear-potentiated startle: Behavioral and anatomic studies. *Journal of Neuroscience, 21*, 9844–9855.

Simcock, G., & Hayne, H. (2002). Breaking the barrier: Children do not translate their preverbal memories into language. *Psychological Science, 13, 225–231.*

Stanton, M. (2000). Multiple memory systems, development and conditioning. *Behavioural Brain Research, 110*, 25–37.

Stanton, M. E., Freeman, J. H. Jr., & Skelton, R. W. (1992). Eyeblink conditioning in the developing rat. *Behavioral Neuroscience, 106*, 657–665.

Supple, W. F., Jr., & Leaton, R. N. (1990). Cerebellar vermis: Essential for classically conditioned bradycardia in the rat. *Brain Research, 509*, 17–23.

Wagner, A. R. (1981). SOP: A model of automatic memory processing in animal behaviour. In N. E. Spear & R. R. Miller (Eds.), *Information processing in animals: Memory mechanisms* (pp. 5–47). Hillsdale, NJ: Erlbaum.

Walker, D. L., & Davis, M. (1997). Involvement of the dorsal periaqueductal gray in the loss of fear-potentiated startle accompanying high footshock training. *Behavioral Neuroscience, 111*, 692–702.

Walker, D. L., & Davis, M. (2002). The role of the amygdala glutamate receptors in fear learning, fear potentiated startle, and extinction. *Pharmacology, Biochemistry, & Behavior, 71*, 379–392.

Weber, M., & Richardson, R. (2001). Centrally administered corticotropin-releasing hormone and peripheral injections of strychnine hydrochloride potentiate the acoustic startle response in preweanling rats. *Behavioral Neuroscience, 115*, 1273–1282.

Weber, M., & Richardson, R. (2004). Pretraining inactivation of the caudal pontine reticular nucleus impairs the acquisition of conditioned fear-potentiated startle to an odor, but not light. *Behavioral Neuroscience, 118*, 965–974.

Weber, M., Watts, N., & Richardson, R. (2003). High illumination levels potentiate the acoustic startle response in preweanling rats. *Behavioral Neuroscience, 117*, 1458–1462.

Wecker, J. R., & Ison, J. R. (1986). Effects of motor activity on the elicitation and modification of the startle reflex in rats. *Animal Learning and Behavior*, 14, 287–292.

Wilensky, A. E., Schafe, G. E., Kristensen, M. P., & LeDoux, J. E. (2006). Rethinking the fear circuit: The central nucleus of the amygdala is required for the acquisition, consolidation, and expression of Pavlovian fear conditioning. *Journal of Neuroscience, 26*, 12387–12396.

Yap, C. S., & Richardson, R. (2005). Latent inhibition in the developing rat: An examination of context-specific effects. *Developmental Psychobiology, 47*, 55–65.

Yap, C. S., & Richardson, R. (2007). Extinction in the developing rat: an examination of renewal effects. . *Developmental Psychobiology, 49, 565–575*

Yap, C. S., Stapinski, L., & Richardson, R. (2005). Behavioral expression of learned fear: Updating of early memories. *Behavioral Neuroscience, 199*, 1467–1476.

Zhao, Z., & Davis, M. (2004). Fear-potentiated startle in rats is mediated by neurons in the deep layer of the superior colliculus/deep mesencephalic nucleus of the rostral midbrain through glutamate non-NMDA receptors. *Journal of Neuroscience, 24*, 10326–10334.

Developmental Neurobiology of Cerebellar Learning

John H. Freeman

Abstract

A fundamental issue in developmental behavioral neuroscience is how learning abilities change ontogenetically. This chapter attempts to address this issue by examining neural mechanisms underlying the ontogeny of eyeblink conditioning. Eyeblink conditioning is a type of associative learning that requires the cerebellum and emerges ontogenetically between postnatal days 17 and 24 in rats. Cerebellar learning emerges developmentally as conditioned stimulus (CS) and unconditioned stimulus (US) neural inputs to the cerebellum develop. The primary developmental change in the CS pathway is an age-related increase in sensory input to the pontine nuclei. Developmental changes in US input include age-related increases in inferior olive input to the cerebellar interpositus nucleus and inhibitory feedback from the cerebellum to the inferior olive. The development of CS and US input pathways to the cerebellum results in the ontogenetic emergence of neuronal plasticity mechanisms that are necessary for eyeblink conditioning.

Keywords: conditioned stimulus, unconditional stimulus, learning abilities, eyeblink conditioning, cerebellar learning, CS pathway, age-related

Introduction

Behavioral studies of the ontogeny of associative learning have focused on long-term retention as well as acquisition. Many of the first animal studies of the ontogeny of associative learning focused on infantile amnesia, the inability to recall experiences that occurred during infancy (Campbell & Spear, 1972). A general finding from these studies is that young rats do not retain associative learning as well as older rats, even when initial learning is equated across ages (Campbell & Spear, 1972). Preweanling rat pups generally cannot retain memories across delays of more than a few hours unless they are given reinstatement training during the retention interval.

Other studies focused on acquisition of associative learning in developing rats. Acquisition of associative learning is limited by the development of sensory systems. In rats and other altricial species, visual function emerges later than the auditory function, which emerges later than olfactory, gustatory, and somatosensory function (Alberts, 1984; Gottlieb, 1971). Within each sensory system, the ability to detect a conditioned stimulus (CS) precedes associative learning (Rudy, 1992). This principle is most clearly demonstrated in studies of associative learning using gustatory, auditory, and visual CSs in Pavlovian conditioning paradigms (Hyson & Rudy, 1984; Moye & Rudy, 1985; Rudy, 1992).

Associative learning using olfactory and gustatory conditioned stimuli has been demonstrated very early in rats. For example, aversive Pavlovian conditioning can be established in the rat fetus with an odor/taste (apple juice) administered into the amniotic fluid as the CS paired with lithium chloride as the unconditioned stimulus (US). Retention tests showed evidence of conditioning during gestation and postnatally (Smotherman, 1982; Smotherman & Robinson, 1985). The Smotherman (1982) study also showed that fetal conditioning to an apple juice CS was specific to the olfactory properties of the stimulus in a postnatal retention test. Earlier studies showed aversive and appetitive Pavlovian conditioning using an odor CS in neonatal rat pups (Haroutunian & Campbell, 1979; Johanson & Teicher, 1980; Rudy & Cheatle, 1977). Taste aversion learning has been demonstrated as early as postnatal day (P)1 (Gemberling & Domjan, 1982) or P12 (Vogt & Rudy, 1984), depending on the specific procedures used during training (Hoffman, Molina, Kucharski, & Spear, 1987). Vogt and Rudy (1984) also demonstrated that the ability to detect and respond to the gustatory CS precedes associative learning. The early emergence of olfactory and gustatory conditioning is consistent with the pattern of sensory system development described above.

Associative learning with auditory and visual CSs emerges considerably later than olfactory and gustatory conditioning. Pavlovian conditioning using an auditory CS has been shown as early as P12 with a train of clicks, but is typically seen between P14 and P21 using continuous or pulsing tones (Hunt & Campbell, 1997; Hyson & Rudy, 1984; Stanton et al., 1992). Hyson and Rudy (1984) also demonstrated that auditory sensation precedes associative learning. Sensory detection of visual stimuli that are typically used in learning experiments can be observed as soon as the eyes open around P14–15, but associative learning using a visual CS does not emerge until P17 or later (Hunt & Campbell, 1997; Moye & Rudy, 1985; Paczkowski, Ivkovich, & Stanton, 1999). More complex or "higher order" forms of learning with auditory or visual stimuli emerge even later than simple associative learning (Chapter 24).

In addition to the development of sensory systems, the development of different response systems also influences the ontogeny of associative learning. This principle is most clearly demonstrated in fear conditioning where conditioned freezing emerges earlier than heart-rate conditioning

and heart-rate conditioning emerges earlier than potentiated startle with olfactory, auditory, or visual CSs (Chapter 25; Hunt & Campbell, 1997; Sananes, Gaddy, & Campbell, 1988). Conditioned freezing with an auditory CS also emerges earlier than eyeblink conditioning (Stanton, 2000). The findings described in the preceding discussion indicate that the mechanisms underlying the ontogeny of associative learning involve interactions of developmental changes in sensory systems, responses systems, and associative processes (see Chapter 25 for a more extensive discussion of these issues).

In the Campbell and Spear (1972) review of experimental work on infantile amnesia, several neural correlates of memory development were discussed. At that time, neurobiological studies of learning had not localized memory to a particular brain system or circuit. As a result, there was no starting point for examining the neural mechanisms underlying the ontogeny of learning. It was not until neurobiological studies began to identify the necessary and sufficient neural circuitry underlying associative learning (Thompson, 1986) that neurobiological approaches could be used to examine the neural mechanisms underlying the *ontogeny* of learning with a high degree of specificity. In this chapter, I review the findings of neurobiological studies of the ontogeny of eyeblink conditioning, which integrate and extend prior behavioral analysis of the ontogeny of associative learning and neural circuit analysis of learning in adult animals.

There are a number of neural mechanisms that could plausibly underlie the ontogeny of learning including (a) development of learning-related neuronal plasticity, (b) development of sensory input to learning systems, and (c) development of memory retrieval systems. My laboratory has endeavored to determine the developmental changes in neural function that are necessary for the ontogenetic transition from nonlearner to learner, and to differentiate changes in learning mechanisms from changes in the ability to detect the relevant stimuli and perform the learned response. This chapter reviews findings from our neurobiological analysis of the ontogeny of eyeblink conditioning that shed light on which of the aforementioned neural mechanisms underlie the development of associative learning.

Eyeblink Conditioning in Developing Organisms

Eyeblink conditioning is a Pavlovian conditioning procedure that involves pairing a stimulus that does not elicit the blink reflex before training, the CS, with a stimulus that *does* elicit the blink reflex before training, the US. The CS comes to elicit a conditioned or learned blink as a result of repeated presentations of the conditioned and unconditioned stimuli (Gormezano, Schneiderman, Deaux, & Fuentes, 1962; Schneiderman, Fuentes, & Gormezano, 1962). The CS typically precedes the US by several hundred milliseconds. Conditioned eyeblinks start before and peak at about the onset time of the US. The eyeblink conditioned response (CR) can, therefore, be considered an anticipatory response that is established based on a predictive relationship between the CS and US. In a general sense, eyeblink conditioning is a well-controlled experimental paradigm for assessing feedforward (i.e., anticipatory) adjustments to movements. Eyeblink conditioning can also be considered a paradigm for assessing behavioral timing because the peak amplitude of the CR occurs at the onset time of the US, and shifts as the interval between the onsets of the CS and US varies (Gormezano, Kehoe, & Marshall, 1983).

Eyeblink conditioning is particularly well suited for developmental studies of learning in that the response does not required limb or trunk control, which avoids the difficulty of differentiating ontogenetic changes in learning from changes in performance. Moreover, performance can be assessed precisely by examining quantitative measures of the unconditioned response.

Behavioral Development of Eyeblink Conditioning

The chapter by Stanton (Chapter 24) in this handbook provides a detailed review of work on the behavioral analysis of eyeblink conditioning in developing rodents and humans. As a result, this section will briefly review the major findings that are relevant to the neurobiological work discussed in subsequent sections.

The ontogeny of eyeblink conditioning in animals was first assessed in 17- and 24-day-old rats (Stanton, Freeman, & Skelton, 1992). Rats given eyeblink conditioning on postnatal day (P) 17 showed very little eyeblink conditioning, whereas rats trained on P24 showed robust conditioning. The developmental difference in conditioning was not due to developmental differences in sensory or motor function, as indicated by strong unconditioned responses to the tone CS and the US at both ages. It was possible that the developmental difference in eyeblink conditioning depended upon

the specific parameters used in the first study. To address this general point, Stanton and colleagues conducted a series of experiments to determine whether parameters that affect eyeblink conditioning in adults such as US intensity, interstimulus interval, level of arousal, and CS salience would eliminate the developmental difference in eyeblink conditioning between P17 and P24 (Stanton & Freeman, 2000; Stanton, this volume). Although variation in these parameters affected conditioning in young rats, the developmental difference in conditioning between P17 and P24 rats was consistent across the various training parameters. The absence of developmental differences in sensory and motor function coupled with the robustness of the developmental difference in conditioning under different training parameters suggested that the ontogeny of eyeblink conditioning is due to the development of the neural mechanisms underlying associative learning. Our experimental analysis of the ontogeny of eyeblink conditioning then turned to an examination of developmental changes within the neural circuitry underlying eyeblink conditioning.

Neural Circuitry Underlying Eyeblink Conditioning in Adults

An exhaustive review of the literature on the neural circuitry underlying eyeblink conditioning is beyond the scope of this chapter. What follows is an abridged review that focuses on the specific components of the eyeblink conditioning circuitry that have been examined in our developmental studies. The neural circuitry underlying delay eyeblink conditioning is illustrated in Figure 26.1.

The cerebellum and several interconnected brain stem nuclei are necessary for delay eyeblink conditioning (Thompson, 2005). Trace conditioning and various higher-order conditioning paradigms require the hippocampus and neocortical areas in addition to the cerebellum (Campolattaro & Freeman, 2006; Galvez, Weible, & Disterhoft, 2007; Galvez, Weiss, Weible, & Disterhoft,, 2006; Kim, Clark, & Thompson, 1995; Moyer, Deyo, & Disterhoft, 1990; Nicholson & Freeman, 2000; Weible, McEchron, & Disterhoft, 2000; Weible, Weiss, & Disterhoft, 2003). Unilateral lesions of the cerebellar interpositus nucleus ipsilateral to the conditioned eye completely prevent acquisition of eyeblink conditioning and abolish CRs established prior to surgery (Clark, McCormick, Lavond, & Thompson, 1984; Lavond, Hembree, & Thompson, 1985; McCormick, Clark, Lavond, & Thompson, 1982a; Steinmetz, Lavond, Ivkovich, Logan, &

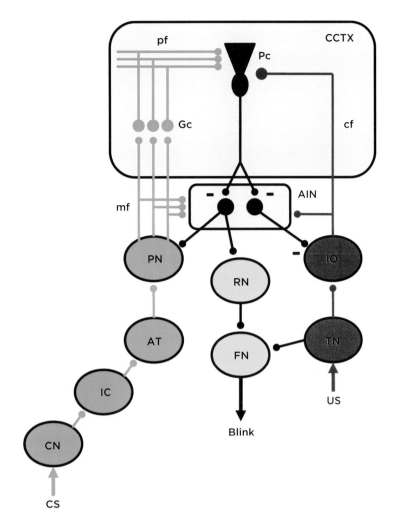

Figure 26.1 Simplified schematic diagram of the neural circuitry underlying eyeblink conditioning. The cerebellar anterior interpositus nucleus (AIN) and Purkinje cells (Pc) in the cerebellar cortex (CCTX) receive convergent input from the conditioned stimulus (CS, green) and unconditioned stimulus (US, red) neural pathways. The auditory CS pathway includes the cochlear nucleus (CN), inferior colliculus (IC), medial auditory thalamus (AT), basilar pontine nuclei (PN), mossy fiber (mf) projection to the AIN and cortical granule cells (Gc), and the parallel fiber (pf) projection to Purkinje cells. The US pathway includes the trigeminal nucleus (TN), dorsal accessory division of the inferior olive (IO), and the climbing fiber (cf) projection to the AIN and Pc. The output pathway for performance of the conditioned response (orange) includes the AIN projection to the red nucleus (RN) and its projection to facial motor nucleus (FN) which causes eyelid closure. The unconditioned response is elicited by activation of the TN, which then activates the FN. Inhibitory synapses are depicted by a minus sign. All other synapses are excitatory.

Thompson, 1992; Yeo, Hardiman, & Glickstein, 1985). Reversible inactivation of the ipsilateral interpositus nucleus with cooling, lidocaine, or muscimol also prevents acquisition of eyeblink CRs (Chapman, Steinmetz, Sears, & Thompson, 1990; Clark, Gohl, & Lavond, 1997; Clark, Zhang, & Lavond, 1992; Freeman et al., 2005; Garcia & Mauk, 1998; Krupa, Thompson, & Thompson, 1993; Krupa & Thompson, 1997). Rabbits or rats given muscimol inactivation show no evidence of retention or savings when subsequently trained without cerebellar inactivation. Lesions of cerebellar cortex have typically produced a severe deficit in acquisition and retention with subsequent relearning in rabbits (Harvey, Welsh, Yeo, & Romano, 1993; Lavond, Steinmetz, Yokaitis, & Thompson, 1987; Lavond & Steinmetz, 1989; McCormick & Thompson, 1984a; Woodruff-Pak, Lavond, Logan,

Steinmetz, & Thompson, 1993). Loss of the cerebellar cortical output by selective depletion of Purkinje cells throughout the cerebellar cortex in Purkinje cell degeneration mice and with OX7-saporin in rats results in impaired acquisition, but most of the rodents with Purkinje cell loss can learn after extensive training (Chen, Bao, Lockard, Kim, & Thompson, 1996; Nolan & Freeman, 2006). Purkinje cell depletion *after* conditioning in rats results in a severe retention deficit with reacquisition after extensive retraining (Nolan & Freeman, 2005). Reversible inactivation of the lateral anterior lobe and lobule HVI in rabbits impairs acquisition, abolishes previously acquired CRs, and impairs consolidation in rabbits (Atwell, Cooke, & Yeo, 2002; Atwell, Rahman, Ivarsson, & Yeo, 1999; Atwell, Rahman, & Yeo, 2001). Pharmacological disconnection of the cerebellar cortex from the deep nuclei with GABA antagonists, however, does not abolish CRs but disrupts the timing of eyeblink CRs, resulting in short latency responses (Bao, Chen, Kim, & Thompson, 2002; Garcia & Mauk, 1998; Ohyama & Mauk, 2001; Ohyama, Nores, & Mauk, 2003; Ohyama, Nores, Medina, Riusech, & Mauk, 2006). The findings of the lesion and inactivation studies suggest that the cerebellar cortex and interpositus nucleus are needed for acquisition and retention of eyeblink conditioning, but the interpositus nucleus can learn slowly in the absence of Purkinje cell input. Purkinje cell input to the cerebellar nuclei is also essential for CR timing.

The respective roles of the cerebellar nuclei and cortex are perhaps best illustrated by the findings from analyses of learning-related changes in neuronal activity. Neurons in the anterior interpositus nucleus exhibit learning-related increases in activity during the CS that mirror the time course and amplitude of the CR in rabbits and rats (Berthier & Moore, 1986, 1990; Freeman & Nicholson, 2000; Gould & Steinmetz, 1994, 1996; McCormick et al., 1982a; McCormick & Thompson, 1984b; Nicholson & Freeman, 2002). The learning-related increase in interpositus nucleus activity develops in parallel with the CR across training trials and precedes the CR consistently within trials. In contrast, activity in the posterior interpositus nucleus follows the onset of the CR (Delgado-Garcia & Gruart, 2005).

Purkinje cells also show learning-related changes in activity during eyeblink conditioning that emerge as CRs are acquired (Berthier & Moore, 1986; Gould & Steinmetz, 1994, 1996; Green & Steinmetz, 2005; Hesslow & Ivarsson, 1994; Jirenhed, Bengtsson, & Hesslow, 2007; McCormick et al., 1982a; McCormick & Thompson, 1984b; Nicholson & Freeman, 2004a). Single-unit analyses of Purkinje cell activity have shown learning-related increases and decreases in simple spike activity (Berthier & Moore, 1986; Gould & Steinmetz, 1996, 2005; Hesslow & Ivarsson, 1994; Jirenhed et al., 2007). Many of the Purkinje cells monitored in the anterior lobe and lobule HVI show decreased simple spike activity as CRs are produced. A subset of the Purkinje cells that show learning-related changes in activity exhibit an initial increase in simple spike activity shortly after the onset of the CS followed by a decrease toward the end of the CS, when CRs occur (Green & Steinmetz, 2005; Hesslow & Ivarsson, 1994). The learning-related changes in Purkinje cell simple spike activity may shape the topography of the CR by inhibiting the

interpositus nucleus early in the CS period and disinhibiting it later in the CS period (Green & Steinmetz, 2005; Medina et al., 2000).

Models of cerebellar learning posit that the memory underlying eyeblink conditioning is established as a result of the convergence of CS and US sensory inputs in the cerebellum (Thompson, 1986). Synaptic convergence of the CS and US occurs in the cerebellar deep nuclei and on Purkinje cells in the cortex. The plasticity mechanisms underlying cerebellar memory are thought to include long-term depression of CS input to Purkinje cells and a facilitation of CS input to the anterior interpositus nucleus (Christian & Thompson, 2003; Kleim et al., 2002; Mauk & Donegan, 1997; Medina & Mauk, 1999, 2000; Ohyama et al., 2006; Thompson, 2005).

The output or behavioral expression of the CR depends on cerebellar efferent projections through the superior cerebellar peduncle (SCP) to the red nucleus and then to the brain stem motor nuclei that innervate eyelid, ocular, and facial muscles. Lesions of the SCP or red nucleus abolish CRs (McCormick, Guyer, & Thompson, 1982b; Rosenfield & Moore, 1983). Reversible inactivation of the SCP or red nucleus also abolishes CRs without affecting acquisition of eyeblink conditioning, as revealed by complete savings during subsequent training in the absence of inactivation (Krupa et al., 1993; Krupa & Thompson, 1995). Moreover, inactivation of the red nucleus does not abolish learning-related activity within the interpositus nucleus (Clark & Lavond, 1993). Inactivation of the interpositus nucleus, in contrast, abolishes CRs and learning-related activity within the red nucleus (Chapman et al., 1990). The findings of the inactivation studies indicate that eyeblink CRs are established in the cerebellum and the red nucleus is necessary for motor output. The red nucleus then activates the motor nuclei that are critical for generating the eyeblink response (Desmond, Rosenfield, & Moore, 1983).

The US pathway to the cerebellum originates in the sensory inputs to the trigeminal nuclei (Harvey, Land, & McMaster, 1984; Schreurs, 1988; van Ham & Yeo, 1996). Some of the trigeminal nuclei send US-related signals to the inferior olive, which then projects to the cerebellum as climbing fibers. Climbing fibers synapse directly on neurons in the cerebellar nuclei and with Purkinje cells (Kitai, McCrea, Preston, & Bishop, 1977; Sugihara, Wu, & Shinoda, 2001; van der Want, Wiklund, Guegan, Ruigrok, & Voogd, 1989). Stimulation of the dorsal accessory division of the inferior olive (DAO) can serve as a sufficient US for conditioning with a peripheral or stimulation CS (Jirenhed et al., 2007; Mauk, Steinmetz, & Thompson, 1986; Steinmetz, Lavond, & Thompson, 1989). In addition, lesions or inactivation of the inferior olive impairs acquisition and retention of eyeblink conditioning (McCormick, Steinmetz, & Thompson, 1985; Welsh & Harvey, 1998; Yeo, Hardiman, & Glickstein, 1986). Inhibition of the inferior olive by stimulating its inhibitory inputs during conditioning produces an extinction-like loss of CRs without disrupting cerebellar activity (Bengtsson, Jirenhed, Svensson, & Hesslow, 2007).

The inferior olive receives an inhibitory feedback projection from the cerebellar nuclei (Andersson, Garwicz, & Hesslow, 1988; Bengtsson & Hesslow, 2006; De Zeeuw, Van Alphen, Hawkins, & Ruigrok, 1997). Cerebellar feedback regulates the rhythmicity of neuronal activity in the inferior olive (Lang, Sugihara, & Llinas, 1996; Nicholson & Freeman, 2003b). As CRs are produced during eyeblink conditioning, cerebellar inhibition significantly inhibits activity in the inferior olive (Bengtsson & Hesslow, 2006; Hesslow & Ivarsson, 1996; Sears & Steinmetz, 1991). CR-related inhibition of the inferior olive virtually shuts down US-elicited complex spikes in Purkinje cells (Bengtsson & Hesslow, 2006; Kim, Krupa, & Thompson, 1998). Inhibition of climbing fiber activity during eyeblink conditioning is thought to be necessary for preventing acquisition of redundant plasticity (noise) and for maintaining learning-related plasticity for extended periods by keeping climbing fiber activity in a state of equilibrium between conditioning trials and sessions (Kenyon, Medina, & Mauk, 1998; Kim et al., 1998; Medina & Mauk, 1999; Medina, Nores, & Mauk, 2002; Thompson, Thompson, Kim, Krupa, & Shinkman, 1998). Cerebellar neurons require input from the inferior olive to support learning-related plasticity and to regulate olivary input, which helps to maintain this plasticity.

The basilar pontine nuclei provide the cerebellum with CS information through their mossy fiber inputs, primarily to the contralateral deep nuclei and granule cell layer of the cerebellar cortex (Mihailoff, 1993; Shinoda, Sugiuchi, Futami, & Izawa, 1992; Steinmetz & Sengelaub, 1992). Lesions, stimulation, and reversible inactivation have been used to show that the pontine mossy fiber projection is an integral part of the necessary and sufficient CS pathway in eyeblink conditioning (Bao, Chen, & Thompson, 2000; Freeman et al., 2005a;

Freeman & Rabinak, 2004; Hesslow, Svensson, & Ivarsson, 1999; Knowlton & Thompson, 1988; Lewis, LoTurco, & Solomon, 1987; Steinmetz, 1990; Steinmetz, Rosen, Chapman, Lavond, & Thompson, 1986; Steinmetz et al., 1987; Tracy et al., 1998). Less is known about the possible contributions of the various sensory structures that send inputs to the pontine nuclei.

Initial studies of the auditory CS pathway in eyeblink conditioning found a monosynaptic projection from the ventral cochlear nucleus to the dorsolateral and lateral pontine nuclei (Steinmetz et al., 1987). The monosynaptic pathway from the cochlear nucleus provides auditory CS information to the pontine nuclei, but it might not be sufficient for acquisition of eyeblink conditioning. Evidence for the involvement of auditory areas other than the cochlear nuclei in eyeblink conditioning initially came from studies that used stimulation of the auditory cortex, cochlear nuclei, inferior colliculus, superior olive, or ventral division of the medial geniculate as a CS for conditioning (Knowlton et al., 1993; Knowlton & Thompson, 1992; Nowak, Kehoe, Macrae, & Gormezano, 1999; Patterson, 1969, 1970). In addition, facilitation of neuronal activity in the medial geniculate was seen during differential auditory trace conditioning in rabbits (O'Connor, Allison, Rosenfield, & Moore, 1997). The stimulation and neurophysiology data suggest that auditory areas that are efferent to the cochlear nuclei might play a role in eyeblink conditioning. Contributions of the auditory cortex to eyeblink conditioning were ruled out by studies that found that acute decerebration rostral to the red nucleus produces only a transient impairment in retention, and decortication does not prevent acquisition or retention (Mauk & Thompson, 1987; Oakley & Russell, 1972, 1977).

A recent series of studies has shed new light on the roles of the inferior colliculus and thalamus in auditory eyeblink conditioning. Halverson and Freeman (2006) found that unilateral lesions of the medial auditory thalamus in rats result in a severe deficit in eyeblink conditioning with a tone CS, but no impairment in conditioning with a light CS. Rats with complete lesions also show no cross-modal savings when switched to the light CS, indicating that subthreshold conditioning is not established during conditioning with the tone CS. Unilateral lesions of the inferior colliculus, which provides most of the input to the auditory thalamus, also impair acquisition of eyeblink conditioning (Freeman, Halverson, & Hubbard, 2007).

A subsequent study found that reversible inactivation of the medial auditory thalamus impairs both acquisition and retention of eyeblink conditioning (Halverson, Poremba, & Freeman, 2008). The sufficiency of thalamic activation as a CS was demonstrated by using electrical stimulation during eyeblink conditioning (Campolattaro, Halverson, & Freeman, 2007). Electrical stimulation of the medial auditory thalamus is a highly effective CS for eyeblink conditioning in rats, producing more rapid acquisition than is seen with a tone. Medial auditory thalamic neurons send auditory information to the basilar pons through a monosynaptic projection to the lateral and medial nuclei (Campolattaro et al., 2007). Our current model of the auditory CS pathway is a serial circuit from the cochlear nuclei to the inferior colliculus (directly and indirectly) and then to the medial auditory thalamus to the pontine nuclei (Figure 26.1). This subcortical CS pathway provides sensory input to the cerebellum via the pontine mossy fiber projection. Neurons within the auditory CS pathway may also undergo learning-related changes in activity that boost CS input to the cerebellum and thereby facilitate eyeblink conditioning.

The detailed and comprehensive analysis of the neural circuitry underlying eyeblink conditioning in adult animals has proven to be advantageous for our developmental studies. We have used the known neural circuitry in adults as a "roadmap" for identifying potential sites of developmental change that might underlie the ontogeny of eyeblink conditioning. That is, knowing where to look in the brain for developmental changes provided a useful framework for our initial experimental approach to elucidating the mechanisms underlying the ontogeny of learning.

Development of Cerebellar Circuitry

The first major issue addressed in our developmental analysis of the neural circuitry underlying eyeblink conditioning was whether there were developmental changes in cerebellar function that correspond to the ontogenetic emergence of conditioning. Disruption of neurogenesis in the cerebellum with methylazoxymethanol or early lesions severely disrupted the ontogeny of eyeblink conditioning (Freeman, Barone, & Stanton, 1995; Freeman, Carter, & Stanton, 1995). Having established that cerebellar development is necessary for the development of eyeblink conditioning, we began a neurophysiological analysis of cerebellar function during eyeblink conditioning in developing rats.

We examined the activity of neurons within the cerebellar anterior interpositus nucleus and cortex during eyeblink conditioning in rats trained on P17–18 and P24–25 (Freeman & Nicholson, 2000; Nicholson & Freeman, 2003a, 2004a). The anterior interpositus nucleus was selected as the first target of our developmental analysis because it is at the center of the neural circuitry underlying eyeblink conditioning. That is, neurons in the anterior interpositus nucleus receive inputs from the CS and US pathways, show learning-related modulation, are influenced by the cerebellar cortex, and their axons form the output pathway for producing the CR. Developmental changes in neuronal activity within the cerebellar cortex were also assessed because, like the anterior interpositus nucleus, it receives inputs from the CS and US pathways and shows learning-related modulation. In addition, the cerebellar cortex is thought to influence the induction of plasticity within the anterior interpositus nucleus (Mauk & Donegan, 1997).

Neurons within the anterior interpositus nucleus and Purkinje cells in the cerebellar cortex exhibited substantial developmental changes in learning-related activity. We observed an age-related increase in the proportion of cerebellar neurons showing learning-related changes in activity during the CS and an increase in the magnitude of activity among the neurons that showed learning-related activity (Figure 26.2). Learning-related activity among neurons in the interpositus nucleus was exclusively excitatory, with increased activity toward the end of the interstimulus interval. Some of the Purkinje cells showed excitatory learning–related activity like the neurons in the interpositus nucleus; other Purkinje cells showed learning–related inhibition that increased toward the end of the interstimulus interval, as seen in adult animals (Green & Steinmetz, 2005; Hesslow & Ivarsson, 1994; Jirenhed et al., 2007). The pups trained on P24–25 also had a higher proportion of neurons that showed greater activity on trials with a CR versus trials with no CR relative to the pups trained on P17–18. A cross-correlation analysis found that the amplitude and time course of neuronal activity among many of the CR-related units were significantly correlated with the eyelid electromyographic (EMG) activity in pups trained on P24–25 but not at P17–18. Moreover, most of the neurons with activity that correlated with the eyelid activity showed changes in activity that preceded eyelid movement within trials, suggesting that the activity of these neurons could be driving

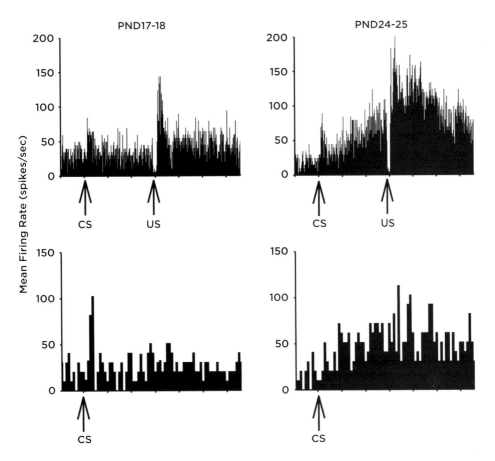

Figure 26.2 Mean firing rate (spikes per second) for single neurons recorded from the anterior interpositus nucleus in infant rats during eyeblink conditioning. The firing frequencies of the neurons recorded from rats trained on P17–18 (left) and P24–25 (right) are displayed. The upper histograms display activity from trials with paired presentations of the conditioned stimulus (CS) and unconditioned stimulus (US). The lower histograms display activity from CS-alone test trials. Arrows indicate the onset times of the CS and US. The gap in unit activity during the US is due to the stimulus artifact, which precludes recording unit activity. Note that the activity is greater on P24–25 relative to P17–18 during the CS and after the US. (Freeman & Nicholson, 2000.)

the eyelid responses through the red nucleus and facial motor nucleus. The proportion of Purkinje cells showing CR-related activity was very high in areas of the cerebellar cortex that were identified as blink zones (Hesslow, 1994). The findings of the unit recording studies suggested that the ontogeny of eyeblink conditioning is related to the development of cerebellar plasticity rather than to developmental changes in motor output or expression of learning. It was important, however, to assess the development of cerebellar output pathways to determine whether the ontogeny of eyeblink conditioning could be, at least partially, accounted for by the development of motor output circuitry.

Developmental changes in the outputs of the cerebellar cortex and anterior interpositus nucleus were assessed using electrical stimulation through the recording electrodes. Stimulation of the anterior interpositus nucleus produced eyeblinks with stimulation intensities as low as 10 µA in pups trained on P17–18 or P24–25. It was also possible to elicit delayed eyeblinks following cerebellar cortical stimulation at both ages (the delay following cortical stimulation is due to inhibition of the interpositus nucleus during stimulation followed by rebound depolarization, which drives the eyelid response). The stimulation findings indicated that the cerebellar cortical and nuclear output circuits are functional at P17–18. The developmental change in eyeblink conditioning is, therefore, not due to development of output or expression mechanisms. Rather, the ontogeny of eyeblink conditioning appears to be more specifically due to the inability to establish robust cerebellar plasticity during training in the younger rats.

Having established that cerebellar neurons exhibit substantial developmental changes in learning-related activity, we focused on determining the basis for these ontogenetic changes. Important clues regarding the mechanisms underlying the developmental changes in cerebellar plasticity came from a developmental analysis of sensory responses to the CS and US in the cerebellum (Freeman & Nicholson, 2000; Nicholson & Freeman, 2000, 2003a, 2004a). Pups with electrodes in the cerebellum were given a pretraining session in which the CS and US were presented separately before sessions with CS–US pairings. The pretraining session was used to assess sensory responses to the CS and US before any conditioning occurred. Purkinje cell responses to the CS and US were weaker in the P17–18 pups in terms of the percentage of units that responded and the magnitude of the activity among responsive units (Figure 26.3). Anterior interpositus neurons showed a longer latency response to the CS and a lower magnitude response to the US. The findings from the pretraining sessions indicated that the development of sensory responsiveness of the cerebellum to the CS and US is an important ontogenetic change in the eyeblink conditioning circuitry.

Weaker inputs from the CS and US pathways might attenuate learning in younger pups by limiting the induction of Hebbian synaptic plasticity in the cerebellum. Indeed, it is well established that the rate and magnitude of eyeblink conditioning are influenced by the intensity of the CS and US (Gormezano et al., 1983). We demonstrated a relationship between US intensity and cerebellar neuronal activity by presenting pups with different US intensities. Increasing US intensity increased the number of activated cerebellar neurons, suggesting that increasing stimulus intensity may increase learning by activating more cerebellar neurons (Freeman & Nicholson, 2000). The developmental change in the strength of stimulus inputs to the cerebellum in younger pups might be functionally equivalent to changing stimulus intensity in adults. As a result, younger pups with weaker CS and US inputs would be less capable of establishing Hebbian synaptic plasticity in the cerebellum during eyeblink conditioning.

Development of the Unconditioned Stimulus Pathway

One of the most striking findings from the neurophysiological analysis of cerebellar development was the ontogenetic change in neuronal response to the US. The first step taken to examine developmental changes in the US pathway was to record the activity of neurons within the DAO in developing rats (Nicholson & Freeman, 2000). The expected outcome of this experiment was that neurons in the DAO would either show no developmental change or would show an age-related increase in response to the US. Neither of these outcomes occurred. Rather, neuronal activity in the DAO exhibited an age-related decrease in activity following the US (Figure 26.4). Purkinje cell complex spikes, which are generated by inferior olive input, also showed an age-related decrease in activity (Nicholson & Freeman, 2004a).

Why would greater activity in the inferior olive result in weaker conditioning in the younger rats? Greater spontaneous and stimulus-elicited activity in the inferior olive leads to a higher level of climbing fiber activity in the cerebellar cortex (Nicholson & Freeman, 2003a, 2003b), which according to some computational models of cerebellar learning (Kenyon et al., 1998; Medina et al., 2002; Medina & Mauk, 1999), leads to disruption of maintenance of learning-related synaptic plasticity in the cerebellum. The elevated climbing fiber activity after the US might also produce widespread activity in the cerebellum that establishes nonadaptive plasticity in neurons not involved in generating or timing the CR (Nicholson & Freeman, 2000, 2003a).

We recognized that the most likely mechanism for the ontogenetic change in inferior olive activity is development of the inhibitory projection from the cerebellar deep nuclei to the inferior olive. The first evidence supporting this hypothesis was that inferior olive neuronal activity and Purkinje cell complex spikes were not modified during CRs in younger pups, but were suppressed during CRs in older pups and adults (Figure 26.5). Cerebellar inhibition of the inferior olive influences the rhythmicity and synchrony of neuronal activity in the inferior olive (Lang et al., 1996). We examined developmental changes in spontaneous and evoked complex spike activity (Nicholson & Freeman, 2003b). Previous studies using adult animals demonstrated that somatosensory stimulation elicits two distinct patterns of complex spike activity: a single short-latency complex spike with no long-latency rhythmic discharge and a long-latency rhythmic discharge with no short-latency complex spike (Bloedel & Ebner, 1984; Llinas & Sasaki, 1989). The rhythmic discharge in long-latency evoked complex spike activity is produced

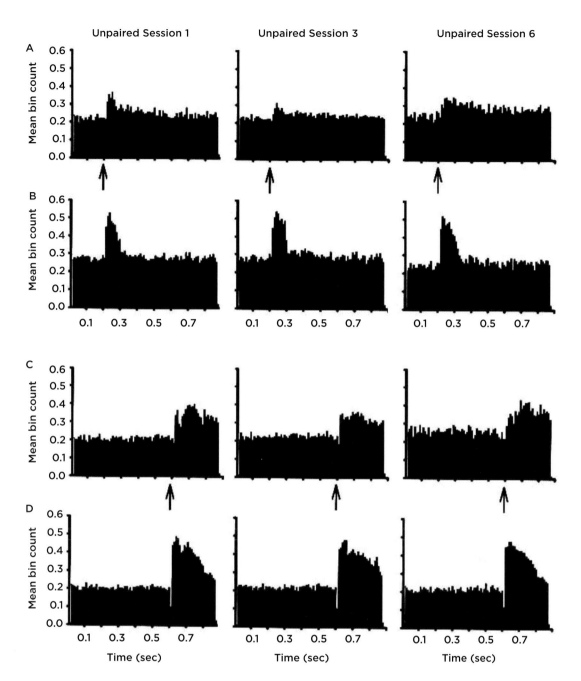

Figure 26.3 Mean neuronal activity for simple spikes recorded from Purkinje cells on P17–18 (A, C) and P24–25 (B, D) during sessions 1, 3, and 6 of unpaired presentations of the conditioned stimulus (A, B) and unconditioned stimulus (C, D). Arrows in (A) indicate CS-onset; arrows in (C) indicate US-onset. Note that the activity is greater following stimulus presentations in the pups trained on P24–25 relative to the activity in pups trained on P17–18 (B and D). (Nicholson & Freeman, 2004a.)

by rhythmic oscillations in the membrane voltage of electrically connected inferior olivary neurons, which are regulated by inhibitory cerebellar feedback (Lang et al., 1996; Llinas, 1974; Llinas, Baker, & Sotelo, 1974; Llinas & Sasaki 1989; Llinas & Yarom, 1981a, 1981b, 1986). Segregation of the

two evoked complex spike response patterns is also regulated by inhibitory feedback (Llinas & Sasaki, 1989; Lang et al., 1996). Evoked complex spike activity in developing rats was monitored to determine whether cerebellar inhibition and excitatory afferent input within the inferior olive exhibit

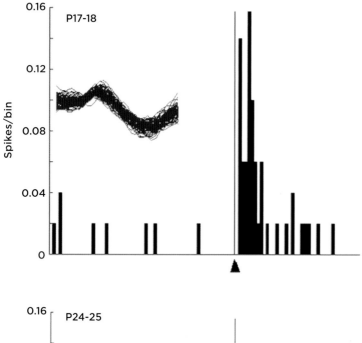

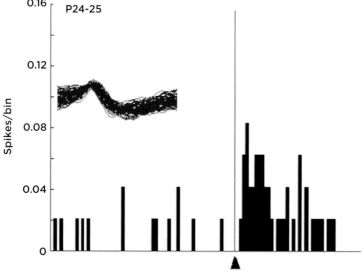

Figure 26.4 Histograms showing neuronal activity during the entire trial length (1 s) for individual inferior olive neurons recorded on P17 (upper) and P24 (lower) during presentations of the unconditioned stimulus (US) during a pretraining session. Arrowheads indicate the offset of the US. Note the greater activity after the US in the neuron recorded on P17 relative to the activity of the neuron recorded on P24. The insets show overlays of the waveforms of the spikes contributing to the histograms.

changes between P17 and P24. Recordings from individual Purkinje cell complex spikes showed that the segregation of short- and long-latency evoked complex spike activity emerged ontogenetically by P24. Pharmacological blockade of cerebellar inhibition by infusion of picrotoxin, a $GABA_A$-receptor antagonist, into the inferior olive abolished the response pattern segregation in the older rats, resulting in an evoked complex spike response pattern similar to that seen on P17 (Figure 26.6). The electrophysiological analysis supports the hypothesis that cerebellar inhibitory feedback to the infe-

rior olive undergoes a substantial change in parallel with the development of eyeblink conditioning.

The hypothesized developmental change in cerebellar inhibition of the inferior olive received further support from a quantitative electron microscopic assessment of the development of inhibitory synapses within the inferior olive (Nicholson & Freeman, 2003a). The physical disector and systematic random sampling (Gundersen, 1986; Geinisman, Gundersen, van der Zee, & West, 1996; Sterio, 1984) were used to obtain unbiased estimates of total number of excitatory axospinous,

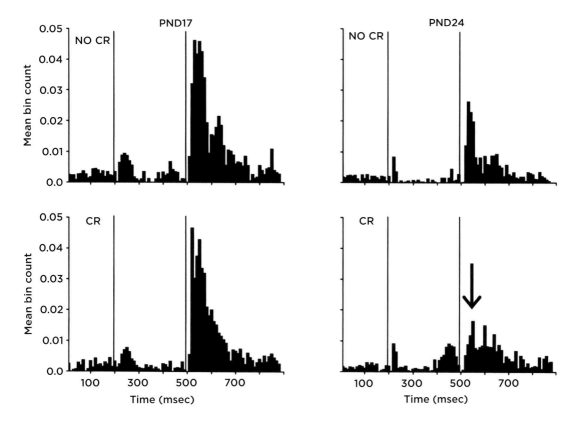

Figure 26.5 Learning-related changes in complex spike responses. Mean neuronal activity for all complex spikes recorded from Purkinje cells in pups trained on P17–18 (left two panels) and P24–25 (right two panels) during trials without (top two panels, No CR) and with (bottom two panels, CR) conditioned responses. Vertical lines indicate the onsets of the CS and US, respectively. Note that the peak of the complex spike activity is diminished during trials with CRs in pups trained on P24–25 (arrow), but not in pups trained on P17–18. (Nicholson & Freeman, 2003a.)

excitatory axodendritic, inhibitory axospinous, and inhibitory axodendritic synapses in the DAO in developing rats (Nicholson & Freeman, 2003a). There was an age-related increase in the number of excitatory axospinous, inhibitory axodendritic, and inhibitory axospinous synapses. The most substantial developmental change was in the number of inhibitory axospinous synapses, which increased nearly threefold between P17 and P24 (Figure 26.7). The age-related increase in inhibitory synapses is a striking morphological substrate that accounts for the greater US-evoked activity in the inferior olive and Purkinje cell complex spikes in younger rats (Nicholson & Freeman, 2000, 2003b, 2004a). The developmental change in inhibitory synapses also accounts for the inability of cerebellar neurons in younger rats to actively inhibit complex spikes during CRs, to regulate climbing fiber rhythmicity, and maintain climbing fiber equilibrium (Nicholson & Freeman, 2003a, 2003b).

Although the studies demonstrating the developmental change in inhibitory feedback to the inferior olive provided valuable information about the development of the eyeblink conditioning circuitry, this finding did not help to explain the ontogenetic increase in US-elicited activity in the interpositus nucleus. It was plausible that the climbing fiber synapses in the interpositus nucleus are weaker in younger rats, even though they exhibit greater olivary and complex spike responses following the US. Development of climbing fiber synaptic input to the interpositus nucleus was examined by recording the field potential in the interpositus nucleus following stimulation of the DAO on P17 and P24. The interpositus nucleus field potential evoked by olivary microstimulation was used to measure the strength of synaptic input to the interpositus nucleus from the DAO. In adult animals, climbing fiber activation of the deep nuclei elicits a short latency

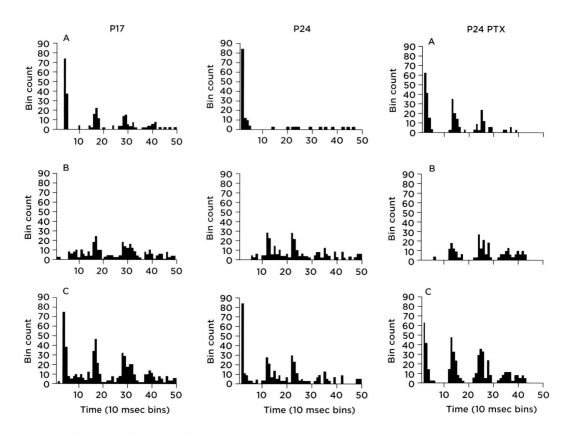

Figure 26.6 Histograms of the activity of representative Purkinje cell complex spikes from a P17 rat (left column), a P24 rat (middle column), and a P24 rat given picrotoxin in the inferior olive (PTX; right column) for trials with short-latency spikes (A), long-latency spikes (B), and both together (C). Note the differences in activity between the P17 complex spike (A, left) and the P24 complex spike (A, middle), and the similarities between the activity of the P17 complex spike (A, left) and the P24 complex spike after picrotoxin infusion in the inferior olive (A, right). (Nicholson & Freeman, 2003b.)

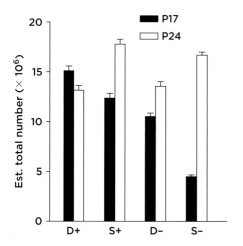

Figure 26.7 Estimated mean total number of excitatory axodendritic (D+) and axospinous (S+) synapses; inhibitory axodendritic (D–) and axospinous (S–) synapses in the dorsal accessory inferior olive on P17 and P24. Note the age-related increase in S+, D–, and S– synapses. (Nicholson & Freeman, 2003a.)

(~ 3 ms) excitatory postsynaptic potential (EPSP), and a longer latency (~ 5 ms) inhibitory postsynaptic potential (IPSP; Delgado-Garcia & Gruart, 1995; Ito, Yoshida, Obata, Kawai, & Udo, 1970; Kitai et al., 1977). Interpositus nucleus field potentials following DAO stimulation were therefore used to assess developmental differences in both the initial EPSP and the Purkinje cell IPSP. Stimulation of the inferior olive in pups on P17 and P24 evoked an adult-like field potential. The negative short latency component was blocked by infusion of the glutamate antagonist kynurenic acid and the positive longer latency component was blocked by infusion of the GABA antagonist picrotoxin (Nicholson & Freeman, 2004b). Substantial ontogenetic increases were found in the initial slope and amplitude of the EPSP (Figure 26.8). However, no developmental change was found in the IPSP (Nicholson & Freeman, 2004b). Thus, the climbing fiber projection to the interpositus

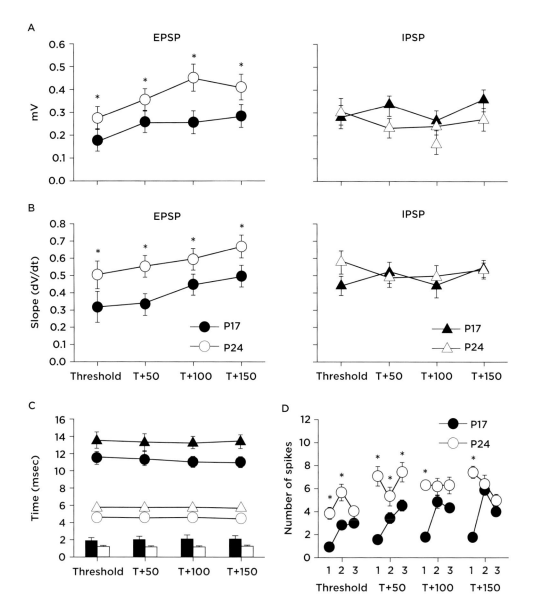

Figure 26.8 Selective developmental increase in the climbing fiber excitatory postsynaptic potential (EPSP) within the anterior interpositus nucleus. (A) Amplitude of the EPSP (circles; left column) and IPSP (triangles; right column) for each of four current levels on P17 (black) and P24 (white). (B) Slope of the EPSP (left column) and IPSP (right column) for each of the four current levels. (C) Peak latencies for the EPSP and IPSP. Plotted along the x-axis is the time between each peak at each of the four current levels for P17 (black) and P24 (white) rats. (D) Mean total number of multiunit spikes evoked in the six trials at each current level for three 4 ms time windows after DAO microstimulation in P17 (black) and P24 (white) rats. Asterisks indicate statistically significant differences. (Nicholson & Freeman, 2004b.)

nucleus undergoes significant development that parallels the ontogenetic emergence of eyeblink conditioning. The developmental change in the DAO projection to the cerebellum might account for the developmental changes in US-elicited activity in the interpositus nucleus and in simple spike activity in the cerebellar cortex.

Development of the Conditioned Stimulus Pathway

As mentioned above, the mossy fiber projection from the basilar pontine nuclei to the cerebellum is the proximal part of the CS pathway in adult animals. The pontine mossy fiber projection is strongest to the granule cell layer of the cerebellar cortex. Granule cells are generated throughout the first few postnatal weeks in rats (Altman, 1982). It therefore seemed likely that developmental changes in mossy fiber input could play an important role in the ontogeny of eyeblink conditioning (Freeman & Nicholson, 2000).

A useful method for examining the efficacy of the pontine mossy fiber projection in conditioning is to assess eyeblink conditioning using mossy fiber stimulation as the CS. If the mossy fiber projection to the cerebellum is weaker or otherwise less effective in younger pups, stimulation should not change the developmental profile of eyeblink conditioning. On the other hand, if the mossy fiber pathway is functional in younger pups, stimulation should produce learning in pups that would otherwise not learn with a peripheral CS.

In our first stimulation experiment, pontine stimulation was used as a CS in rat pups trained on P17–18 or P24–25 (Freeman et al., 2005b). Pups were implanted with a bipolar stimulating electrode in or just dorsal to the basilar pontine nuclei. A 300 ms train of 0.1 ms current pulses presented at 200 Hz was used as the CS. The intensity of the stimulation was set by first determining the level of current that produced blinks or other movements and then adjusting it to half the threshold intensity. Unpaired control groups were also used to assess nonassociative changes in eyeblink responses during training. We were astonished to find that pups trained on P17 with a pontine stimulation CS conditioned as rapidly as the pups trained on P24 (Figure 26.9). This was the first manipulation of

any kind that produced learning at P17 that was equivalent to the learning seen at P24.

It was possible that the conditioning seen with pontine stimulation was established through an extracerebellar mechanism. For example, pontine stimulation could have activated another downstream target of the pontine nuclei or caused antidromic activation of a pontine afferent and established learning-related plasticity in one of these other areas. We used cerebellar inactivation with muscimol to show that conditioning established with pontine stimulation in rat pups was cerebellum-dependent. Pups were trained with a pontine stimulation CS on P17–18 or P24–25, as described above, followed by an infusion of muscimol into the cerebellar interpositus nucleus. CRs were severely impaired by muscimol in both age groups, showing that the conditioning established with pontine stimulation was cerebellum-dependent (Figure 26.10). This finding indicates that the conditioning seen in the rat pups that were given pontine stimulation was due to activating the mossy fiber projection to the cerebellum and the resulting induction of cerebellar plasticity.

The findings of the first two pontine stimulation experiments suggest that the mossy fiber projection to the cerebellum is fully capable of supporting associative learning as early as P17. It was possible, however, that developmental changes in the efficacy of mossy fiber input to the cerebellum could have been masked by the use of a supersalient CS (200 Hz). A less intense CS might have revealed developmental changes in the rate or asymptote of

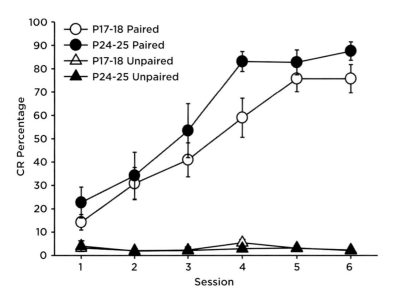

Figure 26.9 Mean conditioned response (CR) percentage for rat pups trained with pontine stimulation as the conditioned stimulus (CS) on P17–18 (white symbols) or P24–25 (black symbols). Pups were given either paired (circles) or unpaired (triangles) presentations of the CS and an unconditioned stimulus. The amount of associative learning in each paired group is determined by the increase in responding across training sessions and by the difference in CR percentage between the paired and unpaired conditions in both age groups. (Freeman et al., 2005.)

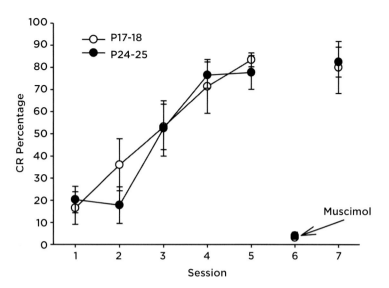

Figure 26.10 Mean conditioned response (CR) percentage for rat pups trained with pontine stimulation as the conditioned stimulus on P17–18 (white symbols) or P24–25 (black symbols). Pups were given paired presentations of pontine stimulation and a shock unconditioned stimulus (US). Muscimol was infused into the cerebellar nuclei prior to session 6 to inactivate the cerebellar nuclei and overlying cortex ipsilateral to the conditioned eye. CRs established by paired training of pontine stimulation and the US were abolished by muscimol inactivation. Response recovery was evident in both groups on session 7. (Freeman et al., 2005.)

conditioning. To address this issue, we conditioned rat pups on P17–18 or P24–25 using pontine stimulation with different pulse frequencies. Pups were given pontine stimulation at 50, 100, or 200 Hz paired with the US. We found no differences in conditioning between the age groups at any of the stimulation frequencies (Figure 26.11). Although our study did not include an exhaustive parametric analysis, the results support the hypothesis that the mossy fiber projection is capable of supporting conditioning in P17 and P24 rats.

We then pushed the limits of this hypothesis by examining whether stimulation of the pontine nuclei could be an effective CS in 12-day-old rats (Campolattaro & Freeman, 2008). Rats at this age have closed eyes and ear canals and therefore cannot show conditioning to visual or auditory stimuli. The main target of the mossy fiber projection, the cerebellar cortical granule cell layer, is also immature at this age, with ongoing neurogenesis and neuronal migration (Altman, 1982). It was possible however that eyeblink conditioning could be induced by direct stimulation the mossy fiber pathway as a CS paired with a peripheral US.

In the first experiment, rat pups were given eyelid conditioning using stimulation of the pontine nuclei as the CS on P12. The eyelids are normally connected at this age in rats. As a result, it was necessary to manually separate the eyelids on P11. Rat pups that were given paired presentations of pontine stimulation and the US showed eyeblink conditioning relative to unpaired controls (Figure 26.12). A second experiment showed

that the conditioning seen in the 12-day-old pups was abolished reversibly by muscimol inactivation of the cerebellum (Figure 26.12). The findings of these experiments indicate that eyeblink conditioning could be established in rat pups as early as P12, even though this is well before the age at which eyelid conditioning is observed using a peripheral CS. It appears that cerebellar neurons are capable of learning-related plasticity early in development, but do not receive sufficient sensory input from the pontine nuclei for conditioning with peripheral CSs until the third postnatal week.

A critical issue to consider on the basis of the findings of the pontine stimulation studies is whether there are developmental changes in the responsiveness of pontine neurons to peripheral CSs. We assessed ontogenetic changes in sensory responses to an auditory CS by recording neuronal activity within the pontine nuclei during eyeblink conditioning in rat pups trained on P17–18 or P24–25 (Freeman & Muckler, 2003). Pontine neurons exhibited a variety of response profiles during tone presentations before conditioning. Neurons with short-latency responses to the tone CS were less prevalent and the magnitude of the response was weaker in the younger pups (Figure 26.13). During training, neurons with later (>100 ms) developing activity during the CS and neurons with short-latency activity that was sustained during the CS showed an increase in activity in the pups trained on P24–25 but not in the pups trained on P17–18. The findings of this study clearly indicate that sensory responsiveness in the pontine nuclei increases substantially

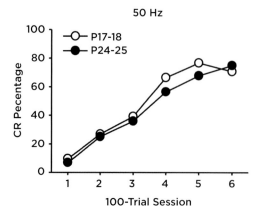

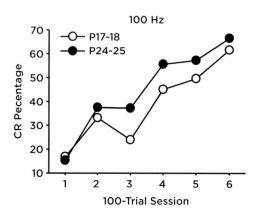

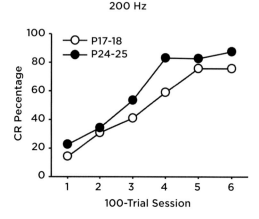

Figure 26.11 Mean conditioned response (CR) percentage in rat pups trained on P17–18 or P24–25 with pontine stimulation as a conditioned stimulus (CS). The CS was presented at either 50, 100, or 200 Hz. Note that there are no significant differences in performance between the age groups, regardless of CS stimulation frequency.

as eyeblink conditioning emerges ontogenetically. Developmental changes in sensory input to the pontine nuclei in turn affect input to cerebellar neurons. Cerebellar neurons that receive weaker input in younger rats will undergo less learning-related modification. Furthermore, weaker learning-related plasticity in the cerebellum will result in less excitatory feedback to the pontine nuclei and thereby provide less excitatory input to the cerebellum during presentations of the CS. Developmental changes in sensory input to the pontine nuclei, therefore, have substantial effects on cerebellar plasticity, and as a result, the ontogeny of eyeblink conditioning.

A goal of our current neurobiological work on the development of eyeblink conditioning is to determine which of the many sensory inputs to the pontine nuclei are changing ontogenetically between P17 and P24. As mentioned above, our work with adult rats indicates that auditory information is projected via a serial circuit from the cochlear nuclei to the inferior colliculus to the medial auditory thalamus and then to the pontine nuclei. The key question for the developmental analysis of cerebellar learning is, which parts of this circuit are changing between P17 and P24 in ways that affect eyeblink conditioning? Our initial approach for answering this question was to use electrical stimulation of different parts of the aforementioned auditory circuit as a CS and to compare acquisition rates among rats trained at different ages. If the stimulation CS produces strong conditioning on P17–18, then the efferent projection to the pontine nuclei is developed enough to support conditioning. On the other hand, if stimulation does not improve conditioning in the younger pups, then some part of the efferent projection to the pontine nuclei is too immature to support conditioning. Although there are clearly alternative interpretations of these hypothetical outcomes, we used this approach as a starting point in our developmental analysis of the cochlear nuclei and medial auditory thalamus.

Medial auditory thalamic input to the pontine nuclei is necessary for eyeblink conditioning in adult rats, as indicated above (Campolattaro et al., 2007; Halverson & Freeman, 2006). We used electrical stimulation of the medial auditory thalamus as a CS in rat pups trained on P17–18, P24–25, or P31–32. The stimulation parameters were the same as those used to stimulate the pontine nuclei (300 ms train, 200 Hz). Rats at each age were given paired or unpaired presentations of thalamic stimulation and a peripheral US. The efficacy of thalamic stimulation in supporting eyeblink conditioning

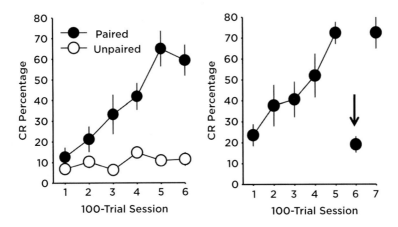

Figure 26.12 Associative eyelid conditioning in rats trained on P12–13. Left, mean conditioned response (CR) percentage across six 100-trial training sessions for rat pups given paired or unpaired presentations of pontine stimulation as a conditioned stimulus (CS) and a peripheral unconditioned stimulus (US). Right, mean conditioned response (CR) percentage for rat pups given paired presentations of pontine stimulation as a CS and a peripheral US before, during (arrow), and after infusion of muscimol into the anterior interpositus nucleus. (Campolattaro & Freeman, 2008.)

in the groups given paired training increased as a function of age (Figure 26.14). Age-related increases in conditioning with thalamic stimulation indicate that the projection from the medial auditory thalamus to the pontine nuclei continues to develop between P17 and P24. A somewhat surprising finding from this study was that the thalamopontine pathway showed further development between P24 and P31. Developmental changes in the efficacy of thalamic stimulation as a CS suggest that the development of thalamic input to the pontine nuclei plays an important role in the ontogeny of eyeblink conditioning. However, the findings do not exclude developmental changes in other inputs to the pontine nuclei or developmental changes in afferent input to the thalamus as factors that contribute to the ontogeny of eyeblink conditioning.

Developmental changes in the cochlea or cochlear nuclei are probably not important factors in the ontogeny of eyeblink conditioning because auditory conditioning and the unconditioned acoustic startle response are seen earlier than P17 (Chapter 25). It is more likely that there are developmental changes in cochlear nucleus projections to the pontine nuclei and thalamus that play a role in the development of auditory eyeblink conditioning. The cochlear nuclei send a predominantly contralateral projection to the pontine nuclei and medial auditory thalamus, in addition to the projections to the inferior colliculus and superior olive (Campolattaro et al., 2007). An experiment was conducted that used the same design as the

thalamic stimulation experiment described above, except that stimulation electrodes were placed in the left or right cochlear nuclei (Freeman & Duffel, 2008). Stimulation of the cochlear nuclei as a CS resulted in an age-related increase in eyeblink conditioning in the pups given paired training (Figure 26.15). The findings of this experiment suggest that the development of projections from the cochlear nuclei to the inferior colliculus, pontine nuclei, and thalamus may play a role in the development of eyeblink conditioning.

Our analysis of the development of the auditory CS pathway has revealed substantial ontogenetic changes in sensory input to the pontine nuclei. The precise origin of these developmental changes is still unclear but the findings of the stimulation studies suggest that developmental changes in thalamic and cochlear projections may play critical roles in the development of pontine input. Neurons in the medial auditory thalamus send direct projections to the pontine nuclei, which may be maturing between P17 and P31. In addition, development of the projections from the cochlear nuclei to the inferior colliculus, medial auditory thalamus, and pontine nuclei may also play a role in the development of auditory input to the pons.

Developmental Changes in Neuronal Interactions Within the Eyeblink Conditioning Circuitry

Cerebellar neurons are capable of supporting associative learning as early as P12 in rats. Cerebellar

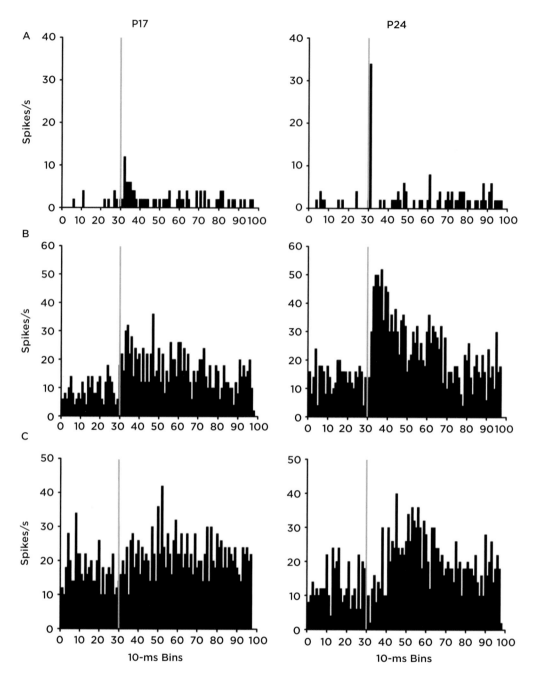

Figure 26.13 Mean firing rate (spikes per second) of representative neurons recorded from the pontine nuclei during presentations of a tone conditioned stimulus (CS) in a pretraining session. The firing frequencies of phasic (A), sustained (B), and late (C) neurons recorded from rats trained on P17 (left column) and P24 (right column) are displayed. The gray lines indicate the onset of the CS. Note the greater activity following CS onset in the phasic (A) and sustained (B) neurons on P24 relative to P17. (Freeman & Muckler, 2003.)

output to premotor and motor nuclei that generate the blink response is sufficiently developed to produce a conditioned response as early as P17. The ontogeny of eyeblink conditioning is, therefore, primarily due to the development of CS and US inputs to the cerebellum (Figure 26.16). The most proximal component of the CS pathway, the basilar pontine nuclei, shows an increase in sensory input between P17 and P24. Origins of the developmental changes in CS input are still under investigation

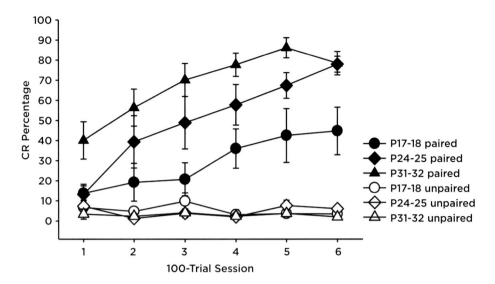

Figure 26.14 Mean conditioned response (CR) percentage for rat pups trained with medial auditory thalamic stimulation as the conditioned stimulus (CS) on P17–18 (circles), P24–25 (diamonds), or P31–32 (triangles). Pups were given either paired (black symbols) or unpaired (white symbols) presentations of the CS and an unconditioned stimulus. Note that the CR percentage increases as a function of age in the paired groups.

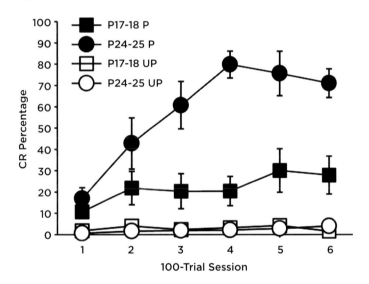

Figure 26.15 Mean conditioned response (CR) percentage for rat pups given paired (black symbols) or unpaired (white symbols) presentations of cochlear nucleus stimulation as the conditioned stimulus and the unconditioned stimulus on postnatal days (P) 17-18 (squares) or P24-25 (circles). The amount of learning in each paired group is determined by the increase in responding across training sessions and greater responding than the unpaired control groups. (Reprinted from *Developmental Psychobiology*, Vol. 50, No. 7, by John H. Freeman and Jessica W. Duffel, Copyright 2008, with permission from Wiley InterScience.)

but probably include development of the thalamo-pontine projection and the contralateral cochlear nucleus projections to the inferior colliculus, medial auditory thalamus, and pontine nuclei. The development of sensory input to the pontine nuclei in turn results in the development of CS input to the cerebellum. To the extent that cerebellar synaptic plasticity (and intrinsic excitability) is driven by excitatory mossy fiber input, developmental changes in CS input to the cerebellum influences the rate and magnitude of conditioning.

Developmental changes in the US pathway also affect the induction and maintenance of learning-related plasticity in the cerebellum. The development of climbing fiber collateral input to the cerebellar nuclei may play a role in the development of learning-related plasticity within the interpositus nucleus. In addition, the development of inhibitory

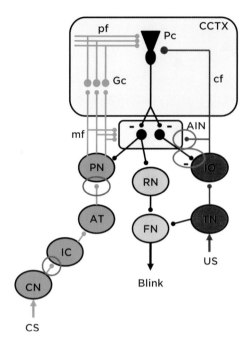

Figure 26.16 Developmental mechanisms underlying the ontogeny of eyeblink conditioning. Blue circles indicate sites of developmental change that affect the ontogeny of eyeblink conditioning. 1, climbing fiber input to the anterior interpositus nucleus (AIN) increases with age. 2, inhibitory feedback regulation of the dorsal accessory inferior olive (IO) increases with age. 3, sensory input to the pontine nuclei (PN) increases with age, resulting in progressively stronger parallel fiber (pf) input to Purkinje cells (Pc) and mossy fiber (mf) input to the AIN. 4, development of projections from the cochlear nucleus (CN) to the inferior colliculus (IC) and perhaps the medial auditory thalamus (AT) also affect conditioned stimulus (CS) input to the cerebellum. Weaker CS (green) and US (red) pathway inputs combined with an unregulated IO leads to weaker synaptic plasticity in the cerebellum (AIN and Pc), and weaker conditioning in younger rats. Abbreviations are the same as in Figure 26.1.

regulation of climbing fiber input to the cerebellar cortex may influence the development of eyeblink conditioning by reducing temporal and spatial noise and maintaining synaptic plasticity between training episodes. As a result, synaptic plasticity that is optimal for conditioned responses emerges developmentally as inhibitory feedback develops.

The ontogeny of eyeblink conditioning can be best characterized as a process that depends upon the development of the neural pathways that provide input from the CS and US to the cerebellum. Cerebellar neurons are capable of plasticity prior to receiving adequate CS input or regulated US input. Developmental mechanisms occurring in parallel within the CS and US pathways limit the

induction of neuronal plasticity in cerebellar neurons. As a result, cerebellar learning continues to develop as the stimulus input pathways develop. The developmental factors that drive the developmental changes in the CS and US pathways are currently unknown.

Role of Early Experience in the Development of the Eyeblink Conditioning Circuitry

The preceding sections of this chapter present our knowledge of *what* is developing within the eyeblink conditioning circuitry but nothing about *how* these developmental changes emerge. Many aspects of early experience may affect the development of sensory input pathways to the cerebellum and feedback to these input pathways.

Prenatally, there is a substantial amount of incidental contact with the face region from the fetus' own paws, fluid movement around the face, and contact with the fetal and uterine membranes (Brumley & Robinson, this volume). Incidental contact with the periocular area of the face may activate the eyelid muscles through what will become the eyeblink reflex. Activation of the reflex pathway could influence the development of cerebellar circuitry by somatosensory and proprioceptive input to the inferior olive and pontine nuclei. The birth process and postbirth maternal grooming could also provide sensory stimulation that influences cerebellar development.

As pups develop in the nest, they continue to receive massive amounts of sensory stimulation (Alberts, 1978; Champagne, this volume). Somatosensory stimulation from maternal care and contact with other pups during huddling and feeding probably provides almost continuous input to the pons and inferior olive. Proprioceptive feedback from the pup's movements during huddling and feeding could also provide critical sensory input for cerebellar development. Prior to ear opening, pups receive auditory input from their own movements and contact with the external ear. After 2 postnatal weeks, pups receive more auditory and visual input as the ear canals and eyes open. Early auditory and visual stimulation is abundant and complex. Pups hear various vocalizations, sounds associated with movement within the huddle and during nipple shifting, and sounds associated with animal husbandry. Visual input will typically include other pups, the dam, the cage, feeder, and human caretakers. The various sources of auditory, proprioceptive, somatosensory, and visual sensation likely influence the development of sensory inputs to the cerebellar circuits involved in eyeblink conditioning.

As mentioned earlier in this chapter, cerebellar learning is necessary for producing anticipatory or feedforward movements. Many of the early experiences described above could drive the development of the cerebellar system to provide feedforward control of the eyelids and other body parts. It would obviously be advantageous for rat pups to be able to make anticipatory eyeblinks to avoid ocular damage. Rat pups can be poked in the eye during huddling, nipple shifting, grooming, and play. We rarely see rats with missing or damaged eyes, which suggests that rat pups do in fact close their eyes in anticipation of damaging stimulation. The somatosensory and proprioceptive sensory inputs experienced during the fetal and early postnatal periods (Chapter 9) may initiate the development of cerebellar learning, which is then further elaborated as the array of threats to the eyeball increases after eye opening. Auditory and visual input can further influence the development of sensory input to the cerebellum. A straightforward prediction that follows from the preceding discussion is that eyeblink conditioning with a somatosensory CS should emerge earlier in development than conditioning with an auditory or visual CS (Rudy, 1992).

The major challenge for future research on the ontogeny of eyeblink conditioning is to elucidate the relationship between early experience and the development of cerebellar learning. To accomplish this goal, we must determine how early experience influences the development of sensory input to the pontine nuclei and the development of feedback regulation of climbing fiber activity.

Summary and Conclusions

This chapter describes the use of eyeblink conditioning to identify developmental changes in the neural mechanisms underlying associative learning. We used eyeblink conditioning to examine developmental changes in learning mechanisms because the neural circuitry underlying this form of associative learning has been characterized extensively in adult animals. The adult neural circuitry has served as a "roadmap" for identifying developmental changes within the neural circuitry that are necessary for the ontogenetic emergence of eyeblink conditioning. In addition, it is relatively straightforward to independently assess learning, sensation, and motor performance in young rats with standard eyeblink conditioning procedures.

Our neurobiological analysis of the ontogeny of eyeblink conditioning has revealed several developmental processes underlying the ontogenetic emergence of associative learning. The analysis of cerebellar neurophysiology indicated that developmental changes in performance do not play a significant role in the ontogeny of eyeblink conditioning. Stimulation studies showed that cerebellar neurons are capable of learning-related plasticity very early in development, well before learning occurs with external stimuli. Moreover, these studies, coupled with the developmental analysis of the US pathway, indicate that developmental changes in sensory inputs to the cerebellum are the primary developmental mechanisms underlying the ontogenetic emergence of eyeblink conditioning. Thus, cerebellar neurons are ready to learn before they have something to learn about. Cerebellar learning can only occur after sensory input pathways to the cerebellum have developed sufficiently.

A future direction for this research is to determine the specific developmental changes in sensory input to the pontine nuclei that are necessary for the ontogeny of cerebellar learning. In addition, it will be important to elucidate the mechanisms underlying the developmental changes in sensory input to the cerebellum. That is, we hope to determine how early experience influences the development of the eyeblink conditioning circuitry.

Acknowledgments

Preparation of this chapter was supported by grant NS38890 from the National Institute for Neurological Disorders and Stroke.

References

Alberts, J. R. (1978). Huddling by rat pups: multisensory control of contact behavior. *Journal of Comparative and Physiological Psychology, 92*, 220–230.

Alberts, J. R. (1984). Sensory-perceptual development in the Norway rat: a view toward comparative studies. In R. Kail & N. Spear (Eds.), *Comparative perspectives on memory development* (pp. 65–101). Hillsdale, NJ: Lawrence Erlbaum.

Altman, J. (1982). Morphological development of the rat cerebellum and some of its mechanisms. In S. L. Palay & V. Chan-Palay (Eds.), *The cerebellum: New vistas* (pp. 8–49). Berlin: Springer-Verlag.

Andersson, G., Garwicz, M., & Hesslow, G. (1988). Evidence for a GABA-mediated cerebellar inhibition of the inferior olive in the cat. *Experimental Brain Research, 72,* 450–456.

Attwell, P. J. E., Cooke, S. F., & Yeo, C. H. (2002). Cerebellar function in consolidation of a motor memory. *Neuron 34*, 1011–1020.

Attwell, P. J. E., Rahman, S., Ivarsson, M., & Yeo, C. H. (1999). Cerebellar cortical AMPA-kainate receptor blockade prevents performance of classically conditioned nictitating membrane responses. *Journal of Neuroscience,* 19, 1–6.

Attwell, P. J. E., Rahman, S., & Yeo, C. H. (2001). Acquisition of eyeblink conditioning is critically dependent on normal function in cerebellar cortical lobule HVI. *Journal of Neuroscience, 21*, 5715–5722.

Bao, S., Chen, L., Kim, J. J., & Thompson, R. F. (2002). Cerebellar cortical inhibition and classical eyeblink conditioning. *Proceedings of the National Academy of Sciences, 99*, 1592–1597.

Bao, S., Chen, L., & Thompson, R. F. (2000). Learning- and cerebellum-dependent neuronal activity in the lateral pontine nucleus. *Behavioral Neuroscience, 114*, 254–261.

Bengtsson, F., Jirenhed, D., Svensson, P., & Hesslow, G. (2007). Extinction of conditioned blink responses by cerebello-olivary pathway stimulation. *NeuroReport*, 18, 1479–1482.

Bengtsson, F., & Hesslow, G. (2006). Cerebellar control of the inferior olive. *Cerebellum*, 5, 7–14.

Berthier, N. E., & Moore, J. W. (1986). Cerebellar Purkinje cell activity related to the classically conditioned nictitating membrane response. *Experimental Brain Research, 63*, 341–350.

Berthier, N. E., & Moore, J. W. (1990). Activity of deep cerebellar nuclear cells during classical conditioning of nictitating membrane extension in rabbits. *Experimental Brain Research, 83*, 44–54.

Bloedel, J. R., & Ebner, T. J. (1984). Rhythmic discharge of climbing fibre afferents in response to natural peripheral stimuli in the cat. *Journal of Physiology, 352*, 129–146.

Campbell, B. A., & Spear, N. E. (1972). Ontogeny of memory. *Psychological Review, 79*, 215–236.

Campolattaro, M. M., & Freeman, J. H. (2006). Perirhinal cortex lesions impair feature-negative discrimination. *Neurobiology of Learning and Memory*, 86, 205–213.

Campolattaro, M. M., & Freeman, J. H. (2008). Eyeblink conditioning in 12-day-old-rats using pontine stimulation as the conditioned stimulus. *Proceedings of the National Academy of Sciences USA, 105*, 8120–8123..

Campolattaro, M. M., Halverson, H. E., & Freeman, J. H. (2007). Medial auditory thalamic stimulation as a conditioned stimulus for eyeblink conditioning in rats. *Learning & Memory, 14*, 152–159.

Chapman, P. F., Steinmetz, J. E., Sears, L. L., & Thompson, R. F. (1990). Effects of lidocaine injection in the interpositus nucleus and red nucleus on conditioned behavioral and neuronal responses. *Brain Research, 537*, 149–156.

Chen, L., Bao, S., Lockard, J. M., Kim, J. J., & Thompson, R. F. (1996). Impaired classical eyeblink conditioning in cerebellar-lesioned and Purkinje cell-degeneration (*pcd*) mutant mice. *Journal of Neuroscience, 16*, 2829–2838.

Christian, K. M., & Thompson, R. F. (2003). Neural substrates of eyeblink conditioning: Acquisition and retention. *Learning and Memory, 10*, 427–455.

Clark, R. E., Gohl, E. B., & Lavond, D. G. (1997). The learning-related activity that develops in the pontine nuclei during classical eye-blink conditioning is dependent on the interpositus nucleus. *Learning and Memory, 3*, 532–544.

Clark, R. E., & Lavond, D. G. (1993). Reversible lesions of the red nucleus during acquisition and retention of a classically conditioned behavior in rabbits. *Behavioral Neuroscience, 107*, 264–270.

Clark, G. A., McCormick, D. A., Lavond, D. G., & Thompson, R. F. (1984). Effects of lesions of cerebellar nuclei on conditioned behavioral and hippocampal neuronal responses. *Brain Research, 291*, 125–136.

Clark, R. E., Zhang, A. A., & Lavond, D. G. (1992). Reversible lesions of the cerebellar interpositus nucleus during acquisition and retention of a classically conditioned behavior. *Behavioral Neuroscience, 106*, 879–888.

Delgado-Garcia, J. M., & Gruart, A. (1995). Signalling properties of deep cerebellar nuclei neurones. In W. R. Ferrel & U. Proske (Eds.), *Neural control of movement* (pp. 225–232). New York: Plenum Press.

Delgado-Garcia, J. M., & Gruart, A. (2005). Firing activities of identified posterior interpositus nucleus neurons during associative learning in behaving cats. *Brain Research Reviews*, 49, 367–376.

Desmond, J. E., Rosenfield, M. E., & Moore, J. W. (1983). An HRP study of the brainstem afferents to the accessory abducens region and dorsolateral pons in rabbit: Implications for the conditioned nictitating membrane response. *Brain Research Bulletin, 10*, 747–763.

De Zeeuw, C. I., Van Alphen, A. M., Hawkins, R. K., & Ruigrok, T. J. H. (1997). Climbing fibre collaterals contact neurons in the cerebellar nuclei that provide a GABAergic feedback to the inferior olive. *Neuroscience*, 80, 981–986.

Freeman, J. H. Jr., Barone, S. Jr., & Stanton, M. E. (1995a). Disruption of cerebellar maturation by an antimitotic agent impairs the ontogeny of eyeblink conditioning in rats. *Journal of Neuroscience, 15*, 7301–7314.

Freeman, J. H. Jr., Carter, C. S., & Stanton, M. E. (1995b). Early cerebellar lesions impair eyeblink conditioning in developing rats: Differential effects of unilateral lesions on postnatal day 10 or 20. *Behavioral Neuroscience, 109*, 893–902.

Freeman, J.H., & Duffel, J. (2008). Eyeblink conditioning using cochlear nucleus stimulation as a conditioned stimulus in developing rats. *Developmental Psychobiology, 50*, 640-646.

Freeman, J. H., Halverson, H. E., & Hubbard, E. M. (2007). Inferior colliculus lesions impair eyeblink conditioning in rats. *Learning & Memory, 14*, 842–846.

Freeman, J. H., Jr., Halverson, H. E., & Poremba, A. (2005a). Differential effects of cerebellar inactivation on eyeblink conditioned excitation and inhibition. *Journal of Neuroscience, 25*, 889–895.

Freeman, J. H., Jr, & Muckler, A. S. (2003). Developmental changes in eyeblink conditioning and neuronal activity in the pontine nuclei. *Learning & Memory, 10*, 337–345.

Freeman, J. H., Jr., & Nicholson, D. A. (2000). Developmental changes in eye-blink conditioning and neuronal activity in the cerebellar interpositus nucleus. *Journal of Neuroscience, 20*, 813–819.

Freeman, J. H., Jr., & Rabinak, C. A. (2004). Eyeblink conditioning in rats using pontine stimulation as a conditioned stimulus. *Integrative Physiological & Behavioral Science, 39*, 180–191.

Freeman, J. H., Jr., Rabinak, C. A., & Campolattaro, M. (2005b). Pontine stimulation overcomes developmental limitations in the neural mechanisms of eyeblink conditioning. *Learning & Memory, 12*, 255–259.

Galvez, R., Weible, A. P., & Disterhoft, J. F. (2007). Cortical barrel lesions impair whisker-CS trace eyeblink conditioning. *Learning & Memory, 14*, 94–100.

Galvez, R., Weiss, C., Weible, A. P., & Disterhoft, J. F. (2006). Vibrissa-signaled eyeblink conditioning induces somatosensory cortical plasticity. *Journal of Neuroscience, 26*, 6062–6068.

Garcia, K. S., & Mauk, M. D. (1998). Pharmacological analysis of cerebellar contributions to the timing and expression of conditioned eyelid responses. *Neuropharmacology, 37*, 471–480.

Geinisman, Y., Gundersen, H. J., van der Zee, E., & West, M. J. (1996). Unbiased stereological estimation of the total number of synapses in a brain region. *Journal of Neurocytology, 25*, 805–819.

Gemberling, G. A., & Domjan, M. (1982). Selective associations in one-day-old rats: Tast-toxicosis and texture-shock aversion learning. *Journal of Comparative and Physiological Psychology, 96*, 105–113.

Gormezano, I., Kehoe, E. J., & Marshall, B. S. (1983). Twenty years of classical conditioning research with the rabbit. *Progress in Psychobiology and Physiological Psychology, 10*, 197–275.

Gormezano, I., Schneiderman, N., Deaux, E. G., & Fuentes, I. (1962). Nictitating membrane: Classical conditioning and extinction in the albino rabbit. *Science, 138*, 33–34.

Gottlieb, G. (1971). Ontogeneis of sensory function in birds and mammals. In E. Tobach, L. Aronson, & E. Shaw (Eds.), *The biopsychology of development* (pp. 211–247). New York: Academic Press.

Gould, T. J., & Steinmetz, J. E. (1994). Multiple-unit activity from rabbit cerebellar cortex and interpositus nucleus during classical discrimination / reversal eyelid conditioning. *Brain Research, 652*, 98–106.

Gould, T. J., & Steinmetz, J. E. (1996). Changes in rabbit cerebellar cortical and interpositus nucleus activity during acquisition, extinction, and backward classical eyelid conditioning. *Neurobiology of Learning and Memory, 65*, 17–34.

Green, J. T., & Steinmetz, J. E. (2005). Purkinje cell activity in the cerebellar anterior lobe after rabbit eyeblink conditioning. *Learning & Memory 12*, 260–269.

Gundersen, H. J. (1986). Stereology of arbitrary particles. A review of unbiased number and size estimators and the presentation of some new ones, in memory of William R. Thompson. *Journal of Microscopy, 143*, 3–45.

Halverson, H. E., & Freeman, J. H. (2006). Medial auditory thalamic nuclei are necessary for eyeblink conditioning. *Behavioral Neuroscience, 120*, 880–887.

Halverson, H. E., Poremba, A., & Freeman, J. H. (2008). Medial auditory thalamus inactivation prevents acquisition and retention of eyeblink conditioning. *Learning & Memory, 15*, 532–538.

Haroutunian, V., & Campbell, B. A. (1979). Emergence of interoceptive and exteroceptive control of behavior in rats. *Science, 205*, 927–929.

Harvey, J. A., Land, T., & McMaster, S. E. (1984). Anatomical study of the rabbit's corneal-VIth nerve reflex: Connections between cornea, trigeminal sensory complex, and the abducens and accessory abducens nuclei. *Brain Research, 301*, 307–321.

Harvey, J. A., Welsh, J. P., Yeo, C. H., & Romano, A. G. (1993). Recoverable and nonrecoverable deficits in conditioned responses after cerebellar cortical lesions. *Journal of Neuroscience, 13*, 1624–1635.

Hesslow, G. (1994). Correspondence between climbing fibre input and motor output in eyeblink-related areas in cat cerebellar cortex. *Journal of Physiology, 476*, 229–244.

Hesslow, G., & Ivarsson, M. (1994). Suppression of cerebellar Purkinje cells during conditioned responses in ferrets. *NeuroReport, 5*, 649–652.

Hesslow, G., & Ivarsson, M. (1996). Inhibition of the inferior olive during conditioned responses in the decerebrate ferret. *Experimental Brain Research*, 110, 36–46.

Hesslow, G., Svensson, P., & Ivarsson, M. (1999). Learned movements elicited by direct stimulation of cerebellar mossy fiber afferents. *Neuron, 24*, 179–185.

Hoffman, H., Molina, J. C., Kucharski, D., & Spear, N. E. (1987). Further examination of ontogenetic limitations on conditioned taste aversion. *Developmental Psychobiology, 20*, 455–463.

Hunt, P., & Campbell, B. A. (1997). Developmental dissociation of the components of conditioned fear. In M. E. Bouton & M. S. Fanselow (Eds.), *Learning, motivation and cognition: The functional behaviorism of Robert C. Bolles* (pp. 53–74). Washington, DC: American Psychological Association.

Hyson, R. L., & Rudy, J. W. (1984). Ontogenesis of leanring: II. Variation in the rat's reflexive and learned responses to acoustic stimulation. *Developmental Psychobiology, 17*, 263–283.

Ito, M., Yoshida, M., Obata, K., Kawai, N., & Udo, M. (1970). Inhibitory control of intracerebellar nuclei by the Purkinje cell axons. *Experimental Brain Research,10*, 64–80.

Jirenhed, D., Bengtsson, F., & Hesslow, G. (2007). Acquisition, extinction, and reacquisition of a cerebellar cortical memory trace. *Journal of Neuroscience*, 27, 2493–2502.

Johanson, I. B., & Teicher, M. H. (1980). Classical conditioning of an odor preference in 3-day-old rats. *Behavioral and Neural Biology, 29*, 132–136.

Kenyon, G. T., Medina, J. F., & Mauk, M. D. (1998). A mathematical model of the cerebellar–olivary system II. Motor adaptation through systematic disruption of climbing fiber equilibrium. *Journal of Computational Neuroscience, 5*, 71–90.

Kim, J. J., Clark, R. E., & Thompson, R. F. (1995). Hippocampectomy impairs the memory of recently, but not remotely, acquired trace eyeblink conditioned responses. *Behavioral Neuroscience, 109*, 195–203.

Kim, J. J., Krupa, D. J., & Thompson, R. F. (1998). Inhibitory cerebello-olivary projections and blocking effect in classical conditioning. *Science, 279*, 570–573.

Kitai, S. T., McCrea, R. A., Preston, R. J., & Bishop, G. A. (1977). Electrophysiological and horseradish peroxidase studies of precerebellar afferents to the nucleus interpositus anterior. I. Climbing fiber system. *Brain Research, 122*, 197–214.

Kleim, J. A., Freeman, J. H., Jr., Bruneau, R., Nolan, B.C., Cooper, N. R., Zook, A., et al. (2002). Synapse formation is associated with memory storage in the cerebellum. *Proceedings of the National Academy of Sciences USA, 99*, 13228–13231.

Knowlton, B. J. & Thompson, R. F. (1988). Microinjections of local anesthetic into the pontine nuclei reduce the amplitude of the classically conditioned eyelid response. *Physiology and Behavior, 43*, 855–857.

Knowlton, B. J., & Thompson, R. F. (1992). Conditioning using a cerebral cortical conditioned stimulus is dependent on the cerebellum and brain stem circuitry. *Behavioral Neuroscience, 106*, 509–517.

Knowlton, B. J., Thompson, J. K., & Thompson, R. F. (1993). Projections from the auditory cortex to the pontine nuclei in the rabbit. *Behavioural Brain Research, 56*, 23–30.

Krupa, D. J., & Thompson, R. F. (1995). Inactivation of the superior cerebellar peduncle blocks expression but not acquisition of the rabbit's classically conditioned eye-blink response. *Proceedings of the. National Academy of Sciences, 92*, 5097–5101.

Krupa, D. J., & Thompson, R. F. (1997). Reversible inactivation of the cerebellar interpositus nucleus completely prevents acquisition of the classically conditioned eye-blink response. *Learning and Memory, 3*, 545–556.

Krupa, D. J., Thompson, J. K., & Thompson, R. F. (1993). Localization of a memory trace in the mammalian brain. *Science, 260*, 989–991.

Lang, E. J., Sugihara, I., & Llinas, R. (1996). GABAergic modulation of complex spike activity by the cerebellar nucleoolivary pathway in rat. Journal of Neurophysiology, *76*, 255–275.

Lavond, D. G., Hembree, T. L., & Thompson, R. F. (1985). Effect of kanic acid lesions of the cerebellar interpositus nucleus on eyelid conditioning in the rabbit, *Brain Research, 326*, 179–182.

Lavond, D. G., Steinmetz, J. E., Yokaitis, M. H., & Thompson, R. F. (1987). Reacquisition of classical conditioning after removal of cerebellar cortex. *Experimental Brain Research, 67*, 569–593.

Lavond, D. G., & Steinmetz, J. E. (1989). Acquisition of classical conditioning without cerebellar cortex. *Behavioural Brain Research, 33*, 113–164.

Lewis, J. L., LoTurco, J. J., & Solomon, P. R. (1987). Lesions of the middle cerebellar peduncle disrupt acquisition and retention of the rabbit's classically conditioned nictitating membrane response. *Behavioral Neuroscience, 101*, 151–157.

Llinas, R. (1974). Eighteenth Bowditch lecture. Motor aspects of cerebellar control. *Physiologist, 17*, 19–46.

Llinas, R., Baker, R., & Sotelo, C. (1974). Electrotonic coupling between neurons in cat inferior olive. *Journal of Neurophysiology, 3*, 560–571.

Llinas, R., & Sasaki, K. (1989). The functional organization of the olivocerebellar system as examined by multiple Purkinje cell recordings. *European Journal of Neuroscience, 1*, 587–602.

Llinas, R., & Yarom, Y. (1981a). Electrophysiology of mammalian inferior olivary neurones *in vitro*. Different types of voltage-dependent ionic conductances. *Journal of Physiology (London), 315*, 549–567.

Llinas, R., & Yarom, Y. (1981b). Properties and distribution of ionic conductances generating electroresponsiveness of mammalian inferior olivary neurones *in vitro*. *Journal of Physiology (London), 315*, 569–584.

Llinas, R., & Yarom, Y. (1986). Oscillatory properties of guinea-pig inferior olivary neurones and their pharmacological modulation: an in vitro study. *Journal of Physiology (London), 376*, 163–182.

Mauk, M. D., & Donegan, N. H. (1997). A model of Pavlovian eyelid conditioning based on the synaptic organization of the cerebellum. *Learning & Memory, 3*, 130–158.

Mauk, M. D., Steinmetz, J. E., & Thompson, R. F. (1986). Classical conditioning using stimulation of the inferior olive as the unconditioned stimulus. *Proceedings of the National Academy of Sciences USA, 83*, 5349–5353.

Mauk, M. D., & Thompson, R. F. (1987). Retention of classically conditioned eyelid responses following acute decerebration. *Brain Research, 403*, 89–95.

McCormick, D. A., Clark, G. A., Lavond, D. G., & Thompson, R. F. (1982a). Initial localization of the memory trace for a basic form of learning. *Proceedings of the National Academy of Sciences USA, 79*, 2731–2735.

McCormick, D. A., Guyer, P. E., & Thompson, R. F. (1982b). Superior cerebellar peduncle lesions selectively abolish the ipsilateral classically conditioned nictitating membrane/eyelid response of the rabbit. *Brain Research, 244*, 347–350.

McCormick, D. A., Steinmetz, J. E., & Thompson, R. F. (1985). Lesions of the inferior olivary complex cause extinction of the classically conditioned eye blink response. *Brain Research, 359*, 120–130.

McCormick, D. A., & Thompson, R. F. (1984a). Cerebellum: essential involvement in the classically conditioned eyelid response. *Science, 223*, 296–299.

McCormick, D. A., & Thompson, R. F. (1984b). Neuronal responses of the rabbit cerebellum during acquisition and performance of a classically conditioned nictitating membrane-eyelid response. *Journal of Neuroscience,11*, 2811–2822.

Medina, J. F., & Mauk, M. D. (1999). Simulations of cerebellar motor learning: computational analysis of plasticity at the mossy fiber to deep nucleus synapse. *Journal of Neuroscience, 19*, 7140–7151.

Medina, J. F., & Mauk, M. D. (2000). Computer simulation of cerebellar information processing. *Nature Neuroscience, 3*, 1205–1211.

Medina, J. F., Nores, W. L., & Mauk, M. D. (2002). Inhibition of climbing fibres is a signal for the extinction of conditioned eyelid responses. *Nature, 416*, 330–333.

Mihailoff, G. A. (1993). Cerebellar nuclear projections from the basilar pontine nuclei and nucleus reticularis tegmenti pontis as demonstrated with PHA-L tracing in the rat. *Journal of Comparative Neurology, 330*, 130–146.

Moye, T. B., & Rudy, J. W. (1985). Ontogenesis of learning: VI. Learned and unlearned responses to visual stimulation in the infant hooded rat. *Developmental Psychobiology, 18*, 395–409.

Moyer, J. R., Deyo, R. A., & Disterhoft, J. F. (1990). Hippocampectomy disrupts trace eye-blink conditioning in rabbits. *Behavioral Neuroscience, 104*, 243–252.

Nicholson, D. A., & Freeman, J. H., Jr. (2000). Developmental changes in eye-blink conditioning and neuronal activity in the inferior olive. *Journal of Neuroscience, 20*, 8218–8226.

Nicholson, D. A. & Freeman, J. H., Jr. (2002). Neuronal correlates of conditioned inhibition of the eyeblink response in the anterior interpositus nucleus. *Behavioral Neuroscience, 116*, 22–36.

Nicholson, D. A, & Freeman, J. H. Jr. (2003a). Addition of inhibition in the olivocerebellar system and the ontogeny of a motor memory. *Nature Neuroscience, 6*, 532–537.

Nicholson, D. A., & Freeman, J. H., Jr. (2003b). Developmental changes in evoked Purkinje cell complex spike responses. *Journal of Neurophysiology, 90*, 2349–2357.

Nicholson, D. A., & Freeman, J. H., Jr. (2004a). Developmental changes in eyeblink conditioning and simple spike activity in the cerebellar cortex. *Developmental Psychobiology, 44*, 45–57.

Nicholson, D. A., & Freeman, J. H., Jr. (2004b). Selective developmental increase in the climbing fiber input to the cerebellar interpositus nucleus in rats. *Behavioral Neuroscience, 118*, 1111–1116.

Nolan, B. C., & Freeman, J. H., Jr. (2005). Purkinje cell loss by OX7-saporin impairs excitatory and inhibitory eyeblink conditioning. *Behavioral Neuroscience, 119*, 190–201.

Nolan, B. C., & Freeman, J. H. (2006). Purkinje cell loss by OX7-saporin impairs acquisition and extinction of eyeblink conditioning. *Learning & Memory, 13*, 359–365.

Nowak, A. J., Kehoe, E. J., Macrae, M., & Gormezano, I. (1999). Conditioning and reflex modification of the rabbit nictitating membrane response using electrical stimulation in auditory nuclei. *Behavioural Brain Research, 105*, 189–198.

Oakley, D. A., & Russell, I. S. (1972). Neocortical lesions and Pavlovian conditioning. *Physiology & Behavior, 8*, 915–926.

Oakley, D. A., & Russell, I. S. (1977). Subcortical storage of Pavlovian conditioning in the rabbit. *Physiology & Behavior, 18*, 931–937.

O'Connor, K. N., Allison, T. L., Rosenfield, M. E., & Moore, J. W. (1997). Neural activity in the medial geniculate nucleus during auditory trace conditioning. *Experimental Brain Research, 113*, 534–556.

Ohyama, T., & Mauk, M. D. (2001). Latent acquisition of timed responses in cerebellar cortex. *Journal of Neuroscience, 21*, 682–690.

Ohyama, T., Nores, W. L., & Mauk, M. D. (2003). Stimulus generalization of conditioned eyelid responses produced without cerebellar cortex: Implications for plasticity in the cerebellar nuclei. *Learning & Memory, 10*, 346–354.

Ohyama, T., Nores, W. L., Medina, J. F., Riusech, F. A., & Mauk, M. D. (2006). Learning-induced plasticity in deep cerebellar nucleus. *Journal of Neuroscience, 26*, 12656–12663.

Paczkowski, C., Ivkovich, D., & Stanton, M. E. (1999). Ontogeny of eyeblink conditioning using a visual conditioned stimulus. *Developmental Psychobiology, 35*, 253–263.

Patterson, M. M. (1969). *The effects of intracranial CS and fluctuating ISI on the classically conditioned rabbit nictitating membrane response.* Dissertation, University of Iowa.

Patterson, M. M. (1970). Classical conditioning of the rabbit's (oryctolagus cuniculus) nictitating membrane response with fluctuating ISI and intracranial CS. *Journal of Comparative and Physiological Psychology, 72*, 193–202.

Rosenfield, M. E., & Moore, J. W. (1983). Red nucleus lesions disrupt the classically conditioned nictitating membrane response in rabbits. *Behavioural Brain Research, 10*, 393–398.

Rudy, J. W. (1992). Development of learning: from elemental to configural associative networks. In C. Rovee-Collier & L. P. Lipsitt (Eds.), *Advances in infancy research* (pp. 247–289). New Jersey: ABLEX Publishing Corporation.

Rudy, J. W., & Cheatle, M. D. (1977). Odor-aversion learning in neonatal rats. *Science, 198*, 845–846.

Sananes, C. B., Gaddy, J. R., & Campbell, B. A. (1988). Ontogeny of conditioned heart rate to an olfactory stimulus. *Developmental Psychobiology, 21*, 117–133.

Schneiderman, N., Fuentes, I., & Gormezano, I. (1962). Acquisition and extinction of the classically conditioning eyelid response in the albino rabbit. *Science, 136*, 650–652.

Schreurs, B. G. (1988). Stimulation of the spinal trigeminal nucleus supports classical conditioning of the rabbit's nictitating membrane response. *Behavioral Neuroscience, 102*, 163–172.

Sears, L. L., & Steinmetz, J. E. (1991). Dorsal accessory inferior olive activity diminishes during acquisition of the rabbit classically conditioned eyelid response. *Brain Research, 545*, 114–122.

Shinoda, Y., Sugiuchi, Y., Futami, T., & Izawa, R. (1992). Axon collaterals of mossy fibers from the pontine nucleus in the cerebellar dentate nucleus. *Journal of Neurophysiology, 67*, 547–560.

Smotherman, W. P. (1982). Odor aversion learning by the rat fetus. *Physiology & Behavior, 29*, 769–771.

Smotherman, W. P., & Robinson, S. R. (1985). The rat fetus in its environment: Behavioral adjustments to novel, familiar, aversive, and conditioned stimuli presented in utero. *Behavioral Neuroscience, 99*, 521–530.

Stanton, M. E. (2000). Multiple memory systems, development and conditioning. *Behavioural Brain Research, 110*, 25–37.

Stanton, M. E., & Freeman, J. H., Jr. (2000). Developmental studies of eyeblink conditioning in a rat model. In D. S. Woodruff-Pak & J. E. Steinmetz (Eds.), *Eyeblink classical conditioning: Animal* (pp. 105–134). Amsterdam: Kluwer Academic.

Stanton, M. E., Freeman, J. H., Jr., & Skelton, R. W. (1992). Eyeblink conditioning in the developing rat. *Behavioral Neuroscience, 106*, 657–665.

Steinmetz, J. E. (1990). Neuronal activity in the rabbit interpositus nucleus during classical NM-conditioning with a pontine-nucleus-stimulation CS. *Psychological Science, 1*, 378–382.

Steinmetz, J. E., Rosen, D. J., Chapman, P. F., Lavond, D. G., & Thompson, R. F. (1986). Classical conditioning of the rabbit eyelid response with a mossy fiber stimulation CS. I. Pontine nuclei and middle cerebellar peduncle stimulation. *Behavioral Neuroscience, 100*, 878–887.

Steinmetz, J. E., Logan, C. G., Rosen, D. J., Thompson, J. K., Lavond, D. G., & Thompson, R. F. (1987). Initial localization of the acoustic conditioned stimulus projection system to the cerebellum essential for classical eyelid conditioning. *Proceedings of The National Academy of Sciences, 84*, 3531–3535.

Steinmetz, J. E., Lavond, D. G., & Thompson, R. F. (1989). Classical conditioning in rabbits using pontine nucleus stimulation as a conditioned stimulus and inferior olive stimulation as an unconditioned stimulus. *Synapse, 3*, 225–233.

Steinmetz, J. E., Lavond, D. G., Ivkovich, D., Logan, C. G., & Thompson, R. F. (1992). Disruption of classical eyelid conditioning after cerebellar lesions: Damage to a memory trace system or simple performance deficit? *Journal of Neuroscience, 12*, 4403–4426.

Steinmetz, J. E., & Sengelaub, D. R. (1992). Possible conditioned stimulus pathway for classical eyelid conditioning in rabbits. *Behavioral and Neural Biology, 57*, 103–115.

Sterio, D. C. (1984). The unbiased estimation of number and sizes of arbitrary particles using the disector. *Journal of Microscopy, 134*, 127–136.

Sugihara, I., Wu, H. S., & Shinoda, Y. (2001). The entire trajectories of single olivocerebellar axons in the cerebellar cortex and their contribution to cerebellar compartmentalization. *Journal of Neuroscience, 21*, 7715–7723.

Thompson, R. F. (1986). The neurobiology of learning and memory. *Science, 233*, 941–947.

Thompson, R. F. (2005). In search of memory traces. *Annual Review of Psychology, 56*, 1–23.

Thompson, R. F., Thompson, J. K., Kim, J. J., Krupa, D. J., & Shinkman, P. G. (1998). The nature of reinforcement in cerebellar learning. *Neurobiology of Learning & Memory, 70*, 150–176.

Tracy, J. A., Thompson, J. K., Krupa, D. J., & Thompson, R. F. (1998). Evidence of plasticity in the pontocerebellar conditioned stimulus pathway during classical conditioning of the eyeblink response in the rabbit. *Behavioral Neuroscience, 112*, 267–85.

Van der Want, J. J. L., Wiklund, L., Guegan, M., Ruigrok, T., & Voogd, J. (1989). Anterograde tracing of the rat olivocerebellar system with Phaseolus vulgaris leucoagglutinin (PHA-L). Demonstration of climbing fiber collateral innervation of the cerebellar nuclei. *Journal of Comparative Neurology, 288*, 1–18.

Van Ham, J. J., & Yeo, C. H. (1996). The central distribution of primary afferents from the external eyelids, conjunctiva, and cornea in the rabbit, studied using WGA-HRP and B-HRP as transganglionic tracers. *Experimental Neurology, 142*, 217–225.

Vogt, M. B., & Rudy, J. W. (1984). Ontogenesis of learning: I. variation in the rat's reflexive and learned responses to gustatory stimulation. *Developmental Psychobiology, 17*, 11–33.

Weible, A. P., McEchron, M. D., & Disterhoft, J. F. (2000). Cortical involvement in acquisition and extinction of trace eyeblink conditioning. *Behavioral Neuroscience, 114*, 1058–1067.

Weible, A. P., Weiss, C., & Disterhoft, J. F. (2003). Activity profiles of single neurons in caudal anterior cingulate cortex during trace eyeblink conditioning in the rabbit. *Journal of Neurophysiology, 90*, 599–612.

Welsh J. P., & Harvey, J. A. (1998). Acute inactivation of the inferior olive blocks associative learning. *European Journal of Neuroscience, 10*, 3321–3332.

Woodruff-Pak, D. S., Lavond, D. G., Logan, C. G., Steinmetz, J. E., & Thompson, R. F. (1993). Cerebellar cortical lesions and reacquisition in classical conditioning of the nictitating membrane response in rabbits. *Brain Research, 608*, 67–77.

Yeo, C. H., Hardiman, M. J., & Glickstein, M. (1985). Classical conditioning of the nictitating membrane response of the rabbit. I. Lesions of the cerebellar nuclei. *Experimental Brain Research, 60*, 87–98.

Yeo, C. H., Hardiman, M. J., & Glickstein, M. (1986). Classical conditioning of the nictitating membrane response of the rabbit. IV. Lesions of the inferior olive. *Experimental Brain Research, 63*, 81–92.

Developmental Neurobiology of Olfactory Preference and Avoidance Learning

Regina M. Sullivan, Stephanie Moriceau, Tania Roth, *and* Kiseko Shionoya

Abstract

Infants from a myriad of species attach to their caregiver regardless of the quality of care received, although the quality of care influences development of the stress system. To better understand this relationship, this chapter characterizes attachment learning and the supporting neural circuit in infant rat pups. During early life, odors paired with pain paradoxically produce subsequent approach responses to the odor and attachment. The neural circuit supporting this attachment learning involves the olfactory bulb encoding the preference learning and suppression of the amygdala to prevent the aversion learning. Increasing the stress hormone corticosterone during acquisition or decreasing endogenous opioids during consolidation prevents this odor approach learning. These data suggest that early life attachment is readily learned and supported by both increased opioids and decreased stress.

Keywords: stress system, attachment learning, odors, pain, olfactory bulb, amygdale, corticosterone, endogenous opioids

Introduction

The altricial infant's helpless and passive appearance is deceptive. Indeed, while parental skills are required, the active participation of the infant is also required for successful mother–infant interactions. For example, the newborn infant rat must learn about the mother's odor for the expression of behaviors critical for survival such as orientation and nipple attachment. While the mother certainly needs to make herself accessible, the infant must successfully express a very specific sequence of behaviors for successful nipple attachment: navigate to the nipple (pushing other pups away at times), grasp the nipple, and suck to procure milk. While this learning-based system may seem like a precarious situation for survival of a species, the robust and rapid neonatal learning system seems presumably evolved to ensure that this life-sustaining learning will occur. Here we describe the learning system of infant rats that is limited during the sensitive period (first 9 days of life), which exhibits potentiated odor preference learning and supports the sequence of behaviors required for survival related behaviors. Additionally, there is an attenuated aversion learning component of this infant learning system, which directs pups to learn to prefer the maternal odor, while preventing them from learning to avoid or inhibit responses to the maternal odor.

Potentiated Odor Preference Learning

The early life of many altricial species is characterized by heightened learning, such as that occuring in imprinting (Bolhuis, 1999; Hess,

1962; Martin, 1978; Salzen, 1970; Wilbrecht & Nottebohm, 2004). Rat pups are no exception and show robust, rapid learning of odors and somatosensory stimuli. Specifically, neonatal pups can learn to prefer an odor within minutes with a wide variety of stimuli functioning as a reward, such as warmth, tactile stimulation (presumably mimics maternal licking of pups), and milk (Alberts & May, 1984; Brake, 1981; Distal & Hudson, 1985; Johanson & Hall, 1982; Johanson & Teicher, 1980; McLean, Darby-King, Sullivan, & King, 1993; Okutani, Zhang, Otsuka, Yagi, & Kaba, 2003; Pedersen, Williams, & Blass, 1982; Polan & Hofer, 1999; Singh & Hofer, 1978; Spear & Rudy, 1991; Sullivan, 2003; Sullivan, Brake, Hofer, & Williams, 1986a; Sullivan & Hall, 1988; Sullivan, Hofer, & Brake, 1986b; Sullivan, McGaugh, & Leon, 1991; Sullivan, Wilson, Wong, Correa, & Leon, 1990; Thoman, Wetzel, & Levine, 1968; Weldon, Travis, & Kennedy, 1991). Once an odor is learned, that odor is capable of functioning as maternal odor and supports approach behaviors, huddling with siblings and nipple attachment. This heightened learning combined with limited sensory (visual or auditory sensory systems emerge after postnatal day PN12) and motor (walking emerges around PN10) function probably limits young pups exposures to extra nest odors while ensuring prolonged exposure to maternal odors (Bolles & Woods, 1965; Hofer, 1981).

The task of learning the maternal odor is lessened by fetal exposure to amniotic fluid, which the fetus tastes and smells during swallowing of the fluid (Bradley & Mistretta, 1973). The overlap in chemical composition of amniotic fluid and maternal odor may ease the abrupt transition from prenatal to postnatal life and prime pups for the postnatal olfactory maternal odor learning (Blass, 1990; Hepper, 1987; Lecanuet & Schaal, 1996; Mennella, Johnson, & Beauchamp, 1995; Pedersen, Steward, Greer, & Shepherd, 1983; Schaal, Marlier, & Soussignan, 1995). The fetus learns about these odors, which will later control the postnatal infant's behaviors (Smotherman, 1982; Spear & Molina, 2005). Furthermore, procedures that retard or inhibit learning in adults (preexposure conditioned stimulus [CS] alone called latent inhibition and uncorrelated presentations of the CS and reward called learned irrelevance) have been found to either enhance or have no effect on the young infant rat's learning (Campbell & Spear, 1972; Hoffmann & Spear, 1989; Rescorla, 1967, 1988; Rescorla & Wagner, 1972; Rush, Robinette, & Stanton, 2001; Siegel &

Domjan, 1971; Spear & Rudy, 1991; Stanton, 2000; Stanton, Fox, & Carter, 1998; Stanton & Freeman, 2000). Additionally, simultaneous presentation of stimuli enhances sensory associations in pups, while sequential presentations are optimal in older pups and adults (Cheslock, Varlinskaya, High, & Spear, 2003; Barr, Marrott, & Rovee-Collier, 2003). Together, pups' limited sensory/motor capabilities, as well as unique learning characteristics, potentiates learning that helps maintain their proximity to the nest and maternal odors and elicit behaviors for attachment to the mother.

This rapid odor learning in early life appears to be coded in the olfactory bulb and occurs with Kucharski & Hall (1987) natural maternal odor, artificial odors experienced in the nest, as well as to odors in controlled learning experiments outside the nest (Johnson, Woo, Duong, Nguyen, & Leon, 1995; Leon, Galef, & Behse, 1977; Moriceau & Sullivan, 2004b, 2006; Roth & Sullivan, 2005; Sullivan et al., 1990; Sullivan & Leon, 1986; Wilson & Leon, 1988; Wilson & Sullivan, 1990, 1991; Wilson, Sullivan, & Leon, 1987; Woo, Coopersmith, & Leon, 1987; Woo, Oshita, & Leon, 1996; Yuan, Harley, McLean, & Knopfel, 2003). The modified olfactory bulb response is characterized by immediate-early gene activity (c-*fos*), intrinsic optical imaging (neural activity sensitive fluorescent probes), enhanced 2-deoxyglucose (2-DG) uptake (Figure 27.1), and modified single-unit response patterns of the bulb's output neurons, mitral/tufted cells. Similarly to the behavioral changes in attachment, the learning occurs during early postnatal life but is retained into adulthood (Pager, 1974; Woo & Leon, 1988; Sevelinges et al., 2007), although the role of the odor changes from attachment to the mothers during infancy to reproduction in adulthood (Fillion & Blass, 1986; Moore, Jordan, & Wong, 1996).

These olfactory-learned behaviors, as well as the olfactory bulb learning–induced changes are dependent on high norepinephrine (NE) levels from the locus coeruleus (LC) (Langdon, Harley, & McLean, 1997; Sullivan, Stackenwalt, Nasr, Lemon, & Wilson, 2000b; Sullivan, Wilson, Lemon & Gerhard, 1994; Sullivan, Zyzak, Skierkowski, & Wilson, 1992; Yuan, Harley, Bruce, Darby-King, & McLean, 2000). NE is not intrinsic to the olfactory bulb but is received from the LC (McLean & Shipley, 1991; Shipley, Halloran, & De la Torre, 1985). Sensory stimulation (i.e., 1-s stroking, shock, or air puff) elicits abundant NE release from

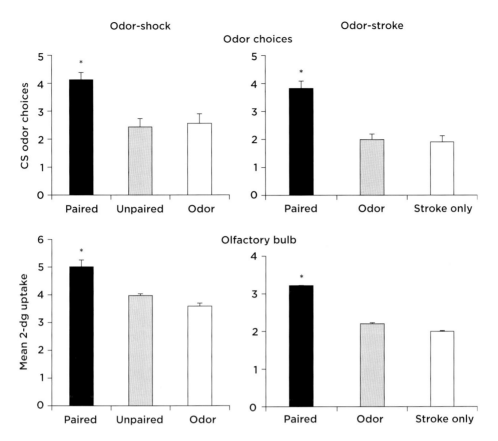

Figure 27.1 (A) After sensitive period (P7) odor–stroke or odor–0.5 mA shock conditioning, paired pups show a preference for the conditioned odor in a Y-maze test. (B) Representative olfactory bulb sections show increased 2-DG in pups receiving paired odor–stroke or odor–0.5 mA shock conditioning compared to control unpaired conditioning (± standard error, * indicates significance at the $p < 0.5$ level).

the neonatal LC due to its prolonged (20–30 s) responses, which is in sharp contrast to the brief millisecond response found in older pups and adults with the same stimulation (Nakamura, Kimura, & Sakaguchi, 1987; Nakamura & Sakaguchi, 1990; Pieribone, Nicholas, Dagerlind, & Hokfelt,1994; Scheinin et al., 1994). Indeed, as measured by olfactory bulb microdialysis, early-life olfactory learning is associated with a dramatic NE increase into the olfactory bulb from the LC (Rangel & Leon, 1995). This high level of NE is both necessary and sufficient for both neonatal somatosensory and olfactory conditioning in young pups (Langdon et al., 1997; Landers & Sullivan, 1999a, 1999b; Sullivan et al., 1992, 1994, 2000b; Yuan et al., 2000). With maturation (>PN10), NE release from the LC is no longer sufficient to produce odor preference learning (Moriceau & Sullivan, 2004a) presumably due to the loss of the prolonged LC response to sensory stimulation (Nakamura et al.,

1987; Nakamura & Sakaguchi, 1990; Scheinin et al., 1994). This difference in odor learning appears to be due to functional changes in the maturing LC associated with emergence of inhibitory $\alpha2$ noradrenergic autoreceptors that quickly terminate the LC's excitatory responses to stimuli. NE now begins to plays a more modulatory role by enhancing or attenuating memories in a manner similar to adults (Harris & Fitzgerald, 1991; Liang, Chen, & Huang, 1995; Moffat, Suh, & Fleming, 1993; Quirarte, Roozendaal, & McGaugh, 1997; Roozendaal, Nguyen, Power, & McGaugh, 1999; Sara, Dyon-Laurent, & Herve, 1995; Selden, Everitt, Jarrard, & Robbins, 1990).

Olfactory bulb NE can be modulated by both serotonin (5-HT) and opiates and both uniquely enhance pup odor preference learning during early life (McLean et al,, 1993; Price, Darby-King, Harley, & McLean, 1998; Roth et al., 2006). Specifically, opioids increase during normal mother–infant interactions (Blass & Fitzgerald, 1988; Gray, Watt, & Blass, 2000; Mooncey, Giannakoulopoulos, & Glover, 1997; Weller & Feldman, 2003) and facilitate pups learning of the maternal odor. The necessity of opioids for odor preference learning was demonstrated both during acquisition and consolidation of odor–stroke (tactile stimulation mimicking maternal grooming of pups) and odor–0.5-mA shock preference conditioning in sensitive period pups. Specifically, disruption of learning was seen when opioid receptor antagonists were injected either systemically or directly into the olfactory bulb, suggesting that opioids facilitate the acquisition and memory consolidation of neonatally learned odors (Roth & Sullivan, 2001, 2003; Roth, Moriceau, & Sullivan, 2006; unpublished observation).

5-HT also appears important in neonatal odor preference learning since depleting the olfactory bulb of 5HT disrupts odor preference learning (McLean et al., 1993). However, while 5-HT without NE is insufficient to support odor learning, it appears to facilitate olfactory bulb NE to support the learning-induced behavioral and olfactory bulb neural changes (Langdon et al., 1997). It should be noted that NE action appears, at least in part, due to suppression of inhibitory GABA (Okutani et al., 2003). Indeed, NE appears to maintain the neural activity of mitral/tufted cells, which are the primary output neurons of the olfactory bulb, both directly and indirectly by blocking the GABA-mediated inhibition of mitral cells. This heightened activity of mitral/tufted cells enables the continued responsiveness to odors that is associated with the olfactory bulb learning–induced neural changes (Wilson et al., 1987).

Attenuation of Aversive /Avoidance/Fear Learning in Early Life

While less understood, learning in early life is also characterized by limitations on aversive learning. For example, during imprinting, chicks do not learn to avoid a surrogate mother paired with shock, rather this procedure enhances following in chicks (Hess, 1962; Salzen, 1970). However, just hours after the sensitive period for imprinting closes, this shock presentation produces an aversion. Similar limitations on learning have been documented in infant dogs that continue to approach a human attendant who shocks or mishandles the puppies (Rajecki, Lamb, & Obmascher, 1978), as well as nonhuman primates that continue to approach caregivers who handle them roughly (Harlow

& Harlow, 1965; Maestripieri, Tomaszycki, & Carroll, 1999; Sanchez, Ladd, & Plotsky, 2001). In young rat pups, inhibitory conditioning and passive avoidance are also attenuated (Blozovski & Cudennec, 1980; Collier, Mast, Meyer, & Jacobs, 1979; Myslivecek, 1997; Stehouwer & Campbell, 1978).

Another example of learning restrictions in infant rats is attenuated avoidance learning and fear conditioning. Specifically, pairing an odor with a painful stimulus (0.5-mA tail or foot shock, or tail pinch) results in pups approaching that odor when it is next encountered (Camp & Rudy, 1988; Haroutunian & Campbell, 1979; Moriceau & Sullivan, 2004a, 2004b; Moriceau, Wilson, Levine, & Sullivan, 2006; Roth & Sullivan, 2001; Spear, 1978; Sullivan, 2003; Sullivan et al., 2000b). This odor–shock conditioning is referred to as fear conditioning, which produces learned freezing responses and odor avoidance in adults with the amygdala being a critical site for learning plasticity (Cahill, McGaugh, & Weinberger, 2001; Davis, Walker, & Myers, 2003; Debiec & LeDoux, 2004; Fanselow & Gale, 2003; Fanselow & Poulas, 2005; Hess, Gall, Granger, & Lynch, 1997; LeDoux, 2003; Rosenkranz & Grace, 2002; Sananes & Campbell, 1989; Schettino & Otto, 2001; Sevelinges et al., 2007; Sevelinges, Gervais, Messaoudi, Granjon, & Mouly, 2004). The failure of pups to avoid an odor previously paired with pain occurs despite a functional pain system. Indeed, 0.5-mA shock elicits escape in neonatal pups and the threshold for responding to shock does not appear to change as fear conditioning emerges (Barr, 1995; Emerich, Scalzo, Enters, Spear, & Spear, 1985; Fitzgerald, 2005; Stehouwer & Campbell, 1978). We have recently replicated these results using a more naturalistic 1-h paradigm where pups were housed with a stressed mother. We used a stress paradigm in which mothers are placed in a novel environment, with too few shavings to build a nest and not given enough time to adapt to the new environment before being given pups (Avishai-Eliner, Gilles, Eghbal-Ahmadi, Bar-El, & Baram, 2001). These mothers spend the hour trying to build a nest for her pups, transporting pups from one potential nest site to the next, trampling on the pups, and failing to nurse. We used this rough behavior as a more natural way of inducing pain in pups in the presence of a novel odor. Other pups received the novel odor and placed

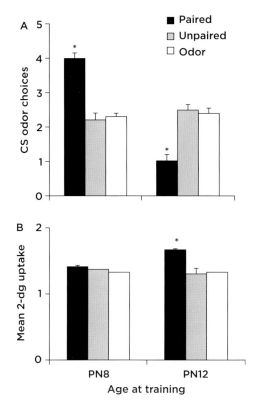

Figure 27.2 (A) After odor–0.5 mA shock conditioning, paired pups show a preference for the conditioned odor in a Y-maze test at P8, although the same conditioning results in an odor aversion in P12 pups. (B) 2-DG autoradiography suggests there is no difference between odor only, paired and unpaired odor–0.5mA shock pups' amygdala neural activity in P8 pups, while the P12 paired odor–0.5 mA shock pups show significantly greater amygdala 2-DG uptake than control unpaired and odor only pups (± standard error, * indicates significance at the $p < 0.5$ level).

with a calm mother (given time to adapt to the new environment with ample shavings for nest building) showing normal pup interactions and frequent nursing. Pups with either the stressed or calm mother showed robust odor preference conditioning, while control groups showed no learning (Roth & Sullivan, 2005). The ecological significance of this effect may relate to the occurrence of rough handling by the mother during normal mother–infant interactions (i.e., stepping on pups while entering/leaving the nest and rough pup retrieval). Considering the necessity of pups learning a preference to their mother's odor for nipple attachment and other related attachment behaviors, it is certainly beneficial for pups *not* to learn an aversion to their mother's odor or inhibit approach responses to nest odors. Perhaps

this attenuated avoidance learning ensures pups continue to only approach/follow the caregiver (Hofer, 1981; Hofer & Sullivan, 2001).

Neural Basis of Attenuated Aversion Learning

In our search for the neural basis for attenuated avoidance learning, we began to focus on the amygdala, a brain area implicated in adult avoidance/fear conditioning (Davis, 1997; Fanselow & LeDoux, 1999; Johnson, Farb, Morrison, McEwen, & LeDoux, 2005; Litaudon, Mouly, Sullivan, Gervais, & Cattarelli, 1997; Maren, 2003; Phelps & Ledoux, 2005; Ressler, Paschall, Zhou, & Davis, 2002). During this early life learning in rat pups when odor and 0.5-mA shock pairings produce an odor preference, the amygdala does not seem to become incorporated into the learning circuit, as determined by 2-DG (Figure 27.2; Sullivan, Landers, Yeaman, & Wilson, 2000a) or c-*fos* (Roth & Sullivan, 2005). In fact, lesioning the amygdala has little effect on infant rat odor preference conditioning (Moriceau & Sullivan, 2006; Sullivan & Wilson, 1993). Indeed, it is not until odor–0.5-mA shock begins to produce odor avoidance that the amygdala seems important in infant odor–0.5-mA shock classical conditioning. Specifically, as illustrated in Figure 27.2, older postsensitive period (PN12) paired odor–0.5-mA shock pups show significantly more 2-DG uptake in the amygdala. Furthermore, similar to adults, temporary amygdala suppression (muscimol) during acquisition disrupts fear conditioning in these older postsensitive period (PN12–14) pups (Cousens & Otto, 1998; Fanselow & Gale, 2003; Maren, 1999; Moriceau & Sullivan, 2006; Muller, Corodimas, Fidel, & LeDoux, 1997; Walker & Davis, 2002).

Opioid and Corticosterone Modulation of the Aversion Learning and the Amygdala

Although immaturity of the amygdala would seem to be the most parsimonious explanation for the amygdala's failure to participate in conditioning, our pharmacological manipulations suggest otherwise. Specifically, systemic or intra-amygdala corticosterone (CORT) infusions during conditioning are sufficient to permit the neonatal-sensitive period pups to learn an odor aversion and the amygdala to participate in odor–0.5-mA shock conditioning (Moriceau et al., 2006; Moriceau & Sullivan, 2004b, 2006). As neonatal sensitive period pups have a "stress hyporesponsive period" when stressful stimuli such as shock fail to elicit a stress-induced CORT release, these data suggest our CORT manipulations produced an amygdala responsive to our odor–0.5-mA shock pairings (Moriceau et al., 2006). A similar role of CORT has been demonstrated for ducklings during imprinting, where the level of CORT controlled the strength of approach behavior, with higher doses of CORT reducing following and blocking CORT increasing following of the surrogate (Martin, 1978). The importance of CORT in neonatal pup attachment behavior and amygdala activity is further suggested by the important role of increasing CORT in the ontogenetic emergence of fear to predator odor and its accompanying amygdala activity (Moriceau, Roth, Okotoghaide, & Sullivan, 2004; Takahashi, 1994; Wiedenmayer & Barr, 2001).

Sensory stimulation pups receive from the mother causes long-term suppression of pups' CORT levels during the sensitive period, although the mother continues to blunt pups' stress-induced CORT response in older pups approaching weaning (Stanton, Wallstrom, & Levine, 1987; Suchecki, Rosenfeld, & Levine, 1993). Indeed, the aversion produced by odor–0.5-mA shock conditioning in older postsensitive period pups can be reversed to the sensitive period odor preference learning simply by having the mother present during the conditioning (Moriceau & Sullivan, 2006). The important role of maternal suppression of shock-induced CORT release in pups odor aversion learning was verified by systemic and intra-amygdala CORT infusions, which permitted pups to learn odor aversions in the presence of the mother. Similar CORT attenuation by social cues have been found in other paradigms and have a dramatic modulatory effect on motivation within social attachments in both infancy and adulthood (Hennessy, Hornschuh, Kaiser, & Sachser, 2006).

Opioids are also important in modulating pups' behavior and nursing elevates pups' opioid levels, which appears to quiet pups, reduce pain threshold, and support nipple attachment (Blass, 1997; Blass, Shide, Zaw-Mon, & Sorrentino, 1995; Goodwin & Barr, 1997; Kehoe & Blass, 1986c; Nelson & Panksepp, 1998; Petrov, Nizhnikov, Varlinskaya, & Spear, 2006; Robinson, Arnold, Spear, & Smotherman, 1993; Robinson & Smotherman, 1997; Shayit, Nowak, Keller, & Weller, 2003). Opioids are also important in pup learning with odor–morphine pairings supporting a conditioned odor preference that can be blocked with the opioid antagonist, naltrexone (Carden, Barr, & Hofer,

1991; Goodwin, Molina, & Spear, 1994; Kehoe & Blass, 1986b; Moles, Kieffer, & D'Amota, 2004; Panksepp, Nelson, & Siviy, 194; Randall, Kraemer, Dose, Carbary, & Bardo, 1992; Roth et al., 2006; Roth & Sullivan, 2003, Shayit et al., 2003). These studies also indicate that blocking opioids (naltrexone) either during or after conditioning prevents odor learning in both classical conditioning procedure (odor-stroking that mimics maternal licking) and natural interactions with the mother. Similarly to CORT, blocking opioids in sensitive period pups can switch odor–0.5-mA shock odor preference learning to odor aversion learning and activate the amygdala, even when limited to the postlearning consolidation period (Roth et al., 2006). This suggests that pups' high levels of opioids can protect pups from learning an odor avoidance to the maternal odor.

Neonatal Pups Can Learn to Avoid Odors

Even as a fetus, rat pups learn to avoid odors when odors are paired with malaise such as that produced by LiCl injection or 1.2-mA shock, which is quite high for neonatal pups (Campbell, 1984; Coopersmith, Lee, & Leon, 1986; Haroutunian & Campbell, 1979; Hennessy & Smotherman, 1976; Hoffman, Hunt, & Spear, 1990; Miller, Molina, & Spear, 1990; Molina, Hoffmann, & Spear, 1986; Richardson & McNally, 2003; Rudy & Cheatle, 1977, 1978, 1983; Shionoya et al., 2006; Smotherman, 1982; Spear, 1978; Spear & Rudy, 1991). However, this early-life odor aversion appears to rely on the olfactory bulb rather than the amygdala until closer to weaning (Figure 27.3; Shionoya et al., 2006). In adults, the amygdala is thought to support taste aversion learning, which involves both taste and smell, although there is some inconsistency (Burt & Smotherman, 1980; Dunn & Everitt, 1988; Kesner, Berman, & Tardif, 1992; Nachman & Ashe, 1974; Sakai & Yamamoto, 1999; Schafe, Thiele, & Bernstein, 1998; Wilkins & Berstein, 2006; Yamamoto, Shimura, Sako, Yasoshima, & Sakai, 1994). However, the amygdala is more consistently implicated in odor–malaise learning (Batsell & Blankenship, 2002; Bermudez-Rattoni, Grijaiva, Klefer, & Garcia, 1986; Ferry, Sandner, & Di Scala,1995 Holland & Gallagher, 2004; Pickens, Saddoris, Gallagher, & Holland, 2005; Touzani & Sclafani, 2005). This experiment also highlights another constraint on pup learning: neonatal pups nursed during odor–LiCl conditioning learned an odor preference, whereas nursing disrupted learning in weanling aged pups (Gubernick

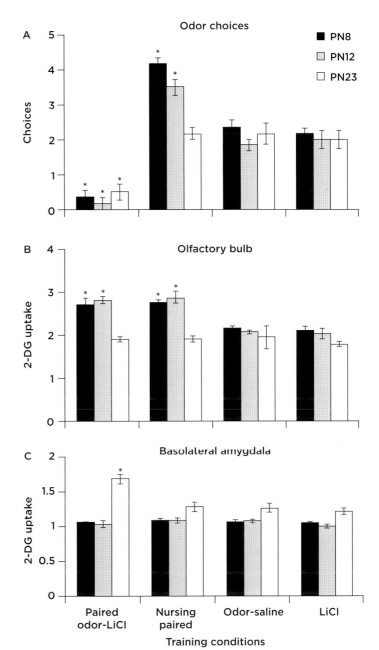

Figure 27.3 The neural basis of odor–malaise learning switches from the olfactory bulb in PN8 and PN12 rats to the amygdala in PN23 pups. (A) Mean number of choices towards conditioned odor in the Y-maze test following odor–LiCl conditioning for Paired odor–LiCl, Nursing Paired odor–LiCl and control odor–saline and LiCl groups. (B) Mean relative olfactory bulb 2-DG uptake during odor–LiCl conditioning. (C) Mean relative basolateral amygdala 2-DG uptake during odor–LiCl conditioning. Asterisks represent significant differences from controls ($p < 0.05$); bars represent the standard error.

& Alberts, 1984; Kehoe & Blass, 1986a; Martin & Alberts, 1979; Melcer, Alberts & Gubernick, 1985; Raineki, Shionoya, Sander, & Sullivan, 2009; Shionoya et al., 2006).

This odor avoidance learning association with olfactory bulb learning–induced changes appears indistinguishable from those induced by odor preference learning. Thus, the olfactory bulb appears to encode aversive and preferred odors in a similar manner, suggesting that it may be identifying an odor as

important but is not encoding the hedonic value of the odor. However, the piriform cortex, which is part of the olfactory cortex, may encode hedonic value since the anterior piriform shows learning-associated changes when an odor preference is learned, while the posterior piriform shows learning-associated changes when an odor aversion is learned (Moriceau et al., 2006; Roth & Sullivan, 2005). This is not consistent with the adult literature on the piriform cortex and learning-associated neural changes, where the learning task and its difficulty appear more important in determining which area of the cortex will show the learning-associated changes (Litaudon et al., 1997; Mouly, Fort, Ben-Boutayab, & Gervais, 2001; Sevelinges et al., 2004; Tronel & Sara, 2002; Wilson, Best & Sullivan, 2004).

Odor Learning Neural Circuit Changes Across Development

As pups mature and walking emerges (~PN10), pups begin to venture outside the nest and begin to eat solid food (Bolles & Woods, 1965). Over the next week-and-a-half, pups must gain the skills necessary for independent living, with maturation as well as experience contributing to these skills. Pups' robust odor preference learning diminishes and the aversion/avoidance learning becomes more robust (Hofer & Sullivan, 2001; Sullivan, 2001, 2003). As would be expected, and reviewed here, the learning neural circuit undergoes corresponding changes to support these behavioral changes with the amygdala supporting aversion learning.

Functional Significance of Pups Changing Learning

The altricial rat is born with a daunting task involving a complex series of behaviors that is initiated by a learned odor guiding pups' approach to the mother, nipple attachment, and nursing. While this behavioral sequence was long thought to be under the control of instinct, we now understand this complex behavioral process is an interaction between a myriad of genetic and environmental factors, requiring complex reciprocal interactions between the mother and infant. This complex mother–infant interaction changes as pups mature and the primary nest environment expands to include the extranest environment. Indeed, as pups become more mobile and independent, new learning capabilities emerge and accommodate the complex contingencies of extranest life and include fear, inhibition, and avoidance learning with the corresponding learning circuit. As described here, as well as other chapters in the "Learning and Memory" section of this book, continued maturation of pups on their way to complete independence and reproductive maturity is further associated with expansion of learning abilities ideally suited to ensure survival. Indeed, taken together, these chapters eloquently illustrate that ontogenetic adaptations at each developmental phase requires unique adaptations to the environment specific to that developmental phase.

Acknowledgment

This work was supported by grants NIH-NICHD-HD33402, NSF-IOB-0544406 and OCAST HR05–114 to R.S.

References

Alberts, J. R., & May, B. (1984). Nonnutritive, thermotactile induction of filial huddling in rat pups. *Developmental Psychobiology, 17*, 161–181.

Avishai-Eliner, S., Gilles, E. E., Eghbal-Ahmadi, M., Bar-El, Y., & Baram, T. Z. (2001). Altered regulation of gene and protein expression of hypothalamic-pituitary-adrenal axis components in an immature rat model of chronic stress. *Journal of Neuroendocrinology, 13*, 799–807.

Barr, G. A. (1995). Ontogeny of nociception and antinociception. *NIDA Research Monograph, 158*, 172–201.

Barr, R., Marrott, R., & Rovee-Collier, C. (2003). The role of sensory preconditioning in memory retrieval by preverbal infants. *Learning and Behavior, 31*, 111–123.

Batsell, W. R., & Blankenship, A. G. (2002). Beyond potentiation: Synergistic conditioning in flavor-aversion learning. *Brain Mind, 3*, 383–408.

Bermudez-Rattoni, F., Grijalva, C. V., Kiefer, S. W., & Garcia, J. (1986). Flavor-illness aversions: The role of the amygdala in the acquisition of taste-potentiated odor aversions. *Physiology & Behavior, 38*, 503–508.

Blass, E. M. (1997) Interactions between contact and chemosensory mechanisms in pain modulation in 10-day-old rats. *Behavioral Neuroscience, 111*, 147–154.

Blass, E. M. (1990). Suckling: determinants, changes, mechanisms, and lasting impressions. *Developmental Psychology, 26*, 520–533.

Blass, E. M., & Fitzgerald, E. (1988). Milk-induced analgesia and comforting in 10-day-old rats: Opioid mediation. *Pharmacology, Biochemistry and Behavior, 29*, 9–13.

Blass, E. M., Shide, D. J., Zaw-Mon, C., & Sorrentino, J. (1995) Mother as shield: differential effects of contact and nursing on pain responsivity in infant rats—evidence for nonopioid mediation. *Behavioral Neuroscience, 109*, 342–353.

Blozovski, D., & Cudennec, A. (1980). Passive avoidance learning in the young rat. *Developmental Psychobiology, 13*, 513–518.

Bolhuis, J. J. (1999). The development of animal behavior: From Lorenz to neural nets. *Naturwissenschaften, 86*, 101–111.

Bolles, R. C., & Woods, P. J. (1965). The ontogeny of behavior in the albino rat. *Animal Behavior, 12*, 427–441.

Bradley, R. M., & Mistretta C. M. (1973). Investigations of taste function and swallowing in fetal sheep. *Symposium on Oral Sensation and Perception, 4*, 185–205.

Brake, S. C. (1981). Suckling infant rats learn a preference for a novel olfactory stimulus paired with milk delivery. *Science, 211*, 506–508.

Burt, G. S., & Smotherman, W. P. (1980). Amygdalectomy induced deficits in conditioned taste aversion: Possible pituitary–adrenal involvement. *Physiology & Behavior, 24*, 651–655.

Cahill, L., McGaugh, J. L., & Weinberger, N. M. (2001). The neurobiology of learning and memory: Some reminders to remember. *Trends in Neuroscience, 24*, 578–581.

Camp, L. L., & Rudy, J. W. (1988). Changes in the categorization of appetitive and aversive events during postnatal development of the rat. *Developmental Psychobiology, 21*, 25–42.

Campbell, B. A. (1984). Reflections on the ontogeny of learning and memory. In R. Kail & N. E. Spear (Eds.), *Comparative perspectives on the development of memory* (pp. 23–35). Hillsdale, NJ: Lawrence Erlbaum.

Campbell, B. A., & Spear, N. E. (1972). Ontogeny of memory. *Psychological Review, 79,* 215–236.

Carden, S. E., Barr, G. A., & Hofer, M. A. (1991). Differential effects of specific opioid receptor agonists on rat pup isolation calls. *Developmental Brain Research, 62,* 17–22.

Cheslock, S. J., Varlinskaya E. I., High, J. M., & Spear, N. E. (2003). Higher order conditioning in the newborn rat: Effects of temporal disparity imply infantile encoding of simultaneous events. *Infancy, 4,* 157–176.

Collier, A. C., Mast, J., Meyer, D. R., & Jacobs, C. E. (1979). Approach-avoidance conflict in preweanling rats: A developmental study. *Animal Learning and Behavior, 7,* 514–520.

Coopersmith, R., Lee, S., & Leon, M. (1986). Olfactory bulb response after odors aversion learning in infancy. *Developmental Brain Research, 24,* 271–277.

Cousens, G., & Otto, T. (1998). Both pre- and posttraining excitotoxic lesions of the basolateral amygdala abolish the expression of olfactory and contextual fear conditioning. *Behavioral Neuroscience, 112,* 1092–1000.

Davis, M. (1997). Neurobiology of fear responses: The role of the amygdala. *Journal of Neuropsychiatry Clinical Neuroscience, 9,* 382–402.

Davis, M., Walker, D. L., & Myers, K. M. (2003). Role of the amygdala in fear extinction measured with potentiated startle. *Annals of the New York Academy of Sciences, 985,* 218–232.

Debiec, J., & LeDoux, J. E. (2004). Disruption of reconsolidation but not consolidation of auditory fear conditioning by noradrenergic blockade in the amygdala. *Neuroscience, 129,* 267–272.

Distal, H., & Hudson, R. (1985). The contribution of the olfactory and tactile modalities to the nipple-search behaviour of newborn rabbits. *Journal of Comparative Physiology, 157,* 1432–1351.

Dunn, L. T., & Everitt, B. J. (1988). Double dissociations of the effects of amygdala and insular cortex lesions on conditioned taste aversion, passive avoidance, and neophobia in the rat using the excitotoxin ibotenic acid. *Behavioral Neuroscience, 102,* 3–23.

Emerich, D. F., Scalzo, F. M., Enters, E. K., Spear, N., & Spear, L. (1985). Effects of 6-hydroxydopamine-induced catecholamine depletion on shock-precipitated wall climbing of infant rat pups. *Developmental Psychobiology, 18,* 215–227.

Fanselow, M. S., & Gale, G. D. (2003). The amygdala, fear, and memory. *Annals of the New York Academy of Science, 985,* 125–134.

Fanselow, M., & LeDoux, J. E. (1999). Why we think plasticity underlying Pavlovian fear conditioning occurs in the basolateral amygdala. *Neuron, 23,* 229–232.

Fanselow, M., & Poulos, A. M. (2005). The neuroscience of mammalian associative learning. *Annual Review of Psychology, 56,* 207–234.

Ferry, B., Sandner, G., & Di Scala, G. (1995) Neuroanatomical and functional specificity of the basolateral amygdaloid nucleus in taste-potentiated odor aversion. *Neurobiology of Learning and Memory, 64,* 169–180.

Fillion, T. J., & Blass, E. M. (1986) Infantile experience with suckling odors determines adult sexual behavior in male rats. *Science, 231,* 729–731.

Fitzgerald, M. (2005). The development of nociceptive circuits. *Nature Reviews Neuroscience, 6,* 507–520.

Goodwin, G. A., & Barr, G. A. (1997). Evidence for opioid and nonopioid processes mediating adaptive responses of infant rats that are repeatedly isolated. *Developmental Psychobiology, 31,* 217–227.

Goodwin, G. A., Molina, V. A., & Spear, L. P. (1994). Repeated exposure of rat pups to isolation-induced ultrasonic vocalization rats: reversal with naltrexone. *Developmental Psychobiology, 27,* 53–64.

Gray, L., Watt, L., & Blass, E. M. (2000). Skin-to-skin contact is analgesic in healthy newborns. *Pediatrics, 105,* 14.

Gubernick, D. J., & Alberts, J. R. (1984). A specialization of taste aversion learning during suckling and its weaning-associated transformation. *Developmental Psychobiology, 17,* 613–628.

Harlow, H. F., & Harlow, M.K. (1965). The affectional systems. In A. Schrier, H. F. Harlow, & F. Stollnitz (Eds.), *Behavior of Nonhuman Primate,* (Vol. 2, pp. 287–334). New York: Academic Press.

Haroutunian, V., & Campbell, B. A. (1979). Emergence of interoceptive and exteroceptive control of behavior in rats. *Science, 205,* 927–929.

Harris, G. C., & Fitzgerald, R. D. (1991). Locus coeruleus involvement in the learning of classically conditioned bradycardia. *Journal of Neuroscience, 11,* 2314–2320.

Hennessy, J. W., & Smotherman, W. P. (1976). Conditioned taste aversion and the pituitary–adrenal system. *Behavioral Biology, 16,* 413–424.

Hennessy, M. B., Hornschuh, G., Kaiser, S., & Sachser, N. (2006). Cortisol responses and social buffering: A study throughout the life span. *Hormones & Behavior, 49,* 383–390.

Hepper, P. G. (1987). The amniotic fluid: An important priming role in kin recognition. *Animal Behavior, 35,* 1343–1346.

Hess, E. H. (1962). Ethology: An approach to the complete analysis of behavior. In R. Brown, E. Galanter, E.H. Hess, & G. Mendler (Eds.), *New directions in psychology* (pp. 159–199). New York: Holt, Rinehart and Winston.

Hess, U. S., Gall, C. M., Granger, R., & Lynch, G. (1997). Differential patterns of c-fos mRNA expression in amygdala during successive stages of odor discrimination learning. *Learning and Memory, 4,* 262–283.

Hofer, M. A. (1981). *The roots of human behavior.* New York: W. H. Freeman & Company.

Hofer, M. A., & Sullivan, R. M. (2001). Toward a neurobiology of attachment. In C.A. Nelson & M. Luciana (Eds.), *Handbook of developmental cognitive neuroscience* (pp. 599–616). Cambridge, MA: MIT Press.

Hoffmann, H., Hunt, P., & Spear, N. E. (1990) Ontogenetic differences in the association of gustatory and tactile cues with lithium chloride and footshock. *Behavioral and Neural Biology, 53,* 441–450.

Hoffman, H., & Spear, N. E. (1989). Facilitation and impairment of conditioning in the preweanling rat after prior exposure to the conditioned stimulus. *Animal Learning & Behavior, 17,* 63–69.

Holland, P. C., & Gallagher, M. (2004). Amygdala–frontal interactions and reward expectancy. *Current Opinions in Neurobiology, 14,* 148–155.

Johanson, I. B., & Hall, W. G. (1982). Appetitive conditioning in neonatal rats: Conditioned orientation to a novel odor. *Developmental Psychobiology, 15,* 379–397.

Johanson, I. B., & Teicher, M. H. (1980). Classical conditioning of an odor preference in 3-day-old rat. *Behavioral Neural Biology, 29*,132–136.

Johnson L. R., Farb, C., Morrison, J. H., McEwen, B. S., & Ledoux, J. E. (2005) Localization of glucocorticoid receptors at postsynaptic membranes in the lateral amygdala. *Neuroscience, 136*, 289–299.

Johnson, B. A., Woo, C. C., Duong, H., Nguyen, V., & Leon, M. (1995). A learned odor evokes an enhanced Fos-like glomerular response in the olfactory bulb of young rats. *Brain Research , 699*, 192–200.

Kehoe, P., & Blass, E. M. (1986a). Conditioned aversions and their memories in 5-day-old rats during suckling. *Journal of Experimental Psychology: Animal Behavior Processes, 12,* 40–47.

Kehoe, P., & Blass, E. M. (1986b). Behaviorally functional opioid system in infant rats I: evidence for olfactory and gustatory classical conditioning. *Behavioral Neuroscience, 100,* 359–367.

Kehoe, P., & Blass, E. M. (1986c). Opioid-mediation of separation distress in 10-day-old rats: Reversal of stress with maternal stimuli. *Developmental Psychobiology, 19,* 385–398.

Kesner, R. P., Berman, R. F., & Tardif, R. (1992). Place and taste aversion learning: role of basal forebrain, parietal cortex, and amygdala. *Brain Research Bulletin, 29,* 345–353.

Kucharski, D., & Hall W. G. (1987). New routes to early memories. *Science, 4828,* 786–788.

Landers, M., & Sullivan, R. M. (1999a). Vibrissae evoked behavior and conditioning before functional ontogeny of somatosensory vibrissae cortex. *Journal of Neuroscience, 19,* 5131–5137.

Landers, M., & Sullivan, R. M. (1999b). Norepinephrine and associative conditioning in the neonatal rat somatosensory system. *Developmental Brain Research, 114,* 261–264.

Langdon, P. E., Harley, C. W., & McLean, J. H. (1997). Increased ß adrenoceptor activation overcomes conditioned olfactory learning induced by serotonin depletion. *Developmental Brain Research, 114,* 261–264.

Lecanuet, J. P., & Schaal, B. (1996). Fetal sensory competencies. *European Journal of Obstetrics and Gynecological Reproductive Biology, 68,* 1–23.

LeDoux, J. (2003). The emotional brain, fear, and the amygdala. *Cellular and Molecular Neurobiology, 23,* 727–738.

Leon, M., Galef, B. G., & Behse, J. H. (1977). Establishment of pheromonal bonds and diet. choice in young rats by odor pre-exposure. *Physiology & Behavior, 18,* 387–91.

Liang, K. C., Chen L. L., & Huang T. E. (1995). The role of amygdala norepinephrine in memory formation: involvement in the memory enhancing effect of peripheral epinephrine. *Chinese Journal of Physiology, 38,* 81–91.

Litaudon, P., Mouly, A., Sullivan, R., Gervais, R., & Cattarelli, M. (1997). Learning-induced changes in rat piriform cortex activity mapped using multisite recording with voltage sensitive dye. *European Journal of Neuroscience, 9,* 1593–1602.

Maestripieri, D., Tomaszycki, M., & Carroll, K. A. (1999). Consistency and change in the behavior of rhesus macaque abusive mothers with successive infants. *Developmental Psychobiology, 34,* 29–35.

Maren, S. (1999). Neurotoxic basolateral amygdala lesions impair learning and memory but not the performance of conditional fear in rats. *Journal of Neuroscience, 19,* 8696–8703.

Maren, S. (2003). The amygdala, synaptic plasticity, and fear memory. *Annals of the New York Academy of Sciences, 985,*106–113.

Martin, J. T. (1978). Imprinting behavior: Pituitary–adrenocortical modulation of the approach response. *Science, 200,* 565–567.

Martin, L. T. & Alberts, J. R. (1979). Taste aversions to mother's milk: The age-related role of nursing in acquisition and expression of a learned association. *Journal of Comparative Physiology and Psychology, 93,* 430–445.

McLean, J. H., Darby-King, A., Sullivan, R. M., & King, S. R. (1993). Serotonergic influences on olfactory learning in the neonatal rat. *Behavioral and Neural Biology, 60,* 152–162.

McLean, J. H., & Shipley, M. T. (1991). Postnatal development of the noradrenergic projection from the locus coeruleus to the olfactory bulb in the rat. *Journal of Comparative Neurology, 304,* 469–477.

Melcer, T., Alberts, J. R., & Gubernick, D. J. (1985). Early weaning does not accelerate the expression of nursing-related taste aversions. *Developmental Psychobiology, 18,* 375–381.

Mennella J. A., Johnson, A., & Beauchamp G. K. (1995). Garlic ingestion by pregnant women alters the odor of amniotic fluid. *Chemical Senses, 20,* 207–209.

Miller, J. S., Molina, J. C., & Spear, N. E. (1990). Ontogenetic differences in the expression of odor-aversion learning in 4- and 8-day-old rats. *Developmental Psychobiology, 23,* 319–330.

Moffat, S. D., Suh, E. J., & Fleming, A. (1993). Noradrenergic involvement in the consolidation of maternal experience in postpartum rats. *Physiology and Behavior, 53,* 805–811.

Moles, A., Kieffer, B. L., & D'Amota, F. R. (2004). Deficit in attachment behavior in mice lacking the μ-opioid receptor gene. *Science, 304,* 1983–1986.

Molina, J. C., Hoffmann, H., & Spear, N. E. (1986). Conditioning of aversion to alcohol orosensory cues in 5- and 10-day rats: subsequent reduction in alcohol ingestion. *Developmental Psychobiology, 19,* 175–183.

Mooncey, S., Giannakoulopoulos, X., & Glover, V. (1997). The effect of mother–infant skin-to-skin contact on plasma cortisol and β-endorphin concentrations in preterm newborns. *Infant Behavior & Development, 20,* 553–557.

Moore, C. L., Jordan, L., & Wong, L. (1996). Early olfactory experience, novelty and choice of sexual partner by male rats. *Physiology & Behavior, 60,* 1361–1367.

Moriceau, S., Roth, T. L., Okotoghaide, T., & Sullivan, R. M. (2004). Corticosterone controls the developmental emergence of fear and amygdala function to predator odors in infant rat pups. *International Journal of Developmental Neuroscience, 22,* 415–422.

Moriceau, S., & Sullivan, R. M. (2004a). Unique neural circuitry for neonatal olfactory learning. *Journal of Neuroscience, 24,* 1182–1189.

Moriceau, S., & Sullivan, R. M. (2004b). Corticosterone influences on mammalian neonatal sensitive period learning. *Behavioral Neuroscience, 118,* 274–281.

Moriceau, S., & Sullivan, R. M. (2006). Maternal presence serves to switch between learning fear and attraction in infancy. *Nature Neuroscience, 9,* 1004–1006.

Moriceau, S., Wilson, D. A., Levine, S., & Sullivan, R. M. (2006). Dual circuitry for odor–shock conditioning during infancy: Corticosterone switches between fear and attraction via amygdala. *Journal of Neuroscience, 26,* 6737–6748.

Mouly, A. M., Fort, A., Ben-Boutayab, N., & Gervais, R. (2001). Olfactory learning induces differential long-lasting changes in rat central olfactory pathways. *Neuroscience, 102*, 11–21.

Muller, J., Corodimas, K. P., Fridel, Z., & LeDoux, J. E. (1997). Functional inactivation of the lateral and basal nuclei of the amygdala by muscimol infusion prevents fear conditioning to an explicit conditioned stimulus and to contextual stimuli. *Behavioral Neuroscience, 111*, 683–689.

Myslivecek, J. (1997). Inhibitory learning and memory in newborn rats. *Progress in Neurobiology, 53*, 399–430.

Nachman, M., & Ashe, J. H. (1974). Effects of basolateral amygdala lesions on neophobia, learned taste aversions, and sodium appetite in rats. *Journal of Comparative Physiology and Psychology, 87*, 622–643.

Nakamura, S. T., & Sakaguchi, T. (1990). Development and plasticity of the locus coeruleus. A review of recent physiological and pharmacological experimentation. *Progress in Neurobiology, 34*, 505–526.

Nakamura, S., Kimura, F., & Sakaguchi, T. (1987). Postnatal development of electrical activity in the locus coeruleus. *Journal of Neurophysiology, 58*, 510–524.

Nelson, E. E., & Panksepp, J. (1998). Brain substrates of infant–mother attachment: Contributions of opioids, oxytocin, and norepinephrine. *Neuroscience and Biobehavioral Review, 22*, 437–452.

Okutani, F., Zhang, J., Otsuka, T., Yagi, F., & Kaba, H. (2003). Modulation of olfactory learning in young rats through intrabulbar GABA$_B$ receptors. *European Journal of Neuroscience, 18*, 2031.

Pager, J. (1974). A selective modulation of olfactory bulb electrical activity in relation to the learning of palatability in hungry and satiated rats. *Physiology and Behavior, 12*, 189–195.

Panksepp, J., Nelson, E., & Siviy, S. (1994). Brain opioids and mother-infant social motivation. *Acta Paediatric Supplement, 397*, 40–46.

Pedersen, P. E., Stewart, W. B., Greer, C. A. & Shepherd, G. M. (1983). Evidence for olfactory function (in) utero. *Science, 4609*, 478–480.

Pedersen, P., Williams, C. L., & Blass, E. M. (1982). Activation and odor conditioning of suckling behavior in 3-day-old albino rats. *Journal of Experimental Psychology: Animal Behavior Process, 8*, 329–341.

Petrov, E. S., Nizhnikov, M. E., Varlinskaya, E. I., & Spear, N. E. (2006). Dynorphin A (1–13) and responsiveness of the newborn rat to a surrogate nipple: Immediate behavioral consequences and reinforcement effects in conditioning. *Behavior Brain Research, 170*, 1–14.

Phelps E. A., & LeDoux J. E. (2005) Contributions of the amygdala to emotion processing: From animal models to human behavior. *Neuron, 48*, 175–87.

Pickens, C. L., Saddoris, M. P., Gallagher, M., & Holland, P. C. (2005). Orbitofrontal lesions impair use of cue–outcome associations in a devaluation task. *Behavioral Neuroscience, 119*, 317–322.

Pieribone, V. A., Nicholas, A. P., Dagerlind, A., & Hokfelt, T. (1994). Distribution of α1 adrenoreceptors in rat brain revealed by in situ hybridization experiments utilizing subtype specific probes. *Journal of Neuroscience, 14*, 4252–4268.

Polan, H. J., & Hofer, M. A. (1999). Psychobiological origins of infant attachment and separation responses. In J. Cassidy & P. R. Shaver (Eds.), *Handbook of attachment: Theory, research, and clinical application* (pp. 162–80). New York: Guilford Press.

Price, T. L., Darby-King, A., Harley, C. W., & McLean, J. H. (1998). Serotonin plays a permissive role in conditioned olfactory learning induced by norepinephrine in the neonate rat. *Behavioral Neuroscience, 112*, 1430–1437.

Quirarte, G. L., Roozendaal, B.. & McGaugh, J. L. (1997). Glucocorticoid enhancement of memory storage involves noradrenergic activation in the basolateral amygdala. *Proceedings of the National Academy of Sciences, 94*, 14048–14053.

Raineki, C,, Shionoya, K., Sander, K., & Sullivan, R. M. (2009). Ontogeny of odor-LiCl vs. odor-shock learning: Similar behaviors but divergent ages of amygdala functional emergence. *Learning & Memory, 16*, 114–121.

Rajecki, D. W., Lamb, M. E., & Obmascher, P. (1978). Towards a general theory of infantile attachment; A comparative review of aspects of the social bond. *Behavioral Brain Sciences, 3*, 417–464.

Randall, C. K., Kraemer, P. J., Dose, J. M., Carbary, T. J., & Bardo, M. T. (1992). The biphasic effect of morphine on odor conditioning in neonatal rats. *Developmental Psychobiology, 25*, 355–364.

Rangel, S., & Leon, M. (1995). Early odor preference training increases olfactory bulb norepinephrine. *Developmental Brain Research, 85*(2), 187–191

Rescorla, R. A. (1967). Pavlovian conditioning and its proper control procedures. *Psychological Review, 74*, 71–80.

Rescorla, R. A. (1988). Behavioral studies of Pavlovian conditioning. *Annual Review of Neuroscience, 11*, 329–352.

Rescorla, R. A., & Wagner, A. R. (1972). A theory of Pavlovian conditioning: Variations in the effectiveness of reinforcement and non-reinforcement. In A. H. Black & W. F. Prokasy (Eds.), *Classical conditioning II: Current research and theory* (pp. 64–69). New York: Appleton. Century. Crofts.

Ressler, K. J., Paschall, G., Zhou, X., & Davis, M. (2002). Regulation of synaptic plasticity genes during consolidation of fear conditioning. *Journal of Neuroscience, 22*, 7892–7902.

Richardson, R., & McNally, G. P. (2003). Effects of an odor paired with illness on startle, freezing, and analgesia in rats. *Physiology & Behavior, 78*, 213–219.

Robinson, S. R., Arnold, H. M., Spear, N. E., & Smotherman, W. P. (1993). Experience with milk and an artificial nipple promote conditioned opioid activity in the rat fetus. *Developmental Psychobiology, 26*, 375–387.

Robinson, S. R., & Smotherman, W. P. (1997). Stimulus contingencies that permit classical conditioning of opioid activity in the rat fetus. *Behavioral Neuroscience, 111*, 1086–1097.

Roozendaal, B., Nguyen, B. T., Power, A, E., & McGaugh, J. L. (1999). Basolateral amygdala noradrenergic influence enables enhancement of memory consolidation induced by hippocampal glucocorticoid receptor activation. *Proceedings of the National Academy of Science, 96*(20), 11642–11647.

Rosenkranz, J. A., & Grace A. A. (2002). Dopamine-mediated modulation of odour-evoked amygdala potentials during Pavlovian conditioning. *Nature, 417*, 282–287.

Roth, T. L., & Sullivan, R. M. (2001). Endogenous opioids and their role in odor preference acquisition and consolidation following odor–shock conditioning in infant rats. *Developmental Psychobiology, 39*, 188–198.

Roth, T. L., & Sullivan, R. M. (2003). Consolidation and expression of a shock-induced odor preference in rat pups is facilitated by opioids, *Physiology & Behavior, 78*, 135–142.

Roth, T. L,, & Sullivan, R. M. (2005). Memory of early maltreatment: Neonatal behavioral and neural correlates of maternal maltreatment within the context of classical conditioning. *Biological Psychiatry, 57*, 823–831.

Roth, T. L., Moriceau, S., & Sullivan, R. M. (2006). Opioid modulation of Fos protein expression and olfactory circuitry plays a pivotal role in what neonates remember. *Learning and Memory, 13*, 590–598.

Rudy, J. W., & Cheatle, M. D. (1977). Odor aversion learning in neonatal rats. *Science, 198*, 845–846.

Rudy, J. W., & Cheatle, M. D. (1978). A role for conditioned stimulus duration in toxiphobia conditioning. *Journal of Experimental Psychology: Animal Behavior Process, 4*, 399–411.

Rudy, J. W., & Cheatle, M. D. (1983). Odor-aversion learning by rats following LiCl exposure: Ontogenetic influences. *Developmental Psychobiolgy, 16*, 13–22.

Rush, A. N., Robinette, B. L., & Stanton, M. E. (2001). Ontogenetic differences in the effects of unpaired stimulus preexposure on eyeblink conditioning in the rat. *Developmental Psychobiology, 39*, 8–18.

Sakai, N., & Yamamoto, T. (1999). Possible routes of visceral information in the rat brain in formation of conditioned taste aversion. *Neuroscience Research, 35*, 53–61.

Salzen, E. A. (1970). Imprinting and environmental learning. In: L. R. Aronson, E. Tobach, J. S. Rosenblatt, & D. S. Lehrman (Eds.), *Development and evolution of behavior* (Vol. 1, pp. 158–178). San Francisco: Freeman.

Sananes, C. B., & Campbell, B. A. (1989). Role of the central nucleus of the amygdala in olfactory heart rate conditioning. *Behavioral Neuroscience, 103*, 519–25.

Sanchez, M. M., Ladd, C. O., & Plotsky, P. M. (2001). Early adverse experience as a developmental risk factor for later psychopathology: Evidence from rodent and primate models. *Developmental Psychopathology, 13*, 419–449.

Sara, S. J., Dyon-Laurent, D., & Herve, A. (1995). Novelty seeking behavior in the rat is dependent upon the integrity of the noradrenergic system. *Cognitive Brain Research, 2*, 181–187.

Schaal, B., Marlier, L., & Soussignan, R. (1995). Responsiveness to the odor of amniotic fluid in the human neonate. *Biology of the Neonate, 67*, 397–406.

Schafe, G. E., Thiele, T. E., & Bernstein, I. L. (1998). Conditioning method dramatically alters the role of amygdala in taste aversion learning. *Learning & Memory. 5*, 481–92.

Scheinin, M., Lomasney, J. W., Hayden-Hixson, D. M., Schambra, U. B., Caron M. G., Lefkowitz, R. J., et al. (1994). Distribution of α2 adrenergic receptor subtype gene expression in rat brain. *Molecular Brain Research, 21*, 133–149.

Schettino, L. F., & Otto, T. (2001). Patterns of Fos expression in the amygdala and ventral perirhinal cortex induced by training in an olfactory fear-conditioning paradigm. *Behavioral Neuroscience, 115*, 1257–1272.

Selden, N. R., Everitt, B. J., Jarrard, L. E., & Robbins, T. W. (1990). Complementary roles for the amygdala and hippocampus in aversive conditioning to explicit and contextual cues. *Neuroscience, 42*, 335–350.

Sevelinges, Y., Moriceau, S., Holman, P., Miner, C., Muzny, K., Gervais, R., et al. (2007). Enduring effects of infant memories: infant odor-shock conditioning attenuates amygdala activity and adult fear conditioning. *Biological Psychiatry, 62*, 1067–1069.

Sevelinges Y., Gervais R., Messaoudi B., Granjon L., & Mouly A. M. (2004). Olfactory fear conditioning induces field potential potentiation in rat olfactory cortex and amygdala. *Learning & Memory, 11*, 761–769.

Shair, N. H., Masmela, J. R., Brunelli, S. A., & Hofer, M. A. (1997). Potentiation and inhibition of ultrasonic vocalization of rat pups: Regulation by social cues. *Developmental Psychobiology, 30*, 195–200.

Shayit, M., Nowak, R., Keller, M., & Weller, A. (2003). Establishment of a preference by the newborn lamb for its mother: The role of opioids. *Behavioral Neuroscience, 117*, 446–454.

Shionoya, K., Moriceau, S., Lunday, L., Miner, C., Roth, T. L., & Sullivan, R. M. (2006). Development switch in neural circuitry underlying odor–malaise learning. *Learning and Memory, 13*, 801–808.

Shipley, M. T., Halloran, F. J., & De la Torre, J. (1985). Surprisingly rich projection from locus coeruleus to the olfactory bulb in the rat. *Brain Research, 239*, 294–299.

Siegel, S., & Domjan, M. (1971). Backward conditioning as an inhibitory procedure. *Learning and Motivation, 2*, 1–11.

Singh, P. J., & Hofer, M. A. (1978). Oxytocin reinstates maternal olfactory cues for nipple orientation and attachment in rat pups. *Physiology & Behavior, 20*, 385–389.

Smotherman, W. P. (1982). Odor aversion learning by the rat fetus. *Physiology & Behavior, 29*, 769–771.

Spear, N. E. (1978). *Processing memories: Forgetting and retention*. Hillsdale, NJ: Erlbaum.

Spear, N. E., & Molina, J. C. (2005). Fetal or infantile exposure to ethanol promotes ethanol ingestion in adolescence and adulthood: A theoretical review. *Alcoholism, Clinical and Experimental Research, 29*, 909–929.

Spear, N. E., & Rudy, J. W. (1991). Tests of the ontogeny of learning and memory: Issues, methods, and results. In H.N. Shair, G.A. Barr, & M.A. Hofer (Eds.), *Developmental psychobiology: New methods and changing concepts* (pp. 84–113). New York: Oxford University Press.

Stanton, M. E. (2000). Multiple memory systems, development, and conditioning. *Behavioral Brain Research, 110*, 25–37.

Stanton, M. E., & Freeman, J. H. Jr. (2000). Developmental psychobiology of eyeblink conditioning in the rat. In D. S. Woodruff-Pak & J. E. Steinmetz (Eds.), *Eyeblink classical conditioning, Volume II: Applications in Animals* (pp. 105–134). Amsterdam: Kluwer.

Stanton, M. E., Fox, G. D., & Carter, C. S. (1998). Ontogeny of the conditioned eyeblink response in rats: Acquisition or expression? *Neuropharmacology, 37*, 623–632.

Stanton, M. E., Wallstrom, J., & Levine, S. (1987). Maternal contact inhibits pituitary–adrenal stress responses in preweanling rats. *Developmental Psychobiology, 20*, 131–145.

Stehouwer, D. J., & Campbell, B. A. (1978). Habituation of the forelimb-withdrawal response in neonatal rats. *Journal of Experimental Psychology and Animal Behavior Processes, 4*, 104–119.

Suchecki, D., Rosenfeld, P., & Levine, S. (1993). Maternal regulation of the hypothalamic-pituitary-adrenal axis in the infant rat: The roles of feeding and stroking. *Developmental Brain Research, 75*, 185–192.

Sullivan, R. M. (2001). Unique characteristics of neonatal classical conditioning: The role of the amygdala and locus coeruleus. *Integrative Physiological and Behavioral Science, 36*, 293–307.

Sullivan, R. M. (2003). Developing a sense of safety: The neurobiology of neonatal attachment. In J. King, C. Ferris, & I. Lederhendler (Eds.), *Roots of mental illness in children*, New York Academy of Sciences, *1008*, 122–132.

Sullivan, R. M., Brake, S. C., Hofer, M. A., & Williams, C. L. (1986). Huddling and independent feeding of neonatal rats can be facilitated by a conditioned change in behavioral state. *Developmental Psychobiology, 19*, 625–635.

Sullivan, R. M., & Hall, W. G. (1988). Reinforcement in infancy: Classical conditioning using tactile stroking or intra-oral milk infusions as UCS. *Developmental Psychobiology, 20*, 215–223.

Sullivan, R. M., Hofer, M. A., & Brake, S. C. (1986b). Olfactory-guided orientation in neonatal rats is enhanced by a conditioned change in behavioral state. *Developmental Psychobiology, 19*, 615–623.

Sullivan, R. M., Landers, M., Yeaman, B., & Wilson, D. A. (2000a). Good memories of bad events in infancy. *Nature, 407*, 38–39.

Sullivan, R. M., & Leon, M. (1986). Early olfactory learning induces an enhanced olfactory bulb response in young rats. *Developmental Brain Research, 27*, 278–282.

Sullivan, R. M., McGaugh, J., & Leon, M. (1991). Norepinephrine-induced plasticity and one-trial olfactory learning in neonatal rats. *Developmental Brain Research, 60*, 219–228.

Sullivan, R. M., Stackenwalt, G., Nasr, F., Lemon, C., & Wilson, D. A. (2000b). Association of an odor with activation of olfactory bulb noradrenergic ß-receptors or locus coeruleus stimulation is sufficient to produce learned approach response to that odor in neonatal rats. *Behavioral Neuroscience, 114*, 957–962.

Sullivan, R. M., & Wilson, D. A. (1993). Role of the amygdala complex in early olfactory associative learning. *Behavioral Neuroscience, 107*, 254–263.

Sullivan, R. M., Wilson, D. A., Lemon, C., & Gerhardt, G. (1994). Bilateral 6-OHDA lesions of the locus coeruleus impair associative olfactory learning in newborn rats. *Brain Research, 643*, 306–309.

Sullivan, R. M., Wilson, D. A., Wong, R., Correa, A., & Leon, M. (1990). Modified behavioral olfactory bulb responses to maternal odors in preweanling rats. *Developmental Brain Research, 53*, 243–247.

Sullivan, R. M., Zyzak, D., Skierkowski, P., & Wilson, D. A. (1992). The role of olfactory bulb norepinephrine in early olfactory learning. *Developmental Brain Research, 70*, 279–282.

Takahashi, L. K. (1994). Organizing action of corticosterone on the development of behavioral inhibition in the preweanling rat. *Developmental Brain Research, 81*, 121–127.

Thoman, E., Wetzel, A., & Levine, S. (1968). Learning in the neonatal rat. *Animal Behavior, 16*, 54–57.

Touzani, K., & Sclafani, A. (2005). Critical role of amygdala in flavor but not taste preference learning in rats. *European Journal of Neuroscience, 22*, 1767–1774.

Tronel, S., & Sara, S. J. (2002). Mapping of olfactory memory circuits: Region-specific c-fos activation after odor-reward associative learning or after its retrieval. *Learning and Memory, 9*, 105–111.

Thoman, E., Wetzel, A., & Levine, S. (1968). Learning in the neonatal rat. *Animal Behavior, 16*, 54–57.

Walker L., & Davis, M. (2002). The role of amygdala glutamate receptors in fear learning, fear-potentiated startle, and extinction. *Pharmacology, Biochemistry and Behavior, 71*, 379–392.

Weldon, D. A., Travis, M. L., & Kennedy, D. A. (1991). Post-training D1 receptor blockade impairs odor conditioning in neonatal rats. *Behavioral Neuroscience, 105*, 450–458.

Weller, A., & Feldman, R. (2003). Emotion regulation and touch in infants: The role of cholecystokinin and opioids. *Peptides, 24*, 779–788.

Wiedenmayer, C. P., & Barr G. A. (2001). Developmental changes in c-fos expression to an age-specific social stressor in infant rats. *Behavioral Brain Research, 126*, 147–157.

Wilbrecht, L., & Nottebohm, F. (2004). Age and experience affect the recruitment of new neurons to the song system of zebra finches during the sensitive period for song learning: Ditto for vocal learning in humans? Adolescent brain development: Vulnerabilities and opportunities. *Annals of the New York Academy of Sciences, 1021*, 404–409.

Wilkins, E. E., & Bernstein, I. L. (2006). Conditioning method determines patterns of c-fos expression following novel taste–illness pairing. *Behavioral Brain Research. 169*, 93–97.

Wilson, D. A., Best, A. R., & Sullivan, R. M. (2004) Plasticity in the olfactory system: Lessons for the neurobiology of memory. *The Neuroscientist, 10*, 513–524.

Wilson, D. A., & Leon, M. (1988). Spatial patterns of olfactory bulb single-unit responses to learned olfactory cues in young rats. *Journal of Neurophysiology, 59*, 1770–1782.

Wilson, D. A., & Sullivan, R. M. (1990). Olfactory associative conditioning in infant rats with brain stimulation as reward. I. Neurobehavioral consequences. *Developmental Brain Research, 53*, 215–221.

Wilson, D. A., & Sullivan, R. M. (1991). Olfactory associative conditioning in infant rats with brain stimulation as reward. II. Norepinephrine mediates a specific component of the bulb response to reward. *Behavioral Neuroscience, 105*, 843–849.

Wilson, D. A., Sullivan, R. M., & Leon, M. (1987). Single-unit analysis of postnatal olfactory learning: Modified olfactory bulb output response patterns to learned attractive odors. *Journal of Neuroscience, 7*, 3154–3162.

Woo, C. C., Coopersmith R., & Leon, M. (1987). Localized changes in olfactory bulb morphology associated with early olfactory learning. *Journal of Comparative Neurology, 263*, 113–125.

Woo, C. C., & Leon, M. (1988). Sensitive period for neural and behavioral responses to learned odors. *Developmental Brain Research, 36*, 309–313.

Woo, C. C., Oshita, M. H., & Leon, M. (1996). A learned odor decreases the number of Fos-immunopositive granule cells in the olfactory bulb of young rats. *Brain Research, 716*, 149–156.

Yamamoto, T., Shimura, T., Sako, N., Yasoshima, Y., & Sakai, N. (1994). Some critical factors involved in formation of conditioned taste aversion to sodium chloride in rats. *Chemical Senses, 19*, 209–217.

Yuan, Q., Harley, C. W., Bruce, J. C., Darby-King, A., & McLean, J. H. (2000). Isoproterenol increases CREB phosphorylation and olfactory nerve-evoked potentials in normal and 5-HT-depleted olfactory bulbs in rat pups only at doses that produce odor preference learning. *Learning and Memory, 7*, 413–421.

Yuan Q., Harley C. W., McLean J. H., & Knopfel T. (2003). Optical imaging of odor preference memory in the rat olfactory bulb. *Journal of Neurophysiology, 87*, 3156–3159.

Development of the Hippocampal Memory System: Creating Networks and Modifiable Synapses

Theodore C. Dumas *and* Jerry W. Rudy

Abstract

The hippocampus is part of a neural system that supports our ability to recall the episodes that make up our past. Because the rat is altricial and its adult characteristics emerge in a relatively short postnatal period, it is possible to use several memory-dependent behavioral tasks that depend on the hippocampus to estimate when its hippocampal-memory system becomes functional. This occurs, around postnatal day 21. This functional maturity of the hippocampus in part appears to be the consequence of changes in the goals of some of the mechanisms of synaptic plasticity. Initially these mechanisms are designed to build synaptic connections that can support a basic infrastructure of interconnected neurons. As this is accomplished, some of the properties of synapses are altered so they become more resolute coincident detectors that can be more strictly modified by experiences that generate memory.

Keywords: hippocampus, synaptic plasticity, synaptic connections, experiences, memory

Introduction

Researchers interested in the biological basis of memory have devoted more time and effort to the study of the hippocampus and its related temporal lobe structures than to any other region of the brain. The hippocampus has been the subject of thousands of reports by researchers interested in memory, brain systems, and neural plasticity. Two major events are responsible for intense interest in this brain region: (a) Brenda Milner's analysis of the amnesic patient, H.M. (1970) and (b) the discovery of long-term potentiation (LTP) by Tim Bliss and Terge Lomo (1973).

The purpose of the chapter is to describe what is known about the development of what, hereafter, we refer to as the hippocampal-dependent memory system. First, we briefly describe the historical foundations that placed the hippocampus at the center

of memory research. We then describe some of the major tasks used to reveal how a neural system in which the hippocampus is situated contributes to memory. A description of the development of this system from a memory/behavioral perspective then follows. The remainder of the chapter focuses on some of what is known about changes in the mechanisms supporting synaptic plasticity that occur during the transition period when the hippocampal memory system becomes functional.

The Case of the Amnesic H.M.

The idea that the hippocampus makes a special contribution to memory is intimately linked to Brenda Milner's (1970) analysis of the now-famous patient, H.M., whose medial temporal lobes were removed to control his epilepsy. Her analysis revealed that H.M.'s short-term memory for recently experienced events was intact, but, if distracted, the memory for recent events was lost. H.M thus had severe anterograde amnesia—after the surgery he could not establish new long-term memories. He also suffered a severe retrograde amnesia; he could not recall events experienced in the approximately 10 years prior to his surgery. In contrast, H.M. was able to learn to perform tasks that depended on perceptual-motor reorganization, such as a mirror tracing task, and motor skills, such as the pursuit rotary task. Even though his performance on these tasks improved with training and was retained, H.M. could not recall the experiences that produced the learning.

An important implication of these results is that damage to the medial temporal lobes did not abolish all memories. The effect was restricted to what most people think of as memory in the common use of the term—the ability to recollect past experiences. It was not important for memories of skills or habits. After comparing H.M.'s performance with that of other patients with damage to different brain regions, Milner suggested that the hippocampus was the critical contributor. Her hypothesis has been supported by more recent results of studies of other amnesic patients with more selective damage to the hippocampus (e.g., Cipolotti et al., 2001; Zola-Morgan, Squire, & Amaral, 1986).

It is difficult to overestimate the impact Milner's work had on memory research. That damage to the medial temporal lobes produced a selective memory impairment marked the beginning of a set of events that led to the modern concept of *multiple memory systems* (see Squire, 2004; Chapter 24). It also made the hippocampus a focal point for hundreds of brain researchers interested in memory.

Discovery of Long-Term Potentiation in the Hippocampus

The second major event that placed the hippocampus in the center of memory research was the discovery of LTP in the dentate gyrus of the hippocampus. Bliss and Lomo (1973) took advantage of the known anatomy of the flow of information through the hippocampus (see Figure 28.1) and focused on the perforant path-dentate gyrus connection. They applied electrical stimulation to the perforant path and recorded field potentials in the dentate gyrus. They discovered that applying a relatively strong stimulus to the perforant-path enhanced or potentiated subsequent responses elicited by the weak stimulus and that this effect lasted hours to days. LTP also is studied by stimulating

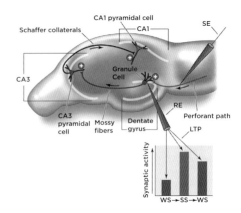

Figure 28.1 Information enters the hippocampus via the perforant path, which synapses on neurons in the dentate gyrus (DG). Mossy fibers connect to the CA3 region and Schaffer collaterals connect CA3 to CA1. Bliss and Lomo stimulated the PP and recorded long term potentiation (LTP) in the DG. Many researchers stimulate the Schaffer collaterals and record LTP in the CA1 region. (Reprinted with permission from Rudy J. W. (2008). The neurobiology of learning and memory. Copyright Sinauer Publishers.)

the Schaffer collaterals connecting CA3 to CA1 pyramidal cells and recording in the CA1 region.

LTP reflects changes in the strength of synaptic connections, and neurobiologists believe that the synapse is the fundamental unit of information storage and memory. Consequently, much of what we know about the biological basis of memory has come from studies of LTP in different subregions of the hippocampus.

Hippocampus Memory System

This chapter will describe the development of the hippocampus-dependent memory system. However, before doing this, it will be useful to more fully characterize the system. As noted, contemporary researchers accept what is called a multiple memory systems view. To illustrate this concept, imagine that you are learning to ride a bike or the facts surrounding some historical event like the death of Abraham Lincoln. The "experience" contains very different kinds of information. It includes information about:

- Where and when you practiced or studied
- Who was there
- The joys, frustrations, and pain that may accompany your efforts
- Specific dates and locations of the historical event
- The motor patterns of the movements you practiced

The multiple memory systems view is that the brain has evolved so that different brain regions are responsible for storing information about the different content of our experiences (see Sherry and Schacter, 1987, for why this may have happened).

The hippocampus is central to what is now commonly referred to as the declarative/episodic memory system. An important attribute of this system is that it stores memories so that the content of experience can be consciously recalled. It allows you to recall where and when you practiced and who was with you. It is also thought to allow you to rapidly and effortlessly store this information and represent it as distinct episodes (Morris et al., 2003; O'Reilly & Rudy, 2001). Thus, you can remember where and what you had for lunch yesterday, even though you made no deliberate effort to store this information.

Animal Models of the Hippocampus Memory System

What we know and can learn about the biological details of the hippocampus and its involvement in memory can only come from the study of animals. Thus, our review will focus on animal studies. However, this choice comes with a problem. It is easy to demonstrate that people with damage to the hippocampus cannot consciously recollect previously experienced events. One can ask them to explicitly recall a prior episode. However, it is impossible to directly assess this feature of memory in nonverbal animals. How can a cat, dog, rodent, or monkey tell you where it has been or what it had for lunch? It cannot because the answer requires both the ability to consciously or intentionally recollect and a verbal response to declare the answer. They might have the former ability, but they do not have the latter. Thus, we have to use what are called implicit behavioral measures (Schacter, 1987) that do not require explicit verbal recall to assess their memory. Given that animals cannot explicitly declare a memory for some experiences, it is difficult to establish a relationship between animal studies and the concept of declarative memory. Thus, we will use the term hippocampal memory system as the umbrella term for the research we will summarize.

For many years after Milner suggested that the hippocampus was critical to some types of memory, researchers studying animals had difficulty in finding learning and memory tasks that required an intact hippocampus for successful performance. In retrospect, this is not surprising

because H.M. was able to gradually acquire habits and most of the tasks that were used could be viewed as being examples of habit learning. His deficit was in recalling his experiences. Beginning in the late 1970s, however, tasks were developed that were sensitive to hippocampus damage in monkeys and in rodents (see Squire, 2004, for historical review). What we know about the details of hippocampus synaptic plasticity come from studies of rodent brains. Thus we will focus on a subset of behavioral tasks that have revealed a contribution of the hippocampus to memory-dependent behaviors of rodents and examine what is known about the development of this system as revealed by behavioral experiments. In the next section, we will describe some of these tasks and why they are used to characterize the hippocampal-dependent memory system.

Assessing the Rodent Hippocampal Memory System

One of the hallmarks of H.M.'s amnesia was that it extended only to some aspects of his memory. His declarative memory was impaired whereas other aspects of his memory were left intact. Consequently, in the search for animal models of the hippocampal memory system, researchers have focused on ones that clearly reveal a pattern of spared and impaired performance associated with damage to the hippocampus. The easy part is finding memory-based behaviors that are spared (see Squire, 2004). Rodents can learn and remember remarkably complex discrimination tasks with complete damage to the hippocampus (see Rudy & Sutherland, 1995). The hard part is finding memory-based tasks that depend on an intact hippocampal formation. Nevertheless, there are several models that reveal a pattern of spared and impaired test performance following damage to the hippocampal formation and have also been used to study memory development. Given that our primary goal will be to determine when the hippocampal memory system becomes functional, we will focus on just three models: (a) spatial versus cued learning in the Morris task, (b) contextual versus cued fear conditioning, and (c) delayed spatial alternation versus position habits.

SPATIAL VERSUS CUED LEARNING
In 1971, John O'Keefe discovered what he called place cells in the hippocampus (O'Keefe & Dostrovsky, 1971). They were cells that fired when

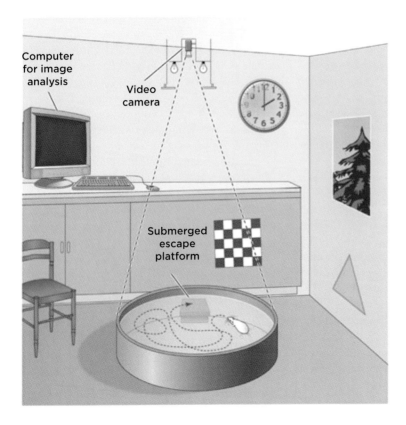

Figure 28.2 An illustration of the spatial location version of the Morris (1981) water escape task. The platform is hidden beneath the surface of the water and is always in the same location relative to the distal cues of the room that surround the tank. Raising the platform above the water's surface and making it visible can create *a cued version* of this task. Rats with damage to the hippocampus cannot learn the spatial location of the platform but can learn to swim to the visible platform. (Copyright Sinauer Publishers, reprinted with permission of the publisher.) (Reprinted with permission from Rudy, J. W. (2008). The neurobiology of learning and memory. Copyright Sinauer Associates.)

Labels in figure: Computer for image analysis; Video camera; Submerged escape platform

the rat was in a particular location of the test environment. Subsequently, O'Keefe and Nadel (1978) proposed that the hippocampus is part of a system that stores map-like representations of the world. This influential hypothesis led researchers to develop spatial learning tasks that would require the acquisition of such a representation. Richard Morris (1981) developed the most widely used task. It is often referred to as the Morris water maze (see Clark et al., 2005 for other examples). As shown in Figure 28.2, the test apparatus consists of a large circular tank filled with water. Two versions of the Morris water-escape task can be constructed. In one version, called the place task, an escape platform is placed into the pool but is hidden beneath the water's surface. The rat is placed into the pool and can escape by finding the hidden platform. It is possible for the rat to learn the platform's location because it is always placed in the same location relative to the visible distal cues in the room that surround the pool. Nevertheless, the solution is not simple and requires the rat to acquire a map-like representation of the room and the location of the platform. Rodents easily learn to swim directly to the platform, and when the platform is removed on

a probe trial, they will search the area of the pool where it was located during training.

The second version of the task is called the cued or visible platform task. In this task, the platform is above the water surface and clearly visible to the rodent. It is moved to a different location on every trial. This task makes the same motivational and motor requirements of the rodent as does the place version. However, the animal only needs to learn to swim toward the visible platform to escape.

Damage to the hippocampal formation severely and permanently disrupts performance on the place version of the task but spares the ability of the rodent to learn the location of the cued platform (Clark et al., 2005; Morris, Garrud, Rawlins, & O'Keefe, 1982; Sutherland & Rudy, 1988; Sutherland, Kolb, & Whishaw, 1982). These results, of course, support O'Keefe and Nadel's cognitive mapping idea. More importantly, however, they reveal a pattern of impaired and spared behavioral performance that is associated with damage to the hippocampus.

CONTEXTUAL AND AUDITORY-CUE FEAR

Variations on what is called fear conditioning have also revealed a pattern of spared and impaired

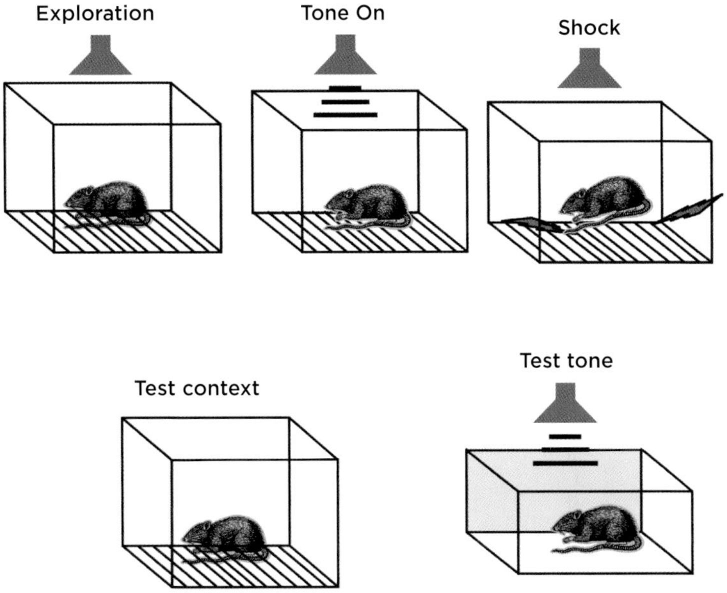

Figure 28.3 Illustration of fear conditioning procedure. Rats are allowed to explore a context for about 2 min. Then a tone is presented for about 15 s. The tone terminates with a brief shock to the rat's feet. Some time later, the rats are tested for their fear of the context in which they were shocked and then for their fear of the tone. A different context is used to test the rat's fear of the tone. Damage to the hippocampus impairs the acquisition of contextual fear conditioning but not acquisition of fear to the tone.

test performance associated with damage to the hippocampus. The basic methodology is illustrated in Figure 28.3. It shows a rodent placed into what is called a conditioning chamber. Sometime after it is placed into the chamber, an auditory stimulus is presented. About 10–15 s after the onset of the auditory stimulus, electrical shock is delivered to the rodent's feet. Training can consist of one or several trials. An innate defensive response called freezing is use to assess the rodent's memory for the experience. In the presence of a danger signal such as the sight or sounds of a predator, rodents become instinctively still or immobile. This behavior has survival advantages because a moving animal is more likely to be detected by a predator than a still one.

Following training, the rodent is tested for its fear of the context/place where it was shocked and for its fear to the auditory cue. Because rodents will freeze in the training context where shock occurred, the auditory cue is typically tested in a novel context that has no association with shock. This allows the experimenter to obtain a relatively pure measure of fear of the tone. Normal rats will freeze in the place where they were shocked and will also freeze when the auditory cue is presented in a novel context.

The value of these two fear conditioning tasks in relationship to the hippocampal memory system became apparent when Kim and Fanselow (1992) and Phillips and LeDoux (1992) reported that damage to the hippocampus following training significantly impaired contextual fear conditioning but had no effect on retention of fear to the auditory cue. Again, the important result was that damage to the hippocampus impaired the contextual fear memory but spared the memory for auditory fear conditioning.

Most researchers now agree that the hippocampus is important for contextual fear conditioning because it is necessary for the rodent to acquire and store a representation of the co-occurring features that make up the context (Fanselow, 2000; Rudy, Huff, & Matus-Amat, 2004). Some researchers call this a configural representation (Fanselow, 2000; Rudy & Sutherland, 1995) and others refer to it as a conjunctive representation (Rudy et al., 2004).

CONDITIONAL DELAYED ALTERNATION VERSUS POSITION HABIT

The procedures for this task are presented in the top of Figure 28.9. A trial consists of two components, a forced run and a choice run. First, the animal is forced to choose one arm of a T maze. On the second part of the trial, it is reinforced for going to another arm. Over a training session, the forced side is randomly varied. Thus, performance on the choice run is conditional upon which side the animal visited on the forced run. This problem can be considered against a second task used to study the acquisition of what is called a position habit. In this task, the animal is rewarded for choosing the left arm or the right arm. Damage to the hippocampus is known to significantly impair performance on the conditional delayed alternation task (Aggleton, Hunt, & Rawlins, 1986) but has no effect on learning a position habit.

Summary

There have been hundreds of experiments examining the effects of damage to the hippocampus on a wide range of behavioral tasks. Research with the three paradigms just described, however, have all produced a pattern of spared and impaired performance on memory-dependent behavioral paradigms, allowing one to see that the hippocampus is more important for some types of memory than for others. Moreover, there is a developmental literature that is isomorphic with these results.

Memory Development

What is known about the neural development of the hippocampus is based on studies of synaptic plasticity using the rodent hippocampus. Thus, we will restrict our brief review of memory development to studies based on the rat. We begin with a general description of the natural development of the rat and its implications for learning and memory.

Rats Are Altricial

Rats are altricial. At birth, they are extremely immature and rely heavily on the dam to meet their basic needs. At birth, they are primarily dependent on their somatosensory and olfactory systems to locate the nipple and nurse. Their gustatory system also is to some extent functional. However, neither the auditory or visual systems are functional at birth. The auditory meatus, the opening to the inner ear, does not occur until about postnatal day (P)12 and their eyelids do not open until about P14. Thus, their sensory systems can be divided into two classes. Members of one class emerge early (the somatosensory, olfaction, and gustatory systems) and participate in the essential behaviors needed to survive in the nest. Members of the other class (the auditory and visual systems) emerge late but are relatively mature when the pups are ready to leave the nest.

A Jacksonian Caudal-to-Rostral Sequence of Development

This pattern of early and late developing systems permits the experimenter to study the emerging learning and memory functions separately for members of each class. Such experiments have

revealed a common organizing developmental principle for each system. Since the writings of Hughlings Jackson (1958), it has been appreciated that the nervous system develops in somewhat caudal-to-rostral sequence with brain stem regions becoming functional in advance of the higher cortical regions. Studies of the development of associative learning capacities across the several sensory systems suggest that the flow of information provided by each sensory system also independently develops in a Jacksonian caudal-to-rostral manner (see Rudy, 1992). Information initially reaches the brain stem regions that support some forms of reflexive reactions, and as the pup ages, it reaches the higher cortical regions where it can be integrated and associated with information coming in through other sensory channels (Hyson & Rudy, 1984; Moye & Rudy, 1985, 1987; Rudy, 1992; Vogt & Rudy, 1984). Basic unlearned or reflexive behavior is the first behavioral capacity a sensory system can support. This outcome is followed by the ability to support elementary associative learning revealed by Pavlovian conditioning procedures. This is followed by the ability of the system to hold a memory of the stimulus for some period of time so that it can associate with other events occurring after its termination. This organizing principle is illustrated in Figure 28.4. Data illustrating this principle for the visual system are also presented in Figure 28.5.

The hippocampus is positioned at the highest level of a neural system that progressively processes information from high-level multimodal neocortical regions to medial temporal lobe cortices, the perirhinal, parahippocampal and entorhinal cortices. Lavenex and Amaral (2000) have described this neural system as being hierarchically organized so that at each higher level in the system, the information becomes more integrated and abstract (see Figure 28.6). Information processed through this system to the hippocampus is then sent back to the sending regions. Given this plan, it follows that for the hippocampus to be fully functional, it must receive the relevant information from all the sending regions. Thus, given the sequential nature of the development of the rat's sensory systems, memory functions that depend on the hippocampus must necessarily be relatively late to develop.

Development of Memories That Depend on the Hippocampus

Based on a number of studies, we know that all the sensory systems are to some degree functional and can support some forms of learning and

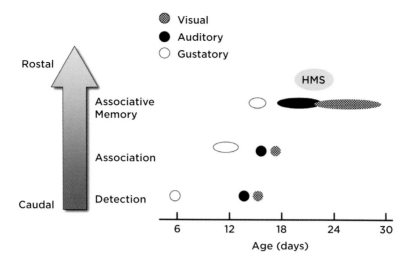

Figure 28.4 The emergence of the rat's learning and memory capacities. The sensory systems of the rat become functional at different times in development. Each system appears to undergo a Jacksonian caudal-to-rostal developmental sequence. So that whether it emerges early or late in development the system goes through the same developmental progression. First, it detects its appropriate stimulus, but only later can it associate that stimulus with some other event. Its capacity to maintain a representation of the stimulus, so that it can support associations over time, develops later. Around postnatal day 21, memories supported by the hippocampal memory system (HMS) emerge.

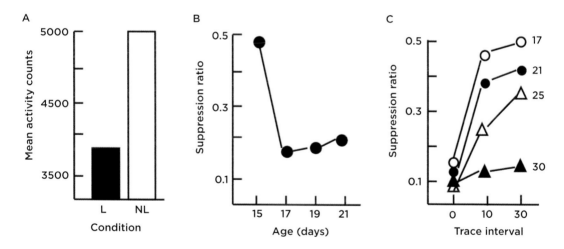

Figure 28.5 An illustration of a "Jacksonian" development sequence. (A) This figure shows that the presentation of a light will suppress ongoing activity in rat pups only 14 days old. (B) However, this same stimulus will not associate with shock until pups are about 17 days. (C) Even though 17-day old pups can associate the light with a shock when the light terminates with shock, pups this age do not associated the light with shock when it terminates prior to shock. Note that the trace interval refers to the time separating the termination of the light form the onset of shock. Pups 30 days old associate the light with shock even when the trace interval is 30 s. The suppression ratio is a measure of the ability of the light to suppress ongoing activity a ratio of 0.50 indicates no suppression. (Redrawn from Moye and Rudy, 1984, 1987.)

memory by P 16–18 (see Rudy, 1992, for summary). However, it is between P 19 and P 23 that one begins to see evidence that memories thought to depend on the hippocampus emerge. We discussed three types of behavioral procedures in which spared and impaired performance were associated with the

hippocampus. Simply stated, rats acquire memories that depend on the hippocampus at a later age than they acquire memories that do not require a contribution from the hippocampus. Thus, when challenged by the two versions of the Morris water escape task, rats learn to swim to a visible platform

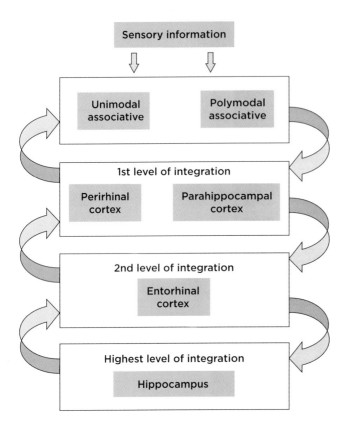

Figure 28.6 A schematic of the hippocampal memory system. Sensory information flows to the hippocampus via unimodal and polymodal associative cortical regions that project to the perirhinal and parahippocampus cortices, which project to the entorhinal cortex. Information is processed in the hippocampus and then projects back to its cortical origins. At each level of integration, the information is believed to become more processed or abstract. Given the sequential development of the rats sensory systems, memory functions that depend on the hippocampus integrating information across sensory systems must necessarily be relatively late to develop. (Redrawn after Lavenex & Amaral, 2000.)

at an earlier age than they can learn the location of the hidden platform (Rudy & Paylor, 1988; Rudy, Stadler-Morris, & Albert, 1987) (see Figure 28.7). Similarly, rats condition to an auditory cue at an earlier age than they condition to the context where the shock occurred (Rudy, 1993) (see Figure 28.8). Finally, as shown in Figure 28.9, rats learn a conditional delayed alternation at a later age than they learn a position habit (Castro, Paylor, & Rudy, 1987; Green & Stanton, 1989).

What is remarkable is that performance on the quite different memory-dependent dependent tasks all emerge around weaning when the rats are about 21 days old. Given that the hippocampal memory system makes a critical contribution to performance on this task, it is reasonable to believe that this convergence signals the functional emergence of this system. Thus, around the time of normal weaning, there is a rather sudden shift from a hippocampal system that cannot support memory to one that does.

Hippocampus Memory Index and Pattern Completion

Around postnatal day 21, the rat's hippocampal memory system comes on-line. What special mnemonic function supported by the hippocampus suddenly emerges that now allows it to make its unique contribution? Consistent with the hierarchical organization of the neural system in which the hippocampus is situated (see Figure 28.6), many theorists believe that the content of our memories are contained in the neocortical regions of the brain that feedforward to the medial temporal lobes. The hippocampus itself contains no content. Instead, it is believed that it binds together co-occurring experience-generated patterns of neocortical activity into what is called a conjunctive representation (e.g., O'Reilly & Rudy, 2003; Squire, 1992) that serves as an index to memories store in the neocortex (Teyler & DiScenna, 1986; Teyler & Rudy, 2007). It can do this because information that is processed through the hippocampus is projected back to the same cortical regions from which it received its inputs (see Figure 28.6), and the index can support the process of pattern completion, whereby a portion of the original experience that established the trace can reproduce the entire experience (see Figure 28.10). In his influential review (see Figure 28.10), Squire (1992, p. 224) concluded that "[i]n the present account the possibility of later retrieval is provided by the hippocampal system

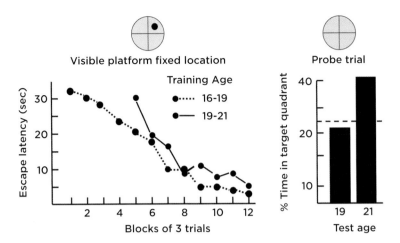

Figure 28.7 Left panel: Rats learn to locate and swim to a visible platform at an earlier age than they learn its spatial location. In this experiment, rats were trained to swim to a visible platform that was always in the same location relative to the distal cues of the training room. By the end of training, rats aged 19 and 21 days were swimming directly to the visible platform. At the completion of training, the platform was removed and rats were given a probe trial. During probe, the 21-day-old rats indicated that they had learned the spatial location of platform because they spent more time searching the target quadrant than they searched the other quadrants. In contrast, the 19-day-old rats did not selectively search the target quadrant. Learning the spatial location of the platform requires the hippocampus. The dashed line indicates the chance search behavior. (Redrawn after Rudy and Paylor, 1988.)

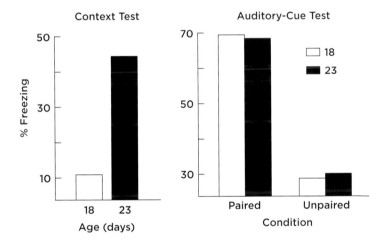

Figure 28.8 Rat 18 and 23 days old display the same level of conditioning to an auditory cue paired with shock but 18-day-olds display an impairment on hippocampus dependent contextual fear conditioning. (Redrawn after Rudy, 1993.)

because it has bound together the relevant cortical sites. A partial cue that is later processed through the hippocampus is able to reactivate all the sites and thereby accomplish the retrieval of the whole memory."

Hippocampus Synapses and Memory

The somewhat abrupt emergence of the hippocampal memory system is likely the product of a large number of gradual changes in its basic anatomy and physiology. They include the development of the intrinsic organization and wiring among the subregions within the hippocampus and their connections to other regions of the brain. In the just described conjunctive/indexing account, the hippocampus participates in memory storage by binding together inputs originating from different cortical sites that support pattern completion. This is where the study of synaptic plasticity interfaces with the hippocampal memory system. In order for such a binding to occur, it is necessary for experience to modify the synaptic connections representing the neocortical inputs onto dendritic fields of the hippocampus neurons. Thus, in the final stages

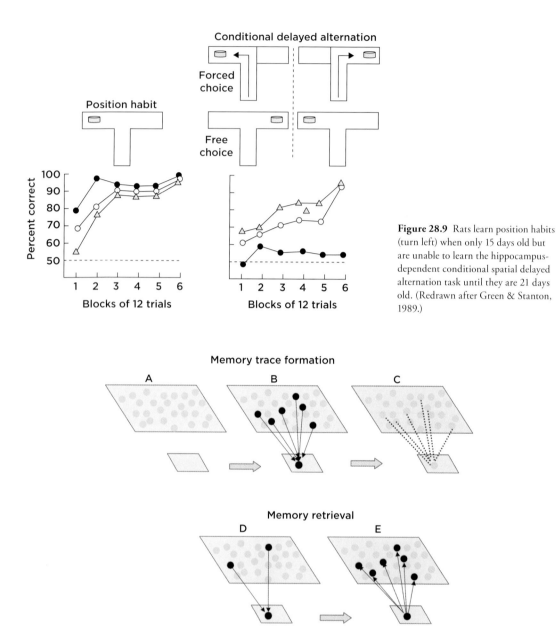

Figure 28.9 Rats learn position habits (turn left) when only 15 days old but are unable to learn the hippocampus-dependent conditional spatial delayed alternation task until they are 21 days old. (Redrawn after Green & Stanton, 1989.)

Figure 28.10 Memory formation: (A) The larger top layer represents potential patterns of neocortical activity; the smaller bottom layer represents the hippocampus. (B) A set of neocortical patterns activated by a particular experience projects to the hippocampus and activates a unique set of synapses. (C) The memory for the experiences is stored as strengthened connections among those hippocampal synapse activated by the input pattern. Memory retrieval: (D) A subset of the initial input pattern can activate the hippocampal representation. (E) When this occurs, output from the hippocampus projects back to the neocortex to activate the entire pattern. Thus the hippocampus stores an index to neocortical patterns that can be used to retrieve the memory.

of development it is likely that there are significant changes in the ability of hippocampal synapses to be modified by experience so they can support the indexing function of the hippocampus.

Thus, in the following sections, we will describe some of the basic changes in pre- and postsynaptic processes that may ultimately lead to functional neural networks in the hippocampus that can support enduring behaviorally induced changes in synaptic strength. What we know about the final stages of these processes comes in large part from studies of synaptic plasticity based on the study of LTP using brain slices taken from rodent hippocampus. Thus, our description will be derived from this literature.

Some Basic Mechanisms of Synaptic Plasticity

Given that the emergence of hippocampal-dependent memories depends on the ability of synapses in the hippocampus to store information about behavioral experiences, it is necessary to understand on a cellular level what developmental processes have to be achieved in order for synapses to store information. Specifically, for example, one needs to know what are the fundamental activity-dependent synaptic plasticity processes that allow the CA3–CA1 neural network to register and store representations of experience? A full review of the mechanisms that support activity-dependent synaptic plasticity is beyond the scope of this chapter (see Malenka & Bear, 2004 for a recent review). However, it is useful to describe the primary events that initiate change and the modifications that result in increased synaptic efficacy.

The basic players are (a) glutamate released from presynaptic neurons and (b) two classes of postsynaptic ionotropic glutamate receptors, *N*-methyl-d-aspartate receptors (NMDARs) and α-amino-3-hydroxy-5-methyl-4-isoxazolepropionate receptors (AMPARs), and (c) the influx of calcium (Ca^{2+}) into the presynaptic terminal and postsynaptic spine (Figure 28.11A). If glutamate binds to the NMDAR when the postsynaptic neuron becomes depolarized, Ca^{2+} enters through the open NMDAR channel. Increases in pre- and postsynaptic Ca^{2+} stimulate biochemical interactions to increase the strength of the synapse. It is generally agreed that these interactions produce many outcomes. They include increased AMPAR conductance, insertion of additional AMPARs into the dendritic spine, increased transmitter release, and formation of new synapses (Figure 28.11B).

Building the Infrastructure

In approaching the problem of how synapses develop the capacity to be modified by experience-induced activity, it is important to keep in mind

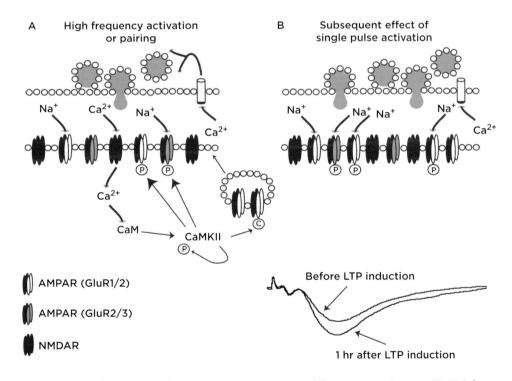

Figure 28.11 LTP arises from numerous alterations in synaptic transmission following patterned activity. (A) High-frequency activation or pairing of presynaptic activation with postsynaptic depolarization activates NMDARs, which allows Ca^{2+} to enter and interact with the Ca^{2+} binding protein, calmodulin (CaM). With Ca^{2+} bound, calmodulin can activate the major kinase in the cascade, Ca^{2+} calmodulin kinase II (CaMKII), which phosphorylates (circled P) numerous target proteins, including itself. (B) CaMKII-dependent phosphorylation of AMPARs already situated in the synapse (GluR1/2 and GluR2/3) increases their conductance. Insertion of additional AMPARs into the synapse (GluR1/2) also enhances postsynaptic sensitivity to glutamate. Certain forms of LTP induction in adult and juvenile animals can result in a lasting increase in transmitter release (Zakharenko, Zablow, & Siegelbaum, 2001; Dumas, unpublished observation). (C) The end result of LTP induction is an activity-dependent and lasting increase in the strength of synaptic contacts.

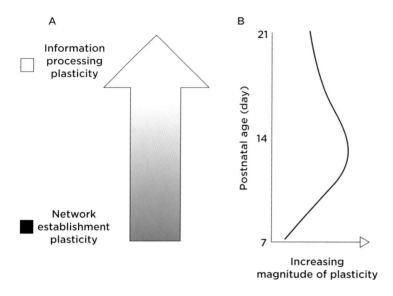

A

☐ Information processing plasticity

■ Network establishment plasticity

B

Postnatal age (day)

21

14

7

Increasing magnitude of plasticity

Figure 28.12 Developing and mature forms of synaptic plasticity overlap during the late postnatal period. (A) As the animal matures, network formation plasticity gives way to information processing plasticity. (B) Measures of lasting synaptic plasticity are greater at 2 weeks of age because plasticity processes involved in forming the hippocampal network overlap with plasticity processes that underlie hippocampal-dependent learning and memory. As developmental forms of plasticity dissipate with increasing age, overall LTP magnitude decreases.

that the brain is solving two general problems. First, a basic synaptic infrastructure connecting neurons in a network that can potentially represent experience has to be created. Thus, some basic synaptic connections have to be put in place so that neurons in the circuit can communicate. Second, synapses have to be produced that can store representations of behavioral experiences. Although these two tasks may share some common requirements (such as glutamate release and NMDA receptors), they are not the same. This means that there likely will be a transition period when some of the intrinsic processes operating that are responsible for laying down the synaptic infrastructure give way to the processes that make it possible for behavioral experiences to modify synaptic strength (Figure 28.12). In the sections that follow, some of the important developmental changes in basic synaptic machinery that occur during the transition period will be described.

Synaptic Development and Hippocampal-Dependent Memory

From the moment of contact, bidirectional communication allows pre- and postsynaptic elements to act in concert to construct a mature synaptic network that can form representations of behavioral experiences (Gerrow & El-Husseini, 2006). As such, it is likely that no single developmental change in synaptic plasticity mechanisms is responsible for the emergence of the hippocampus memory system. Instead, the emergence of synapses that can support memory is likely the result of coregulated developmental changes in both pre- and postsynaptic

processes. However, because the synapse is such a complex device, for analytical purposes, it is useful to consider some of the changes in pre- and postsynaptic processes separately.

DEVELOPMENTAL CHANGES IN PRESYNAPTIC FUNCTION

During the development of the hippocampus memory circuit, it is necessary to establish and maintain a synaptic infrastructure that connects neurons in the network, so that they can be modified by experience. Glutamate release from the presynaptic neurons is a prerequisite to the formation of this network. Beginning at the second postnatal week, when the infrastructure is still being built and begins to receive input from late-developing sensory systems, there is a shift in the level of synaptic glutamate release from relatively low to relatively high levels. On average, immature synapses release less transmitter per action potential than mature synapses (Figure 28.13) (Dumas & Foster, 1995).

It is also the case that during this period, Schaffer collateral-CA1 (SC-CA1) synapses are more sensitive to presynaptic potentiation. Given an identical LTP induction pattern, indices of increased presynaptic function are greater at immature synapses than at mature synapses (Dumas, unpublished observation; McNaughton, Shen, Rao, Foster, & Barnes, 1994; Williams et al., 1993). The increase in presynaptic strength reflects that the activated presynaptic neurons release more neurotransmitter than they did before the potentiating stimulus was presented.

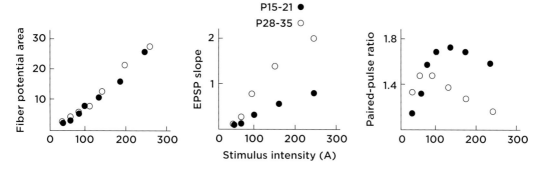

Figure 28.13 Presynaptic function at SC-CA1 synapses increases from P15–21 to P28–35. (A) The fiber potential, a measure of the number of input fibers that are activated by the electrical impulse is not different between rats aged P15–21 and P28–35, indicating no alteration in afferent input across this period of development. (B) An increase in the slope of the excitatory postsynaptic potential (EPSP), in the absence of a change in the fiber potential, reflects an increase in the efficacy of excitatory synaptic transmission between CA3 and CA1 pyramidal cells. (C) When two stimulus pulses are delivered in rapid succession (50 ms interstimulus interval in this case), the response to the second pulse is increased relative to the response to the first pulse. This phenomenon is termed paired pulse facilitation (PPF) and has a presynaptic locus. The decrease in the paired-pulse ratio in the older group suggests that the increase in synaptic efficacy across this period of development is due, in part, to an increase in transmitter release. (Dumas and Foster, 1995.)

The initial low level of transmitter release may be important for presynaptic modifications (Larkman, Hannay, Stratford, & Jack, 1992). If basal transmitter release is low, then it may be relatively easy for synaptic activity to induce processes that result in an increase in glutamate release. Presynaptic potentiation may act to stabilize CA3–CA1 pyramidal cell contacts in pairs where the CA3 neuron is active (Haydon & Drapeau, 1995). Moreover, a differential increase in glutamate release at SC-CA1 synapses across the CA3–CA1 network may be an important signal for establishing the basic connectivity necessary to support memory.

One possible contributor to increased release of neurotransmitter associated with presynaptically mediated LTP is adenylate cyclase type-1 (AC1). When the presynaptic terminal is activated at a high frequency, enough Ca^{2+} accumulates to bind to the Ca^{2+}-binding protein, calmodulin, and activate AC1. AC1 expression in the hippocampus peaks at 2 weeks of age and then declines to adult levels (Matsuoka, Suzuki, Defer, Nakanishi, & Hanoune, 1997). Activation of ACs in general produces an intracellular signal that begins with an increase in the level of cyclic AMP and results in increased transmitter release. When forskolin, a known activator of AC is applied to slices taken from rats in the 15- to 21-day-old range, the resulting population excitatory postsynaptic potential (EPSP) produced by the test stimulus is more greatly enhanced compared to when the drug is applied to slices from 28- to 35-day-old rats (Figure 28.14A) (Dumas, 2005a). Greater changes in presynaptically mediated short-term plasticity during forskolin application in slices from 3-week-old rats supported a greater presynaptic effect of the drug (Figure 28.14B). Additionally, application of forskolin occluded the subsequent induction of LTP by high-frequency stimulation in juvenile but not young adult rats (Yasuda, Barth, Stellwagen, & Malenka, 2003). These observations suggest that the response of AC1 to synaptic activity produced by an LTP-inducing stimulus may produce a lasting increase in glutamate release when the network is being formed.

The age-related reduction in the ability of AC1 to increase presynaptic function is likely due to two events: (a) a decrease in AC1 expression (Matsuoka et al., 1997) and (b) an increase in the effects of a Ca^{2+}-insensitive AC2 (Feinstein et al., 1991), which upregulates transmitter release in a more constitutive fashion. As AC2 increases baseline transmitter release in an activity-insensitive manner, it occludes the diminishing effects of AC1 and the ability of activity to produce lasting changes in presynaptic function. It is possible that during the transition period, AC1 maintains higher transmitter release levels at immature synapses of active CA3 pyramidal cells, and then AC2 relieves AC1 as the synapse becomes stable. The decrease in the activation properties of AC1 may then contribute to the shift away from LTP that is expressed as an increase in glutamate release.

The ramping up of presynaptic release at mature synapses also may be important for the subsequent production of LTP that depends on changes in postsynaptic mechanisms. It is possible that endogenous activity-dependent synaptic activity in immature

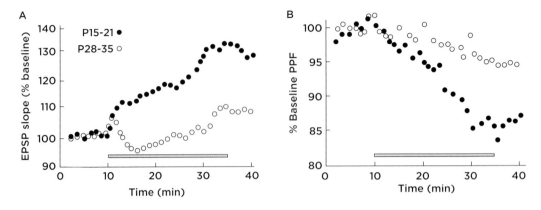

Figure 28.14 Application of the AC activator, forskolin, to hippocampal slices increases transmitter release at SC-CA1 synapses more at P15–21 than at P28–35. (A) After the establishment of a stable response to electrical impulses delivered once every 20 s, forskolin was washed across the slice (duration of drug application is indicated by the solid horizontal bar). Forskolin increased the EPSP slope indicating an increase in synaptic efficacy. (B) A greater decrease in PPF during application of forskolin at P15–21 than at P28–35 suggests that activation of AC increases transmitter release more at SC–CA1 synapses in the younger animals. (See Figure 28.12 for a description of PPF.)

synapses may contribute to the development of the mature network by increasing the number of synapses that can release enough glutamate to support the induction of postsynaptic LTP.

PRESYNAPTIC NMDAR-INDEPENDENT TO POSTSYNAPTIC NMDAR-DEPENDENT LTP

At immature and mature synapses, NMDAR-dependent LTP is present and is expressed postsynaptically. However, NMDAR-independent LTP is also observed in slices from 15- but not 30-day-old rats (Velisek, Moshe, & Stanton, 1993). Thus, during the transition period when the hippocampus is developing the capacity to support memory, LTP might be produced by modifications in both pre- and postsynaptic processes. Consequently, immature synapses in the hippocampus may be more easily modified by activity, but the information they collectively contain might be reduced. This is because increases in synaptic efficacy that do not depend on the coincidence detection properties of NMDARs might not represent behavioral experience (Figure 28.15). Thus, the contribution from presynaptic changes could mask the critical content contained in synapses that were strengthened via NMDAR-dependent receptors. Alternatively, during this transition period, there may be too few synapses present that contain all of the components necessary for coincidence detection, or transmitter release levels may be too low to transmit information through the entire hippocampus (Waters, Klintsova, & Foster, 1997). In either case

the neural memory representation of the experience in an immature networr may be degraded compared to the representation captured by a more mature network.

Thus, during development, one might expect a shift from LTP induction that depends on activity-dependent changes in presynaptic release mechanisms to LTP induction that is produced by activity-dependent enhancement of postsynaptic processes. So, during the transition period, in addition to increasing transmitter release from presynaptic terminals, dendritic spines must acquire the right balance of NMDA and AMPA receptors needed to produce a degree of coincidence detection that is optimal to represent experience. There are two classes of developmental events that may contribute to this outcome: (a) a developmental decrease in silent synapses and (b) a shift in the composition of the subunits of the NMDA receptor.

Silent Synapses Diminish During Postnatal Development

The coincidence detection property of the NMDAR is derived from the fact that passage of Ca^{2+} into the postsynaptic spine requires two events: (a) the binding of glutamate to the NMDAR outside the plasma membrane and (b) the depolarization of the postsynaptic membrane to remove an Mg^{2+} blockade of the ion channel. Depolarization of mature postsynaptic neurons depends heavily on glutamate binding to AMPARs. Thus, when enough AMPAR channels on enough spines open to permit

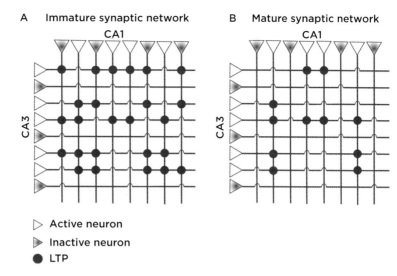

Figure 28.15 The distribution of alterations in synaptic strength during activity is different in the immature hippocampal network due to the presence of a nonassociative presynaptic component to LTP. (A) In the immature network, presynaptic LTP is not restricted by the coincidence detection properties of the NMDAR and occurs everywhere there is presynaptic activity. (B) In contrast, in the mature synaptic network, the number of synapses that undergo LTP is reduced because the pre- and postsynaptic neurons must be coactive. (Dumas, 2005a.)

a critical level of Na⁺ into the cell, the postsynaptic neuron will depolarize enough to allow Ca^{2+} entry through NMDARs. Consequently, developmental changes in AMPAR function will affect NMDAR-dependent synaptic plasticity.

The hippocampus contains what are called silent synapses. These synapses display no AMPAR responses and are silent near resting membrane potential (because NMDARs are blocked by Mg^{2+}). Silent synapses are identified in single-cell recordings where the postsynaptic neuron can be depolarized by the recording pipette, which unmasks and enables recording of NMDAR responses (Figure 28.16A2 and 16B1). After pairing of presynaptic stimulation with postsynaptic depolarization, AMPAR responses can subsequently be observed at resting membrane potential and the previously silent synapse is said to be induced (Figure 28.16B2) (Isaac, Nicoll, & Malenka, 1995; Liao, Hessler, & Malinow, 1995). However, the mechanisms that induce silent into active synapses are not fully understood.

Currently, two classes of silent synapses have been described. The first class of silent synapses contains only NMDARs. Cooperative action of other AMPAR-containing synapses on the same postsynaptic neuron can depolarize the silent synapse while glutamate is being released from the presynaptic neuron to fully activate NMDARs. Such activity causes AMPARs to be inserted into the postsynaptic density of the silent synapse (Figure 28.16A1) (Liao, O'Brien, Ehlers, & Huganir, 1999). Since the synapse now contains AMPARs, it is no longer silent during low-frequency activity at resting

membrane potential (Figure 28.16A2). The second class of silent synapses contain both NMDARs and AMPARs but are silent because the rate of glutamate release is too low to affect the lower affinity AMPARs (Figure 28.16B1). An increase in the rate of glutamate release produced by LTP-inducing stimulation permits the activation of AMPARs (Figure 28.16B2) (Choi, Klingauf, & Tsien, 2003; Renger, Egles, & Liu, 2001).

During the final transition week leading up to the formation of the mature hippocampal synaptic infrastructure, silent synapse numbers remain elevated relative to adult levels (Durand, Kovalchuk, & Konnerth, 1996). An increase in the number of synapses that cannot produce large and fast excitatory AMPAR responses (especially synapses lacking AMPARs) presents a problem for the induction of NMDAR-dependent LTP because fewer synapses can contribute to the cooperative postsynaptic depolarization process. Since NMDAR-dependent increases in synaptic strength store information about behavioral experiences, the number of synapses that can participate in memory storage in the immature hippocampus may be reduced, compared to the mature hippocampus. Additionally, the spatial distribution of synaptic strengthening would be different in a system where new synapses are turned "on" compared to a system where "on" synapses are turned up, which would likely result in synaptic representations of behavioral experience that are dramatically different. Thus, it is not surprising that during the transition to a mature hippocampus, there are developmental processes at work that result in a decrease in silent synapses.

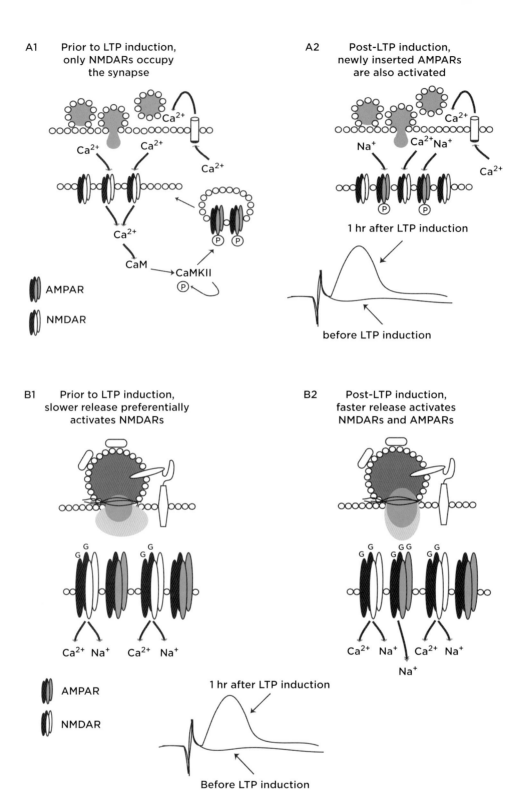

Figure 28.16 Two types of silent SC-CA1 synapses exist in the developing hippocampus. (A1) In the first case, there are no AMPAR in the postsynaptic density prior to LTP induction. During high-frequency stimulation or pairing of pre- and postsynaptic activity, AMPARs are inserted into the synapse. (A2) After LTP induction, single activating pulses produce fast AMPAR synaptic responses because AMPARS have physically moved into the synapse (Liao et al., 1999). (B1) In the second case, silent synapses lack fast depolarizing responses near resting membrane potential because the rate of neurotransmitter release is too low to activate AMPARs already present in the synapse. (B2) After LTP inducing stimulation, an increase in the rate of neurotransmitter permits activation of AMPARs, producing large fast AMPAR synaptic response. (Renger et al., 2001; Choi et al., 2003.)

Changes in NMDAR Receptor Subtype

Both activity-dependent synaptic modifications that result in a mature hippocampal neuronal network and changes in synaptic efficacy that represent behavioral experience depend on the activation of NMDARs (Kandel & O'Dell, 1992). However, there are different subtypes of NMDARs in the hippocampus, leaving open the possibility that different types of NMDARs are responsible for synaptic modifications related to development of the infrastructure and storage of information. Moreover, the basic composition of NMDARs changes substantially during the transition period just preceding the age at which hippocampal-dependent behaviors are first observed (Dumas, 2005b).

Forebrain NMDARs are primarily heterodimers. They contain two pairs of identical subunits. The most common types found in the mature hippocampus are those that contain NR1 and NR2A subunits and those that contain NR1 and NR2B subunits. Early in development, however, the vast majority of synaptic NMDARs are composed of the NR1/NR2B combination (Monyer, Burnashev, Laurie, Sakmann, & Seeburg, 1994). It is during the second and third postnatal week that the balance of NMDAR subtypes at hippocampal SC-CA1 synapses shifts so that the NR1/NR2A combination is more prevalent. At 2 weeks of age, when the NR2A/NR2B content is high, post-synaptic plasticity processes, including LTP, are enhanced (Dudek & Bear, 1993; Dumas, unpublished observations). However, as the NR1/NR2A combination occupies more synaptic territory, synaptic plasticity is reduced (Figure 28.17).

The Ca^{2+} channel conductance properties (the opening and closing of the receptor ion pore) of the two NMDAR subtypes are quite different. Conductance decays more slowly following activation of the NR1/NR2B subtype than activation of the NR1/NR2A subtype, resulting in increased entry of Ca^{2+} via the NR1/NR2B compared to the NR1/NR2A subtype (Barria & Malinow, 2002; Kirson & Yaari 1996; Monyer et al., 1992). It is possible that the more slowly decaying conductance property of the NR1/NR2B subtype may be especially important for initially endowing synaptic contacts with the plasticity necessary to establish stability. However, the continued abundance of the NR1/NR2B subtype might work against achieving a neural network that needs to store the content of a behavioral experience. So it is possible that it is the shift in the ratio of synaptic NR1/NR2B to NR1/NR2A that is critical for the hippocampal synapse to support the detailed information contained in a behavioral experience (Quinlan, Lebel, Brosh, & Barkai, 2004; Roberts & Ramoa, 1999).

The decrease in Ca^{2+} conductance that accompanies increased synaptic NR1/NR2A content may be responsible for age-related decreases in synaptic plasticity and improvement in hippocampal-

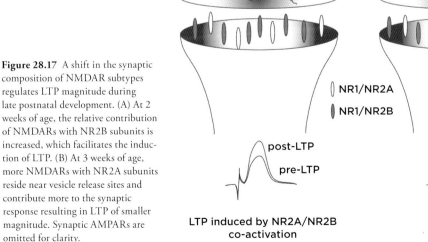

Figure 28.17 A shift in the synaptic composition of NMDAR subtypes regulates LTP magnitude during late postnatal development. (A) At 2 weeks of age, the relative contribution of NMDARs with NR2B subunits is increased, which facilitates the induction of LTP. (B) At 3 weeks of age, more NMDARs with NR2A subunits reside near vesicle release sites and contribute more to the synaptic response resulting in LTP of smaller magnitude. Synaptic AMPARs are omitted for clarity.

dependent memories. However, there are other age-related differences between the NMDAR subtypes that also may be important. They include (a) where the different subtypes reside in the synapse, which affects how they respond to presynaptically released glutamate, and (b) the intracellular signaling cascades they activate, which dictate the direction of change in synaptic efficacy. For instance, it is thought that the developmental decrease in synaptic NMDAR response duration reflects the displacement of the synaptic NR1/NR2B subtype with the NR1/NR2A subtype. This relocation places the NR1/NR2A subtype closer to the site of transmitter release (Steigerwald et al., 2000). As a consequence of this relocation, activity generated at the NR1/NR2A subtype might supersede NR1/NR2B activity because the NR1/NR2A subtypes receive higher concentrations of glutamate. In addition, the two subtypes communicate with different sets of intracellular signaling proteins to differentially regulate synaptic efficacy (Li, Tian, Hartley, & Feig, 2006). Given all of these differences between the two NMDAR subtypes, it may be the case that no single change is responsible for the differences in synaptic plasticity and memory that occur during the transition period.

Whether or not any of these scenarios is correct, there is behavioral evidence that supports the idea that the NR1/NR2A combination in the hippocampus is more critical for memory than is the NR1/NR2B combination. For example NR2A-deficient mice exhibit reduced hippocampal LTP and impaired learning in the spatial water maze (Ito, Akashi, Sakimura, Mishina, & Sugiyama, 1998; Sakimura et al., 1995) and an increased threshold for LTP induction (Kiyama et al., 1998). In contrast, pharmacological blockade of hippocampal NR2B subunits in the hippocampus does not alter LTP (Bartlett et al., 2006; Liu et al., 2004) or performance in the Morris water maze (Guscott et al., 2003; Higgins, Ballard, Huwyler, Kemp, & Gill, 2003).

Conclusions

The hippocampus is part of a neural system that supports our ability to recall our past. Because the rat is altricial and its adult characteristics emerge in a relatively short postnatal period, it has been possible to use several memory-dependent behavioral tasks that depend on the hippocampus to estimate when its hippocampal-memory system becomes functional. Studies of place learning, contextual fear conditioning, and conditional delayed

alternation all converge to indicate that just about the age rats are weaned, around postnatal day 21, the hippocampal memory system begins to function. Our review of the changes in the mechanisms of synaptic plasticity in the hippocampus occurring during the transition period leading up to the emergence of this system reveal several complementary changes in synaptic function. These changes revolve around a shift from synaptic plasticity mechanisms needed to generate a basic neural network to mechanisms that have the potential to support behaviorally-induced, lasting changes in synaptic strength. They include an increase in transmitter release levels, a loss of silent synapses, and a change in the composition of synaptic NMDARs. Together these changes produce a stable infrastructure containing mature synapses that express moderate levels of functional plasticity and are highly attuned to coincidence detection. With the establishment of these synaptic properties and the waning of developmental plasticity processes that are not involved in information coding, at approximately 3 weeks of age, the hippocampus reaches a level of maturity that enables it influence cognitive function and behavior.

References

Aggleton, J. P., Hunt, P. R., & Rawlins, J. N. P. (1986). The effects of hippocampal lesions on spatial and nonspatial test of working memory. *Behavioral Brain Research, 19,* 133–146.

Barria, A. & Malinow, R. (2002). Subunit-specific NMDA receptor trafficking to synapses. *Neuron, 35,* 345–353.

Bartlett, T. E., Bannister, N. J., Collett, V. J., Dargan, S. L., Massey, P. V., Bortolotto, Z. A., et al. (2006). Differential roles of NR2A and NR2B-containing NMDA receptors in LTP and LTD in the CA1 region of two-week old rat hippocampus. *Neuropharmacology*.

Bliss, T. V., & Lomo, T. (1973). Long lasting potentiation of synaptic transmission in the dentate area of the anaesthetized rabbit following stimulation of the perforant path. *Journal of Physiology, 232,* 331–356.

Castro, C. A., Paylor, R., & Rudy, J. W. (1987). A developmental analysis of the learning and short-term memory processes mediating performance in conditional–spatial discrimination problems. *Psychobiology, 15,* 308–316.

Choi, S., Klingauf, J., & Tsien, R. W. (2003). Fusion pore modulation as a presynaptic mechanism contributing to expression of long-term potentiation. *Philosophical Transactions of the Royal Society of London B Biological Sciences, 358,* 695–705.

Cipolotti, L., Shallice, T., Chan, D., Fox, N., Scahill, R., Harrison, G., et al. (2001). Long-term retrograde amnesia…the crucial role of the hippocampus. *Neuropsychologia, 39,* 151–72.

Clark R. E., Broadbent N. J., & Squire L. R. (2005). Hippocampus and remote spatial memory in rats. *Hippocampus, 15*(2), 260–72.

Dudek, S. M., & Bear, M. F. (1993). Bidirectional long-term modification of synaptic effectiveness in the adult and immature hippocampus. *Journal of Neuroscience, 13*, 2910–2918.

Dumas, T. C. (2005a). Late postnatal maturation of excitatory synaptic transmission permits adult-like expression of hippocampal-dependent behaviors. *Hippocampus, 15*, 562–578.

Dumas, T. C. (2005b). Developmental regulation of cognitive abilities: Modified composition of a molecular switch turns on associative learning. *Progress in Neurobiology, 76*, 189–211.

Dumas, T. C., & Foster, T. C. (1995). Developmental increase in CA3–CA1 presynaptic function in the hippocampal slice. *Journal of Neurophysiology, 73*, 1821–1828.

Durand, G. M., Kovalchuk, Y., & Konnerth, A. (1996). Long-term potentiation and functional synapse induction in developing hippocampus. *Nature, 381*, 71–75.

Fanselow, M. S. (2000). Contextual fear gestalt memories, and the hippocampus. *Behavioral Brain Research, 110*, 73–81.

Feinstein P. G., Schrader, K. A., Bakalyar, H. A., Tang, W. J., Krupinski J., Gilman. A. G., Reed, R. R. (1991). Molecular cloning and characterization of a Ca2+/calmodulin-insensitive adenylyl cyclase from rat brain. *Proceedings of the National Academy of Sciences, 88*, 10173–10177.

Gerrow, K., & El-Husseini, A. (2006). Cell adhesion molecules at the synapse. *Frontiers in Biosciences, 11*, 2400–2419.

Green, R. J., & Stanton, M. E. (1989). Differential ontogeny of working memory and reference memory in the rat. *Behavioral Neuroscience, 103*, 98–105.

Guscott, M. R., Clarke, H. F., Murray, F., Grimwood, S., Bristow, L. J., & Hutson, P. H. (2003). The effect of ( )-CP-101,606, an NMDA receptor NR2B subunit selective antagonist, in the Morris watermaze. *Journal of Pharmacology, 476*, 193–199.

Haydon, P. G., & Drapeau, P. (1995). From contact to connection: Early events during synaptogenesis. *Trends in Neuroscience, 18*, 196–201.

Higgins, G. A., Ballard, T. M., Huwyler, J., Kemp, J. A., & Gill, R. (2003). Evaluation of the NR2B-selective NMDA receptor antagonist Ro 63-1908 on rodent behavior: Evidence for an involvement of NR2B NMDA receptors in response inhibition. *Neuropharmacology, 44*, 324–341.

Hyson, R. L. & Rudy, J. W. (1984). Ontogenesis of learning. II. Variation in the rat's reflexive and learned responses to acoustic stimulation. *Developmental Psychobiology, 17*, 263–283.

Isaac, J. T. R., Nicoll, R. A., & Malenka, R. C. (1995). Evidence for silent synapses: implications for the expression of LTP. *Neuron, 15*, 427–434.

Ito, I., Akashi, K., Sakimura, K., Mishina, M., & Sugiyama, H. (1998). Distribution and development of NMDA receptor activities at hippocampal synapses examined using mice lacking the epsilon 1 subunit gene. *Neuroscience Research, 30*, 119–123.

Jackson, J. H. (1958). Evolution and dissolution of the nervous system. In J. Taylor (Ed), *Selected writings of John Hughlings Jackson* (Vol. 2, pp. 45–75). New York: Basic Books.

Jackson, J. H. (2001). Evolution and dissolution of the nervous system. In J. Taylor (Ed.), *Selected writings of John Hughlings Jackson* (Vol. 2 pp 45-75). New York: Basic Books.

Kandel, E. R., & O'Dell, T. J. (1992). Are adult learning mechanisms also used for development? *Science, 258*, 243–245.

Kim, J. J., & Fanselow, M. (1992). Modality-specific retrograde amnesia of fear. *Science, 256*, 675–676.

Kirson, E. D., & Yaari, Y. (1996). Synaptic NMDA receptors in developing mouse hippocampal neurones: Functional properties and sensitivity to ifenprodil. *Journal of Physiology, 497*, 437–455.

Kiyama, Y., Manabe, T., Sakimura, K., Kawakami, F., Mori, H., & Mishina, M. (1998). Increased thresholds for long-term potentiation and contextual learning in mice lacking the NMDA-type glutamate receptor epsilon 1 subunit. *Journal of Neuroscience, 18*, 6704–6712.

Larkman, A., Hannay, T., Stratford, K., & Jack, J. (1992). Presynaptic release probability influences the locus of long-term potentiation. *Nature, 360*, 70–73.

Lavenex, P., & Amaral, D.G. (2000). Hippocampal–neocortical interaction: A hierarchy of associativity. *Hippocampus, 10*, 420–430.

Li, S., Tian, X., Hartley, D. M., & Feig, L. A. (2006). Distinct roles for Ras-guanine nucleotide-releasing factor 1 (Ras-GRF1) and Ras-GRF2 in the induction of long-term potentiation and long-term depression. *Journal of Neuroscience, 26*, 1721–1729.

Liao, D., Hessler, N. A., & Malinow, R. (1995). Activation of postsynaptically silent synapses during pairing-induced LTP in CA1 region of hippocampal slice. *Nature, 375*, 400–404.

Liao, D., O'Brien, R., Ehlers, M. D., & Huganir, R. (1999). Regulation of morphological postsynaptic silent synapses in developing hippocampal neurons. *Nature Neuroscience, 2*, 37–43.

Liu, L., Wong, T. P., Pozza, M. F., Lingenhoehl, K., Wang, Y., Sheng, M., et al. (2004). Role of NMDA receptor subtypes in governing the direction of hippocampal synaptic plasticity. *Science, 304*, 1021–1024.

Malenka, R. M., & Bear, M. F. (2004). LTP and LTD: An embarrassment of riches. *Neuron, 44*, 5–21.

Matsuoka, I., Suzuki, Y., Defer, N., Nakanishi, H., & Hanoune, J. (1997). Differential expression of type I, II, and V adenylyl cyclase gene in the postnatal developing brain. *Journal of Neurochemistry, 68*, 498–506.

McNaughton, B. L., Shen, J., Rao, G., Foster, T. C., & Barnes, C. A. (1994). Temperature, NMDA receptor, and nitric oxide synthase dependent increase in CA1 axon terminal excitability following repetitive stimulation. *Proceedings of the National Academy of Science USA, 91*, 4830–4834.

Milner, B. (1970). Memory and the medial temporal lobe regions of the brain. In K. H. Pribram & D. E. Broadbent (Eds.), *Biology of memory* (pp 29–50). New York; Academic Press.

Misane, I., Tovote, P., Meyer, M., Spiess, J., Ogren, S. O., & Stiedl, O. (2005). Time-dependent involvement of the dorsal hippocampus in trace fear conditioning in mice, *Hippocampus, 15*, 418–426.

Monyer, H., Sprengel, R., Schoepfer, R., Herb, A., Higuchi, M., Lomeli, H., et al. (1992). Heteromeric NMDA receptors: molecular and functional distinction of subtypes. *Science, 256*, 1217–1221.

Monyer, H., Burnashev, N., Laurie, D. J., Sakmann, B., & Seeburg, P. H. (1994). Developmental and regional expression in the rat brain and functional properties of four NMDA receptors. *Neuron, 12*, 529–540.

Morris, R. G. M. (1981). Spatial localisation does not depend on the presence of local cues. *Learning and Motivation, 12*, 239–260.

Morris, R. G. M., Garrud, P., Rawlins, J. N. P., & O'Keefe, J. (1982). Place-navigation impaired in rats with hippocampal lesions. *Nature, 297*, 681–683.

Morris, R. G. M., Moser, E. I., Riedel, G., Martin, S. J., Sandin, J., et al. (2003). Elements of a neurobiological theory of the hippocampus: The role of activity-dependent synaptic plasticity in memory. *Philosophical Transactions of the Royal Society of London B Biological Sciences, 358*, 773–786.

Moye, T. B., & Rudy, J. W. (1985). Ontogenesis of learning. VI. Learned and unlearned responses to visual stimulation in the infant hooded rat. *Developmental Psychobiology, 18*, 395–409.

Moye, T. B., & Rudy, J. W. (1987). Ontogenesis of trace conditioning in young rats: Dissociation of associative and memory processes. *Developmental Psychobiology, 20*, 405–414.

O'Keefe, J., & Dostrovsky, J. (1971). The hippocampus as a spatial map. *Brain Research, 34*, 171–175.

O'Keefe, J. and Nadel, L. (1978). *The hippocampus as a cognitive map*. Oxford: Clarendon Press.

O'Reilly, R. C., & Rudy, J. W. (2001). Conjunctive representations in learning and memory: Principles of cortical and hippocampal function. *Psychological Review, 108*, 311–345.

Phillips, R. G., & LeDoux, J. E. (1992). Differential contribution of amygdala and hippocampus to cued and contextual fear conditioning. *Behavioral Neuroscience, 106*, 274–285.

Quinlan, E. M., Lebel, D., Brosh, I., & Barkai, E. A. (2004). A molecular mechanism for stabilization of learning-induced synaptic modifications. *Neuron, 41*, 185–192.

Renger, J. J., Egles, C., & Liu, G. (2001). A developmental switch in neurotransmitter flux enhances synaptic efficacy by affecting AMPA receptor activation. *Neuron, 29*, 469–484.

Roberts, E. B., & Ramoa, A. S. (1999). Enhanced NR2A subunit expression and decreased NMDA receptor decay time at the onset of ocular dominance plasticity in the ferret. *Journal of Neurophysiology, 81*, 2587–2591.

Rudy, J. W. (1992). Development of Learning: From elementistic to configural association systems. In C. Rovee-Collier & L. Lipsitt (Eds.), *Advances in infancy research* (pp. 247–290). Norwood, NJ: Ablex Publishing Corp.

Rudy, J. W. (1993). Contextual conditioning and auditory cue conditioning dissociate during development. *Behavioral Neuroscience, 107*, 887–891.

Rudy, J. W. (2008). *The neurobiology of learning and memory*. Sunderland, MA: Sinauer Associates.

Rudy, J. W., Huff, N., & Matus-Amat, P. (2004). Understanding contextual fear conditioning: Insights from a two process model. *Neuroscience and Biobehavioral Reviews, 28*, 675–685.

Rudy, J. W., & Paylor, R. (1988). Reducing the temporal demands of the Morris place learning task fails to ameliorate the place-learning impairment in preweanling rats. *Psychobiology, 16*, 152–156.

Rudy, J. W., Stadler-Morris, S., & Albert, P. A. (1987). Ontogeny of spatial navigation behaviors in the rat: Dissociation of "proximal-" and "distal-cue" based behaviors. *Behavioral Neurosciences, 101*, 62–73.

Rudy, J. W. & Sutherland, R. J. (1995). Configural association theory and the hippocampal formation: An appraisal and reconfiguration. *Hippocampus, 5*, 375–389.

Sakimura, K., Kutsuwada, T., Ito, I., Manabe, T., Takayama, C., Kushiya, E., et al.. (1995). Reduced hippocampal LTP and spatial learning in mice lacking NMDA receptor e1 subunit. *Nature, 373*, 151–155.

Schacter, D. L. (1987). Implicit memory: History and current status. *Journal of Experimental Psychology: Learning, Memory and Cognition, 13*, 501–518.

Sherry, D. F., & Schacter, D. L. (1987). The evolution of multiple memory systems. *Psychological Review, 94*, 439–454.

Squire, L. R. (1992). Memory and the hippocampus: A synthesis from findings with rats, monkeys, and humans. *Psychological Review, 99*, 195–231.

Squire, L. R. (2004). Memory systems of the brain: A brief history and current perspective. *Neurobiology of Learning and Memory, 82*, 171–177.

Steigerwald, F., Schulz, T. W., Schenker, L. T., Kennedy, M. B., Seeburg, P. H., & Kohr, G. (2000). C-Terminal truncation of NR2A subunits impairs synaptic but not extrasynaptic localization of NMDA receptors. *Journal of Neuroscience, 20*, 4573–4581.

Sutherland, R. J., Kolb, B., & Whishaw, I, Q. (1982). Spatial mapping: Definitive disruption by hippocampal or medial frontal cortical damage in the rat. *Neuroscience Letters, 31*, 271–276.

Sutherland, R. J., & Rudy, J. W. (1988). Place learning in the Morris place learning task is impaired by damage to the hippocampal formation even if the temporal demands are reduced. *Psychobiology, 16*, 157–163.

Teylor, T. J., and DiScenna, P. (1986). The hippocampal memory indexing theory. *Behavioral Neuroscience, 100*, 147–154.

Teyler, T. J., & Rudy, J. W. (2007). The hippocampal indexing theory and episodic memory. Updating the index. *Hippocampus, 17*, 1158–1169.

Velisek, L., Moshe, S. L., & Stanton, P. K. (1993). Age-dependence of homosynaptic non-NMDA mediated long-term depression in field CA1 of rat hippocampal slices. *Brain Research: Developmental Brain Research, 75*, 253–260.

Vogt, M. B., & Rudy, J. W. (1984). Ontogenesis of learning. I. Variation in the rat's reflexive and learned responses to gustatory stimulation. *Developmental Psychobiology, 17*, 11–33.

Waters, N. S., Klintsova, A. Y., & Foster, T. C. (1997). Insensitivity of the hippocampus to environmental stimulation during postnatal development. *Journal of Neuroscience, 17*, 7967–7973.

Williams, J. H., Li, Y. G., Nayak, A., Errington, M. L., Murphy, K. P. S. J., & Bliss, T. V. P. (1993). The suppression of long-term potentiation in rat hippocampus by inhibitors of nitric oxide synthase is temperature and age dependent. *Neuron, 11*, 877–884.

Yasuda, H., Barth, A. L., Stellwagen, D., & Malenka, R. C. (2003). A developmental switch in the signaling cascades for LTP induction. *Nature Neuroscience, 6*, 15–16.

Zakharenko, S. S., Zablow, L., & Siegelbaum, S. A. (2001). Visualization of changes in presynaptic function during long-term synaptic plasticity. *Nature Neuroscience, 4*, 711–717.

Zola-Morgan, S., Squire, L. R., & Amaral, D. G. (1986). Human amnesia and the medial temporal region: Enduring memory impairment following a bilateral lesion limited to field CA1 of the hippocampus. *Journal of Neuroscience, 6*(10), 2950–2967.

Development of Medial Temporal Lobe Memory Processes in Nonhuman Primates

Alyson Zeamer, Maria C. Alvarado, *and* Jocelyne Bachevalier

Abstract

The declarative memory system, which supports "explicit" memory for facts and events, is known to be mediated by an integrated neural network including the medial temporal lobe, diencephalon, and the prefrontal cortex. This chapter focuses on the development of those declarative memory processes mediated by the medial temporal lobe structures, specifically, the hippocampus, entorhinal cortex, and perirhinal cortex. This chapter examines what we currently know about the morphological maturation of these structures in monkeys, as well as how these maturational patterns map onto the development of two types of declarative memory: recognition memory and relational memory. The current evidence indicates that the infant brain may use alternate neural pathways to support memory functions observed in adulthood.

Keywords: recognition memory, relational memory, hippocampus, perirhinal cortex, parahippocampal cortex

There has been a great deal of progress in the last half century in our understanding of the neural substrates involved in memory processing in human and nonhuman primates. Through the course of examining patients with damage restricted to the medial temporal lobe (Corkin, Amaral, Gonzalez, Johnson, & Hyman, 1997; Scoville & Milner, 1957), as well as more recent animal models with rodents (Eichenbaum, 1992, 2003) and nonhuman primates (Alvarado & Bachevalier, 2007), memory processes have classically been divided into two major types: nondeclarative and declarative memory (Squire, 1992; Tulving, 1972).

The nondeclarative system supports "implicit" forms of memory, such as conditioning to neutral stimuli as well as the acquisition and retention of skill learning, and is mediated by the neostriatum and cerebellum (see for review, Eichenbaum, 2003). The declarative system supports "explicit"

forms of memory that can further be divided into semantic and episodic memories. Semantic memory encompasses our general knowledge of the world and contains information that can be used in many different contexts, including such facts as "Washington DC is the capital of the United States" or "strawberries are red." Episodic memory encompasses memories that are autobiographical in nature and contains information that can be localized to a specific time and place, such as remembering what song played at your wedding, and when and where it took place. The declarative memory system is supported by an integrated neural network including the medial temporal lobe (Eichenbaum, Yonelinas, & Ranganath, 2007), the diencephalon (Aggleton & Brown, 1999; Squire, Amaral and Press, 1990; Vann & Aggleton, 2004), and the prefrontal cortex (Braver et al., 2001; Dudukovic & Wagner, 2007; Fernandez

& Tendolkar, 2001; Petrides, 2005; Ranganath, Johnson, & D'Esposito, 2003). This chapter will focus on the development of declarative memory processes, and, more specifically, of memory processes mediated by the medial temporal lobe structures (see Bachevalier, 2008, for a recent review of the nondeclarative memory processes).

The chapter will begin with a brief review of our knowledge of the morphological maturation of the structures within the medial temporal lobe in monkeys, followed by a section summarizing how these maturational patterns map onto the development of medial temporal lobe memory processes; more specifically, recognition memory and relational memory. The final section is devoted to a discussion on how these developmental studies in monkeys can shed light onto the development of memory processes in humans.

Medial Temporal Lobe Structures and Memory

The medial temporal lobe includes a set of cortical areas that receives highly processed multimodal information (Figure 29.1). These temporal cortical areas are involved in the storage and retrieval of stimulus representations, and are viewed as storing information or knowledge independently of the context in which they are learned (fact or semantic memory). Recent anatomical studies in rodents (Burwell & Witter, 2002) and monkeys (Suzuki & Amaral, 2004) have shown that multimodal inputs reaching these medial temporal cortical areas appear to be loosely segregated. Thus, the parahippocampal cortex (TH and TF) receives more extensive spatial information about objects, mainly from the parietal cortex and lateral prefrontal cortex, and is known to support spatial memory. The perirhinal (PRh) cortex by contrast receives perceptual information about objects from sensory cortical areas (such as visual areas TEO and TE) and mediates item-specific memory, as well as learning of stimulus–stimulus, cross-modal, and stimulus–reward associations. Finally, both TH/TF and PRh project to the entorhinal (ERh) cortex, which represents the final station before these inputs reach the hippocampal formation (dentate gyrus, CA fields, and subicular complex). It is believed that the hippocampal formation is needed to acquire, store, and recollect interitem relations and their context and supports recollection of specific episodes or events (Brown & Aggleton, 2001; Eichenbaum, 2003; Lavenex & Amaral, 2000; Mishkin, Suzuki, Gadian, & Vargha-Khadem, 1997; O'Reilly &

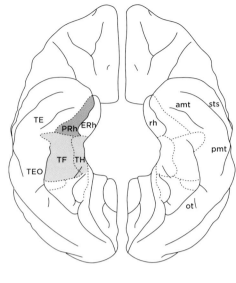

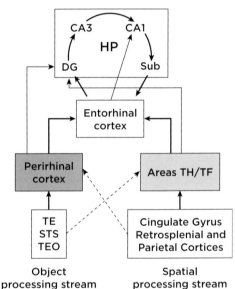

Figure 29.1 Anatomy of the medial temporal lobe. Ventral view of the monkey brain (top) defining the cytoarchitectonic borders of the different medial temporal cortical areas (left) and the major sulci (right). Schematic drawing of the hierarchical organization of cortical inputs reaching the hippocampal formation (bottom). Abbreviations: amt, anterior medial temporal sulcus; CA1 and CA3, cornus ammoni fields; DG, dentate gyrus; ERh, entorhinal cortex; HP, hippocampal formation; ot, occipitotemporal sulcus; pmt, posterior medial temporal sulcus; PRh, perirhinal cortex; rh, rhinal sulcus; sts, superior temporal sulcus; TH/TF, temporal cortical areas on the parahippocampal gyrus; TE and TEO, visual temporal areas as defined by von Bonin and Bailey (1947).

Rudy, 2001; Yonelinas, 2002). Although the evidence in humans and animals suggests that each of these medial temporal lobe (MTL) structures may contribute to declarative memory processes in a specific and integrative way, their contribution to the emergence of MTL memory processes during development is still poorly understood.

Maturation of MTL Structures

Detailed knowledge of the morphological, neurochemical, and functional maturation of the MTL structures is still very scarce. However, the available data indicate that the maturation of the hippocampal formation may lag behind that of the medial temporal cortical areas (see for review Alvarado & Bachevalier, 2000). Thus, most of the neurogenesis in medial temporal cortical areas occurs prenatally, although there are several morphological and neurochemical changes occurring in the first few months postnatally. The rhinal sulcus, which divides the entorhinal from the perirhinal cortex (see Figure 29.1), is still only a small indent on the cortical surface by the last quarter of gestation (Berger & Alvarez, 1994). At birth, the cytoarchitectonic and chemoanatomical characteristics of the perirhinal and entorhinal cortex in the primate can be clearly identified and appear adult-like (Berger & Alvarez, 1994), whereas those of areas TH and TF are still unknown. By contrast, the connectional system between these cortical areas continues to be refined after birth. Thus, afferent projections from temporal cortical area TEO to area TF are present in the 1-week-old infant but are absent in the adult, and those from temporal cortical area TE to the perirhinal cortex are more widespread in the 1-week-old infant than in the adult (Webster, Ungerleider, & Bachevalier, 1991, 1995). These transient connections retract between 2 and 6 months postnatally (Webster, Bachevalier, & Ungerleider, unpublished data), indicating that maturation of the medial temporal cortical areas becomes complete and fully mature in the first postnatal months in monkeys.

By contrast, synaptogenesis and myelination of the hippocampal formation continue throughout the first postnatal year. Indeed, a recent longitudinal structural neuroimaging study revealed an increase in overall hippocampal volume as well as changes in the ratio of gray to white matter from birth to 11 months of age in monkeys (Machado, Babin, Jackson, & Bachevalier, 2002). This is consistent with recent findings showing that the volume of the dentate gyrus remains relatively the same between 3 weeks and 3 months of age, but nearly doubles by adulthood (Lavenex, Lavenex, & Amaral, 2007a). Thus, significant synaptic changes occur within the hippocampal formation during the first year postnatally. As for the medial temporal cortical areas,

neurogenesis of the CA fields as well as the dentate gyrus occurs mostly during prenatal life. However, many morphological and neurochemical changes as well as fine-tuning of the synaptic connections continue in the hippocampal formation for several years after birth. In the monkey (see for review, Alvarado & Bachevalier, 2000; Lavenex et al., 2007a; Seress & Ribak, 1995a, 1995b), neurogenesis in the dentate gyrus is approximately 80% complete at birth, but nearly 20% of neurons are added postnatally (Lavenex et al., 2007a). In addition, in the second half of the first postnatal year, CA3 neurons increase in number and in size, and their spines increase in complexity. Throughout the first postnatal year, synapses from axons of dentate neurons contacting the dendrites of the CA3 cells (mossy fiber pathway) are formed and there is an increase in the myelination of hippocampal afferent and efferent fibers. Finally, whereas the neurotransmitter systems within the hippocampus, both cholinergic and GABAergic, are present at birth, they undergo considerable changes postnatally (Lavenex et al., 2007a).

To summarize, the basic trisynaptic pathway of the hippocampal formation (ERh → dentate gyrus → CA3 → CA2 → CA1→ subiculum) demonstrates a protracted postnatal maturation. Although afferent projections from the entorhinal cortex to the dentate gyrus are present by 3 weeks of age (Lavenex et al., 2007a), the dentate gyrus continues to mature during the first postnatal year. Similarly, the CA3 pyramidal cells (the second station of the trisynaptic pathway) show synaptic changes beyond the first postnatal year. By contrast, afferent projections from the ERh to the CA1, the so-called "direct pathway" (Sybirska, Davachi, & Goldman-Rakic, 2000), are present at birth and mature over the first few months of life. Thus, the two main cortical–hippocampal pathways that are linked to memory processes appear to develop at different rates. It is tempting to suggest that memory processes supported by the entorhinal–CA1 pathway may emerge earlier than those supported by the trisynaptic pathway (Alvarado & Bachevalier, 2000).

Development of Recognition Memory Abilities

Although declarative memory processes are usually measured in humans by asking a subject to recall and describe verbally an event or episode that had occurred earlier, measuring similar memory processes in animals (or young preverbal infants) is more problematic and memory is usually inferred by observing a change in the subject's behavior. Thus, although we cannot determine whether an animal can recall a specific memory, we can determine (a) whether animals can recognize a previously seen memorandum and use that information to guide behavior, (b) whether animals forget newly learned information more rapidly as a result of brain damage or brain immaturity, and (c) whether only information learned in a specific context (i.e., episode) is forgotten, or if the processes that allow encoding of context are somehow impaired. Several recognition and relational tasks have been developed in animals to assess memory processes mediated by the medial temporal lobe structures (see for review Alvarado & Bachevalier, 2007).

One memory paradigm that has been shown to be sensitive to damage to the medial temporal lobe structures is the visual paired comparison (VPC) task (also known as "preferential looking"). VPC takes advantage of an animal's natural preference for looking toward a novel stimulus over a familiar one (Figure 29.2) and indexes recognition memory (Fagan, 1970); more specifically, an incidental recognition-based memory since the animal is not required to learn any rules to solve the task. Several studies have now demonstrated that preference for novelty is significantly reduced or abolished by selective damage to either the medial temporal cortical areas (Nemanic, Alvarado, & Bachevalier, 2004) or the hippocampal formation in both monkeys (Nemanic et al., 2004; Zola et al., 2000) and humans (McKee & Squire, 1993; Pascalis, Hunkin, Holdstock, Isaac, & Mayes, 2004).

Earlier studies in infant monkeys have demonstrated the presence of preference for novelty as early as the first postnatal month, even after long delays between familiarization and retention tests (Bachevalier, Brickson, & Hagger, 1993; Gunderson & Sackett, 1984, Gunderson & Swartz, 1985, 1986). In a recent longitudinal study, a group of infant rhesus macaques were tested in the VPC task at 1, 6, and 18 months of age (Zeamer, Resende, Heuer, & Bachevalier, 2006). As shown in Table 29.1 (see Group Neo-C), preference for novelty was present at the youngest age (1 month), averaging 64% looking at novel stimuli at the shortest delay of 10 s and 64% at the longest delay of 120 s, but became more robust by 6 months of age (72% at 10 s and 74% at 120 s). By 18 months of age, however, a delay-dependent effect emerged with preference for novelty averaging 74% at the shortest delay of 10 s and decreasing to 65% at the longest delay of 120 s. This pattern of results is interesting because

it may suggest critical changes within the neural substrate supporting this ability during maturation as described below. To investigate whether this delay-dependent effect in novelty preference reflected changes within the medial temporal lobe structures, novelty preference was also assessed at 1, 6, and 18 months of age in monkeys that had received selective bilateral neurotoxic lesions of the hippocampus between 10 and 12 days of age (Bachevalier & Vargha-Khadem, 2005; Zeamer et al., 2006). Preference for novelty in monkeys with neonatal hippocampal lesions (see Table 29.1, Group Neo-H) was similar to that of controls at 1 and 6 months of age, suggesting that structures other than the hippocampal formation could support this function in the first postnatal months. Thus, in early infancy this type of recognition memory could be mediated by the medial temporal lobe cortical areas thought to be critical for familiarity judgments in adults (Brown & Aggleton, 2001; Murray, 2000; Nemanic et al., 2004; Yonelinas, 2002). However, by 18 months of age, whereas the monkeys with neonatal hippocampal lesions did not differ from controls at the short delays, at 120 s delay, they showed significantly weaker preference for novelty (56%) than controls (65%). This pattern of impairment suggests that with maturation the animals with neonatal hippocampal lesions grow into a recognition memory deficit. Thus, the delay-dependent recognition memory observed in the controls at 18 months of age together with the

Table 29.1 Preference for Novelty as a Function of Delay and Age

| Age | Delay (s) | Percent Looking at Novel | |
		Group Neo-C	Group Neo-H
1 Month	10	63.59	61.40
	30	68.80	64.83
	60	65.81	64.84
	120	64.22	61.68
6 Months	10	71.73	67.74
	30	74.89	75.65
	60	70.56	68.86
	120	74.29	73.25
18 Months	10	73.65	66.25
	30	68.69	63.97
	60	68.47	71.75
	120	65.11	56.16*

Note: Group Neo-C: monkeys that received sham-operation; Group Neo-H: monkeys that received bilateral neurotoxic lesions of the hippocampal formation in infancy. * denotes Group × Delay, $p < 0.05$

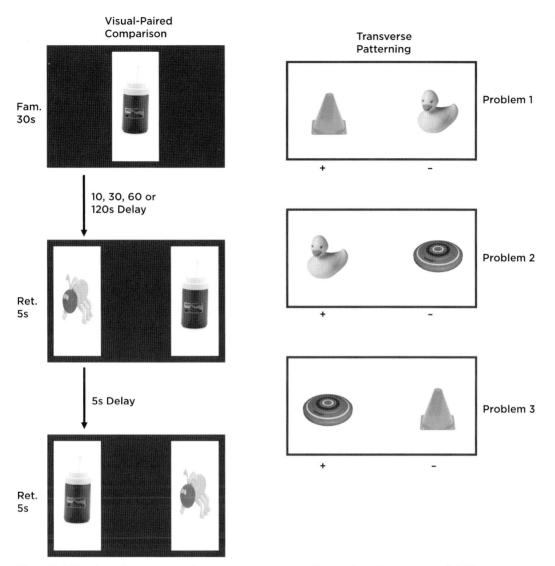

Figure 29.2 Visual paired comparison and transverse patterning tasks. The visual paired comparison task (left) measures recognition of a previously seen stimulus. First, the animal passively views a visual stimulus for familiarization (Fam.), often lasting 30 s. Following familiarization, there is a delay period, which can vary for 1 s to several minutes, and then the familiar stimulus reappears on the screen side-by-side with a novel stimulus for two retention tests (Ret.) of 5 s each, separated by a 5 s interval. Longer time spent fixating one of the stimuli (normally the novel one) during the retention tests indicates recognition memory. The transverse patterning task (Spence, 1952) includes three discrimination problems (right) formed by three objects. The animal is rewarded for selecting one of the 2 objects in each problem, as indicated by the symbol "+," and has to learn these three problems concurrently.

appearance of an impairment in incidental recognition-based memory in the animals with neonatal hippocampal lesions at the same age suggest that in infancy, the medial temporal cortical areas can mediate recognition memory processes in which the hippocampus will ultimately participate.

Development of Relational Memory Abilities

Several different paradigms have been used in animals to assess relational memory abilities mediated by the medial temporal lobe structures and have provided evidence for both spatial and nonspatial deficits in animals and humans with hippocampal or medial temporal cortical damage (see for review, Alvarado & Bachevalier, 2007). These paradigms have also been used to follow the development of memory abilities and have shown that relational memory has a more protracted development than recognition memory.

In the transverse patterning problem (Figure 29.2), the animal must learn concurrently a set of three discrimination problems (A+ B–; B+ C–; C+ A–). Because the individual stimuli (A, B, and C) are associated with reward (+) and nonreward (–), a representation of the three conjunctions <AB>, <BC>, and <CA> allows for the disambiguation of the individual stimuli. In a longitudinal study (Málková et al., 1999), infant monkeys were tested in this task at 3, 6, 12, 24, and 36 months. Performance scores to solve transverse patterning problems increased steadily with age, reaching 53% correct responses in the last hundred trials at 3 months of age, 72% correct at 6 months, 78% correct at 12 months, 81% correct at 24 months, and finally 90% correct (criterion performance) at 36 months. Although the abilities to solve this task emerged at about 1 year of age, they did not reach adult proficiency until 3 years. Similarly, the ability to solve a biconditional discrimination task, in which an animal learns to discriminate between two rewarded and two unrewarded pairs of objects (e.g. AB+, CD+, AD–, CB–) is absent in infant monkeys at 6 months and 1 year of age (Killiany, Rehbein, & Mahut, 2005). Finally, monkeys do not show adult levels of proficiency on the oddity task until 3–4 years of age (Harlow, 1959). In the oddity task, animals are presented with three objects (two similar and one odd) and receive a reward for displacing the odd object. Thus, the ability to solve relational tasks is not evident before 2–3 years of age in monkeys, although it is still unknown whether immaturity of the hippocampal formation is the limiting factor for this protracted development. However, our preliminary data using an oddity task have shown significant impairment in the task in monkeys with neonatal hippocampal lesions (Alvarado, Kazama, & Bachevalier, unpublished data).

Finally, spatial memory, which measures the ability to use spatial relationships among cues to recollect specific locations within an environment, has also been shown to be mediated by the hippocampal formation (see for review Alvarado & Bachevalier, 2007) and the parahippocampal areas TH/TF (Alvarado & Bachevalier, 2005; Málková & Mishkin, 2003) in monkeys. There has been no investigation of the development of spatial memory abilities in monkeys. Recently, however, Lavenex and Lavenex (2006) used a foraging memory task known to be impaired after damage to the hippocampal formation and parahippocampal cortex in adult monkeys (Lavenex, Amaral, & Lavenex, 2006) to assess spatial memory abilities in infant

monkeys. Nine-month-old monkeys showed that they could remember locations in which they had previously found food and these abilities were not disrupted by neonatal damage to the hippocampal formation (Lavenex, Lavenex, & Amaral, 2007b). These findings suggest that other areas, such as parahippocampal cortex, could support these spatial memory abilities in early infancy and it will thus be interesting to see whether, as is the case for recognition memory measured by VPC (see above), impairment in this spatial task emerges at a time when the trisynaptic circuit becomes fully mature, i.e., 2–3 years in monkeys.

Relationship to Memory Development in Humans

The data reviewed in this chapter provide several insights into the development of medial temporal lobe memory processes in monkeys that could have direct implications for our understanding of the development of these processes in humans.

First, the accumulation of anatomical and behavioral data from the developmental studies reviewed above does not show a single pattern of development for memory processes supported by the medial temporal lobe structures. Thus, whereas the maturation of the temporal cortical areas as well as the circuit connecting the entorhinal cortex to the CA1 field of the hippocampal formation becomes functional within the first months postnatally, the trisynaptic circuit of the hippocampal formation does not reach full maturity before 2 years of age. Concomitantly, incidental recognition-based memory processes, as measured by VPC, are present as early as the first postnatal month, whereas relational memory abilities develop over the first 2 postnatal years (see Alvarado & Bachevalier, 2000; Bachevalier & Vargha-Khadem, 2005). A similar developmental pattern exists in humans (Table 29.2). Thus, whereas preference for novelty is present as early as 3 days of age (Pascalis & de Schonen, 1994) and become more robust during the first years of age (for review see Nelson, 1995, 1997), the ability to solve relational memory tasks, such as transverse patterning (Rudy, Keith, & Georgian, 1993), oddity (Overman, Bachevalier, Miller, & Moore, 1996a) and spatial (i.e., human versions of the Morris water maze and radial arm maze, Overman, Pate, Moore, & Peuster, 1996b) tasks does not reach adult proficiency before 5 years of age. It is also interesting to note that in human as well, the hippocampal formation appears to have

Table 29.2 Development of MTL Memory Processes in Monkeys and Humans

Memory Processes/Tasks	Monkeys	Humans
Recognition tasks		
Visual paired comparison	2 weeks (earliest age tested)	3 days[a]
Relational tasks		
Spatial	9 months	4–5 years[b]
Biconditional discrimination	2–3 years	
Transverse patterning	2–3 years	4–5 years[c]
Oddity	3–4 years	7 years[b,d]

Note: For visual functions, 1 week of development in monkeys corresponds roughly to 1 month of development in humans.

[a]Nelson, 1995; [b]Overman, Pate, Brooke, and Peuster, 1996b; [c]Rudy, Keith, and Georgen, 1993; [d]Overman, Bachevalier, Miller, and Moore, 1996a.

a protracted morphological development (Benes, Turtle, Khan, & Farol, 1994; Giedd et al., 1996; Seress, 2001). Thus, it is possible that the earliest types of memories available in infancy are those that are context-free and that could be supported by the early developing medial temporal cortical areas and the ERh-CA1 pathway. By contrast, context-rich memory process (Tulving, 1995) may develop more slowly, mirroring the protracted development of the hippocampal formation and its interactions with other cortical areas, such as temporal and prefrontal cortex (Bachevalier & Vargha-Khadem, 2005; Mishkin et al., 1997; Mishkin, Vargha-Khadem, & Gadian, 1998).

Second, the data also suggest that neonatal damage to the hippocampal formation yields significant sparing of memory functions that is not seen after the same lesions in adulthood. Thus, in the absence of a functional hippocampal formation at birth, infant monkeys could still display incidental recognition-based memory (Zeamer et al., 2006) as well as spatial abilities (Lavenex et al., 2007b), though these abilities, at least those measured by VPC at 18 months of age, were not as robust as those measured in the control animals (see Table 29.1). These data suggest that, in the absence of a functional hippocampal formation at birth, the medial temporal cortical areas could remain committed to these memory processes. It is interesting that children with damage to the hippocampal formation occurring perinatally or in childhood show verbal and nonverbal recognition (measuring context-free memory processes) within the normal range, but marked impairment in recall taxing context-reach memory processes (Baddeley, Vargha-Khadem, & Mishkin, 2001; Duzel, Vargha-Khadem, Heinze, & Mishkin, 2001). Thus, the existence of preserved recognition abilities in human developmental

amnesia may, as in the monkeys, be maintained by the early developing medial temporal cortical areas.

The final and significant comment with which we would like to conclude this chapter is that the monkey data clearly demonstrate that the neural structures within the medial temporal lobe that support the early types of memory processes in infancy are not necessarily the same structures that will be committed to the same functions in adulthood. Thus, finding that an infant monkey or a preverbal human infant can perform well on a memory task known to be mediated by the hippocampal formation in adulthood does not necessarily mean that the hippocampal formation is fully functional at this early age since different brain structures may be committed to performance on the same tasks. This notion has already been discussed for the development of working memory in monkeys (Goldman & Rosvold, 1972) and for the development of language abilities in humans (Bates, 2004).

To sum up, whereas significant progress has been made in our understanding of the development of the neural circuits underlying declarative memory processes, there is still much more to be learned. Given growing evidence indicating that the infant brain may possess alternate pathways to support cognitive functions observed in adulthood (Bates, 2004; Goldman & Rosvold, 1972; Webster et al., 1995), additional morphological and functional studies in nonhuman primates will be critical for defining the neural substrate available at different time points in development to support memory functions. Of particular interest will be studies aimed at evaluating the age, if any, at which neonatal hippocampal damage may severely impact relational memory processes. Is it possible that, as with recognition memory, relational memory processes may, at least in part, be supported by other neural structures before full maturation of the trisynaptic circuit within the hippocampal formation? Finally, longitudinal studies that take advantage of tasks and paradigms that can be used across species will be most important for furthering our understanding of the functional maturation of declarative memory processes in humans.

Acknowledgment

Preparation of this chapter was supported in part by grants from the National Institute of Mental Health, MH58846, the Yerkes Base Grant NIH RR00165 and the Center for Behavioral Neuroscience grant NSF IBN-9876754.

References

Aggleton, J. P., & Brown, M. W. (1999). Episodic memory, amnesia, and the hippocampal–anterior thalamic axis. *Behavioural Brain Science, 22,* 425–444.

Alvarado, M. C., & Bachevalier, J. (2000). Revisiting the maturation of medial temporal lobe memory functions in primates. *Learning and Memory, 7,* 244–256.

Alvarado, M., & Bachevalier, J. (2005). Selective neurotoxic damage to the hippocampal formation impairs acquisition and performance of the transverse patterning task and location memory in rhesus macaques. *Hippocampus, 15,*118–131.

Alvarado, M. C., & Bachevalier, J. (2008, in press). Animal models of amnesia. In: J. Byrne (ed.) *Learning and Memory: A Comprehensive Reference* (Vol 3, pp. 143–167). New York: Elsevier.

Bachevalier, J., & Vargha-Khadem, F. (2005). The primate hippocampus: Ontogeny, early insult and memory. *Current Opinion in Neurobiology, 15,* 168–174.

Bachevalier, J. (2008). Non-human primate models of memory development. In: C. Nelson, & M. Luciana (Eds.), *Handbook of developmental cognitive neuroscience,* 2nd ed., (pp. 499–508). Cambridge, MA: MIT Press.

Bachevalier, J., Brickson, M., & Hagger, C. (1993). Limbic-dependent recognition memory in monkeys develops early in infancy. *NeuroReport, 4,* 77–80.

Baddeley, A., Vargha-Khadem, F., & Mishkin, M. (2001). Preserved recognition in a case of developmental amnesia: implications for the acquisition of semantic memory? *Journal of Cognitive Neuroscience, 13,* 357–369.

Bates, E. A. (2004). Explaining and interpreting deficits in language development across clinical groups: Where do we go from here? *Brain and Language, 88,* 248–253.

Benes, F. M., Turtle, M., Khan, Y., & Farol, P. (1994). Myelination of a key relay zone in the hippocampal formation occurs in the human brain during childhood, adolescence, and adulthood. *Archives of General Psychiatry, 51,* 477–484.

Berger, B., & Alvarez, C. (1994). Neurochemical development of the hippocampal region in the fetal rhesus monkey II. Immunocytochemistry of peptides, calcium-binding proteins, DARPP-32, and monoamine innervation in the entorhinal cortex by the end of gestation. *Hippocampus, 4,* 84–114.

Braver, T. S., Barch, D. M., Kelley, W. M., Buckner, R. L., Cohen, N. J., Miezin, F. M., et al. (2001). Direct comparison of prefrontal cortex regions engaged by working and long-term memory tasks. *NeuroImage, 14,* 48–59.

Brown, M. W., & Aggleton, J. P. (2001). Recognition memory: What are the roles of the perirhinal cortex and hippocampus? *Nature Review of Neuroscience, 2,* 51–61.

Burwell, R. D., & Witter, M. P. (2002). Basic anatomy of the parahippocampal region in monkeys and rats. In: M. Witter, & F. Wouterlood (Eds.), *The parahippocampal region: Organization and role in cognitive function* (pp. 35–60). New York: Oxford University Press.

Corkin, S., Amaral, D.G., Gonzalez, R.G., Johnson, K.A., & Hyman, B.T. (1997). H. M.'s medial temporal lobe lesion: Findings from magnetic resonance imaging. *Journal of Neuroscience, 17,* 3964–3979.

Dudukovic, N.M., & Wagner, A.D. (2007) Goal-dependent modulation of declarative memory: Neural correlates of temporal recency decisions and novelty detection. *Neuropsychologia, 45,* 2608–2620.

Duzel, E., Vargha-Khadem, F., Heinze, H. J., & Mishkin, M. (2001). Brain activity evidence for recognition without recollection after early hippocampal damage. *Proceedings of the National Academy of Science USA , 98,* 8101–8106.

Eichenbaum, H. B. (1992). The hippocampal system and declarative memory in animals. *Journal of Cognitive Neuroscience, 4,* 217–231.

Eichenbaum, H. B. (2003). Learning and memory: Brain systems. In: L. R. Squire, F. E. Bloom, S. K. McConnell, J. L. Roberts, N. C. Spitzer, & M. J. Zigmond (Eds.), *Fundamental neuroscience* (pp. 1299–1328). New York: Academic Press.

Eichenbaum, H. B., Yonelinas, A. R., & Ranganath, C. (2007). The medial temporal lobe and recognition memory. *Annual Review of Neurosciences, 30,* 123–152.

Fagan, J. F. (1970). Memory in the infant. *Journal of Experimental Child Psychology, 9,* 217–226.

Fernandez, G., & Tendolkar, I. (2001). Integrated brain activity in medial temporal and prefrontal areas predicts subsequent memory performance: Human declarative memory formation at the system level. *Brain Research Bulletin, 55,* 1–9.

Giedd, J. N., Vaituzis, A. C., Hamburger, S. D., Lange, N., Rajapakse, J. C., Kaysen, D., et al. (1996). Quantitative MRI of the temporal lobe, amygdala, and hippocampus in normal human development: Ages 4–18 years. *Journal of Comparative Neurology, 366,* 223–227.

Goldman, P. S., & Rosvold, H. E. (1972) The effects of selective caudate lesions in infant and juvenile rhesus monkeys. *Brain Research, 43,* 53–66.

Gunderson, V. M., & Sackett, G. P. (1984). Development of pattern recognition in infant pigtailed macaques (*Macaca nemestrina*). *Developmental Psychology, 20,* 418–426.

Gunderson, V. M., & Swartz, K. B. (1985). Visual recognition in infant pigtailed macaques after 24-hour delay. *American Journal of Primatology, 8,* 259–264.

Gunderson, V. M., & Swartz, K. B. (1986). Effects of familiarization time on visual recognition memory in infant pigtailed macaques (*Macaca nemestrina*). *Developmental Psychology, 22,* 477–480.

Harlow, H. F. (1959). The development of learning in the rhesus monkey. *American Scientist, Winter,* 459–479.

Killiany, R., Rehbein, L., & Mahut, H. (2005). Developmental study of the hippocampal formation in rhesus monkeys (*Macaca mulatta*): II. Early ablations do not spare the capacity to retrieve conditional object–object associations. *Behavioral Neuroscience, 119,* 651–661.

Lavenex, P., & Amaral, D. G. (2000). Hippocampal–neocortical interaction: a hierarchy of associativity. *Hippocampus, 10,* 420–430.

Lavenex, P., & Lavenex, P. B. (2006). Spatial relational memory in 9-month-old macaque monkeys. Learning and Memory, 13, 84–96.

Lavenex, P., Amaral, D. G., & Lavenex, P. (2006). Hippocampal lesion prevents spatial relational learning in adult macaque monkeys. *Journal of Neuroscience, 26,* 4546–4558.

Lavenex, P., Lavenex, P. B., & Amaral, D. G. (2007a). Postnatal development of the primate hippocampal formation. *Devolpmental Neurobiology, 29,* 179–192.

Lavenex, P., Lavenex, P. B, & Amaral, D. G. (2007b). Spatial relational learning persists following neonatal hippocampal lesions in macaque monkeys. *Nature Neuroscience, 10,* 234–240.

Machado, C. J., Babin, S. L., Jackson, E. F., & Bachevalier, J. (2002). Use of MRI techniques to investigate the maturation of the nonhuman primate temporal lobes. *Society for Neuroscience Abstracts, 29,* 183.1.

Málková, L., Alvarado, M. C., Pixley, E. L., Belcher, A. M., Mishkin, M., & Bachevalier J. (1999). Maturation of relational memory processes in monkeys. *Society for Neuroscience Abstracts, 25,* 88.

Málková, L., & Mishkin, M. (2003). One-trial memory for object-place associations after separate lesions of hippocampus and posterior parahippocampal region in the monkey. *Journal of Neuroscience, 23,* 1956–1965.

McKee, R. D., & Squire, L. R. (1993). On the development of declarative memory. *Journal of Experimental Psychology: Learning, Memory, Cognition, 19,* 397–404.

Mishkin, M., Suzuki, W. A., Gadian, D. G., & Vargha-Khadem, F. (1997). Hierarchical organization of cognitive memory. *Philosophical Transactions of the Royal Society of London B352,* 1461–1467.

Mishkin, M., Vargha-Khadem, F., & Gadian, D. G. (1998). Amnesia and the organization of the hippocampal system. *Hippocampus, 8,* 212–216.

Murray, E. A. (2000). Memory for objects in nonhuman primates. In: M. S. Gazzaniga (Ed.) *The new cognitive neurosciences* (pp. 753–764). Cambridge, MA: MIT Press.

Nelson, C. A. (1995). The ontogeny of human memory: A cognitive neuroscience perspective. *Developmental Psychology, 31,* 723–738.

Nelson, C. A. (1997). The neurobiological basis of early memory development. In: N. Cowan (Ed.), *The development of memory in childhood* (pp. 41–82). Hove East Sussex, UK: Psychology Press.

Nemanic, S., Alvarado, M. C., & Bachevalier, J. (2004). The hippocampal/ parahippocampal regions and recognition memory: Insights from visual paired comparison versus object delayed nonmatching in monkeys. *Journal of Neuroscience, 24,* 2013–2026.

O'Reilly, R. C., & Rudy, J. W. (2001). Conjunctive representations in learning and memory: Principles of cortical and hippocampal function. *Psychological Review, 108,* 311–345.

Overman, W. H., Bachevalier, J., Miller, M., & Moore, K. (1996a). Children's performance on "animal tests" of oddity: Implications for cognitive processes required for tests of oddity and delayed non-match to sample. *Journal of Experimental Child Psychology, 62,* 223–242.

Overman, W. H., Pate, B. J., Moore, K., & Peuster, A. (1996b). Ontogeny of place learning in children as measured in the radial arm maze, Morris search task, and open field task. *Behavioral Neuroscience, 110,* 1205–1228.

Pascalis, O., & de Schonen, S. (1994). Recognition memory in 3- to 4-day-old human neonates. *NeuroReport, 5,* 1721–1724.

Pascalis, O., Hunkin, N. M., Holdstock, J. S., Isaac, C. L., & Mayes, A. R. (2004). Differential performance on recognition memory tests and the visual paired comparison task in a patient with selective hippocampal lesion. *Neuropsychologia, 42,* 1293–1300.

Petrides, M. (2005). Lateral prefrontal cortex: Architectonic and functional organization. *Philosophical Transactions of the Royal Society of London, B 360,* 781–795.

Ranganath, C., Johnson, M. K., & D'Esposito, M. (2003). Prefrontal activity associated with working memory and episodic long-term memory. *Neuropsychologia, 41,* 378–389.

Rudy, J. W., Keith, J., & Georgian, K. (1993). The effect of age on children's learning of problems that require a configural association solution. *Developmental Psychobiology, 26,* 171–184.

Scoville, W. B., & Milner, B. (1957). Loss of recent memory after bilateral hippocampal lesions. *Journal of Neurology, Neurosurgery and Psychiatry, 20,* 11–21.

Seress, L. (2001). Morphological changes of the human hippocampal formation from midgestation to early childhood. In: C. Nelson, M. Luciana (Eds.), *Handbook of developmental cognitive neuroscience* (pp. 45–58). Cambridge, MA: MIT Press.

Seress, L., & Ribak, C. E. (1995a) Postnatal development of CA3 pyramidal neurons and ther afferents in the Ammon's horn of Rhesus monkeys. *Hippocampus, 5,* 217–231.

Seress, L., & Ribak, C. E. (1995b). Postnatal development and synaptic connections of hilar mossy cells in the hippocampal dentate gyrus of rhesus monkeys. *Journal of Comparative Neurology, 355,* 93–110.

Spence, K. W. (1952). The nature of the response in discrimination learning. *Psychological Review, 59,* 89–93.

Squire, L. R. (1992). Declarative and nondeclarative memory: Multiple brain systems supporting learning and memory. *Journal of Cognitive Neuroscience, 4,* 232–243.

Squire, L. R., Amaral, D. G., & Press, G. A. (1990). Magnetic resonance imaging of the hippocampal formation and mammillary nuclei distinguish medial temporal lobe and diencephalic amnesia. *Journal of Neuroscience, 10,* 3106–3117.

Suzuki, W. A., & Amaral, D. G. (2004). Functional neuroanatomy of the medial temporal lobe memory system. *Cortex, 40,* 220–222.

Sybirska, E., Davachi, L., & Goldman-Rakic, P. S. (2000). Prominence of direct entorhinal-CA1 pathway activation in sensorimotor and cognitive tasks revealed by 2-DG functional mapping in nonhuman primate. *Neuroscience, 20,* 5827–5834.

Tulving, E. (1972). Episodic and semantic memory. In E. Tulving & W. Donaldson (Eds.), *Organization of memory* (pp. 381–403). New York: Academic Press.

Tulving, E. (1995). Organization of memory: Quo vadis? In M.S. Gazzaniga (Ed.), *The cognitive neurosciences* (pp. 839–847). Cambridge, MA: The MIT Press.

Vann, S. D., & Aggleton, J. P. (2004). The mammillary bodies: Two memory systems in one? *Nature Reviews of Neuroscience, 5,* 35–44.

von Bonin, G., & Bailey, P. (1947). *The neocortex of* Macaca mulatta. Urbana, IL: The University of Illinois Press.

Webster, M. J., Ungerleider, L. G., & Bachevalier, J. (1991). Connections of inferior temporal areas TE and TEO with medial–temporal lobe structures in infant and adult monkeys. *Journal of Neuroscience, 11,* 1095–1116.

Webster, M. J., Ungerleider, L. G., & Bachevalier, J. (1995). Development and plasticity of the neural circuitry underlying visual recognition memory. *Canadian Journal of Physiology and Pharmacology, 73,* 1364–1371.

Yonelinas, A. P. (2002). The nature of recollection and familiarity: A review of 30 years of research. *Journal of Memory and Language, 46,* 441–517.

Zeamer, A. E., Resende, M., Heuer, E., & Bachevalier J. (2006). The development of infant monkeys' recognition-memory abilities in the absence of a functional hippocampus. *Society for Neuroscience Abstracts, 32,*195.8.

Zola, S. M., Squire, L. R., Teng, E., Stefanacci, L., Buffalo, E. A., & Clark, S. K. (2000). Impaired recognition memory in monkeys after damage limited to the hippocampal region. *Journal of Neuroscience, 20,* 451–463.

Episodic Memory: Comparative and Developmental Issues

Michael Colombo *and* Harlene Hayne

Abstract

The term episodic memory is used to refer to the recollection of personal, past experiences. More recently, the term has also been used to refer to the ability to use past experience to make plans for the future. According to Tulving, episodic memory is a uniquely human ability; no other animal has the ability to scan the past or plan for the future and, in humans, episodic memory does not emerge until approximately the age of 4. This chapter reviews the literature on episodic memory. Despite some elegant experimental procedures, no single study to date yields conclusive evidence for episodic memory in animals, infants, or very young children. Instead, the data can be reinterpreted in terms of simpler mechanisms that do not require episodic memory.

Keywords: episodic memory, recollection, past experiences, Tulving

Human beings possess a form of memory (episodic memory) and a form of consciousness (autonoetic consciousness, or "autonoesis") that no other animals do. Thus, the thesis is that these two aspects of the mind are unique in humans, in the sense that the mental capacities that define them do not exist in quite the same full-fledged form in other species. They do not exist in insects, in birds, in mice or rats, in cats or dogs, and not even in gorillas and chimps.

—*Tulving* (2005)

Most modern theorists of memory agree that our ability to remember the past does not rely on a single memory system, but rather a series of different memory systems that are comprised of different neural substrates and which operate according to different principles (for recent reviews, see Gold, 2004; McDonald, Devan, & Hong, 2004; Squire, 2004). Although a large number of theoretical distinctions have been proposed, one of the most influential distinctions has been Squire's distinction between *nondeclarative* (nee procedural) and *declarative* memory (Squire, 1987, 1994). According to Squire's theory, the nondeclarative memory system supports the retention of skills and habits, priming, perceptual learning, simple classical conditioning, and nonassociative learning. The declarative memory system, on the other hand, is required for the conscious recollection of facts and events and allows for rapid, one-trial learning.

Within the declarative memory system, a further distinction has been drawn between episodic and semantic memory (Tulving, 1972, 1983). In formal terms, episodic memory refers to the recollection of personal experiences (e.g., what "I" did to celebrate my birthday last year), while semantic memory involves the recollection of facts (e.g., My birthday sometimes falls near Easter). In more col-loquial terms, episodic memory allows us to take a trip down memory lane, revisiting the past in our mind's eye and, as we will show later, allowing us to consider future possibilities that have yet to occur.

Although there is now little debate that nonhu-man animals (for review, see Squire & Schacter, 2002) and preverbal infants (for review, see Hayne, 2004, 2007) exhibit at least some declarative mem-ory skills, the question we address in this chapter is whether there is similar evidence that animals, infants, or young children also exhibit episodic memory. In short, do animals, infants, and chil-dren exhibit the kind of mental time travel that is such a pervasive part of human, adult cognition?

Tulving Sets the Bar

Much like Descartes over 500 years ago, Tulving sets the bar between humans and all other species quite high. As illustrated in the quote at the begin-ning of this chapter, Tulving argues that episodic memory is a recently evolved memory system. According to his view, not even our closest ani-mal relatives possess the kind of episodic memory that allows human adults to relive the good ol' days or to plan for the future—not rats, pigeons, or the family cat, not even gorillas or chimps. In fact, Tulving has recently argued that infants and young children also lack episodic memory skill. He proposes that episodic memory emerges late in the course of human development and that it is the first memory system to decline during the course of normal aging (Tulving, 2005).

Tulving first made the claim that only humans could imagine themselves in past and future scenar-ios in his 1983 book, *Elements of Episodic Memory*. Since the publication of this book, there has been an explosion of research on episodic memory, and more recently, on the more general issue of mental time travel. In the current chapter, we review the evidence for episodic memory in both nonhuman animals and human infants and young children.

Obstacles to Investigation

Perhaps the biggest obstacle to determining whether nonhuman animals or infants and chil-dren possess the kind of episodic memory described by Tulving is that, unlike verbal adults, animals, infants, and very young children cannot tell us what they remember. For this reason, we are always in the invidious position of inferring episodic memory on the basis of some kind of nonverbal behavior, while at the same time drawing analogies to the kind of complex, verbal memory skills that are exhibited by human adults. In doing so, we must avoid mak-ing some fundamental mistakes in interpretation. For example, in order to conclude that a memory (even a verbal memory) is episodic, we must ensure that the dependent variable clearly reflects episodic memory rather than semantic memory or general knowledge.

For example, if someone asks you what you had for breakfast, your verbal report might constitute an episodic memory (cf., Zentall, 2005). In order to answer the question, you might think back to the activities of that particular morning, recalling the fight that you had with your son, the smell of your wife's new perfume, as well as what you grabbed from the pantry on your way out of the door. If, on the other hand, someone asks you what you had for breakfast every day, and in anticipation of being asked that question, you rehearsed the information over and over again on your way to work, then your verbal report about your breakfast would not meet the criterion for an episodic memory because your answer to this question would be based on a well-rehearsed working memory, or semantic prospec-tion. This example illustrates that verbal reports are not immune to semantic prospection, but the issue of semantic prospection is critically important when we try to evaluate whether a particular non-verbal behavior reflects episodic memory.

In the case of nonhuman animals, many experts agree that the delayed matching-to-sample task requires declarative memory (for review, see Rovee-Collier, Hayne, & Colombo, 2001), but does it also require the kind of episodic memory described by Tulving? In the matching-to-sample task, the sub-ject is presented with a sample stimulus. Following a delay, the subject is presented with two compari-son stimuli, one that is the same as the sample and one that is different from the sample. The correct response in this task is to choose the test stimulus that matches the sample stimulus after the delay.

If we think of the test trial in the matching-to-sample task as a memory question, "which one of these stimuli served as the sample?" then a cor-rect response might constitute evidence of a non-verbal, episodic memory (see Figure 30.1, top) in much the same way that the description of our breakfast might constitute evidence of episodic memory for the events of a particular morning. If, on the other hand, the subject has been rehearsing the answer to the question throughout the delay, then the correct choice during the test would have been achieved through the use of semantic

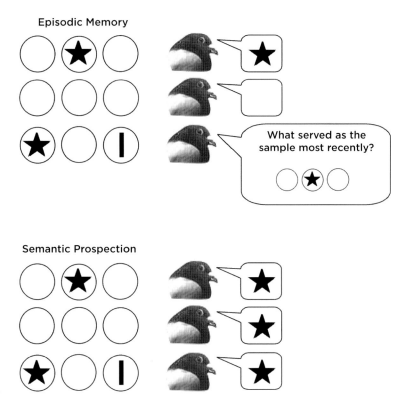

Figure 30.1 An illustration of the two hypothetical ways in which an animal might solve a delayed matching-to-sample task. The circles represent displays on which the stimuli are presented. The top row in each display represents the sample phase. During the sample phase, the sample stimulus is presented on the center display. The middle row represents the delay phase during which no stimuli are presented and the animal must remember the sample stimulus. The bottom row represents the comparison phase. During the test phase, two stimuli are presented. The correct choice is to select the stimulus that matches the stimulus that was presented as the sample, in this case the star. The top diagram illustrates a solution based on a hypothetical episodic memory. The bottom diagram illustrates a solution based on hypothetical semantic prospection.

prospection (see Figure 30.1, bottom). One way that experimenters have tried to get around the problem of semantic prospection is to test subjects following very long delays. Although it is difficult to know at what point semantic prospection is abandoned in favor of episodic memory, at least over the delays that are commonly used in this task (e.g., seconds or minutes), it is very likely that semantic prospection is the basis of performance in the matching-to-sample task (Colombo & Graziano, 1994).

Episodic Memory in Nonhuman Animals
The Seminal Experiment with Scrub Jays

Episodic memory was initially characterized as memory for the *what, when*, and *where* of a particular experience (Tulving, 1972)—what is now colloquially referred to as WWW-memory. For this reason, initial attempts to study episodic memory in nonhuman animals focussed on animals' ability to remember information about the *what, when*, and *where* of a particular learning experience. Given some of the problems inherent in interpreting performance on the standard matching-to-sample task described earlier, researchers began to develop new experimental procedures that capitalized on

the animal's behavior in the wild—behavior they hoped would yield evidence of nonverbal episodic memory.

The now-classic study of episodic memory in nonhuman animals was originally published by Clayton and Dickinson (1998). In their task, Clayton and Dickinson capitalized on the food-storing tendency of scrub jays. In the wild, scrub jays cache their food and their recovery strategies for their cache vary as a function of the perishability of the food item they have hidden. In the laboratory, Clayton and Dickinson provided jays the opportunity to hide and then to find certain food items that varied in terms of palatability as well as in terms of perishability. For example, although scrub jays prefer waxworms over peanuts, waxworms degrade faster than peanuts once they have been hidden.

The basic procedure that was used by Clayton and Dickinson (1998) is illustrated in Figure 30.2. In the experiment, there were two trial types, a 4-h trial and a 124-h trial. On 4-h trials, the scrub jays were forced to cache the less preferred peanuts on one side of an ice cube tray; 120 h later, they were then forced to cache the more preferred waxworms on the other side of the ice cube tray. Four hours after the second caching opportunity, the scrub jays were presented with the ice cube tray and they were allowed to recover the peanuts and the worms. The same procedure was used in the 124-h trials except that the waxworms were cached first and the peanuts were cached second.

When the waxworms were cached second, and were still fresh at the time of recovery, the birds concentrated their searches on the side of the ice cube tray that contained the worms. In contrast, when the worms were cached first, and thus had degraded by the time of the recovery phase, the birds concentrated their searches on the side of the ice cube tray that contained the peanuts. According to the authors, "…the cache recovery pattern of scrub jays fulfils the three, *what*, *where*, and *when* criteria for episodic recall and thus provides, to our knowledge, the first conclusive behavioral evidence of episodic-like memory in animals other than humans." Given the very long retention intervals between the cache and recovery phases of the experiment, it is highly unlikely that the animals' performance was based on semantic prospection alone. As such, we agree with the authors that their study provides the best evidence to date for episodic (or episodic-like) memory in a nonhuman species. Since the publication of Clayton and Dickinson's (1998) seminal study, the

basic findings have been replicated and extended under a wide range of different experimental conditions (Clayton, Bussey, & Dickinson, 2003; de Kort, Dickinson, & Clayton, 2005). In addition, the demonstration of episodic-like memory in scrub jays launched new research on episodic memory in a wide range of different species.

Pigeons

Given that the seminal demonstration of episodic-like memory was shown with scrub jays, is there any evidence that other species of birds show similar episodic-like memory? To examine this question, Skov-Rackette, Miller, and Shettleworth (2006) examined pigeons' capacity for episodic memory. In their first experiment, pigeons were trained on a *what–when–where* version of the delayed matching-to-sample task. The sample stimulus consisted of either a red circle or a green triangle that was presented in one of eight positions around the periphery of a computer screen (see Figure 30.3). The sample was presented for at least 3 s, after which the first peck resulted in the disappearance of the sample and the start of either a 2- or 6-s retention interval.

At the end of the retention interval, an X appeared in the center of the screen and a peck to

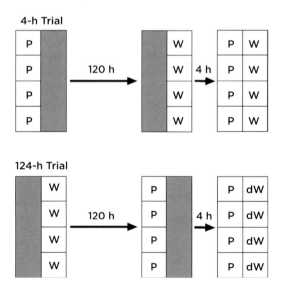

Figure 30.2 The design of the classic Clayton and Dickinson (1998) experiment. W refers to waxworms, the scrub jays' preferred food, P refers to peanuts, the scrub jays' less preferred food, and dW refers to degraded waxworms. In the 4-h trial (top), the peanuts are cached first, whereas in the 124-h trial (bottom), the worms are cached first.

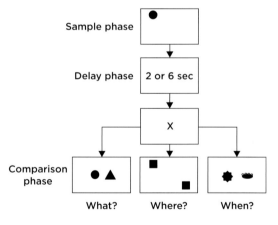

Figure 30.3 The design of the Skov-Rackette et al. (2006) study. The sample stimulus consisted of either a red circle or green triangle. After the delay, an X was presented and a peck to it initiated either a what trial (left), where trial (middle), or a when trial (right). In the current example, the correct choice on what trials was to respond to the red circle. The correct choice on the where trials was to respond to the position where the red circle had appeared as the sample stimulus, the upper left square. The correct choice on when trials was to respond to the yellow star if the delay had been 6 s or the blue paw if the delay had been 2 s.

it resulted in either a *what, when,* or *where* comparison phase. On *what* trials, both the red circle and green triangle were presented at the center of the screen and the subject had to respond to the stimulus that had served as the sample. On *where* trials, two gray squares were presented, one that occupied the position of the sample stimulus, and the other that occupied one of the remaining 7 positions. A correct response consisted of pecking the square that occupied the position that the sample had occupied. On *when* trials, a blue paw stimulus and a yellow star stimulus appeared in the center. The subject was required to peck the blue paw stimulus if the just-experienced delay was 2 s in length and the yellow star if the just-experienced delay was 6 s in length.

The pigeons performed surprisingly well on this complex task. While the data are impressive and suggest episodic-like memory in pigeons, it is possible, given the short delays, that the birds could have used semantic prospection to solve the task, particularly in light of the amount of training that was required for the birds to learn the task in the first place. Furthermore, Skov-Rackette et al. (2006) conducted a subsequent series of clever probe tests to determine whether the *what, where,* and *when* information was bound together into a single memory representation. Consider, for example, the *what* trial that is shown in Figure 30.3. On this trial, the sample stimulus is a red circle that appears in the upper left of the screen, and the comparison stimuli, a red circle and green triangle, both appear in the center of the screen. Effectively, for this *what* trial, the *where* information has been eliminated. Skov-Rackette et al. refer to this as an unbound test of *what* memory. In contrast, in the bound test of *what* memory, the red circle was presented in its correct spatial position (upper left) next to the green triangle. This stimulus configuration still constitutes a *what* test, but in this bound condition, the correct alternative dimension (spatial position) is preserved. Similarly, in the bound *where* trial, the correct shape would be presented in the correct spatial position.

Using these new test configurations, Skov-Rackette et al. (2006) hypothesized that if the *what* and *where* information about the sample were bound into a single representation, as would be expected in the case of episodic memory, then the birds' performance should be better on the bound trials relative to the unbound trials. Instead, the authors noted no difference in performance between the two trial types. On the basis of this

finding, the authors concluded that the *what* and *where* of the task were not bound together into a unified memory representation, challenging the episodic basis of the animals' performance.

Rats

Several studies of episodic memory have been conducted with rats. In many of them, rats are required to hide food in the arms of a radial arm maze and are then given the opportunity to retrieve the food after a delay. In one of the first studies of this kind, Bird, Roberts, Abroms, Kit, and Crupi (2003) trained rats to hide cheese and pretzels, their preferred and less preferred food, respectively, in four of the eight arms of a radial arm maze. After a 45-min delay, the rats were allowed to retrieve the food. Bird et al. found that the rats tended to retrieve the cheese before the pretzels, suggesting that they may have had *what* and *where* memory. To test the animals' memory for the *when* component of the hiding event, rats were tested after delays of 1 and 24 h. The cheese was degraded for one group of animals and not for the other. Overall, there was no evidence that rats retained a memory for *when* in this task. That is, they failed to alter their search strategy in the degraded condition.

Babb and Crystal (2005) also assessed *what–where–when* memory in a study conducted with rats trained to forage for food in a radial arm maze. The design of their experiment is illustrated in Figure 30.4. Each trial consisted of two phases. In Phase 1, the rats were forced to enter four arms of the maze and the remaining four arms were blocked. Three of the arms were baited with pellets, and one was baited with a more preferred food, chocolate. Phase 2 of this task took place after a delay of either 30 min or 4 h. If the delay was 30 min, then the four arms that had not been baited in Phase 1 were baited with pellets in Phase 2—there was no chocolate present in any arm when rats were tested after a 30-min delay. If the delay had been 4 h, then pellets were available in the arms that had not baited in Phase 1, but chocolate was replenished in the arm in which it had appeared in Phase 1. Thus, after the 30-min delay, chocolate was not available, whereas after the 4-h delay it was. The authors predicted that, if rats retained a unified representation of the *what, when,* and *where* of this task, then they should return to the chocolate arm when they were tested after a 4-h delay, but not when they were tested after a 30-min delay. The data confirmed this prediction insofar as the rats revisited the previously baited chocolate arm 25%

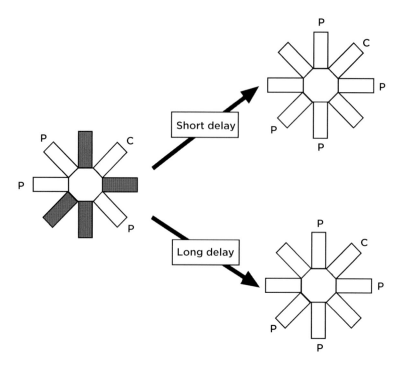

Figure 30.4 The design of the Babb and Crystal (2005) study. In Phase 1, the rats were trained to enter four arms (light color) by blocking entry to the other arms (dark color). In Phase 2, the rats were given the opportunity to search for food in all eight arms. P refers to pellets, C to chocolate. The short delay was 30 min, the long delay was 4 h.

of the time when they were tested after the short delay, and they revisited the previously baited chocolate arm 54% of the time when they were tested after the long delay.

On the surface, these data appear impressive, but interpretation of the study is complicated by the fact that the percentages were calculated on the basis of the revisit rate *across* the first four choices that rats made during the test. On the basis of these calculations, it is possible to generate the percentages obtained by Babb and Crystal without concluding that the rat's behavior was guided by episodic memory. In fact, it is possible to generate the same percentages and conclude that the rats have no idea where the chocolate is when they are tested after the long delay.

The best way to illustrate this interpretive problem is to use the hypothetical data set shown in Table 30.1. Although the data from the Babb and Crystal (2005) study were collected across 17 days of testing, for simplicity's sake, our hypothetical data set was collected across 4 days of testing. P and C refer to selection of the arms that contain pellets and chocolate, respectively. The top part of Table 30.1 refers to choices after the short delay and the bottom part of the Table 30.1 refers to choices after the long delay. On the basis of our hypothetical data set, we can generate the exact same percentages that were reported by Babb and Crystal (2005), yet our

interpretation of the data is dramatically different. In our example, the rats overwhelmingly return to arms with pellets (i.e., select new arms over those visited in Phase 1). Occasionally, on their fourth choice, they return to the arm that had chocolate in Phase 1.

The data shown in Table 30.1 yield the exact same percentages that were reported by Babb and Crystal (2005). The probability of hitting a chocolate arm in the first four choices across the 4 days after the short delay is $(0+1+0+0)/4 = .25$ and $(0+1+1+0)/4 = .5$ after the long delay. These hypothetical data illustrate the fundamental problems with the Babb and Crystal study. First, it is possible that the rats always chose pellets first, then chocolate, a pattern we would not expect if rats used episodic memory to find their preferred food. Second, a score of .5 (.54 in Babb and Crystal study) represents nothing more than chance performance. Across 2 days in which a rat make four choices on each day, the chance that it hits the chocolate arm is 1 in 8, which is exactly what the rats in the Babb and Crystal study were doing; they selected the chocolate arm once over the 8 choices across a block of 2 days.

Although Babb and Crystal (2005) recognized that the different choice patterns in their study (.25 and .54) may simply reflect "more forgetting of the forced-choice locations after the [long delay] than

Table 30.1 A Hypothetical Data Set Illustrating an Alternative Interpretation of the Babb and Crystal (2005) Study

Choices on Day 1	Choices on Day 2	Choice on Day 3	Choice on Day 4
Choices made after the short delay			
P	P	P	P
P	P	P	P
P	P	P	P
P	C	P	P
0 Chocolate revisit	1 Chocolate revisit	0 Chocolate revisit	0 Chocolate revisit
Choices made after the long delay			
P	P	P	P
P	P	P	P
P	P	P	P
P	C	C	P
0 Chocolate revisit	1 Chocolate revisit	1 Chocolate revisit	0 Chocolate revisit

C refers to chocolate, a highly preferred food for rats, and P refers to pellets, a less preferred food.

the [short delay]" (p. 183), they argue against this possibility on the basis of the fact that the rats are 91% accurate in retrieving pellets after the long delay. Granted, memory for the pellets is very high, but this finding says nothing about the rats' memory for the location of chocolate. In fact, our hypothetical data set also shows that memory for the pellets remains high after the long delay. In our example, the rats return to 7/8 (87.5%) arms with pellets, a score not that different from the score (91%) that is reported in the paper, illustrating that it is possible to maintain high levels of performance on the pellets while being completely unaware of the location of the chocolate. If our analysis is correct, then the rats in the Babb and Crystal (2005) study might have *where* memory (because they go to arms in Phase 2 that were not baited in Phase 1), and they may have *what* memory, but they do not have *when* memory. As such, the Babb and Crystal study, like so many others, fails to show the full complement of *what*, *where*, and *when* required for episodic memory.

Using yet another experimental procedure, Ergorul and Eichenbaum (2007; see also Eichenbaum, Fortin, Ergorul, Wright, & Agster, 2005) examined *what–where–when* memory in rats. The task used by Ergorul and Eichenbaum is outlined in Figure 30.5. In the sample phase of the task, the rat was first presented with odor A (an odor mixed in sand) in a distinct location within a test arena. The rat was trained to approach this

odor and to dig for a hidden piece of fruit loop cereal. The rat was then returned to the home cage and, 7 s later, it was allowed to approach odor B, which occupied a different location in the test arena. In a similar way, the rat was also exposed to odor C and odor D. After a further 7-s delay, the rat was tested with all possible pairwise combinations of the odors. During a standard test trial, a correct response consisted of selecting the odor that had occurred earlier in the series relative to the other test odor. In the example shown in Figure 30.5, the correct response was to approach odor B first because it had been encountered prior to odor C during the sample phase. During standard test trials, the odors were located in the same positions during the test that they had occupied during the sample phase.

Overall, the rats performed above 70% correct on these standard test trials. The animals' test performance was further scored in terms of the initial visit to a location (where did the rat go first) and on the final choice behavior (where did the rat dig). On the basis of the standard test trial illustrated in Figure 30.5, the correct response is to approach and dig at B. Given where the rat was placed in the arena at the beginning of the test (see Figure 30.5, black circle), it could not smell either test odor, so the decision to initially approach B is based exclusively on spatial cues. When we consider these initial visit scores, rats approached the correct spatial position 69% of the time. On this basis, Ergorul and Eichenbaum conclude that the rats have *when* and *where* memory; they remember that B was presented earlier than C (*when*), and they remember where B was located (*where*).

Ergol and Eichenbauem further argue that the rats in their study also demonstrated memory for *what*. This argument is based on the finding that although rats were 69% correct on their first approach during the test, when they actually began to dig, they were correct 76% of the time. The authors argue that the 7% increase in final choice behavior was due to the fact that the rats corrected their initial mistakes on the basis of the odor (*what*) that they encountered. In other words, when they approached the initial (incorrect) location, the rats said "No, this is not the correct location because the odor is not right." If the rats in this study actually solved the task in the manner described by Ergorul and Eichenbaum, then it is possible that their experiment yields some evidence of episodic-like, WWW-memory. It is also possible, however, that the additional 7% increase in performance

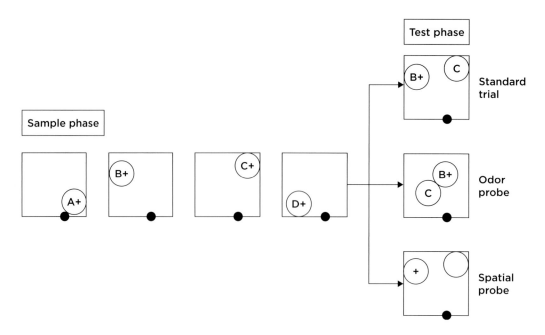

Figure 30.5 The design of the Ergorul and Eichenbaum (2007) study. A, B, C, and D denote different odors. The black circle indicates the release point of the rat. On Standard Trials, the odors were presented in their original spatial locations. A correct response consisted of selecting the odor that had occurred earlier in the series. On Odor Probe trials, the odors were presented in new, neutral locations. On Spatial Probe trials, the reward was located in the original spatial location, but no odors were present.

was due to the fact that the rats corrected their spatial position during the test. In other words, on approaching the initial (incorrect) location, the rats might have said, "No, this is not the right place." For obvious reasons, it is impossible to disentangle these two competing interpretations of the data.

Ergorul and Eichenbaum (2007) also argue that the finding that the rats perform well on probe trials in which they were confronted with two odors at neutral locations (see Figure 30.5, Odor Probe) yields further evidence that the rats have *what* memory. Unfortunately, however, just because the rats selected the proper odor on the odor probe trials does not mean that they used this same information to guide their choice on the standard test trial. Likewise, the fact that the rats performed at chance on spatial probe trials (see Figure 30.5, Spatial Probe) was also used by the authors to support their argument that the rats had *what* memory. Chance performance on spatial probe trials, however, is exactly what we would expect irrespective of what the rats remember. Because the odors were not present on spatial probe trials, a rat that approaches the correct position but smells nothing would naturally try a new location. At the very best, Ergorul and Eichenbaum's data provide some evidence for *where* and *when* memory, but

they provide no evidence for *what* memory of the same event.

Monkeys

Using a task that was similar to the task originally pioneered by Clayton and Dickinson (1998), Hampton, Hampstead, and Murray (2005) trained monkeys to search for food at two different locations within an enclosure. One of the locations contained a preferred food and the other contained a less preferred food. Once the monkeys had found both food items, they were tested after two retention intervals, first after 1 h and then after 24 h. The monkeys were taught that, after 1 h, both the preferred and less preferred foods were still fresh (e.g., they had been replenished at their respective foraged locations during the delay). In contrast, after 24 h, the less preferred food remained fresh, but the preferred food had degraded.

Each monkey completed one trial per day over a total of 30 days. Across the 30 days of training, the monkeys should learn that after the 1-h retention interval, the preferred food item was still available and in good condition, so they should first search in the location of the preferred food item. Therefore, when tested after the 1-h delay, the proportion of searches at the preferred food location should remain high and, in fact, might actually increase over trials. Across the 30 days of training, the monkeys should also learn that after the 24-h retention interval, the preferred food is degraded. As such, searches to the preferred food location after the long delay interval should decrease across successive days of training.

The results of the experiment yielded no evidence that the monkeys learned to avoid the location of the preferred food when they were tested after a 24-h retention interval. The authors concluded that monkeys exhibited memory for *what* and *where*, but not *when* of the food-hiding event. Furthermore, although the hippocampus is thought to play an important role in episodic memory (Tulving, 2002; Vargha-Khadem, Gadian, & Mishkin, 2001), in the Hampton et al. (2005) study, monkeys with hippocampal lesions performed identically to control, unoperated monkeys, raising additional questions about the basis of their performance on the task.

Gorillas

In an experiment designed to examine episodic memory in the gorilla, Schwartz and his colleagues trained a gorilla named "King" on a task in which one of two experimenters gave King a piece of food (Schwarts, Colon, Sanchez, Rodriguez, & Evans, 2002). After a delay, King was presented with a number of cards. He was required to select the card that contained a picture of both the experimenter who had given King the food (*who*) and the item of food that King had been given (*what*). Although King performed this task with a high degree of accuracy, because he knew what question was coming, it is impossible to know whether his performance was based on episodic memory of the original event or whether his choice was based on semantic prospection.

In an attempt to circumvent the problem of semantic prospection, Schwartz and his colleagues conducted another experiment in which King witnessed a unique event and was then required to select a photograph of either *what* the event was or *who* participated in the event (Schwartz, Meissner, Hoffman, Evans, & Frazier, 2004). This test procedure made it impossible for King to anticipate which "question" the experimenter was going to ask, making it more difficult for him to rehearse the "answer" over the delay. Although King's performance on this version of the task was statistically higher than would be expected by chance alone, overall, his performance was generally poor.

In two studies described above, King was only tested on *what* or *who* information about the target event. In a subsequent series of experiments, however, Schwartz, Hoffman, and Evans (2005) extended the task to include information about *where* and *when*. In the *when* aspect of the task, King was required to recall the order in which he received three food items. During the presentation phase, King received Food 1 at Time 1, followed by Food 2 at Time 2, and then by Food 3 at Time 3. After a delay that ranged from 5 to 23 min, King was required to respond to pictures of the food items in the reverse order to which they had been presented to him in the first place. That is, he was required to select the picture of Food 3 first, the picture of Food 2 second, and the picture of Food 1 last. During the test, King was presented with five pictures of food items. King scored 90%, 50%, and 60% on the first, second, and third selections, respectively. On the basis of King's performance, Schwartz et al. (2005) concluded that he demonstrates an "episodic-like organization of events" (p. 237).

On closer inspection, however, King's performance on the task may not reflect episodic memory at all. The authors' interpretation of King's behavior was based on how he performed relative to chance. According to Schwartz et al. (2005), chance on the first selection would be 20% (1 out of 5 pictures), 25% on the second selection (1 out of 4 pictures; once removed, the pictures were not replaced), and 33% on the third selection (1 out of 3). But is this the appropriate way to calculate chance in this task? For example, it is not unreasonable to assume that within a particular trial, King remembers the three food items that he has just consumed. Therefore, although he was presented with 5 cards during the test, he could easily eliminate 2 from the pile on the basis of familiarity alone. If King uses this strategy, chance performance for the first, second, and third selections would be 33%, 50%, and 50% respectively.[1] If we reevaluate King's performance relative to these new chance statistics, his performance on the second selection, and very likely the third selection, is no different from chance. Thus, beyond the first item selected, which by itself is not evidence of episodic memory, King demonstrates no episodic knowledge of the order of food item presentation.

In addition to *when* information, Schwartz et al. (2005) also tested whether King could recall *where* information about a particular event. Using a method very similar to that described above,

King was allowed to witness a novel event at one of three distinct locations. After an average delay of 6 min, King was presented with three pictures of the possible locations. Chance performance on this task is 33% (1 out of 3). Across 60 trials, King did perform significantly above chance, but his average score was only 45% correct, and this score differed from chance on the basis of only a single response according to binomial probabilities. In addition, the delay in this task may have been too short and thus King, who was certainly well trained in the matching tasks by this point, may have solved the task by using semantic prospection rather than retrieving an episodic memory of a past event. Furthermore, even if we put aside the issue of semantic prospection and the issue of how best to calculate chance in this task, the authors still failed to show that King exhibited the cardinal feature of episodic memory—a bound representation of *what-where-AND-when* memory. Although many of the studies we have reviewed thus far show that animals can recall *what*, *where*, and *when* information separately, the cardinal feature of episodic memory is a unified memory that reflects all three kinds of information. At no point did Schwartz et al. (2005) demonstrate that King possessed an integrated *what–where–when* memory of the target events.

Evidence of Episodic Memory Beyond the What–Where–When Criterion

On the basis of our review of the literature so far, the original Clayton and Dickinson (1998) study stands as the best evidence of episodic-like memory in nonhuman animals. In all of the other research reviewed here, alternative interpretations of the data are possible and there is little or no evidence that animals, irrespective of species, form an integrated memory representation of the *what*, *where*, and *when* elements of the target event.

Although the data reported by Clayton and Dickinson (1998) have paved the way for dozens of different experiments, this study is also not without its critics (see Roberts, 2002; Suddendorf & Busby, 2003). For example, in the Clayton and Dickinson study, like most others conducted with animals, the subjects received extensive training in the task before they took part in the critical test. In this way, the animals may have learned to expect a particular "test question," and may have solved the task using semantic prospection rather than episodic memory. In fact, even the Clayton and Dickinson task may be open to this criticism (Zentall, Clement,

Bhatt, & Allen, 2001). For this reason, some investigators have abandoned the standard hiding and finding tasks that were pioneered by Clayton and Dickinson in favor of new test procedures that they argue might yield less ambiguous evidence of episodic memory in nonhuman animals.

Surprise Questions

According to Zentall et al. (2001), the key to revealing episodic memory is to ask an unexpected question. If the subject cannot anticipate the question, its answer is more likely to be based on episodic memory than on overly rehearsed, semantic information. In an attempt to develop a surprise question procedure for use with animals, Zentall et al. (2001) conducted an experiment with pigeons (see also Zentall, 2005, 2006). In Phase 1 of the task, pigeons were trained on a conditional matching task in which they were required to peck at a vertical line and to refrain from pecking at a horizontal line (see Figure 30.6). The pigeons were then presented with two comparison stimuli, red and green. The comparison stimuli were used as surrogate nonverbal answers to the question "What did you do most recently?" A peck to red indicated that "I pecked most recently" whereas a peck to green indicated "I did not peck most recently."

In Phase 2 of this experiment, the pigeons were trained on an autoshaping procedure in which a yellow stimulus was followed by food, and a blue stimulus was not. In Phase 2, the birds pecked at the stimulus that predicts food (yellow) and refrained from pecking at the stimulus that does not predict food (blue).

Phase 3 represented the critical test. After pecking the yellow stimulus, or not pecking to blue stimulus, the birds were given a surprise choice between the red and green stimuli. The correct response after a yellow stimulus would be to peck the red stimulus, indicating that "I pecked most recently." On the other hand, after the blue stimulus, the correct choice would be to peck the green stimulus, indicating "I did not peck most recently." Across the 96-trial test phase, the birds' performed about 70% correct. This high level of responding was also present across the first four exposures to the surprise question. On the basis of these surprise question data, the authors conclude that the birds exhibited episodic memory.

As interesting as this experiment is, there is a potential confound. Although the authors assume that the animals treat Phase 3 as a surprise question, it is also possible that their performance in Phase 3

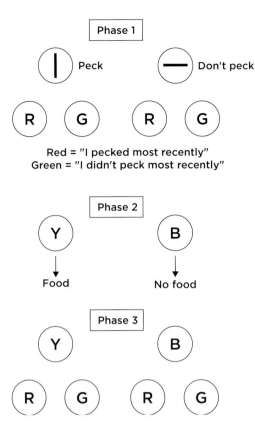

Figure 30.6 The design of the Zentall et al. (2001) study. R, G, Y, and B refer to red, green, yellow, and blue stimuli projected onto response keys. If the pigeons pecked, the correct response was to respond to red. The correct response following the absence of pecking was to respond to green. Phase 2 was an autoshaping procedure in which the yellow and blue stimuli were and were not followed by food, respectively.

represents simple generalization to the conditions that were present in Phase 1. If this is the case, then the transfer seen in Phase 3 is to be expected given that, from the birds' perspective, Phase 3 is identical to Phase 1.

In another study using the surprise-question technique, Mercado, Murray, Uyeyama, Pack, and Herman (1998) taught dolphins that a specific gestural command meant "repeat the action you have just performed." According to the authors, "[a]n animal's short-term memory for its own actions can be interpreted as a type of metaknowledge; self reports based on such memories can be used to measure an animal's ability to explicitly recall past behaviors" (p. 210). Initially, the dolphins were trained to apply the repeat command to four different types of behaviors. Once they could apply the repeat command to the original four behaviors, they were given a formal test in which they were asked to repeat 32 other behaviors from their behavioral repertoire. One of the dolphins scored almost as high with these new 32 behaviors (90% correct) as she had during training with the original four behaviors (94%).

In the Mercado et al. (1998) study, the dolphins were asked, "What did you just do" and they answered by repeating their last behavior. It is unlikely, however, that this constitutes a surprise question to the dolphin. As we indicated above, the dolphins had been trained to respond to the repeat command with four original target behaviors. It is true that they did apply the repeat command to 32 other behaviors from their behavioral repertoire, but it is very likely that by this point they had come to expect that the repeat command might be asked. This, plus the fact that the delay between when they executed a behavior and when the question to repeat that behavior was made was almost zero, makes it more than likely that the dolphins came to expect that a repeat command would be asked and so maintained a representation of what they had just done. If true, this would be another example of impressive semantic prospection, but it would not constitute evidence of episodic memory.

Metamemory

Another critical feature of episodic memory is that as we recall a particular personal experience, we are often aware of the state of our knowledge. When we travel back in time and imagine an event, we have an accompanying feeling that that event has happened in our past. Tulving (1985) refers to this phenomenological experience as autonoetic consciousness, which is related to metamemory, or a knowledge of the state of one's memory. Is there any evidence that nonhuman animals exhibit evidence of metamemory skills? Hampton (2001) explored the issue of metamemory in monkeys using a matching task. The design of the experiment is shown in Figure 30.7. Monkeys were first shown a sample stimulus that was followed by a delay. After the delay, the monkeys were allowed to make a choice. Two-thirds of the test trials were Free-choice trials in which the monkeys saw two stimuli. In Figure 30.7, these stimuli are designated as R and F for ease of exposition (the actual stimuli were geometric shapes). Selecting the R stimulus resulted in the presentation of a test phase in which the sample stimulus and three other distractor stimuli were shown. There is a certain risk involved in selecting this test phase because although choosing the stimulus that matches the sample results in

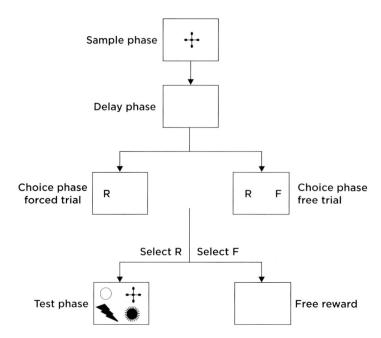

Figure 30.7 The design of the Hampton (2001) study. One third of the trials were forced-choice trials, and two thirds were free-choice trials. On free-choice trials, the monkeys could choose to take the test by selecting R or they could avoid the test by selecting F. On forced-choice trials, the monkeys had to take the test. A correct response after selecting R yielded a large reward, whereas selecting F yielded a free small free reward.

a substantial reward, an incorrect response results in no reward at all. Selecting the F stimulus, on the other hand, results in a small, but guaranteed, free reward. The authors reasoned that the monkeys should select the R stimulus only if they are aware that they remember the sample stimulus. If they have no memory of the sample stimulus, then the best option is to select the F stimulus.

To ensure that the monkeys did not simply opt for the small, but free, reward by default, one-third of the trials in the Hampton (2001) study were Forced-choice trials in which only the R stimulus appeared, and the only option was to select it and take the test. The logic behind this aspect of the design was that performance on Free-choice trials should be better than performance on Forced-choice trials; this is exactly what Hampton (2001) found. On the basis of these data, Hampton concluded that monkeys know when they remember. While this study does not show episodic memory per se, it does show that monkeys are aware of their memory state, which is a critical ingredient of episodic memory.

Tulving Weighs in Again: The Spoon Test

Although Tulving initially characterized episodic memory as the *what*, *where*, and *when* of an experience, it soon became apparent that it is possible to recall this kind of information even in the absence of episodic recollection of a personal experience.

For example, you may know that the Titanic (*what*) sank in 1912 (*when*) in the North Atlantic (*where*), yet you have no personal experience of having been there. Likewise, it is highly likely that you know that you were born (*what*) on a certain date (*when*) in a certain city (*where*), yet it is highly unlikely that this knowledge is based on your personal recollection of the actual event. For this reason, Tulving (1985) modified the requirement for episodic memory to include another phenomenological experience—autonoetic consciousness—or the feeling that the WWW-memory has happened to you in the past.

The notion of autonoetic consciousness is a particularly thorny issue for researchers who study animals or infants and young children—in the absence of verbal report, it is hard to imagine how an organism could ever demonstrate the feeling of "pastness" that soon became central to Tulving's definition of episodic memory. Many researchers accused Tulving of using this semantic sleight of hand to, by definition alone, rule out episodic memory in any thing other than verbally competent human beings.

Over time, however, Tulving responded to his critics, providing an example of nonverbal episodic memory that he believed would meet the criterion for autoneoetic consciousness. His example is based on an Estonian children's story. In the story, a little girl goes to sleep and dreams about a friend's birthday party. At the party, the guests are served a wonderful chocolate pudding, which just happens to be the girl's favorite dessert. Unbeknownst to the little girl, however, guests were required to bring their own spoons to the party. Because she does not have a spoon, the little girl must stand by and watch as others enjoy the pudding. The next night when this same little girl goes to bed, she tucks a spoon under her pillow, just in case she returns to the party in her dreams. According to Tulving (2005), taking the spoon to bed provides a hallmark measure of episodic memory—it signals the little girl's ability to travel both forward and backward in mental time, using a prior experience to plan for a future event. Tulving argued that variations of this "spoon test" could be used as a nonverbal marker for mental time travel and for conscious awareness of a past event—the two essential ingredients for an episodic memory.

Tulving's Spoon Test soon became the new benchmark for research on nonverbal episodic memory as researchers began to shift from studies of animals' memory for the past, to new studies that focussed on their ability to use the past to plan for the future. In one of the first experiments of this kind, Mulcahy and Call (2006) examined the future planning abilities of bonobos and orangutans. The task they used was modeled on Tulving's (2005) Spoon Test.

In the Mulcahy and Call (2006) experiment, bonobos and orangutans were first taught to use a particular tool to procure a reward from an apparatus. One at a time, each primate was then placed in a room where they could see the baited, but otherwise inaccessible, apparatus. Two suitable and 6 unsuitable tools were also placed in the room. After a 5-min period, the animals were moved into a waiting room where they remained for 1 h. After 1 h, they were allowed back into the test room where the apparatus was now accessible. The

critical question was whether the primates would carry the appropriate tool into the waiting room so that they could use it when they were returned to the test room 1 h later. Each animal was given a total of 16 trials. The results are shown in Table 30.2.

It is important to note that the animals did not transport a tool into the waiting room on every trial, and even if they did take a tool into the waiting room, they did not always bring it with them into the test room. Nevertheless, when they did select a tool, both bonobos and orangutans selected suitable tools (i.e., tools that were identical to or similar to the tools they had learned to use initially) significantly more often than they selected unsuitable tools. The authors argued that the data provide evidence for a "genuine case of future planning" in nonhuman primates (p. 1039). In Tulving's terms, Mulcahy and Call (2006) believed that they had clear evidence of nonverbal episodic memory by nonhuman primates.

In our view, however, some of the selections that the animals made could have been guided by mechanisms other than episodic memory or future planning. For example, it is hard to envision how an animal could possibly choose the correct tool on Trial 1, *before* knowing it would be returned to the test room where it would be given access to the apparatus. At least on Trial 1, the selection must occur on the basis of some other factor, such as a preference for a particular tool. This interpretation is further strengthened by the fact that the animals had successfully used a given tool on multiple occasions prior to this particular manipulation. If selecting the correct tool on Trial 1 does not constitute future planning, then how do we know that selecting the correct tool on subsequent trials reflects future planning either?

In another line of research, Janmaat, Byrne, and Zuberbuhler (2006) used the natural foraging

Table 30.2 Results of Experiment 1 of Mulcahy and Call (2006)

	1	2	3	4	5	6	7	8	9	10	11	12	13	14	15	16
Bonobo #1							X	X		X			X	X	X	X
Bonobo #2	X												X			
Bonobo #3							X			X	X		X			X
Orangutan #1				X	X	X	X	X						X		
Orangutan #2	X		X			X				X	X	X	X			
Orangutan #3	X		X	X	X	X	X	X	X	X	X	X	X	X	X	X

Each animal was given 16 test trials. The X refers to trials in which the animals carried the suitable tool into the waiting room and then back into the test room, and does not include trials in which one of these actions was omitted (see text).

patterns of mangabeys to argue that, in this species, foraging decisions reflect future planning based on weather conditions. In fact, these authors conclude that "…monkeys make foraging decisions based on episodic-like memories of whether or not a tree previously carried fruit, combined with a more generalized understanding of the relationship between temperature and solar radiation and the maturation rate of fruit and insect larvae." Despite the bold nature of this claim, we fail to see how a simpler interpretation based on increased searching on sunny days could not also account for the same data.

Clayton and her colleagues have also examined prospective episodic memory in scrub jays (Raby, Alexis, Dickinson, & Clayton, 2007). Each morning, birds were placed in one of two compartments. In one compartment, the birds always received breakfast, whereas in the other compartment they did not. On the night of the sixth day, the scrub jays were given food to cache. If they were able to plan for the future, then they should selectively cache the food in the compartment in which breakfast was never available. This is exactly what the scrub jays did; they cached more food in the no-breakfast compartment than they did in the breakfast compartment.

One possible interpretation of the data was that the birds were planning for the future. An alternative interpretation that was raised by the authors themselves was that the scrub jays were simply caching food in the compartment that had been associated with hunger, which does not necessarily require planning for the future. To distinguish between the hunger-context account and the future planning account of the data, the authors conducted an additional experiment. The procedure for this experiment was similar to the original experiment except that, rather than having breakfast and no-breakfast compartments, the animals always received kibble in one compartment and peanuts in the other. Again, on the night of the sixth day, the scrub jays were allowed to cache both kibble and peanuts. Raby et al. reasoned that if the birds were planning for the future (and if they prefer to have a choice of foods for breakfast), they should cache peanuts in the kibble compartment, and kibble in the peanuts compartment. Once again, this is exactly what they did. According to the authors, these findings "challenge the assumption that the ability to anticipate and take action for future needs evolved only in the hominid lineage."

Episodic Memory in Infants and Young Children

On the basis of the data reviewed thus far, we conclude that there is little or no evidence that nonhuman animals exhibit the kind of episodic memory that was originally described by Tulving. This does not necessarily mean that animals do not have episodic memory, but at this stage in the research, we cannot refute Tulving's claim that episodic memory is a uniquely human ability. But what about infants and young children? They clearly meet the "human" criterion, but do they have episodic memories that allow them to reflect on the past and plan for the future? Tulving has made his view on this issue very clear arguing that not only is episodic memory a uniquely human skill, but that it does not emerge prior to the age of 4 years (Tulving, 2005). Do we have any evidence to the contrary?

WWW-Memory in Infants and Young Children

The issue of episodic memory captured the attention of researchers working with nonhuman animals long before it captured the attention of researchers working with infants and young children. For this reason, the data base on the development of episodic memory is relatively slim. Research with very young infants has shown that even 3-month-olds remember the *what* of their past experiences. In fact, infants' highly precise memory for *what* places serious constraints on their ability to use their past experiences in similar, but novel situations. For example, Rovee-Collier and her students have shown that when 3-month-olds are trained to kick their feet to produce movement in a particular 5-item mobile, their memory is highly specific to the original training stimulus—infants exhibit no retention whatsoever when they are tested with a different mobile (for review, see Rovee-Collier et al., 2001). Similarly infants also remember the *where* of their past experiences retrieving the target memory if and only if they are returned to the original training context. These same findings have been replicated and extended in numerous studies of deferred imitation by toddlers (Hayne, 2004).

Taken together, studies conducted using the mobile conjugate reinforcement and deferred imitation paradigms indicate that infants exhibit declarative memory skills very early in development. But is there any evidence to suggest that infants or young children also form and retain the kind of integrated, episodic representations originally described by Tulving? Many studies of age-related changes in episodic memory during childhood have employed experimental tasks that are extremely language-laden (e.g., Atance & O'Neill, 2005; Guajardo & Best, 2000; Kliegel & Jager, 2007; Perner & Ruffman, 1995). Across these studies, younger children consistently perform more poorly than older children, and more often than not, 2- and 3-year-olds fail the tasks altogether. Although these data are used to draw strong conclusions about the development of episodic memory, we suspect that the findings tell us as much about language development as they do about memory development. What we really need is a nonverbal, or a minimally verbal task that can be used with children whose language skills are still extremely immature.

In an attempt to overcome the language barrier, we have developed a hide-and-seek procedure that can be used with young children. In many ways, this task is analogous to the procedure originally developed by Clayton and Dickinson (1998). Although our task does require some degree of linguistic comprehension and production, the language requirements of the task are far less than those in other studies. In the most recent version of our task, 3- and 4-year-olds were tested in their own homes during a single session that lasted approximately 30 min. At the beginning of the session, the experimenter familiarized the child with seven soft toys (Bert, Ernie, the Count, Mickey Mouse, Donald Duck, Ronald McDonald, and Cookie Monster) and then instructed the child to choose five toys from the original group of seven. Once the child made his or her selections, the experimenter and the child hid the toys in different rooms throughout the child's house. As the experimenter and the child entered each room, the child was instructed to watch carefully as a toy was hidden in a specific location such as under a bed or behind a chair. This sequence of events continued until all five of the toys were hidden.

Following the hiding portion of the task, the experimenter and the child returned to a central location in the house (e.g., the living room), and to prevent the child from overtly rehearsing the hiding locations, the experimenter read the child two books. At the end of the 5-min retention interval, the child was asked to name one of the rooms in which a toy was hidden. Once the child provided the name of a room (e.g., the bedroom), he/she was asked to name the toy (e.g., Bert) that was hiding

in that room and then to name the specific hiding place (e.g., under the bed). The same sequence of questions was repeated until the child could provide no further information.

For each hidden item, a child could recall a total of three pieces of information: The room, the toy, and the exact location of the toy within that room (i.e., under the bed). For each child, verbal recall was expressed as the number of items that the child correctly recalled. As shown in Figure 30.8, children's overall accuracy was very high ($M = 77.7\%$). Importantly, there was no age-related difference in the number of *what* or *where* items that children recalled. That is, children as young as 3 performed as well on this task as children who were 4.

On the basis of our hiding and finding task, we tentatively conclude that, at least by the age of 3, children are beginning to acquire rudimentary episodic memory skills. In our task, children were highly accurate at recalling the *what* and *where* of the event. We have recently modified the task to yield a measure of *when,* by asking children to recall the items in the order in which they were originally hidden; data collection in this task is currently in progress. Unfortunately, the verbal nature of the instructions and test in this task, although simple, still preclude using it with preverbal participants. We are, however, currently using the task with 2-year-olds, relying on their behavioral search, rather than on their verbal report during the test.

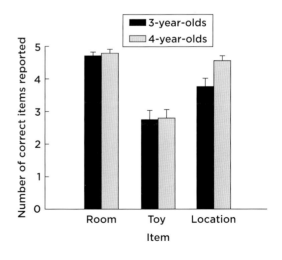

Figure 30.8 Correct verbal recall scores for 3- and 4-year-old children tested in a hide-and-seek task in which 5 unique toys were hidden in 5 specific locations in 5 different rooms.

The Spoon Test

In addition to measures of WWW-memory in young children, some researchers have begun to examine children's performance on variations of Tulving's Spoon Test. In one of these studies, Suddendorf and Busby (2005) tested 3-, 4-, and 5-year old children on a Rooms Task, which is a variant of the spoon test. The children were brought into the "empty room" where they encountered a puzzle board without the puzzle pieces (Experimental condition) or nothing (Control condition). Children remained in this room for a few minutes. Next, they were brought into the "active room" where they played various games. After 5 min in the "active room," the experimenter announced that they were going to return to the "empty room." The experimenter then presented the child with four items, one of which was puzzle pieces. The experimenter told the child that he or she could take any of the four items into the "empty room."

Suddendorf and Busby (2005) found that the same number of 3-year olds chose the puzzle pieces irrespective of whether the "empty room" contained a puzzle board (experimental condition) or not (control condition). In contrast, none of the 4- and 5-year-olds in the control condition chose the puzzle pieces. Although significantly more 4- and 5-year-old children in the experimental condition chose the puzzle pieces than did 4- and 5-year-old children in the control condition, Suddendorf and Busby do not report the data for the 4- and 5-year-olds in the experimental condition. Thus, it is possible that performance did not change as a function of the age in the experimental condition. Furthermore, the age-related differences that Suddendorf and Busby found in the control condition suggest that children's spontaneous preference for the puzzle pieces changed with age, making it virtually impossible to draw meaningful conclusions about age-related changes in the experimental condition, if indeed there were any.

Rate-Limiting Steps
Language

By now, some readers may be wondering whether the rate-limiting step in episodic memory is language. Here, we have argued that our ability to develop nonverbal episodic memory tasks is plagued with complex problems, but maybe these problems reflect a more fundamental limitation—maybe you need language in order to have an episodic memory. Although this issue remains highly controversial, episodic memory should not, by definition, require linguistic ability. In the absence of data to the contrary, it is possible that nonverbal organisms reflect on their past in nonverbal terms, travelling back in time to a particularly stressful experience or forward in time to an anticipated foraging site or social interaction. By the same token, verbal report per se is not sufficient evidence for episodic memory. When a verbal adult tells us that a cat is a mammal, we have a measure of what that person knows (semantic memory), but no measure of what that same person remembers. Similarly, we also know that it is relatively easy to implant false memories, leading verbal adults to retrieve and report episodic-like memories for events that never actually took place (for review, see Garry & Hayne, 2006). Thus, although verbal ability appears to be neither a necessary nor a sufficient condition for episodic memory, in our view, researchers have yet to develop a suitable nonverbal test of episodic memory that could be used in studies with animals, infants, and young children. Clearly, this is an important avenue for future research.

Neural Basis of Episodic Memory

Given the difficulty that researchers have encountered in developing tasks that might tap episodic memory in nonverbal organisms, is it possible that animals, infants, and children lack the fundamental neural structures that are required for this specialized memory skill? Researchers have hypothesized that a number of neural structures may be important for episodic memory. One key structure is the hippocampus (Tulving & Markowitsch, 1998). The importance of the hippocampus can be traced back to the original study of the severely amnesic patient H.M. who was studied extensively by Scoville and Milner (1957). In order to relieve the symptoms of his epilepsy, H.M. received bilateral resection of substantial portions of the medial temporal lobe which rendered him profoundly amnestic. Although he could no longer form episodic memories, H.M. and other patients like him could learn to perform nondeclarative tasks (Corkin, 1968; Tulving, 2005), and patients with more limited damage restricted to the hippocampus but sparing adjacent cortex can even learn to perform semantic memory tasks (Vargha-Khadem et al., 1997). More recently, Hassabis, Kumaran, Van, and Maguire (2007) have also shown that patients with hippocampal damage are unable to imagine new, future situations, providing evidence for the view that the hippocampus is involved in both forward and backward mental time travel.

Given the importance of the hippocampus in episodic memory, what would we predict about episodic memory ability in animals and young humans on the basis of the status of their hippocampal neuroanatomy? First, it is not the case that humans alone have a hippocampus. If anything, the input and output connections of the hippocampus in humans are remarkably similar to those of other primates, and they are also similar to those of rats as well (Amaral, 1987). Second, the size of the hippocampus (relative to the rest of the brain) is not dramatically different across humans, monkeys, rats, and birds. If anything, the relative size of the hippocampus is larger in rats and birds than in primates (Jatzko et al., 2006; Kalisch et al., 2006; Rehkämper, Haase, & Frahm, 1988). Finally, for decades, researchers assumed that the hippocampus was extremely immature during the infancy period, precluding infants from exhibiting higher order memory skills. More recent research on the human infant brain, however, has shown that the hippocampus matures much faster than was originally envisaged (Seress, 2001) and that infants can solve a wide range of declarative memory tasks very early in development (Hayne, 2004). Thus, from the perspective of the hippocampus, there is no a priori reason why we should not see evidence for episodic memory in animals and infants.

Tulving (2005; see also Wheeler, Stuss, & Tulving, 1997) has recently argued that the prefrontal cortex may be the region of the brain that is required for episodic memory skill. In contrast to the hippocampus, the prefrontal cortex in adult humans is considerably larger than it is in other species (Wheeler et al., 1997; but see Semendeferi, Lu, Schenker, & Damasio, 2002). Furthermore, the prefrontal cortex has a very long developmental trajectory in humans and may not reach full functional maturity until early in the third decade of life (Dahl & Spear, 2004). On the surface, these data could be used to argue that we would not see much evidence of episodic memory in other members of the animal kingdom or in younger members of our species.

Unfortunately, this argument is complicated by the fact that humans do not have the largest prefrontal cortex in the animal kingdom; that honor belongs to the spiny anteater, a monotreme (Divac, Holst, Nelson, & McKenzie, 1987). Some have argued that the large prefrontal cortex of this beast evolved because it does not engage in rapid eye movement (REM) sleep (Siegel, Manger, Nienhuis, Fahringer, & Pettigrew, 1996) and that, whatever sleep affords memory, the spiny anteater does in an awake what we humans accomplish from the comfort of our beds. More recent research suggests that spiny anteaters do engage in REM sleep (Nicol, Anderson, Phillips, & Berger, 2000), leaving the purpose of their large prefrontal cortex a mystery. Nevertheless, it is probably premature to rule out episodic memory in other species on the basis of the prefrontal cortex alone. Perhaps the species of choice in understanding the neural basis of episodic memory should not be the rodent or monkey, but rather the much neglected spiny anteater.

It is somewhat odd, given that consciousness or autonoetic awareness is one of the distinguishing features of episodic memory, little emphasis has been placed on the neural basis of consciousness. Here again, however, we run into trouble if we try to claim that human adults are the only ones who posses the neural structures that might be involved in this process. At least two candidate mechanisms for consciousness have been proposed. Consciousness might be the product of synchronized cell assemblies (Singer, 1998) and/or the activity of the reticular complex of the thalamus might serve as an attentional searchlight directing attention to certain aspects of a scene (Crick, 1984). At this stage, there is no reason to believe that these neural mechanisms are not available to any of the animals in which episodic memory has been studied thus far.

Summary and Conclusions

Our understanding of memory processing by animals, infants, and young children has increased substantially over the past 30 years. On the basis of this research, no one doubts that animals, infants, and young children retain information they have learned in the past—in this sense, they all exhibit memory. Furthermore, each new claim about the human or developmental uniqueness of a particular form of memory has been met with experimental challenges which have shown that animals, infants, and young children exhibit many of the highly sophisticated memory skills that are exhibited by their human, adult counterparts. Given this, do animals, infants, and young children also exhibit episodic memory or have we finally identified a truly unique human memory skill that sets us apart from the rest of the animal kingdom and from the youngest members of our own species? In other words, are animals, infants, and young children "stuck in time" (Roberts, 2002), or can they travel back in time to relive a personal episode or travel forward in time to imagine a future scenario?

At this stage, all undisputed evidence for episodic memory has been confirmed through the use of language. Despite some very elegant experimental procedures, research with animals, infants, and young children falls short of demonstrating the kind of episodic memory that is easily elicited by asking an adult, "what did you do last weekend?" In the studies reviewed in this chapter, many of the researchers failed to show clear evidence of episodic memory because (a) the study failed to demonstrate one of the components of episodic memory, usually *when*, (b) there was no evidence that the *what*, *where*, and *when* components were bound together in a single, unified representation, or (c) the study can be reinterpreted on the basis of simpler mechanisms that do not require episodic memory. At present, the best nonverbal evidence for episodic memory has been obtained with the scrub jay, but even the scrub jay data are open to alternative explanations that do not require the birds to travel back in time to imagine what food was hidden where and how long ago. Furthermore, if scrub jays actually do exhibit episodic memory, then we would also have to explain why this skill has leapfrogged over all other primates on the way to humans.

To some, it might seem that our critique of the literature is reminiscent of the "repression by behaviorism" (Griffin, 2001). Are we just a couple of killjoys? We think not. Studies of the cognition of nonhuman animals and preverbal humans have a long history of overinterpreting the behavior of their experimental subjects. Our attention is grabbed much more by studies showing that horses or infants have mathematical ability than by studies showing that they do not (for similar arguments see Haith, 1998). Although we naturally want to side with the enthusiastic protagonist, it is important to remain objective, always keeping in mind that similar looking behaviors do not necessarily imply similar underlying processes.

In conclusion, we argue that most, if not all of the studies that purport to shown evidence of episodic memory can be explained in terms of simpler noncognitive mechanisms, or a failure to show all three *what*, *where*, and *when* components of episodic memory (see also, Suddendorf & Corballis, 2007). We conclude that the richness of human episodic memory has not yet been captured in nonhuman animals or preverbal infants and young children. We fall short of concluding that we will never find evidence of episodic memory in these groups and we encourage researchers to continue to explore this fascinating, if not recalcitrant, issue.

Acknowledgments

Preparation of this manuscript was supported by a Marsden grant to H. Hayne and M. Colombo, and a Neurological Foundation of New Zealand Grant to M. Colombo. We thank Arii Watanabe and Damian Scarf for assistance with the preparation of this manuscript.

References

Amaral, D. G. (1987). Memory: Anatomical organization of candidate brain regions. In V. B. Mountcastle, F. Plum, & S. R. Geiger (Eds.), *Handbook of physiology: The nervous system, Volume V: Higher functions of the brain, Part 1* (pp. 211–294). Bethesda, MD: American Physiological Society.

Atance, C. M., & O'Neill D. K. (2005). The emergence of episodic future thinking in humans. *Learning and Motivation*, *36*, 126–144.

Babb, S. J., & Crystal, J. D. (2005). Discrimination of what, when, and where: Implications for episodic-like memory in rats. *Learning and Motivation, 36*, 177–189.

Bird, L. R., Roberts, W. A., Abroms, B., Kit, K. K., & Crupi, C. (2003). Spatial memory for food hidden by rats (*Rattus norvegicus*) on the radial maze: Studies of memory for where, what, and when. *Journal of Comparative Psychology*, *117*, 176–187.

Clayton, N. S., & Dickinson, A. (1998). Episodic-like memory during cache recovery by scrub jays. *Nature, 395*, 272–274.

Clayton, N. S., Bussey, T. J., & Dickinson, A. (2003). Can animals recall the past and plan for the future? *Nature Reviews Neuroscience, 4*, 685–691.

Colombo, M., & Graziano, M. (1994). Effects of auditory and visual interference on auditory–visual delayed matching-to-sample in monkeys (*Macaca fascicularis*). *Behavioral Neuroscience, 108*, 636–639.

Corkin, S. (1968). Acquisition of motor skill after bilateral medial temporal-lobe excision. *Neuropsychologia, 6*, 255–265.

Crick, F. (1984). Function of the thalamic reticular complex: The searchlight hypothesis. *Proceedings of the National Academy of Sciences USA, 81*, 4586–4590.

Dahl, R., E., & Spear, L., P. (2004) (Eds.). *Adolescent brain development: Vulnerabilities and opportunities*. New York: New York Academy of Sciences.

de Kort, S. R., Dickinson, A., & Clayton, N. S. (2005). Retrospective cognition by food-catching western scrub-jays. *Learning and Motivation, 36*, 159–176.

Divac, I., Holst, M. -C., Nelson, J., & McKenzie, J. S. (1987). Afferents of the frontal cortex in the echidna (*Tachyglossus aculeatus*). Indication of an outstandingly large prefrontal area. *Brain, Behavior and Evolution, 30*, 303–320.

Eichenbaum, H., Fortin N. J., Ergorul, C., Wright S. P., & Agster K. L. (2005). Episodic recollection in animals: "If it walks like a duck and quacks like a duck...." *Learning and Motivation, 36*, 190–207.

Ergorul, C., & Eichenbaum, H. (2007). The hippocampus and memory for "what," "where," and "when." *Learning and Memory, 11*, 397–405.

Garry, M., & Hayne, H. (Eds.) (2006). *Do justice and let the sky fall: Elizabeth F. Loftus and her contributions to science, law, and academic freedom.* Hillsdale, NJ: Erlbaum.

Gold, P. E. (2004). Coordination of multiple memory systems. *Neurobiology of Learning and Memory, 82,* 230–242.

Griffin, D. R. (2001). Animals know more than we used to think. *Proceedings of the National Academy of Science USA, 98,* 4822–4834.

Guajardo, N. R., & Best, D. L. (2000). Do preschoolers remember what to do? Incentive and external cues in prospective memory. *Cognitive Development, 15,* 75–97.

Haith, M. M. (1998). Who put the cog in infant cognition? Is rich interpretation too costly? *Infant Behavior and Development, 21,* 167–179.

Hampton, R. R. (2001). Rhesus monkeys know when they remember. *Proceedings of the National Academy of Science USA, 98,* 5359–5362.

Hampton, R. R., Hampstead B. M., & Murray, E. A. (2005). Rhesus monkeys (*Macaca mulatta*) demonstrate robust memory for what and where, but not when, in an open-field test of memory. *Learning and Motivation, 36,* 245–259.

Hassabis, D., Kumaran, D., Vann, S. D., & Maguire, E. A. (2007). Patients with hippocampal amnesia cannot imagine new experiences. *Proceedings of the National Academy of Sciences, 104,* 1726–1731.

Hayne, H. (2004). Infant memory development: Implications for childhood amnesia. *Developmental Review, 24,* 33–73.

Hayne, H. (2007). Infant memory development: New questions, new answers. In L. Oakes & P. Bauer (Eds.), *Short- and long-term memory in infancy and early childhood: Taking the first steps toward remembering* (pp. 209–239). New York: Oxford University Press.

Janmaat, K. R. L., Byrne, R. W., & Zuberbuhler, K. (2006). Primates take weather into account when searching for fruits. *Current Biology, 16,* 1232–1237.

Jatzo, A., Rothenhöfer, S., Schmitt, A., Gaser, C., Demirakca, T., Weber-Fahr, W., et al. (2006). Hippocampal volume in chronic posttraumatic stress disorder (PTSD): MRI study using two different evaluation methods. *Journal of Affective Disorders, 94,* 121–126.

Kalisch, R., Schubert, M., Jacob, W., Keβler, M. S., Hemauer, R., Wigger, A., et al. (2006). Anxiety and hippocampus volume in rats. *Neuropsychopharmacology, 31,* 925–932.

Kliegel, M., & Jager, T. (2007). The effects of age and cue–action reminders on event-based prospective memory performance in preschoolers. *Cognitive Development, 22,* 33–46.

McDonald, R. J., Devan, B. D., & Hong, N. S. (2004). Multiple memory systems: The power of interactions. *Neurobiology of Learning and Memory, 82,* 333–346.

Mercado III., E., Murray, S. O., Uyeyama, R. K., Pack, A. A., & Herman, L. M. (1998). Memory for recent actions in the bottlenosed dolphin (*Tursiops truncatus*): Repetition of arbitrary behaviors using an abstract rule. *Animal Learning & Behavior, 26,* 210–218.

Mulcahy, N. J., & Call, J. (2006). Apes save tools for future use. *Science, 312,* 1038–1040.

Nicol, S. C., Andersen, N. A., Phillips, N. H., & Berger, R. J. (2000). The echidna manifests typical characteristics of rapid eye movement sleep. *Neuroscience Letters, 283,* 49–52.

Perner, J., & Ruffman, T. (1995). Episodic memory and autonoetic consciousness: Developmental evidence and a theory of childhood amnesia. *Journal of Experimental Child Psychology, 59,* 516–548.

Raby, C. R., Alexis, D. M., Dickinson, A., & Clayton, N. S. (2007). Planning for the future by western scrub-jays. *Nature, 445,* 919–921.

Rehkämper, G., Haase, E., & Frahm, H. D. (1988). Allometric comparison of brain weight and brain structure volumes in different breeds of domestic pigeons, *Columba livia f.d.* (fantails, homing pigeons, strassers). *Brain, Behavior and Evolution, 31,* 141–149.

Roberts, W. A. (2005). Are animals stuck in time? *Psychological Bulletin, 128,* 473–489.

Rovee-Collier, C., Hayne, H., & Colombo, M. (2001). *The development of implicit and explicit memory.* Amsterdam: John Benjamins Publishing Co.

Schwartz, B. L., Colon, M. R., Sanchez, I. C., Rodriguez, I. A., & Evans, S. (2002). Single-trial learning of "what" and "who" information in a gorilla (*Gorilla gorilla gorilla*): Implications for episodic memory. *Animal Cognition, 5,* 85–90.

Schwartz, B. L., Hoffman, M. L., & Evans, S. (2005). Episodic-like memory in a gorilla: A review and new findings. *Learning and Motivation, 36,* 226–244.

Schwartz, B. L., Meissner, C. M., Hoffman, M., Evans, S., & Frazier, L. D. (2004). Event memory and misinformation effects in a gorilla (*Gorilla gorilla gorilla*). *Animal Cognition, 7,* 93–100.

Scoville, W. B., & Milner, B. (1957). Loss of recent memory after bilateral hippocampal lesions. *Journal of Neurology, Neurosurgery, and Psychiatry, 20,* 11–21.

Semendeferi, K., Lu, A., Schenker, N., & Damasio, H. (2002). Humans and great apes share a large frontal cortex. *Nature Neuroscience, 5,* 272–276.

Seress, L. (2001). Morphological changes of the human hippocampal formation from midgestation to early childhood. In C. A. Nelson & M. Luciana (Eds.), *Handbook of developmental cognitive neuroscience* (pp. 45–58). Cambridge, MA: The MIT Press.

Siegal, J. M., Manger, P. R., Nienhuis, R., Fahringer, H. M., & Pettigrew, J. D. (1996). The echidna *Tachyglossus aculeatus* combines REM and non-REM aspects in a single sleep state: Implications for the evolution of sleep. *Journal of Neuroscience, 16,* 3500–3506.

Singer, W. (1998). Consciousness and the structure of neuronal representations. *Philosophical Transactions of the Royal Society of London, 353B,* 1829–1840.

Skov-Rackette, S. I., Miller, N. Y., & Shettleworth, S. J. (2006). What-where-when memory in pigeons. *Journal of Experimental Psychology: Animal Behavior Processes, 32,* 345–358.

Squire, L. R. (1987). *Memory and brain.* New York: Oxford University Press.

Squire, L. R. (1994). Declarative and nondeclarative memory: Multiple brain systems supporting learning and memory. In D. L. Schachter & E. Tulving (Eds.), *Memory systems 1994* (pp. 203–232). Cambridge, MA: MIT Press.

Squire, L. R. (2004). Memory systems of the brain: A brief history and current perspective. *Neurobiology of Learning and Memory, 82,* 171–177.

Squire, L. R., & Schacter, D. L. (2002) (Eds.). *Neuropsychology of memory* (3rd ed.). New York: Guilford Press.

Suddendorf, T., & Busby, J. (2003). Mental time travel in animals? *Trends in Cognitive Science, 9,* 391–396.

Suddendorf, T., & Busby, J. (2005). Making decisions with the future in mind: Developmental and comparative identification of mental time travel. *Learning and Motivation, 36,* 110–125.

Suddendorf, T., & Corballis, M. C. (2007). The evolution of foresight: What is mental time travel, and is it unique to humans? *Behavioral and Brain Sciences, 30,* 299–351.

Tulving, E. (1972). Episodic and semantic memory. In E. Tulving & W. Donaldson (Eds.), *Organization of memory* (pp. 382–403). New York: Academic Press.

Tulving, E. (1983). *Elemental of episodic memory.* Oxford: Clarendon Press.

Tulving, E. (1985). Memory and consciousness. *Canadian Psychology, 26,* 1–12.

Tulving, E. (2002). Episodic memory: From mind to brain. *Annual Review of Psychology, 53,* 1–25.

Tulving, E. (2005). Episodic memory and autonoesis: Uniquely human? In H.S. Terrace & J. Metcalfe (Eds.), *The missing link in cognition: Origins of self-reflective consciousness* (pp. 3–56). Oxford: Oxford University Press.

Tulving, E., & Markowitsch, H. J. (1998). Episodic and declarative memory: Role of the hippocampus. *Hippocampus, 8,* 198–204.

Vargha-Khadem, F., Gadian, D. G., & Mishkin, M. (2001). Dissociations in cognitive memory: the syndrome of developmental amnesia. *Philosophical Transactions of the Royal Society of London, 356B,* 1435–1440.

Vargha-Khadem, F., Gadian, D. G., Watkins, K. E., Connelly, A., Van Paesschen, W., & Mishkin, M. (1997). Differential effects of early hippocampal pathology on episodic and semantic memory. *Science, 277,* 376–380.

Wheeler, M. A., Stuss, D. T., & Tulving, E. (1997). Toward a theory of episodic memory: The frontal lobes and autonoetic consciousness. *Psychological Bulletin, 121,* 331–354.

Zentall, T. R., Clement, T. S., Bhatt, R. S., & Allen, J. (2001). Episodic-like memory in pigeons. *Psychonomic Bulletin & Review, 8,* 685–690.

Zentall, T. R. (2005). Animals may not be stuck in time. *Learning and Motivation, 36,* 208–225.

Zentall, T. R. (2006). Mental time travel in animals: A challenging question. *Behavioural Processes, 72,* 173–183.

Note

1 A score of 50% for the third choice is an artifact of the testing procedure of terminating the trial if an incorrect response was made: On half of the trials, King is going to be correct on the second choice and thus performance on the third choice is 100%, whereas on the other half of the trials, King is going to be incorrect on the second choice and thus have a score of 0% because no third choice is available.

PART 7

Communication

Hormones and the Development of Communication-Related Social Behavior in Birds

Elizabeth Adkins-Regan

Abstract

Avian communication and social behavior have been a rich source of insights into the epigenetic nature of development. Hormones are both mechanisms permitting behavior to occur in appropriate contexts and also one of the physiological responses to engaging in social behavior. Hormones are important for some of the changes in behavior that occur as birds experience life transitions such as hatching, juvenile dispersal, onset of adulthood, and senescence. Hormones are part of the developmental process producing sex differences in communication and its neural substrates in response to sexual selection. Avian communication research has the potential to elucidate the developmental basis of the evolutionary changes that have led to species differences in communication and sociality.

Keywords: avian communication, avian social behavior, hormones, hatching, juvenile dispersal, adulthood, senescence

Introduction and Conceptual Background
Why Focus on Birds?

Birds have long been important in the science of behavioral and neural development. Imprinting by ducks and motor development in chick embryos, for example, are classics of interest to both psychologists and biologists. Birds will continue to be essential to the integrative approach to neuroscience that focuses on adaptive mechanisms of ecologically relevant behavior. With over 9000 species, they are the largest class of terrestrial vertebrates. Because they are primarily diurnal, often highly vocal, and esthetically pleasing, the lives of marked individuals of a number of species have been observed intensively in nature. Such observations are increasingly accompanied by genotyping to establish relatedness, parentage, and reproductive success. Among vertebrates, birds are the predominant subjects at the cutting edges of behavioral ecology and evolutionary biology. Contrary to popular belief, their brains are not necessarily smaller than those of mammals (relative to body size), and some have relative brain sizes in the primate range (Iwaniuk, Dean, & Nelson, 2005; Striedter, 2005).

As developmental and comparative neuroscience grapples increasingly with complex social behavior, yet another advantage of birds becomes evident. Birds, both captive and free-living, are also key subjects for the study of such socially interesting phenomena as mating systems, mate choice, and the interactional and kin structure of groups (bird societies and extended families). The current combination of state-of-the-art theory of social life and rich data sets from marked individuals throughout their years of life forms an excellent foundation for discovering how this behavior comes about developmentally and neurally. Birds are where we can best hope to reveal both the ultimate and proximate causes of communication-related social behavior in an integrated fashion, achieving all four of Tinbergen's aims for understanding behavior: development, physiology, function, and phylogeny (Tinbergen, 1963).

Birds are a highly diverse group as well, socially and otherwise. A few brief descriptions of the social life of species to appear in this chapter will give a flavor of this diversity. The zebra finch is a songbird (songbirds are oscine passerines) that lives in the arid interior of Australia and breeds opportunistically in response to unpredictable rainfall. Zebra finches are gregarious, living in flocks (Zann, 1996). Birds are nomadic when not breeding, traveling in search of water and seeds. The subunit of the flock is the male–female pair. All adults are paired, and pairs are stable, terminating only if a bird dies. Paired birds sit close together when perched, preen each other, and call back and forth frequently. Only the males sing, however. When and if it rains, birds build their nests colonially, several to a bush or tree. The chicks are altricial and fed by both parents. Once fledged (after about 16–18 days), young birds often perch together. As they get older, they spend more time away from the parents, flocking with other juveniles, and in short order (hatching to sexual maturity occurs as fast as 60 days) find a partner and enter their adult pair relationship. Thus the social life course of this species is marked by a high degree of sociality at all times (birds are always in close proximity to and interacting with a number of other birds) and an adult life characterized by a behaviorally distinctive close affiliative relationship with an opposite-sex bird punctuated by one or more bouts of coparental chick rearing.

The social lives of many north temperate zone seasonally breeding songbirds such as the white-crowned sparrow (Chilton, Baker, Barrentine, & Cunningham, 1995; Wingfield & Farner, 1978) look different. Many species have separate winter and summer ranges, migrating between the two twice a year, and many are territorial during the breeding season. Males often arrive first in the spring, claim a territory, and form pairs as the females arrive. Typically only the male sings to defend the territory (and attract a mate), but both sexes aggressively keep other birds away from their territory, so that the mated pairs are widely spaced. During the breeding season, social interaction with nonpair mates appears to be limited to aggressive vocalization and the occasional foray to obtain an extrapair copulation. Such extrapair matings, which generate deviations from genetic monogamy, are why male–female pair mating systems are referred to as "social monogamy" instead of just "monogamy." Either the female alone, or the female and male together, depending on the species, care for the young. Later in the season, the territories dissolve, and both juveniles and adults may live and migrate in flocks in autumn and winter. Spring migration brings the males back to where they were the previous year, but they do not necessarily have the same female mate in successive years. Thus, these birds' lives are marked by dramatic seasonal changes in social life and in the frequency and function of singing and displaying.

Yet another pattern is seen in nonpasserine birds such as wandering albatrosses, pairs of which produce a single chick every other year, if they are successful (Angelier, Shaffer, Weimerskirch, & Chastel, 2006). The chick does not reach sexual maturity until it is 8 years old or older. Birds spend long periods of time over the open ocean, seemingly alone except when breeding, and live for 40 years or more. These singleton chicks, who develop very slowly and are completely dependent on the parents for an extended period, are very different from the young of quail of the *Coturnix* genus, which hatch in clutches of up to 10 or more, are highly precocial, cared for mainly by the mother, and can begin to reproduce themselves by 8 weeks of age (Madge & McGowan, 2002).

The social lives of birds, then, are a reflection of their life histories (short vs. long lives, large vs. small clutches), their developmental modes (altricial vs. precocial at hatching, rapid vs. slow posthatching development), ecological factors such as predation pressure and food distribution that select for greater or lesser degrees of sociality, and sexual selection (mate competition and mate choice). A search for neuroendocrine mechanisms or developmental processes of communication behavior should take these evolutionary origins (ultimate causes) of social life into account through an integrative approach.

What Are the Questions?

Social behavior requires communication, and much of avian communication is accessible to humans. Few birds seem to communicate through chemosensory systems, such as odors (see Hagelin, Jones, & Rasmussen [2003] for an interesting exception). Instead, they rely heavily on vocalizations and displays, with the latter often enhanced by ornaments such as special plumage forms, colors, or markings. In close relationships—those between parents and offspring, mated pairs, or cooperatively breeding group members—perching in direct physical contact or allopreening (preening of one bird by another) may occur, raising the additional possibility of somatosensory communication.

The production and reception of signals, and their interpretation in order to make adaptive decisions, are an important part of a bird's social developmental life course. Such a life course is marked by change as the bird goes from one developmental stage to another (from egg to chick, from nest-bound chick to flying juvenile, from prereproductive juvenile to breeding adult) and by some differences between males and females, as when only males sing or only females perform a special copulation solicitation display. These developmental changes and sex differences raise important questions about the underlying mechanisms at work. What is producing these changes and sex differences? This is where hormones come into the picture. Hormones and the neural mechanisms upon which they act are obvious candidates to be part of the answer, especially when hormone levels also change during development and differ between the sexes, as they so often do. To the extent that hormones are involved, we need to know the underlying processes upon which they have acted to produce developmental changes and sex differences, and through what brain regions. These effects occur in a social context, so we can ask how association with other individuals might affect hormone levels and responses to hormones. Given the diversity of adult developmental outcomes with respect to overall sociality and social systems, we also can ask how those species differences evolve from a hormonal perspective, that is, how hormone–social behavior relationships change during evolution. Finally, because evolution is based on changes in development, we need to ask what has changed about development to produce species differences.

What Concepts and Theories Might Be Important for Seeking Answers?
SEXUAL SELECTION AND SIGNALING

Evolutionary approaches distinguish between two sources of sex differences in signaling (natural and sexual selection) and two forms of sexual selection (intrasexual and intersexual selection). If females have a special vocalization to warn their chicks of danger, it would likely have resulted from natural selection. But if a vocalization serves to threaten other females in the context of competing for a nest site, or serves to attract a male mate,

it would be regarded as resulting from intrasexual (competition with members of one's own sex) or intersexual (mate choice) selection, respectively. In reality, it is not always possible to cleanly distinguish between results of the two kinds of sexual selection, as, for example, when male song serves both to defend the territory and to attract a female. Upon closer study, however, it might be found that the songs are slightly different in the two contexts, as has been shown in several species (Catchpole & Slater, 1995).

From an evolutionary perspective, "communication" and "signal" mean that the signaler is doing something (or has some trait like a plumage color) that has evolved for the purpose of generating an effect in other individuals that is (or was in the past) beneficial for the signaler, increasing its fitness (Searcy & Nowicki, 2005). An important distinction is made between such *signals* and *cues*. Both are stimuli with respect to the receiver's sensory systems, but cues are stimuli that would be given off regardless of whether there was any receiver present and that have not evolved for the purpose of communicating. For example, if a bird flees from attempted predation, other birds may see that flight and use that information to decide to fly away as well, but that does not mean that flight has evolved in order to communicate. Receivers are simply capitalizing on some useful information that evolved for other purposes (escape in the case of flight). But bird song is a signal: it can be shown experimentally that the function of a male bird singing is to alter the behavior of receivers.

It takes two parties to communicate, signaler and receiver, but selection acts on individuals, not dyads. The two individuals are usually not genetically identical, and while their interests and genes may overlap (as with parents and offspring), they do not always (as with males competing for a territory). This raises interesting issues about who is benefiting from the communication and how, or whether, signals are entirely reliable ("honest"), somewhat reliable, or downright deceptive (Searcy & Nowicki, 2005). Is the signaler conveying accurate information to the receiver for their mutual benefit? This would be a cooperative arrangement, evolutionarily speaking. Or is the signaler sending false information in order to manipulate the receiver, so that only the signaler benefits? If so, why have not the receivers evolved to detect such dishonesty and resist being manipulated? If not, what is it that keeps the signaling honest? This and many other domains of social behavior involving individuals whose interests and genes differ raise pressing theoretical issues of how and why the cooperative elements have evolved, and what the mixture of cooperation and conflict is. Male–female interactions are an interesting case, because the two parties are normally genetically distinct yet have a reproductive interest in common that requires some degree of behavioral cooperation. Why should females choose males on the basis of their ability to show off? What attribute of the male that is important to the female is indicated by this showiness? If all he is contributing is sperm (as in species with no male contribution to nesting or parenting), could his signals indicate something about his genetic quality? If so, what keeps males from faking their quality in order to gain copulations?

Current theory draws on Zahavi's (1975) handicap principle and Hamilton and Zuk's (1982) hypothesis that a male's appearance might reflect his parasite status. It proposes that male courtship signaling is kept honest by the costs of the signals, which are greater (a heavier burden that is less likely to be bearable) for males in poorer condition (Grafen, 1990; Johnstone, 1997). Only the best quality males can afford to express high signal levels, and quality will reflect in part genetic quality (pathogen resistance, ability to forage effectively, etc.) but also the male's developmental environment and experience (quality of parenting received, degree of sibling competition, etc.). The link to hormones was then made by Folstad and Karter (1992) in the immunocompetence handicap hypothesis. According to this hypothesis, the immune suppressing effects of testosterone are the significant costs of testosterone-stimulated male-specific signaling that help keep such signals honest by making it impossible for poor-quality males to perform them at a high level. The evidence for the hypothesis that the cost of testosterone lies in immune suppression is somewhat mixed, and it is possible that corticosterone (the primary adrenal glucocorticoid in birds) is more important than testosterone for causing immune suppression and keeping signaling honest (Hillgarth, Ramenofsky, & Wingfield, 1997; Roberts, Buchanan, & Evans, 2004). Even if the testosterone version of the hypothesis does not turn out to be correct, it is stimulating much research on the behavioral endocrinology of wild birds and many lively theoretical debates, hallmarks of a valuable idea.

A distinction can be made between static and dynamic signals (Bradbury & Vehrencamp, 1998). Dynamic signals should be particularly good indicators of the current state of the signaler (whether it is ill, starving, incompetent). Behavioral signals (displays, vocalizations) are the epitome of dynamic signals, and have the additional virtue of potentially revealing something about the current and past state of the signaler's brain, not just its body. If the display is performed in an unskilled manner, that might indicate lack of overall intelligence (learning ability), a poor upbringing (the developmental stress hypothesis, in which poor early nutrition or disease puts the young at a future disadvantage by affecting the brain: Buchanan, Spencer, Goldsmith, & Catchpole, 2003; MacDonald, Kempster, Zanette, & MacDougall-Shackleton, 2006; Nowicki, Searcy, & Peters, 2002), or simply immaturity or lack of experience, all of which would indicate an undesirable mating partner or a foe that could be easily vanquished.

As mentioned above, social relationships between males and females, like those between parents and offspring, are now recognized to involve elements of conflict as well as cooperation, and communication between the two parties could include deceptive as well as honest elements (Arnqvist & Rowe, 2005; Parker, 2006; Wedell, Kvarnemo, Lessells, & Tregenza, 2006). The conflict may not be obvious to the researcher (would not necessarily involve any overt aggression), but might require experimentation to be revealed. For example, in a study of zebra finches, removal of the male parent, combined with halving the number of eggs in the nest to maintain the same number of chicks per parent, resulted in greater female investment per chick than when coparenting, revealing hidden conflict between the two parents over parental investment (Royle, Hartley, & Parker, 2002).

CONCEPTS FROM BEHAVIORAL ENDOCRINOLOGY

Social relationships have a developmental course, forming, continuing, and (in many cases) dissolving to be replaced by new relationships. There are important precedents in the literature on hormones and social behavior, especially in research on dominance relationships and parental behavior, for distinguishing between the formation and maintenance of such relationships. The formation stage, like developmental transitions generally, seems especially subject to hormonal influence and more likely to require some kind of special hormonal or other mechanisms to get it going. Once the relationship is established, a kind of "social inertia" (produced in part by stimuli from the other party and possibly by conditioning as well) seems to keep it going without the continuing need for the special mechanism to be active. Thus the testosterone status of males may predict rank when strangers are introduced to each other but not when the animals are already familiar with each other (Harding, 1983). The maternal behavior of rodents requires a particular circulating hormonal milieu to begin when the first litter is born, but is relatively independent of those hormones once the litter is a few days old (Bridges, 1996). This does not mean that there are no hormone-like mechanisms maintaining the behavior and the relationships, because neurohormones could be involved, but rather that whatever they are, they are not peripheral circulating hormones.

A second important principle of hormones and behavior relevant to understanding social and communicative behavior is that hormone levels change in dynamic fashion in response to social encounters and outcomes. The causal relationship between hormones and behavior goes in both directions. The function and fitness consequences of hormonal changes in response to other individuals is sometimes obvious, as when they cause a female to ovulate when paired with a male or a male to experience elevated glucocorticoids during an aggressive encounter. It is not so obvious, however, when an aggressive encounter produces elevated testosterone, because until recently little attention had been paid to whether that elevated testosterone had any consequences in the short- or long-term, and how there could be short-term benefits (benefits during the encounter itself) when the known mechanisms of action of testosterone take hours or days to play out (Adkins-Regan, 2005b).

An important distinction in the hormones and behavior literature that is essential for thinking about social behavior development is that between hormonal activation and organization. These concepts date back to a classic 1959 paper by Phoenix, Goy, Gerall, and Young. In current parlance, activational effects are those typically occurring at puberty or in adulthood, in which hormones facilitate the expression of behavior in a manner that is reversible (the behavioral facilitation goes away if the hormone level goes down), can occur at any time in adult life (rather than being limited to a particular age), and does not fundamentally change the behavioral sex of the animal. Organizational effects, on the other hand, are those that typically occur early in development (even before birth or hatching), are limited to a critical period, are permanent,

and establish the behavioral sex of the animal (the capacities that can then be expressed in adulthood if activational hormones are present). Whether the nervous system is altered by the hormones is not part of this conceptual distinction, but the existence of critical periods for organizational effects clearly has something to do with ways in which the developing nervous system differs from the adult nervous system. Also, "activational" should not be taken to mean that hormones are deterministic with respect to behavior. Animals normally require both the hormone and some appropriate social context to perform a hormone-dependent behavior, so that hormones are necessary but not sufficient for expression of the behavior.

It is interesting to ask whether organization is possible in adulthood and whether there might be some connection between the organization–activation distinction and the formation–maintenance concepts. Do hormonal changes occurring at the onset of new relationships produce long-term changes of an organizational nature that account for subsequent hormone independence? Also of interest is whether hormonal changes at key developmental transitions such as the onset of sexual maturity, which lie outside the conventional early critical period, have permanent organizational effects. There is evidence for pubertal organization in hamsters (Sisk & Zehr, 2005), but its existence in birds is still an open question.

Social relationships manifest themselves through the overt behavioral acts of the animals, but their essence lies not in what the animals are doing, but in the targets for their behavior, the choices of individuals to be receivers. This higher level of behavioral organization has two implications for the search for physiological mechanisms. With respect to hormones, we cannot assume without evidence that we know what the relevant hormones are based on their effects on specific motor acts. For example, if we know that estradiol is important for female receptivity during mating, this does not mean we know that estradiol is important for a female's preference for the male with the largest song repertoire, or for how faithful she is to her male mate with respect to extrapair copulations. In searching for neural mechanisms, this higher level of behavioral organization, involving preferences, choices, and decisions about communication partners, suggests focusing the search on so-called higher parts of the brain, especially the telencephalon, rather than the brain stem, the site of important copulation centers and motor pattern generators for some signaling.

Hormonal and Neurohormonal Mechanisms in Relation to Life Stages of Social Development
Life as a Chick: Begging Behavior

It has been known for many years that avian communication begins even before hatching. Late-stage embryos of precocial species vocalize, and such vocalizations have important consequences, such as synchronizing hatching among the chicks in the clutch, signaling to the mother that hatching is imminent, and eliciting vocal responses from her that begin the processes of acoustic species identification and individual recognition (Beecher, 1988; Gottlieb, 1974; Vince, 1973). After hatching, chicks of some species are highly vocal, giving off loud distress calls when cold or separated from others, or, especially in altricial young, begging for food. Food begging can be visual (posture, colorful markings in the mouth) or acoustic (vocalizations) or both together. Begging is an excellent case of a communication system that is best understood by viewing it from the fitness perspectives of both parties (chicks and parents), whose interests overlap but are not identical (Beecher, 1988). They overlap in that both the parents and each chick want at least one chick to survive. Because they are genetic relatives, no special new theoretical tricks are required to understand how cooperation in signaling has evolved to ensure the survival of one chick. And indeed chick begging does appear to reliably signal hunger (short-term need for food) (Searcy & Nowicki, 2005). Where the parents' and offsprings' interests do not overlap is that each individual chick's agenda is to beg to get food for itself; the others in the clutch are not its concern and it might even benefit if they died (then it would get more food for itself). The parents may have a different agenda, however, with a goal of rearing multiple chicks and allocating food more equally across them. A chick might benefit by exaggerating its need at relatively low cost to itself, but the parents should guard against such a possibility when there are multiple young chicks (Searcy & Nowicki, 2005). In two recent research developments, these evolutionary views of begging have been linked to hormones.

In one of these developments, the focus is on hormone-mediated maternal effects viewed as strategies for the mother's fitness interests. The yolks of bird eggs contain hormones from the mother, and the developing embryo is exposed to these hormones as it absorbs the yolk. Schwabl (1993) found significant amounts of androgens in the yolks of

canary eggs, with increasing levels as laying order increased from first laid to last laid eggs in a clutch. Later hatched birds in a clutch are usually thought to be at a disadvantage because they are smaller than their older siblings. Schwabl (1993) hypothesized that these yolk androgens reflected a maternal strategy to enhance the vigor of the later-hatched chicks so as to make the chicks more equal. This highly original hypothesis has stimulated a great deal of research with a variety of wild and domestic species, some of which has found that injecting freshly laid eggs with testosterone increases the vigor or duration of begging behavior (reviewed in Groothuis, Müller, von Engelhardt, Carere, & Eising, 2005). Such treatment has also been observed to increase the loudness of late embryonic vocalization (Boncoraglio, Rubolini, Romano, Martinelli, & Saino, 2006).

Cases where yolk hormones affect begging or late embryonic vocalizations raise questions about how the hormones are having this effect. Is it the brain mechanisms for begging that have been affected, or the muscle strength required to hold the head up to beg (similar to the effect of yolk testosterone on hatching muscle strength, see Lipar & Ketterson, 2000), or both? There is evidence that maternal hormones in the yolk are largely gone after just a few days of embryonic development (Pilz, Adkins-Regan, & Schwabl, 2005), suggesting that yolk hormone effects on begging might be organizational. What, therefore, has been organized? The brain itself? Or are the gonads or adrenals altered, so that the effects of yolk hormones on begging are mediated by the chick's hormonal state at the time of begging?

In the other research development, the focus has been on the chick's own hormones during the begging period, after the maternal yolk hormones are gone. Groothuis and Ros (2005) found that giving testosterone to black-headed gull chicks after hatching reduced begging and increased aggressive displays (Figure 31.1). This is a species in which elevation of yolk testosterone increases, not decreases, begging, indicating that testosterone's effects on begging depend importantly on the bird's stage of development. Hungry (food deprived) seabirds experience elevated corticosterone and beg more, suggesting that this hormone could be mediating the effect of hunger on begging behavior. Kitaysky, Kitaiskaia, Piatt, and Wingfield (2003) found that well-fed kittiwake chicks given corticosterone begged more, supporting this hypothesis. It would appear that testosterone and corticosterone

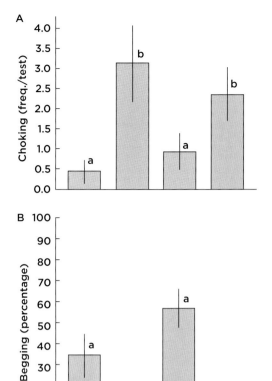

Figure 31.1 Mean frequency (± S.E.M.) of nest-oriented choking displays (an aggressive display) (top panel) and mean (± S.E.M.) percentage of birds begging (bottom panel) in four tests of black-headed gull chicks with control implants (C) or implants of dihydrotestosterone (DHT), 17β-estradiol (E), or testosterone (T). Sample sizes are in parentheses. Groups with different letters are significantly different. Testosterone and DHT decreased begging but increased aggression; estradiol did not affect either behavior. (Reproduced with permission from Groothuis & Ros, 2005. © 2005 Elsevier Inc.)

administered experimentally after hatching have opposite effects on begging. Also, once again, there seems to be a contrast between effects of experimentally elevated yolk versus chick hormone, because elevated yolk corticosterone mainly reduces begging as well as late embryonic vocalization (Rubolini et al., 2005).

Juvenile Dispersal

After days, weeks, or months of daily interaction with and dependence on the parent(s) for food and other survival necessities, the young of many species disperse, terminating the communicative relationship with the parents and leaving the natal territory or home range. Dispersal is thought to have benefits for future reproductive success that outweigh (on average) its costs. One potentially large cost is increased mortality during dispersal. Dispersal is a dramatic developmental life stage. Yet surprisingly little is known about the hormonal and neural basis of this critical event.

If dispersal coincides with the onset of reproductive maturity, as it does in some mammals, it is natural to hypothesize that increasing levels of sex steroids might underlie dispersal. This hypothesis does not appear to have been tested in any bird (and seldom in any mammal either). In chickens, it has been shown that male chicks imprinted to a rubber ball (a hen surrogate) increasingly detach from it beginning at age 5–7 weeks because of an increase in circulating testosterone (Gvaryahu, Snapir, Robinzon, & Goodman, 1986); this detachment could reflect an increased dispersal tendency. When dispersal occurs prior to the onset of reproductive maturity, it is possible that a hormone related to energetics or body condition, such as corticosterone, is responsible. Willow tits implanted with corticosterone in the late summer, when winter flocks are beginning to form, were more likely to disappear than controls, who integrated into winter flocks, or than birds treated in late autumn after joining a winter flock, although whether those that disappeared dispersed or died is unclear (Silverin, 1997). Captive juvenile western screech owls show peak levels of both locomotor activity and corticosterone at around the time dispersal would have occurred in the wild (Belthoff & Dufty, 1998).

Onset of Adult Behavior

The transition from late juvenile to adult social life is likely to vary depending on whether the birds are seasonal breeders and whether they are migratory. In seasonal breeders, the timing of initial reproductive maturation will be determined by the time of year and the age of the bird. For example, north temperate zone birds hatched in the spring or early summer may not transition to reproductive adulthood until the following spring, because the same influences of day length that cause gonadal regression in adults in late summer will also prevent gonadal maturation in juveniles (Wingfield & Farner, 1993). Some birds spend years as juveniles before becoming reproductively mature.

How are the behavioral changes of this new developmental stage related to hormones? From a mammalian perspective, it might seem obvious that hormonal puberty is responsible. Yet remarkably little is known about the hormonal profiles of the juvenile-early adult period of birds except in a few domestic or captive species. Birds cannot be assumed to undergo the same kind of endocrine puberty that mammals do. Old World primates and apes (including humans), for example, have low levels of sex steroids throughout juvenile life that then rise dramatically at the onset of reproductive maturity. Those few avian studies that have measured hormones throughout juvenile development, however, find different profiles. Either sex steroids are present in quantities only slightly below those of adults (e.g., zebra finches: Adkins-Regan, Abdelnabi, Mobarak, & Ottinger, 1990), or hormones rise gradually over a substantial period (e.g., ducks and chickens: Yang, Medan, Watanabe, & Taya, 2005), or, in species that require more than 1 year to mature, hormones rise somewhat and then fall multiple times on an annual basis before finally reaching adult levels (e.g., black-headed gulls: Groothuis & Meeuwissen, 1992). Nor would the critical hormonal changes have to lie in the gonads. In rats and hamsters, the pubertal onset of adult aggression is due to maturation of the hypothalamic-pituitary-adrenal axis (Delville, Newman, Wommack, Taravosh-Lahn, & Cervantes, 2006).

Hormone measurements of free-living birds at multiple juvenile ages are rare. Silverin and Sharp (1996) found high levels of circulating testosterone and estradiol at hatching in great tits that then declined over the next week and remained low up to 40 days of age. Williams, Dawson, Nicholls, and Goldsmith (1987) measured plasma hormones in starlings from hatching to 12 weeks of age, and found that prolactin rose during the nestling period, then fell during the next weeks. Luteinizing hormone levels were similar to those of adults in a photorefractory state (regressed gonads due to sustained long days), but testosterone was nearly at the level of breeding adults during the entire period.

In male domestic Japanese quail housed on reproductively stimulatory daylengths, circulating androgens rise steadily after 10 days of age, reaching about 75% of adult male levels by age 24 days. Crowing and mating attempt frequencies begin to rise at 30 days (Ottinger & Bakst, 1981; Ottinger & Brinkley, 1979). Here, it is clear that the behavioral change is caused in part by the hormonal change. If very young chicks are given adult levels of testosterone, they too crow (Yazaki, Matsushima, & Aoki, 1999). Similarly, juvenile gulls treated with testosterone show adult displays and vocalizations prematurely (Groothuis &

Meeuwissen, 1992; Terkel, Moore, & Beer, 1976). Such precocially induced behavior indicates that the brain mechanisms are already in place or can rapidly be induced by hormones. Male chickens, quail, and ducks castrated as juveniles never begin to crow or show courtship displays, strengthening the evidence that changes in testicular hormones are causing the onset of adult-typical signaling in normal individuals (Balthazart, 1983). Similarly, female ducklings given estradiol show premature sexual receptivity. Such precocious behavior is not quite like the normal adult version, however, and may require supraphysiological doses of hormone, suggesting that additional brain maturation or experience is required (Balthazart, 1983).

Recent years have brought several new twists to this story. The discovery that steroids can be made in the brain as well as gonads and adrenals (Tsutsui & Schlinger, 2001) has inspired new hypotheses about the hormonal basis of signaling and other social behavior when it occurs outside the breeding season. For example, male song sparrows sing and aggressively defend a territory all year long, even though the gonads are regressed and circulating sex steroid levels are low in the winter. Giving winter birds an estrogen synthesis inhibitor reduces this behavior, confirming that it is still sex steroid–dependent, and suggesting that estrogen produced in the brain is supporting it (Soma, 2006).

Another new development is an increased interest in birds from regions other than the north temperate zone, especially tropical birds. Because tropical species are numerous and many are from different branches of the phylogenetic tree from north temperate birds, they are critical to assessing the generality of principles derived from temperate species. Studies of spotted antbirds, which defend a territory year round even when not breeding, suggest the intriguing possibility that dehydroepiandrosterone (DHEA) might be supporting territorial behavior outside the breeding season by acting as a precursor to more potent sex steroids (Hau, Stoddard, & Soma, 2004). Male golden-collared manakins, like other manakin species, perform elaborate and lively displays, with striking visual and acoustic components, on a lek, a multimale courting arena. Treatment of young males (those still in their juvenile plumage, who do not display on leks) with testosterone implants resulted in significant increases in display behavior (Day, McBroom, & Schlinger, 2006), suggesting that this hormone is responsible for the normal onset of mature male displaying.

In seasonal breeders, each bird, not just the juveniles, experiences an onset of reproductive behavior at the beginning of each breeding season. This raises questions about whether and how the behavioral changes at these annual onsets, and their hormonal and neural bases, differ in birds breeding for the first time compared to older birds who have been through this process before. A number of studies of free-living birds have found that birds breeding for the first time are less successful than second time and older birds (Clutton-Brock, 1988; see Angelier et al. [2006] for a recent example). There is obviously a potentially large role for behavioral and other experience to make a difference, but without experiments, such effects cannot be separated from age per se. In addition, any organizational effects of hormones at the onset of reproductive maturity could magnify the difference. Little research has addressed these issues. Sockman, Williams, Dawson, and Ball (2004) found a priming effect of photostimulation in the first reproductive year in female starlings on subsequent gonadal responses to photostimulation and proposed that this might be one mechanism responsible for an increase in reproductive performance with age. The behavioral consequences of such priming are not yet known.

A number of avian species show delayed maturation, in which young birds do not attempt to breed even though their hypothalamic-pituitary-gonadal axes appear to be physiologically capable. For example, Williams (1992) found that macaroni penguins on Bird Island, South Georgia, did not breed until they were 6–8 years old, even though some 3- to 5-year-olds had testosterone levels in the breeding adult range. Young male satin bowerbirds retain juvenile plumage and do not build bowers or display to females. If they are given testosterone, however, they begin showing full adult male-typical aggression, bower building, and display (Collis & Borgia, 1992, 1993). This raises the question of why they delay hormonal and behavioral maturation. The authors suggest that with this kind of highly competitive mating system, in which a male's skill in bower building and displaying might be critical to females, young males are simply too inexperienced to have any chance of success and are better off putting their energy into survival. Subsequent research using robotic females has confirmed that the male's skill in dynamically varying his display intensity in response to her feedback is indeed crucial for his success (Patricelli, Uy, Walsh, & Borgia, 2002).

In some seasonally breeding songbirds, not only do the gonads wax and wane seasonally, but so do

the telencephalic song system nuclei (Ball, Riters, & Balthazart, 2002; Nottebohm, 1981). The behavioral functions of these seasonal changes in the song system are not clear and more than one hypothesis has received limited support (Brenowitz & Kroodsma, 1996). How they occur (through what mechanisms) has been studied experimentally in several species, especially in starlings and for nucleus HVC (Ball et al., 2002). Photoperiod (daylength) is a major influence. Some but not all of the effect of photoperiod is mediated by gonadal testosterone. Melatonin is also involved, levels of which in birds as in other vertebrates are higher when lights are off and therefore higher more of the time on short days (Bentley, Van't Hof, & Ball, 1999). In addition, males that own a nest box and sing from it show greater HVC enlargement than males not engaging in such behavior (Sartor & Ball, 2005). This suggests the fascinating possibility that the bird's own singing behavior might be able to affect the size of song nucleus HVC through some kind of feedback (proprioceptive or otherwise) (Adkins-Regan, 2005a; Sartor & Ball, 2005).

Female birds have been relatively neglected. Estradiol is commonly administered to female songbirds to elicit a high level of copulation solicitation display in response to song playback, but the estradiol levels that result are supraphysiological, and complementary estrogen-blocking experiments have seldom been done. In one exception, Leboucher, Beguin, Mauget, and Kreutzer (1998) found that fadrozole, an estrogen synthesis inhibitor, lowers copulation solicitation by female canaries, but only when the behavior is just getting underway following photostimulation, as if it has a low estrogen threshold that is easily exceeded. Belle, Sharp, and Lea (2005) found that fadrozole eliminates the nest-soliciting display from both male and female ring doves. Ketterson, Nolan, and Sandell (2005) carried out a comparative analysis of female testosterone levels and found that females of socially monogamous species have more testosterone. This intriguing result should help direct increased attention to the role of this androgen in female social behavior and the role of females in generating mating systems.

In another welcome departure from this earlier neglect of females, new research is uncovering some of the neurohormonal mechanisms for the copulation solicitation display of estrogen-primed white-crowned sparrow females. Using intracranial cannulas placed in the third ventricle to deliver treatments, it has been found that copulation solicitation can be stimulated by chicken GnRH-II and inhibited by the newly discovered gonadotropin inhibitory hormone (Bentley et al., 2006; Maney, Richardson, & Wingfield, 1997b). Oxytocin family peptides are also being explored, and Maney, Goode, and Wingfield (1997a) found that administering arginine vasotocin (AVT) into the third ventricle made estrogen-primed female white-crowned sparrows sing, a behavior sometimes seen in wild females.

Onset and Maintenance of Pairing

Socially monogamous birds, which are many, choose a partner not only for copulation, but for a more extended relationship involving physical proximity, frequent social interaction (sometimes with mutual displaying, singing, or aggression toward outsiders). and coparenting. Such relationships are especially obvious in birds such as pigeons and doves, parrots, and estrildid finches, because mated pairs spend much time in the nest together or preening (grooming) each other or making beak contact ("billing"). These behaviors (signals? their communicative functions are unclear) seem to have great significance for the birds. Zebra finches, the best studied estrildid finches, do not pair without having this kind of direct bodily contact (Silcox & Evans, 1982), as if somatosensory cues are important along with visual and auditory cues.

Avian pair relationships have been well studied by ethologists, and the ultimate causes of social monogamy as a mating system have received much attention from behavioral ecologists. Pairing is a critical life event for an individual's fitness, especially when birds pair for life and extrapair fertilization rates are low. Until recently, however, little work had been directed at the proximate hormonal and neurohormonal mechanisms of pairing. Major advances in discovering some of the mechanisms behind socially monogamous pairing in prairie voles have sparked new interest in this subject. One of the more practical avian "models" for the study of pairing is the zebra finch. The birds breed well in captivity, pair at a young age, have pair bonds that are permanent in the wild and often in captivity as well, and demonstrate the pair relationship through the easily observed behaviors of clumping (sitting with bodies in direct contact), allopreening (mutual preening), and spending periods of time in a nest box together (Zann, 1996).

When unpaired birds are introduced into an aviary together, a flurry of singing and dancing (male courtship display) ensues, following the desired partner around, and aggression to keep potential rivals away or defend a nest box. Some pairs form almost immediately and others require several days or more to develop. Both sexes appear to exercise choice, and both compete aggressively with same-sex rivals, as would be expected in a socially monogamous system (Adkins-Regan & Robinson, 1993). Relatively little is known about preferences of males for individual females other than that they prefer females that eat a diet which produces more eggs (Jones, Monaghan, & Nager, 2001). Studies of females' preferences and choices have shown that a male's song is quite important. Females prefer males with higher song rates (Collins, Hubbard, & Houtman, 1994), and males raised normally have greater reproductive success than males raised without adult male song tutors (Williams, Kilander, & Sotanski, 1993). Untutored males sing abnormal songs that lack correct learned syllables, but they differ from normal males in other social behavior as well (Adkins-Regan & Krakauer, 2000). A recent experiment applied a more direct experimental approach to females' choices of males singing songs of different quality (Tomaszycki & Adkins-Regan, 2005). Females were placed in aviaries along with (a) males surgically manipulated to be unable to sing (air sac punctured males), (b) males surgically manipulated to sing songs that were normal in every respect except for the frequency structure of the learned syllables (males with one tracheosyringeal nerve cut), (c) sham-operated control males, and (d) unmanipulated males. Among the first three groups, the control males were the first to be chosen as pairing partners by the females, so that after five days all controls were paired but only one vocally distorted male was paired. With additional time, a few of the vocally distorted males paired. Clearly females were initially relying heavily on one trait, singing, for their decision.

In contrast to the importance of singing for getting the pair relationship going (for its formation), the maintenance of the already established pair relationship does not seem to depend on the male's singing ability, at least not over periods of a few weeks. When the same surgical manipulations described above were performed on males in established pairs, there was no change in the behavior of the males' female partners, and no greater likelihood of pairs dissolving compared to control pairs (Tomaszycki & Adkins-Regan, 2006).

It is easy to assume that sex steroids must surely have something to do with pairing, but so far there is little experimental evidence for this. When unpaired adult zebra finches were treated with drugs to lower sex steroid action (flutamide as an androgen receptor antagonist plus an estrogen synthesis inhibitor), neither males nor females so treated were any less likely to pair successfully than control birds (Tomaszycki, Banerjee, & Adkins-Regan, 2006). Combined with the fact that birds normally pair as they reach sexual maturity, these negative results suggest that either (a) sex steroids are not responsible for the onset of pairing as reproductive maturity is reached or (b) the hormonal environment at the early onset of reproductive maturity stimulates an interest in pairing in a permanent (organizational?) manner, so that hormone action is no longer needed for pairing to be expressed. With respect to this second possibility, the behaviors shown by paired birds such as clumping and being in a nest together are shown by zebra finches throughout their nestling and juvenile lives. What changes as they head toward reproductive maturity is that the behaviors become directed toward a pair partner rather than family members, a change in social preference (Adkins-Regan & Leung, 2006). Any role for hormones would more likely be on the preference (the targets for the behavior), not the behaviors themselves—on motivation to affiliate closely with one opposite-sex bird.

Zebra finches are not seasonal breeders, and are continuously paired even when not actively breeding. While thus far sex steroid actions do not seem to be required for pairing, such actions could be important in species that pair seasonally.

In socially monogamous prairie voles, oxytocin family peptide mechanisms are important for pairing (Carter, DeVries, & Getz, 1995; Young, Young, & Hammock, 2005). Several studies have pointed to V1a receptors in the ventral pallidum in particular as key for a male's tendency to affiliate with the familiar female partner (one with which he has cohabited for 24 hours) rather than a novel female. The parallel avian peptides to oxytocin and vasopressin, mesotocin and vasotocin, have not yet been found to affect social preferences or pairing by zebra finches when experimentally manipulated (Goodson, Lindberg, & Johnson, 2004). Further research is needed to know whether this represents a difference between birds and mammals in mechanisms of pairing or in the nature of pairing.

Paired zebra finches are never very far from each other and are in regular vocal contact (Zann, 1996). If pairs are separated into different rooms, mimicking loss through accident or predation, the birds increase their locomotor activity and calling,

as if searching for the missing partner (Butterfield, 1970). The corticosterone levels of both sexes rise; when reunited, the levels fall (Remage-Healey, Adkins-Regan, & Romero, 2003). This adrenal glucocorticoid response to separation and reunion of animals that have a close affiliative social relationship has also been observed in several kinds of mammals, and such hormonal changes have been used to infer attachment (Mason & Mendoza, 1998; von Holst, 1998).

Onset and Maintenance of Parental Behavior

Newly hatched chicks usually need immediate care, and in a substantial majority (more than 80%) of avian species, they get it from both parents (Cockburn, 2006). Parents need to brood them (keep them warm, because they cannot yet thermoregulate), feed them if they are altricial (altricial birds have very steep growth curves requiring prodigious amounts of food), and lead them to food and warn them of predators if they are precocial. They need to respond appropriately to the begging of the chicks (see section "Life as a Chick: Begging Behavior"). A body of work has examined how hormonal changes contribute to the onset of parental behavior, and how stimuli from the mate (in biparental species), nest, eggs, and chicks are critical for the onset and maintenance of the behavior, in part because they stimulate changes in levels of hormones such as prolactin. Such effects have been best studied in ring doves and chickens, and those research programs are classics in hormones and behavior (Buntin, 1996; Lehrman, 1965; Richard-Yris, Garnier, & Leboucher, 1983; Sharp, MacNamee, Talbot, Sterling, & Hall, 1984).

The role of prolactin in chick-directed behavior is best understood in ring doves. Ring doves, like other pigeons and doves, are biparental, and both sexes produce crop "milk" from the crop sac that is fed to the chicks. Elevated posthatching prolactin stimulates feeding of the chicks both by acting peripherally, on the crop, and by acting directly on the brain (Buntin, 1996). Prolactin is elevated during the early posthatching period in a number of other kinds of birds with altricial young as well, including passerines (Wingfield & Farner, 1993), but there is little experimental work to establish a role in chick care. In birds with precocial young, prolactin tends to fall when the chicks hatch, suggesting that its contribution to interaction with the chicks, if any, lies in priming the behavior to appear at hatching, rather than in maintaining it thereafter (Buntin, 1996; El Halawani, Burke, Millam, Fehrer, & Hargis, 1984).

Relatively little is known about the specific brain regions involved in parental behavior in birds. The distribution of prolactin-containing neurons and prolactin receptors has been determined in the ring dove and turkey, and changes in steroid receptor expression during the breeding cycle have been described (Buntin, Ruzycki, & Witebski, 1993; Lea, Clark, & Tsutsui, 2001; Ramesh, Kuenzel, Buntin, & Proudman, 2000), providing a number of candidate sites for actions of these hormones. Preoptic lesions in ring doves prevent prolactin from stimulating chick feeding (Slawski & Buntin, 1995). Female Japanese quail induced to brood by brief exposures to chicks show increased neuronal activity (as indicated by labeling for the immediate early gene product C-FOS) in the medial portion of the bed nucleus of the stria terminalis and in the ectostriatum (Ruscio & Adkins-Regan, 2004).

Several recent developments concern the parental behavior of wild birds. One line of research looks at cases where one or both parents leave the chick(s) for long periods of time (days or weeks) but still respond with parental behavior upon return (Figure 31.2). Penguins are famous for this parental style. Is prolactin elevated during the parent's absence? If so, what is keeping it elevated in the absence of stimuli from the chick? (Such stimulation is required in other kinds of birds, and prolactin falls if chicks are predated or experimentally removed.) Measurements of prolactin in several penguin species indicate that parental prolactin remains elevated during the time spent at sea fishing, suggesting an endogenous prolactin cycle rather than one dependent on stimuli from the chick (Figure 31.2; Lormée, Jouventin, Chastel, & Mauget, 1999; Vleck, Ross, Vleck, & Bucher, 2000).

Another line of research asks if testosterone is mediating a trade-off between mating effort and parental effort in males (Wingfield, Hegner, Dufty, & Ball, 1990; Ketterson & Nolan, 1999). A common pattern in north temperate songbirds is for males' testosterone levels to fall as parental phases of breeding begin (Wingfield & Farner, 1993). In several species, administration of testosterone to males so that they sustain the higher levels of the egg-laying and mating period into the chick rearing phase causes the males to feed the chicks less and to spend more time singing and behaving aggressively or pursuing extrapair matings (De Ridder, Pinxten, & Eens, 2000; Dittami, Hoi, & Sageder, 1991; Hegner & Wingfield, 1987; Raouf, Parker, Ketterson, Nolan, & Ziegenfus, 1997; Silverin, 1980; Wingfield, 1984). It is as if mating and parental effort are incompatible behaviorally and hormonally, and testosterone falls to ensure a transition from the one to the other at the right time. Not all males' testosterone levels fall when they become parents, however, and elevating testosterone does not always interfere with paternal care.

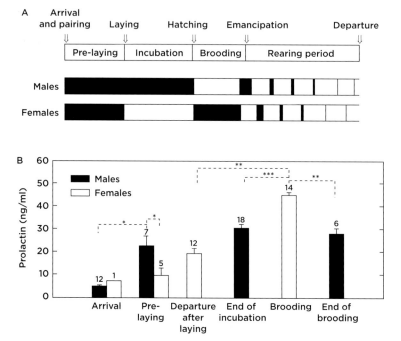

Figure 31.2 (A) The breeding cycle of the emperor penguin and (B) mean (± S.E.M.) plasma prolactin levels in birds sampled at different times in the cycle. The breeding cycle is eight months long; dark portions of the bars in (A) indicate that birds are present at the breeding colony and light portions indicate that birds are absent. In (B) prolactin levels of females returning to brood after an absence of 2 months (while the male was incubating) were elevated. $^{*} = P < 0.05$, $^{**} = P < 0.01$, $^{***} P < 0.001$. Sample sizes are given above the bars. [Reproduced with permission from: Lormée, Jouventin, Chastel, & Mauget, 1999. © 1999 Academic Press (Elsevier).]

This raises important questions about when and why such trade-offs occur and how best to interpret species differences in males' testosterone profiles. Studies of the clade of songbirds that includes the longspurs and the *Plectrophenax* buntings support the hypothesis that elevated testosterone is more likely to interfere with paternal care when such care is not critical for chick survival (Lynn, Walker, & Wingfield, 2005).

In cooperatively breeding species of birds, conspecific individuals other than the biological parents also feed the young (in contrast to brood parasitic species, in which the young are fed by a different species). Another line of research asks about the hormonal correlates and causes of such "alloparenting." In several species, alloparents have been found to have elevated prolactin, and prolactin becomes elevated before the chicks hatch (Brown & Vleck, 1998; Schoech, Reynolds, & Boughton, 2004), but the necessary manipulation experiments have not yet been done to show a causal relationship to the alloparenting behavior. Alloparents are usually socially subordinate to the parents, and can have either lower or higher corticosterone levels depending on whether being dominant or subordinate is a more energetically demanding rank (Goymann & Wingfield, 2004). Again, it is not known whether the birds' corticosterone levels are causally related to their chick-directed behavior.

Middle and Older Life Stages

Birds tend to be longer-lived than mammals of comparable body size, and adults may live to breed for many years. On theoretical grounds, reproductive effort is expected to increase with age (Roff, 2001). Long-term studies of marked populations have shown a strong tendency for breeding success to rise with age, and for birds (both males and females) looking for a new mate to prefer older individuals as partners (Black 1996; Clutton-Brock 1988). There are several possible reasons for this age trend, including possible hormonal changes with age and improvements due to experience. Most interesting from a social behavior and communication standpoint would be if birds improve in their interactional skills with age or experience.

Until recently, there was virtually no information about hormone levels across the adult life span in free-living birds from either cross-sectional or longitudinal samples. This is now changing, with rich data sets emerging from, for example, albatrosses and terns (Figure 31.3; Angelier et al., 2006; Heidinger, Nisbet, & Ketterson, 2006). Disentangling experience from chronological aging requires a kind of experimentation that has not yet been done and is probably better suited to captive populations.

Senescence is not as obvious (to humans) in birds as in mammals, but there is now evidence that reproductive success does begin to drop in very old birds (Angelier et al., 2006). Domestic Japanese quail, a relatively short-lived species, show pronounced reproductive senescence in both behavior and fertility after 2.5 years of age and are a good laboratory model for studying neuroendocrine mechanisms of senescence (Ottinger et al., 2004). Although senescence involves progressive failure of the hypothalamic-pituitary-gonadal axis,

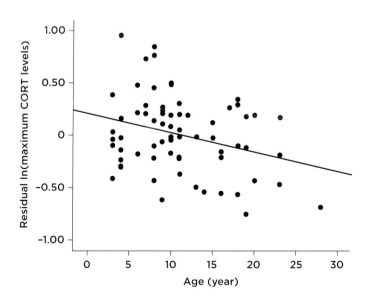

Figure 31.3 Corticosterone elevation in response to a standard stressor (human handling and blood sampling) in common terns of different ages. The *Y*-axis is residual natural log-transformed maximum corticosterone from a multiple regression including tern weight and date (time in the year). In this analysis, maximum corticosterone in response to the stressor declined with age. (Reproduced with permission from: Heidinger, Nisbet, & Ketterson, 2006. © 2006 The Royal Society.)

behavior declines before male testosterone levels drop, caused by brain changes on the receiving end of the hormones (Balthazart, Turek, & Ottinger, 1984). The focus thus far has been on the mating behavior of the males, but it will be interesting to see if birds show declines in communicative behavior (production or reception of signals) as they age that could be contributing to reduced reproductive success.

What is the Role of Hormonal and Neurohormonal Mechanisms in the Generation of Sex Differences in Social Behavior?
Sex Differences in Vocal and Visual Displays

As a result of sexual selection, one sex (usually males) may have elaborate songs or courtship displays that females do not exhibit, or the sexes may sing different songs or have different displays. Where do such sex differences come from developmentally? Are they based on sex differences in the brain, and if so, what are those brain differences? These questions have inspired a substantial body of research in birds as well as in mammals. The two principal avian models have been Japanese quail and zebra finches. Both species show some obvious sex differences in signaling behavior. Male quail crow and strut; females do not, but do emit "cricket calls." Male zebra finches sing and dance; females do not, but do solicit copulation from males by tail quivering.

SEX DIFFERENCES IN QUAIL

In Japanese quail, sex differences in vocal and visual displays seem to result largely from activational hormone effects, that is, they are produced by adult sex differences in circulating steroid levels (Balthazart & Adkins-Regan, 2002). Males have more circulating testosterone, and females have more circulating estradiol (Balthazart, Delville, Sulon, & Hendrick, 1986). If adult females that are gonadectomized or have regressed ovaries are administered testosterone to raise their levels, they begin to crow and strut. If males that are gonadectomized or have regressed testes are given estradiol, they emit cricket calls. So qualitatively, these systems do not appear to be hormonally organized to be sexually dimorphic. Similarly, testosterone treatment of females of a number of species from diverse avian clades stimulates singing and/or male-like displaying (Balthazart & Adkins-Regan, 2002).

Quantitatively, however, testosterone-treated female quail do not reach the level of males; their crowing and strutting frequencies are lower, and their crows are not as loud. Thus there is some potential for an organizational contribution to the normal adult sex differences. Indeed, there is a consistent tendency for males hatched from eggs injected with estradiol to have slightly lower crowing and strutting frequencies than control males. Such a result is consistent with the pattern of hormonal organization that has been well established for the development of sexual dimorphism in mating behavior (Balthazart & Adkins-Regan, 2002). In this pattern, embryonic treatment with sex steroids demasculinizes behavior (makes males more like females), and blocking sex steroids in embryos masculinizes behavior (makes females more like males), the opposite pattern from mammalian organization. This conclusion that the adult sex difference results from both activational and organizational hormone actions also seems to apply to crowing in chickens. Adult hens given testosterone crow, but feebly. Male chickens hatched from eggs treated with estradiol crow less and with less acoustic energy and duration, and females hatched from eggs treated with the estrogen synthesis inhibitor fadrozole crow more than normal females (Marx, Jurkevich, & Grossmann, 2004).

Where are the hormones acting to determine whether the bird will crow and strut like a male or a female? Nothing seems to be known about brain mechanisms of strutting even though most domestic male galliform birds have a version of this distinctive display and much attention has been paid to its role in mate choice in species such as peacocks. With respect to crowing, a study by Yazaki et al. (1999) has identified the midbrain intercollicular nucleus as a possible brain target producing the sex difference. Neurons in the male nucleus had more dendrites than those in the female nucleus, electrical stimulation of the male but not female nucleus produced crows, and when females were given testosterone, electrical stimulation of their nucleus also produced crows. Prior work by other researchers had established this nucleus as the one rich in sex steroid receptors (Ball & Balthazart, 2002).

The same early hormonal manipulations that alter crowing, strutting, and mating behavior in Japanese quail also change the sexually dimorphic vasotocinergic system of the medial preoptic nucleus in an exactly parallel manner (Figure 31.4; Panzica et al., 1998). Exposure of embryos to estradiol changes a male system to a female-typical one,

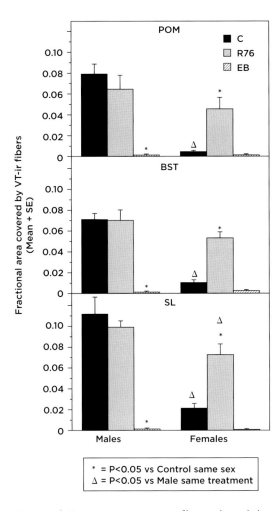

Figure 31.4 Vasotocin immunoreactive fibers in the medial preoptic nucleus (POM), bed nucleus of the stria terminalis (BST), and lateral septum (SL) of male and female Japanese quail hatched from eggs injected on day 9 of incubation with vehicle (C, control), an estrogen synthesis inhibitor (R76 = R76713), or estradiol benzoate (EB). Vasotocinergic innervation in all three regions is markedly sexually dimorphic in control birds, is masculinized in females by R76, and is demasculinized in males by EB, in parallel with the effects of these same treatments on mating behavior. (Reprinted with permission from: Panzica et al. 1998. © 1998 John Wiley & Sons, Inc. Reprinted with permission of Wiley-Liss, Inc., a subsidiary of John Wiley & Sons, Inc.)

and treatment with an estrogen synthesis inhibitor changes a female system to a male-typical one. Sexual dimorphism in vasotocinergic systems is surprisingly conserved in vertebrates, and vasotocin has been linked to vocal communication in a number of vertebrates (Goodson & Bass, 2001; De Vries & Panzica, 2006), and so hormonal organization of this system in quail could conceivably underlie sex differences in crowing and strutting along with mating behavior.

Peripheral actions of hormones could also be involved. Perhaps testosterone treated females do not crow as loudly as males because the relevant muscles are not as strong. Galliform birds have extrinsic but not intrinsic syringeal muscles, the largest of which are the sternotrachealis muscles. These muscles have been reported to be heavier in males (Balthazart, Schumacher, & Ottinger, 1983). In a recent study, however, males, females, and testosterone-treated females did not differ in either muscle volume or muscle fiber number (Burke, Adkins-Regan, & Wade, 2007). Instead, both sexes had more fibers in the muscle on the right side, the functional significance of which is unclear.

SEX DIFFERENCES IN ZEBRA FINCHES

The most striking sex differences in this species are found in the neural song system and singing behavior (Schlinger & Brenowitz, 2002). Males sing, and have relatively large telencephalic song nuclei containing more or larger neurons. Adult females never sing, even when given testosterone, and have smaller telencephalic song nuclei that do not enlarge to any major extent in response to adult testosterone (Arnold, 1980). These are signs pointing to a sex difference established earlier in development through hormonal organization. And indeed, early work supported such a hypothesis. Beginning with Gurney and Konishi (1980), research by several laboratories found that females treated with estradiol during the early posthatching stage (as nestlings) were dramatically masculinized behaviorally and neurally (reviewed in Balthazart & Adkins-Regan, 2002). Their telencephalic song system nuclei were substantially increased in volume and neuron numbers or soma sizes (see Figure 31.5 for an example). Some of these females sang remarkably good songs as adults. Estradiol was more effective than testosterone, and the critical period for the effect of estradiol seemed to lie during the first 2 weeks posthatching (the nestling period), and especially in week one (Adkins-Regan, Mansukhani, Seiwert, & Thompson, 1994). These results suggested a pattern of sexual differentiation very different from that seen in quail, and instead similar to what occurs in mammals, in which development of the female phenotype occurs without the addition of sex steroids, and exposure to sex steroids produces a male phenotype. This is what Gurney and Konishi (1980) proposed.

Since that time, however, compelling evidence has accumulated that such a mammalian scenario cannot be correct (Arnold & Schlinger, 1993;

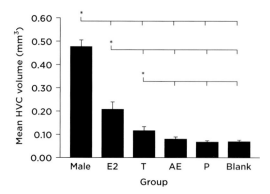

Figure 31.5 Mean ± S.E.M. volume of zebra finch song system nucleus HVC in males and in females implanted on the day of hatching with estradiol (E2), testosterone (T), androstenedione (AE), progesterone (P), or empty implants (BLANK). Estradiol produced greater masculinization of HVC volume than any of the other sex steroids administered, but even estradiol did not fully masculinize volumes. (Reprinted with permission from: Grisham & Arnold, 1995. © 1995 John Wiley & Sons, Inc.)

Wade, 1999). For example, partial or near-complete sex reversal of the gonads of zebra finches does not prevent the development of a neural song system and singing that is typical of a bird's genetic sex, arguing against an important role for gonadal hormones in organizing the system. Nor does administration of a drug that blocks estrogen synthesis in body and brain prevent male-typical development in genetic males. Instead, it is as if the system is organized by something nongonadal that is produced more locally, in the telencephalon, and that is not estrogen. According to this alternative hypothesis (Arnold, 2002), the telencephalic nuclei differentiate in response to products of genes on the sex chromosomes that are expressed in or near those nuclei. Some progress has been made in finding out what those genes or their products might be (Akutagawa & Konishi, 2001; Wade, Tang, Peabody, & Templeman, 2005). For the present, however, how male and female zebra finches come to have their dimorphic brains and vocal signals remains a problem in need of a solution.

Also unclear is whether the zebra finch developmental process, whatever it might turn out to be, will generalize to other taxonomic families of songbirds. A number of other songbirds have primarily activational sex differences in singing (summarized in Balthazart & Adkins-Regan, 2002), so the most promising cases to compare with zebra finches would be those with dimorphic neural song systems where testosterone-treated females still do not sing. When starling nestlings were treated with estrogen,

only very slight masculinization of the song system occurred in the females (Casto & Ball, 1996), but female starlings (even untreated ones) do sing.

Sex Differences in Mate Choice and Sexual Preferences

Animals court and mate neither randomly nor indiscriminately, but instead demonstrate preferences that lead to particular mating or pairing combinations (choices, outcomes). There are preferences for the animal's own species, for the opposite sex, and for particular individuals of the opposite sex. These all involve perception and assessment of the cues and signals given off by others, and selective responding to some but not others. Much of the mate choice literature focuses on females' preferences for particular males, testing hypotheses about why and how it promotes the fitness interests of the females to choose males that sing more, display more, etc. In socially monogamous mating systems where pair bonds are formed, it behooves both sexes to make fitness-promoting choices, although less is known about what males prefer in females aside from age and fecundity.

Recent studies of two types have examined some hormonal underpinnings of females' choices of males. In one type, testosterone levels of intact (nongonadectomized) males are manipulated, and the hypothesis is tested that females will prefer those with higher testosterone, because those males are expressing higher signal levels and can afford to do so despite the putative costs of testosterone. This hypothesis has been supported by experiments with jungle fowl (from which domestic chickens are derived) and dark-eyed juncos (Enstrom, Ketterson, & Nolan, 1997; Zuk, Johnsen, & Mclarty, 1995). In the other type of study, it is the females' hormones that are manipulated. Female dark-eyed juncos with elevated testosterone were less discriminating than control females when given a choice between testosterone-treated and control males (McGlothlin, Neudorf, Casto, Nolan, & Ketterson, 2004). Males have been found to be less "choosy" than females in a number of animals, and so this experiment suggests that such a sex difference could have an activational hormone basis.

Males and females have different preferences; the attractiveness of cues and signals depends importantly on the sex of the receiver. Most obviously, males prefer females and females prefer males. Females may prefer males with particular kinds of songs, but if the females do not sing, males cannot have song quality as one of their mate choice criteria. Where do these kinds of sex differences come from, and are any of them hormonally organized in early development?

Experiments with Japanese quail have confirmed an organizational hormonal basis for the sex difference in sexual interest in female stimuli. Sexually experienced males are very motivated to look at females, and will spend more than half of their test time looking through a small high window if there is a female on the other side of the wall (Domjan & Hall, 1986). Females are not interested in looking at other females in this way, even if they are given testosterone. Females hatched from eggs treated with an estrogen synthesis inhibitor, however, are quite masculinized, showing male-typical levels of looking at female stimuli (Balthazart, Castagna, & Ball, 1997). This is the same result found for mating behavior itself, one indicating that male-typical behavioral development results from an estrogen-poor embryonic hormonal milieu and female-typical behavioral development results from an estrogen-rich milieu (Balthazart & Adkins-Regan, 2002). The male's interest in females also shows an important learning component. Naïve males are much less discriminating and respond to both sexes. Males come to direct their attention to females in the course of repeated trials (Domjan & Ravert, 1991). Both the right embryonic hormonal environment (low estrogen) and learning from experience enter into the development of the male's preference for females.

Japanese quail have additional sexually dimorphic mate preferences, but their hormonal bases have not yet been studied. For example, males are averse to females they have seen brooding chicks, whereas females prefer males they have seen brooding chicks (Adkins-Regan, Zhou, & Leung, 2004; Ruscio & Adkins-Regan, 2003). Females prefer a male they have seen mating with another female (exhibit mate choice copying), whereas males avoid a female they have seen with another male (White & Galef, 2000). Both these sex differences make sense, that is, can readily be interpreted as adaptive mate choice strategies.

Mate Choice and Sexual Preferences: Studies with Zebra Finches

There have many studies of mate preferences in zebra finches but few have looked for any hormonal bases. Sex differences in sexual partner preference (preference for opposite sex partners) are clearly not a product of adult activational hormone effects alone. Adult females that were ovariectomized and given testosterone still attempted to pair with males (were still attracted to male cues and signals), and adult males that were castrated and given estradiol still attempted to pair with females (Adkins-Regan & Ascenzi, 1987). Adults treated with a combination of an androgen receptor antagonist (flutamide) and an estrogen synthesis inhibitor (ATD) paired as successfully as controls did with the opposite sex, as if they were still responding positively to those signals and still had sufficient signaling value themselves (Tomaszycki et al., 2006). Presumably such treated birds would not be able to attract as high-quality partners as controls, however.

A recent experiment examined whether hormones are involved in the onset of the expression of sexual partner preference as juvenile birds reach sexual maturity (at about 60 to 90 days of age posthatching) (Adkins-Regan & Leung, 2006). In this study, the social and sexual preferences of birds were assessed throughout juvenile life (from 30 to 90 days) with three-choice proximity tests. The choices were the family members, unpaired males, and unpaired females. Subjects were chronically treated with supplemental testosterone, supplemental estradiol, or the same flutamide plus ATD combination referred to above that is designed to lower sex steroid action. Males given supplemental testosterone showed a premature interest in the unpaired females and loss of interest in the family compared to control males. Females given flutamide plus ATD failed to show the increased interest in males toward the end of testing that the control females showed. These results suggest some sex steroid involvement in the timing of the adult onset of expression of preferences for opposite-sex birds. The result for the females also contrasts with the inability of the same flutamide plus ATD treatment to suppress the expression of sexual partner preference when given to females that are already adults (summarized above). One interpretation is that expression of sexual partner preference is subject to hormonal influence only at the point of onset, while undergoing a developmental transition, and that once already established its continued maintenance is hormonally insensitive. This could conceivably represent some kind of pubertal organizational hormone effect, but the experiments required to directly test this hypothesis have not been done.

The direction, as opposed to expression, of sexual partner preference (whether the bird prefers males vs. females) was not affected in any of the experiments just described. Instead, other experiments point to an earlier stage of development, during the nestling period, when the direction of the preference is shaped. Females treated with estradiol for the first 2 weeks posthatching (a treatment that masculinizes singing and the neural song system) show a marked tendency to try to pair with other females, not males, and some of them succeed in pairing with females (Figure 31.6; Adkins-Regan & Ascenzi, 1987; Mansukhani, Adkins-Regan, & Yang, 1996). Females hatched from eggs injected with the estrogen synthesis inhibitor fadrozole, who have testes or ovotestes, also prefer to pair with other females as adults (Adkins-Regan & Wade, 2001). Males treated with fadrozole as nestlings, however, show the normal male preference for males (Adkins-Regan, Yang, & Mansukhani, 1996). As happens all too often with this species, there are puzzles and contradictions in these results. If nestling treatment with estradiol masculinizes females, why does not fadrozole feminize males? Why do both estradiol and an estrogen synthesis inhibitor produce the same outcome in genetic females? As with the puzzles of song system differentiation, it is as if estradiol is working not because it is the natural hormonal signal for sexual differentiation, but because it alters something else that is the signal. More secure is the conclusion that the sex difference in direction of sexual partner preference is somehow established early in development and is not altered by hormonal manipulations thereafter.

The masculinizing effect of early estrogen treatment on partner preference is seen only if the females have spent their juvenile life (time from independence from the parents, at 45–50 days, to testing in young adulthood at 100 or more days) in an all-female aviary (Figure 31.6; Mansukhani et al., 1996). A combination of a particular physiological milieu and a particular social environment is required to produce females that prefer other females. What is it about this all-female social environment that contributes to the outcome? Zebra finches require direct physical contact through activities like allopreening and being in a nest box together in order to pair (Silcox & Evans, 1982). If the females are prevented from such contact during the juvenile period by placing barriers between their individual housing compartments within the aviary, then early estrogen treatment no longer produces any shift in partner preference even though the birds are still in an all-female aviary (Adkins-Regan, 2005c). This suggests that engaging in physical contact with other females (the only birds available for contact in all-female aviaries) is consolidating the masculinization produced by the hormone treatment.

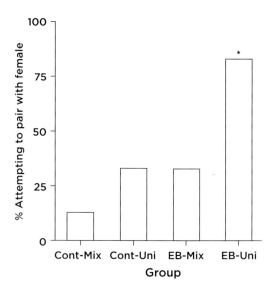

Figure 31.6 Percentage of female zebra finches attempting to pair with another female when tested as adults in aviaries following implantation with testosterone propionate. Females were injected with vehicle (Cont = control) or estradiol benzoate (EB) daily for the first two weeks posthatching; between independence from the parents and testing they were housed in mixed sex (Mix) or all-female (Uni = unisex) aviaries. Estrogen treatment masculinized the females' pairing partner preferences, but only if they had spent the juvenile period in an all-female aviary. * $P < 0.05$ compared with Cont-Mix. (From: Mansukhani, Adkins-Regan, & Yang, 1996.)

Even in the absence of hormonal manipulations, the social environment during development seems to contribute to the development of sexual partner preference in this species. Removal of all adult males from breeding aviaries when the chicks are very young results in birds that are equally inclined to pair with either sex, that is, do not show a sexual partner preference (Adkins-Regan & Krakauer, 2000). Evidently the young birds learn something important about the formation of male–female pairs by growing up in social environment that includes both sexes.

Although there is still much to learn about how the mating preferences of zebra finches develop, it is already apparent that the processes underlying sexual partner preference fit squarely into the kind of epigenetic framework that is a longstanding tradition in developmental behavioral neuroscience. Behavior that some would write off as "instinctive" and therefore not in need of explanation turns out to much richer and more scientifically intriguing once it is accepted that development is always something to be explained.

Sex-Specific Aggression and Sex-Biased Dispersal

Sexual partner preference is an unusually widespread and robust sex difference in positive sexual and affiliative reactions to cues and signals from conspecifics. Its analog in the realm of agonistic behavior is sex-specific aggression, in which males target their aggressive behavior mainly at other males, and females target theirs mainly at other females. Here the "preferred" stimuli are from the same sex. This kind of aggression is relatively common in birds. Although the phenomenon of sex-specific aggression can be elicited in birds in the laboratory (e.g., Adkins-Regan & Robinson, 1993), little is known about its hormonal basis or development. It is conceivable that the developmental processes leading to this sex difference might overlap with those producing sexual partner preference, but with the "polarity" reversed (attraction to the opposite sex, antagonism to the same sex). Clearly some kind of sex recognition has to be involved in both.

Sex differences in dispersal tendency are also widespread. A fairly common pattern in birds is for the males to remain in the natal area, or return to it from migration, and for the females to change locations (Pusey, 1987). Several hypotheses such as inbreeding avoidance have been considered for the function of such sex-biased dispersal, but the developmental processes producing the avian pattern are unknown. The most common pattern in mammals is for males to disperse and females to remain in the natal area. In at least one mammalian species, Belding's ground squirrel, hormonal organization is responsible for the sex bias in dispersal (Holekamp, Smale, Simpson, & Holekamp, 1984), but this hypothesis does not seem to have been tested in any bird.

What Are the Processes and Brain Areas Responsible for These Effects of Hormones on Communication-based Social Behavior?

A common way to approach such a question is to view behavior as responses to stimuli and then categorize processes as sensory, motor, or an intervening type such as perception, attention, motivation, or emotion. During much of its history, the field of hormones and behavior has tended to focus on the motor end (e.g., sound producing organs and their associated musculature) and on motivation (e.g., sexual arousal). This continues to be a gold mine of new discoveries, for example, the sex difference in manakins in spinal cord testosterone accumulation associated with an elaborate male wing-snapping display (Schultz & Schlinger, 1999) and the

importance of the medial preoptic area for a songbird's motivation to sing (Riters & Ball, 1999).

Thinking about social behavior and mate preferences as based on communication systems involving receivers as well as signalers, however, highlights the desirability of giving equal attention to the receiving end—the sensory, perceptual, and attentional processes. When a male zebra finch is attracted to a female for pairing, and a female is attracted to a male, the pairing behavior (the motor acts of allopreening and clumping) is not sexually dimorphic and not necessarily hormone-based (because it occurs in birds of all postfledging ages). Instead, it is the reaction to the cues and signals from other birds that differs between the sexes.

Is there any evidence that sensory or perceptual processes involved in communication-based social behavior are hormonally influenced in birds? The peripheral sensory organs and their first-order projections have not been reported to contain either steroid receptors or steroid metabolizing enzymes in either adult or developing birds. Further upstream, testosterone alters oxidative metabolism in visual regions of the male Japanese quail brain along with many other regions, but the function of this regulation is unknown (Balthazart, Stamatakis, Bacola, Absil, & Dermon, 2001).

Higher parts of the auditory system are a promising place to look for hormone effects. Many birds are quite vocal, and birds may respond differently to song and other vocalizations as a function of their hormonal status. Females are more likely to respond to song playback with a copulation solicitation display if they have been primed with estradiol first (see, for example, Maney et al., 1997b). Castrated male zebra finches learn to discriminate their own song from that of another male faster if they are given testosterone (Cynx & Nottebohm, 1992). Such effects could of course be on motivation rather than sensory or perceptual processes, but there is some evidence pointing to hormone effects on higher-order auditory processing. The song system nucleus HVC, which in males contains many neurons that fire preferentially to the bird's own song, is located in a part of the telencephalon, the caudomedial nidopallium, that is rich in aromatase (estrogen synthase) (Margoliash & Konishi, 1985; Schlinger & Brenowitz, 2002). Female canaries prefer certain male song syllables, and neurons in the female's HVC respond differently to these syllables when females are on long days compared to short days (Del Negro, Kreutzer, & Gahr, 2000). The zebra finch NCM, an auditory projection area in the telencephalon thought to be the homolog

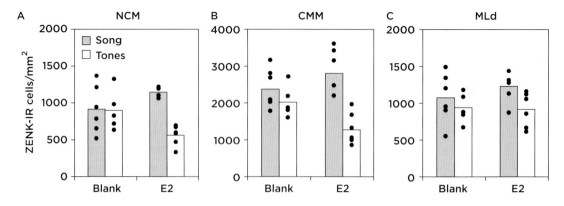

Figure 31.7 Number of cells immunoreactive for the immediate early gene product ZENK in two higher auditory system areas, NCM (A) and CMM (B) and one brainstem auditory region, MLd (C), in female white-throated sparrows given blank or estradiol filled implants and exposed to song or synthetic tones. Only estradiol treated females had significantly more ZENK-immunoreactive neurons in NCM and CMM following song exposure. (Reproduced with permission from: Maney, Cho, & Goode, 2006. © 2006 Federation of European Neuroscience Societies and Blackwell Publishing Ltd.)

of part of the mammalian auditory cortex, has high levels of aromatase and is sexually dimorphic; the male NCM has twice the number of a specific subset of GABAergic neurons (Pinaud, Fortes, Lovell, & Mello, 2006; Saldanha et al., 2000). Using the immediate-early gene product ZENK as a marker of neuronal activity, estradiol treatment was found to be required for female white-throated sparrows housed on winter daylengths to show song-selective activity in the caudomedial nidopallium (NCM) and caudomedial mesopallium (CMM) (another higher auditory area) (Figure 31.7; Maney, Cho, & Goode, 2006).

Studies of mammalian brain regions involved in social behavior have identified a network consisting of six bidirectionally connected nodes: the extended amygdala (medial amygdala plus medial portion of the bed nucleus of the stria terminalis), the lateral septum, the preoptic area, the anterior hypothalamus, the ventromedial hypothalamus, and a portion of the midbrain (the periaqueductal gray and parts of the tegmentum) (Newman, 2002). These nodes contain sex steroid receptors and other neuroendocrine mechanisms, and are all involved in the principal forms of social behavior, whether aggressive, parental, sexual, affiliative, etc. What differs as a function of the category of social behavior is the relative amounts of activity in the six nodes, as indicated by, for example, immediate-early gene expression during the behavior. Homologs of all six nodes are present in bird brains, and evidence is accumulating from multiple approaches (tract-tracing, lesions, neurochemical stimulation, immediate-early gene expression,

studies of steroid receptors) that this network is also present in birds (Figure 31.8; Goodson, 2005; see also section "Evolutionary Changes in Sociality"). The anatomical distribution of the neuropeptides that have been linked to social behavior is also similar in birds and mammals (Blahser, 1984). Research to identify the social behavior contributions of the avian nodes is still in its early stages, but some important steps have already been taken. It has been shown that aggressive responses to male stimuli are related to vasotocinergic mechanisms in the lateral septum (as shown in several species of songbirds) (Goodson, 1998a, 1998b; Goodson & Adkins-Regan, 1999). Engaging in maternal behavior (brooding chicks) increases the density of C-FOS positive neurons in the medial portion of the bed nucleus of the stria terminalis of female quail (Ruscio & Adkins-Regan, 2004). The preoptic area and ventral tegmentum may regulate sexually motivated singing by male starlings in the presence of females (Heimovics & Riters, 2005).

An important issue for the future is how these processes and mechanisms and their responses to hormones might be changing during the bird's lifetime to account for changes in social behavior at different life stages. Also remaining to be discovered are the emotional and cognitive processes involved in hormone effects on communication-based social behavior.

How Do Species Differences in Hormone-Related Social Behavior Arise?

Birds show interesting diversity in social behavior related to communication. In some species, both

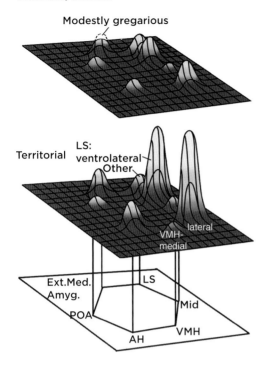

Figure 31.8 Schematic diagram representing counts of neurons expressing immediate-early gene products in six brain regions in response to same-sex conspecifics in four species of estrildid finches differing in sociality. The six regions are the preoptic area (POA), anterior hypothalamus (AH), ventromedial hypothalamus (VMH), midbrain (Mid), lateral septum (LS), and extended medial amygdala (Ext.Med.Amyg.). Such results suggest that Newman's (2002) social behavior network model is applicable to birds as well as mammals, and that internodal differences in relative neuronal activity underlie species differences in sociality in birds. (Reproduced with permission from: Goodson, 2005. © 2005 Elsevier Inc.)

sexes sing; in others, only the male sings. Some have relatively monomorphic displays; others have sex-specific displays. Some species have a socially monogamous mating system, some are polygynous, and yet others have "reversed" sex roles. Some are territorial and others are colonial. The behavioral characters that underpin these social systems are often hormone modulated. The social systems themselves, especially mating systems, are correlated with different male testosterone profiles and with variation in sex differences in circulating testosterone levels (little or no sex difference in socially monogamous species, larger sex differences in polygynous species) (Ketterson et al., 2005; Wingfield et al., 1990). How do changes from one character state to another occur? While little is known about this thus far, new developments in

genomics, phylogenetics, and evolutionary developmental biology promise the dawn of a new era of progress in understanding how related species come to diverge in brain mechanisms for social behavior.

Evolutionary Changes in Song

Birds show interesting diversity in whether both sexes or only males sing, and evolutionary changes appear to have occurred in both directions numerous times. In tropical species, males and females may sing together in a skillfully coordinated manner called duetting. The functions of duetting are still unclear, but the behavior occurs in association with year-round joint defense of a territory by a mated pair. Neotropical wrens of the genus *Thryothorus* vary with respect to whether both sexes sing, and the degree of song dimorphism is correlated with the degree of dimorphism in the neural song system (Brenowitz & Arnold, 1986; Farabaugh, 1982; Levin, 1996; Nealen & Perkel, 2000). A molecular phylogeny of these birds has recently become available that makes it possible to infer which state is ancestral and how many times duetting evolved in this genus (Mann, Barker, Graves, Dingess-Mann, & Slater, 2006). It suggests that duetting is derived in this clade and arose once. As progress is made determining the genetics and neurochemistry of song system, sexual differentiation (see section "Sex Differences in Zebra Finches"), it will be possible to propose realistic hypotheses for the developmental mechanisms that have been altered to produce this evolutionary change to singing females. Such hypotheses would likely be inspired by the work with zebra finches, and could be applied to understanding the diversity in song dimorphism in the estrildid finch family as well. Although female zebra finches, Bengalese finches, and spice finches never sing, female strawberry finches do. One of the proteins that is expressed mainly in the song system is found in both sexes of strawberry finches but only in males of the zebra finch (Akutagawa & Konishi, 2001), making the gene for this protein or the genes that regulate its expression candidates for the locus of an evolutionary change from singing by males only to singing by both sexes.

Evolutionary Changes in Mating Systems

An impressive body of work with free-living birds has shown that males of socially monogamous species tend to have testosterone levels that are at their annual peak for only a short time (during the nest building and copulation part of the breeding cycle), and then fall during the incubation and chick rearing periods (Wingfield et al., 1990). Males of polygynous species, however, sustain peak levels of testosterone for a considerably longer time, and are less likely to contribute to any incubation or chick care. This suggests that an evolutionary change in the annual testosterone profile could be a mechanistic basis of an evolutionary change in mating system. In support of this hypothesis, males of two species of socially monogamous sparrows were likely to acquire a second or even a third female mate when given supplemental testosterone (Wingfield, 1984), as if monogamous species had been turned into polygynous ones. This raises interesting questions about why the monogamous males have not evolved polygyny, but also the developmental question of what produces adult males with different testosterone profile types. If the testosterone levels during incubation and chick rearing are lower in monogamous males because they are engaging in parental care (i.e., if the hormones drop as a consequence, not a cause, of paternal care), then the question becomes, why do some males mature to be interested in caring for chicks (to be sensitive to stimuli from eggs and chicks) while others do not? Is some kind of organizational hormone effect responsible for evolutionary gains or losses in paternal behavior? As is now well-known, oxytocin family peptidergic mechanisms, and especially a duplication in the gene for one of the vasopressin receptors (V1a), have been found to be part of the story of how monogamous voles have diverged from polygynous voles (Young et al., 2005). The developmental mechanisms responsible for species differences between monogamous and polygynous birds, however, are completely unknown.

Also obscure is how sex role "reversal" comes about (Eens & Pinxten, 2000). In a small percentage of avian species, including jacanas, phalaropes, painted snipes, and buttonquail, the females are more brightly colored, do the fancy displaying, and aggressively compete for males, whereas the males do all the incubation and chick rearing. In buttonquail (Turnicidae) of the genus *Turnix*, females, but not males, produce frequent loud low-pitched advertisement calls with a specialized vocal organ (Madge & McGowan, 2002). It has long been hypothesized that such reversed sex roles (which include reversed signaling and responses to signals) might be produced by reversed adult sex steroid profiles. Studies of phalaropes have not supported this hypothesis, however (Fivizzani, Oring, El Halawani, & Schlinger, 1990; Schlinger, Fivizzani,

& Callard, 1989). Evidently the sexes respond differently to the adult hormone levels than they do in nonrole-reversed species, as if the hormone response mechanisms in the nodes of the social behavior network have developed differently. A role for organizational hormone actions in producing such reversed developmental trajectories is a possibility, but this hypothesis has not yet been tested.

Evolutionary Changes in Sociality

Gannets nest "cheek by jowl" with each other in huge, dense, noisy colonies. Owls, on the other hand, vocally defend large territories, and are distributed sparsely as a result. This kind of diversity in social life also occurs among more closely related birds. The behavioral and emotional processes that underpin this variation in sociality include, among others, variation in the birds' willingness to tolerate others nearby, that is, in their responsiveness to cues and signals from neighbors with respect to approach, withdrawal, aggression and fear. Progress is being made in discovering the neurohormonal basis for these kinds of species differences through comparative studies of finches and sparrows (Goodson, 2005). In comparisons of multiple species of estrildid finches ranging from territorial to colonial, immediate-early gene responses in the nodes of the social behavior network were correlated with sociality (Figure 31.8; Goodson, Evans, Lindberg, & Allen, 2005), as were binding densities of the receptors for corticotropin releasing factor (CRF), vasoactive intestinal polypeptide (VIP), and AVT in some of the nodes (Goodson, Evans, & Wang, 2006). In comparative studies of the territorial field sparrow (an emberizid finch), territorial violet-eared waxbill (an estrildid finch), and the colonial zebra finch (also an estrildid), sociality best predicted the direction of effects on aggressive behavior of two kinds of manipulations of the lateral septum: lesions, and infusions of AVT (Goodson, 1998a, 1998b; Goodson & Adkins-Regan, 1999). The developmental mechanisms and processes that produce these adult species differences are as yet unknown, but clearly these birds will be important for understanding how evolutionary changes in communication-based sociality occur.

Conclusions

Studies of hormones in relation to communication-based social behavior in birds have been a rich source of new ideas and insights into the development of this behavior and its neural substrates.

Important advances have been made in understanding the development of sex differences in signaling behavior and in responses to other individuals on the basis of their sex. There have been new discoveries about the neuroendocrinology of female signaling and of sociality itself. There is now a greater awareness of the involvement of hormones in behavior during the early posthatching period. Yet it is also apparent that there is much that is poorly understood. The brain mechanisms involved in non-vocal displays and their development have seldom been explored, in spite of their significance for sexual selection. Potential hormonal influences on the perceptual and attentional processes of the receiving end of communication have been relatively neglected. The entire juvenile period of behavioral development, including the entry into adulthood, is poorly understood with respect to its underlying hormonal and brain substrates. The species represented in research are limited to a small number of avian clades. As further progress is made in reconstructing avian phylogeny, it will be important to select species from currently unrepresented clades with the greatest potential to elucidate the developmental bases of evolutionary transitions, convergences, and divergences in social life and the social brain.

References

Adkins-Regan, E. (2005a). Activity dependent brain plasticity: Does singing increase the volume of a song system nucleus? Theoretical comment on Sartor and Ball (2005). *Behavioral Neuroscience, 119*, 346–348.

Adkins-Regan, E. (2005b). *Hormones and animal social behavior.* Princeton: Princeton University Press.

Adkins-Regan, E. (2005c). Tactile contact is required for early estrogen treatment to alter the sexual partner preference of female zebra finches. *Hormones and Behavior, 48*, 180–186.

Adkins-Regan, E., Abdelnabi, M., Mobarak, M., & Ottinger, M. A. (1990). Sex steroid levels in developing and adult male and female zebra finches (*Poephila guttata*). *General and Comparative Endocrinology, 78*, 93–109.

Adkins-Regan, E., & Ascenzi, M. (1987). Social and sexual behaviour of male and female zebra finches treated with oestradiol during the nestling period. *Animal Behaviour, 35*, 1100–1112.

Adkins-Regan, E., & Krakauer, A. (2000). Removal of adult males from the rearing environment increases preference for same sex partners in the zebra finch (*Taeniopygia guttata*). *Animal Behaviour, 60*, 47–53.

Adkins-Regan, E., & Leung, C. H. (2006). Sex steroids modulate changes in social and sexual preference during juvenile development in zebra finches. *Hormones and Behavior, 50*, 772–778.

Adkins-Regan, E., Mansukhani, V., Seiwert, C., & Thompson, R. (1994). Sexual differentiation of brain and behavior in the zebra finch: Critical periods for effects of early estrogen treatment. *Journal of Neurobiology, 25*, 865–877.

Adkins-Regan, E., & Robinson, T.M. (1993). Sex differences in aggressive behavior in zebra finches (*Poephila guttata*). *Journal of Comparative Psychology, 107*, 223–229.

Adkins-Regan, E., & Wade, J. (2001). Masculinized sexual partner preference in female zebra finches with sex-reversed gonads. *Hormones and Behavior, 39*, 22–28.

Adkins-Regan, E., Yang, S., & Mansukhani, V. (1996). Behavior of male and female zebra finches treated with an estrogen synthesis inhibitor as nestlings. *Behaviour, 133*, 847–862.

Adkins-Regan, E., Zhou, M. X., & Leung, C. H. (2003). *How does male brooding behavior affect female mate choice in Japanese quail?* Unpublished honors thesis, Cornell University.

Akutagawa, E., & Konishi, M. (2001). A monoclonal antibody specific to a song system nuclear antigen in estrildine finches. *Neuron, 31*, 545–556.

Angelier, F., Shaffer, S. A., Weimerskirch, H., & Chastel, O. (2006). Effect of age, breeding experience and senescence on corticosterone and prolactin levels in a long-lived seabird: The wandering albatross. *General and Comparative Endocrinology, 149*, 1–9.

Arnold, A. P. (1980). Effects of androgens on volumes of sexually dimorphic brain regions in the zebra finch. *Brain Research, 185*, 441–444.

Arnold, A. P. (2002). Concepts of genetic and hormonal induction of vertebrate sexual differentiation in the twentieth century, with special reference to the brain. In D. W. Pfaff, A. P. Arnold, A. M. Etgen, S. E. Fahrbach, & R. T. Rubin (Eds.), *Hormones, Brain and Behavior* (Vol. 4, pp. 105–136). Amsterdam: Academic Press (Elsevier).

Arnold, A. P., & Schlinger, B. A. (1993). Sexual differentiation of brain and behavior: The zebra finch is not just a flying rat. *Brain Behavior and Evolution, 42*, 231–241.

Arnqvist, G., & Rowe, L. (2005). *Sexual conflict.* Princeton: Princeton University Press.

Ball, G. F., & Balthazart, J. (2002). Neuroendocrine mechanisms regulating reproductive cycles and reproductive behavior in birds. In D. W. Pfaff, A. P. Arnold, A. M. Etgen, S. E. Fahrbach, & R. T. Rubin (eds.), *Hormones, brain and behavior* (Vol. 2, pp. 649–798). Amsterdam: Academic Press (Elsevier).

Ball, G. F., Riters, L. V., & Balthazart, J. (2002). Neuroendocrinology of song behavior and avian brain plasticity: Multiple sites of action of sex steroid hormones. *Frontiers in Neuroendocrinology, 23*, 137–178.

Balthazart, J. (1983). Hormonal correlates of behavior. In D. S. Farner, J. R. King, & K. C. Parkes (Eds.), *Avian Biology* (Vol. VII, pp. 221–366). New York: Academic Press.

Balthazart, J., & Adkins-Regan, E. (2002). Sexual differentiation of brain and behavior in birds. In D. W. Pfaff, A. P. Arnold, A. M. Etgen, S. E. Fahrbach, & R. T. Rubin (Eds.), *Hormones, brain and behavior* (Vol. 4, pp. 223–301). Amsterdam: Academic Press (Elsevier).

Balthazart, J., Castagna, C., & Ball, G. F. (1997). Aromatase inhibition blocks the activation and sexual differentiation of appetitive male sexual behavior in Japanese quail. *Behavioral Neuroscience, 111*, 381–397.

Balthazart, J., Delville, Y., Sulon, J., & Hendrick, J. C. (1986). Plasma levels of luteinizing hormone and of five steroids in photostimulated, castrated and testosterone-treated male and female Japanese quail (*Coturnix coturnix japonica*). *General Endocrinology*, 5, 31–36.

Balthazart, J., Schumacher, M., & Ottinger, M. A. (1983). Sexual differences in the Japanese quail: Behavior, morphology, and intracellular metabolism of testosterone. *General and Comparative Endocrinology*, 51, 191–207.

Balthazart, J., Stamatakis, A., Bacola, S., Absil, P., & Dermon, C. R. (2001). Effects of lesions of the medial preoptic nucleus on the testosterone-induced metabolic changes in specific brain areas in male quail. *Neuroscience*, 108, 447–466.

Balthazart, J., Turek, R., & Ottinger, M. A. (1984). Altered brain metabolism of testosterone is correlated with reproductive decline in aging quail. *Hormones and Behavior*, 18, 330–345.

Beecher, M. D. (1988). Kin recognition in birds. *Behavior Genetics*, 18, 465–482.

Belle, M. D., Sharp, P. J., & Lea, R. W. (2005). Aromatase inhibition abolishes courtship behaviours in the ring dove (*Streptopelia risoria*) and reduces androgen and progesterone receptors in the hypothalamus and anterior pituitary gland. *Molecular and Cell Biochemistry*, 276, 193–204.

Belthoff, J. R., & Dufty, A. M. (1998). Corticosterone, body condition and locomotor activity: A model for dispersal in screech-owls. *Animal Behaviour*, 55, 405–415.

Bentley, G. E., Jensen, J. P., Kaur, G. J., Wacker, D. W., Tsutsui, K., & Wingfield, J. C. (2006). Rapid inhibition of female sexual behavior by gonadotropin-inhibitory hormone (GnIH). *Hormones and Behavior*, 49, 550–555.

Bentley, G. E., Van't Hof, T. J., & Ball, G. F. (1999). Seasonal neuroplasticity in the songbird telencephalon: A role for melatonin. *Proceedings of the National Academy of Sciences USA*, 96, 4674–4679.

Black, J. M. (Ed.). (1996). *Partnerships in birds: The study of monogamy*. Oxford: Oxford University Press.

Blahser, S. (1984). Peptidergic pathways in the avian brain. *Journal of Experimental Zoology*, 232, 397–403.

Boncoraglio, G., Rubolini, D., Romano, M., Martinelli, R., & Saino, N. (2006). Effects of elevated yolk androgens on perinatal begging behavior in yellow-legged gull (*Larus michahellis*) chicks. *Hormones and Behavior*, 50, 442–447.

Bradbury, J. W., & Vehrencamp, S. L. (1998). *Principles of animal communication*. Sunderland, MA: Sinauer.

Brenowitz, E. A., & Arnold, A. P. (1986). Interspecific comparisons of the size of neural song control regions and song complexity in duetting birds: Evolutionary implications. *Journal of Neuroscience*, 6, 2875–2879.

Brenowitz, E. A., & Kroodsma, D. E. (1996). The neuroethology of birdsong. In D. E. Kroodsma, & E. H. Miller (Eds.), *Ecology and evolution of acoustic communication in birds* (pp. 285–304). Ithaca, NY: Cornell University Press.

Bridges, R. S. (1996). Biochemical basis of parental behavior in the rat. In J. S. Rosenblatt, & C. T. Snowdon (Eds.), *Parental care: Evolution, mechanisms, and adaptive significance, Advances in the study of behavior* (Vol. 25, pp. 215–242). San Diego: Academic Press.

Brown, J. L., & Vleck, C. M. (1998). Prolactin and helping in birds: Has natural selection strengthened helping behavior? *Behavioral Ecology*, 9, 541–545.

Buchanan, K. L., Spencer, K. A., Goldsmith, A. R., & Catchpole, C. K. (2003). Song as an honest signal of past developmental stress in the European starling (*Sturnus vulgaris*). *Proceedings of the Royal Society* (London) B, 270, 1149–1156.

Buntin, J. D. (1996). Neural and hormonal control of parental behavior in birds. In J. S. Rosenblatt, & C. T. Snowdon (Eds.), *Parental care: Evolution, mechanisms, and adaptive significance, Advances in the study of behavior* (Vol. 25, pp. 161–214). San Diego: Academic Press.

Buntin, J. D., Ruzycki, E., & Witebsky, J. (1993). Prolactin receptors in dove brain: Autoradiographic analysis of binding characteristics in discrete brain regions and accessibility to blood-borne prolactin. *Neuroendocrinology*, 57, 738–750.

Burke, M. R., Adkins-Regan, E., & Wade, J. (2007). Laterality in syrinx muscle morphology of the Japanese quail (*Coturnix japonica*). *Physiology and Behavior*, 90, 682–686 .

Butterfield, P. A. (1970). The pair bond in the zebra finch. In J. H. Crook (Ed.), *Social behavior in birds and mammals* (pp. 249–278). London: Academic Press.

Carter, C. S., DeVries, A. C., & Getz, L. L. (1995). Physiological substrates of mammalian monogamy: The prairie vole model. *Neuroscience and Biobehavioral Reviews*, 19, 303–314.

Casto, J. M., & Ball, G. F. (1996). Early administration of 17β-estradiol partially masculinizes song control regions and α_2-adrenergic receptor distribution in European starlings (*Sturnus vulgaris*). *Hormones and Behavior*, 30, 387–406.

Catchpole, C. K., & Slater, P. J. B. (1995). *Bird song: Biological themes and variations*. Cambridge: Cambridge University Press.

Chilton, G., Baker, M. C., Barrentine, C. D., & Cunningham, M. A. (1995). White-crowned Sparrow (*Zonotrichia leucophrys*). In A. Poole, & F. Gill (Eds.), *The birds of North America*, No. 183. Philadelphia: The Academy of Natural Sciences and Washington, D.C.: The American Ornithologists' Union.

Clutton-Brock, T. H. (Ed.). (1988). *Reproductive success: Studies of individual variation in contrasting breeding systems*. Chicago: University of Chicago Press.

Cockburn, A. (2006). Prevalence of different modes of parental care in birds. *Proceedings of the Royal Society* (London) B, 273, 1375–1383.

Collins, S. A., Hubbard, C., & Houtman, A. M. (1994). Female mate choice in the zebra finch—The effect of male beak colour and male song. *Behavioral Ecology and Sociobiology*, 35, 21–25.

Collis, K., & Borgia, G. (1992). Age-related effects of testosterone, plumage, and experience on aggression and social dominance in juvenile male satin bowerbirds (*Ptilonorhynchus violaceus*). *Auk*, 109, 422–434.

Collis, K., & Borgia, G. (1993). The costs of male display and delayed plumage maturation in the satin bowerbird (*Ptilonorhynchus violaceus*). *Ethology*, 94, 59–71.

Cynx, J., & Nottebohm, F. (1992). Testosterone facilitates some conspecific song discriminations in castrated zebra finches (*Taeniopygia guttata*). *Proceedings of the National Academy of Sciences USA*, 89, 1376–1378.

Day, L. B., McBroom, J. T., & Schlinger, B. A. (2006). Testosterone increases display behaviors but does not stimulate growth of adult plumage in male golden-collared manakins (*Manacus vitellinus*). *Hormones and Behavior*, 49, 223–232.

De Ridder, E., Pinxten, R., & Eens, M. (2000). Experimental evidence of a testosterone-induced shift from paternal to mating behaviour in a facultatively polygynous songbird. *Behavioral Ecology and Sociobiology*, 49, 24–30.

De Vries, G. J., & Panzica, G. C. (2006). Sexual differentiation of central vasopressin and vasotocin systems in vertebrates: Different mechanisms, similar endpoints. *Neuroscience*, *138*, 947–955.

Del Negro, C., Kreutzer, M., & Gahr, M. (2000). Sexually stimulating signals of canary (*Serinus canaria*) songs: Evidence for a female-specific auditory representation in the HVc nucleus during the breeding season. *Behavioral Neuroscience*, *114*, 526–542.

Delville, Y., Newman, M. L., Wommack, J. C., Taravosh-Lahn, K., & Cervantes, M. C. (2006). Development of aggression. In R. J. Nelson (Ed.), *Biology of aggression* (pp. 327–350). Oxford: Oxford University Press.

Dittami, J., Hoi, H., & Sageder, G. (1991). Parental investment and territorial/sexual behavior in male and female reed warblers: Are they mutually exclusive? *Ethology*, *88*, 249–255.

Domjan, M., & Hall, S. (1986). Determinants of social proximity in Japanese quail (*Coturnix coturnix japonica*): Male behavior. *Journal of Comparative Psychology*, *100*, 59–67.

Domjan, M., & Ravert, R. D. (1991). Discriminating the sex of conspecifics by male Japanese quail (*Coturnix coturnix japonica*). *Journal of Comparative Psychology*, *105*, 157–164.

Eens, M., & Pinxten, R. (2000). Sex-role reversal in vertebrates: Behavioural and endocrinological accounts. *Behavioural Processes*, *51*, 135–147.

El Halawani, M. E., Burke, W. H., Millam, J. R., Fehrer, S. C., & Hargis, B. M. (1984). Regulation of prolactin and its role in gallinaceous bird reproduction. *Journal of Experimental Zoology*, *232*, 521–529.

Enstrom, D. A., Ketterson, E. D., & Nolan, V. (1997). Testosterone and mate choice in the dark-eyed junco. *Animal Behaviour*, *54*, 1135–1146.

Farabaugh, S. M. (1982). The ecological and social significance of duetting. In D. E. Kroodsma, & E. H. Miller (Eds.), *Acoustic communication in birds* (Vol. 2, pp. 85–124). New York: Academic Press.

Fivizzani, A. J., Oring, L. W., El Halawani, M. E., & Schlinger, B. A. (1990). Hormonal basis of male parental care and female intersexual competition in sex-role reversed birds. In M. Wada, S. Ishii, & Scanes, C. G. (Eds.), *Endocrinology of birds: Molecular to behavioral* (pp. 273–286). Tokyo: Japan Scientific Societies Press and Berlin: Springer-Verlag.

Folstad, I., & Karter, A. J. (1992). Parasites, bright males, and the immunocompetence handicap. *American Naturalist*, *139*, 603–622.

Goodson, J. L. (1998a). Territorial aggression and dawn song are modulated by septal vasotocin and vasoactive intestinal polypeptide in male field sparrows (*Spizella pusilla*). *Hormones and Behavior*, *34*, 67–77.

Goodson, J. L. (1998b). Vasotocin and vasoactive intestinal polypeptide modulate aggression in a territorial songbird, the violet-eared waxbill (Estrildidae: *Uraeginthus granatina*). *General and Comparative Endocrinology*, *111*, 233–244.

Goodson, J. L. (2005). The vertebrate social behavior network: Evolutionary themes and variations. *Hormones and Behavior*, *48*, 11–22.

Goodson, J. L., & Adkins-Regan, E. (1999). Effect of intraseptal vasotocin and vasoactive intestinal polypeptide infusions on courtship song and aggression in the male zebra finch (*Taeniopygia guttata*). *Journal of Neuroendocrinology*, *11*, 19–25.

Goodson, J. L., & Bass, A. H. (2001). Social behavior functions and related anatomical characteristics of vasotocin/vasopressin systems in vertebrates. *Brain Research Reviews*, *35*, 246–265.

Goodson, J. L., Evans, A. K., Lindberg, L., & Allen, C. D. (2005). Neuro-evolutionary patterning of sociality. *Proceedings of the Royal Society (London) B*, *272*, 227–235.

Goodson, J. L., Evans, A. K., & Wang, Y. (2006). Neuropeptide binding reflects convergent and divergent evolution in species-typical group sizes. *Hormones and Behavior*, *50*, 223–236.

Goodson, J. L., Lindberg, L., & Johnson, P. (2004). Effects of central vasotocin and mesotocin manipulations on social behavior in male and female zebra finches. *Hormones and Behavior*, *45*, 136–143.

Gottlieb, G. (1974). On the acoustic basis of species identification in wood ducklings (*Aix sponsa*). *Journal of Comparative and Physiological Psychology*, *87*, 1038–1049.

Goymann, W., & Wingfield, J. C. (2004). Allostatic load, social status and stress hormones: The costs of social status matter. *Animal Behaviour*, *67*, 591–602.

Grafen, A. (1990). Biological signals as handicaps. *Journal of Theoretical Biology*, *144*, 517–546.

Grisham, W., & Arnold, A. P. (1995). A direct comparison of the masculinizing effects of testosterone, androstenedione, estrogen, and progesterone on the development of the zebra finch song system. *Journal of Neurobiology*, *26*, 163–170.

Groothuis, T., & Meeuwissen, G. (1992). The influence of testosterone on the development and fixation of the form of displays in two age classes of young black-headed gulls. *Animal Behaviour*, *43*, 189–208.

Groothuis, T. G., Müller, W., von Engelhardt, N., Carere, C., & Eising, C. (2005). Maternal hormones as a tool to adjust offspring phenotype in avian species. *Neuroscience and Biobehavioral Reviews*, *29*, 329–352.

Groothuis, T. G. G., & Ros, A. F. H. (2005). The hormonal control of begging and early aggressive behavior: Experiments in black-headed gull chicks. *Hormones and Behavior*, *48*, 207–215.

Gurney, M. E., & Konishi, M. (1980). Hormone-induced sexual differentiation of brain and behavior in zebra finches. *Science*, *208*, 1380–1383.

Gvaryahu, G., Snapir, N., Robinzon, B., & Goodman, G. (1986). The gonadotropic-axis involvement in the course of the filial following response in the domestic fowl chick. *Physiology and Behavior*, *38*, 651–656.

Hagelin, J. C., Jones, I. L., & Rasmussen, L. E. (2003). A tangerine-scented social odour in a monogamous seabird. *Proceedings of the Royal Society* (*London*) *B*, *270*, 1323–1329.

Hamilton, W. D., & Zuk, M. (1982). Heritable true fitness and bright birds: A role for parasites? *Science*, *218*, 384–387.

Harding, C. F. (1983). Hormonal influences on avian aggressive behavior. In B. B. Svare (Ed.), *Hormones and aggressive behavior* (pp. 435–468). New York: Plenum Press.

Hau, M., Stoddard, S. T., & Soma, K. K. (2004). Territorial aggression and hormones during the non-breeding season in a tropical bird. *Hormones and Behavior*, *45*, 40–49.

Hegner, R. E., & Wingfield, J. C. (1987). Effects of experimental manipulation of testosterone levels on parental investment and breeding success in male house sparrows. *Auk*, *104*, 462–469.

Heidinger, B. J., Nisbet, I. C., & Ketterson, E. D. (2006). Older parents are less responsive to a stressor in a long-lived seabird: A mechanism for increased reproductive performance with age? *Proceedings of the Royal Society (London) B*, *273*, 2227–2231.

Heimovics, S. A., & Riters, L. V. (2005). Immediate early gene activity in song control nuclei and brain areas regulating motivation relates positively to singing behavior during, but not outside of, a breeding context. *Journal of Neurobiology, 65*, 207–224.

Hillgarth, N., Ramenofsky, M., & Wingfield, J. (1997). Testosterone and sexual selection. *Behavioral Ecology, 8*, 108–112.

Holekamp, K. E., Smale, L., Simpson, H. B., & Holekamp, N. A. (1984). Hormonal influences on natal dispersal in free-living Belding's ground squirrels (*Spermophilus beldingi*). *Hormones and Behavior, 18*, 465–483.

Iwaniuk, A. N., Dean, K. M., & Nelson, J. E. (2005). Interspecific allometry of the brain and brain regions in parrots (Psittaciformes): Comparisons with other birds and primates. *Brain Behavior and Evolution, 65*, 40–59.

Johnstone, R. A. (1997). The evolution of animal signals. In J. R. Krebs, & N. B. Davies (Eds.), *Behavioural ecology: An evolutionary approach* (4th ed., pp. 155–178). Oxford: Blackwell Science.

Jones, K. M., Monaghan, P., & Nager, R. G. (2001). Male mate choice and female fecundity in zebra finches. *Animal Behaviour, 62*, 1021–1026.

Ketterson, E. D., & Nolan, V. (1999). Adaptation, exaptation, and constraint: A hormonal perspective. *American Naturalist, 154*, S3–S25.

Ketterson, E. D., Nolan, V., & Sandell, M. (2005). Testosterone in females: Mediator of adaptive traits, constraint on sexual dimorphism, or both? *American Naturalist, 166*, S85–S98.

Kitaysky, A. S., Kitaiskaia, E. V., Piatt, J. F., & Wingfield, J. C. (2003). Benefits and costs of increased levels of corticosterone in seabird chicks. *Hormones and Behavior, 43*, 140–149.

Lea, R. W., Clark, J. A., & Tsutsui, K. (2001). Changes in central steroid receptor expression, steroid synthesis, and dopaminergic activity related to the reproductive cycle of the ring dove. *Microscopy Research and Technique, 55*, 12–26.

Leboucher, G., Beguin, N., Mauget, R., & Kreutzer, M. (1998). Effects of fadrozole on sexual displays and reproductive activity in the female canary. *Physiology and Behavior, 65*, 233–240.

Lehrman, D. S. (1965). Interaction between internal and external environments in the regulation of the reproductive cycle of the ring dove. In F. A. Beach (Ed.), *Sex and behavior* (pp. 344–380). New York: Wiley.

Levin, R. (1996). Song behaviour and reproductive strategies in a duetting wren, *Thryothorus nigricapillus*: I. Removal experiments. *Animal Behaviour, 52*, 1093–1106.

Lipar, J. L., & Ketterson, E. D. (2000). Maternally derived yolk testosterone enhances the development of the hatching muscle in the red-winged blackbird *Agelaius phoeniceus*. *Proceedings of the Royal Society (London) B, 267*, 2005–2010.

Lormée, H., Jouventin, P., Chastel, O., & Mauget, R. (1999). Endocrine correlates of parental care in an Antarctic winter breeding seabird, the emperor penguin, *Aptenodytes forsteri*. *Hormones and Behavior, 35*, 9–17.

Lynn, S. E., Walker, B. G., & Wingfield, J. C. (2005). A phylogenetically controlled test of hypotheses for behavioral insensitivity to testosterone in birds. *Hormones and Behavior, 47*, 170–177.

MacDonald, I. F., Kempster, B., Zanette, L., & MacDougall-Shackleton, S. A. (2006). Early nutritional stress impairs development of a song-control brain region in both male and female juvenile song sparrows (*Melospiza melodia*) at the onset of song learning. *Proceedings of the Royal Society (London) B, 273*, 2559–2564.

Madge, S., & McGowan, P. (2002). *Pheasants, partridges, and grouse*. Princeton: Princeton University Press.

Maney, D. L., Cho, E., & Goode, C. T. (2006). Estrogen-dependent selectivity of genomic responses to birdsong. *European Journal of Neuroscience, 23*, 1523–1529.

Maney, D. L., Goode, C. T., & Wingfield, J. C. (1997a). Intraventricular infusion of arginine vasotocin induces singing in a female songbird. *Journal of Neuroendocrinology, 9*, 487–491.

Maney, D. L., Richardson, R. D., & Wingfield, J. C. (1997b). Central administration of chicken gonadotropin-releasing hormone-II enhances courtship behavior in a female sparrow. *Hormones and Behavior, 32*, 11–18.

Mann, N. I., Barker, F. K., Graves, J. A., Dingess-Mann, K. A., & Slater, P. J. B. (2006). Molecular data delineate four genera of "*Thryothorus*" wrens. *Molecular Phylogenetics and Evolution, 40*, 750–759.

Mansukhani, V., Adkins-Regan, E., & Yang, S. (1996). Sexual partner preference in female zebra finches: The role of early hormones and social environment. *Hormones and Behavior, 30*, 506–513.

Margoliash, D., & Konishi, M. (1985). Auditory representation of autogenous song in the song system of white-crowned sparrows. *Proceedings of the National Academy of Sciences USA, 82*, 5997–6000.

Marx, G., Jurkevich, A., & Grossmann, R. (2004). Effects of estrogens during embryonal development on crowing in the domestic fowl. *Physiology and Behavior, 82*, 637–645.

Mason, W. A., & Mendoza, S. P. (1998). Generic aspects of primate attachments: Parents, offspring and mates. *Psychoneuroendocrinology, 23*, 765–778.

McGlothlin, J. W., Neudorf, D. L., Casto, J. M., Nolan, V., & Ketterson, E. D. (2004). Elevated testosterone reduces choosiness in female dark-eyed juncos (*Junco hyemalis*): Evidence for a hormonal constraint on sexual selection? *Proceedings of the Royal Society (London) B, 271*, 1377–1384.

Nealen P. M., & Perkel, D. J. (2000). Sexual dimorphism in the song system of the Carolina wren *Thryothorus ludovicianus*. *Journal of Comparative Neurology, 418*, 346–360.

Newman, S. W. (2002). Pheromonal signals across the medial extended amygdala: One node in a proposed social behavior network. In D. W. Pfaff, A. P. Arnold, A. M. Etgen, S. E. Fahrbach, & R. T. Rubin (Eds.), *Hormones, brain and behavior* (Vol. 2, pp. 17–32). Amsterdam: Academic Press (Elsevier).

Nottebohm, F. (1981). A brain for all seasons: Cyclical anatomical changes in song control nuclei of the canary brain. *Science, 214*, 1368–1370.

Nowicki, S., Searcy, W. A., & Peters, S. (2002). Brain development, song learning and mate choice in birds: A review and experimental test of the "nutritional stress hypothesis". *Journal of Comparative Physiology A, 188*, 1003–1014.

Ottinger, M. A., Abdelnabi, M., Li, Q., Chen, K., Thompson, N., Harada, N., et al. (2004). The Japanese quail: A model for studying reproductive aging of hypothalamic systems. *Experimental Gerontology, 39*, 1679–1693.

Ottinger, M. A., & Bakst, M. R. (1981). Peripheral androgen concentrations and testicular morphology in embryonic and young male Japanese quail. *General and Comparative Endocrinology, 43*, 170–177.

Ottinger, M. A., & Brinkley, H. J. (1979). The ontogeny of crowing and copulatory behavior in Japanese quail (*Coturnix coturnix japonica*). *Behavioural Processes, 4*, 43–51.

Panzica, G. C., Castagna, C., Viglietti-Panzica, C., Russo, C., Tlemçani, O., & Balthazart, J. (1998). Organizational effects of estrogens on brain vasotocin and sexual behavior in quail. *Journal of Neurobiology, 37*, 684–699.

Parker, G. A. (2006). Sexual conflict over mating and fertilization: An overview. *Philosophical Transactions of the Royal Society (London) B 361*, 235–259.

Patricelli, G. L., Uy, J. A., Walsh, G., & Borgia, G. (2002). Male displays adjusted to female's response. *Nature, 415*, 279–280.

Phoenix, C. H., Goy, R. W., Gerall, A. A., & Young, W. C. (1959). Organizing action of prenatally administered testosterone propionate on the tissues mediating mating behavior in the female guinea pig. *Endocrinology, 65*, 369–382.

Pilz, K. M., Adkins-Regan, E., & Schwabl, H. (2005). No sex difference in yolk steroid concentrations of avian eggs at laying. *Biology Letters, 1*, 318–321.

Pinaud, R., Fortes, A. F., Lovell, P., & Mello, C. V. (2006). Calbindin-positive neurons reveal a sexual dimorphism within the songbird analogue of the mammalian auditory cortex. *Journal of Neurobiology, 66*, 182–195.

Pusey, A. E. (1987). Sex-biased dispersal and inbreeding avoidance in birds and mammals. *Trends in Ecology and Evolution, 2*, 295–299.

Ramesh, R., Kuenzel, W. J., Buntin, J. D., & Proudman, J. A. (2000). Identification of growth-hormone- and prolactin-containing neurons within the avian brain. *Cell and Tissue Research, 299*, 371–383.

Raouf, S. A., Parker, P. G., Ketterson, E. D., Nolan, V., & Ziegenfus, C. (1997). Testosterone affects reproductive success by influencing extra-pair fertilizations in male dark-eyed juncos (Aves: *Junco hyemalis*). *Proceedings of the Royal Society (London) B, 264*, 1599–1603.

Remage-Healey, L., Adkins-Regan, E., & Romero, L. M. (2003). Behavioral and adrenocortical responses to mate separation and reunion in the zebra finch. *Hormones and Behavior, 43*, 108–114.

Richard-Yris, M. A., Garnier, D. H., & Leboucher, G. (1983). Induction of maternal behavior and some hormonal and physiological correlates in the domestic hen. *Hormones and Behavior, 17*, 345–355.

Riters, L. V., & Ball, G. F. (1999). Lesions to the medial preoptic area affect singing in the male European starling (*Sturnus vulgaris*). *Hormones and Behavior, 36*, 276–286.

Roberts, M. L., Buchanan, K. L., & Evans, M. R. (2004). Testing the immunocompetence handicap hypothesis: A review of the evidence. *Animal Behaviour, 68*, 227–239.

Roff, D. A. (2001). *Life history evolution*. Sunderland, MA: Sinauer.

Royle, N. J., Hartley, I. R., & Parker, G. A. (2002). Sexual conflict reduces offspring fitness in zebra finches. *Nature, 416*, 733–736.

Rubolini, D., Romano, M., Boncoraglio, G., Ferrari, R. P., Martinelli, R., Galeotti, P., et al. (2005). Effects of elevated egg corticosterone levels on behavior, growth, and immunity of yellow-legged gull (*Larus michahellis*) chicks. *Hormones and Behavior, 47*, 592–605.

Ruscio, M. G., & Adkins-Regan, E. (2003). Effect of female brooding behavior on male mate choice in Japanese quail, *Coturnix japonica*. *Animal Behaviour, 65*, 397–403.

Ruscio, M. G., & Adkins-Regan, E. (2004). Immediate early gene expression associated with induction of brooding behavior in Japanese quail. *Hormones and Behavior, 46*, 19–29.

Saldanha, C. J., Tuerk, M. J., Kim, Y. H., Fernandes, A. O., Arnold, A. P., & Schlinger, B. A. (2000). Distribution and regulation of telencephalic aromatase expression in the zebra finch revealed with a specific antibody. *Journal of Comparative Neurology, 423*, 619–630.

Sartor, J. J., & Ball, G. F. (2005). Social suppression of song is associated with a reduction in volume of a song-control nucleus in European starlings (*Sturnus vulgaris*). *Behavioral Neuroscience, 119*, 233–244.

Schlinger, B. A., & Brenowitz, E. A. (2002). Neural and hormonal control of birdsong. In D. W. Pfaff, A. P. Arnold, A. M. Etgen, S. E. Fahrbach, & R. T. Rubin (Eds.), *Hormones, brain and behavior* (Vol. 2, pp. 799–840). Amsterdam: Academic Press (Elsevier).

Schlinger, B. A., Fivizzani, A. J., & Callard, G. V. (1989). Aromatase, 5α- and 5β-reductase in brain, pituitary and skin of the sex-role reversed Wilson's phalarope. *Journal of Endocrinology, 122*, 573–581.

Schoech, S. J., Reynolds, S. J., & Boughton, R. K. (2004). Endocrinology. In W. D. Koenig, & J. Dickenson (Eds.), *Ecology and evolution of cooperative breeding in birds* (pp. 128–141). Cambridge: Cambridge University Press.

Schultz, J. D., & Schlinger, B. A. (1999). Widespread accumulation of [(3)H]testosterone in the spinal cord of a wild bird with an elaborate courtship display. *Proceedings of the National Academy of Sciences USA, 96*, 10428–10432.

Schwabl, H. (1993). Yolk is a source of maternal testosterone for developing birds. *Proceedings of the National Academy of Sciences USA, 90*, 11446–11450.

Searcy, W. A., & Nowicki, S. (2005). *The evolution of animal communication: Reliability and deception in signaling systems*. Princeton: Princeton University Press.

Sharp, P. J., MacNamee, M. C., Talbot, R. T., Sterling, R. J., & Hall, T. R. (1984). Aspects of the neuroendocrine control of ovulation and broodiness in the domestic hen. *Journal of Experimental Zoology, 232*, 475–483.

Silcox, A. P., & Evans, S. M. (1982). Factors affecting the formation and maintenance of pair bonds in the zebra finch, *Taeniopygia guttata*. *Animal Behaviour, 30*, 1237–1243.

Silverin, B. (1980). Effects of long-acting testosterone treatment on free-living pied flycatchers, *Ficedula hypoleuca*, during the breeding period. *Animal Behaviour, 28*, 906–912.

Silverin, B. (1997). The stress response and autumn dispersal behaviour in willow tits. *Animal Behaviour, 53*, 451–459.

Silverin, B., & Sharp, P. (1996). The development of the hypothalamic-pituitary-gonadal axis in juvenile great tits. *General and Comparative Endocrinology, 103*, 150–166.

Sisk, C. L., & Zehr, J. L. (2005). Pubertal hormones organize the adolescent brain and behavior. *Frontiers in Neuroendocrinology, 26*, 163–174.

Slawski, B. A., & Buntin, J. D. (1995). Preoptic area lesions disrupt prolactin-induced parental feeding behavior in ring doves. *Hormones and Behavior, 29*, 248–266.

Sockman, K. W., Williams, T. D., Dawson, A., & Ball, G. F. (2004). Prior experience with photostimulation enhances photo-induced reproductive development in female European starlings: A possible basis for the age-related increase in avian reproductive performance. *Biology of Reproduction, 71*, 979–986.

Soma, K. K. (2006). Testosterone and aggression: Berthold, birds, and beyond. *Journal of Neuroendocrinology, 18,* 543–551.

Striedter, G. F. (2005). *Principles of brain evolution.* Sunderland, MA: Sinauer.

Terkel, A. S., Moore, C. L., & Beer, C. G. (1976). The effects of testosterone and estrogens on the rate of long-calling vocalization in juvenile laughing gulls, *Larus atricilla. Hormones and Behavior, 7,* 49–57.

Tinbergen, N. (1963). On aims and methods of ethology. *Zeitschrift für Tierpsychologie, 20,* 410–433.

Tomaszycki, M. L., & Adkins-Regan, E. (2005). Experimental alteration of male song quality and output affects female mate choice and pair bond formation in zebra finches. *Animal Behaviour, 70,* 785–794.

Tomaszycki, M. L., & Adkins-Regan, E. (2006). Is male song quality important in maintaining pair bonds? *Behaviour, 143,* 549–567.

Tomaszycki, M. L., Banerjee, S. B., & Adkins-Regan, E. (2006). The role of sex steroids in courtship, pairing and pairing behaviors in the socially monogamous zebra finch. *Hormones and Behavior, 50,* 141–147.

Tsutsui, K., & Schlinger, B. A. (2001). Steroidogenesis in the avian brain. In A. Dawson, & C. M. Chaturvedi (Eds.), *Avian endocrinology* (pp.59–77). New Delhi: Narosa Publishing.

Vince, M. A. (1973). Some environmental effects on the activity and development of the avian embryo. In G. Gottlieb (Ed.), *Behavioral embryology* (pp. 285–323). New York: Academic Press.

Vleck, C. M., Ross, L. L., Vleck, D., & Bucher, T. L. (2000). Prolactin and parental behavior in Adelie penguins: Effects of absence from nest, incubation length, and nest failure. *Hormones and Behavior, 38,* 149–158.

von Holst, D. (1998). The concept of stress and its relevance for animal behavior. *Advances in the Study of Behavior, 27,* 1–131.

Wade, J. (1999). Sexual dimorphisms in avian and reptilian courtship: Two systems that do not play by mammalian rules. *Brain Behavior and Evolution, 54,* 15–27.

Wade, J., Tang, Y. P., Peabody, C., & Tempelman, R J. (2005). Enhanced gene expression in the forebrain of hatchling and juvenile male zebra finches. *Journal of Neurobiology, 64,* 224–238.

Wedell, N., Kvarnemo, C., Lessells, C. M., & Tregenza, T. (2006). Sexual conflict and life histories. *Animal Behaviour, 71,* 999–1011.

White, D. J., & Galef, B. G. (2000). Differences between the sexes in direction and duration of response to seeing a potential sex partner mate with another. *Animal Behaviour, 59,* 1235–1240.

Williams, H., Kilander, K., & Sotanski, M. L. (1993). Untutored song, reproductive success and song learning. *Animal Behaviour, 45,* 695–705.

Williams, T. D. (1992). Reproductive endocrinology of macaroni (*Eudyptes chrysolophus*) and gentoo (*Pygoscelis papua*) penguins. II. Plasma levels of gonadal steroids and LH in immature birds in relation to deferred sexual maturity. *General and Comparative Endocrinology, 85,* 241–247.

Williams, T. D., Dawson, A., Nicholls, T. J., & Goldsmith, A. R. (1987). Reproductive endocrinology of free-living nestling and juvenile starlings, *Sturnus vulgaris*; an altricial species. *Journal of Zoology, 212,* 619–628.

Wingfield, J. C. (1984). Androgens and mating systems: Testosterone-induced polygyny in normally monogamous birds. *Auk, 101,* 665–671.

Wingfield, J. C., & Farner, D. S. (1978). The endocrinology of a natural breeding population of the White-crowned Sparrow (*Zonotrichia leucophrys pugetensis*). *Physiological Zoology, 51,* 188–205.

Wingfield, J. C., & Farner, D. S. (1993). Endocrinology of reproduction in wild species. In D. S. Farner, J. R. King, & K. C. Parkes (Eds.), *Avian Biology* (Vol. IX, pp. 164–328). London: Academic Press.

Wingfield, J. C., Hegner, R. E., Dufty, A. M., & Ball, G. F. (1990). The "challenge hypothesis": Theoretical implications for patterns of testosterone secretion, mating systems, and breeding strategies. *American Naturalist, 136,* 829–846.

Yang, P., Medan, M. S., Watanabe, G., & Taya, K. (2005). Developmental changes of plasma inhibin, gonadotropins, steroids hormones, and thyroid hormones in male and female Shao ducks. *General and Comparative Endocrinology, 143,* 161–167.

Yazaki, Y., Matsushima, T., & Aoki, K. (1999). Testosterone modulates stimulation-induced calling behavior in Japanese quails. *Journal of Comparative Physiology A, 184,* 13–19.

Young, L. J., Young, A. Z. M., & Hammock, E. A. D. (2005). Anatomy and neurochemistry of the pair bond. *Journal of Comparative Neurology, 493,* 51–57.

Zahavi, A. (1975). Mate selection—A selection for a handicap. *Journal of Theoretical Biology, 53,* 205–214.

Zann, R. A. (1996). *The zebra finch: A synthesis of field and laboratory studies.* Oxford: Oxford University Press.

Zuk, M., Johnsen, T. S., & Maclarty, T. (1995). Endocrine-immune interactions, ornaments and mate choice in red jungle fowl. *Proceedings of the Royal Society (London) B, 260,* 205–210.

Development of Antipredator Behavior

Jill M. Mateo

Abstract

Among birds and mammals, vocalizations warning of predators serve an important survival function, especially for young animals particularly vulnerable to predation. Because natural selection may favor plasticity in survival strategies, allowing adjustments to temporal or spatial variation in predators, antipredator behaviors are often learned rather than fully formed when young first encounter predators. The mechanisms shaping the ontogeny of survival skills are surveyed here, in particular the development of responses to alarm calls. These include social, acoustic, and hormonal factors as well as direct and indirect experiences with predators. In addition, the communicative functions of alarm-call systems are discussed, such as referential signaling and response urgency. Finally, the sources of plasticity in the development of antipredator behavior and the costs and benefits of such plasticity in a range of species are discussed.

Keywords: vocalization warnings, survival, predation, antipredator behavior, alarm calls, referential signaling

In many species of birds and mammals, predators elicit vocal responses from potential prey that can alert conspecifics (and heterospecifics) of impending danger. Such vocalizations are labeled "alarm calls," "warning calls," "distress calls," and "mobbing calls," among other terms, and they likely serve different functions depending on the context and the species (Klump & Shalter, 1984; Owings & Hennessy, 1984). The term "alarm call" is used here in a purely descriptive manner to refer to a vocalization elicited by a predator, without inferring a function or motivation on the part of the caller. Alarm calls are important for those individuals who have not already detected the predator because the calls indicate that danger is imminent and that quick action might be required to reduce the likelihood of capture. Responding properly to alarm calls can be especially important for immature

young, since they are generally more vulnerable to predators than adults (e.g., Caro, 1994; Cheney & Seyfarth, 1990; Coss, Guse, Poran, & Smith, 1993; Hoogland, 1995; Mateo, 1996a; Rasa, 1986). One might expect antipredator reactions to be fully developed in young animals and effective upon first encounter with a predator, as young would be unlikely to survive to correct suboptimal or ineffective responses for their next encounter (Bolles, 1970; Darwin, 1859; Galef, 1976). However, if predator contexts change temporally or spatially, then learned or acquired responses, shaped by individual experiences with local environments, can be favored by natural selection (Johnston, 1982; Shettleworth, 1998). This raises the question of when and how young develop adaptive antipredator behaviors. This chapter will survey the evolutionary and ecological pressures shaping the ontogeny of antipredator strategies in birds and mammals, as well as the social and hormonal mechanisms contributing to the plasticity of such behaviors, and will then focus on ground-dwelling squirrels, a group whose alarm-call response development has been particularly well studied.

For alarm calls to have communicative value, the recipient must perceive and interpret the information in the sender's signal (Dawkins & Krebs, 1978; Guilford & Dawkins, 1991; Owings & Hennessy, 1984; Wiley, 1983), and if alarm calls are to have adaptive value (e.g., Davis, 1984b; Sherman, 1977), recipients must be able to respond appropriately to the calls. Appropriate responsiveness involves a cumulative four-stage process (Figure 32.1; see also Mateo, 1996a), as a listener must (1) detect the call, (2) discriminate the call from other nonalarm vocalizations produced by conspecifics and heterospecifics, (3) exhibit a response to "important" stimuli and to ignore stimuli unrelated to predators, and finally (4) determine the form and duration of its response (e.g., simply raising its head briefly or remaining hidden for an extended period). In general, these four stages are expected to occur sequentially across development, although the ways in which an animal responds can change over time with changes in vulnerability. In addition, behavioral discrimination might precede the development of appropriate motor patterns under some conditions, but if experience is necessary for discrimination, then this order can be interrupted if the particular experience is withheld (Mateo, 1995). The ontogeny of alarm-call response behavior occurs at all four of these stages, with each stage contributing to the next, as sensory, perceptual, and motor systems develop independently and then integrate. To place behavioral development in an appropriate context, any analysis of antipredator behavior must take into account the young animal's particular developmental niche, including its stage of development, its current level of vulnerability, and its interactions with the immediate physical and social environments (Alberts, 1987; Johnston, 1987; Lehrman, 1970; West & King, 1987; Williams, 1966).

Several elegant studies have been conducted on the development of antipredator behavior to identify the specific factors influencing the expression of unfolding traits. Some investigators have proposed that survival behavior, such as squirrel-monkey alarm calls or fish antipredator tactics, is preprogrammed or innate so that the behavior emerges independent of environmental input (e.g., Buitron & Nuechterlein, 1993; Curio, 1975; Heaton, Miller, & Goodwin, 1978; Herzog & Hopf, 1984; Impekoven, 1976). In contrast, some have argued that antipredator behavior, including vervet-monkey alarm-call responses and mobbing by scrub jays, is acquired or learned, through either direct or indirect experiences with predators and conspecifics (e.g., Cheney & Seyfarth, 1990; Ferrari, Trowell, Brown, & Chivers, 2005; Francis, Hailman, & Woolfenden, 1989; Hauser, 1988; Macedonia, 1990; Mateo, 1996a; Rydén, 1982; Schwagmeyer & Brown, 1981; Tulley & Huntingford, 1987; Vitale, 1989). This nature–nurture dichotomous thinking is still evident despite acknowledgments by most scholars that behavior is not innate or acquired per se, but instead develops epigenetically, through interactions between the organism and the series of environments it encounters throughout its life span. In addition to this epigenetic or interactionist view of development, other researchers have viewed development as a series of ontogenetic adaptations, with each stage functionally complete for that period of development and contributing to successive stages (e.g., Alberts, 1987; Johnston, 1987; Lehrman, 1970; Miller, 1988; West & King, 1987; Williams, 1966). These two approaches to the study of development are complementary rather than competitive, however, as their interpretations focus to some extent on different levels of analysis (Tinbergen, 1963; see also Stamps, 2003).

Many research programs have studied the nature and function of adults' responses to alarm

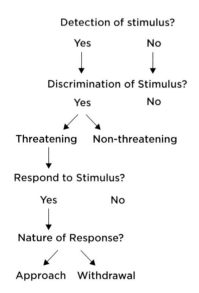

Figure 32.1 Four stages of the development of alarm-call response behavior. Stages also apply broadly to the development and expression of other antipredator behaviors.

calls (e.g., Evans, Evans, & Marler, 1993; Harris, Murie, & Duncan, 1983; Leger & Owings, 1978; Macedonia, 1990; Masataka, 1993; Schwagmeyer & Brown, 1981; Weary & Kramer, 1995), but few have focused explicitly on the responses of developing animals. There are a few notable studies of developing antipredator behavior, however. Miller and his colleagues studied extensively the epigenesis of responses to maternal alarm calls by mallard ducklings (*Anas platyrhynchos*). They investigated a variety of factors that influence the expression of duckling responses to maternal vocalizations, such as call structure (e.g., frequency modulation, repetition rate), the social environment during rearing and testing, and prehatching auditory exposure. Maternal assembly calls elicit behavioral excitation and following, whereas maternal alarm calls lead to behavioral inhibition including freezing and cessation of vocalizations by ducklings. Responses to both maternal calls are well formed at hatching, and the specificity of responses to acoustic stimuli is affected by social rearing (Blaich & Miller, 1986; Miller, 1994; Miller & Blaich, 1984; Miller, Hicinbothom, & Blaich, 1990).

That some animals respond appropriately to acoustic stimuli the first time they are heard does not imply that the behavior is innate or instinctual. Gottlieb's elegant series of studies with ducklings illustrates this point well. Mallard and wood ducklings (*A. platyrhynchos* and *Aix sponsa*, respectively) reared in incubators preferentially approach maternal contact calls of their own species, despite never having heard them before. Maternal contact calls and vocalizations that ducklings make in the egg are acoustically similar, and if ducklings are devocalized and incubated in isolation, they fail to show a preference for their own species' contact calls, and can even develop a preference for another species' maternal call (reviewed in Gottlieb, 1981). In other words, exposure to their own vocalizations prior to hatching is sufficient to induce a preference for their mother's contact calls. Gottlieb's demonstration that normal species-typical experiences can canalize behavioral development underscores the importance of considering all forms of experiential input shaping developing phenotypes, including antipredator strategies.

As part of their research on alarm-call production and responses in adult vervet monkeys (*Cercopithecus aethiops*), Seyfarth and Cheney (1986) reported preliminary data on the development of responses by infants and juveniles. Vervets are preyed upon by a variety of predators, including leopards (*Panthera pardus*), pythons (*Python sebae*), and martial eagles (*Polemaetus bellicosus*). Adults typically (but not always) run up a tree in response to leopard alarm calls, scan the ground in response to snake calls, and look up and/or run into brush after hearing eagle calls. Infants initially run to their mothers when an alarm call is heard, despite having the motor ability to exhibit species-typical responses. As they get older, young cease running to the mother and begin to exhibit adult-like responses, but also exhibit inappropriate, potentially risky responses to calls (e.g., run out of a tree after a leopard call). Finally, by 6 or 7 months of age, most young respond as adults do. The development of infant responses might be socially facilitated, as young are more likely to make an appropriate response if they observe the response of an adult or juvenile monkey before responding.

A behavioral system that required each young animal to learn independently how to recognize and respond to predators would consume time and energy and be prone to fatal errors in learning (Bolles, 1970; Darwin, 1859; Galef, 1976). Reliance on experience, whether it be practice or learning, might at first appear less than optimal, given the vulnerability of young to predators, but a flexible developmental program might be beneficial when predator contexts vary among age groups and among populations, favoring plasticity of species-typical behavior (Johnston, 1982; Shettleworth, 1998). For example, young animals need not spend energy responding to calls that warn of predators that pose no risk to them, such as predators that cannot reach the nest where young are confined (e.g., Magrath, Platzen, & Kondo, 2006), predators which do not inhabit their geographic region (e.g., Coss et al., 1993), or predators which currently do not pose a threat (e.g., a perched raptor; Cheney & Seyfarth, 1990; Robinson, 1980). Likewise, populations that are sympatric with predatory snakes do need to develop antisnake behavior (e.g., tail flagging, throwing dirt; Coss & Biardi, 1997; Hersek & Owings, 1994), whereas populations that do not encounter snakes do not need to learn these responses. Such behavior, then, would not necessarily be present upon first encounter with predators, but would be acquired rapidly with additional exposure (see below).

Development of Antipredator Behavior in Ground Squirrels

Ground-dwelling squirrels (prairie dogs: genus *Cynomys*; marmots: *Marmota*; and ground squirrels: *Spermophilus*) provide an excellent opportunity to examine the conditions that affect the development of alarm-call responses. First, the ecological and social contexts in which adults produce and respond to alarm calls have been well documented. Second, several taxonomic groups prey on ground squirrels, including terrestrial (e.g., bears, coyotes, weasels, martens, venomous snakes) and aerial (e.g., hawks, eagles) predators, and the particular predators ground squirrels face can change temporally and spatially, favoring a plastic learning process. Finally, all mammals face a series of challenges from environmental factors that change markedly during early development; the challenges faced by ground squirrels are especially apparent as young move from the safety of an underground natal burrow to an independent life above ground.

Because ground-dwelling squirrels are vulnerable to both aerial and terrestrial predators, most species produce vocal signals warning of danger from predators (reviewed in Owings & Hennessy, 1984). The complexity of juvenile alarm-call response development will reflect the number of alarm calls in a species' repertoire. Some species produce two or more acoustically distinct calls, which can indicate different predator classes (see below for more on the "meaning" of calls). If each type of alarm call elicits a different, adaptive escape response, then juveniles must not only recognize and discriminate among the calls, they must also acquire the responses that are appropriate to each call. Thus the development of alarm-call responses in juvenile *S. beldingi*, *S. beecheyi*, *S. richardsonii*, *S. parryi*, and *S. armatus*, for example, that have two different alarm calls, might be more complex than in *S. tridecemlineatus*, *S. columbianus*, *S. tereticaudus*, or *C. ludovicianus*, that have a single alarm call (Balph & Balph, 1966; Betts, 1976; Davis, 1984a; Dunford, 1977; Hoogland, 1995; Melchior, 1971; Owings & Virginia, 1978; Schwagmeyer, 1980; Sherman, 1985). Detailed analyses of the development of antipredator behavior are available for few sciurid species (see Davis, 1984a; MacWhirter, 1992; Schwagmeyer & Brown, 1981 for short descriptions of juvenile alarm-call production and responses, and Holmes, 1984; Owings & Loughry, 1985; Owings & Owings, 1979; Poran & Coss, 1990; Randall & Stevens, 1987 for reports of juvenile–predator interactions). Belding's ground squirrels are perhaps the best-studied species, and below I describe the ontogeny of their antipredator repertoires.

Behavioral Ecology of Belding's Ground Squirrels

Belding's ground squirrels (*S. beldingi*) are 200–500 g, group-living, diurnal rodents found in alpine and subalpine regions throughout the western United States. They are socially active above ground between April and August and hibernate alone in the remainder of the year. Mothers mate with multiple males shortly after emerging from torpor, and after ~25 days give birth to a litter of 4–8 pups, which are reared in an underground natal burrow. In this burrow, pups experience a relatively dark, quiet environment, and do not begin to hear alarm calls routinely until just before they first come above ground at around 25 days of age (their "natal emergence"). When young emerge as nearly weaned juveniles, they leave their quiet, well-protected natal burrow and enter a drastically different environment, one that includes increased auditory and visual stimulation, predators, and other ground squirrels that both produce and respond to alarm calls. A few days after natal emergence, young begin to explore the surrounding area that includes other burrows, although the natal burrow will remain the activity center for juveniles for about 2 weeks. During the next month, juveniles must achieve independence from their mother, undergo natal dispersal, establish a hibernaculum, and gain adequate weight to survive the winter, all while avoiding predators, which can account for over 60% of juvenile mortality (Holekamp, 1984; Jenkins & Eshelman, 1984; Mateo, 1996a; Sherman, 1976; Sherman & Morton, 1984).

Belding's ground squirrels emit two sonographically and auditorily distinct alarm calls, whistles and trills, that elicit different behavioral responses and reportedly serve different functions (Leger, Berney-Key, & Sherman, 1984; Mateo, 1996a; Robinson, 1980; Sherman, 1977, 1985). Trills are composed of a series of five or more short duration notes and are elicited by slow-moving predators, primarily terrestrial animals such as coyotes and badgers or other predators that pose no immediate threat (e.g., a perched raptor). Trills usually cause others to post (a bipedal stance accompanied by visual scanning), with or without changing location (Mateo, 1996a). Whistles are single, nonrepetitive high-frequency notes and are elicited by fast-moving, typically aerial, predators or other predators that do pose an immediate threat (e.g., an ambushing coyote). Listeners show evasive behavior such as running to and/or entering a burrow and scanning the area only after reaching safety. Adults produce whistles while running, but emit trills after reaching a safe vantage point. Trills are also elicited in social contexts, such as when a ground squirrel intrudes onto a female's territory, requiring juveniles to learn the difference between predator- and conspecific-elicited trills. The two types of trills can be distinguished acoustically, however, based on fundamental frequency and internote intervals, so that once young learn to discriminate the two, they need not expend energy responding to socially elicited trills.

Alarm-call responses reflect not only the type of call that was emitted, but also the number and age class of callers (Robinson, 1981). Adults are more responsive to trills elicited by predators than by social interactions or nonpredatory animals (such as yellow-bellied marmots, *Marmota flaviventris* or mule deer, *Odocoileus hemionus*). Adults prefer multiple-entrance rather than single-entrance burrows when responding to trills, because terrestrial predators such as badgers (*Taxidea taxus*) and weasels (*Mustela* spp.) can pursue individuals into the tunnel system. Individuals often bypass a closer single-entrance burrow in favor of a burrow with multiple openings that is more distant. Conversely, *S. beldingi* run to the nearest burrow, regardless of its structure, in response to whistles, as the call often signals a fast-moving, stooping avian predator that can approach quickly but cannot enter a burrow (Turner, 1973). Developing juveniles therefore not only have to learn which behavioral responses are associated with each alarm call, but also the spatial configuration of nearby refugia and which burrows to use for each type of alarm call.

Trills are commonly produced by resident adult females with kin, yet there are no effects of age, sex, reproductive status, or kinship on whistle production. Ground squirrels farthest from refuge (and therefore most vulnerable) are more likely to whistle at a distant hawk than those close to refuge, and callers are better able to escape capture by aerial predators than by terrestrial predators (Sherman, 1985). Whistles are difficult to localize because of their acoustic characteristics (Klump & Shalter, 1984; Marler, 1955) and frequently prompt other squirrels to whistle ("whistle chorus"); as a result, whistling imposes little cost on individual callers. By emitting a whistle, the individual most at risk induces other ground squirrels to scatter to burrows, which may "confuse" the predator and increases the caller's likelihood of escape (Leger, Owings, & Gelfand, 1980; Sherman, 1985). Trills, on the other hand, are acoustically easily localized

by conspecifics and predators, and the caller is often visually conspicuous as well (posting upright with mouth open and chest heaving), so the caller is at a much higher risk of capture. The indirect fitness benefits accrued by alerting close kin to possible danger can offset the potentially fatal cost to the triller, and as such females with close kin are more likely to trill than females without close kin and are more likely to trill than males, who disperse and often do not live near kin. In summary, whistles are considered selfish calls that benefit callers as much as receivers, whereas trills are considered nepotistic because of the potential cost to the caller at the benefit of kin (Sherman, 1977, 1985). For trills to have adaptive value, relatives, including young offspring, must respond appropriately to them, again highlighting the need to understand how antipredator repertoires develop.

The "Meaning" of Alarm Calls

Much discussion has been generated concerning the nature of the information that is transmitted by alarm calls (Klump & Shalter, 1984; Macedonia & Evans, 1993; Owings, 1994; Owings & Hennessy, 1984; Seyfarth, Cheney, & Marler, 1980; Sherman, 1985). For instance, in functionally referential signaling systems, vocalizations represent specific external referents (e.g., the "leopard" alarm call warns vervet monkeys of a nearby leopard rather than a nearby snake; Seyfarth et al., 1980). Response-urgency systems, on the other hand, signal the immediacy of danger or constraints on the time available to exhibit a response, such as a "low-urgency" call given by Arctic ground squirrels (*S. parryii*) when a hawk is walking on the ground, and a "high-urgency" call given if a hawk is flying overhead (e.g., Melchior, 1971; Robinson, 1981; reviewed in Owings & Hennessy, 1984). Although some researchers have inferred that referential systems are more cognitively sophisticated than response-urgency systems, and are thus more "evolved", we should instead consider what signaling system will best serve to protect an animal (and/or its kin), depending on its habitat and the hunting style of its predators. In other words, evolution will favor a communication system based on a species' particular needs, and not its phylogenetic group (e.g., Macedonia, 1990).

Marler and his colleagues (1992) suggested two criteria to determine if a species' calls are part of a referential-signaling system. First, calls must be elicited by specific predator classes and should rarely be produced in other contexts ("production specificity"). Second, recipients of the signals must be able to respond appropriately without the benefit of additional cues, such as the nonvocal behavior of the sender or the eliciting stimulus itself ("perception specificity"). In response-urgency systems, a high-urgency call will be given when danger is imminent, regardless of predator type. A review of the data available at the time suggested that the alarm-call systems of two species of primates (vervet monkeys; ring-tailed lemurs, *Lemur catta*) have production specificity whereas those of ground-dwelling squirrels do not (Macedonia & Evans, 1993). However, a closer examination of the original literature indicates that in both primates and sciurids, adults give the "correct" call when they encounter a predator 80%–100% of time (Leger et al., 1984; Macedonia, 1990; Robinson, 1980, 1981; Seyfarth & Cheney, 1980; Sherman, 1985; Turner, 1973), indicating fairly high production specificity.

However, the responses of vervet monkeys to alarm-call playbacks fail to suggest high perceptual specificity, as animals often give "incorrect" behavioral responses or look toward the speaker before responding, indicating that the acoustic stimulus itself is not always sufficient to elicit appropriate escape behavior. In contrast, adult *S. beldingi* show distinct behavioral responses to whistles and trills (Mateo, 1996a; Sherman, 1985). Moreover, adults reliably run to the nearest burrow in response to whistles but might bypass the closest burrow in favor of a more distant two-entrance burrow in response to trills (Mateo, 1995; Turner, 1973), indicating that the calls denote, without additional context, a fast-moving predator posing a significant threat (typically raptors) and a slower-moving predator that might follow the animal into a burrow (e.g., weasel), respectively. Thus the alarm-call system of *S. beldingi* appears to be functionally referential, with whistles referring to aerial predators and trills referring to terrestrial threats, although populations differ in the degree of production specificity (compare Robinson, 1981, with Sherman, 1985 and Turner, 1973).

Ontogeny of *S. beldingi* Antipredator Responses

During their first few days above ground, *S. beldingi* juveniles typically hear alarm calls throughout the day, and at least one predator appears in the area on most days (Robinson, 1980; Sherman, 1976; Mateo 1996a). Despite the regular appearance of predators in ground-squirrel habitat, researchers rarely observe successful predation (Robinson, 1980;

Sherman, 1976; Mateo, personal observations). The high frequency of both predator sightings and the resulting alarm calls, together with the low occurrence of successful hunts, might provide a relatively low-risk opportunity for newly emergent juveniles to observe the responses of adults to alarm calls and to develop their own age-appropriate responses, at a time when they might not be motorically capable of escaping from predators. Newly emergent juveniles are physically uncoordinated, with awkward gaits, poor balance, and tentative movements, and do not appear to distinguish between threatening and nonthreatening visual and auditory stimuli. For example, they might dive below ground if an insect flutters by, but a patient researcher can easily capture them by hand at the burrow entrance (personal observations).

Despite the obvious survival advantage of evading a hunting predator, young need to learn from which animals to flee, to which warning calls to respond, and in what manner. Prior to emerging aboveground for the first time at about 1 month of age, *S. beldingi* pups exhibit different physiological responses to the two alarm calls. Specifically, 20- to 24 day-old pups react with decreased heart rates to playbacks of whistles and increased rates to trills (Mateo, 1996b). However, after natal emergence, juveniles do not discriminate behaviorally between these calls, or even among alarm calls and other conspecific and heterospecific vocalizations. It takes approximately 1 week for juveniles to learn to respond selectively to alarm calls and to ignore calls not associated with threatening stimuli (Figure 32.2, upper panel). During these initial days, juveniles also learn the correct motoric response for each type of call, although behavioral responses continue to change quantitatively over the next several weeks (Mateo, 1996a).

During this early period after natal emergence, up to 60% of juveniles disappear, many to predation (Mateo, 1996a). The frequency of observed predation attempts is often too low to determine what response, if any, the intended victim exhibited and how successful or unsuccessful the response was. However, despite the lack of direct empirical verification that alarm calls reduce the likelihood of successful predation, the advantage of age-appropriate alarm-call responses can be inferred from the significant effect of predation on ground-squirrel populations, especially juveniles (Coss et al., 1993; Hoogland, 1995; Luttich, Rusch, Meslow, & Keith, 1970; Owings & Loughry, 1985; Sherman, 1976). For example, 82 % of aerial-predator hunts

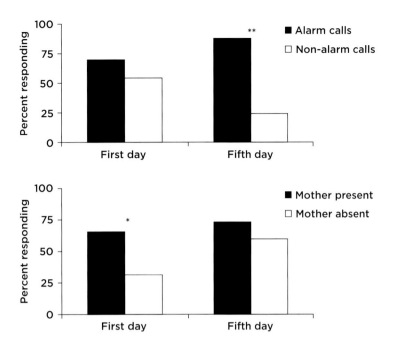

Figure 32.2 Development of alarm-call responses by newly emergent juvenile *S. beldingi*. *Upper panel*: Percentage of juveniles exhibiting a response to alarm-call and nonalarm-call playbacks on their first and fifth day above ground. (Reprinted from Mateo, 1996a.) *Lower panel*: Percentage of juveniles exhibiting a response to alarm-call playbacks on their first and fifth day above ground as a function of their mother's presence (within 5 m) at the time of the playback. Asterisks represent a significant difference (*P < .05, **P < .001) in responsivity.

witnessed by Sherman (1976) were directed toward juveniles. Although there are no data on the relative threat of aerial and terrestrial predators on juveniles, the frequency of hunts by raptors and their fast attack style suggest that juveniles would benefit from developing responses to whistles before responses to trills (which denote slower-moving predators and are also emitted in social encounters; Robinson, 1981; Sherman, 1977). Accordingly, on the first day after natal emergence, juveniles respond reliably to a fast-moving overhead visual stimulus and are more likely to respond to playbacks of whistles than trills (Mateo, 1996a). Altogether, the major source of juvenile mortality is predation by conspecifics and heterospecifics (accounting for 89% of active-season deaths reported by Sherman, 1976). Thus natural selection would favor a rapid acquisition of age-appropriate alarm-call responses by young juveniles.

With respect to age differences in the production of alarm calls, adults give trills and whistles to known predators, whereas young juveniles are likely to give calls to both predators and harmless animals, suggesting a lack of juvenile discrimination in call production (Robinson, 1981; personal observations). Adults are more likely to respond to trills emitted by adults than by juveniles, whereas juveniles responded regardless of a caller's age class (Robinson, 1981; see also Hanson & Coss, 2001; Hersek & Owings, 1994; Seyfarth & Cheney, 1986). Juveniles are equally responsive to playbacks

of their mother's alarm calls and calls of other adults (Mateo & Holmes, 1997).

Factors Influencing the Acquisition of Antipredator Repertoires

That juveniles do not emerge with fully formed alarm-call responses begs the question of how young prey learns to avoid predators. In *S. beldingi*, this learning is facilitated by experience hearing the calls as well as observations of adult reactions. Juveniles attend to and model adult responses, particularly those of their mother rather than those of other nearby females. Juveniles are more likely to respond to alarm calls on their first day above ground if their mother is nearby at the time, but her presence no longer modulates juvenile responsivity by their fifth day, when behavioral discrimination is largely developed (Figure 32.2, lower panel). Furthermore, juveniles adopt a response style similar to their mothers', remaining alert for extended periods if she does, and showing more exaggerated vigilance responses if she does, even when the mother is not visible at the time (Mateo, 1996a; Mateo & Holmes, 1997). Newly emergent juveniles are also more likely to exhibit socially facilitated responses than older juveniles, in which a juvenile does not respond to a call until another ground squirrel exhibits a response, or a juvenile resumes vigilance if nearby individuals continue their vigilant behavior. By attending to the responses of alarm-call experienced adults, juveniles can develop species-appropriate responses to the auditory stimuli earlier than if they do not observe others' responses (Mateo, 1996a).

Juveniles reared in seminatural outdoor enclosures without their mothers after the age of emergence eventually exhibit species-typical responses to alarm calls, but it takes on average 1 day longer for them to show behavioral discrimination of alarm calls and nonalarm calls (Mateo & Holmes, 1997), suggesting that mothers facilitate rather than induce (sensu Gottlieb, 1976) the development of antipredator behavior by their juvenile offspring. This 1-day acceleration in behavioral discrimination might seem trivial, but recall that it takes juveniles up to 5 days to acquire this discrimination and during this period, up to 60% die (Mateo, 1996a). In this light, attending to and modeling mother's responses results in a 20% increase in the rate at which relatively predator-inexperienced juveniles acquire a skill critical to survival.

Natural selection would favor copying of maternal styles if mother's responses are locally adapted to the degree of predation threat in the natal area. Mothers who locate their natal burrows at the edge of meadows are more reactive to alarm calls and remain alert longer than those from the center of a meadow (Mateo, 1996a), which can reflect increased vulnerability to predators near the edge (Elgar, 1989). A mother's reactions, which serve as a model for her offsprings' responses, might reflect her own vulnerabilities, or can be a form of maternal care, becoming more vigilant if she locates her natal burrow, and thus her offspring, in a dangerous area (edge) and less vigilant if in a safer region (center). Note that parents can even teach appropriate responses to their offspring, adjusting their behavior as the competency of their offspring improves (e.g., Caro & Hauser, 1992; Swaisgood, Rowe, & Owings, 2003; Tulley & Huntingford, 1987; White & Berger, 2001). Because juveniles model their responses after their mother's, they are also more alert if reared on the edge of a meadow than in the center (Mateo, 1996a). By acquiring responses that are appropriate for a given microhabitat, *S. beldingi* can optimize both their foraging and antipredator efforts, allowing juveniles (and adults) to gain adequate bodyweight before hibernation without expending energy on unnecessary vigilance (Mateo & Holmes, 1999b). In addition, daughters often nest near their mothers in subsequent years (personal observations), so adopting location-specific responses would be favored across generations.

Plasticity in antipredator behavior is also seen in Rock and California ground squirrels (*S. variegatus, S. beecheyi*), which commonly encounter venomous predatory snakes, including western diamondback rattlesnakes (*Crotalus atrox*) and northern Pacific rattlesnakes (*Crotalus viridis oreganus*). In *S. beecheyi*, predation by snakes accounts for about 40% of pup and juvenile deaths (Fitch, 1948). Animals that are sympatric with venomous snakes need to develop and maintain antisnake behavior, such as tail flagging and substrate throwing toward the snake. In contrast, populations not exposed to venomous snakes fail to exhibit responses to snakes (Coss et al., 1993; Coss & Owings, 1985; Owings, Coss, McKernon, Rowe, & Arrowood, 2001). Population differences in the presence of antisnake tactics suggest that such responses would not necessarily be present upon first encounter with predators, but would be acquired rapidly with additional experience, perhaps through observational learning of their mother's behavior (e.g., Swaisgood, Owings, & Rowe, 1999).

Adult *S. beecheyi* are largely resistant to rattlesnake venom, with resistance higher in populations with high rattlesnake densities. Newly emergent juveniles are also resistant, but because of their small size cannot sufficiently neutralize the venom to survive an attack (Poran & Coss, 1990; Poran, Coss, & Benjamini, 1987). When confronted with a snake, pups and juveniles exhibit snake-directed behavior similar to adults, despite their vulnerability to venom. Coss and his colleagues have suggested that this early onset of risky behavior prior to full development of venom resistance would be favored because the costs of not responding to snakes would be too high (Coss et al., 1993; Coss & Owings, 1978; Poran & Coss, 1990).

Mechanisms and Functions of Plasticity

Juvenile *S. beldingi* born in captivity and housed in a large outdoor enclosure after the age of natal emergence are more responsive to both alarm calls and nonalarm calls, maintain alert behavior longer, exhibit more vigilant postures, and are more likely to run to a refuge than free-living juveniles. Free-living juveniles also begin to discriminate between alarm and nonalarm calls sooner than captive juveniles. These differences in the expression of antipredator behavior are evident within the first week after emergence and persist at least until the age of natal dispersal (Mateo & Holmes, 1999b). A series of studies was conducted to identify the developmental processes contributing to these differences between captive and free-living juveniles (Mateo & Holmes, 1999a). First, because captive ground squirrels did not have to make a trade-off between foraging and vigilance, this may have permitted them to "afford" to be more responsive to playbacks, including spending more time alert (and thus not eating) and expending more energy in their responses, such as running to a burrow rather than posting in place (e.g. Bachman, 1993; Lima, 1998). Yet a comparison of two field-born groups of juveniles and their mothers placed in enclosures after natal emergence, with both groups able to forage on grass but one group also provisioned with chow, yielded no significant differences in alarm-call responses. Second, being in the enclosure with its high walls may have made animals more vigilant, as the walls prevent detection of approaching predators yet at the same time do not provide protective cover (Lazarus & Symonds, 1992; Lima, 1998). A comparison of two additional groups of field-born juveniles, one which was placed in an enclosure and the other which remained in the field, failed to yield any differences in responses. Thus neither foraging pressure nor visual obstructions explained the differences between free-living and captive juveniles reported in Mateo and Holmes (1999b).

Lastly, the effects of preemergent experience on subsequent alarm-call responses were investigated by comparing two more groups of juveniles. Captive-born and reared juveniles experience frequent auditory, visual, and tactile stimulation, as mothers and older juveniles vocalize frequently, lights are on 14 h per day, and pups are handled periodically to monitor their growth. Furthermore, captive mothers are likely in better nutritional condition, as they are provisioned with chow and do not incur the costs of foraging. In contrast, pups in the field experience a relatively quiet, dark natal burrow for about 1 month, exposed only to their littermates' and mother's tactile, thermal, olfactory, and auditory cues. Alarm-call responses of field-born and captive-born juveniles placed in separate enclosures after the age of natal emergence (Mateo & Holmes, 1999a) mirrored those originally described for those living in the field and those living in captivity (Mateo & Holmes, 1999b). Thus differences in antipredator repertoires are attributable to pre- rather than postemergent environments; it is unclear which particular experiences affect future antipredator responses, but they likely include differential exposure to both species-specific and nonspecific auditory stimulation. In captivity, pups and mothers rarely trill or whistle inside their nestboxes (personal observations), but it remains unknown whether ground squirrels vocalize within their burrow systems. This variation in preemergence stimulation might help explain population differences in antipredator behavior (see below).

The heightened responsiveness to auditory stimuli by captive ground squirrels may result from stimulation of all sensory modalities prior to natal emergence. Experiential enhancement, or early stimulation at greater-than-species-typical levels, can influence the later expression of behavioral traits (Miller, 1981). For example, quail chicks (*Colinus virginianus*) exposed to enhanced auditory stimulation prior to hatching exhibited increased visual (but not auditory) responsiveness after hatching (Lickliter & Stoumbos, 1991). Rat pups reared in a quiet laboratory environment during the pre- or postweaning period (similar to natural *S. beldingi* natal burrows) defecate less frequently in open-field tests than pups reared in standard laboratory rooms (Denenberg et al., 1966). Great-tit nestlings (*Parus major*) exposed to higher-than-normal levels of alarm calls paired with a model predator were subsequently more responsive to alarm calls (as evidenced by their cessation-of-begging response; Rydén, 1978). Thus the amount of exposure to auditory, visual, and tactile cues may have influenced the ontogeny of alarm-call responses by *S. beldingi* pups, causing them to be more reactive to auditory stimuli they experienced as juveniles.

Alternatively, the timing rather than the type of stimulation may modulate alarm-call response development, much as it influences the development of bird song (Marler, 1987). For example, premature stimulation of a later-developing sensory system can influence the functioning of earlier-developing systems (Turkewitz & Kenny, 1982). Ducklings (*A. platyrhynchos*) must hear conspecific vocalizations prior to hatching (their own or siblings' vocalizations) if they are to respond appropriately to hens' alarm calls after hatching (e.g. Blaich & Miller, 1988; Miller & Blaich, 1984). Early experience with predators, with predator-experienced parents or with agonistic adult conspecifics, affects later responses by young fish, particularly those from high-predation populations (Goodey & Liley, 1986; Magurran, 1990; Tulley & Huntingford, 1987; but see Wright & Huntingford, 1993). Late prehatching experience with alarm calls attenuates posthatching responsivity of chicks to those calls

(Impekoven, 1976; Vince, 1980). In *S. beldingi*, differences in preemergent, but not postemergent, environments affect the development of responses to conspecific alarm vocalizations (Mateo & Holmes, 1999a, 1999b).

One possible function of *S. beldingi* pups' sensitivity to their early environment would be to prepare juveniles in sites with high predation risk for increased vigilance, and prepare juveniles in low-risk sites for reduced vigilance and, perhaps, increased foraging effort. Populations differ in how frequently they produce alarm calls (Mateo, 2007), and as a result developing pups will be differentially exposed to calls, particularly in the last few days before emergence when young are spending time in their natal burrow near the exit. Ground squirrels can thus adjust their postemergent vigilance according to their preemergent auditory exposure to conspecific alarm calls. The selective advantage to this experiential "priming" is rapid acquisition of location-appropriate alarm-call responses and an optimal trade-off between vigilance and foraging efforts.

Although the above discussion focused on external stimuli and their influence on juvenile response development, the rearing effects found in Mateo and Holmes (1999a, 1999b) could also have physiological causes. For example, in addition to serving as a model for appropriate antipredator responses (Mateo & Holmes, 1997), a mother can indirectly affect her offsprings' physiology, such as adrenal functioning, that can further modulate responses to predators. For seasonally breeding ground squirrels, the first emergence of young from natal burrows is fairly synchronous; in *S. beldingi* 100–200 juveniles typically emerge within a 10-day period (personal observations). Not surprisingly, this natal emergence draws predators, and direct encounters with predators, observations of sudden, rapid responses of nearby adults, and experience with hearing loud alarm calls likely cause changes in circulating glucocorticoids of adults and offspring alike. The range of acute cortisol responses to these events depends on the particular stressor as well as an individual's hypothalamic-pituitary-adrenal (HPA) axis (Mateo & Cavigelli, 2005; unlike rats and mice, most rodents produce both cortisol and corticosterone, with one being the predominant circulating glucocorticoid). Maternal stress responses can affect the HPA functioning of their offspring, and thus a mother's hormonal patterns can have long-lasting effects on those of her offspring (e.g., Barbazanges, Piazza, Le Moal, & Maccari, 1996;

Catalani, 1997; Maccari, Piazza, Barbazanges, Simon, & Le Moal, 1995; Smith, Seckl, Evans, Costall, & Smythe, 2004).

In this manner, variation in adrenal functioning can be transmitted across generations nongenetically (e.g., Liu et al., 1997; Meaney, 2001) and can have adaptive consequences for offspring. Mothers and their young living near the edge of meadows are more vigilant and exhibit prolonged alarm-call responses, and they have lower basal cortisol levels compared with *S. beldingi* from the center of the meadow (Mateo, 1996a, 2008). At a larger scale, *S. beldingi* living in sites where they experience greater predation risk spend more time vigilant and less time feeding, and show longer and more exaggerated alarm-call responses, compared with those living in other sites with less predation risk. At the high-risk site, both juveniles and adults have lower basal cortisol than *S. beldingi* at the lower-risk sites (Mateo, 2006, 2007). This lower basal cortisol allows animals to mount large acute responses, mobilizing energy for quick escapes from ambushing predators (Mateo, 2007).

Maternal glucocorticoids can affect the rate at which young acquire important behavioral repertoires. In laboratory rodents, the influence of glucocorticoids on learning and memory has an inverted-U shaped function. Very low or very high levels of corticoids can lead to hypo- or hyperarousal and poor selective attention to input and thus impair consolidation of new memories. Moderate levels of corticoids are optimal for attention to and consolidation of memories (reviewed in Lupien & McEwen, 1997). Maternal glucocorticoids transmitted to offspring during gestation or lactation can have long-term effects on offspring hormones, and this "set point" might promote learning of antipredator responses, particularly in animals inhabiting areas with high predation risk. There have been few investigations of how glucocorticoids affect learning in free-living animals (see Pfeffer, Fritz, & Kotrschal, 2002; Pravosudov, 2003; Saldanha, Schlinger, & Clayton, 2000), and there have been no studies of their effects on antipredator behavior. However, in recent experiments with *S. beldingi*, maternal cortisol was noninvasively manipulated during lactation to affect offspring HPA functioning. Juveniles were tested for their spatial and associative-learning abilities, simulating how they would learn their mother's burrow system and the location of refugia, as well as how they would learn to associate vocalizations with the appropriate escape response.

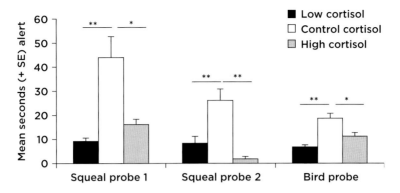

Figure 32.3 Effects of cortisol on acquisition and retention of multiple-trial and single-trial associative learning. Newly emergent juveniles with naturally elevated cortisol ("Control"; mean cortisol 648.70 ng/g dried feces + 42.38) or experimentally decreased ("Low"; 404.87 + 47.18) or increased ("High"; 768.68 + 72.59; significantly higher than the Control group) cortisol experienced pairings of a *S. beldingi* squeal vocalization (typically made during play) with a frisbee on Days 1–5, simulating an aerial predator and warning call. During these training trials all ground squirrels responded to the squeal as if it warned of an aerial predator, running to a burrow and often going belowground. Day 6 was Probe 1 with the call itself, testing for retention of the association; Day 10 (Probe 2) was the second retention trial. Later Day 10 a blackbird call was paired once with the frisbee, and memory of the pairing was tested Day 11 with a Bird Probe. Data show duration of alert behavior following onset of playback of probes. Asterisks represent significant differences (*$P < .05$, **$P < .001$) in time spent alert based on Bonferroni-adjusted post-hoc pairwise t-test comparisons for significant ANOVAs on log-transformed data. Both low and high cortisol interfered with acquisition and retention of the associations, whereas moderate elevation of cortisol promoted learning. (Reprinted from *Neurobiology of Learning and Memory*, Vol. 89, by Jill M. Mateo, "Inverted—U shape relationship between cortisol and learning in ground squirrels, pages 582–590, Copyright 2008, with permission from Elsevier.)

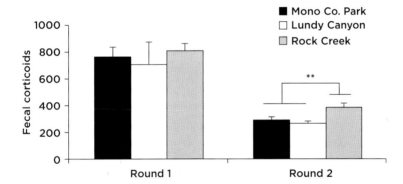

Figure 32.4 Patterns of developmental and geographic variation in fecal corticoids (mean ng/g dried feces + SE) of free-living juvenile *S. beldingi* from three populations in the eastern Sierra of California. Unadjusted fecal cortisol levels are shown; analyses were based on log-transformed data, with asterisks representing significant differences (**$P < .001$) in cortisol. Round 1 represents fecal sampling during the first 5 days after natal emergence and Round 2 occurred approximately 2 weeks later. (Reprinted from Mateo, 2006.)

Consistent with the inverted-U shaped relationship between glucocorticoids and learning in inbred strains of laboratory rodents, juvenile *S. beldingi* with moderately elevated cortisol after emergence acquire the two tasks faster than those with low or very high basal cortisol (e.g., Figure 32.3; Mateo, 2008). In all *S. beldingi* populations studied to date, cortisol increases in juveniles just after their natal emergence, and remains elevated for about 5 days (Figure 32.4; see also Mateo, 2006), corresponding with when they are learning their alarm-call

responses and the spatial configurations of their mother's territory (Mateo, 1996a).

Concluding Remarks

When juvenile Belding's ground squirrels first emerge above ground at about 1 month of age, they are not armed with a fixed, well-established antipredator repertoire. Instead, it takes them almost 1 week to discriminate between alarm calls and nonthreatening calls, and to learn which behavioral responses are appropriate for each alarm-call type. Although young squirrels are most susceptible to predation at this age, this lack of behavioral discrimination at emergence could be favored by natural selection if the local predator environment changes spatially or temporally within or across different populations of *S. beldingi*. This can include changes in predator species, numbers of predators, type of habitat, and availability of refuges (Mateo, 2007). Prey species must be able to modify their antipredator response repertoires to such changes, and a plastic developmental program is one mechanism by which animals can adjust their behavior in response to the unique features of the local predator environment (Mateo & Holmes, 1999a, 1999b).

Animals can receive many benefits from group living, including a reduction of time spent on vigilance by individuals as group size increases (Alexander, 1974). Another benefit for *S. beldingi* is that young can develop survival skills at a faster rate by observing nearby conspecifics, which therefore increases their likelihood of successfully escaping from predators. Adults do not directly guide juvenile responses, such as by running to young when an alarm call is heard or by herding young into a safe burrow. Instead, adults indirectly facilitate (sensu Gottlieb, 1976) response development, as their own alarm-call responses serve as models of appropriate reactions for juveniles (Mateo & Holmes, 1997).

Accordingly, the process of antipredator behavioral development will vary with the costs of learning as well as with opportunities for learning (see also Mateo, 2009). First, plasticity will be favored when the costs of learning (e.g. fatal mistakes during learning or formation of "incorrect" associations) do not outweigh its benefits (Johnston, 1982). For instance, high predation pressure will discourage variable developmental pathways to antipredator behavior whereas populations experiencing low predation can exhibit more plastic behavior during development (e.g., compare defensive responses of nestling black-headed gulls and kittiwakes; Cullen, 1957). The particular habitat in which an organism develops can also attenuate the costs of learning. As an example, trial-and-error learning might be less dangerous for terrestrial animals than for arboreal animals, as the risks incurred by inappropriate escape movements will differ in the two niches.

Second, the developmental process will be influenced by opportunities to observe the responses of experienced individuals, as animals that incorporate the behavior of others might commit fewer, potentially fatal, errors than those that independently acquire such behavior (Galef, 1976; Mateo

& Holmes, 1997). These opportunities vary with relative degrees of precocity in sensory and motor abilities as well as with periods of dependence upon adults. For instance, spider monkeys (*Ateles paniscus*) do not move independently until over 1 year of age (Symington, 1988), and thus can safely observe their mother's reactions to predators and alarm calls longer than vervet monkeys, which are carried less frequently after 4 months of age (Cheney & Seyfarth, 1990). Likewise, the antipredator behavior of altricial young that follow or are carried by their mothers (e.g., reindeer, *Rangifer tarandus*: Espmark, 1971; ring-tailed lemurs: van Schaik & Kappeler, 1993) might be facilitated by social factors more than those that are "hidden" or "parked" by their mothers during daily foraging periods (e.g. roe deer, *Capreolus capreolus*: Espmark, 1969; ruffed lemurs, *Varecia variega*: van Schaik & Kappeler, 1993). Brown (1984) studied the development of antipredator behavior in two bass species differing in the length of time fathers guard their young. Recently hatched young of a species with limited paternal care (*Ambloplites rupestris*) show predator-avoidance behavior sooner than young of a species with extended care (*Micropterus salmoides*). Mexican jays (*Aphelocoma ultramarina*) with prolonged associations with experienced adults exhibit mobbing behavior at a later age than less social scrub jays (*Aphelocoma coerulescens*) that fledge at an earlier age (Culley & Ligon, 1976). Finally, delayed natal dispersal can provide young with more opportunities to observe conspecifics and subsequently practice their responses with fewer costs than early dispersing species, particularly for less urgent antipredator behavior such as mobbing (e.g., Culley & Ligon, 1976).

Historically, developmental studies of antipredator behavior have been predominated by research on fish and reptile species (reviewed in Burghardt, 1978; Endler, 1995; Huntingford & Wright, 1993). Studies of the ontogeny of communicative behavior have also largely ignored mammals, with most research on vocal development concentrated on birds (e.g., Kroodsma, 1988; Marler, 1987) and a limited number of primates (e.g., Cheney & Seyfarth, 1990; Snowdon, 1988). In addition, detailed studies on the ontogeny of responses to alarm calls have been largely limited to young birds or vervet monkeys (e.g., Buitron & Nuechterlein, 1993; Cheney & Seyfarth, 1990; Curio, 1993; Miller et al., 1990), and the development of responses to predator odors (e.g., Brown & Chivers, 2006) or to visual displays associated with predators (such as mobbing reactions) have been well studied in a few species (e.g., Curio, 1975; Culley & Ligon, 1976; Owings & Coss, 1977). The ground-squirrel studies described above are some of the first to examine the development of antipredator behavior in a mammal from before birth to adulthood. For all taxonomic groups, more research is needed incorporating multiple levels of analysis (Tinbergen, 1963) to understand how social environments interact with endocrinological and neural processes to mediate plasticity in antipredator repertoires, and how those mechanisms are shaped by ecological factors and, ultimately, evolutionary forces.

References

Alberts, J. R. (1987). Early learning and ontogenetic adaptation. In N. A. Krasnegor, E. M. Blass, M. A. Hofer & W. P. Smotherman (Eds.), *Perinatal development: A psychobiological perspective* (pp. 11–37). Orlando: Academic Press.

Alexander, R. D. (1974). The evolution of social behavior. *Annual Review of Ecology and Systematics, 5*, 325–383.

Bachman, G. C. (1993). The effect of body condition on the trade-off between vigilance and foraging in Belding's ground squirrels. *Animal Behaviour, 46*, 233–244.

Balph, D. M., & Balph, D. F. (1966). Sound communication of Uinta ground squirrels. *Journal of Mammalogy, 47*, 440–450.

Barbazanges, A., Piazza, P. V., Le Moal, M., & Maccari, S. (1996). Maternal glucocorticoid secretion mediates long-term effects of prenatal stress. *Journal of Neuroscience, 16*, 3943–3949.

Betts, B. J. (1976). Behaviour in a population of Columbian ground squirrels. *Spermophilus columbianus columbianus. Animal Behaviour, 24*, 652–680.

Blaich, C. F., & Miller, D. B. (1986). Alarm call responsivity of mallard ducklings (*Anas platyrhynchos*). IV. Effects of social experience. *Journal of Comparative Psychology, 100*, 401–405.

Blaich, C. F., & Miller, D. B. (1988). Alarm call responsivity of mallard ducklings (*Anas platyrhynchos*): VI. Effects of sibling and self-produced auditory stimulation. *Journal of Comparative Psychology, 102*, 56–60.

Bolles, R. C. (1970). Species-specific defense reactions and avoidance learning. *Psychological Reviews, 77*, 32–48.

Brown, J. A. (1984). Parental care and the ontogeny of predator-avoidance in two species of centrarchid fish. *Animal Behaviour, 32*, 113–119.

Brown, G. E., & Chivers, D. P. (2006). Learning about danger: chemical alarm cues and the assessment of predation risk by fishes. In C. Brown, K. Laland & J. Krause (Eds.), *Fish cognition and behavior* (pp. 49–69). Oxford: Blackwell Publishing.

Buitron, D., & Nuechterlein, G. L. (1993). Parent–young vocal communication in eared grebes. *Behaviour, 127*, 1–20.

Burghardt, G. M. (1978). Behavioral ontogeny in reptiles: Whence, whither and why. In G. M. Burghardt & M. Bekoff (Eds.), *The development of behavior: Comparative and evolutionary aspects* (pp. 149–174). New York: Garland STPM Press.

Caro, T. M. (1994). *Cheetahs of the Serengeti plains: Group living in an asocial species*. Chicago: University of Chicago Press.

Caro, T. M., & Hauser, M. D. (1992). Is there teaching in non-human animals? *Quarterly Review of Biology, 67*, 151–174.

Catalani, A. (1997). Neonatal exposure to glucocorticoids: Long-term endocrine and behavioral effects. *Developmental Brain Dysfunction, 10*, 393–404.

Cheney, D. L., & Seyfarth, R. M. (1990). *How monkeys see the world*. Chicago: University of Chicago Press.

Coss, R. G., & Biardi, J. E. (1997). Individual variation in the antisnake behavior of California ground squirrels (*Spermophilus beecheyi*). *Journal of Mammalogy, 78*, 294–310.

Coss, R. G., Guse, K. L., Poran, N. S., & Smith, D. G. (1993). Development of antisnake defenses in California ground squirrels (*Spermophilus beecheyi*): II. Microevolutionary effects of relaxed selection from rattlesnakes. *Behaviour, 124*, 137–164.

Coss, R. G., & Owings, D. H. (1978). Snake-directed behavior by snake naive and experienced California ground squirrels in a simulated burrow. *Zeitschrift für Tierpsychologie, 48*, 421–435.

Coss, R. G., & Owings, D. H. (1985). Restraints on ground squirrel antipredator behavior: Adjustments over multiple time scales. In T. D. Johnston & A. T. Pietrewicz (Eds.), *Issues in the Ecological Study of Learning* (pp. 167–200). Hillsdale, NJ: Lawrence Erlbaum Associates.

Cullen, E. (1957). Adaptations in the kittiwake to cliff nesting. *Ibis, 99*, 275–302.

Culley, J. F., Jr., & Ligon, J. D. (1976). Comparative mobbing behavior of scrub and Mexican jays. *Auk, 93*, 116–125.

Curio, E. (1975). The functional organization of anti-predator behaviour in the pied flycatcher: A study of avian visual perception. *Animal Behaviour, 23*, 1–115.

Curio, E. (1993). Proximate and developmental aspects of antipredator behavior. In P. J. B. Slater, J. S. Rosenblatt, C. T. Snowdon & M. Milinski (Eds.), *Advances in the study of behavior* (Vol. 22, pp. 135–238). New York: Academic Press.

Darwin, C. (1859). *On the origin of species*. London: J. Murray.

Davis, L. S. (1984a). Alarm calling in Richardson's ground squirrels (*Spermophilus richardsonii*). *Zeitschrift für Tierpsychologie, 66*, 152–164.

Davis, L. S. (1984b). Kin selection and adult female Richardson's ground squirrels: a test. *Canadian Journal of Zoology, 62*, 2344–2348.

Dawkins, R., & Krebs, J. R. (1978). *Animal signals: Information or manipulation*. Paper presented at the Behavioural Ecology, Sunderland, MA.

Denenberg, V. H., Schell, S. F., Karas, G. G., & Haltmeyer, G. C. (1966). Comparison of background stimulation and handling as forms of infantile stimulation. *Psychological Reports, 19*, 943–948.

Dunford, C. A. N., (1977). Kin selection for ground squirrel alarm calls. *American Naturalist, 111*, 782–785.

Elgar, M. A. (1989). Predator vigilance and group size in mammals and birds: A critical review of the empirical evidence. *Biological Review, 64*, 13–33.

Endler, J. A. (1995). Multiple-trait coevolution and environmental gradients in guppies. *Trends in Ecology and Evolution, 10*, 22–29.

Espmark, Y. (1969). Mother–young relations and development of behaviour in roe deer (*Capreolus capreolus* L.). *Swedish Wildlife Research, 6*, 461–540.

Espmark, Y. (1971). Mother–young relationship and ontogeny of behaviour in reindeer (*Rangifer tarandus* L.). *Zeitschrift für Tierpsychologie, 29*, 42–81.

Evans, C. S., Evans, L., & Marler, P. (1993). On the meaning of alarm calls: Functional reference in an avian vocal system. *Animal Behaviour, 46*, 23–38.

Ferrari, M. C. O., Trowell, J. J., Brown, G. E., & Chivers, D. P. (2005). The role of learning in the development of threat-sensitive predator avoidance by fathead minnows. *Animal Behaviour, 70*, 777–784.

Fitch, H. S. (1948). Ecology of the California ground squirrel on grazing lands. *American Midland Naturalist, 39*, 513–596.

Francis, A. M., Hailman, J. P., & Woolfenden, G. E. (1989). Mobbing by Florida scrub jays: Behaviour, sexual asymmetry, role of helpers and ontogeny. *Animal Behaviour, 38*, 795–816.

Galef, B. G., Jr. (1976). Social transmission of acquired behavior: A discussion of tradition and social learning in vertebrates. In J. S. Rosenblatt, R. A. Hinde, S. E. & C. Beer (Eds.), *Advances in the study of behavior* (Vol. 6, pp. 77–100). New York: Academic Press.

Goodey, W., & Liley, N. R. (1986). The influence of early experience on escape behaviour in the guppy. *Canadian Journal of Zoology, 64*, 885–888.

Gottlieb, G. (1976). The roles of experience in the development of behavior and the nervous system. In G. Gottlieb (Ed.), *Studies on the development of behavior and the nervous system. Vol. 3 Neural and behavioral specificity* (pp. 25–53). New York: Academic Press.

Gottlieb, G. (1981). Roles of early experience in species-specific perceptual development. In R. N. Aslin, J. R. Alberts & M. R. Petersen (Eds.), *Development of perception* (Vol. 1, pp. 5–44). New York: Academic Press.

Guilford, T., & Dawkins, M. S. (1991). Receiver psychology and the evolution of animal signals. *Animal Behaviour, 42*, 1–14.

Hanson, M. T., & Coss, R. G. (2001). Age differences in the response of California ground squirrels (*Spermophilus beecheyi*) to conspecific alarm calls. *Ethology, 107*, 259–275.

Harris, M. A., Murie, J. O., & Duncan, J. A. (1983). Responses of Columbian ground squirrels to playback of recorded calls. *Zeitschrift für Tierpsychologie, 63*, 318–330.

Hauser, M. D. (1988). How infant vervet monkeys learn to recognize starling alarm calls: The role of experience. *Behaviour, 105*, 187–201.

Heaton, M. B., Miller, D. B., & Goodwin, D. G. (1978). Species-specific auditory discrimination in bobwhite quail neonates. *Developmental Psychobiology, 11*, 13–21.

Hersek, M. J., & Owings, D. H. (1994). Tail flagging by young California ground squirrels, *Spermophilus beecheyi*: Age-specific participation in a tonic communicative system. *Animal Behaviour, 48*, 803–811.

Herzog, M., & Hopf, S. (1984). Behavioral responses to species-specific warning calls in infant squirrel monkeys reared in isolation. *American Journal of Primatology, 7*, 99–106.

Holekamp, K. E. (1984). Natal dispersal in Belding's ground squirrels (*Spermophilus beldingi*). *Behavioral Ecology and Sociobiology, 16*, 21–30.

Holmes, W. G. (1984). Predation risk and foraging behavior of the hoary marmot in Alaska. *Behavioral Ecology and Sociobiology, 15*, 293–301.

Hoogland, J. L. (1995). *The black-tailed prairie dog: Social life of a burrowing mammal.* Chicago: University of Chicago Press.

Huntingford, F. A., & Wright, P. J. (1993). The development of adaptive variation in predator avoidance in freshwater fishes. *Marine Behaviour & Physiology, 23*, 45–61.

Impekoven, M. (1976). Responses of laughing gull chicks (*Larus atricilla*) to parental attraction- and alarm-calls, and effects of prenatal auditory experience on the responsiveness to such calls. *Behaviour, 56*, 250–277.

Jenkins, S. H., & Eshelman, B. D. (1984). *Spermophilus beldingi. Mammalian Species, 221*, 1–8.

Johnston, T. D. (1982). Selective costs and benefits in the evolution of learning. In J. S. Rosenblatt, R. A. Hinde, C. Beer & M.-C. Busnel (Eds.), *Advances in the study of behavior* (Vol. 12, pp. 65–106). New York: Academic Press.

Johnston, T. D. (1987). The persistence of dichotomies in the study of behavioral development. *Developmental Review, 7*, 149–182.

Klump, G. M., & Shalter, M. D. (1984). Acoustic behaviour of birds and mammals in the predator context. II. The functional significance and evolution of alarm signals. *Zeitschrift für Tierpsychologie, 66*, 206–226.

Kroodsma, D. E. (1988). Contrasting styles of song development and their consequences among passerine birds. In R. C. Bolles & M. D. Beecher (Eds.), *Evolution and learning* (pp. 157–184). Hillsdale, NJ: Lawrence-Erlbaum Associates.

Lazarus, J. & Symonds, M. (1992). Contrasting effects of protective and obstructive cover on avian vigilance. *Animal Behaviour, 43*, 519–521.

Leger, D. W., Berney-Key, S. D., & Sherman, P. W. (1984). Vocalizations of Belding's ground squirrels (*Spermophilus beldingi*). *Animal Behaviour, 32*, 753–764.

Leger, D. W., & Owings, D. H. (1978). Responses to alarm calls by California ground squirrels: Effects of call structure and maternal status. *Behavioral Ecology and Sociobiology, 3*, 177–186.

Leger, D. W., Owings, D. H., & Gelfand, D. L. (1980). Single-note vocalizations of California ground squirrels: Graded signals and situation-specificity of predator and socially evoked calls. *Zeitschrift für Tierpsychologie, 52*, 227–246.

Lehrman, D. S. (1970). Semantic and conceptual issues in the nature–nurture problem. In L. R. Aronson, E. Tobach, D. S. Lehrman & J. S. Rosenblatt (Eds.), *Development and evolution of behavior* (pp. 17–52). San Francisco: W. H. Freeman.

Lickliter, R., & Stoumbos, J. (1991). Enhanced prenatal auditory experience facilitates species-specific visual responsiveness in bobwhite quail chicks (*Colinus virginianus*). *Journal of Comparative Psychology, 105*, 89–94.

Lima, S. L. (1998). Stress and decision making under the risk of predation: Recent developments from behavioral, reproductive, and ecological perspectives. *Advances in the Study of Behavior, 27*, 215–290.

Liu, D., Diorio, J., Tannenbaum, B., Caldji, C., Francis, D., Freedman, A., Sharma, S., Pearson, D., Plotsky, P. M., & Meaney, M. J. (1997). Maternal care, hippocampal glucocorticoid receptors, and hypothalamic-pituitary-adrenal responses to stress. *Science, 277*, 1659–1662.

Lupien, S. J., & McEwen, B. S. (1997). The acute effects of corticosteroids on cognition: Integration of animal and human model studies. *Brain Research Reviews, 24*, 1–27.

Luttich, S., Rusch, D. H., Meslow, E. C., & Keith, L. B. (1970). Ecology of red-tailed hawk predation in Alberta. *Ecology, 51*, 190–203.

Maccari, S., Piazza, P. V., Barbazanges, A., Simon, H., & Le Moal, M. (1995). Adoption reverses the long-term impairment in glucocorticoid feedback induced by prenatal stress. *Journal of Neuroscience, 15*, 110–116.

Macedonia, J. M. (1990). What is communicated in the antipredator calls of lemurs: Evidence from playback experiments with ringtailed and ruffed lemurs. *Ethology, 86*, 177–190.

Macedonia, J. M., & Evans, C. S. (1993). Variation among mammalian alarm call systems and the problem of meaning in animal signals. *Ethology, 93*, 177–197.

MacWhirter, R. B. (1992). Vocal and escape responses of Columbian ground squirrels to simulated terrestrial and aerial predator attacks. *Ethology, 91*, 311–325.

Magrath, R. D., Platzen, D., & Kondo, J. (2006). From nestling calls to fledgling silence: adaptive timing of change in response to aerial alarm calls. *Proceedings of the Royal Society of London. Series B: Biological Sciences, 273*, 2335–2341.

Magurran, A. E. (1990). The inheritance and development of minnow anti-predator behaviour. *Animal Behaviour, 39*, 834–842.

Marler, P. (1955). Characteristics of some animal calls. *Nature, 176*, 6–8.

Marler, P. (1987). Sensitive periods and the roles of specific and general sensory stimulation in birdsong learning. In J. P. Rauschecker & P. Marler (Eds.), *Imprinting and cortical plasticity* (pp. 99–135). New York: Wiley & Sons.

Marler, P., Evans, C. S., & Hauser, M. (1992). Animal signals: motivational, referential or both? In H. Papousek, U. Jurgens & M. Papousek (Eds.), *Non-verbal vocal communication: Comparative and developmental approaches* (pp. 66–86). Cambridge: Cambridge University Press.

Masataka, N. (1993). Effects of experience with live insects on the development of fear of snakes in squirrel monkeys, *Saimiri sciureus. Animal Behaviour, 46*, 741–746.

Mateo, J. M. (1995). *The development of alarm-call responses in free-living and captive Belding's ground squirrels, Spermophilus beldingi.* Unpublished doctoral dissertation, University of Michigan.

Mateo, J. M. (1996a). The development of alarm-call response behaviour in free-living juvenile Belding's ground squirrels. *Animal Behaviour, 52*, 489–505.

Mateo, J. M. (1996b). Early auditory experience and the ontogeny of alarm-call discrimination in Belding's ground squirrels (*Spermophilus beldingi*). *Journal of Comparative Psychology, 110*, 115–124.

Mateo, J. M. (2006). Developmental and geographic variation in stress hormones in wild Belding's ground squirrels (*Spermophilus beldingi*). *Hormones and Behavior, 50*, 718–725.

Mateo, J. M. (2007). Ecological and physiological correlates of anti-predator behaviors of Belding's ground squirrels (*Spermophilus beldingi*). *Behavioral Ecology and Sociobiology, 62*, 37–49.

Mateo, J.M. (2008). Inverted-U shape relationship between cortisol and learning in ground squirrels. *Neurobiology of Learning and Memory, 89*, 582–590.

Mateo, J. M. (2009). Maternal influences on development, social relationships and survival behaviors. In D. Maestripieri & J. M. Mateo (Eds.), *Maternal effects in mammals*. Chicago: University of Chicago Press.

Mateo, J. M., & Cavigelli, S. A. (2005). A validation of extraction methods for non-invasive sampling of glucocorticoids in free-living ground squirrels. *Physiological and Biochemical Zoology, 78*, 1069–1084.

Mateo, J. M., & Holmes, W. G. (1997). Development of alarm-call responses in Belding's ground squirrels: The role of dams. *Animal Behaviour, 54*, 509–524.

Mateo, J. M., & Holmes, W. G. (1999a). How rearing history affects alarm-call responses of Belding's ground squirrels (*Spermophilus beldingi*, Sciuridae). *Ethology, 105*, 207–222.

Mateo, J. M., & Holmes, W. G. (1999b). Plasticity of alarm-call response development in Belding's ground squirrels (*Spermophilus beldingi*, Sciuridae). *Ethology, 105*, 193–206.

Meaney, M. J. (2001). Maternal care, gene expression, and the transmission of individual differences in stress reactivity across generations. *Annual Review of Neuroscience, 24*, 1161–1192.

Melchior, H. R. (1971). Characteristics of Arctic ground squirrel alarm calls. *Oecologia, 7*, 184–190.

Miller, D. B. (1981). Conceptual strategies in behavioral development: Normal development and plasticity. In K. Immelmann, G. W. Barlow, L. Petrinovich & M. Main (Eds.), *Behavioral development* (pp. 58–85). New York: Cambridge University Press.

Miller, D. B. (1988). Development of instinctive behavior: An epigenetic and ecological approach. In E. M. Blass (Ed.), *Handbook of behavioral neurobiology* (Vol. 9, pp. 415–444). New York: Plenum Press.

Miller, D. B. (1994). Social context affects the ontogeny of instinctive behaviour. *Animal Behaviour, 48*, 627–634.

Miller, D. B., & Blaich, C. F. (1984). Alarm call responsivity of mallard ducklings: The inadequacy of learning and genetic explanation of instinctive behavior. *Learning and Motivation, 15*, 417–427.

Miller, D. B., Hicinbothom, G., & Blaich, C. F. (1990). Alarm call responsivity of mallard ducklings: Multiple pathways in behavioural development. *Animal Behaviour, 39*, 1207–1212.

Owings, D. H. (1994). How monkeys feel about the world: A review of *How monkeys see the world. Language & Communication, 14*, 15–30.

Owings, D. H., & Coss, R. G. (1977). Snake mobbing by California ground squirrels: Adaptive variation and ontogeny. *Behaviour, 62*, 50–69.

Owings, D. H., Coss, R. G., McKernon, D., Rowe, M. P., & Arrowood, P. C. (2001). Snake-directed antipredator behavior of rock squirrels (*Spermophilus variegatus*): Population differences and snake-species discrimination. *Behaviour, 138*, 575–595.

Owings, D. H., & Hennessy, D. F. (1984). The importance of variation in sciurid visual and vocal communication. In J. O. Murie & G. R. Michener (Eds.), *The biology of ground-dwelling squirrels: Annual cycles, behavioral ecology, and sociality* (pp. 169–200). Lincoln, NE: University of Nebraska Press.

Owings, D. H., & Loughry, W. J. (1985). Variation in snake-elicited jump-yipping by black-tailed prairie dogs: Ontogeny and snake-specificity. *Zeitschrift für Tierpsychologie, 70*, 177–200.

Owings, D. H., & Owings, S. C. (1979). Snake-directed behavior by black-tailed prairie dogs (*Cynomys ludovicianus*). *Zeitschrift für Tierpsychologie, 49*, 35–54.

Owings, D. H., & Virginia, R. A. (1978). Alarm calls of California ground squirrels (*Spermophilus beecheyi*). *Zeitschrift für Tierpsychologie, 46*, 58–70.

Pfeffer, K., Fritz, J., & Kotrschal, K. (2002). Hormonal correlates of being an innovative greylag goose, *Anser anser*. *Animal Behaviour, 63*, 687–695.

Poran, N. S., & Coss, R. G. (1990). Development of antisnake defenses in California ground squirrels (*Spermophilus beecheyi*): I. Behavioral and immunological relationships. *Behaviour, 112*, 222–245.

Poran, N. S., Coss, R. G., & Benjamini, E. (1987). Resistance of California ground squirrels (*Spermophilus beecheyi*) to the venom of the Northern Pacific rattlesnake (*Crotalus viridis oreganus*): A study of adaptive variation. *Toxicon, 25*, 767–777.

Pravosudov, V. V. (2003). Long-term moderate elevation of corticosterone facilitates avian food-caching behaviour and enhances spatial memory. *Proceedings of the Royal Society of London. Series B: Biological Sciences, 270*, 2599–2604.

Randall, J. A., & Stevens, C. M. (1987). Footdrumming and other anti-predator responses in the bannertail kangaroo rat (*Dipodomys spectabilis*). *Behavioral Ecology and Sociobiology, 20*, 187–194.

Rasa, O. A. E. (1986). Coordinated vigilance of dwarf mongoose family groups: The "Watchman's Song" hypothesis and the costs of guarding. *Ethology, 71*, 340–344.

Robinson, S. R. (1980). Antipredator behaviour and predator recognition in Belding's ground squirrels. *Animal Behaviour, 28*, 840–852.

Robinson, S. R. (1981). Alarm communication in Belding's ground squirrels. *Zeitschrift für Tierpsychologie, 56*, 150–168.

Rydén, O. O. (1978). The significance of antecedent auditory experiences on later reactions to the "seeet" alarm-call in great tit nestling *Parus major*. *Zeitschrift für Tierpsychologie, 47*, 396–409.

Rydén, O. O. (1982). Selective resistance to approach: A precursor to fear responses to an alarm calls in great tit nestlings (*Parus major*). *Developmental Psychobiology, 15*, 113–120.

Saldanha, C. J., Schlinger, B. A., & Clayton, N. S. (2000). Rapid effects of corticosterone on cache recovery in mountain chickadees (*Parus gambeli*). *Hormones and Behavior, 37*, 109–115.

Schwagmeyer, P. L. (1980). The function of alarm calling behavior in *Spermophilus tridecemlineatus*, the thirteen-lined ground squirrel. *Behavioral Ecology and Sociobiology, 7*, 195–200.

Schwagmeyer, P. L., & Brown, C. H. (1981). Conspecific reaction to playback of thirteen-lined ground squirrel vocalizations. *Zeitschrift für Tierpsychologie, 56*, 25–32.

Seyfarth, R. M., & Cheney, D. L. (1980). The ontogeny of vervet monkey alarm calling behaviour: A preliminary report. *Zeitschrift für Tierpsychologie, 54*, 37–56.

Seyfarth, R. M., & Cheney, D. L. (1986). Vocal development in vervet monkeys. *Animal Behaviour, 34*, 1640–1658.

Seyfarth, R. M., Cheney, D. L., & Marler, P. (1980). Monkey responses to three different alarm calls: Evidence for predator classification and semantic communication. *Science, 210*, 801–803.

Sherman, P. W. (1976). *Natural selection among some group-living organisms*. Unpublished doctoral dissertation, University of Michigan.

Sherman, P. W. (1977). Nepotism and the evolution of alarm calls. *Science, 197*, 1246–1253.

Sherman, P. W. (1985). Alarm calls of Belding's ground squirrels to aerial predators: Nepotism or self-preservation? *Behavioral Ecology and Sociobiology, 17*, 313–323.

Sherman, P. W., & Morton, M. L. (1984). Demography of Belding's ground squirrels. *Ecology, 65*, 1617–1628.

Shettleworth, S. (1998). *Cognition, evolution, and behavior*. New York: Oxford University Press.

Smith, J. W., Seckl, J. R., Evans, A. T., Costall, B., & Smythe, J. W. (2004). Gestational stress induces post-partum depression-like behaviour and alters maternal care in rats. *Psychoneuroendocrinology, 29*, 227–244.

Snowdon, C. T. (1988). Communications as social interaction: Its importance in ontogeny and adult behavior. In D. Todt, P. Goedeking & D. Symmes (Eds.), *Primate vocal communication* (pp. 108–122). New York: Springer-Verlag.

Stamps, J. (2003). Behavioural processes affecting development: Tinbergen's fourth question comes of age. *Animal Behaviour, 66*, 1–13.

Swaisgood, R. R., Owings, D. H., & Rowe, M. P. (1999). Conflict and assessment in a predator-prey system: Ground squirrels versus rattlesnakes. *Animal Behaviour, 57*, 1033–1044.

Swaisgood, R. R., Rowe, M. P., & Owings, D. H. (2003). Antipredator responses of California ground squirrels to rattlesnakes and rattling sounds: the roles of sex, reproductive parity, and offspring age in assessment and decision-making rules. *Behavioral Ecology and Sociobiology, 55*, 22–31.

Symington, M. M. (1988). Demography, ranging patterns, and activity budgets of black spider monkeys (*Ateles paniscus chamek*) in the Manu National Park, Peru. *American Journal of Primatology, 15*, 45–67.

Tinbergen, N. (1963). On the aims and methods of ethology. *Zeitschrift für Tierpsychologie, 20*, 410–433.

Tulley, J. J., & Huntingford, F. A. (1987). Parental care and the development of adaptive variation in anti-predator responses in sticklebacks. *Animal Behaviour, 35*, 1570–1572.

Turner, L. W. (1973). Vocal and escape responses of *Spermophilus beldingi* to predators. *Journal of Mammalogy, 54*, 990–993.

Turkewitz, G., & Kenny, P. A. (1982). Limitations on input as a basis for neural organization and perceptual development: A preliminary theoretical statement. *Developmental Psychobiology, 15*, 357–368.

van Schaik, C. P., & Kappeler, P. M. (1993). Life history, activity period and lemur social systems. In P. M. Kappeler & J. Ganzhorn (Eds.), *Lemur social systems* (pp. 243–263). New York: Plenum Press.

Vince, M. A. (1980). The posthatching consequences of prehatching stimulation: Changes with amount of prehatching and posthatching exposure. *Behaviour, 75*, 36–53.

Vitale, A. F. (1989). Changes in anti-predator responses of wild rabbits, *Oryctolagus cuniculus* (L.), with age and experience. *Behaviour, 110*, 47–61.

Weary, D. M., & Kramer, D. L. (1995). Response of eastern chipmunks to conspecific alarm calls. *Animal Behaviour, 49*, 81–93.

West, M. J., & King, A. P. (1987). Settling nature and nurture into an ontogenetic niche. *Developmental Psychobiology, 20*, 549–562.

White, K. S., & Berger, J. (2001). Antipredator strategies of Alaskan moose: Are maternal trade-offs influenced by offspring activity? *Canadian Journal of Zoology, 79*, 2055–2062.

Wiley, R. H. (1983). The evolution of communication: Information and manipulation. In T. R. Halliday & P. J. B. Slater (Eds.), *Animal behaviour, Vol. 2. Communication* (pp. 156–215). New York: W. H. Freeman.

Williams, G. C. (1966). *Adaptation and natural selection.* Princeton: Princeton University Press.

Wright, P. J., & Huntingford, F. A. (1993). Agonistic interactions in juvenile sticklebacks (*Gasterosteus aculeatus*) in relation to local predation risk. *Ethology, 94*, 248–256.

Comparative Perspectives on the Missing Link: Communicative Pragmatics

Julie Gros-Louis, Meredith J. West, *and* Andrew P. King

Abstract

A common assumption is that communicative competence simply flows from some possibly innate by-product of vocal development. Understanding the dimensions of competence, or what in this chapter is called "communicative pragmatics," can be summed up as answering the "wh" questions, the "who," "what," "where," "when," and "why" of vocal performance. This chapter shows that songbirds and infants have to (a) learn how to use their signals though social modeling and social operant learning and (b) learn to lengthen their attention span so as to be able to acquire critical feedback from social companions. Of particular importance is the convergence of directed attention and vocalizations because individuals are able to receive both vocal and visual feedback to their behaviors.

Keywords: communicative competence, vocal development, communicative pragmatics, songbirds, social modeling, social operant learning, attention span

Overview

The basic plan for a journalist writing a newspaper article is to assemble facts, beginning with "who," followed by "what," "when," and "where," progressing to "why" and ending with "how." Here, we introduce the journalistic plan to define the major variable in this chapter, communicative pragmatics. The idea is simple—we are asking how an individual correctly identifies to whom to convey information in a timely fashion and in a correct context. Further, we ask what biological or psychological means facilitate the act of communicating. An effective communicative act, one that answers the questions cited above, can be compared to an effective newspaper article. We argue that many of the parameters of successful pragmatic performance are still unknown in even seemingly well-studied species. The consequence of the missing answers is that stories are formed that may sound good but are inaccurate, leaving the usually more complex account untold.

We have chosen two organisms, brown-headed cowbirds and humans, because much is known about their communication system, i.e., the structuring and meaning of information. The use of the information, the pragmatics, is less well studied than ordering or meaning because it is more difficult to measure and frequently taken for granted. The mode of communication is generally vocal, although we will see that dividing communication by reference to single senses does not always work. The time period of most interest is early in postnatal development, although one cannot ignore the life span. The function of the vocalizations ("why") also are considered but not stressed as we have written about this topic often (King & West, 2002; West & King, 2001). And, we do not focus on the "how" in detail because the biology of the communicative system has been explained extensively by other labs (Zeigler & Marler, 2004).

Our research perspective originated in reaction to traditional views that development is guided by automated maturational programs. Studies of development during the 1960s and 1970s were guided by the simplified dichotomous view of nature (genes) dictating the end product with nurture (environment/experience) passively triggering the developmental process toward that predetermined end point. In this view, the developing organism and the environmental experience are separable entities. Traditional studies of vocal development in songbirds, for example, removed individuals from the natural developmental context and examined what experience was necessary to trigger the innate developmental program. Young males were housed in isolation to control their exposure to auditory stimulation and experimenters selected what the males heard and how much they heard to determine the influence of auditory experience on development. Or, alternatively, deprivation experiments were conducted to see what developed in the absence of any stimulation, thus revealing what was thought to be the innate blueprint for song (e.g., Marler et al., 1972). Although the research approach was well-intentioned—individuals were removed from their social environment to control external variables—it actually created a novel developmental environment because the absence of companionship introduced its own effects on development (Kuo, 1967). Comparable naturalistic studies of human vocal development at the time were those that examined infants with sensory impairments. Early babbling, when examined for phonetic properties of speech, seemed to be similar in deaf and hearing infants, thus suggesting that early experience had no influence on prelinguistic vocal development (Lenneberg, 1967).

A fundamental flaw of the false dichotomy of nature and nurture as separable entities is the implicit assumption that contributions of environment to development can be controlled like measurable quantities in a recipe. Adding or excluding certain experiences was thought to have predictable outcomes because the fluidity of the interaction of genes and environment was construed to be minimal at best: an environmental trigger of a predetermined genetic program (e.g., "reaction range" proposed by Gottesman, 1963; Scarr-Salapatek, 1976). Thus, environment was seen as a static influence rather than dynamically shaping the organisms' development. However, rather than development being a passive unfolding of preprogrammed pathways through exposure to the environment, interactions with the environment, particularly the social environment, are key to directing behavioral development (Gottlieb, 1976; Lickliter & Gottlieb, 1985; Moore, 1984). Individuals' early experiences have a cascading effect in structuring the pattern of further development, with a fluid interaction of what was traditionally viewed as "nature" and "nurture." Therefore, there is no explanatory value in distinguishing the contribution of "nature" and "nurture" in development, as there is no boundary between the two—they are interdependent and inseparable. Furthermore, with the recognition of the inheritance of environments, the ontogenetic niche, one could no longer distinguish genes and environment on the basis of what is preexisting before development occurs (Oyama, 2000; West & King, 1987, 1988). The social surroundings and interactions of a young organism are part of its heritage just as are genes and proteins in the body.

In this chapter, our goals stem from this theoretical framework underscored at all times by the idea that communicative development is an interactive process involving social partners. Mere exposure to environmental or social variables is not sufficient; individuals must be active participants in their environment to learn. Organisms acting and behaving elicit social responses that shape an organism's perception, affecting what there is to be learned ("performatory feedback": Gibson, 1966). To exemplify this idea, we present evidence for a social gateway, which is the role of ecology in making stimulation available in the environment. Proximity to and interactions with social partners offer different opportunities for interactions, thus mediating the communicative behaviors that individuals produce and feedback they receive (West et al., 2003; White et al., 2002a). For example, for young individuals the degree of access to adults—a social gateway—predicts cultural guidance and thus what is available to be learned. Therefore, instead of considering exposure to all potential stimulation in the environment as relevant for development, we focus on the bioavailability of social stimulation: that portion that is accessible via the social gateway.

Traditional Studies of Communicative Development

Studies of early vocal development do not often focus on the development of pragmatics, that is, putting correct acoustic form into effective use; rather, most studies focus on the development of mature acoustic forms of vocalizations or speech sounds, with the assumption that there is a predetermined linkage between producing the appropriate vocal forms and knowing how to use them. This assumption is a historic result of the widely held viewpoint that vocal development in humans and songbirds can be explained through the action of innate modules (Bloom, 1993; Chomsky, 1965; Konishi, 1965; Lenneberg, 1967; Marler, 1967; Marler & Nelson, 1992). Additionally, original comparisons made between birdsong and speech development focused on acoustic form rather than pragmatic use (Marler, 1970), as both were thought to be based on similar innate mechanisms. Included in such predeterminism is the pragmatic component of communication, which is simply assumed to follow the development of functional vocalizations: once a bird sings, or a human produces their first protoword, correct usage comes in tow. A result of a reliance on innate explanations is that development becomes oversimplified because environmental influences are overlooked and underestimated.

However, a closer examination of the studies of communicative development (Payne & Payne, 1993), and many studies that have been performed in our laboratory, suggests that such simplistic views of development of acoustic form and usage cannot be supported. Studies of cowbirds have revealed that the development of song structure and communicative competence is dependent upon the nature of interactions between young males and their social partners. Females provide nonvocal social feedback that shapes fine acoustic structure of male song and that influences the rate of vocal development (King & West, 1988; King et al., 2005; Smith et al., 2000; West & King, 1988). Adult males provide the interactions through which males develop effective use of song (White et al., 2002b). Similarly, we have evidence in humans that differential responses to vocalizations may influence vocal development and usage similar to what we have seen in cowbirds (Goldstein et al., 2003; Goldstein & Schwade, 2008; Gros-Louis, 2006; Gros-Louis et al., 2006a, in preparation-b). Thus, in contrast to the view that early "babbling" in both songbirds and infants is merely motor practice (Bloom, 1993; Oller, 2000); contingent stimulation by social partners in response to early vocalizations actually drives development. The demonstration that social stimulation shapes developmental change makes it necessary to view the ontogeny of communication as part of a broader developmental ecology. The task that we face as researchers is to figure out the aspects of the social environment and social contingencies within that environment that operate to influence different components of communicative behavior.

Pragmatics Defined

To clarify the way in which we use the terms "pragmatics" and what we mean by "vocal usage" in this chapter, we provide a brief overview of three different analytic levels of communication that stem from early semiotic and linguistic theory (Chomsky, 1965; Morris, 1946) and its extension to ethology (Sebeok, 1962, 1965). The first two levels, syntactic and semantic, examine what message potentially could be contained in a signal or display rather than its use in the context of an interaction. Syntactic analysis abstracts signals from their communicative context to investigate their potential for communicating meaning alone and in combination with other signals, asking such questions as what constitutes a signal and how the potential meaning of a signal changes in combination with other signals (Chomsky, 1965; Smith, 1977). Semantics, on the other hand, investigates what kind of information is contained in a signal, asking whether a signal carries meaning through association with particular objects or behaviors; however, although semantics examine the predictable association of a signal and potential referents, this association is divorced from social context to strip away any potential contextual "cues" for meaning.

The pragmatic level of analysis considers use of signals in social interactions. Therefore, it is both the signal and the contextual production of it that results in a signal's function. For this reason, the same signals in different contexts may have different meanings or functional outcomes (Smith, 1977). And, this leads us to an important point of comparison of pragmatics to syntax or semantics. Syntax involves specific structures, semantics involves specific meanings, but because of variation across contexts, pragmatics is not predictable and predefined in the same way as syntax or semantics. To illustrate this point, Dore states "The function of interrogative structures, for example, is to ask questions. But this tells us little about the experienced regularities of what, where, when, why, how, and with whom questions are used" (Dore, 1986, p. 6). The analogy in the present chapter is that although the function of birdsong or prelinguistic behaviors may be recognized, the development of the content of a signal is not predictive of the development of its pragmatic usage. Furthermore, pragmatic usage is essential for the functional effectiveness of signals.

Table 33.1 Excerpts of Definitions of Communication from a Variety of Theoretical Perspectives of Different Academic Disciplines

Academic Discipline	Definition
Behavioral ecology	"…signals or displays to modify the behaviour of reactors…" (Krebs & Davies, 1993, p. 349)
Cognitive psychology	"…internal representation and symbolic behaviour that conveys that representation…the interpretation of the symbolic behaviour." (Johnson-Laird, 1990, pp. 2–4)
Ethology	"…the transfer of information via signals…between sender and receiver" (Hailman, 1977, p. 52)
Linguistics	"…vocal and nonvocal gestures as we interact…" (Lindblom, 1990, p. 220)
Neuropsychology	"…behaviors of one member of a species conveys information to another member of the species…" (Kimura, 1993, p. 3)
Sensory ecology	"…behavior generates a signal that mediates interaction…" (Dusenbery, 1992, p. 37)
Sociobiology	"…action or cue given by one organism to another…" (Wilson, 1975, p. 111)

Source: Adapted from Hauser (1996).

Although the early semiotic distinction of the three components of the communicative process included syntax, semantics, and pragmatics, an examination of definitions of communication from different theoretical perspectives indicates that definitions do not explicitly include pragmatics (Hauser, 1996; Table 33.1). Such an omission reiterates the fact that pragmatics are often inherently taken for granted, assumed to follow from the production of vocalizations (but see Dore, 1979 who argues that function precedes form and can derive from separate sources ontogenetically). Thus, the differential focus across academic disciplines is the structure or content of the signal but not the delivery of the signal. Ethology and sociobiology view signals as inherent in the behaviors of individuals (e.g., Smith, 1977; Wilson, 1975), whereas cognitive psychology views signals with discrete meaning and an underlying mental representation (Johnson-Laird, 1990).

In addition, in our view, definitions of communication provide the description for the end point, a successful communicative act, rather than the necessary precursors of communicative behavior or the process that results in a communicative act. For example, the "prerequisites" for describing vocal interactions in songbirds are indicated to be the "who," "what," and "why," leaving out the "when" (Dabelsteen & McGregor, 1996).

Nonetheless, pragmatics are implied in the definitions of communication in that they either explicitly include a signaler and a recipient of a signal, or the premise that information is transmitted between two individuals. Definitions that focus on behavioral interaction as communication, rather than those that focus specifically on the *content* of signals, are most useful in comparative studies of communication across species. In particular, when comparing prelinguistic communication in humans to communication in other animals, an ethological perspective is a valuable approach, as both communication systems share more similarities with one another than human language: "information is a feature of an interaction between sender and perceiver" (Hauser, 1996) or communication is a "process of signaling and eliciting responses" (Smith, 1977).

It is probably no accident that definitions of communication and studies of communicative development lack explicit focus on the correct delivery or usage of signals. Popular experimental designs employed in studies of nonhuman vocal development involve solitary individuals. In such a design, pragmatics are inherently absent, as pragmatics involve social partners. Furthermore, there is no need to explain origins of behavior when relying on a nativist explanation: ghosts in the machine provide the blueprint for development and connect form with function. Thus, end points serve as a starting point from which researchers work backward to explain development rather than prospective studies considering the process to get to the end point. The danger in a retrospective approach is that it fails to capture the origins of behavior, as researchers have certain preconceptions of early behaviors and their potential plasticity (cf., Reddy, 1999). The use and significance of sounds, or their directedness to a social partner (defined by visual gaze), are overlooked because they will be supplanted by mature song or words. We provide examples from studies of both cowbirds and infants that demonstrate that understanding the origins of behavior is necessary to understanding its function and that communicative development needs to be studied in a prospective manner in order to appreciate the role of socially gated stimulation to construct behavior.

Absence of Pragmatics in Developmental Studies
Birdsong Development

Researchers have noted recently that although the historical emphasis has been on strictly auditory influences on song learning, the next few decades will be devoted to analyses of social factors (Beecher & Brenowitz, 2005; Beecher & Burt, 2004). An early consideration of social influences was rooted in the finding in the mid-1980s that live tutors could facilitate imitation beyond that seen with a tape tutor (Baptista & Petrinovich, 1984). At the same time, studies by King and West revealed that nonvocal social stimulation of females influenced vocal development in male cowbirds (King & West, 1983, 1988; West & King, 1988). The newly recognized role of social interactions in development ultimately led to a greater focus on the behavior of singers and recipients in the form of "action-based" learning (Marler & Peters, 1982). However, because of the strong hold of innate underpinnings in developmental theory, social influences were viewed as experiential contributions to divergent pathways of predetermined vocal end points. Song variants were winnowed during development via feedback between senders and receivers, rather than feedback contributing to song origins (Marler & Nelson, 1993; Nelson & Marler, 1994). Furthermore, social feedback was generally considered to be of an acoustic nature, such as song matching to a tutor or through interactions between neighboring males (Beecher et al., 2000). This is not to say that pragmatics is not part of birdsong, as birds must decide whether and when to match songs or repertoires with neighbors (Beecher, Burt, O'Loghlen, Templeton, & Campbell, 2007) and from whom to learn song (Kroodsma, 2004). However, an important point is that this research considers the role of pragmatics in *vocal* development rather than pragmatic development itself.

The focus on acoustic variables may account for the fragmented state of the field as a whole. Kroodsma (1996), in calling for more serious attention to the ecology of song, has characterized the field of song learning as composed of "myriad

facts…largely unconnected, bits of a grand evolutionary picture" (p. 3). The fragmentation of the field of birdsong may be tolerable for those interested in only part of the communication process, e.g., the mechanisms of motor or hormonal control underlying song production and seasonal neuronal plasticity (Brenowitz, 2004). But for those seeking to understand the development and evolution of communication, knowledge about the dynamical nature of interactions between communicators is essential (McGregor & Peake, 2000; Nowicki et al., 2001; Payne & Payne, 1993). Acoustic variables are insufficient because they neglect the actual social interactions in which song use is embedded. Thus, research over the past decades on the development of acoustic structure of song in birds have made significant discoveries into the potential mechanisms of vocal development, ranging from neurobiological to external social influences, but the research has overlooked the fact that effective song may not bring with it effective use in social interactions.

The oversight of pragmatics in vocal studies has several root causes. First and foremost, investigators have simply assumed that evidence of the presence of a communicative signal is also evidence that its use will be appropriate. Second, the contexts studied, often isolates or small groups of songbirds, may not reveal the absence of pragmatic skills. Third, investigators may unwittingly substitute their own actions for the behaviors that animals must perform in nature. For example, in playback work, experimenters expose male-deprived females to recorded songs and measure whether she adopts a copulatory posture to the songs. The focus is on discovering song function and it has been used in diverse songbird species (Searcy, 1992). The appeal of this unambiguous response is its objectivity and quantifiability, but its simplicity can be deceiving because it completely obscures the realm of pragmatics. It is the investigator, not the singing bird, who determines what, where, when, and to whom recorded vocalizations are directed. In reality, however, males must not only know what to sing, but they must also know where, when, and to whom to sing.

Such an omission is critical when we consider the instrumental importance of pragmatics of singing behavior in natural contexts. By removing the playback context previously engineered by humans, a series of experiments revealed that the development of biologically effective song does not automatically result in the reproductive success that is suggested by song efficacy in playback experiments.

Young male cowbirds were housed first with adult female cowbirds or canaries and then were exposed to a new set of female cowbirds or canaries to provide a more "freestyle" social context of courting and mating behavior (Freeberg et al., 1995; West et al., 1996). The "where" component of communicating was varied by first having males meet their new companions in a flight cage and then in a large aviary populated by female cowbirds from three populations, canaries of different color morphs, and starlings, a novel species. In the flight cage setting, the male cowbirds, who had been housed with female cowbirds, looked normal: they sang to female cowbirds and ignored the canaries. But in the aviaries, the female-housed cowbirds sang primarily to themselves or one another, ignoring the often-solicitous female cowbirds. Even after observing the mating behavior of adult male models in the aviaries, the male cowbirds still ignored females of their own species. The data from the canary housed males was more dramatic. In both contexts, the canary-housed males courted new canaries and ignored female cowbirds.

Returning to the journalistic framework, males in these studies collectively showed deviations in "who," "what," "where," and "when." Males who developed effective songs, but not appropriate "pragmatic" skills, did not achieve copulations. These results provided experimental evidence for the idea that form and usage do not automatically develop concurrently. More importantly, it pointed to the need for researchers to consider the inherited environment of development and emphasized the need for multiple contexts for assessment of the end point of functional behaviors such as singing. Had the experiments stopped with playback experiments or with the flight cage test, male's development would have appeared normal. And, in fact, these would have been potential stopping points for many researchers without access to the complex social context of a flock, the context where song is actually used.

Infant Development

Most studies of early infant vocal development, like those of songbirds, historically have focused on auditory influences on vocal learning, such as the influence of exposure to speech sounds of the primary language on structural variation in phonemes during the first year (e.g, de Boysson-Bardies & Vihman, 1991; Vihman et al., 1986). Thus, vocal behavior is examined to document and explain stage-like changes at the phonemic level rather than

communicative use of vocalizations (Locke, 1983; Oller, 2000; Stoel-Gammon & Otomo, 1986). However, just as in songbirds, vocal development is not only about producing more phonologically advanced sounds, but is also about learning the pragmatics of communication: how to use vocalizations for effective social and communicative interactions (Dore, 1974). The social-pragmatic approach to language development recognizes the importance of pragmatic *comprehension* scaffolding language development toward the end of the first year (Akhtar & Tomasello, 2000; Baldwin & Tomasello, 1998; Tomasello, 1997). However, few studies examine the development of pragmatics of *productive* communicative behavior (Carpenter et al., 1983; but see Dore, 1983; Smith, 1998). Studies more often provide descriptions of predetermined pragmatic abilities, which are labeled "intentional communication" or "communicative intentions" rather than examining their developmental origins (e.g., Carpenter et al., 1983; e.g., Wetherby et al., 1988). By examining an expected end point, as suggested by the term "communicative intentions," researchers fail to notice the potential communicative function of combined vocal, attentional, and gestural behaviors. Not all infants will develop similar pragmatic behaviors, as some infants will use more gesture, tone, or protowords (Dore, 1974) and thus it is important to study their convergent development.

One reason that few studies have explored prelinguistic communicative development may be that there is often a conflation of language and communication (Golinkoff & Gordon, 1983). The designation of the term "pre" linguistic indicates that language is the end point rather than broader communicative competence. Thus, language researchers have often approached the study of the prelinguistic period in a retrospective manner, focusing on month-by-month or stage-by-stage changes to bridge the gap between babbling and first words by identifying precursors to formal language (e.g., Kent & Miolo, 1995 and references therein). Studies that do consider social influences on language development attempt to predict behavioral changes over many months, e.g., from 8 to 14 months. Often, infants' abilities or behaviors at time y (14 months) are then retrospectively related to their abilities at time x (8 months) to determine the relative influence of particular communicative measures on developmental linguistic milestones (Bornstein et al., 1992; Tamis-LeMonda et al., 2001). The result is that the development of pragmatics is taken for granted just as in songbirds, in that development of a communicative signal (language) brings with it the development of its appropriate use. This may be a result of early views of not only innate behaviors, but also a "hereditary teaching mechanism" responsible for connecting behaviors to function (Lorenz, 1965). The machine supplies the pragmatic connection in an automatic fashion not requiring learning. Pragmatics is simply doing what comes naturally or nativistically. Development is of the "plug and play" variety.

Prelinguistic behaviors originally were identified relative to their mode of production, and thus viewed as distinct channels of communication (Stern, 1974): affective (vocal and facial expression), attentional (eye gaze, gestures), and vocal (babbling) (see also Barratt et al., 1992; Stern, 1974). A number of studies have explored the temporal relationship among communicative behaviors, such as visual gaze, vocalizing, and/or smiling (D'Odorico & Cassibba, 1995; Keller & Scholmerich, 1987; Schaffer et al., 1977; Striano & Rochat, 1999), although the perspective has been to study their co-occurrence or sequential nature. Thus the structural timing, rather than communicative significance, has been the focus of many studies. What is needed is a study that documents when and how phonologically different vocal behaviors converge with other modes of communication and how that results in broader communicative competency.

We propose that combining studies of vocal behavior with those of sociocognitive behavior is the starting point for understanding the development of communication because sociocognitive abilities contribute to the attentional components of prelinguistic communication. It is the integration of directed attentional focus (toward objects or social partners), vocal behaviors, and nonverbal gestures (though not considered in detail in this chapter) that gives rise to the pragmatic function of early communicative behaviors (cf., Bates, 1976; Ninio & Bruner, 1978). Bringing attentional and vocal behaviors together is a key, as suggested for later language and apt for our journalist metaphor: integrating gaze and linguistic channels tells a recipient the when, where, and what use to give the gazing activity in relation to language (Kasher & Meilijson, 1996; Schieffelin, 1983). Compounded behaviors are especially apparent in the second 6 months of life when infants bring together new skills: babbling, socially directed behaviors such as social referencing, establishing joint attention episodes, and attentional-sharing behaviors such

as protodeclarative pointing. A quote from Bates (1976) exemplifies the communicative capacity of combined prelinguistic behaviors at the end of the first year: "...combinations of apparent imperative intention: stretching forth the arms with an open-and-shut gesture of the hand, pointing, reiterated and insistent vocalizations, and intermittent eye contact with the adult" (Bates, 1976, pp. 55–56; Bruner, 1975; see also Ninio & Bruner, 1978). Also, a point alone may orient caregivers' attention, but if the point is accompanied by a vocalization, there is more indication of the infants' goal (Jones & Zimmerman, 2003). In particular, it is the coordination of behavioral and attentional focus on objects and people in interactions, i.e., joint attention or secondary intersubjectivity (Bakeman & Adamson, 1984; Trevarthen & Hubley, 1979), that is thought to form the basis of preverbal communication because it "encodes" infants' intentions (Sugarman, 1984, p. 60).

Though the parallel development of vocal and sociocognitive behaviors are the basis of more complex communication, at present, there is a disconnect between studies of early vocal development and social and cognitive development. In contrast to a handful of studies in the 1970s and 1980s that examined the potential communicative function of combined behaviors (e.g., Dore, 1974; Sugarman, 1984), current studies of sociocognitive abilities focus on the ages at which these abilities emerge, rather than consider these abilities in combination with emerging vocal skills. This is tantamount to the documentation of phonological achievements in studies of early speech development and how they may contribute to language learning (Baldwin & Tomasello, 1998; Pruden et al., 2006). Often times, it is not until after a child has referential language that vocal behavior and skills such as joint attention are considered together for their communicative potential (termed "verbalizations"—Carpenter et al., 2002; but see Wetherby et al., 1988). Clearly sociocognitive skills play a role in language development, but we stress the need to consider the convergence of prelinguistic vocalizations and emerging sociocognitive skills during development as the beginning of communicative pragmatics. As infants begin to produce directed vocalizations in the context of social referencing, for example, caregiver responsiveness is likely to be influenced by both the phonological quality of the infants' vocalization in addition to their attentional focus or activity (Rochat & Striano, 1999). A fruitful line of research would be to explore the significance and effectiveness of "re-engagement vocalizations" and "re-engagement activities" that have been observed in dyadic interactions in which adults adopt a still face (Striano & Rochat, 1999). And, further, researchers should explore how caregiver responsiveness to such vocalizations shape pragmatic development.

The main studies that examine pragmatic development concurrently with vocal development are those of children with sociocommunicative disorders. In these cases, dissociations in the form and function of communicative behavior make the significance of pragmatics apparent. For example, most relevant to our comparative work with songbirds, children with autism spectrum disorder, in particular Asperger's syndrome, may show deficits in the pragmatics of language although they show few deficits in vocabulary or grammar (e.g, Surian et al., 1996; Tanguay et al., 1998). In fact, high-functioning autistic children develop referential language, i.e. words, before they begin producing protodeclarative gestures, such as pointing or showing to share or direct (although they do produce protoimperative gestures: Baron-Cohen, 1989); thus, they can produce words before becoming communicatively competent, which is the opposite of typically developing children (Carpenter et al., 2002). Also, although apparent later in development, children with attention deficit hyperactivity disorder (ADHD) and Williams syndrome show deficits in pragmatic aspects of language rather than in other areas (Purvis & Tannock, 1997), such as inappropriate initiation of conversation and conversational rapport (Laws & Bishop, 2004). In cases where grammatical or semantic deficits are present, these are likely linked to pragmatic deficits that negatively impact learning (Camarata & Gibson, 1999).

In sum, the "why," "when," and "who" of communicative interactions are most impaired in children with social communicative disorders, while the "what" is less impaired. Although there are obviously other significant differences, through a comparative lens, we see a parallel with male cowbirds that lack the ability to sustain attention in social interactions, thus developing potent song but never engaging in successful pragmatics of song production (White et al., 2002b). Therefore, there is compelling evidence in both songbirds and human infants that the linkage between structure and function is not inherent in the system and that pragmatic development needs to be integrated with vocal development.

Mechanisms of Communicative Development
Contingent Stimulation and the Development of Attention

Our research has shown that from the beginning of vocal production, young songbirds produce variable vocalizations, akin to infant "babbling," and nonvocal, social feedback is bounced back to them, a process termed "behavioral sonar" (King & West, 1988; Skoyles, 1998; West et al., 1990). This process is an extension of "performatory" feedback (Gibson, 1966) because young males can learn what notes to keep and what notes to drop by attending to feedback from females who cannot sing (West & King, 1988). This finding was provocative because prior research had assumed that auditory input and feedback was the necessary and sufficient experiential variable for song development. However, for behavioral sonar to work, males must produce directed song (oriented toward a social partner, in this case the female; see Figure 33.1) rather than undirected song (no song recipient) and attend to the consequences of their singing. The attention span of the singing male delimits the opportunities to receive social feedback that shapes acoustic form and connects form and function. Thus, the songs that receive feedback from females during development are those that elicit copulatory postures from those same females (White et al., 2006).

In the most extensive studies of the social shaping of avian babbling, Smith et al. (2000), West and King (1988), and King et al. (2005) found that the nonsinging female companions of immature male cowbirds provided different forms of nonvocal feedback that influenced the rate of vocal development and phonological quality of male song. Frame-by-frame measurements of male–female

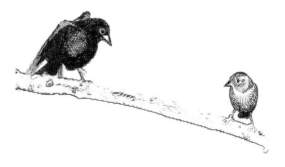

Figure 33.1 Illustration from a single frame of a video recording of a male cowbird directing a song to a female cowbird.

interactions revealed that female wing strokes and gapes are performed in reaction to songs that are directed to females. A wing stroke is a rapid flick of the wing that by definition must occur coincident with song delivery and a gape is rapid opening of the beak accompanied by raising of the head (Figure 32.2A,B). These behaviors led males to repeat the sounds and behaviors that produced social responses from companions and eventually to drop sounds that did not produce reactions. Furthermore, social feedback shaped the attention span of the males, as measured by looking (King et al., 2005) and the length and content of social interactions (King, unpublished data). Directed song, a proxy for attentional focus, predicts the acquisition of articulate and attractive song, as wing strokes and gapes correlated with the earlier onset of stereotyped song and higher song quality as measured by playback (King et al., 2005). Greater social feedback led to a faster rate of development and faster progress toward stable articulation of the phonemic-like structures of their vocalizations. Males producing more directed song have an advantage entering the breeding season: having developed song at a faster rate and having better song repertoires, they court earlier and more successfully (Smith et al., 2000). Thus, proper use of directed song and accompanying attentional skills are a critical pragmatic dimension of communication in cowbirds and should be considered a "prelinguistic" milestone that drives further development.

Different social responses of females also affect neural development. Males housed with more socially interactive females, compared to those housed with less interactive females, had a greater volume and higher number of neurons in one of the visual nuclei located in the thalamus that is thought to process information about form and motion (Freeberg et al., 2002; Hamilton et al., 1998). As males were randomly assigned to conditions, the differences in their repertoires and neural structures must reflect the differential influence of their female companions' social stimulation. Males learn to read visual signals from females to modify their own vocal signals and they do so on-line while interacting with females. Thus, it is likely that the neural differences between males housed with responsive compared to unresponsive females stem from the demands of males sustaining their attention in cross-modal tasks. Further indication that attention is a significant component of communicative interaction comes from research showing that differential ZENK gene expression is associated with the use of directed but not undirected song (Jarvis et al., 1998). Therefore, the attentional aspect of social interaction is important for communicative development from social, neural, and molecular perspectives. And, we believe, it is this attentional aspect that is the basis of the pragmatic dimension of communication.

Directed vocalizations in infants, just as in cowbirds, are the critical pragmatic dimension of communication between caregivers and infants and provide the opportunity for learning through responding by social partners. Similar to our findings in songbirds, there is an implied behavioral sonar mechanism in infant vocal development. Locke (2001) suggests that vocalizations and other expressive behaviors are part of a developmental system that necessitates that "signals be sent in order for information to be received" (p. 302). Infants produce variable vocal or social behaviors and feedback to these behaviors is "bounced" back to them, providing a potential source of information about the effectiveness of infants' behaviors, a first step in learning what sounds to produce and how to use them. For example, at around 4 months of age, infants can shift their gaze and exhibit more varied vocalizations. Particular patterns of vocalizing, or

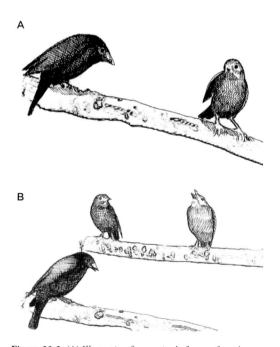

A

B

Figure 33.2 (A) Illustration from a single frame of a video recording of a female cowbird reacting to a directed male song with a wingstroke. (B) Illustration of a female cowbird reacting to a directed male song with a gape.

vocalizations occurring concurrently with attentional focus on an object, are initially coincidences rather than being under voluntary control (cf., Collis, 1979). Nonetheless, regardless of the intentionality on the part of the infant to communicate, the vocalizations elicit responses from caregivers (Bates et al., 1975; Locke, 1996). The responses can bootstrap the infant to behaviors that appear more "intentional," thus connecting form and function, by commenting on or manipulating the object that the infant is vocalizing to (Collis, 1979; Halliday, 1979; Siegel, 1999).

An example of behavioral sonar in infants comes from Lawrence's 1986 study of 20 mother–infant pairs when the children were 9 months of age. Lawrence (1986) found that different dyads produced different combinations of communicative gestures, tones, or protowords (see also Dore, 1974). These gestures, tones, and protowords are the initial behaviors emitted as "sonar." The mother's decisions about which behaviors were communicative led to differential feedback and thus her reactions represent a potential source for vocal shaping (Papousek, 1992). Infants may, therefore, take different developmental pathways and progress at different rates in their communicative skills due to individual variation in early vocal and attentional behaviors and caregiver responses to these behaviors. Such variability has been shown to predict the development of language and coordinated joint attention in the second year (Markus et al., 2000), indicating that infants' behaviors drive their own development through interaction with the environment as in other domains such as locomotion (Thelen et al., 1996; Thelen & Ulrich, 1991) and as we have seen in cowbirds.

Contingent responses during social interactions provide the mechanism for infant phonological development similar to the social shaping that we discovered in cowbirds (King et al., 2005; West & King, 1988). Specifically, differential feedback from caregivers provided in moment-to-moment social interactions plays a central role in creating developmental pathways. The intonational quality of infant vocalizations, in addition to their acoustic structure, influences how caregivers respond (Beaumont & Bloom, 1993; Bloom et al., 1993; Gros-Louis et al., 2006a; Papousek, 1989). The timing and nature of feedback has now been shown to be important in both vocal and pragmatic development (Goldstein et al., 2003; Goldstein & Schwade, 2008; Gros-Louis & Ables, 2006; Gros-Louis et al., in preparation-b). Goldstein et al. (2003) documented a

significant increase in infants' well-formed, speech-like syllables ("canonical syllables," Oller, 2000) when mothers provided contingent, nonvocal social feedback (smiles, touches) in response to their infants' vocalizations. Furthermore, infants continued to increase production of these vocalizations after the period of structured maternal responding. By contrast, infants who received the same amount of noncontingent stimulation did not increase their production of speech-like syllables.

To follow up on Goldstein et al.'s (2003) experimental evidence of social shaping, we examined uninstructed maternal responsiveness during freeplay interactions in 10 mother–infant pairs (Gros-Louis et al., 2006a). Mothers responded to infant vocalizations with more vocal responses than nonvocal, interactive responses, such as making eye contact and smiling or touching the infant. Of these vocal responses, mothers delivered significantly more differentiated feedback to vocalizations that were acoustically more mature. Mothers responded with more imitations and acknowledgments ("oh really?", "mmm-hmmm") to phonologically advanced, syllable-like sounds ("bah") compared to vowel-like sounds ("ah"). Mothers' differential, contingent feedback may shape the structure of vocalizations, in addition to their usage, as acknowledgments provide a conversational-like framework for vocalizing.

To explore the relationship between contingent stimulation and the development of communicative behaviors, we conducted a longitudinal study of 12 infants over a period of 6 months starting when they were 8 months of age. Infants showed variation in their attentional focus in relation to caregiver responses when they vocalize, similar to males directing songs to females in cowbirds (Gros-Louis et al., in preparation-b). Directed vocalizations included those produced to a parent or a toy (defined by direction of visual gaze), while undirected vocalizations occurred when infants appeared not to be focused on any person or object, such as when looking around the room. Mothers showed variation in how they responded to their infants' vocalizations, with most offering information about the object of infants' attentional focus but many also ignoring a fairly large proportion of vocalizations. Mothers whose responses focused in on infants' attentional focus had infants who scored higher on vocal comprehension and gesture on the MacArthur Communicative Development Inventory (Gros-Louis et al., in preparation-b). Similar associations have been found for following of infants' attentional focus and language development (Dunham et al., 1993; Rollins, 2003; Tamis-LeMonda et al., 2001; Tomasello & Farrar, 1986).

We also found suggestive evidence that maternal responsiveness to prelinguistic vocalizations influenced the development of infants' pragmatic behavior. Infants who received more responses to their vocalizations from their mothers showed a larger relative increase in vocalizations that they directed toward their mothers between 8 and 14 months of age than infants who received fewer responses (Gros-Louis et al., in preparation-b; Figure 32.3). Therefore, infants who received more contingent feedback increased their pragmatic use of vocalizations.

Results from our prelinguistic infant studies suggest a bidirectional influence on communicative development that is embedded in real-time social interactions, just as we have documented in developmental studies of cowbirds. Bidirectional effects of infant–caregiver interactions on development, often termed transactional processes, have been suggested previously (Bruner, 1977, 1983; Papousek & Papousek, 1975; Sameroff, 1975; Vygotsky, 1962), but not at the level of identifying the specific mechanism whereby feedback shapes structural form and pragmatic force. Our research demonstrates that infants learn about the relative effectiveness of different behaviors through

social interactions in which they are embedded (cf., Bruner, 1978; Gibb Harding, 1983; Papousek, 2007), suggesting a dynamic process of social shaping, where infants modify their behaviors in keeping with changing feedback from their ecology (e.g., Locke, 1993, 1996). At the heart of the social interactions are the behavioral contingencies that the infant receives to particular behaviors or joint behaviors (vocalizing and attentional focus). It is this contingent feedback that leads the infant to produce behaviors with more specificity in terms of their production, thus resulting in more precise pragmatics in terms of the "when," "who," and the "why" of communicative interactions.

Not Too Much, Not Too Little: the Perfect Level of Contingent Responding

The finding that socially contingent responding leads to infants producing sounds with more complex phonological features suggests that, as in studies of social, emotional, and cognitive development (Rochat & Striano, 1999; Stern, 2000; Watson, 1985), contingency may play a role in vocal development (see also Locke, 2001; Papousek & Bornstein, 1992). This fact is not surprising given the early sensitivity that infants show to perfect contingency, which later shifts to a preference for imperfect or "social" contingency (Bigelow, 1999; Bigelow & DeCoste, 2003; Gergely & Watson, 1999) and forms the basis for social expectations in interactions with people compared to objects (Ellsworth et al., 1993; Legerstee et al., 1987). Studies indicate that just the right amount of contingent responding is necessary to be effective in driving development (Bigelow & Birch, 1999), a suggestion that is supported with our studies of cowbird and infant vocal development (Gros-Louis et al., in preparation-b; Miller et al., 2008). In particular, variable contingent responding rather than predictable delivery of responses is likely to be more powerful for shaping behavior based on basic mechanisms of operant conditioning (cf., Neuringer et al., 2000).

In cowbirds, females differ substantially in their level of responsiveness, although group trends are reliably present. For example, local females respond more to local than distant song and permit more directed songs to be sung by local males because they remain in close proximity to the singing male (King et al., 2005). Female cowbirds also range considerably in their degree of responsiveness to song playback with some females showing much more choosiness than others (King & West, 1989). The variation in female behavior suggests that the

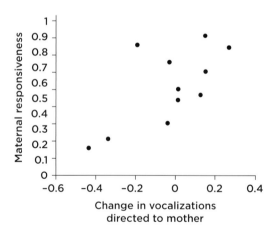

Figure 33.3 The relationship between maternal responsiveness and relative change in the proportion of vocalizations that infants directed to their mothers from 8 to 14 months old (*n* = 11). A negative change in directed vocalizations indicates a decrease over time. Maternal responsiveness of 0.1 = response to every sixth vocalization; 1 = response to every vocalization.

birds may display different communicative phenotypes, with parallels to different styles of maternal responsiveness in humans (discussed below).

The effect of variable female responsivity on male vocal development is highlighted in a recent study, with levels of contingent stimulation correlating with improvisation (Miller et al., 2008). Young males were more likely to improvise and develop variable songs when they were housed with adult females who were more discriminating in their interactions, and thus less responsive. By contrast, young males were more likely to copy one another's song and showed less diversity in their song repertoires when they were housed with juvenile females who interacted indiscriminately and were therefore extremely responsive. Furthermore, when the males were switched between aviaries, they showed a new pattern of vocal development consistent with the responsiveness of the social environment: juvenile males who had been with extremely responsive juvenile females showed a dramatic increase in the number of note clusters that they produced in songs compared to when they were placed with less responsive adult females (Miller et al., 2008; Figure 32.4). In addition, the juvenile males now housed with adult females showed an increase in improvisation, likely related to the combinatorial possibilities introduced by the increase in note clusters in their repertoires. Although individual variation in female responsiveness to different song variants exists (White et al., 2006), it cannot account for the results of this study, as the level of interactivity of juvenile females and adult females with juvenile males showed distinct, nonoverlapping distributions (Freed-Brown et al., 2006). Clearly, females cannot be entirely unresponsive, as there would be no feedback available to males when they sing; however, these results indicate that the level of contingent stimulation can be too high. If any and all vocalizations receive feedback, the pattern of contingent stimulation is not informative, thus losing some efficacy in the ability to elicit variable vocal behavior.

The findings of the important role of female feedback in male vocal development are consistent with studies in other songbirds. Generally, there is a relation between variable vocal behavior and variable social contexts, which we propose may be related to the level of predictability of social partners. For example, nomadic sedge wrens show improvisation, whereas marsh wrens who are site faithful do not (Kroodsma & Pickert, 1984). In addition, male zebra finches show different strategies for song

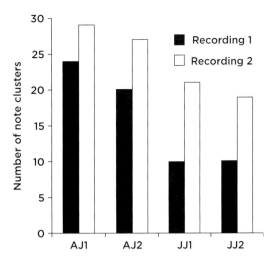

Figure 33.4 Number of note clusters in 4 flocks of juvenile males who were housed with adult females (AJ1 & AJ2) or juvenile females (JJ1 & JJ2) during development. Recording 1 was performed with males in their original flocks (AJ vs. JJ). Recording 2 was performed after males had However, recording 2 was performed after AJ1 and JJ1 males were switched and AJ2 and JJ2 males were switched so that the juvenile males originally housed with adult females were housed with juvenile females and the juvenile males originally housed with juvenile females were housed with adult females.

learning relative to the group size they are in during development (Liu et al., 2004). And, directly related to our findings, male zebra finches improvise more when they are housed with deafened females compared to hearing females, suggesting that males are sensitive to feedback of female companions (Williams, personal communication). Thus, our research fits with theoretical and experimental studies that have recognized the role of *variability* in female preferences in the development of male traits and behaviors (Coleman et al., 2004; Jennions & Petrie, 1997). Furthermore, it can be speculated that the prevalence of markings and color patterns in many avian species—wing-bars, eye-rings, stripes on the face—are likely effective in providing contextual information about body posture, head orientation, direction of gaze, etc., which are exactly the sorts of signals that would be useful in providing social feedback.

Similar to the patterns observed in female cowbirds, early during development human mothers sometimes ignore sounds or behaviors altogether because they do not infer communicative intent or simply are not attending closely to their infant. Mothers' ignoring of signals, like the adult female cowbird's selective inattention to song, may make infants more aware of what needs to occur for their behavior to be taken seriously. Thus, infants' vocal repertoire development and variability may be tied to caregiver responsiveness. At this point, we do not have a clear idea of what proportion of infant acts is treated as communicative and how this varies across individuals. However, results from our longitudinal study of 12 infants indicate wide variation across caregivers. Mothers verbally responded to 17%–83% of their infants' prelinguistic vocalizations. Similar to the findings in the cowbirds, there is probably a level of contingent stimulation that is ideal. For instance, we know from studies of depressed mothers that too little feedback is detrimental to multiple aspects of communicative development. Depressed mothers may show less affect in their voices, with fewer temporal and intonational patterns of infant-directed speech to which infants attend (Kaplan et al., 2002). These infants are exposed to fewer of the important prosodic cues available in infant-directed speech that are thought to assist language learning (Kemler Nelson et al., 1989) and they experience fewer contingency-based interactions or less appropriately timed responses (Cohn et al., 1986; Field, 1998). As a result, these infants show communicative disorders in the first year of life, exhibiting less optimal interactive patterns and becoming withdrawn (Field et al., 1988; Jones et al., 1997). Furthermore, these infants show differential frontal lobe activation and neurotransmitter levels (Dawson & Ashman, 2000; Jones et al., 1997), which is reminiscent of neural differences in male cowbirds housed with females that differed in their levels of responsiveness. Although we do not have parallel evidence for extremely responsive caregivers, the findings for the extreme example of low levels of responsiveness of depressed mothers indicate that optimal levels of contingent stimulation within social interactions are necessary for communicative development from social and neural perspectives.

Caregivers differ not only in their level, or frequency, of responses, but also in their style of responding. One of the primary characterizations of caregiving styles identified in studies of infant attachment, maternal sensitivity, may be familiar to many readers. Measures of maternal sensitivity bring together a wide variety of maternal characteristics, including maternal warmth and appropriate responding to emotional, attentional, and communicative aspects of infants' behavior using a numbered scale (Ainsworth et al., 1974, 1978). Here, however, we use terms that focus on one dimension of maternal sensitivity that refer specifically to how caregivers respond to infants' attentional focus. Caregiver responses range between two extremes, which have been labeled "directive" and "follow-in" (Baldwin et al., 1996; Tomasello & Farrar, 1986). "Directive" behavior involves caregivers attempting to lead or direct infants' attention away from their current attentional focus (i.e., introducing or commenting on a toy that is not the infant's current focus). "Follow-in" behavior involves caregivers following in to the infants' attentional focus (i.e., commenting on or labeling a toy that the infant is currently engaged with). There is experimental and observational evidence that follow-in responses that are sensitive to infant's attentional focus facilitate vocabulary learning and language development, whereas directive responses that redirect infants' attention to objects outside of their current focus have a negative impact on language learning (Baldwin & Tomasello, 1998; Baumwell et al., 1997; Tamis-LeMonda et al., 2001; Tomasello & Farrar, 1986).

Recent studies in our laboratory revealed the impact of these different response styles on infants' prelinguistic attentional and communicative behaviors. The first study explored short-term effects of infants' interactions with unfamiliar adults who either followed-in to or redirected the infants' attentional focus (sensitive vs. redirective responses). Infants shifted their attentional focus more often in the redirective condition than in the sensitive condition not only to toys that the experimenter introduced, but also more frequently to toys that the experimenter had not introduced. Also, in the redirective condition infants focused their attention on their social partner or the toy with which they were interacting for shorter amounts of time than in the sensitive condition. This difference in duration of attentional engagement was also apparent when infants were looking away from their social partner or to other toys in the room. Thus, when interactive with the redirective individual, infants had shorter attention periods of attentional engagement both during social interaction and outside of the social interaction. The results indicate that the style of social partners' interaction can shape infants' attentional engagement, which could have effects no only on communicative development, but also on exploration and information (Miller et al., in press; Figure 32.5).

The second, longitudinal study revealed that over time, such different response styles can impact vocal usage, possibly related to infants not sustaining attention in social interactions. For illustrative

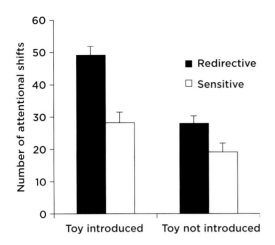

Figure 33.5 Average duration and frequency of attentional shifts in engaged and disengaged sequences with the sensitive and redirective individuals (mean seconds + SEM). (From Miller et al., in press.)

purposes, we provide examples from two mother–infant pairs, representing the two extremes of responsiveness: "follow-in" and "directive." The infant whose mother displayed the most follow-in behavior at 8 months, responding to her infant's vocalizations by attending to her attentional focus, increased her percentage of directed vocalizations by 14 months more than the infant whose mother was most directive, leading her infant's attention away from her current attentional focus. Specifically, the infant of the mother who followed-in more increased vocalizations directed to her mother by 39%, whereas the infant whose mother was directive decreased vocalizations directed to her mother by 63%, thus appearing disengaged in interactions with her mother (Gros-Louis, unpublished data). These data suggest that caregiver responses early in the prelinguistic phase influence the development of communicative behavior, including pragmatics, prior to the advent of language.

Gating Contingent Stimulation

Given that feedback in social interactions lies at the heart of learning about both acoustic structure and pragmatics, West, King, and colleagues have examined the effects of different social environments, particularly the availability of social partners, on development. It was discovered that wide variation in singing behavior of young male cowbirds was dependent on the social contexts in which they were housed (e.g., Smith et al., 2000; White et al., 2002a, 2002b). Young males showed very different outcomes in their singing behavior

(including song structure, song usage, repertoire size and rate of development) that varied consistently with the age and sex of individuals housed with them. Different environments resulted in different patterns of social associations and singing interactions, which in turn led to different facultative developmental trajectories of young males in their vocal production and communicative competency (vocal usage) as measured by reproductive success. These results led to consideration of a mechanism termed the "social gateway": different social environments offer different opportunities for interactions, thus metering the communicative behaviors that individuals produce and the feedback they receive (West et al., 2003; White et al., 2002a). The existence of a social gateway is consistent with the observations in several songbird species that indicate a relationship between social responsiveness of the environment and vocal and social learning. More specifically, access to and interactions with experienced individuals at specific points in development are key to acquiring communicative competence (Beecher, 1996).

We propose that a social gateway provides a useful construct for examining how social interactions between infants and social partners (caregivers, parents, siblings) affect vocal development and vocal usage. We believe that human infants interacting with different social partners in different environments are vulnerable to influences on development, just as we have observed in songbirds. The structure of social interactions serves a "gatekeeping" function, modulating the information available to infants through differential attention and feedback. Future studies in our laboratory aim to document the variability of social contingencies available in interactions with different social partners and how these impact infants' communicative behavior.

Research that demonstrates that the social gateway is the critical predictor of pragmatic competence bears on the nature–nurture question that often accompanies research in cowbirds. As brood parasites, the young are never raised by their own species but instead by over 200 different species and subspecies, leaving the question of ultimate outcome open: how do they recognize their own species and what if they mistakenly mate with the wrong species? This circumstance has led many theorists to suppose the hardwiring of directed behaviors such as singing to females or males serves as a genetic safety net. What better species to have innate modules than a brood parasite, as relying on postnatal learning experience to guide development could have disastrous consequences?

Cowbirds were thought to be the model species for a closed developmental program (Lehrman, 1971; Mayr, 1974, 1979), but research by West and King has found precisely the opposite: lack of social experience leads to communicative and reproductive incompetence. Even if isolate birds learn songs that are effective in eliciting copulatory postures of females in playback experiments, there is no endogenous connection between form and function. These same birds cannot successfully mate even if their songs elicit copulatory postures. Thus, given that social experience is necessary to develop proper usage of vocalizations, the safety net is external to the individual, rather than existing in innate developmental programs. The social interactions that an individual experiences during development are the safety net that ensures correct pragmatic function of communicative behavior. It is possible that cowbirds, being brood parasites, are unusual in their reliance on social feedback as juveniles in part because they lack early conspecific experience. Unfortunately, to our knowledge, there is no evidence available from other avian species that confirms the importance of social feedback in shaping the pragmatics of vocal communication because the research has not been done.

Coordinated Communicative Behaviors

Thus far, we have been discussing relatively simple communicative behaviors such as the act of singing or babbling. Can we see the role for pragmatics in more complex behaviors? An example of such a behavior is countersinging (CS) in male cowbirds, i.e., exchanges of directed songs by males (Figure 32.6). CS highlights another dimension of the journalistic frame of questioning as two males must simultaneously make the same decision about to whom and when and where to sing. This behavior can only be studied when males live in flocks, as it requires at least the cooperation of two males and sometimes more. Adult males differ in how much they CS, varying from very frequently to not at all. The data show an underlying pragmatic dimension that differs as a result of early experience with or without adults (White et al., 2002b).

To examine how early interactions shape development, we conducted two studies which revealed that the level of CS can be culturally transmitted, representing an excellent example of a cultural trait that is not genetically controlled, but sustained through learning (White et al., 2007). In the first

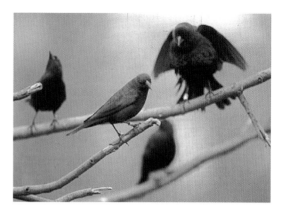

Figure 33.6 Male cowbirds engaged in a countersinging bout. The male performing a wingspread display is the one singing. The recipient directly in front of him then sings a song in return. Songs are exchanged until one of the two males flies away.

study, we exposed two groups of juvenile males to adults who had exhibited different levels of male competition via CS in the prior year. In the second study, we gave two new groups of juvenile males either social access to competitive males or only visual and auditory access to them. In addition, the juveniles in the second study were exposed to the competitive males only for a brief period in the fall months when CS is *not* occurring. In both studies, juvenile males developed behaviors that matched that of their adult "models," but only if they had social access, that is, housed in the same flock within an aviary. They also exhibited other behavioral differences regarding courtship even though they had no opportunity to witness adult males performing courtship behaviors in either study.

The form of social influence on behavior depicted here for pragmatic forms differs from traditional concepts of cultural transmission where a behavior is directly copied. Because juveniles in the second study learned to CS even when they were with adult males not engaging in CS, it is clear that the juveniles were not merely copying an observed behavior. How had the juvenile males come to exhibit behaviors of "models" whom they did not see perform the target behaviors? We propose that the juveniles had learned to sustain their attention span via social interactions. Learning what to attend to, rather than observation of model behavior, shaped future interactions, resulting in the compounded behavior of CS later in development. Adults' behavior set the early conditions for the group's pattern of social engagement (see also White et al., 2002a), which put juveniles on a different developmental pathway.

This study highlights the importance of considering how learning occurs in a social environment. These data tell us that cultural transmission occurs for pragmatic dimensions and that it happens within a group network where individuals may influence one another in nonobvious ways. The importance of the group dynamic must be emphasized. Males needed physical contact, not just visual and acoustic stimulation, in order to learn adult behaviors. This is suggested from further findings in aviary studies: birds in adjacent aviaries, who can see and hear one another, do not share song types, something that occurs routinely within aviaries and in the wild (White et al., 2007). Males appear to need first-hand experience within interactions, receiving reactions to their own behavior rather than just observing other males' interactions. Through particular interactions information becomes accessible. In our words, the bioavailability of information is metered by the social gateway.

A rough parallel to CS in cowbirds is early protoconversation in caregiver–infant interactions. Infants primarily must learn when to respond in interactions, and later in development, they must learn to whom to respond when they start to engage in triadic interactions with multiple social partners or caregivers and objects (Striano & Rochat, 1999). Protoconversations develop in the first 2–3 months of life and involve the exchange of mutual gaze and affect (Bateson, 1975; Trevarthen, 1979). Although protoconversations often focus on socioemotional aspects of interaction, such as affect attunement (e.g., Stern, 2000; Stern et al., 1985), a key component important to our discussion here is the coordinated timing of infants and social partners. The rhythm of vocal exchanges is a key predictor of attachment and cognitive development in the first year (Jaffe et al., 2001) and, we propose, turn-taking within interactions forms the initial pragmatic basis of communication.

As with CS interactions in cowbirds, infants do not learn by observation, but by being an active social partner. It is the structural aspect of early interactions, not their content per se, that contributes to infant learning by modulating infants' attention (Menyuk et al., 1995; Papousek, 2007). In particular, early games and social routines contribute to learning about the *pragmatics* of conversational exchange, because infants learn turn-taking and turn-giving in social interactions (Bruner, 1979; Mayer & Tronick, 1985; Ratner & Bruner, 1978; Snow, 1984; Watson, 1972). Studies that show that infants become sensitive to the timing of

social responses within games such as peekaboo at about 4 months of age (Rochat et al., 1999) indicate that infants are learning about the temporal patterning of social exchanges (see also Ninio & Bruner, 1978). "Communicating about communicating" in these early interactions (Bateson, 1956) thus provides information about the structuring of social exchanges, a first step in learning about the effectiveness of communicative behaviors.

It is after infants learn to sustain attention in interactions that specific feedback between caregivers and infants gives infants feedback about the effectiveness of their own behaviors. "Shared meaning" develops in caregiver–infant dyads, which contributes to learning the significance of particular behaviors (Halliday, 1975; Newson, 1979). Differentiated responses to variable behaviors across contexts can provide the infant with information about the communicative function of behaviors in social interactions (e.g., Gros-Louis et al., in preparation-a). Communication thus shifts from "communication by action to communication by symbol" (Camaioni, 1993, p. 161). What is needed is a study that investigates the contributions to this shift during development. Therefore, in addition to the many studies that investigate the temporal coordination and sequencing of behaviors in infant–caregiver exchanges (e.g., Hsu et al., 2001; Stevenson et al., 1992; Yale et al., 2003), studies must explore the development of pragmatic significance of conversational exchanges (e.g., Dore, 1979).

Pragmatics and Evolutionary Implications

In our laboratory, we have looked at evolutionary consequences by studying reproductive outcomes of different developmental trajectories and associated social skills. Parentage analysis of 1071 eggs from ten flocks (32 males and 57 females) documented longitudinal reproductive histories over a 4-year period as birds experienced different social contexts (unfamiliar males and females). We were surprised to discover that dominant males who are characterized by aggressive behavior (e.g., displacements, fights, etc.) sired only 1/4 as many eggs as the most successful males. The dominant males typically sing the most potent songs, a finding we have replicated numerous times. This leaves social pragmatics in the form of song use to distinguish individuals. Thus, traditional measures of song quality or status are misleading in understanding reproductive success because they leave out many pragmatic dimensions. The most successful males may be more attentive to their potential mates or rivals and know they must integrate their behavior, not dominate another's behavior.

An example of a critical constructor of successful reproductive behavior is the behavior of staying or leaving when approached by another individual male. Juvenile males tend to leave when adults sing to them whereas adults tend to stay. The juveniles must learn not to leave so that social negotiations such as CS can develop, which is correlated with increased levels of reproductive success (Gros-Louis et al., 2006b; King et al., 2003; West et al., 2002). Juveniles learn the pragmatic aspect of staying versus leaving through interactions with experienced males. For example, in White et al. (2007), direct social experience with competitive adults led juveniles to interact socially more often. Under these conditions, juveniles experienced different learning environments where different types of information were available and different contingencies connected their behaviors. For example, early in the fall when housed with adult males, these juveniles sang to adult males who, in turn, rarely left in response to the juveniles' songs. As a result, the first significant difference between the two groups of juveniles after adult males were removed from physical or visual and acoustic proximity was in the behavior of leaving to song. Juveniles who had been housed with adult males, and thus had experienced direct contact with adults, learned to respond to song by staying, whereas juveniles who could only observe adults in another aviary, seemed by default to leave to a song directed to them and thus rarely experienced the consequences of singing. In effect, these observer juveniles constructed a condition of self-imposed social isolation. They rarely engaged in male social interactions, rarely showed the development of CS with other males, and in turn developed higher potency song, which is a characteristic of males developing in experimentally imposed male social isolation (West & King, 1980).

Until we discovered the role of pragmatics we were led to conclude, as many researchers do, that males with high-potency songs, as tested by playback, would be the most successful in an aviary setting. Although females are attracted to potent song, only some males can withstand the social pressure that comes with singing such songs, in particular, aggression from other males. Thus, they must learn that what they sing depends on to whom they direct their song and that the conditions for potent song may be rare, whereas the conditions for moderate song sung repeatedly to males

and females may take them farther. The story about playback song potency is an example of a de-pragmatized narrative. The result is a good story but an inaccurate one. We initially assumed that playback potency always correlated with copulatory success but we were using the female's copulatory posture as a proxy for copulation, an assumption we do not now make. One of the biggest lessons is that males with good songs as judged by playback may not use their song in an effective manner. Males have to learn song content but this learning is inadequate without understanding the social conditions in which to sing it.

Similar to our identification of cultural transmission in cowbirds that differs from the traditional view, Tomasello (2001) has indicated a similar process in language development in infants that he terms cultural learning (see also Trevarthen, 1988). Though he focuses on learning within an individual, he points out implications for evolutionary origins of communicative behavior. The parallel with the mechanism that we identified in the development of CS behavior is that children do not learn by directly emulating behaviors of caregivers or attending to specific associations that are made clear to them by their caregivers; rather, they learn through ongoing interactions with their caregivers. For example, most of the words learned by children do not come from direct attentional focus and labeling by a caregiver. In fact, this could only work for concrete nouns and some action verbs. Therefore, it is through social conventions and being a participant in an interaction that infants can learn the meaning of words by attending to nonverbal and paralinguistic cues (Tomasello & Barton, 1994; Tomasello et al., 1996). And, most importantly, similar to what we have concluded from our research on cowbirds, children inherit ontogenetic niches that bring with them patterns of interactions and contexts of learning that ensure cultural transmission.

Conclusion

Our research with both human infants and songbirds provides us with a comparative framework from which to examine communicative development. Songbirds provide a good parallel to infants because of similar developmental stages, and social and neural influences (Doupe & Kuhl, 1999; Kuhl, 2003). Until recently, the conspicuous period of production termed "babbling" in both systems had been considered to be motor practice for the goal of stereotyped song repertoires or speech with limited or no social/communicative function (Bloom, 1993; but see Locke, 2001 where a "relational" function of babbling is proposed; Oller, 2000). However, our experience with vocal development in birds and infants demonstrate a strong social interactive component of early vocal interactions that influences communicative development (Goldstein et al., 2003; King & West, 1988).

Both animal studies and human communicative pathologies indicate that different mappings between vocal and pragmatic development can occur (Locke, 1993). Vocal learning (of birdsong or referential language) can progress without correct usage of vocal forms in social interactions. The emergence of directed attention while producing vocalizations provides a platform for pragmatic learning in both human and avian communicative development (Miller et al., 2006). We believe that the emphasis on the innate basis of vocal development, and the focus on the role of copying signals, has obscured the importance of pragmatic development. For example, although most of the focus in bird song learning is on imitation, improvisation is also a documented route, and one used by cowbirds. Improvisation occurs not only with song content, but song use. Thus, in the studies of CS, the young birds exposed to adults in the fall could not copy appropriate adult courtship behavior because they never saw it. But those with social contact ended up pragmatically competent because their social development created a pathway toward knowing how to respond to song, i.e., by staying and responding to social partners.

In both birds and babies, the use of copied versus improvised vocalizations coupled with directedness creates different learning opportunities. Specifically the use of directed improvised vocalizations may accelerate learning the relationship between vocal structure and its function because it provides varied contingent feedback to a range of vocalizations. Preliminary data support this view in cowbirds: in two flocks where we have followed juvenile males that were high or low improvisers, the high improvisers sang more directed song to males and females during the fall than the low improvisers and 6 months later were more successful courting females during their first breeding season (Miller, unpublished data). Thus, to return to the theme of the journalistic practice or reporting "who," followed by "what," "when," and "where," progressing to "why" and ending with "how," we propose that vocal improvisation may represent an important engine of pragmatic learning, which

informs about these issues. Because vocal development in nonmimicking birds is rooted in copying (Beecher, 1996; Nordby, Campbell, & Beecher, 2007), improvisation is often treated as copying errors and thus obscures the possibility of programmatic adaptive learning.

With respect to human vocal development, contrary to early views that imitation is the primary mechanism of development, it is through contingent stimulation in interactions that communicative behavior develops. Starting in the 1970s, researchers began to recognize the potential extent of the relationship between vocalizations used in social exchanges and the development of language (e.g., Bates et al., 1979; Bruner, 1977). It is the basic functional understanding of early prelinguistic communicative behaviors that is thought to provide the sociocognitive structures necessary for the development of language. An important point in prelinguistic infants and nonlinguistic species is that it is through the responses of social partners that behaviors are shaped and acquire functionality (Dore, 1979; Halliday, 1975). There need not be intentionality on the part of a young organism to communicate but, through interactions, functional communication emerges (Cheney & Seyfarth, 1996; Smith, 1977; Sugarman, 1984). For example, as noted previously, infants will begin to disengage their gaze and look around the room at about 4 months of age. Caregivers view this as intentional or communicative and respond accordingly, providing feedback to the infant about the function of gazing (cf., Siegel, 1999). Thus, throughout development, infants' production of novel vocalizations or actions provides new opportunities for caregivers to respond and to respond differentially, thus potentially providing potent feedback about the effectiveness of infants' behaviors (Papousek, 1992; Snow, 1984).

The overarching purpose of our comparative research program is to discover principles of development through the investigation of the ontogeny of experience. We define the ontogeny of experience as the process by which an organism progressively creates and selects stimulation from a rich ecology. We believe that by maximizing the extent to which the organism can select information from its ecology, the opportunity to uncover common denominators of developmental systems becomes apparent. For example, understanding the role for attentional development to filter stimulation will be predictive of both social and cognitive outcomes across taxa. Our studies of the cowbird demonstrate the limitations of a reliance on innate modules to predict functional outcomes and suggest the even supposedly "closed" developmental systems are inherently sensitive to developmental ecology. The avian work has been predictive of our human prelinguistic work, as similar processes appear to be functioning. Thus, the evidence suggests than developmental explanations of communicative behavior will rely on an understanding of the recurring opportunities for social experience, and the role of contingency-based learning within interactions, to understand the role of the developmental ecology to shape functional outcomes.

References

Ainsworth, M. D. S., Bell, S. M., & Stayton, D. J. (1974). Infant–mother attachment and social development: "socialization" as a product of reciprocal responsiveness to signals. In M. P. M. Richards (Ed.), *The intergration of a child into a social world* (pp. 99–135). Cambridge: Cambridge University Press.

Ainsworth, M. D. S., Blehar, M., Waters, E., & Wall, S. (1978). *Patterns of attachment*. Hillsdale, NJ: Erlbaum.

Akhtar, N., & Tomasello, M. (2000). The social nature of words and word learning. In R. M. Golinkoff, K. Hirsh-Pasek, L. Bloom, L. B. Smith, A. Woodward, N. Akhtar, M. Tomasello & G. Hollich (Eds.), *Becoming a word learner: A debate on lexical acquisition* (pp. 115–135). New York: Oxford University Press.

Bakeman, R., & Adamson, L. (1984). Coordinating attention to people and objects in mother–infant and peer–infant interactions. *Child Development, 55*, 1278–1289.

Baldwin, D. A., Markman, E. M., Bill, B., Desjardins, R. N., Irwin, J. M., & Tidball, G. (1996). Infants' reliance on a social criterion for establishing word–object relations. *Child Development, 67*, 3135–3153.

Baldwin, D. A., & Tomasello, M. (1998). Word learning: a window on early pragmatic understanding. In E. V. Clark (Ed.), *The Proceedings of the Twenty-Ninth Annual Child Language Research Forum* (pp. 3–23). Stanford: Center for the Study of Language and Information.

Baptista, L. F., & Petrinovich, L. (1984). Social interaction, sensitive periods, and the song template hypothesis in the white-crowned sparrow. *Animal Behaviour, 36*, 1752–1764.

Baron-Cohen, S. (1989). Perceptual role taking and protodeclarative pointing in autism. *British Journal of Developmental Psychology, 7*, 113–127.

Barratt, M. S., Roach, M. A., & Leavitt, L. A. (1992). Early channels of mother–infant communication: Preterm and term infants. *Journal of Child Psychology and Psychiatry, 33*, 1193–1204.

Bates, E. (1976). *Language and context: The acquisition of pragmatics*. New York: Academic Press.

Bates, E., Benigni, L., Bretherton, I., Camaioni, L., & Volterra, V. (1979). *The emergence of symbols: Cognition and communication in infancy*. New York: Academic Press.

Bates, E., Camaioni, L., & Volterra, V. (1975). The acquisition of performatives prior to speech. *Merrill-Palmer Quarterly, 21*, 205–226.

Bateson, G. (1956). The message: "This is play." In B. Schaffner (Ed.), *Group processes: Transactions of the Second Conference* (pp. 145–242). New York: Josiah Macy Foundation.

Bateson, G. (1975). Mother–infant exchanges: The epigenesis of conversational interaction. In D. Aaronson & R. W. Rieber (Eds.), *Developmental psycholinguistics and communicative disorders* (Vol. 263, pp. 101–113). New York: New York Academy of Sciences.

Baumwell, L., Tamis-LeMonda, C. S., & Bornstein, M. H. (1997). Maternal verbal sensitivity and child language comprehension. *Infant Behavior and Development, 20*, 247–258.

Beaumont, S. L., & Bloom, K. (1993). Adults' attributions of intentionality to vocalizing infants. *First Language, 13*, 235–247.

Beecher, M. D. (1996). Birdsong learning in the laboratory and field. In D. E. Kroodsma & E. H. Miller (Eds.), *Ecology and evolution of acoustic communication in birds* (pp. 61–78). Ithaca, NY: Cornell University Press.

Beecher, M. D., & Brenowitz, E. A. (2005). Functional aspects of song learning in songbirds. *Trends in Ecology and Evolution, 20*, 143–149.

Beecher, M. D., & Burt, J. M. (2004). The role of social interaction in bird song learning. *Current Directions in Psychological Science, 13*, 224–228.

Beecher, M. D., Burt, J. M., O'Loghlen, A. L., Templeton, C. N., & Campbell, S. E. (2007). Bird song learning in an eavesdropping context. *Animal Behaviour, 73*, 929–935.

Beecher, M. D., Campbell, S. E., Burt, J. M., Hill, C. E., & Nordby, J. C. (2000). Song-type matching between neighbouring song sparrows. *Animal Behaviour, 59*, 21–27.

Bigelow, A. E. (1999). Infants' sensitivity to imperfect contingency in social interaction. In P. Rochat (Ed.), *Early social cognition* (pp. 137–154). Hillsdale, NJ: Erlbaum.

Bigelow, A. E., & Birch, S. A. J. (1999). The effects of contingency in previous interactions on infants' preference for social partners. *Infant Behavior and Development, 22*(3), 367–382.

Bigelow, A. E., & DeCoste, C. (2003). Sensitivity to social contingency from mothers and strangers in 2-, 4-, and 6-month-old infants. *Infancy, 4*(1), 111–140.

Bloom, K., D'Odorico, L., & Beaumont, S. (1993). Adult preferences for syllabic vocalizations: Generalizations to parity and native language. *Infant Behavior and Development, 16*, 109–120.

Bloom, L. (1993). *The transition from infancy to language: Acquiring the power of expression*. Cambridge, England: Cambridge University Press.

Bornstein, M. H., Tamis-LeMonda, C. S., Tal, J., Ludemann, P., Toda, S., Rahn, C. W., et al. (1992). Maternal responsiveness to infants in three societies: The United States, France, and Japan. *Child Development, 63*, 808–821.

Brenowitz, E. A. (2004). Plasticity of the adult avian sound control system. In: P. Zeigler & P. Marler, (Eds.), *Behavioral neurobiology of bird song, Annals of the New York Academy of Science*, 1016, 560–585.

Bruner, J. (1977). Early social interaction and language acquisition. In H. R. Schaffer (Ed.), *Studies in mother–infant interaction* (pp. 271–289). London: Academic Press.

Bruner, J. (1978). Berlyne Memorial Lecture acquiring the uses of language. *Canadian Journal of Psychology, 32*(4), 204–218.

Bruner, J. (1979). The organization of action and the nature of the adult–infant transaction. In E. Tronick (Ed.),

Social interchange in infancy (pp. 23–35). Baltimore, MD: University Park Press.

Bruner, J. (1983). *Child's talk: Learning to use language*. New York: Norton.

Bruner, J. S. (1975). From communication to language: a psychological perspective. *Cognition, 3*, 255–287.

Camaioni, L. (1993). The development of intentional communication: A re-analysis. In *New perspectives in early communicative development* (pp. 82–96). London: Routledge.

Camarata, S. M., & Gibson, T. (1999). Pragmatic language deficits in attention-deficit hyperactivity disorder (ADHD). *Mental Retardation and Developmental Disabilities Research Reviews, 5*(3), 207–214.

Carpenter, M., Pennington, B. F., & Rogers, S. J. (2002). Interrelations among social-cognitive skills in young children with autism. *Journal of Autism and Developmental Disorders, 32*(2), 91–106.

Carpenter, R. L., Mastergeorge, A. M., & Coggins, T. E. (1983). The acquisition of communicative intentions in infants eight to fifteen months of age. *Language and Speech, 26*(2), 101–116.

Cheney, D. L., & Seyfarth, R. M. (1996). Function and intention in the calls of non-human primates. *Proceedings of the British Academy of Sciences, 88*, 59–76.

Chomsky, N. (1965). *Syntactic structures*. The Hague: Mouton.

Cohn, J. F., Matias, R., Tronick, E. Z., Connell, D., & Lyons-Ruth, K. (1986). Face-to-face interactions of depressed mothers and their infants. In E. Z. Tronick & T. Field (Eds.), *Maternal depression and infant disturbance* (Vol. 24). San Francisco: Jossey-Bass.

Coleman, S. W., Patricelli, G. L., & Borgia, G. (2004). Variable female preferences drive complex male displays. *Nature, 428*, 742–745.

Collis, G. (1979). Describing the structure of social interaction in infancy. In M. Bullowa (Ed.), *Before speech: the beginning of interpersonal communication* (pp. 111–130). Cambridge, UK: Cambridge University Press.

D'Odorico, L., & Cassibba, R. (1995). Cross-sectional study of coordination between infants' gaze and vocalization towards their mothers. *Early Development & Parenting, 4*, 11–19.

Dabelsteen, T., & McGregor, P. K. (1996). Dynamic acoustic communication and interactive playback. In D. E. Kroodsma & E. H. Miller (Eds.), *Ecology and evolution of acoustic communication in birds* (pp. 398–408). Ithaca, NY: Cornell University Press.

Dawson, G., & Ashman, S. B. (2000). On the origins of a vulnerability to depression: the influence of the early social environment on the development of psychological systems related to the risk of affective disorder. In C. A. Nelson (Ed.), *The effects of early adversity on neurobehavioral development* (Vol. 31, pp. 245–279). Mahwah, NJ: Lawrence Erlbaum Associates.

de Boysson-Bardies, B., & Vihman, M. M. (1991). Adaptation to language: Evidence from babbling and first words in four languages. *Language, 67*(2), 297–319.

Dore, J. (1974). A pragmatic description of early language development. *Journal of Psycholinguistic Research*, 3(4), 343–350.

Dore, J. (1979). Conversational acts and the acquisition of language. In E. Ochs & B. B. Schieffelin (Eds.), *Developmental pragmatics* (pp. 359–361). New York: Academic Press, Inc.

Dore, J. (1986). The development of conversational competence. In R. L. Schiefelbusch (Ed.), *Language competence:*

Assessment and intervention (pp. 3–60). San Diego: College-Hill Press, Inc.

Dore, M. (1983). Feeling, form and intention in the baby's transition to language. In R. M. Golinkoff (Ed.), *The transition for prelinguistic to linguistic communication* (pp. 167–190). Hillsdale, NJ: Lawrence Erlbaum Associates.

Doupe, A. J., & Kuhl, P. K. (1999). Birdsong and human speech: Common themes and mechanisms. *Annual Review of Neuroscience, 22*, 5567–5631.

Dunham, P. J., Dunham, F., & Curwin, A. (1993). Joint-attentional states and lexical acquisition at 18 months. *Developmental Psychology, 29*, 827–831.

Dusenbery, D. B. (1992). *Sensory ecology: How organisms acquire and respond to information*. New York: W. H. Freeman.

Field, T. (1998). Maternal depression effects on infants and early interventions. *Preventive Medicine, 27*, 200–203.

Field, T., Healy, B., Goldstein, S., Perry, S., Bendell, D., Schanberg, S., et al. (1988). Infants of depressed mothers show "depressed" behavior even with nondepressed adults. *Child Development, 59*, 1569–1579.

Freeberg, T. M., King, A. P., & West, M. J. (1995). Social malleability in cowbirds (*Molothrus ater artemisiae*): Species and mate recognition in the first 2 years of life. *Journal of Comparative Psychology, 109*, 357–367.

Freeberg, T. M., West, M. J., King, A. P., Duncan, S. D., & Sengelaub, D. R. (2002). Cultures, genes, and neurons in the development of song and singing in brown-headed cowbirds (*Molothrus ater*). *Journal of Comparative Physiology A, 188*, 993–1002.

Freed-Brown, S. G., King, A. P., Miller, J. L., & West, M. J. (2006). Uncovering sources of variation in female sociality: Implications for the development of social preferences in female cowbirds (*Molothrus ater*). *Behaviour, 143*, 1293–1315.

Gergely, G., & Watson, J. (1999). Early socio-emotional development: Contingency perception and the social-biofeedback model. In P. Rochat (Ed.), *Early social cognition: understanding others in the first months of life* (pp. 101–136). Mahwah, NJ: Lawrence Erlbaum Associates, Inc.

Gibb Harding, C. (1983). Setting the stage for language acquisition: Communication development in the first year. In R. M. Golinkoff (Ed.), *The transition for prelinguistic to linguistic communication* (pp. 93–113). Hillsdale, NJ: Lawrence Erlbaum Associates.

Gibson, J. J. (1966). *The senses considered as perceptual systems*. Boston: Houghton-Mifflin.

Goldstein, M. H., King, A. P., & West, M. J. (2003). Social interaction shapes babbling: Testing parallels between birdsong and speech. *Proceedings of the National Academy of Science, 100*, 8030–8035.

Goldstein, M. H., & Schwade, J. A. (2008). Social feedback to infants' babbling facilitates rapid phonological learning. *Psychological Science, 19*, 515–523.

Golinkoff, R. M., & Gordon, L. (1983). In the beginning there was word: A history of the study of language acquisition. In R. M. Golinkoff (Ed.), *The transition from prelinguistic to linguistic communication*. Hillsdale, NJ: Lawrence Erlbaum Associates, Inc.

Gottesman, I. I. (1963). Genetic aspects of intelligent behavior. In N. Ellis (Ed.), *The handbook of mental deficiency* (pp. 253–296). New York: McGraw-Hill.

Gottlieb, G. (1976). Roles of early experience in the development of behavior and the nervous system. In G. Gottlieb

(Ed.), *Studies in the development of behavior and the nervous system* (pp. 25–54). New York: Academic Press.

Gros-Louis, J. (2006, June). *The role of prelinguistic vocalizations in vocal and social development*. Poster presented at the 5th International Conference on Development and Learning, Bloomington, IN.

Gros-Louis, J., & Ables, E. (2006, October 2). *Contextual influences on caregiver responsiveness*. Paper presented at the 39th Annual Meeting of the International Society for Developmental Psychobiology, Atlanta, GA.

Gros-Louis, J., Ables, E., King, A. P., & West, M. J. (Manuscript in preparation-a). *Consistency and differentiation of caregiver responses across contexts*.

Gros-Louis, J., West, M. J., Goldstein, M. H., & King, A. P. (2006a). Mothers provide differential feedback to infants' prelinguistic sounds. *International Journal of Behavioral Development, 30(6),* 509–516.

Gros-Louis, J., West, M. J., & King, A. P. (Manuscript in preparation-b). *Caregiver responses influence the development of communicative behaviors*.

Gros-Louis, J., White, D. J., King, A. P., & West, M. J. (2006b). Do juvenile males affect adult males' reproductive success in brown-headed cowbirds (*Molothrus ater*)? *Behaviour, 143,* 219–237.

Hailman, J. P. (1977). *Optical signals: Animal communication and light*. Bloomington: Indiana University Press.

Halliday, M. (1979). One child's protolanguage. In M. Bullowa (Ed.), *Before speech: The beginning of interpersonal communication* (pp. 149–170). Cambridge, UK: Cambridge University Press.

Halliday, M. A. K. (1975). *Learning how to mean: Explorations into the development of language*. London: Edward Arnold.

Hamilton, K. S., King, A. P., Sengelaub, D. R., & West, M. J. (1998). Visual and song nuclei correlated with courtship skills in brown-headed cowbirds. *Animal Behaviour, 56,* 973–982.

Hauser, M. D. (1996). *The evolution of communication*. Cambridge, MA: MIT Press.

Hsu, H. C., Fogel, A., & Messinger, D. S. (2001). Infant non-distress vocalization during mother–infant face-to-face interaction: factors associated with quantitative and qualitative differences. *Infant Behavior and Development, 24,* 107–128.

Jaffe, J., Beebe, B., Feldstein, S., Crown, C. L., & Jasnow, M. (2001). *Rhythms of dialogue in infancy: Coordinated timing in development*. Boston, MA: Blackwell Publishers.

Jarvis, E. D., Scharff, C., Grossman, M., Ramos, J. A., & Nottebohm, F. (1998). For whom the bird sings: Context-dependent gene expression. *Neuron, 21,* 775–788.

Jennions, M. D., & Petrie, M. (1997). Variation in mate choice and mating preferences: A review of causes and consequences. *The American Naturalist, 72,* 283–327.

Johnson-Laird, P. N. (1990). Introduction: What is communication? In D. H. Mellor (Ed.), *Ways of communicating* (pp. 1–13). Cambridge: Cambridge University Press.

Jones, N. A., Field, T., Fox, N. A., Davalos, M., Malphurs, J., Carraway, K., et al. (1997). Infants of intrusive and withdrawn mothers. *Infant Behavior and Development, 20,* 175–186.

Jones, S. E., & Zimmerman, D. H. (2003). A child's point and the achievement of intentionality. *Gesture, 3*(2), 155–185.

Kaplan, P. S., Bachorowski, J.-A., Smoski, M. J., & Hudenko, W. J. (2002). Infants of depressed mothers, although competent learners, fail to learn in response to their own moth-

ers' infant-directed speech. *Psychological Science, 13*(3), 268–271.

Kasher, S., & Meilijson, A. (1996). Autism and pragmatics of language. *Incontri Cita Aperta, 4/5,* 37–54.

Keller, H., & Scholmerich, A. (1987). Infant vocalizations and parental reactions during the first four months of life. *Developmental Psychology, 23,* 62–67.

Kemler Nelson, D. G., Hirsh-Pasek, K., Jusczyk, P. W., & Cassidy, K. W. (1989). How the prosodic cues in motherese might assist language learning. *Journal of Child Language, 16,* 55–68.

Kent, R. D., & Miolo, G. (1995). Phonetic abilities in the first year of life. In P. Fletcher & B. MacWhinney (Eds.), *The handbook of child language* (pp. 303–334). Cambridge: Blackwell Publishers.

Kimura, D. (1993). *Neuromotor mechanisms in human communication*. Oxford: Oxford University Press.

King, A. P., & West, M. J. (1983). Epigenesis of cowbird song: A joint endeavor of males and females. *Nature, 305,* 704–706.

King, A. P., & West, M. J. (1988). Searching for the functional origins of cowbird song in eastern brown-headed cowbirds (*Molothrus ater ater*). *Animal Behaviour, 36,* 1575–1588.

King, A. P., & West, M. J. (1989). Presence of female cowbirds (*Molothrus ater ater*) affects vocal improvisation in males. *Journal of Comparative Psychology, 103,* 39–44.

King, A. P., & West, M. J. (2002). Ontogeny of competence. In D. J. Lewkowicz & R. Lickliter (Eds.), *Conceptions of development* (pp. 77–104). New York: Psychology Press.

King, A. P., West, M. J., & Goldstein, M. (2005). Nonvocal shaping of avian song development: Parallels to human speech development. *Ethology, 111,* 101–117.

King, A. P., White, D. J., & West, M. J. (2003). Female proximity stimulates development of male competition in juvenile brown-headed cowbirds, *Molothrus ater. Animal Behaviour, 66,* 817–828.

Konishi, M. (1965). The role of auditory feedback in the control of vocalization in the white-crowned sparrow. *Zeitscrift fur Tierpsychologie, 22,* 770–783.

Krebs, J. R., & Davies, N. B. (1993). *Introduction to behavioural ecology*. Oxford: Blackwell Scientific.

Kroodsma, D. E. (1996). Ecology of passerine song development. In D. E. Kroodsma & E. H. Miller (Eds.), *Ecology and evolution of acoustic communication in birds* (pp. 3–19). Ithaca, NY: Cornell University Press.

Kroodsma, D. E. (2004). The diversity and plasticity of birdsong. In P. Marler & H. Slabbekoorn (Eds.), *Nature's music: The science of birdsong* (pp. 108–131). San Diego: Elsevier Academic Press.

Kroodsma, D. E., & Pickert, R. (1984). Sensitive phases for song learning: effects of social interaction and individual variation. *Animal Behaviour, 32,* 389–394.

Kuhl, P. (2003). Human speech and birdsong: Communication and the social brain. *Proceedings of the National Academy of Sciences, 100*(17), 9645–9646.

Kuo, Z. Y. (1967). *The dynamics of behavioral development: An epigenetic view*. New York: Random House.

Lawrence, B. (1986). *Parent's perceptions of communication with prelinguistic children*. Unpublished PhD Dissertation, University of North Carolina, Chapel Hill, NC.

Laws, G., & Bishop, D. V. M. (2004). Verbal deficits in Down's syndrome and specific language impairment: a comparison. *International Journal of Language & Communication Disorders, 39*(4), 423–451.

Lehrman, D. S. (1971). Conceptual and semantic issues in the nature–nurture problem. In L. R. Aronson, E. Tobach, D. S. Lehrman & J. S. Rosenblatt (Eds.), *Development and the evolution of behaviour: Essays in the memory of T. C. Schneirla* (pp. 17–52). San Francisco: W. H. Freeman.

Lenneberg, E. (1967). *Biological foundations of language*. New York: Wiley.

Lickliter, R., & Gottlieb, G. (1985). Social interaction with siblings is necessary for visual imprinting of species-specific maternal preferences in ducklings. *Journal of Comparative Psychology, 99*, 371–379.

Lindblom, B. (1990). On the communication process: Speaker-listener interaction and the development of speech. In K. Fraurud & U. Sundberg (Eds.), *AAC augmentative and alternative communication* (pp. 220–230). London: Williams & Wilkins.

Liu, W., Gardner, T. J., & Nottebohm, F. (2004). Juvenile zebra finches can use multiple strategies to learn the same song. *Proceedings of the National Academy of Sciences, 101*, 18177–18182.

Locke, J. L. (1983). *Phonological acquisition and change*. New York: Academic Press.

Locke, J. L. (1993). *The child's path to spoken language.* Cambridge, MA: Harvard University Press.

Locke, J. L. (1996). Why do infants begin to talk? Language as an unintended consequence. *Journal of Child Language, 23*, 251–268.

Locke, J. L. (2001). First communion: the emergence of vocal relationships. *Social Development, 10*(3), 294–308.

Lorenz, K. (1965). *Evolution and modification of behavior.* Chicago: University of Chicago Press.

Markus, J., Mundy, P., Morales, M., Delgado, C. E. F., & Yale, M. (2000). Individual differences in infant skills as predictors of child–caregiver joint attention and language. *Social Development, 9*(3), 302–315.

Marler, P. (1967). Animal communication signals. *Science, 157*, 769–774.

Marler, P. (1970). Birdsong and speech development: Could there be parallels? *American Scientist, 58*, 669–673.

Marler, P., Mundinger, P., Waser, M. S., & Lutjen, A. (1972). Effects of acoustical deprivation on song development in redwing blackbirds (*Agelaius phoeniceus*). *Animal Behaviour, 20*, 586–606.

Marler, P., & Nelson, D. (1992). Neuroselection and song learning in birds: Species universals in a culturally transmitted behavior. *Seminars in the Neurosciences, 4*, 415–423.

Marler, P., & Nelson, D. A. (1993). Action-based learning: A new form of developmental plasticity in bird song. *Netherlands Journal of Zoology, 43*(1–2), 91–103.

Marlter, P., & Peters, S. (1982). Action-based learning—a new form of developmental plasticity in bird song. *Netherlands Journal of Zoology, 43*, 91–103.

Mayer, N. K., & Tronick, E. Z. (1985). Mothers' turn-giving signals and infant turn-taking in mother–infant interaction. In T. M. Field & N. A. Fox (Eds.), *Social perceptions in infants* (pp. 199–216). Norwood, NJ: Ablex Publishing Co.

Mayr, E. (1974). Behavioral programs and evolutionary strategies. *American Scientist, 62*, 650–659.

Mayr, E. (1979). Concepts in the study of animal behavior. In J. S. Rosenblatt & B. R. Komisaruk (Eds.), *Reproductive behavior and evolution* (pp. 1–16). New York: Plenum Press.

McGregor, P. K., & Peake, T. M. (2000). Communication networks: social environments for receiving and signaling behavior. *Acta Ethology, 2*, 71–81.

Menyuk, P., Liebergott, J. W., & Schultz, M. C. (1995). *Early language development in full-term and premature infants*. Hillsdale, NJ: Lawrence Erlbaum.

Miller, J. L., Ables, E., King, A. P., & West, M. J. (in press). Different patterns of contingent stimulation differentially affect attention span in prelinguistic infants. *Infant Behavior and Development.*

Miller, J. L., Freed-Brown, S. G., White, D. J., King, A. P., & West, M. J. (2006). Developmental origins of sociality in brown-headed cowbirds (*Molothrus ater*). *Journal of Comparative Psychology, 120*, 229–238.

Miller, J. L., King, A. P., & West, M. J.. (2008) *Female social networks influence male vocal development in brown-headed cowbirds (Molothrus ater). Animal Behaviour, 76*, 931–941.

Moore, C. L. (1984). Maternal contributions to the development of masculine sexual behavior in laboratory rats. *Developmental Psychobiology, 17*, 347–356.

Morris, C. W. (1946). *Signs, language, and behavior.* New York: Braziller. Prentice Hall Reprint (1955).

Nelson, D. A., & Marler, P. (1994). Selection-based learning in bird song development. *Proceedings of the National Academy of Science, 91*, 10498–10501.

Neuringer, A., Dreiss, C., & Olson, G. (2000). Reinforced variability and operant learning. Journal of Experimental Psychology: *Animal Behavior Processes, 26*, 98–111.

Newson, J. (1979). The growth of shared understandings between infant and caregiver. In M. Bullowa (Ed.), *Before speech: The beginning of interpersonal communication* (pp. 207–222). Cambridge: Cambridge University Press.

Ninio, A., & Bruner, J. (1978). The achievement and antecedents of labelling. *Journal of Child Language, 5*, 1–15.

Nordby, J. C., Campbell, S. E., & Beecher, M. D. (2007). Selective attrition and individual song repertoire development in song sparrows. *Animal Behaviour, 74*, 1413–1418.

Nowicki, S., Searcy, W. A., Hughes, M., & Podos, J. (2001). The evolution of bird song: Male and female response to song innovation in swamp sparrows. *Animal Behaviour, 62*, 1189–1195.

Oller, D. K. (2000). *The emergence of the speech capacity.* Mahwah, NJ: Lawrence Erlbaum.

Oyama, S. (2000). *The ontogeny of information: Developmental systems and evolution* (2nd ed.). Durham, NC: Duke University Press.

Papousek, H., & Bornstein, M. H. (1992). Didactic interactions: Intuitive parental support of vocal and verbal development in human infants. In H. Papousek, U. Jurgens & M. Papousek (Eds.), *Nonverbal vocal communication: Comparative and developmental approaches* (pp. 209–229). New York: Cambridge University Press.

Papousek, H., & Papousek, M. (1975). Cognitive aspects of preverbal social interactions between human infants and adults. In *Parent–infant interaction* (pp. 241–269). Amsterdam: Associated Scientific Publishers.

Papousek, M. (1989). Determinants of responsiveness to infant vocal expression of emotional state. Infant *Behavior and Development, 12*, 507–524.

Papousek, M. (1992). Early ontogeny of vocal communication in parent–infant interactions. In H. Papousek, U. Jurgens

& M. Papousek (Eds.), *Nonverbal vocal communication: Comparative and developmental approaches* (pp. 230–261). New York: Cambridge University Press.

Papousek, M. (2007). Communication in early infancy: An arena of intersubjective learning. *Infant Behavior and Development, 30*, 258–266.

Payne, R. B., & Payne, L. L. (1993). Song copying and cultural transmission in indigo buntings. *Animal Behaviour, 46*, 1045–1065.

Pruden, S. M., Hirsh-Pasek, K., & Golinkoff, R. M. (2006). The social dimension in language development: a rich history and a new frontier. In P. J. Marshall & N. A. Fox (Eds.), *The development of social engagement: Neurobiological perspectives* (pp. 118–152). Oxford: Oxford University Press.

Purvis, K. L., & Tannock, R. (1997). Language abilities in children with attention deficit hyperactivity disorder, reading disabilities, and normal controls. *Journal of Abnormal Child Psychology, 25*, 133–144.

Ratner, N., & Bruner, J. (1978). Games, social exchange, and the acquisition of language. *Journal of Child Language, 5*, 391–402.

Reddy, V. (1999). Prelinguistic communication. In M. Barrett (Ed.), *The development of language* (pp. 25–50). Hove, East Sussex: Psychology Press.

Rochat, P., Querido, J. G., & Striano, T. (1999). Emerging sensitivity to the timing and structure of protoconversation in early infancy. *Developmental Psychology, 35*, 950–957.

Rochat, P., & Striano, T. (1999). Social-cognitive development in the first year. In P. Rochat (Ed.), *Early social cognition: Understanding others in the first months of life* (pp. 3–34). Mahwah, NJ: Lawrence Erlbaum Associates, Inc.

Rollins, P. R. (2003). Caregivers' contingent comments to 9-month-old infants: Relationships with later language. *Applied Psycholinguistics, 24*, 221–234.

Sameroff, A. J. (1975). Early influences on development: fact or fancy? *Merrill-Palmer Quarterly, 21*, 267–294.

Scarr-Salapatek, S. (1976). Genetic determinants of infant development: an overstated case. In L. Lipsitt (Ed.), *Developmental psychobiology: The significance of infancy* (pp. 59–79). Hillsdale, NJ: Erlbaum.

Schaffer, H. R., Collis, G. M., & Parsons, G. (1977). Vocal interchange and visual regard in verbal and pre-verbal children. In H. R. Schaffer (Ed.), *Studies in mother–infant interaction* (pp. 291–324). London: Academic Press.

Schieffelin, B. B. (1983). Looking and talking: the functions of gaze direction in the conversations of a young child and her mother. In E. Ochs & B. B. Schieffelin (Eds.), *Acquiring conversational competence* (pp. 50–65). Boston: Routledge and Kegan Paul.

Searcy, W. A. (1992). Measuring responses of female birds to male song. In P. K. McGregor (Ed.), *Playback and studies of animal communication* (pp. 175–189). New York: Plenum Press.

Sebeok, T. A. (1962). Coding in the evolution of signaling behavior. *Behavioral Science, 7*, 430–442.

Sebeok, T. A. (1965). Animal communication. *Science, 147*, 1006–1014.

Siegel, D. J. (1999). *The developing mind: Toward a neurobiology of interpersonal experience*. New York: The Guilford Press.

Skoyles, J. R. (1998). Child development and autism: a cerebellar prefrontal model [electronic version]. Cogprints. Retrieved May 23, 2006 from http://web.archive.org/web/20071017181851/cogprints.org/791/0/autism.htm

Smith, L. (1998). Predicting communicative competence at 2 and 3 years from pragmatic skills at 10 months. *International Journal of Language & Communication Disorders, 33*, 127–148.

Smith, V. A., King, A. P., & West, M. J. (2000). A role of her own: female cowbirds, Molothrus ater, influence the development and outcome of song learning. *Animal Behaviour, 60*, 599–609.

Smith, W. J. (1977). *The behavior of communicating*. Cambridge, MA: Harvard University Press.

Snow, C. E. (1984). Parent–child interaction and the development of communicative ability. In R. L. Schiefelbusch & J. Pickar (Eds.), *The acquisition of communicative competence* (pp. 69–107). Baltimore: University Park Press.

Stern, D. N. (1974). Mother and infant at play: The dyadic interaction involving facial, vocal, and gaze behaviors. In M. Lewis & L. A. Rosenblum (Eds.), *The effect of the infant on its caregiver* (pp. 187–213). New York: John Wiley & Sons.

Stern, D. N. (2000). *The interpersonal world of the infant* (2nd ed.). New York: Basic Books.

Stern, D. N., Hofer, L., Haft, W., & Dore, J. (1985). Affect attunement: the sharing of feeling states between mother and infant by means of intermodal fluency. In T. M. Field & N. A. Fox (Eds.), *Social perception in infants* (pp. 249–268). Norwood, NJ: Ablex Publishing Corporation.

Stevenson, M. B., Roach, M. A., & Leavitt, L. A. (1992). Early channels of mother–infant communication: preterm and term infants. *Journal of Child Psychology and Psychiatry, 33*, 1193–1204.

Stoel-Gammon, C., & Otomo, K. (1986). Babbling development of hearing-impaired and normally hearing subjects. *Journal of Speech and Hearing Disorders, 51*, 33–41.

Striano, T., & Rochat, P. (1999). Developmental link between dyadic and triadic social competence in infancy. *British Journal of Developmental Psychology, 17*, 551–562.

Sugarman, S. (1984). The development of preverbal communication: Its contribution and limits in promoting the development of language. In R. L. Schiefelbusch & J. Pickar (Eds.), *The acquisition of communicative competence* (pp. 23–67). Baltimore: University Park Press.

Surian, L., Baron-Cohen, S., & Van der Lely, H. (1996). Are children with autism deaf to Gricean maxims? *Cognitive Neuropsychiatry, 1*, 55–71.

Tamis-LeMonda, C. S., Bornstein, M. H., & Baumwell, L. (2001). Maternal responsiveness and children's achievement of language milestones. *Child Development, 72*(3), 748–767.

Tanguay, P. E., Robertson, J., & Derrick, A. (1998). A dimensional classification of autism spectrum disorder by social communication domains. *Journal of the American Academy of Child & Adolescent Psychiatry, 37*, 271–277.

Thelen, E., Corbetta, D., & Spencer, J. P. (1996). Development of reaching during the first year: role of movement speed. *Journal of Experimental Psychology: Human Perception and Performance, 22*(5), 1059–1076.

Thelen, E., & Ulrich, B. D. (1991). Hidden skills: a dynamic systems analysis of treadmill stepping during the first year. *Monographs of the Society for Research in Child Development, 56*(1, Serial No. 223).

Tomasello, M. (1997). The pragmatics of word learning. *Cognitive Studies: Bulletin of Japanese Cognitive Science Society, 4*, 59–74.

Tomasello, M. (2001). Cultural transmission: A view from chimpanzees and human infants. *Journal of Cross-Cultural Psychology, 32*, 135–146.

Tomasello, M., & Barton, M. (1994). Learning words in non-ostensive contexts. *Developmental Psychology, 30*, 639–650.

Tomasello, M., & Farrar, M. J. (1986). Joint attention and early language. *Child Development, 57*, 1454–1463.

Tomasello, M., Strosberg, R., & Akhtar, N. (1996). Eighteen-month old children learn words in non-ostensive contexts. 23, *Journal of Child Language*, 157–176.

Trevarthen, C. (1979). Communication and cooperation in early infancy: A description of primary intersubjectivity. In M. Bullowa (Ed.), *Before speech: The beginning of interpersonal communication* (pp. 321–347). Cambridge: Cambridge University Press.

Trevarthen, C. (1988). Universal cooperative motives: How infants begin to know language and skills of culture. In G. Jahoda & I. M. Lewis (Eds.), *Acquiring culture: Ethnographic perspectives on cognitive development* (pp. 37–90). London: Croom Helm.

Trevarthen, C., & Hubley, P. (1979). Secondary intersubjectivity: Confidence, confiding and acts of meaning in the first year. In A. Lock (Ed.), *Action gesture and symbol* (pp. 183–229). London: Academic Press.

Vihman, M. M., Ferguson, C. A., & Elbert, M. (1986). Phonological development from babbling to speech: common tendencies and individual differences. *Applied Psycholinguistics, 7*, 3–40.

Vygotsky, L. S. (1962). *Thought and language.* Cambridge, MA: MIT Press.

Watson, J. S. (1972). Smiling, cooing and "the game." *Merrill-Palmer Quarterly, 18*, 323–339.

Watson, J. S. (1985). Contingency perception in early social development. In T. M. Field & N. A. Fox (Eds.), *Social perception in infants* (pp. 157–177). Norwood, NJ: Ablex Publishing Corporation.

West, M. J., & King, A. P. (1987). Settling nature and nurture into an ontogenetic niche. *Developmental Psychobiology, 20*, 549–562.

West, M. J., & King, A. P. (1988). Female visual displays affect the development of male song in the cowbird. *Nature, 334*, 244–246.

West, M. J., & King, A. P. (2001). Science lies its way to the truth…really. In E. M. Blass (Ed.), *Developmental psychobiology* (Vol. 13, pp. 587–614). New York: Kluwer Academic/ Plenum Publishers.

West, M. J., King, A. P., & Duff, M. A. (1990). Communicating about communicating: when innate is not enough. *Developmental Psychobiology, 23*, 585–598.

West, M. J., King, A. P., & Freeberg, T. M. (1996). Social malleability in cowbirds: New measures reveal new evidence of plasticity in the Eastern subspecies (*Molothrus ater ater*). *Journal of Comparative Psychology, 110*, 15–26.

West, M. J., King, A. P., & White, D. J. (2003). The case for developmental ecology. *Animal Behaviour, 66*, 617–622.

West, M. J., White, D. J., & King, A. P. (2002). Female brown-headed cowbirds' (*Molothrus ater*) organization and behaviour reflects male social dynamics. *Animal Behaviour, 64*, 377–385.

Wetherby, A. M., Cain, D. H., Yonclas, D. G., & Walker, V. G. (1988). Analysis of intentional communication of normal children from the prelinguistic to the multiword stage. *Journal of Speech and Hearing Research, 31*, 240–252.

White, D. J., Gros-Louis, J., King, A. P., Papakhian, M., & West, M. J. (2007). Constructing culture in cowbirds (*Molothrus ater*). *Journal of Comparative Psychology, 121*(113–123).

White, D. J., Gros-Louis, J., King, A. P., & West, M. J. (2006). A method to measure the development of song preferences in female cowbirds. *Animal Behaviour, 72*, 181–188.

White, D. J., King, A. P., Cole, A., & West, M. J. (2002a). Opening the social gateway: Early vocal and social sensitivities in brown-headed cowbirds (*Molothrus ater*). *Ethology, 108*, 23–37.

White, D. J., King, A. P., & West, M. J. (2002b). Facultative development of courtship and communication in juvenile male cowbirds (Molothrus ater). *Behavioral Ecology, 13*, 487–496.

Wilson, E. O. (1975). *Sociobiology.* Cambridge, MA: Harvard University Press.

Yale, M. E., Messinger, D. S., Cobo-Lewis, A. B., & Delgado, C. F. (2003). The temporal coordination of early infant communication. *Developmental Psychology, 39*(5), 815–824.

Zeigler, H. P. & Marler, P. (2004). Behavioral neurobiology of bird song. *Annals of the New York Academy of Science, 1016*.

From Birds to Words: Perception of Structure in Social Interactions Guides Vocal Development and Language Learning

Michael H. Goldstein *and* Jennifer A. Schwade

Abstract

Infant songbirds and humans face a similar task: to produce a functional repertoire of sounds that operates within the communication system of conspecifics. The mechanisms by which infants learn to talk and birds learn to sing share parallels at the neural, behavioral, and social levels of organization. By making immature sounds and observing the reactions of others, infants of both taxa learn the acoustic structures and temporal contingencies that define communicative interaction. Social and vocal learning, however, are rarely investigated as part of the same system. This chapter uses avian song learning as a model for socially guided vocal learning in human infants. It then discusses socially guided learning in the development of speech and language.

Keywords: vocal development, language learning, songbirds, conspecifics, immature sounds, reactions, acoustic structures, temporal contingencies

Introduction

In a backyard, near the window of a house, a young bird alights on a branch and sings. His song is immature; its structure bears little resemblance to the rapid sequences of clearly articulated notes that he will produce during the breeding season in a few months. A nearby female, however, listens to his infantile sounds and responds with a quick movement of her wings. The male catches her subtle signal, and repeats the cluster of notes that he just sang.

In the house, a 9-month-old infant watches the birds through a window. She utters a stream of babbling sounds. Her babbling could not be mistaken for mature speech, as she has no words in her productive vocabulary, and her sounds do not follow the phonology of the language that surrounds her. Her mother, however, reacts to her babbling by pointing at the singing bird and saying "that's a birdy." As the infant continues to babble, her mother keeps taking vocal turns

with her, and over the next few minutes, the infant's sounds become more speech-like, with more resonant vowels and faster consonant–vowel transitions.

Both of these scenes describe powerful moments of learning, in which the responsiveness of social partners to immature behavior is perceived and used by the young learner to generate more advanced forms of vocalization. Such a socially mediated system of vocal learning relies on specific mechanisms of perception and action in both the infant and the adult. Adults' behavior must be sensitive to acoustic characteristics of vocal precursors, and infants must be capable of using adults' feedback to modify their vocalizations. These mechanisms, described in detail below, play strong roles in the development of song, speech, and language.

The development of birdsong and human speech share parallels at the neural, behavioral, and social levels of organization (Doupe & Kuhl, 1999;

Goldstein, King, & West, 2003; King, West, & Goldstein, 2005; Marler, 1970; Petrinovich, 1972; Wilbrecht & Nottebohm, 2003). Though much of the research described below focuses on humans, our theoretical perspective and even some of the experimental paradigms derive from studies of songbird vocal development. We link research on the two taxa by way of an ecological approach to understanding development. An ecological approach emphasizes connections between opportunities for action that the environment affords and the learner's ability to perceive those affordances (Gibson, 1979; Gibson & Pick, 2000). In this view, the behavioral capacities of animals are best studied in the environmental contexts in which they evolved and developed. Thus an ecological approach to learning and development, in both birds and babies, considers developmental phenomena such as the ability to sing or talk as a product of both the young organism and specific environmental opportunities for learning (Green & Gustafson, 1997; Johnston, 1981; West & King, 1985).

We focus on the role of early vocal precursors in the construction of both birdsong and human speech. In our ecological framework, vocal precursors are not just something that an infant has in its possession, rather they get used as instruments of learning. When the responsiveness of social partners is considered along with infants' ability to perceive changes in others' behavior, babbling becomes part of an active process in which infants' actions contribute to their own development. In this view, the possible functional significance of immature song and speech can best be assessed in a social context. Thus we take a microgenetic approach to social learning. In our infant research, we observe and manipulate parent–offspring interactions at moment-to-moment timescales to understand mechanisms of developmental change. By studying social interaction and learning as they occur from moment to moment, we can connect specific mechanisms of perceptual and cognitive development with social influences on the acquisition of speech and language.

Such an approach stands in contrast to the mainstream of research on communicative and linguistic development. Most work focuses on infant capacities or on the nature of the input, but not both *at the same time*. The studies we describe below integrate the perceptual and cognitive mechanisms by which infants pick up information with the structure available in adult reactions to infant behavior. Data from these studies indicate that

the development of intelligent behavior is embedded in social processes. Infants, like many organisms, must rely on the brains and bodies of others as an alternative to evolving specific capacities for surviving in a complex environment. Socially distributed intelligence is evidenced by the foraging and nest-building activities of termites, ants, and bees (e.g., Seeley, 1995), in the movements of rat pups as they huddle to collectively thermoregulate (Alberts, 1978; Schank & Alberts, 1998), and in the vocal development of male cowbirds that rely on the visual reactions of females to shape their immature sounds into functional song (West & King, 1988). In our view, caregivers and infants constitute a system of distributed intelligence, one in which maternal behavior and infant sensory capacities interact to construct more advanced infant behavior. Thus we focus on patterns of interaction between caregivers and infants as a source of developmental change. In this chapter, we will start by describing the implications of social learning for vocal development in songbirds and then show what our research has revealed about the role of social learning for communicative development in human infants.

Social Influences on Vocal Learning in Songbirds

In songbirds, strong evidence indicates that the social environment is crucial for vocal development (Beecher & Brenowitz, 2005; Beecher & Burt, 2004). Vocal learning has long been assumed to depend on early memorization of adult song, followed by a period of vocal development in which the young bird attempts to imitate the memorized song (see Marler, 1997 for review). However, there are multiple models of social influences on vocal learning. For example, in several species, socially guided learning is an important mechanism driving the development of complex articulatory patterns and auditory learning that catalyzes production of well-formed, species-typical song. Social learning also facilitates the selective attrition of functional elements from immature vocalizations (Marler & Nelson, 1993). Investigations of animal communication have shown that responses of conspecifics to the vocal precursors of young songbirds influence developmental outcomes and thus constitute a social mechanism of vocal learning (Doupe & Kuhl, 1999; Marler & Nelson, 1993; West & King, 1988).

An instructive example of the role of immature vocalizations in the socially guided learning of song comes from studies of the brown-headed cowbird (*Molothrus ater*). Cowbirds are brood parasites; the females lay their eggs in the nests of other species, so a young cowbird is not likely to hear the songs of conspecifics early in life (Friedman, 1929). Despite their lack of early species-specific experience, males sing to females during the breeding season (May–June) and a mature song is necessary for successful courtship and copulatory success (Chapter 33). Thus cowbirds were long assumed to have an innate, unmodifiable program of song development (Mayr, 1974). The reasons for such a closed developmental program are easy to understand: Since song is necessary for reproductive success, there is too much at stake for species survival to leave song development to the vagaries of individual experience, especially in a brood parasite. A cowbird being reared by another species might learn the wrong song or court the wrong species.

Evidence that learning played a crucial role in song production came from studies that focused on the early stages of song development. The ontogeny of song in cowbirds is gradual, lasting from 2 to 12 months of age, and can be broken down into several stages (Smith, King, & West, 2000; see also Chapter 33). Subsong, the initial stage, is characterized by low amplitude and high variability in structure and timing. Plastic song, beginning at approximately 60–75 days of age, is composed of poorly articulated notes that are sung in varying, unstable sequences. Formatted song, beginning at approximately 200 days, has elements with stable ordering and timing, but with variable content. Finally, stereotyped song typically develops at 250–300 days. These are mature, stable songs, and a male's repertoire typically consists of 2–6 song types (Rothstein, Yokel, & Fleischer, 1988).

To assess the relative influences of nature and nurture on song production, West and King (1988) housed individual males over the winter and spring in 1.3 m³ sound attenuating chambers. Each male was housed with a female, so the males would have a social companion but would still live in acoustic isolation, as females do not sing. Results showed that being housed with a female was a vocally enriching experience. Males housed in acoustically impoverished conditions developed song that had high potency, as measured by females' responses to playbacks of the song (West & King, 1988). What were the females doing to create males with high song potency? Video analyses showed that the females were using small,

infrequent wing movements (called wingstrokes) to selectively reinforce elements of the male's plastic song. Females produced wingstrokes either during or immediately after songs, which often were 1 s in duration. Wingstrokes were typically under 200 ms in duration and were infrequent, occurring once for every 100 songs. Males that received a wingstroke were, on average, three times more likely to repeat the element that they just sang (West & King, 1988).

Were the females responding to more advanced vocalizations, thus shaping the males in a developmentally advanced direction? To test the functional value of wingstrokes, West and King took immature songs from the early spring that preceded, elicited, and followed wing strokes, and played them back to a new set of females. They used a female bioassay procedure (West, King, Eastzer, & Staddon, 1979) in which females during the breeding season respond with copulatory postures to immature songs, as long as those songs contain some functional elements. They found that females were most responsive to plastic songs that had earlier elicited wing strokes. In addition, songs that followed wingstrokes received higher responding than songs that preceded wingstrokes (West & King, 1988).

Thus the immature vocalizations of young male cowbirds elicit orientation and wing movements from adult females, and this feedback facilitates the development of more advanced forms of song (King et al., 2005; Smith et al., 2000; West & King, 1988). The functional significance of plastic song only became apparent in social contexts; the value of early vocalizing would not have been discovered if the males had been studied in isolation. Later studies showed that females from different regions, with differing levels of responsiveness, create differences in the acoustics of plastic song, the rate of song development, and the potency of song (King et al., 2005; Smith et al., 2000; West & King 1988). A focus on the functional significance of vocal precursors has been successfully employed in studies of vocal learning in multiple species (Marler & Nelson, 1993; Snowdon & Hausberger, 1997; West, King, & Duff, 1990).

Socially Guided Vocal Learning in Human Infants

Those who study the vocal precursors of songbirds and human infants face similar challenges. Like the subsong and plastic song of songbirds, the early noncry vocalizations of human infants are highly variable and immature in acoustic form. In both taxa, mechanisms of social learning have often taken a backseat to a focus on innate templates guiding vocal development. When social learning has been found, processes of imitation are usually invoked to explain the results. Our work on vocal learning and development in human infants was a direct result of the cowbird work described above. If vocal precursors in songbirds could have functional significance in social settings, the babbling of human babies might also be a strong force in socially guided vocal learning.

Infant sounds have been extensively studied from a taxonomic perspective, in which vocal development has been described in terms of universal and invariant stages (Oller, 1980, 1985, 2000; Oller & Lynch, 1992; Stark, 1979, 1980). The aim of these studies was not to consider the effects of social context or other environmental influences on vocal production, but rather to map out the species-typical course of vocal development. In our vocal learning studies, we quantify babbling using Oller's categories of prelinguistic production, as they describe early sounds in terms of their "infraphonology" or the acoustic prerequisites of well-formed speech. The infraphonological acoustic

classification system incorporates both acoustic parameters (e.g. fundamental frequency [F_0], formant transitions) and qualitative descriptors (e.g. phonetic categories). From 1 to 4 months of age (primitive articulation stage), vocal production incorporates articulator movements at the back of the vocal tract using tongue and epiglottal contact with the soft palate to produce some consonant stops. Combinations of stops with quasi-resonant nuclei produce the first "goo"- and "coo"-type syllables. At 3–8 months (Expansion/Exploratory stage), the vocal tract becomes more open and fully resonant sounds are produced. Infants produce marginal syllables, which are slow sequences of consonant–vowel articulation, with long transitions between consonant and vowel. From 5 to 10 months (Canonical Syllable stage), infants begin to produce fully resonant sounds and faster formant transitions, resulting in canonical syllables (e.g., [ba], [da]), a language-general unit of mature vocal production (Figure 34.1).

What are the underlying mechanisms mediating transitions to new vocal forms? At the level of the articulators, there are constraints imposed by the developing vocal tract. The nasalized quasi-resonant vocalizations of the primitive articulation stage are

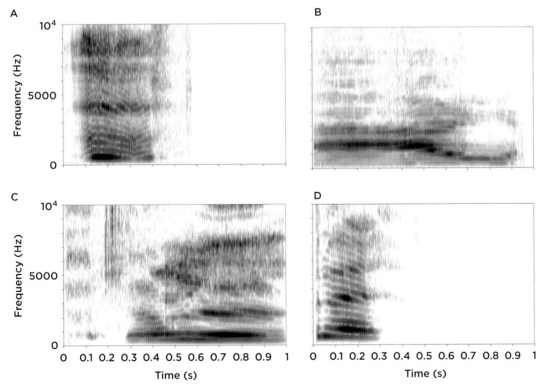

Figure 34.1 Spectrograms of the four vocal types. (A) Quasi-resonant vowel. (B) Fully resonant vowel. (C) Marginal syllable. (D) Canonical syllable.

due to the overlapped larynx and nasopharynx at the back of the vocal tract, which forces infants to breathe nasally. Also, the small size of the oral cavity restricts tongue movement (Kent, 1981a, 1981b). As the larynx descends into the throat, the fully resonant vowels of the expansion/exploratory stage can be produced. These physiological constraints are most important in the first months of life. By approximately 7 months of age, a new type of articulatory pattern, rhythmic jaw oscillations, emerges and permits reduplicated canonical syllables (Iverson, Hall, Nickel, & Wozniak, 2007; Iverson & Thelen, 1999; MacNeilage, 1998; MacNeilage & Davis, 2000; Meier, 1997). MacNeilage attributes the oscillatory pattern to evolutionary forces that shaped the physiology and neuroanatomy of jaw control, while Iverson shows that rhythmic behavior is a global, whole-organism event, occurring in limbs at the same time as the jaw (Iverson et al., 2007).

While the presence of rhythmic, reduplicated vocalizations is a ubiquitous feature of vocal development after 7 months of age, there are also large individual differences in early vocal development. For example, there are large age overlaps across the stages of vocal development discussed above. Data from deaf and hearing-impaired infants reveal that their babbling is acoustically different from that of hearing infants from 6 months onward, with abnormalities in marginal syllables and a marked delay in onset of canonical syllables (Locke, 1993; Locke & Pearson, 1992; Oller, 1985; Oller & Eilers, 1988; Oller, Eilers, Bull, & Carney, 1985; Stoel-Gammon & Otomo, 1986). These studies suggest that typical vocal development requires environmental input.

The phonology of prelinguistic vocalizations also shows effects of the ambient language on early vocalizing. The "babbling drift" hypothesis emphasizes the influence of the ambient language on babbling. By approximately 8 months of age, several suprasegmental features of vocalizing have come to resemble that of the ambient language. For example, the intonation patterns (rising and falling pitch) and rhythm (final syllable lengthening) of 7–11-month-old French and English infants resemble those of their ambient languages (Levitt & Wang, 1991; Whalen, Levitt, & Wang, 1991). Segmental features, such as the patterns of vowels and consonants that comprise syllables, are also influenced by experience. Nigerian infants are exposed to Yoruba, a language in which many words begin with a vowel. The babbling of 10- to 12-month-old Nigerian infants has a typical disyllable structure of vowel–consonant–vowel (VCV),

in contrast to the typical CVCV disyllable pattern found in the babbling of French infants (Boysson-Bardies, 1993). In comparisons of French, English, Japanese, and Swedish infants, the modes of consonant production are similar in distribution to that of the ambient language (Boysson-Bardies & Vihman, 1991), and comparisons of French, English, Chinese, and Algerian 10-month-old infants has revealed that the distribution of vowels in their babbling is similar to that of the ambient language (Boysson-Bardies, Halle, Sagart, & Durand, 1989). Nine-month-old infants can change their babbling to reflect sound patterns in their mothers' speech within minutes (Vihman & Miller, 1988). Though these studies reveal a gradual shift toward the phonology of the ambient language, they do not shed light on the nature of the interactions that lead to phonological learning.

The ambient language also exerts a strong influence on speech perception. Studies of environmental influence on speech perception yield clues as to the mechanisms that might be involved in vocal learning. By 8–10 months of age, infants form categories corresponding to the phonemic contrasts of their language environment (e.g., Best, 1994, 2002; Jusczyk, 1992; Werker & Tees, 1984). Social interaction facilitates the development of categorical speech perception (Kuhl, 2007a, 2007b; Kuhl, Tsao, & Liu, 2003). Social feedback may focus attention on relevant features of the speech signal and/or provide additional sources of information that specify perceptual categories (Kuhl, 2007a, 2007b). Categorical speech perception is negatively impacted when infants attend to speech to learn word–object associations (Fennell, Byers-Heinlein, & Werker, 2007; Stager & Werker, 1997; Werker & Curtin, 2005). Social interaction may be beneficial for speech perception because its attention-organizing effects buffer the increased cognitive load of word learning. Social interaction may benefit vocal learning in similar ways.

Given the important role of language experience in the development of speech perception and production, what mechanisms incorporate the phonology of the ambient language into babbling? Infants develop in a responsive, structured social environment, and can perceive regularities in others' behavior (Baldwin, Baird, Saylor, & Clark, 2001). Structured and consistent social responses to babbling, if present, can create opportunities for infants to learn from the consequences of their vocalizing and acquire an understanding of the contingencies defining communicative interaction. Socially

scrambled transcripts. We found that the amount of infant vocal imitation was not different from chance levels. The kinds of sounds that infants produced shared phonological rules but not phonetic characteristics with their mothers' speech. This means that vocal learning is a nonimitative process.

Thus the form and timing of maternal behavior influenced the learning of specific acoustic parameters of babbling. Changes in the sounds mirrored acoustic changes that occur during development. Infant imitation is not a likely explanation for these data. Though these infants produced sounds with more resonance or CV syllables, they did not produce the same phonemes their mothers modeled. Because mothers produced a diversity of phonemes, the underlying infraphonological patterns became more salient. Previous research on statistical learning, using an auditory discrimination task, has shown that 9-month-old infants can rapidly learn to recognize phonological patterns (Gerken, 2006; Saffran & Thiessen, 2003). In an artificial grammar learning task, greater variability in the input results in infants learning higher-order patterns across nonadjacent elements in the input (Gómez, 2002). We believe that variability in the input plays an important role in determining the speech patterns that infants incorporate into their vocal repertoires, as infants who receive repetitions of the same utterance produce sounds that imitate the input (Kuhl & Meltzoff, 1996). If infants' prelinguistic vocalizations are guided by statistical learning, input consisting of repetitions of a single syllable would lead to infants' learning of the phonetic surface features rather than learning the underlying CV structure. As a result, infants would not have a phonological framework with which to generalize to new combinations of sounds. Thus vocal production resulting from repeated exposure to a single syllable would not show evidence of generalization beyond the phonemes the infants heard, yielding sounds that seemed imitative but were really the output of a statistical learning mechanism that is operating on input with no variability. Current studies in our laboratory are systematically manipulating the amount of phonological and phonetic variability in the input to understand the role of variability in vocal learning.

Infants in the YC Resonance and CV groups, who were exposed to the same maternal vocalizations and behaviors as Contingent infants, did not show changes in vocal quality. These data suggest that the timing of feedback is important, as mere exposure to their mothers' utterances was not enough to get infants to change their sounds. Why is contingency crucial for vocal learning? In studies of statistical learning in speech perception, infant learning does not require contingent presentations of stimuli. There are several reasons why contingency is important for learning new forms of vocal production. The learning task is more difficult because infants are creating, rather then recognizing, utterances that obey phonological rules. Thus focused attention and increased arousal, which may be facilitated by social contingency (Kuhl, 2007a, 2007b), should have stronger effects on tasks in which the infant is required to produce as well as to recognize new phonological patterns. Contingent vocal responses also tend to be prompt (within 5 s), which means that the utterances of infants and adults are contiguous in time. Such temporal proximity may facilitate infants' detection of differences between their own and adults' utterances. Computer models of unsupervised language learning rely on the perception of utterances that are partially redundant to learn grammatical structure (e.g., Solan, Horn, Ruppin, & Edelman, 2005). For these models, temporal contiguity between utterances would enhance the distillation of structure in the input. We are currently testing the role of contingency by manipulating the promptness of social feedback in new studies of vocal learning.

In summary, infants learned new patterns of vocalizing by recognizing phonological patterns in caregivers' contingent speech and using those patterns to restructure their own babbling. Infants can learn from social feedback as they vocalize; vocal learning is guided in real time by phonological patterns in caregivers' speech. Thus the activity of babbling, in combination with caregivers' responsiveness to vocal precursors, creates a process of socially guided vocal learning. Taken together, our studies support socially guided learning as an important mechanism in early vocal development. Prelinguistic vocal learning may lay the foundation for later advances in language acquisition, as discussed below.

Role of Social Feedback in the Transition from Babbling to Words

How do infants learn that their sounds map onto objects in the world around them? Observations of infants in our laboratory have revealed new patterns of infant actions and social reactions that accompany babbling. These patterns of interaction provide a source of nonimitative learning of correspondences between sounds and objects. Infants often babble while looking at or manipulating an object, and we are currently studying the effect of these "object-directed" sounds on the behavior of caregivers. By investigating the effects of directed versus undirected babbling on caregiver behavior, we can elucidate the earliest social interactions that support the association of sounds and referents.

Maternal Responses to Babbling are Related to Later Lexical Development

Patterns of parental responsiveness to infant behavior have been linked to long-term language development (e.g. Hart & Risley, 1995; Tamis-LeMonda & Bornstein, 2002; Tamis-LeMonda, Bornstein, & Baumwell, 2001). Social interaction clearly plays an important role in language development, but what role does responsiveness to babbling play in later language learning? There is strong acoustic continuity between babbling and early words, so that socially guided learning during the babbling phase may carry over into early lexical development. Observations of language development indicate that babbling blends into word production (Stoel-Gammon, 1992; Vihman, Macken, Miller, Simmons, & Miller, 1985). The onset of first words is correlated with the onset and number of syllable types of canonical babbling (Stoel-Gammon, 1992).

Given prior demonstrations of the sensitivity of babbling to caregiver feedback, what are the effects on language of different styles of caregiver responses to babbling? Mothers and their 9-month-old infants were recorded as they played together in our large playroom. The room contained toys and pictures. Mothers were asked to play as they would at home. We coded and categorized several styles of caregiver behavior based upon their contingent verbal responses to the babbling of their 9-month-old infants (Table 34.2). We then assessed the long-term effects of those response styles on early vocabulary acquisition at 15 months.

We focused on mother's responses to their infants' object-directed vocalizations (ODVs) during naturalistic play. An ODV is one that is emitted when the infant is looking at an object that is within reach or being held. We found several stable categories of contingent verbal responses to ODVs. We then used the MacArthur Communicative Development Inventory (CDI; Fenson et al., 1994) to examine vocabulary when infants were approximately 15 months old (mean age 15;11, range 14;11–16;25). The CDI is a parental report measure of productive and receptive vocabulary that has been validated with laboratory measures of vocabulary development (Bornstein & Haynes, 1998). In addition, the CDI shows long-term stability in predictive value for later language and cognitive development (Fenson et al., 2000).

We obtained correlations between two categories of maternal response to babbling and later vocabulary. We found a significant positive linear association between the proportion of *proximal object labeling* and later productive vocabulary, r (11) = .81, *p* < .01. A proximal object label occurs when the mother says the name of an object that infant was touching or looking at when he/she vocalized. We also found a negative curvilinear relationship between proportion of *phonological resemblance* responses and later receptive vocabulary, r (11) = −.68, *p* < .01. A phonological resemblance response occurs when the mother utters a word that sounded like the infant's vocalization, for example, infant utters "ba," for which the mother says "ball."

Table 34.2 Categories of Mothers' Verbal Responses to Infant Vocalizations

Maternal Response	Description
Proximal object label	Name of object that infant was touching or looking at when he or she vocalized, e.g., "cup," "ball"
Phonological resemblance	Word that sounded like the infant's vocalization, e.g., infant utters "da," mother says "dog", but no dog is present
Conversational placeholder	An utterance that does not convey information, e.g., "uh-huh," "oh really"
Internal state	Description of infant's emotional state or needs, e.g., "happy," "up," "thirsty"
Imitation	Mother imitated her infant's vocalization
Object/property descriptor	Word describing an aspect of an object that the infant was touching or looking at when s/he vocalized, e.g., "red," "big," "round"
Object action	Word describing an action could be done on an object that the infant was touching or looking at when s/he vocalized, e.g., "roll," "throw," "eat"
Other	Other vocal maternal responses, e.g., laughing

Overall maternal responsiveness at 9 months was not significantly correlated with either vocabulary measure at 15 months [comprehension r (11) = .06, p = .86, production, r (11) = .39, p = .19].

Thus mothers' spontaneous verbal responses to their infants' ODVs were related to their children's later vocabulary. Mothers who used more proximal object labels in response to their infants' ODVs at 9 months had children with larger vocabularies at 15 months. Mothers who responded with more phonologically similar (but contextually irrelevant) words at 9 months had children with smaller vocabularies at 15 months. Other response types (e.g., conversational placeholders) and overall amount of maternal responsiveness were not related to later vocabulary development.

What factors explain the relationships between social responses to ODVs and vocabulary? Mothers who respond to their infants' ODVs by providing object labels may facilitate word learning by helping their infants recognize the connection between sounds and objects present in the environment. When mothers label the objects their infants are attending to in response to their babbling, they provide structure that may promote associative learning of word–object pairings. In contrast, mothers who react with words that are similar to their infants' sounds, but unrelated to the context of infants' ODVs, may be inhibiting later word learning because they are providing inconsistent word–object pairings.

Mothers who provide labels for nearby objects may also be more verbal, or interact with their infants in other ways that facilitate infants' language development. Mothers' verbal skills are a significant predictor of their children's language development (e.g., Bornstein, Tamis-LeMonda, & Haynes, 1999; Hart & Risley, 1995; Hoff-Ginsberg, 1986). Mothers who respond to their infants' ODVs with an object label may also be more likely to later report that their infant understands more words and produces more words. However, the CDI correlates with laboratory and observational measures of vocabulary for children in this age range (Fenson et al., 1994). Given the CDI's validity and the strong negative correlation between phonological resemblance responses and later vocabulary, we believe the positive correlation between proximal object labeling and child vocabulary arises from the opportunities for associative learning created when mothers label objects in response to ODVs.

Though the manner in which caregivers responded to babbling predicted later language development, the overall quantity of mothers'

responsiveness does not. This finding stands in contrast to the results of previous research (e.g., Tamis-LeMonda & Bornstein, 2002). Perhaps the reason that higher maternal responsiveness has been correlated with positive language outcomes in previous studies is that increased responding in general is related to more responses to ODVs. The present research focused on mothers' responses to ODVs rather than to all infant vocalizations. Narrowing the type of vocalizations considered has uncovered more specific underlying relations between maternal responsiveness and later language. Future longitudinal studies relating caregiver responsiveness to language learning could be informed by including caregiver behaviors that relate to mechanisms of real-time infant learning.

This study represents a first step in establishing links between prelinguistic vocal development and early word learning. The link is illustrated only by examining caregivers and infants together, as a system. Specific forms of feedback from caregivers may provide reliable cues about the relationship between sounds and objects, thus serving as a source of learning for infants, facilitating the transition between babbling and words.

Perceptual Learning While Vocalizing

What infant learning mechanisms explain the correlations between maternal responses to ODVs and lexical development that were found in the study above? In combination with our vocal learning studies, the findings suggest that prelinguistic vocalizing occurs when an infant is in a state conducive to learning. We hypothesize that ODVs signal a state of focused attention, so that maternal responses to those sounds occur when an infant is in an optimal state for learning the properties of an object. In addition to learning about the speech acoustics of mothers' contingent vocal responses to their vocalizations, infants may also be learning about the objects at which they vocalize. To test this idea, we investigated whether infants learned more about the visual features of the objects to which they were attending when they produced ODVs (Briesch, Schwade, & Goldstein, 2008; Goldstein, Schwade, Briesch, & Syal, 2009). Twelve-month-old infants explored a set of 12 novel objects, each for 40 s. For each infant, we determined the object that elicited the highest (HV) and lowest number (LV) of vocalizations. In a subsequent preferential looking task, each infant was presented with pictures pairing the original HV and LV objects with shape-distorted versions of each (6 s trials, 2 trials each, counterbalanced for side and order). We predicted that infants would learn more about the objects that elicited vocalizations than about objects that did not.

Infants looked significantly longer at the distorted version of the HV object than to the original. In contrast, infants did not differ in looking times to distorted versus original LV objects. We interpret the looking times to mean that infants learned the visual features of the HV object, thus their attention was drawn to the distorted, novel version during the test trials. Infants did not learn the features of the LV object, so the familiar and distorted versions were equally interesting during the test trials. The amount of looking and handling of objects during object exploration was not different for HV and LV objects (Briesch et al., 2008; Goldstein et al., 2009). In a second experiment, we extended the findings to word learning by investigating the effect of labeling novel objects contingently on infant vocalizing or on infant looking (Goldstein et al., 2009). Twelve-month-old infants learned associations between novel words and objects more readily when the words were presented contingently on an ODV. Data from these studies have thus linked prelinguistic vocal learning and language learning, phenomena that are usually studied as separate entities.

Thus prelinguistic infants might be especially sensitive to perceptual information just after vocalizing. Mothers who respond contingently to babbling do so at exactly the time when their infants are ready to learn and remember new information. Specific forms of feedback from caregivers may provide reliable cues about the relationship between sounds and objects, thereby serving as a source of information for infants, facilitating the transition between babbling and words.

Socially Guided Learning of Words and Syntax

As infants' vocal, social, and cognitive skills develop, so do opportunities for socially guided learning of more advanced forms of communication. In word learning outside of laboratory experiments, children usually associate labels and objects after multiple experiences with the words and objects. Often, an adult pairs the words and objects during several social interactions with the child. Acquiring a novel word outside of an experiment has advantages for children. Learning new nouns and verbs is accomplished with fewer trials when an adult provides the new words over

several play sessions than when the adult provides the word many times within a single play session (Childers & Tomasello, 2002). Word learning is possible even when the objects and labels are not presented in isolation. Children typically see many objects when hearing a new object name, and the problem of associating the new label with the correct object is thus logically complex (Quine, 1960). When given a variety of objects and novel labels for those objects, adults are able to correctly associate the labels with the correct objects given the cross-situational regularities present across *several* exposures, even when the words and objects are never paired in isolation (Yu & Smith, 2007). Experiments on word learning show that children are capable of similar cross-situational learning (Smith & Yu, 2008). This type of learning is possible given only the statistics present in the input, without the benefit of additional social information. Two recently developed computational models are capable of extracting words from speech and correctly correlating those words with raw visual information; learning was facilitated with the additional of social information such as pointing or the adult's eye gaze (Roy & Pentland, 2002; Yu, Ballard, & Aslin, 2005).

Children are also capable of using social information when learning words. Many explanations of word learning focus on children's interpretation of an adult's behavior while learning the association between an object and a word. In these accounts, the argument is made that children rely on a parent's intention in naming new objects in order to discern the referent of a parent's label (Akhtar & Tomasello, 2000; Baldwin, 1993, Baldwin et al., 1996). Children's task while learning words would thus be to determine the parent's intention, then to associate the object label with the thing to which the parent intended to refer. These approaches often test the ability of children to learn words when the object and word are not present at the same time so as to evaluate children's reliance on adult intention (e.g., Akhtar, Carpenter, & Tomasello, 1996; Baldwin & Moses, 1996).

However, children's performance on theory-of-mind tasks is poor at the onset of word learning, then improves over the first few years (Flavell, 2004). Rather than incorporating children's inferences about adult intentions into an explanation of word learning, other approaches have sought to identify structure in social interactions, especially in the predictable behaviors of caregivers, that children could detect and use for word learning.

Children's sensitivity to such adult behaviors could serve as a foundation for the development of theory of mind (Moore & Povinelli, 2007). In their interactions with infants and young children, adults create a highly structured environment of co-occurrences between speech, movement, and objects that facilitates associative learning (Gogate & Bahrick, 2001; Graf Estes, Evans, Alibali, & Saffran, 2007).

One such study on the social context of word learning observed mothers as they labeled objects and actions for their toddlers (Yu, Smith, Christensen, & Pereira, 2007). During their interaction, mothers and children each wore a head-mounted camera to capture an approximation of what they saw during the interaction. The study found that word-object pairings were disambiguated, in part, through mothers' and children's actions on the objects. Parents labeled objects while holding them, or as children closely examined them. Thus, parents' timing in labeling objects and actions allows children to coordinate visual and auditory perception to learn labels, rather than forcing them to rely on reading parents' intentions while labeling. Other studies of naturalistic parent–child interaction have discovered additional sources of information about word–object pairings. Parents spontaneously move objects in synchrony with their voices as they label (Gogate, Bahrick, & Watson, 2000). Experiments have shown that such intersensory redundancy of label and object improves object–label associative learning in infants (Gogate & Bahrick, 2001). Thus, in the course of social interactions, parents provide multiple sources of information to infants about the associations between words and objects. As parents label objects, they do so in ways that match children's perceptual abilities, which facilitates word learning. The ways in which adults organize the attention of infants and children is an effective mechanism of socially guided word learning.

The size of children's productive vocabularies increases dramatically, beginning around 18 months of age (Bloom, 1973; McMurray, 2007). Around the same time, children begin combining words (around 18–24 months of age), and can produce complex sentences by about 3–5 years of age (Bloom, 2000; Huttenlocher, Vasilyeva, Cyrnerman, & Levine, 2002). The acquisition of syntax, in which children learn to combine words according to the grammatical rules of their native language, is more complex than word learning and has been subject to more debate. The debate has centered on whether syntax is too complex to be learnable, or whether there is instead sufficient reliable information about syntax that children can detect and use to learn the grammatical rules of their language.

Language acquisition is a species-typical human behavior; all neurologically typical humans with a normal social upbringing learn language. Given the universal acquisition and the complexity of syntax, Chomsky (1957) famously argued that that syntax is not learnable and therefore must be innately specified (see also Lenneberg, 1967; Pinker, 1991; Pinker & Jackendoff, 2005). In recent years, an increasing number of linguists, psychologists, and computational modelers have argued against the necessity of innate specifications for syntactic acquisition (e.g., Bates & Goodman, 1999; Edelman, 2008; Elman et al., 1996; Goldberg, 2006; MacWhinney, 2004; Tomasello, 2003). They argue that the impossibility of learning of syntax has been overstated (e.g., Edelman, 2008; MacWhinney, 1999), that not all native speakers acquire syntax with the same degree of competence, reflecting in part differences in input, especially differences in parents' child-directed speech (e.g., Dabrowska & Street, 2006; Hoff, 2003), and that the trajectory of syntactic development is predictable from a combination of the information available to children in the input and a statistical learning mechanism (e.g., Bates & Goodman, 1999; Chater & Manning, 2006; MacWhinney, 2004; Regier & Gahl, 2004).

As discussed above, caregivers' speech to infants is structured in ways that facilitate word learning. Child learners also have many sources of information about syntax from caregivers' child-directed speech. Adults model correct forms of children's ungrammatical utterances, often in the next conversational turn (e.g., Chouinard & Clark, 2003). In infant-directed speech, mothers change their pitch and shorten their sentences, but they also include repetitions and partial repetitions of their utterances (Masters & McRoberts, 2001; Newport, Gleitman, & Gleitman, 1977). Although exact repetitions have a negative effect language development (Newport et al., 1977), partial repetitions have beneficial effects on language learning.

Variation Sets

Child-directed speech often contains partial repetitions, either within parents' own speech (e.g., "Go walky! Want to go walky? Go walky! Walky") or as expansions of children's utterances (e.g., *Child*: "Disappear," *Mother* "It disappeared," *Child*: "Yes, it did disappear," Waterfall, 2006). Such clusters of related utterances are called variation sets. Variation sets are common in parents' speech directed to children between 5 and 30 months of age; approximately 17%–21% of parents' child-directed speech occurs as part of variation sets (Küntay & Slobin, 1996; Waterfall, 2006, 2009a).

Variation sets contain related utterances that are contiguous in time (Waterfall, 2009a). Utterances are related in having the same nonlinguistic content and similar lexical items. Although the sentences contain similar lexical items, they also contain differences within a set. Parents can form variation sets by inserting an item in a previous sentence (e.g., "A hat. A *funny little* hat"), by deleting an item (e.g., "*You* dance. Dance."), by substituting an item in the sentence (e.g., "Let *me* see. Let *Mommy* see"), or by restructuring an item (e.g., "Is this it? This is it," Waterfall, 2009b). Because of their temporal contiguity and their structural similarity, variation sets are structured as to assist children's comparison of sentences. The similarities in topic and structure allow children to discover classes of words or phrases that have equivalent roles in a sentence. For example, in the variation set "Put it in the basket. Throw it in the basket," a child can compare the two sentences and discover that "put" and "throw" can play the same role in a sentence. Harris (1946, 1954) argued that one method for finding lexical classes is to compare similar sentences to determine what words or strings of words can be substituted for each other. This process of comparing similar utterances has been used successfully in computational approaches to extract syntactic patterns and generate new utterances (Solan et al., 2005).

Variation sets promote child language learning, thus it is likely that children can detect the structure available in variation sets. Children are disproportionately likely to learn nouns and verbs that appeared in parents' variation sets (Waterfall, 2009a). In addition, parents' use of variation sets is correlated with children's acquisition of particular syntactic structures, such as use of direct objects and grammatical subjects in commands (Waterfall, 2009b).

Construction-Based Grammar

Parents and children often engage in routines during play, such as peekaboo, book reading, tickling games, etc. (Ninio & Bruner, 1978; Ratner & Bruner, 1978). Bruner (1983) argued that routines provide a context that supports language learning. Because the social content of the interaction is predictable and familiar, infants learn to predict what mothers say and associate her speech with objects and actions. In a longitudinal observational study of picture-book reading in a single parent–child dyad, Ninio and Bruner (1978) observed that the mother used many predictable sentence frames when looking at picture books with her child, such as "Where's the X?" and "Look at the X." These frames could enhance word learning by providing familiar sentence frames with only one unfamiliar element. Recent theories of syntactic development have analyzed language acquisition in terms of these common frames or items (e.g., Cameron-Faulkner, Lieven, & Tomasello, 2003; Tomasello, 2000). These item-based analyses successfully predict children's language production and generalization of new forms.

Frames are very common in parents' child-directed speech; 51% of parents' utterances directed to their 12-month-old children began with one of 52 frames (e.g., *Look at…*, *It's a…*; Cameron-Faulkner et al., 2003). In addition, when children began combining words, they produced utterances that began with these sentence frames. Their rate of use of particular sentence frames was correlated with the rate of parents' use of those frames. Children's production of more complex syntactic structure can also be predicted from the patterns present in parents' speech. For example, the extent to which children produce generalizations of verbs and phrases depends on the extent to which they heard these patterns generalized in parents' speech (e.g., Goldberg, 2006; Tomasello, 2003). Taken together, these findings suggest that children's word learning and syntax are closely tied to the language they hear in social interactions.

Neural Mechanisms of Socially Guided Learning

Scientists who have argued for an innate predisposition for language, especially for syntax acquisition, have sought to identify brain regions responsible for the human language capacity (see Pinker, 1994 for a review). Brain regions implicated in adult language processing were usually identified through studies of brain-injured adults, who had already acquired language and, later, imaging studies of adult language processing. However, developmental studies have identified additional neural mechanisms recruited for language *learning* (e.g., Bates & Roe, 2001, Thomas & Karmiloff-Smith, 2005).

Though the experiments presented in this chapter focus on the behavioral level, there are important parallels between avian and human vocal learning at the neural level. Data on avian socially guided vocal learning have influenced neural analyses by showing that regions of the brain involved in social perception and learning are fundamental to birdsong learning, and thus possibly to human language learning (Freeberg, West, King, Duncan, & Sengelaub, 2002; Hamilton, King, Sengelaub, & West, 1997, 1998; Jarvis, Scharff, Grossman, Ramos, & Nottebohm, 1998; also see Chapter 35). Vocal learning in songbirds is mediated by the anterior frontal pathway (AFP), a neural loop connecting cortical, thalamic, and basal ganglia areas (e.g., Brenowitz & Beecher, 2005). The AFP is homologous to circuitry connecting cortical and basal ganglia areas in primates, including humans (Doupe & Kuhl, 1999; Doupe, Perkel, Reiner, & Stern, 2005).

The basal ganglia may play a particularly important role in socially guided vocal learning, as these structures are involved in reward-based learning of acoustic patterns. When adults receive feedback for performance on a phonological learning task, the caudate nucleus is activated (Tricomi, Delgado, McCandliss, McClelland, & Fiez, 2006). The caudate is involved in the reinforcement of actions that lead to a reward (Tricomi, Delgado, & Fiez, 2004). In addition, the striatum of the basal ganglia, which forms part of the cortical–basal ganglia–cortical loop in primates, is involved in the recognition and control of patterned behavioral sequences and may be important in syntax learning (see review in Osterhout, Kim, & Kuperberg, in press).

The basal ganglia are necessary for attaching value to sound patterns and can influence the organization of auditory cortex (Gao & Suga, 2000). Such structures allow for close associations to be made between forms of vocalizing and emotional state (Cheng, 2003; Cheng & Durand, 2004). Basal ganglia mediation of vocal learning would thus allow an infant bird or baby to have differential reactions to similar auditory stimuli based on emotional value, such as the interaction history between an infant and adult (Martinez-Garcia, Novejarque, & Lanuza, 2007). Thus the basal ganglia are likely to be important substrates of socially guided vocal learning. The robust effects of socially guided learning in multiple aspects of language development indicate that the basal ganglia should be considered in future studies of the neurobiology of language.

Conclusions: From Birds to Words to Language

In summary, our research, grounded in an ecological framework, has shown that social learning is a crucial part of vocal development. Caregivers use the babbling of infants to inform their reactions to the infants (Goldstein & West, 1999). At the same time, vocal learning is sensitive to social feedback (Goldstein et al., 2003; Goldstein & Schwade, 2008). When a new type of sound is produced in the context of contingent social interaction, there are thus multiple processes—both in the parent and in the infant—that support the ability of the infant to retain the new sound form in his or her repertoire. Taken together, these findings suggest that social responses to prelinguistic vocalizations have functional significance for vocal development. Infants learn how to make well-formed syllables, and learn how to order those syllables, as a result of social feedback. Such a system of mutually engaged infants and receivers constitutes an active feedback mechanism that plays a strong role in vocal learning (Figure 34.4). Recent research on cowbird song development has continued the ecological tradition and has moved beyond the dyad to focus on patterns of interaction and learning at the level of the flock (Miller, 2007; Miller, King, & West, 2008). Studying cowbirds and humans in seminaturalistic settings allows them to express species-typical

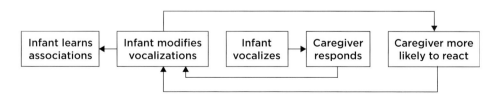

Figure 34.4 A schematic of a socially distributed mechanism of vocal development. When an infant vocalizes, observational studies and our playback studies show that caregivers provide consistent responses to the infant's babbling. Our vocal learning studies show that caregiver responses cause infants to modify their vocalizations; the modifications make the vocalizations more speech-like, which (as shown by our playback studies) elicit stronger responses from caregivers. In addition, infants who receive responses after object-directed vocalizing are more likely to learn from those responses, thus facilitating the learning of word–object associations.

degrees of behavioral freedom and demonstrate multiple forms of socially guided learning.

In both songbirds and human infants, vocal precursors take on functional significance for the development of more advanced forms of vocalizing, but only when the immature sounds are studied in a social context. In both taxa, adults provide rapid, real-time feedback for infants' vocalizations. Infants learn to construct new, more developmentally advanced vocal forms from the reactions of adults to their immature sounds. The processes that create communicative competence from social feedback to vocal precursors are grounded in general learning mechanisms. Learning from contingent responses (social shaping) and learning from recognizing patterns in adults' speech (statistical learning) are both effects of mechanisms that are also used in domains outside of vocal communication. In addition, vocal learning in infants is guided by contingency rather than the perception of intentionality in social partners. We have shown that babbling can be shaped by contingent feedback from an inanimate vehicle.

In our view, learning while babbling lays the foundation for later advances in language. Our findings blur the boundary between prelinguistic and linguistic learning, as phonological and lexical development are necessary components of language. The connections between social learning of phonology, words, and syntax need to be better explored so we can determine how perceptual and statistical mechanisms contribute to the development of language. For example, the role of statistical learning in speech segmentation and grammar learning is well-understood, but there is little research on the statistical learning of patterns in the behavior of social partners. Understanding mechanisms by which infants build expectations of social feedback would help connect socially guided vocal learning with later, more traditionally linguistic advances such as syntax. Caregivers' speech to children as they learn language continues to provide important sources of information about individual lexical items and larger syntactic structures; we need to better characterize the mechanisms by which infants perceive and use that information.

We conclude that socially guided learning is a fundamental characteristic of vocal development. In humans, this includes phonological, lexical, and syntactic development. Taken together, our studies show that the infant's social world is a crucial component of the learning process. When studied as a form of social interaction, babbling is an important stage in the development of communication. The social environment is structured by consistent behavior that captures infants' attention and increases arousal. Infants are active participants in these interactions, creating new patterns of vocalizing that catalyze developmental changes in speech and language.

Acknowledgments

We thank Shimon Edelman and Heidi Waterfall for stimulating discussions on speech and language development. We thank Jennifer Miller and Ambrose Gosling for their helpful comments on the manuscript. The preparation of this manuscript was supported by grants from the Cornell Population Program and the Institute for the Social Sciences at Cornell University.

References

Akhtar, N., Carpenter, M., & Tomasello, M. (1996). The role of discourse novelty in early word learning. *Child Development, 67*, 635–645.

Akhtar, N., & Tomasello, M. (2000). The social nature of words and word learning. In R. M. Golinkoff, K. Hirsh-Pasek, L. Bloom, L. B. Smith, A. L. Woodward, N. Akhtar, M. Tomasello, & G. Hollich (Eds.), *Becoming a word learner: A debate on lexical acquisition* (pp. 114–135). New York: Oxford University Press.

Alberts, J. R. (1978). Huddling by rat pups: Group behavioral mechanisms of temperature regulation and energy conservation. *Journal of Comparative and Physiological Psychology, 92*(2), 231–246.

Anderson, B. J., Vietze, P., & Dokecki, P. R. (1977). Reciprocity in vocal interactions of mothers and infants. *Child Development, 48*, 1676–1681.

Baldwin, D. A. (1993). Infants' ability to consult the speaker for clues to word reference. *Journal of Child Language, 20*(2), 395–418.

Baldwin, D. A., Baird, J. A., Saylor, M. M., & Clark, M. A. (2001). Infants parse dynamic action. *Child Development, 72*, 708–717.

Baldwin, D. A., Markman, E. M., Bill, B., Desjardins, R. N., Irwin, J. M., & Tidball, G. (1996). Infants' reliance on a social criterion for establishing word–object relations. *Child Development, 67*, 3135–3153.

Baldwin, D. A., & Moses, L. J. (1996). The ontogeny of social information gathering. *Child Development, 67*, 1915–1939.

Bates, E., & Roe, K. (2001). Language development in children with unilateral brain injury. In C. A. Nelson & M. Luciana (Eds.) *Handbook of developmental cognitive neuroscience* (pp. 281– 308). Cambridge, MA: MIT Press.

Bates, E., & Goodman, J. C. (1999). On the emergence of grammar from the lexicon. In B. MacWhinney (Ed.), *The emergence of language* (pp. 29–80). Hillsdale, NJ: Lawrence Erlbaum Associates.

Beaumont, S. L., & Bloom, K. (1993). Adults' attributions of intentionality to vocalizing infants. *First Language, 13*, 235–247.

Beecher, M. D., & Brenowitz, E. A. (2005). Functional aspects of song learning in songbirds. *Trends in Ecology and Evolution, 20*, 143–149.

Beecher, M. D., & Burt, J. M. (2004). The role of social interaction in bird song learning. *Current Directions in Psychological Science, 13*, 224–228.

Best, C. T. (1994). The emergence of native-language phonological influences in infants: A perceptual assimilation model. In J. C. Goodman & H. C. Nusbaum (Eds.), *The development of speech perception: The transition from speech sounds to spoken words* (pp. 167–224). Cambridge, MA: MIT Press.

Best, C. T. (2002). Revealing the mother tongue's nurturing effects on the infant ear. *Infant Behavior and Development, 25*, 134–139.

Bloom, K., D'Odorico, L., & Beaumont, S. (1993). Adult preferences for syllabic vocalizations: Generalizations to parity and native language. *Infant Behavior and Development, 16*, 109–120.

Bloom, K., & Lo, E. (1990). Adult perceptions of vocalizing infants. *Infant Behavior and Development, 13*, 209–219.

Bloom, K., Russell, A., & Wassenberg, K. (1987). Turn taking affects the quality of infant vocalizations. *Journal of Child Language, 14*, 211–227.

Bloom, L. (1973). *One word at a time: The use of single word utterances before syntax.* The Hague: Mouton.

Bloom, P. (2000). *How children learn the meanings of words.* Cambridge, MA: MIT Press.

Bornstein, M. H., & Haynes, O. M. (1998). Vocabulary competence in early childhood: Measurement, latent construct, and predictive validity. *Child Development, 69*(3), 654–671.

Bornstein, M. H., Tamis-LeMonda, C. S., & Haynes, O. M. (1999). First words in the second year: Continuity, stability, and models of concurrent and predictive correspondence in vocabulary and verbal responsiveness across age and context. *Infant Behavior and Development, 22*, 65–85.

Boysson-Bardies, B. (1993). Ontogeny of language-specific syllabic productions. In B. Boysson-Bardies, S. Schonen, P. Jusczyk, P. MacNeilage & J. Morton (Eds.), *Developmental neurocognition: Speech and face processing in the first year of life* (pp. 353–363). Dordrecht: Kluwer.

Boysson-Bardies, B., Halle, P., Sagart, L., & Durand, C. (1989). A cross-linguistic investigation of vowel formants in babbling. *Journal of Child Language, 16*, 1–17.

Boysson-Bardies, B., & Vihman, M. M. (1991). Adaptation to language: Evidence from babbling and first words in four languages. *Language, 67*, 297–320.

Brenowitz, E. A., & Beecher, M. D. (2005). Song learning in birds: Diversity and plasticity, opportunities and challenges. *Trends in Neuroscience, 28*, 127–132.

Briesch, J., Schwade, J. A., & Goldstein, M. H. (2008). *Responses to prelinguistic object-directed vocalizations facilitate word learning in 11-month-olds.* Poster presented at the International Conference on Infant Studies, Vancouver, BC.

Bruner, J. S. (1983). *Child's talk: Learning to use language.* New York: W.W. Norton.

Cameron-Faulkner, T., Lieven, E., & Tomasello, M. (2003). A construction based analysis of child directed speech. *Cognitive Science, 27*, 843–873.

Chater, N., & Manning, C. D. (2006). Probabilistic models of language processing and acquisition. *Trends in Cognitive Sciences, 10*, 335–344.

Cheng, M. F. (2003). Vocal self-stimulation: From the ring dove story to emotion-based vocal communication. *Advances in the Study of Behavior, 33*, 309–353.

Cheng, M. F., & Durand, S. E. (2004). Song and the limbic brain: A new function for the bird's own song. *Annals of the New York Academy of Sciences, 1016*, 611–627.

Childers, J. B., & Tomasello, M. (2002). Two-year-olds learn novel nouns, verbs, and conventional actions from massed or distributed exposures. *Developmental Psychology, 38*, 967–978.

Chomsky, N. (1957). *Syntactic structures.* The Hague: Mouton.

Chouinard, M. M., & Clark, E. V. (2003). Adult reformulations of child errors as negative evidence. *Journal of Child Language, 30*, 637–669.

Dabrowska, E., & Street, J. (2006). Individual differences in language attainment: Comprehension of passive sentences by native and non-native English speakers. *Language Sciences, 28*, 604–615.

Doupe, A. J., & Kuhl, P. K. (1999). Birdsong and human speech: Common themes and mechanisms. *Annual Review of Neuroscience, 22*, 567–631.

Doupe, A. J., Perkel, D. J., Reiner, A., & Stern, E. A. (2005). Birdbrains could teach basal ganglia research a new song. *Trends in Neurosciences, 28*(7), 353–363.

Edelman, S. (2008). *Computing the mind: How the mind really works.* New York: Oxford University Press.

Elman, J., Bates, E. A., Johnson, M. H., Karmiloff-Smith, A., Parisi, D., & Plunkett, K. (1996). *Rethinking innateness: A connectionist perspective on development.* Cambridge, MA: MIT Press.

Fennell, C. T., Byers-Heinlein, K., & Werker, J. F. (2007). Using speech sounds to guide word learning: The case of bilingual infants. *Child Development, 78*(5), 1510–1525.

Fenson, L., Bates, E., Dale, P., Goodman, J., Reznick, J. S., & Thal, D. (2000). Measuring variability in early child language: Don't shoot the messenger. *Child Development, 71*(2), 323–328.

Fenson, L., Dale, P. S., Reznick, J. S., Bates, E., Thal, D. J., & Pethick, S. J. (1994). Variability in early communicative development. *Monographs of the Society for Research in Child Development, 59*(5, Serial No. 242), 1–173.

Flavell, J. H. (2004). Theory-of-mind development: Retrospect and prospect. *Merril-Palmer Quarterly, 50*(3), 274–290.

Freeberg, T. M., West, M. J., King, A. P., Duncan, S. D., & Sengelaub, D. R. (2002). Cultures, genes, and neurons in the development of song and singing in brown-headed cowbirds (*Molothrus ater*). *Journal of Comparative Physiology, A, 188*, 993–1002.

Friedmann, H. (1929). *The cowbirds: A study in the biology of social parasitism.* Springfield, Ill: C. C. Thomas.

Gao, E., & Suga, N. (2000). Experience-dependent plasticity in the auditory cortex and the inferior colliculus of bats: Role of the corticofugal system. *Proceedings of the National Academy of Science USA, 97*, 8081–8086.

Gerken, L. A. (2006). Decisions, decisions: Infant language learning when multiple generalizations are possible. *Cognition, 98*, B67–B74.

Gibson, E. J., & Pick, A. D. (2000). *An ecological approach to perceptual learning and development.* Oxford: Oxford University Press.

Gibson, J. J. (1979). *The ecological approach to perception.* Boston: Houghton Mifflin.

Gogate, L. J., & Bahrick, L. E. (2001). Intersensory redundancy and 7-month-old infants' memory for arbitrary syllable-object relations. *Infancy, 2*(2), 219–231.

Gogate, L. J., Bahrick, L. E., & Watson, J. D. (2000). A study of multimodal motherese: The role of temporal synchrony between verbal labels and gestures. *Child Development, 71*(4), 878–894.

Goldberg, A. E. (2006). *Constructions at work: The nature of generalization in language.* Oxford: Oxford University Press.

Goldstein, M. H., King, A. P., & West, M. J. (2003). Social interaction shapes babbling: Testing parallels between birdsong and speech. *Proceedings of the National Academy of Sciences, 100*(13), 8030–8035.

Goldstein, M. H., & Schwade, J. A. (2008). Social feedback to infants' babbling facilitates rapid phonological learning. *Psychological Science, 19,* 515-523.

Goldstein, M. H., Schwade, J., Briesch, J., & Syal, S. (2009). *Learning while babbling: Prelinguistic object-directed vocalizations facilitate learning about objects and words.* Manuscript submitted for publication.

Goldstein, M. H., & West, M. J. (1999). Consistent responses of human mothers to prelinguistic infants: The effect of prelinguistic repertoire size. *Journal of Comparative Psychology, 113*(1), 52–58.

Gómez, R. (2002). Variability and detection of invariant structure. *Psychological Science, 13,* 431–436.

Graf Estes, K., Evans, J. L., Alibali, M. W., & Saffran, J. R. (2007). Can infants map meaning to newly segmented words? Statistical segmentation and word learning. *Psychological Science, 18*(3), 254–260.

Green, J. A., & Gustafson, G. E. (1983). Individual recognition of human infants on the basis of cries alone. *Developmental Psychobiology, 16*(6), 485–593.

Green, J. A., & Gustafson, G. E. (1997). Perspectives on an ecological approach to social communicative development in infancy. In P. Zukow-Goldring & C. Dent-Read (Eds.), *Evolving explanations of development: Ecological approaches to organism-environment systems* (pp. 515–546). Washington, DC: American Psychological Association.

Gros-Louis, J., West, M. J., Goldstein, M. H., & King, A. P. (2006). Mothers provide differential feedback to infants' prelinguistic sounds. *International Journal of Behavioral Development, 30*(6), 509–516.

Gustafson, G. E., & Harris, K. L. (1990). Women's responses to young infants' cries. *Developmental Psychology, 26*(1), 144–152.

Hamilton, K. S., King, A. P., Sengelaub, D. R., & West, M. J. (1997). A brain of her own: A neural correlate of song assessment in a female songbird. *Neurobiology of Learning and Memory, 68*(3), 325–332.

Hamilton, K. S., King, A. P., Sengelaub, D. R., & West, M. J. (1998). Visual and song nuclei correlate with courtship skills in brown-headed cowbirds. *Animal Behaviour, 56,* 973–982.

Harris, Z. S. (1946). From morpheme to utterance. *Language, 22,* 161–183.

Harris, Z. S. (1954). Distributional structure. *Word, 10,* 140–162.

Hart, B., & Risley, T. (1995). *Meaningful differences in the everyday experience of young American children.* Baltimore, MD: Brookes.

Hoff, E. (2003). The specificity of environmental influence: Socioeconomic status affects early vocabulary development via maternal speech. *Child Development, 74,* 1368–1378.

Hoff-Ginsberg, E. (1986). Function and structure in maternal speech: Their relation to the child's development of syntax. *Developmental Psychology, 22,* 155–163.

Hsu, H., & Fogel, A. (2003). Social regulatory effects of infant nondistress vocalization on maternal behavior. *Developmental Psychology, 39*(6), 976–991.

Huttenlocher, J., Vasilyeva, M., Cymerman, E., & Levine, S. (2002). Language input and child syntax. *Cognitive Psychology, 45,* 337–374.

Iverson, J. M., Hall, A. J., Nickel, L., & Wozniak, R. H. (2007). The relationship between reduplicated babble onset and laterality biases in infant rhythmic arm movements. *Brain and Language, 101,* 198–207.

Iverson, J. M., & Thelen, E. (1999). Hand, mouth, and brain: The dynamic emergence of speech and gesture. *Journal of Consciousness Studies, 6,* 19–40.

Jaffe, J., Beebe, B., Feldstein, S., Crown, C. L., & Jasnow, M. D. (2001). Rhythms of dialogue in infancy. *Monographs of the Society for Research in Child Development, 66*(2, Serial No. 265), 1–132.

Jarvis, E. D., Scharff, C., Grossman, M. R., Ramos, J. A., & Nottebohm, F. (1998). For whom the bird sings: Context-dependent gene expression. *Neuron, 21*(4), 775–788.

Johnston, T. D. (1981). Contrasting approaches to a theory of learning. *Behavioral and Brain Sciences, 4,* 125–173.

Jusczyk, P. W. (1992). Developing phonological categories from the speech signal. In C. A. Ferguson, L. Menn & C. Stoel-Gammon (Eds.), *Phonological development: Models, research, implications* (pp. 17–64). Timonium, MD: York Press.

Keller, H., & Scholmerich, A. (1987). Infant vocalizations and parental reactions during the first 4 months of life. *Developmental Psychology, 23*(1), 62–67.

Kent, R. D. (1981a). Articulatory-acoustic perspectives on speech development. In R. E. Stark (Ed.), *Language behavior and early childhood* (pp. 105–126). New York: Elsevier.

Kent, R. D. (1981b). Sensorimotor aspects of speech development. In R. N. Aslin, J. R. Alberts & M. R. Petersen (Eds.), *Development of perception* (Vol. 1, pp. 161–189). New York: Academic Press.

King, A. P., West, M. J., & Goldstein, M. H. (2005). Nonvocal shaping of avian song development: Parallels to human speech development. *Ethology, 111,* 101–117.

Kuhl, P. K. (2007a). Cracking the speech code: How infants learn language. *Acoustical Science and Technology, 28*(2), 71–83.

Kuhl, P. K. (2007b). Is speech learning "gated" by the social brain? *Developmental Science, 10,* 110–120.

Kuhl, P. K., & Meltzoff, A. N. (1996). Infant vocalizations in response to speech: Vocal imitation and developmental change. *Journal of the Acoustical Society of America, 100,* 2425–2438.

Kuhl, P. K., Tsao, F. M., & Liu, H. M. (2003). Foreign-language experience in infancy: Effects of short-term exposure and social interaction on phonetic learning. *Proceedings of the National Academy of Sciences USA, 100,* 9096–9101.

Küntay, A., & Slobin, D. (1996). Listening to a Turkish mother: Some puzzles for acquisition. In D. Slobin, J. Gerhardt, A. Kyratzis, & J. Guo (Eds.), *Social interaction, social context, and language: Essays in honor of Susan Ervin-Tripp* (pp. 265–286). Hillsdale, NJ: Lawrence Erlbaum Associates.

Legerstee, M. (1990). Infants use multimodal information to imitate speech sounds. *Infant Behavior and Development, 13,* 343–354.

Lenneberg, E. (1967). *Biological foundations of language.* New York: Wiley.

Levitt, A., & Wang, Q. (1991). Evidence for language-specific rhythmic influences in the reduplicative babbling of French- and English-learning infants. *Language and Speech, 34,* 235–249.

Locke, J. L. (1993). *The child's path to spoken language*. Cambridge, MA: Harvard University Press.

Locke, J. L. (2001). First communion: The emergence of vocal relationships. *Social Development, 10*(3), 294–308.

Locke, J. L., & Pearson, D. M. (1992). Vocal learning and the emergence of phonological capacity: A neurobiological approach. In C. A. Ferguson, L. Menn & C. Stoel-Gammon (Eds.), *Phonological development: Models, research, implications* (pp. 91–129). Timonium, MD: York Press.

MacNeilage, P. F. (1998). The frame/content theory of evolution of speech production. *Behavioral and Brain Sciences, 21*, 499–546.

MacNeilage, P. F., & Davis, B. L. (2000). On the origin of the internal structure of word forms. *Science, 288*, 527–531.

MacWhinney, B. (1999). *The emergence of language*. Mahwah, NJ: Lawrence Erlbaum.

MacWhinney, B. (2004). A multiple process solution to the logical problem of language acquisition. *Journal of Child Language, 31*, 883–914.

Marler, P. (1970). Birdsong and speech development: Could there be parallels? *American Scientist, 58*, 669–673.

Marler, P. (1997). Three models of song learning: Evidence from behavior. *Journal of Neurobiology, 33*, 501–516.

Marler, P., & Nelson, D. A. (1993). Action-based learning: A new form of developmental plasticity in bird song. *Netherlands Journal of Zoology, 43*(1–2), 91–103.

Martinez-Garcia, F., Novejarque, A., & Lanuza, E. (2007). Evolution of the amygdala in vertebrates. In J. H. Kaas (Ed.), *Evolution of nervous systems: A comprehensive reference* (Vol. 2, pp. 255–334). Oxford: Academic Press.

Masataka, N. (2003). *The onset of language*. Cambridge: Cambridge University Press.

Masters, R., & McRoberts, G. W. (2001, April). *Verbal repetition in speech to infants*. Poster presented at the Biennial Meeting of the Society for Research in Child Development, Minneapolis, MN.

Mayr, E. (1974). Behavior programs and evolutionary strategies. *American Scientist, 62*, 650–659.

McMurray, B. (2007). Defusing the childhood vocabulary explosion. *Science, 317* (3), 631.

Meier, R. P. (1997). Silent mandibular oscillations in vocal babbling. *Phonetica, 54*, 153–171.

Miller, J. L. (2007, November). *Vocal strategies in brown-headed cowbirds* (Molothrus ater) *are sensitive to social ecology*. Paper presented at the International Society for Developmental Psychobiology, San Diego, CA.

Miller, J. L., King, A. P., & West, M. J. (2008). Female social networks influence male vocal development in brown-headed cowbirds (*Molothrus ater*). *Animal Behaviour, 76*, 931–941.

Moore, C., & Povinelli, D. J. (2007). Differences in how 12- and 24-month-olds interpret the gaze of adults. *Infancy, 11*, 215–231.

Narayan, A. J., Goldstein, M. H., & Schwade, J. A. (2008). *What characteristics of social interaction facilitate early learning? Effects of animacy and contingency on vocal learning in prelinguistic infants*. Poster presented at the International Conference on Infant Studies, Vancouver, BC.

Newport, E. L., Gleitman, H., & Gleitman, L. (1977). Mother, I'd rather do it myself: Some effects and noneffects of maternal speech style. In C. E. Snow & C. A. Ferguson (Eds.), *Talking to children: Language input and acquisition* (pp. 109–150). Cambridge: Cambridge University Press.

Ninio, A., & Bruner, J. (1978). The achievement and antecedents of labeling. *Journal of Child Language, 5*(1), 1–15.

Oller, D. K. (1980). The emergence of the sounds of speech in infancy. In G. Yemi-Komshian, J. Kavanagh & C. Ferguson (Eds.), *Child phonology*. New York: Academic Press.

Oller, D. K. (1985). Infant vocalizations: Traditional beliefs and current evidence. In S. Harel & N. J. Anastasiow (Eds.), *The at-risk infant: Psycho/socio/medical aspects* (pp. 333–339). Baltimore, MD: Paul H. Brookes.

Oller, D. K. (2000). *The emergence of the speech capacity*. Mahwah, NJ: Lawrence Erlbaum Associates.

Oller, D. K., & Eilers, R. E. (1988). The role of audition in infant babbling. *Child Development, 59*, 441–449.

Oller, D. K., Eilers, R. E., & Basinger, D. (2001). Intuitive identification of infant vocal sounds by parents. *Developmental Science, 4*(1), 49–60.

Oller, D. K., Eilers, R. E., Bull, D. H., & Carney, A. E. (1985). Prespeech vocalizations of a deaf infant: A comparison with normal metaphonological development. *Journal of Speech and Hearing Research, 28*, 47–63.

Oller, D. K., & Lynch, M. P. (1992). Infant vocalizations and innovations in infraphonology: Toward a broader theory of vocal development and disorders. In C. A. Ferguson, L. Menn & C. Stoel-Gammon (Eds.), *Phonological development* (pp. 509–536). Timonium, MD: York Press.

Osterhout, L., Kim, A., & Kuperberg, G. (in press). The neurobiology of sentence comprehension. In M. Spivey, M. Joannisse & K. McRae (Eds.), *The Cambridge handbook of psycholinguistics*. Cambridge: Cambridge University Press.

Papoušek, M. (1989). Determinants of responsiveness to infant vocal expression of emotional state. *Infant Behavior and Development, 12*, 507–524.

Papoušek, M. (1991). Early ontogeny of vocal communication in parent–infant interactions. In H. Papoušek, U. Jergens & M. Papoušek (Eds.), *Nonverbal vocal communication: Comparative and developmental approaches* (pp. 230–261). Cambridge: Cambridge University Press.

Papoušek, M., & Papoušek, H. (1989). Forms and functions of vocal matching in interactions between mothers and their precanonical infants. *First Language, 9*, 137–158.

Papoušek, M., Papoušek, H., & Bornstein, M. H. (1985). The naturalistic vocal environment of young infants: On the significance of homogeniety and variability in parental speech. In T. Field & N. Fox (Eds.), *Social perception in infants* (pp 269–297). Norwood, NJ: Ablex.

Petitto, L. A., Holowka, S., Sergio, L. E., Levy, B., & Ostry, D. J. (2004). Baby hands that move to the rhythm of language: Hearing babies acquiring sign languages babble silently on the hands. *Cognition, 93*, 43–73.

Petrinovich, L. P. (1972). Psychobiological mechanisms in language development. In G. Newton & A. H. Riesen (Eds.), *Advances in psychobiology* (Vol. 1, pp. 259–285). New York: Wiley-Interscience.

Pinker, S. (1991). Rules of language. *Science, 253*, 530–535.

Pinker, S, (1994). *The language instinct*. New York: Harper Collins.

Pinker, S., & Jackendoff, R. (2005). The faculty of language: What's special about it. *Cognition, 95*, 201–236.

Poulson, C. (1983). Differential reinforcement of other-than-vocalization as a control procedure in the conditioning of infant vocalization rate. *Journal of Experimental Child Psychology, 36*, 471–489.

Quine, W. V. O. (1960). *Word and object*. Cambridge: MIT Press.

Ratner, N., & Bruner, J. (1978). Games, social exchange and the acquisition of language. *Journal of Child Language, 5*(5), 391–401.

Regier, T., & Gahl, S. (2004). Learning the unlearnable: The role of missing evidence. *Cognition, 93*, 147–155.

Rheingold, H. L., Gewirtz, J. L., & Ross, H. W. (1959). Social conditioning of vocalizations in the infant. *Journal of Comparative and Physiological Psychology, 52*, 68–73.

Rothstein, S. I., Yokel, D. A., & Fleischer, R. C. (1988). The agonistic and sexual functions of vocalizations of male brown-headed cowbirds (*Molothrus ater*). *Animal Behaviour, 36*, 73–86.

Routh, D. K. (1969). Conditioning of vocal response differentiation in infants. *Developmental Psychology, 1*(3), 219–226.

Roy, D. K., & Pentland, A. P. (2002). Learning words from sights and sounds: A computational model. *Cognitive Science, 26*, 113–146.

Saffran, J. R., & Thiessen, E. D. (2003). Pattern induction by infant language learners. *Developmental Psychology, 39*, 484–494.

Schank, J. C., & Alberts, J. (1997). Self-organized huddles of rat pups modeled by simple rules of individual behavior. *Journal of Theoretical Biology, 189*, 11–25.

Schwartz, J.-L., Berthommier, F., & Savariaux, C. (2004). Seeing to hear better: Evidence for early audio-visual interactions in speech identification. *Cognition, 93*, B69–B78.

Seeley, T.D. (1995). *The wisdom of the hive*. Boston: Harvard University Press.

Smith, L. & Yu, C. (2008). Infants rapidly learn word-referent mappings via cross-situational statistics. *Cognition, 106*, 1558–1568.

Smith, V. A., King, A. P., & West, M. J. (2000). A role of her own: Female cowbirds, *Molothrus ater*, influence the development and outcome of song learning. *Animal Behaviour, 60*, 599–609.

Snowdon, C. T., & Hausberger, M. (Eds.). (1997). *Social influences on vocal development*. Cambridge: Cambridge University Press.

Solan, Z., Horn, D., Ruppin, E., & Edelman, S. (2005). Unsupervised learning of natural languages. *Proceedings of the National Academy of Sciences USA, 102*, 11629–11634.

Stager, C. L., & Werker, J. F. (1997). Infants listen for more phonetic detail in speech perception than in word-learning tasks. *Nature, 388*(6640), 381–382.

Stark, R. E. (1979). Prespeech segmental feature development. In P. Fletcher & M. Garman (Eds.), *Language acquisition*. Cambridge: Cambridge University Press.

Stark, R. E. (1980). Stages of speech development in the first year of life. In G. Yeni-Komshian, J. Kavanagh & C. Ferguson (Eds.), *Child phonology*. New York: Academic Press.

Stoel-Gammon, C. (1992). Prelinguistic vocal development: Measurement and predictions. In C. A. Ferguson, L. Menn & C. Stoel-Gammon (Eds.), *Phonological development: Models, research, implications* (pp. 439–456). Timonium, MD: York Press.

Stoel-Gammon, C., & Otomo, K. (1986). Babbling development of hearing-impaired and normally hearing subjects. *Journal of Speech and Hearing Disorders, 51*, 33–41.

Tamis-LeMonda, C. S., & Bornstein, M. H. (2002). Maternal responsiveness and early language acquisition. *Advances in Child Development and Behavior, 29*, 89–127.

Tamis-LeMonda, C. S., Bornstein, M. H., & Baumwell, L. (2001). Maternal responsiveness and children's achievement of language milestones. *Child Development, 72*(3), 748–767.

Thelen, E. (1986). Treadmill-elicited stepping in seven-month-old infants. *Child Development, 57*, 1498–1506.

Thomas, M. S. C., & Karmiloff-Smith, A. (2005). Can developmental disorders reveal the component parts of the human language faculty? *Language Learning and Development, 1*, 65–92.

Tomasello, M. (2000). The item-based nature of children's early syntactic development. *Trends in Cognitive Sciences, 4*, 156–163.

Tomasello, M. (2003). *Constructing a language: A usage-based theory of language acquisition*. Cambridge, MA: Harvard University Press.

Tricomi, E., Delgado, M. R., McCandliss, B. D., McClelland, J. L., & Fiez, J. A. (2006). Performance feedback drives caudate activation in a phonological learning task. *Journal of Cognitive Neuroscience, 18*(6), 1029–1043.

Tricomi, E. M., Delgado, M. R., & Fiez, J. A. (2004). Modulation of caudate activity by action contingency. *Neuron, 41*(2), 281–292.

Vihman, M. M., Macken, M. A., Miller, R., Simmons, H., & Miller, J. (1985). From babbling to speech: A reassessment of the continuity issue. *Language, 61*, 397–446.

Vihman, M. M., & Miller, R. (1988). Words and babble at the threshold of language acquisition. In M. D. Smith & J. L. Locke (Eds.), *The emergent lexicon: The child's development of a linguistic vocabulary* (pp. 151–183). San Diego: Academic Press.

Waterfall, H. R. (2006). *A little change is a good thing: Feature theory, language acquisition and variation sets*. Unpublished doctoral dissertation, University of Chicago.

Waterfall, H. R. (2009a). *The relation of variation sets to children's noun and verb use*. Manuscript submitted for publication.

Waterfall, H. R. (2009b). *Things change for the better: The relation of variation sets to syntactic development*. Manuscript submitted for publication.

Watson, J. S. (1972). Smiling, cooing, and "the game." *Merrill-Palmer Quarterly, 18*, 323–329.

Weisberg, P. (1963). Social and nonsocial conditioning of infant vocalizations. *Child Development, 34*, 377–388.

Werker, J. F., & Curtin, S. (2005). PRIMIR: A developmental framework of infant speech processing. *Language Learning and Development, 1*, 197–234.

Werker, J. F., & Tees, R. C. (1984). Cross-language speech perception: Evidence for perceptual reorganization during the first year of life. *Infant Behavior and Development, 7*, 49–63.

West, M. J., & King, A. P. (1985). Learning by performing: An ecological theme for the study of vocal learning. In T. D. Johnston & A. T. Pietriwicz (Eds.), *Issues in the ecological study of learning* (pp. 245–272). Hillsdale, NJ: LEA Press.

West, M. J., & King, A. P. (1988). Female visual displays affect the development of male song in the cowbird. *Nature, 334*(6179), 244–246.

West, M. J., King, A. P., & Duff, M. A. (1990). Communicating about communicating: When innate is not enough. *Developmental Psychobiology, 23*(7), 585–598.

West, M. J., King, A. P., Eastzer, D. H., & Staddon, J. E. R. (1979). A bioassay of isolate cowbird song. *Journal of Comparative and Physiological Psychology, 93*, 124–133.

Whalen, D. H., Levitt, A., & Wang, Q. (1991). Intonational differences between the reduplicative babbling of French- and English-learning infants. *Journal of Child Language, 18*, 501–516.

Wilbrecht, L., & Nottebohm, F. (2003). Vocal learning in birds and humans. *Mental Retardation and Developmental Disabilities Research Reviews, 9*, 135–148.

Wood, R. M., & Gustafson, G. E. (2001). Infant crying and adults' anticipated caregiving responses: Acoustic and contextual influences. *Child Development, 72*(5), 1287–1300.

Yu, C., Ballard, G. A., & Aslin, R. N. (2005). The role of embodied intention in early lexical acquisition. *Cognitive Science, 29*, 961–1005.

Yu, C., & Smith, L. B. (2007). Rapid word learning under uncertainty via cross-situational statistics. *Psychological Science, 18*, 414–420.

Yu, C., Smith, L. B., Christensen, M., & Pereira, A. (2007). *Two views of the world: Active vision in real-world interaction.* Paper presented at the Proceedings of the 29th annual meeting of the Cognitive Science Society, Nashville, TN.

Relaxed Selection and the Role of Epigenesis in the Evolution of Language

Terrence W. Deacon

Abstract

It is generally assumed that there is a positive correlation between the complexity of functional adaptive systems and the intensity and duration of natural selection driving their evolution. Although the role of selection is unquestionable, especially with respect to functional correspondences between organism and environment, the correlation with functional complexity is not so clear. The recent resurgence of interest in the contribution of epigenetic processes to the course of evolutionary change, popularly known as evodevo, has begun to focus attention on other potential sources of complex integration: that is, the self-organizing and intraselection processes that are recruited by evolution to serve epigenetic functions. This chapter reviews evidence for a general evolutionary logic that the chapter calls the "Lazy Gene" effect, which suggests that genes will tend to offload control of morphogenetic processes to epigenetic mechanisms in evolution whenever reliable extragenomic constraints or influences can induce the same effect. The chapter also explores an example of this effect that is particularly relevant to language evolution: a case of birdsong change under the influence of artificial breeding for an unrelated trait.

Keywords: adaptive systems, epigenetic processes, evodevo, Lazy Gene, morphogentic processes, extragenomic constraints, birdsong

The Evodevo Perspective

Historically, theories attempting to explain the evolution of brain organization and neural complexity have not ascribed a significant role to developmental processes, other than carrying out the implementation of genetic instructions for neural differentiation and adapting neural circuits to receptor and effector systems of the body. This is understandable from the point of view of what might be called classical neo-Darwinism. To the extent that the mechanism of natural selection is classically framed in post hoc terms and new variations of structure and function are understood as arising irrespective of any eventual functional consequence, the specific mechanisms producing these variations tend to be considered irrelevant with respect to their adaptive consequences.

This classical perspective has, however, come to be seen as a special case of a more general paradigm, popularly known as evodevo (see for example, Alberch, 1989; Carroll, 2000; Gilbert, 2003). In this augmentation of neo-Darwinian theory, constraints on the development and differentiation of organism features are understood to introduce an independent source of structure into the evolutionary process. This approach does not assume any violation of the neo-Darwinian doctrine that the ultimate sources of the variations presented to natural selection only derive from chance genetic mutations and sexual recombination. But, it additionally recognizes that those variations, which ultimately get expressed at the whole organism level, are products of developmental mechanisms that are themselves highly structured, indirect, and systemically interdependent. In this respect, past adaptations, and specifically the mechanisms underlying their developmental expression, serve as the context in which unprecedented genetic variations get expressed. Thus, otherwise randomly generated genetic variations do not necessarily have uncorrelated developmental consequences. To invert a famous aphorism about computing: genetic garbage *in* does not necessarily produce phenotypic garbage *out*.

More importantly, these developmental constraints and biases contribute an organizing influence on the variant traits presented to natural selection; an influence that is independent of genetic variation, and which indirectly reflects constraints of past adaptations. One of the more counterintuitive consequences of this epigenetic contribution to evolutionary design is that its effects can become more marked under conditions of relaxed selection,[1] precisely because the systematic biases these mechanisms contribute are not constrained by the demands of adaptive fit. This introduces a non-Darwinian mechanism, which acts as a complement to natural selection in the generation of functional synergies, because its form-generating properties derive from the self-organizing tendencies of molecular and cellular interactions rather than from relationships to environmental conditions. Paradoxically, this suggests that selection may actually hinder the evolutionary "exploration" of alternative functional synergies, and that the relaxation of selection may play an important role in the evolution of increased functional complexity. This possibility will be explored below.

In as much as the architecture of the central nervous system is generated via the operation of many more levels of developmental interactions than most other tissues—including contributions from such uniquely neuronal mechanisms as activity-based modification of connectivity and axonal extension linking distal cell populations—there is an enormous opportunity for developmental mechanisms to contribute to brain evolution (e.g., Chapter 18). This greater degree of developmental and functional interdependency should make brain evolution particularly susceptible to epigenetic influences.

This susceptibility is particularly relevant for understanding some of the more enigmatic and unprecedented events in brain evolution, such as the evolution of language. But to understand how epigenetic processes can contribute to patterns of evolution, even in the absence of the effects of natural selection (or, as we will see below, precisely because of its absence), we first need to step back from the neuroanatomical details to reconsider more generally how such entanglements of evolution with epigenesis and behavior can occur and how this may alter the simple predictions of neo-Darwinian theory.

In this chapter, then, we begin with a brief overview of the contemporary view of the role of development in brain evolution and outline the historical development of ideas about this entanglement of levels of formative processes in biology. Next we consider some counterintuitive implications of the role of developmental processes in evolution, as contrasted to natural selection processes, and offer a few paradigm examples of these general principles at work at multiple levels of organic structure and function. In the final sections of the chapter, we will turn to a particularly counterintuitive example of increased neural and functional complexity emerging in the absence of natural selection, and finally show how many features of human cognition and language function also exhibit analogous features.

There is little doubt that many features of human brain evolution relevant to the language capacity have evolved under the influence of natural selection, and identifying these effects and their causes have been the focus of nearly all theories of human brain evolution (Deacon, 1997). But here we focus on the possibility that certain, perhaps crucial, contributors to the human difference may have arisen as a consequence of epigenetic constraints and biases rather than selection favoring adaptive improvement. Indeed, an adequate account of language origins depends on it. By refocusing attention on this otherwise ignored component of the evolutionary process, I do not intend to suggest that natural selection mechanisms are incorrect or subordinate to these epigenetic contributions. Instead, I believe that epigenetic constraints and biases contribute critical formative principles that must be considered an integral component of a complete natural selection theory.

Developmental Influences Affecting Mammalian Brain Evolution

The starting point for any exploration of brain evolution is the recognition that brain organization in all bilateral animals shares deep commonalities, and that these are largely the result of highly conserved developmental mechanisms. The segmental organization of the brain is a consequence of the neuromeric partitioning of the embryonic neural tube by rostrocaudally distributed bands of gene expression that determine regional cell fates. At this level of differentiation, one can observe a remarkably conserved plan of organization characteristic of many animal phyla. Thus, the homeotic gene expression in developing flies and mice exhibit a generic segmental organization that likely antedates their common ancestor. Vertebrate brain organization is a variation on this general theme, with more subdomains and dorsoventral differentiation contributed by paralogues of these homeotic genes, creating mosaic patterns of concentric and intersecting expression domains (Rubenstein et al., 1994; Lumsden & Krumlauf, 1996). Within vertebrates (though excluding the most primitive transitional forms), this patterning is ubiquitous, resulting in a shared brain plan in which there are local regional structural variations, but effectively no significant variation in the topology of major brain segments (e.g., telencephalon, diencephalon, mesencephalon, etc.). The most common variations involve differences in the relative sizes and differentiation of these major structures (for a general overview see Butler & Hodos, 1996; Striedter, 2005).

The major clades of the vertebrate radiation are distinguished by sharing distinctive patterns of subdivision organization within this global segmental architecture. The degree of structural variation of brains within any given clade of species is also roughly correlated with its phyletic age (Striedter, 1997). Consequently, there is considerable diversity of regional brain structure size and specialization in different fish species due to the cumulative effect of long separate evolutionary histories in distinct ecological domains demanding highly specialized sensory-motor adaptations (Figure 35.1). This size correlation of brain structure with functional importance or with peripheral organ development has led to a general expectation that relative deviation of subdivision size and differentiation, with respect to the average for the clade, reflects a computational rule of brain evolution, in which differential elaboration of a given structure with respect to others roughly reflects relative computational power dedicated to that function.

Compared to such ancient vertebrate classes as teleost fishes, or sharks and rays, mammalian brains are remarkably uniform in structural organization from species to species (Striedter, 2005), reflecting the fact that the terrestrial vertebrate radiation is but a tiny terminal branch of the tree of vertebrate evolution and the mammalian radiation is a tiny branch of this branch (as shown in Figure 35.2).

So, while there can be orders of magnitude difference in the sizes of mammal brains, their regional organization generally shares highly invariant patterns of relative growth. Among mammalian species, for instance, there are remarkable quantitative correlations linking the sizes of different major brain segments. Allometric studies of primate and insectivore brains, for example, have shown that the relative sizes of most of the major divisions of the brain are predictable from the single variable of brain size (see for example an early study by Sacher, 1970; and a recent approach by Finlay & Darlington, 1995). There appear to be subtle clade-specific trends (e.g., between insectivores and primates, and between prosimians and anthropoid primates) but remarkably high correlations within mammalian orders despite large body and brain size ranges. These striking quantitative regularities

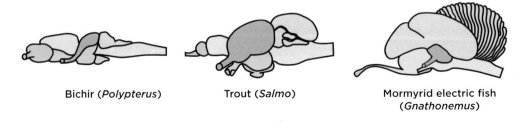

Bichir (*Polypterus*) Trout (*Salmo*) Mormyrid electric fish (*Gnathonemus*)

Figure 35.1 Comparison of three teleost fish brains demonstrates considerable regional size diversity correlated with distinctive sensory and motor specializations. (Modified from Striedter 2005.)

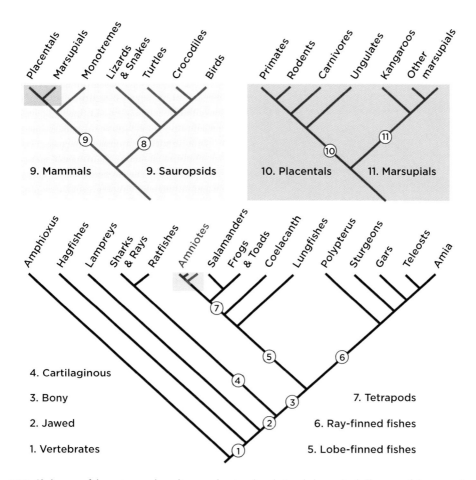

Figure 35.2 Cladogram of the major vertebrate lineages showing the relative phylogenetic shallowness of the tetrapod and mammal lineages as compared to other groups, such as teleost fish. (Modified from Striedter 2005.)

almost certainly reflect highly conserved mechanisms for the control of early stem cell multiplication and neuronal differentiation throughout the brain.

But this comparative uniformity of regional growth patterns in mammal brains has not limited the capacity for mammals to evolve highly distinctive specializations of sensory and motor adaptation, which are reflected both in structural size effects and in relative differentiation of the relevant brain structures. Though much of this specialization can be attributed to divergent organization of peripheral structures, such as the eyes, the olfactory system, or musculature, there is also considerable brain reorganization possible at the subdivision level. The most obvious expression of this is in the distribution of functionally distinct subdivisions of the cerebral cortex (see a recent review by Krubitzer & Kaas, 2005). Cerebral cortex is, however, peculiar to mammals and is one of the more anomalous

variants of vertebrate telencephalic organization (Karten, 1969). Although the vertebrate telencephalon is the outgrowth of a surface sheet of cells, in most vertebrates the multiplication of telencephalic stem cells lining the ventricular wall and their eventual production of neurons within this embryonic forebrain structure tends to enlarge the ventral and lateral walls of each telencephalic "bubble" so that they expand into the ventricular space to form nucleated structures. Only in mammals does the dorsal half expand in a highly laminar fashion, due to the mostly radial migration of newly produced neuroblasts through layers of cells produced in previous waves of neurogenesis. So unlike the telencephalic nuclei of other vertebrate brains, the resulting laminar and columnar organization of mammalian cerebral cortex maintains a uniform sheet topology that is well suited to maintain discretely separated map-like representations of its input–output connections with other structures, particularly with sensory receptor systems like the retina, the skin surface, and the organ of corti within the cochlea.

Whereas mammalian brains lack the large-scale quantitative variations between brain regions that are characteristic of much older vertebrate clades, they do exhibit considerable quantitative variation of cortical subregions. In this way, despite the relatively limited phylogenetic depth of the mammalian radiation, mammal brains have evolved highly distinctive and divergent adaptive organizations. This evolvability is aided by two additional features characteristic of mammalian brains.

The first of these is the comparatively larger size of many mammalian brains, both compared to other species' averages of gross brain sizes and with respect to average brain/body proportions; or encephalization (e.g., Jerison, 1973). Since significant differences in vertebrate brain sizes are not correlated with a corresponding enlargement of neuronal soma sizes, larger brains have more opportunity for regional differentiation (Killackey, 1990; Deacon, 1990). This general rule is reflected across brain structures in all vertebrate species, but is particularly evident when comparing numbers of functionally distinguishable cortical regions in mammalian brains of different sizes. Moreover, the segmental scaling trend for mammalian brains is not isometric with respect to gross brain size. The telencephalon scales with positive allometry with respect to most other brain structures (e.g., diencephalon and brain stem) and so with size increase the relative proportion of the brain comprising cerebral cortex increases disproportionately (Sacher, 1970). Thus the "opportunity" for regional differentiation of cerebral cortex significantly increases with size as well.

The second of these features of mammalian brains that contributes to their heightened evolvability, despite their conservative global organization, is the potential for developmental processes—such as cell–cell interaction and functional activity—to play a role in subregional organization of connections and neuronal differentiation. Afferent–efferent determined modifiability of connectivity pattern and even of neuronal survival is a generic feature of the developing vertebrate central nervous system (CNS; see Cowan et al., 1984; Deacon, 1990; Finlay et al., 1987; Holliday & Hamburger, 1976; Oppenheim, 1981; Purves & Lichtman, 1980; Wilczynski, 1984). It is, for example, responsible for the matching of central versus peripheral cell populations and establishing topographic mapping between them, in the case of spinal neurons and peripheral target cells, such as muscle cells (Purves, 1988). But mammalian cerebral cortex offers a highly responsive forebrain arena for this mechanism to influence global brain function as well. Thus both the relative sizes and the organization of cortical regions associated with distinct peripheral specializations and analytic processes can be significantly influenced by the numbers of afferent axons projecting to them and the level and patterning of signals conveyed by these projections (Deacon, 1990). This is demonstrated by the responsiveness of cortical patterns to manipulations of projections and afferent signals during brain development. Over the past three decades, developmental manipulations have demonstrated afferent–efferent-dependent differentiation of cortical functional differentiation in many cortical domains (e.g., Frost, 1981; Stanfield & O'Leary, 1985; Sur et al., 1988; and recent studies reviewed in Kubitzer & Kaas, 2005)

The interaction between extrinsic activity-dependent influences and intrinsic genetic mechanisms that establish cell fate and guide axon growth have demonstrated that cortical regionalization is a multilevel process. A once lively debate between researchers who argued that cortical area distinctions were expressions of a locally controlled protomap (e.g., Rakic, 1988) versus those who argued that they were the result of competition between peripheral influences conveyed by afferent axons (e.g., O'Leary, 1989) has mostly been resolved by recognizing their necessary interdependence (Mallamaci & Stoykova 2006; O'Leary & Nakagawa, 2002). Relatively conserved "generic" cell differentiation and axon guidance mechanisms are generated by the overlap of gene expression and growth factor gradients across cortex. These constrain and bias the subsequent topographic biases of axonal invasion, which in turn bias activity-dependent competitive interactions between afferent axons to determine the final fine-scale topography and the relative sizes of cortical subdivisions.

Evidence contributing to this general conclusion comes from many different research paradigms. Cross-species fetal neuronal transplantation studies have shown that initial axon guidance mechanisms are largely shared across species (e.g., Balaban, 1997; Isacson & Deacon, 1996). Manipulations of gene expression and regional growth factor production in the developing cortex has also shown that although there may not be protomap determination of functional area positioning in cerebral cortex, the relative concentration gradients of these molecular cues distributed in different and overlapping patterns set up a continuous "grid" defined by the different relative concentrations of these morphogens (Mallamaci & Stoykova, 2006; O'Leary & Nakagawa, 2002). As a result, experimental modification of these gradients by increasing or blocking expression of a particular molecular cue can distort the eventual functional topography, and ectopic introduction of one of these morphogens can fractionate this topology, producing mirror-image duplication of distinctive cortical areas. Finally, very early loss of specific sensory afferents or peripheral degeneration of specific receptor systems can also cause significant changes in cortical area differentiation, including significant size effects and the failure to form distinctive boundaries between cortical areas (e.g., Krubitzer & Kass 2005).

So we can roughly summarize the process of cortical regional differentiation in terms of three general levels of developmental processes that ensue largely independent of cortical stem cell production and neurogenesis (which do not predetermine cortical subregionalization). The first phase is due to locally generated molecular gradients and their overlapping patterns of distribution, which function analogous to a coordinate grid. The second phase is characterized by afferent invasion from thalamic neurons influenced by afferent population differences. The third phase is characterized by synaptic competition between afferent axons, which is strongly influenced by activity-dependent signal correlation mechanisms. By this means the sizes, organization, and functioning of distal brain and peripheral structures all contribute to central organization. Additionally, the particularities of peripheral receptor organization and the invariants of stimulation imposed by extrinsic sources (such as the systematic visual map differences of the two retinas) also influence the organization of cortical function and differentiation.

To summarize, a significant fraction of the structural information embodied in mammalian brains emerges from self-organizing and Darwinian epigenetic processes, and is not "coded" in the genes. The role of genetic information might thus be described as guaranteeing the maintenance of the boundary conditions necessary to support the reliable emergence of these spontaneous organizing processes.

Can Behavior Influence Brain Evolution?

Epigenetic influences on normal brain development, and especially peripheral stimulation and environmental invariants, open the possibility that behavior itself might directly influence the course of brain evolution. This possibility has been considered of central significance by many researchers interested in human brain evolution over the last century (including the present author, whose 1997 book *The Symbolic Species* explored this possibility).

The classic attempt to explain how behavioral interaction with the environment could shape the course of evolution was the use-inheritance theory of Jean Baptiste de Lamarck (1809). He argued that animals acquired adaptations in response to environmental conditions and that these adaptations were inherited by offspring. He thus reasoned that acquired traits could be combined, adjusted, and honed by feedback trial and error and in this way convey considerable adaptive flexibility and exploration of alternatives, potentially aiding both optimality and integration of interdependent systems. Lamarck's ideas were later championed by Herbert Spencer during Darwin's time, but evidence against this mechanism of inheritance was presented by August Weismann and others toward the end of the nineteenth century, and additional contrary evidence for the transmission of acquired characters has accumulated since (though limited inheritance of other acquired traits has also been demonstrated).

In the late nineteenth century, a non-Lamarckian mechanism was described that appeared able to produce an analogous evolutionary effect. Almost simultaneously Baldwin (1896) and two other researchers, Conwy Lloyd Morgan (1896) and Henry Osborne (1896), independently described a theoretical mechanism whereby acquired traits might influence natural selection in such a way as to increase the probability that parallel inherited traits might emerge spontaneously. Each of these theorists independently published papers that proposed such a mechanism. They argued that although Lamarckian inheritance is unlikely, Darwinian mechanisms might be able to produce analogous consequences by virtue of the fact that learning and plasticity can change the effects of selection imposed by the environment.

Though this theoretical mechanism has come to be called the Baldwin effect, Baldwin himself called the effect "organic selection." He argued that the Lamarckian-like consequence could be produced if an acquired trait, such as a learned habit, could block the effects of natural selection. The ability to use the flexibility of developmental and learning processes to persist and reproduce in conditions that are not optimal preserves a lineage. This would protect the organism's lineage from being eliminated in the reproductive lottery. This "umbrella effect" would also thereby increase the probability that some members of the lineage would additionally acquire a fortuitous variation that would more efficiently accomplish that which behavioral flexibility previously accomplished. Over time, this would aid the accumulation of inherited variants that would lighten the load imposed by trial and error learning and enable fortuitous mutations to arise and replace the original acquired capacity. Baldwin called this process organic selection because it occurs at the organism level as a result of what an individual organism does during its lifetime. It is not something that is initially transmitted genetically and yet it can indirectly bias the direction of evolution, according to Baldwin, in such a direction as to lead it to become more genetically inherited.

About 50 years later, a developmental biologist, Conrad Waddington (1942), proposed a related process that he called "genetic assimilation." This process also appeared to produce an apparent path from environmentally acquired traits to congenitally generated traits. But in this case, it was not just a theoretical possibility. Waddington (1953) demonstrated by experiment that stress-induced trait-expression could eventually come to breed true. He showed that a trait that in one generation was only expressed under special atypical environmental conditions could become an ineluctably expressed trait independent of the environment, merely by selectively breeding for that environmentally induced trait. Waddington's experiments with fruit flies raised in atypical environments (e.g., unusually high temperatures) showed that traits initially expressed by some individuals only when in these special environments could nevertheless be selectively bred to become expressed under normal conditions. He argued that this involved a kind of coassortment effect in which multiple genetic contributors are collected together over generations by selectively breeding individuals with these environmental sensitivities, producing a synergistic epigenetic effect that independently parallels the environmental contribution. Recent, genetic analysis of this effect largely supports this combinatorial genetic–epigenetic explanation (e.g., Rutherford & Lindquist, 1998).

It is a common error to see these two theoretical mechanisms—organic selection and genetic assimilation—as variants of the same process (Deacon, 2003). But aside from the fact that only

Waddington's claims had direct empirical support, organic selection and genetic assimilation only share a superficial similarity. And neither actually provides even a pseudo-Lamarckian mechanism.

Crucial to both mechanisms is the fact that many expressed physical and behavioral traits may have no reproductive consequence for generations. For example, nose shape, chin shape, earlobe shape, and many other human physiognomic traits may be below the threshold of having a reproductive consequences and so are effectively neutral with respect to natural selection. Neutral traits can almost freely vary in form over the course of evolution until for some reason they rise above this threshold. Until this happens, however, their probability of expression also drifts randomly from individual to individual and generation to generation. With respect to the differential susceptibility of traits to selection, Waddington's and Baldwin's mechanisms are in fact inverses of each other. Waddington's mechanism assumes that certain previously neutral traits become newly subject to natural selection due to changing environmental conditions. In contrast, Baldwin's mechanism assumes that reducing selection due to behavioral or physiological flexibility can create "space" for better variants to emerge.

This difference has significant implications for the two mechanisms and what they are likely to produce over generations. The basis of Waddington's effect is an exposure (or "unmasking") of features that were previously hidden from selection, and he showed that this produces an organizing effect influencing who mates with whom by virtue of these unmasked traits. The basis of Baldwin's claimed effect is that learning and other types of environmentally responsive plasticity shield the organism from selection. This hides (or masks) many variations that were previously exposed to selection, with the result that less and less is selectively stabilized, more drift is possible, and thus more variation eventually shows up. This difference matters.

The first step in gaining perspective on these mechanisms is to abandon the Lamarckian framing of the issue. Rather than attempting to frame a Darwinian means to achieve a Lamarckian end, we can simply ask what Baldwin's mechanism would likely produce. Many problems with the Baldwin effect have been identified over the years but are often not generally acknowledged. For example, the phenotypic plasticity that the Baldwin effect depends upon will increase variability but will not necessarily favor selection for new adaptations to replace it. The very plasticity that favors an increase in variation will also mask (i.e., partially shield the organism from) the very forces of selection that would be necessary to shape up or stabilize any of the congenitally produced surrogates that by chance could have supplanted this acquired adaptation. This shielding would not only inhibit their evolution, it would likely also degrade any *existing* congenital analogues to the acquired adaptation due to a failure to eliminate mutations affecting it. So reduced selection is a double-edged sword.

In 1953 the evolutionary biologist George Gaylord Simpson wrote a critique of the Baldwin effect (in which the phrase "Baldwin effect" was coined) that pursued some of the implications of this problem. Simpson argued that indeed it did not violate the strictures of strict neo-Darwinian logic, but that it may be only trivially important in evolution because it can only occur in very special conditions. These constraints have been more rigorously explored by computer simulation studies (e.g., Yamauchi, 2004). First, it requires that there is a high cost–benefit ratio between the acquired and highly canalized alternatives of a trait. For example, if trial and error learning is associated with high error costs (e.g., likely getting eaten by predators), then an inherited stereotypic behavior that is easy to produce (e.g., a tendency to automatically hide when startled) and not particularly costly (e.g., does not impair exploration for food or mates) will tend to be favored. This can be viewed as merely two competing adaptations, though it puts considerable weight on the probability of such a coincidental mutation occurring. But even if such a coincidental variant were to arise, the cost-differential between the acquired and inherited trait would be self-limiting for selection. Because of the flexibility of an acquired trait, if a highly heritable variant came to coexist alongside it, the effect will be to reduce the costs of its acquisition, and so will reduce selection favoring it. The result is that evolution will stall somewhere in between.

A second condition that limits the Baldwin effect is more troublesome. For the replacement effect to work, there also has to be a high correlation between the acquired trait (also sometimes called a phenocopy, following Waddington) and the ineluctable highly canalized version. This is most likely when alleles of the same genes are involved in producing both the acquired and congenitally generated adaptations (a condition that is probably highly unlikely for complex traits). As a result, it is most likely in cases of simple genotype–phenotype correspondences and less likely where multigenic and epistatic factors are involved.

A third restrictive condition, related to the first, is that the presence of an acquired adaptation sufficient to preserve the lineage that expresses it, creates conditions that limit forces of selection that would be necessary to select among initially crude versions of an alternative congenitally produced adaptation to make it progressively more suited to its context. This is especially significant if the adaptation in question must be integrated with other functions or responsive to variable environmental conditions. Thus models of the Baldwin effect that postulate "hopeful monster" mutations (i.e., which produce a fully functional "innate" alternative phenotype) have shown the most promise, but make unrealistic epigenetic assumptions.

Despite these constraints on a Lamarckian outcome, however, traits becoming shielded from selection by virtue of acquired adaptations should be quite common. The Baldwinian mechanism is therefore important even if its predicted effects might not be what Baldwin envisioned (Deacon, 2003). Are some of these other consequences of the Baldwinian masking effect relevant to evolution? The answer is yes, and as I will argue below, they may be far more significant than Baldwin could have imagined. They just turn out to be, paradoxically, the reverse of what Baldwin claimed, and yet perhaps more important in evolution than Baldwin's predicted outcome.

Evolutionary Cycle of Duplication–Masking–Degeneration–Complementation

There is a parallel to the Baldwinian masking of the effects of selection in a well-studied genomic effect: gene duplication. Gene duplication is a common occurrence in the evolution of genomes (Ohno, 1970; Ohta, 1994; Van de Peer et al., 2001). It is probably the major source of new genes in the course of evolution. It is also a major means by which cooperative protein complexes arise in evolution (Orgel, 1977; Zhang, 2003). Thus, multiple occurrences of gene duplication over the course of evolution have produced large "families" of structurally and functionally related genes. Indeed, most genes can be recognized as members of larger families of genes sharing a common ancestral gene (Walsh, 1995; Zhang, 2003).

During gene duplication, a length of DNA is literally copied and spliced into the chromosome nearby, possibly as a result of uneven crossover events during meiotic replication, viral gene insertion and excision, or some other intrinsic or extrinsic mechanism that modifies gene replication. The result of such events is that a nucleotide sequence may be duplicated that contains intact regulatory and coding segments for production of a functional protein. The functional consequence is that there is now two ways of producing the same phenotypic effect. This redundancy can provide masking of selection on the duplicate gene's function, much as learning can mask selection on phenotypic adaptations in the case of the Baldwin effect. Thus if one of two duplicated genes acquires a mutation that alters its protein product in a way that modifies or degrades its function, this mutation would not necessarily impact the reproduction of the organism so long as the other copy remains intact. Moreover, the now mutated gene can continue to acquire mutational changes without negatively impacting organisms that inherit it, so long as this slightly modified phenotypic contribution is not somehow deleterious. Such mutations will thus be effectively or nearly neutral.

The typical consequence of this sort of neutrality with respect to selection can be described as a "random walk" away from the original function. The result is the accumulation of arbitrary sequence changes at the genetic level and a progressively degraded or dedifferentiated contribution to the phenotype. Presumably, persistent shielding from any selection effects will eventually lead to complete loss of function, as in pseudogenes that no longer produce any RNA transcripts. Accumulation of a very large number of mutations, or of mutations that stop the translation of its sequence information, can in this way ultimately produce complete loss of function. This has been the fate of a very large number of genes in the human genome, which were once associated with a more acute olfactory sense (e.g., Rouquier, 1998). It is estimated that a typical mammal has on the order of 1300 genes encoding distinct olfactory receptor molecules. This number was radically reduced both in primate and in human evolution. The human species has had roughly 60% of these genes degrade to become pseudogenes (Gilad et al., 2003). This clearly reflects very weak, to nearly nonexistent, selection to maintain the numbers and diversity of these receptor molecules.

But degradation to pseudogene status is not inevitable for gene duplicates. Precisely because gene duplication can involve an already functional segment of DNA, slight degradations of its sequence will only incrementally alter the structure of its coded protein. So long as the changes do not involve an essential binding site or some other critical structure, its functional links to other molecular components are also likely to degrade in noncatastrophic ways. This often means a progressive loss of specificity, with some functional associations being lost but other related interactions becoming possible that were previously prevented by the stabilizing selection that sustained the original function. In this sense, the progressive drift in genetic sequence is at the same time an exploration of the "phase space" of interactions "near" an original function. And whereas a single protein may require structural compromises to accommodate its multiple associations to others, multiple variant forms may provide a "have your cake and eat it too" option with each variant able to evolve greater specificity for one or another of these capacities. In other words, the duplication, masking, and random walk can provide a kind of exploration of the space of possible synergistic relationships that lie, in effect, in the "function space" just adjacent to an existing function. This is a recipe for increasing functional complexity (Lynch & Conery, 2003).

If the prevalence of gene duplication in animal and plant genomes is any indication, the probability that a given duplication will achieve functional integration is far from zero. Gene families, consisting of large numbers of paralogous genes (e.g., derived from a common ancestral gene), are widespread in complex organisms and are often responsible for similar or even synergistic phenotypic functions. One incidental advantage for genomic research has been that identification of a functional correlate of one genetic sequence often provides a probe sequence that can be used for searching out other members of its family that have related functions. To illustrate this, let me describe two well-known examples.

The first is the globin gene family, and specifically the hemoglobins. The hemoglobin protein complex contained in red blood cells comprises two varieties of the hemoglobin protein—alpha and beta hemoglobin—each coded by a distinct gene. The structure of the protein makes it possible to bind a special molecular formation within which an iron atom is suspended. It is this iron atom that provides the oxygen-binding capacity. Two alpha and two beta hemoglobin proteins fit together to form a tetrahedral complex made possible due to the complementary shapes of the molecular surfaces forming the interior of the tetramer. The two forms of hemoglobin arose from a gene duplication event, and the ancestral hemoglobin itself arose as one of two duplicates from the common ancestral gene for both hemoglobin and myoglobin. The alpha and beta hemoglobin duplicates each acquired independent changes in shape but only minimal changes in oxygen binding capacity in their separate divergent "degradation." Changes that increased the stability of tetrameric binding appear to have been favored by natural selection with respect to one another, probably because of the superior oxygen transport capacity of the tetrahedral form. In other words, in their random walks through different three-dimensional configurations, the duplicates retained their oxygen-binding function while effectively "sampling" functional consequences of this secondary feature of molecular shape.

This particular combination of alpha and beta hemoglobins is not, however, present at all stages of the mammalian life cycle. In the fetus of a placental mammal, additional variant beta-hemoglobin forms are expressed, three of which are termed gamma, delta, and epsilon hemoglobin. These variants are expressed at different stages of gestation, and are each coded by a different variant duplicate of the beta form of the gene, with the entire family present in a continuous segment of the chromosome. These beta-hemoglobin duplication events, which occurred during the course of placental mammal evolution, have also given rise to two pseudo–beta hemoglobin genes, which no longer produce a corresponding protein. In effect, these variants acquired mutations that inactivated gene translation in their random walk away from the original sequence. The remaining four beta-hemoglobin genes are expressed at slightly different times during development in the order epsilon-gamma-delta-beta. The functional value of this is related to the fetus's need to acquire oxygen from mother's hemoglobin and yet still transfer it from blood to somatic cells. So in order to be able to "steal" oxygen from maternal hemoglobin, fetal hemoglobin requires a slightly higher oxygen-binding affinity than mother's hemoglobin. It then must diffuse oxygen out of its own hemoglobin into its tissues, which ideally requires yet a higher oxygen-binding affinity than its own hemoglobin. Between these values there is an optimal balance, but this will change as the fetus grows larger in size and its oxygen needs change. The result is that the different beta-hemoglobin variants expressed during different phases of gestation each have a slightly different affinity for oxygen that allows the fetus to progressively adapt to this challenge, until at birth the beta-hemoglobin becomes the predominant form produced.

So in this case, analogous to the shape complementarities "discovered" consequent to alpha/beta duplication, these parallel random walks of beta-hemoglobin gene duplicates led to synergies of timing and molecular affinities, as certain variant mutations, which modified the different redundant genes' oxygen-binding properties, became subject to selection with respect to each other in the context of internal gestation.

Perhaps the most dramatic example of the duplication, masking, random walk, and functional complementation effect is demonstrated by duplication of genes that code for proteins that bind to DNA and regulate the expression of yet other genes. One consequence of this hierarchic recursive genetic relationship is that changes in one gene can influence a large number of other genes in concert. So the functional divergence and interaction effects that result from duplication of such regulatory genes can be global and systemic.

The classic example of regulatory gene duplication effects involves a family of genes containing a nucleotide sequence coding for a DNA binding domain called the homeodomain. A class of such genes called homeobox genes are responsible for the large scale segmental organization of animal body plans (independently discovered by McGinnis, Levine, Hafen, Kuroiwa, & Gehring, 1984; Scott & Weiner, 1984). In the fruit fly, they are called HOM genes and their homologues in mammals are called Hox genes (though there are a very large number of more distantly related regulatory genes as well). These underwent a number of duplications in the common ancestry, leading up to the separation of the arthropod and vertebrate lineages. Because these genes affect coordinated expression of large suites of other genes (many of which also have further regulatory functions), they play a role in producing slightly variant forms of whole body structures in these animals. This was first demonstrated by recognizing that mutations of these genes produce systematic variations of body segments in flies, causing out-of-place expression of structures that normally are segment-specific, such as legs expressed where antennae are normally produced. The discovery that the theme-and-variation logic of the different insect body segments was correlated with the expression of different HOM gene duplicates in that segment has revolutionized the study of development and served as the keystone insight solidifying the value of the evodevo paradigm.

But the fact that homeotic gene duplication expresses itself as organ duplication demonstrates that the logic of duplication, masking, divergence, and complementation is general. In arthropods such as centipedes the corresponding organs (e.g., legs) of adjacent segments are highly similar, but since adjacent legs serve almost identical functions they can also partially mask selection on the functional specificity of one another. This reduction of the effects of stabilizing selection can lead to drift of features on one segment away from those on another. The structural–functional redundancy provided by adjacent segments minimizes the probability of catastrophic loss of function, and also increases the likelihood that complementary functions might develop on other segments. In various arthropods, such as grasshoppers, spiders, lobsters, flies, and so forth, the different appendages with leg-like form have evolved into specialized antennae, spinnerets, claws, and many other structures sharing the same jointed architecture, but modified to serve quite distinct functions.[2]

In each of these cases, and despite their different levels of function, the redundancy of function that results from duplications significantly reduces the improbability of evolving synergistic functional linkages. Because they share a common ancestral function, randomly variant duplicated features of an organism potentially "explore" the diverse dimensions of the original function. Their underlying commonalities also increase the probability that variant duplicates will fractionate the original function, each assuming greater roles with on but not another aspect of the original, thereby increasing synergistic organization. By fractionating an originally unitary and poorly optimized adaptation, variant duplicates can also be independently expressed in response to critical variables, and thus provide greater flexibility of function with respect to uncertain environments.

This interplay between duplicated genetic epigenetic factors borrows features from both Baldwinian and Waddingtonian mechanisms, and yet it does not involve, even superficially, a Lamarckian logic. The way that duplication reduces the constraints of natural selection on a particular structure or function is analogous to the way acquired adaptations produce what Baldwin thought of as protection from selective elimination. But unlike Baldwin's hypothesized effect, this more often contributes to degradation of epigenetic constraint than the reverse. The way that the resulting functional interactions exploit combinatorial relationships that were previously hidden (or inaccessible because intense selection prevented variation) is analogous

to Waddington's logic of canalization, in which epigenetic interdependencies can emerge to become selected in their own right. Like Waddington's notion of a "phenocopy," a novel functional capacity that emerges from complementary combinatorial relationships can become selectively favored for the synergy that results. Together these effects not only "explore" adjacent functional possibilities and "capture" novel higher-order synergistic relationships, but they provide an evolutionary cycle that can generate progressively more complex forms of adaptation, as each stabilized synergistic relationship can supply the substrates for new duplication effects.

Extrinsic Factors and the Lazy Gene Hypothesis

But this interplay between Baldwinian and Waddingtonian mechanisms suggest an even more general application of this principle, which is particularly relevant to brain evolution. This is the possibility that redundancy and masking effects can be generated extrinsically, and maintained irrespective of specific genetic inheritance, by virtue of redistributing selection fractionally onto highly diverse, and previously independent, genetic loci and extragenomic mechanisms. A classic example that bridges between genetic and environmental duplication-masking effects is the evolution of ascorbic acid (vitamin C) dependency in anthropoid primates.

Monkeys and apes, including humans, are among some of the very few mammals that must obtain ascorbic acid from dietary sources (Chatterjee, 1973). Most mammals synthesize their own ascorbic acid. This is the case for rats. In 1994, a group of Japanese researchers (Nishikimi et al., 1994) sequenced the gene on chromosome 8 of the rat that codes for the final catalyst in the metabolic pathway that endogenously produces ascorbic acid (called l-gulano-lactone oxidase, abbreviated GULO). They then used the sequence from this gene to probe the genomes of other species. One of the first species they probed was *Homo sapiens*. What they found was surprising. Although humans are unable to synthesize their own ascorbic acid, the human genome includes a pseudogene that is homologous to the rat GULO. The GULO pseudogene in humans has accumulated considerable mutational damage, including the deletion of large coding regions (exons) and the random insertion of "stop" codons (see Figure 35.3A). This is evidence that it has long been freed from the stabilizing influence of natural selection, and that the sequence has effectively taken a random walk, resulting in complete loss of function. So what masked its functionality and allowed it to degrade to this extent?

Although phylogenetic analysis of the variants of the GULO pseudogene in other anthropoid primates is still incomplete, it is likely that all share a GULO pseudogene with divergent mutations. A reasonable estimate of the date in the evolution of primates when this gene began to accumulate damaging mutations is suggested by the comparative fossil evidence. Changes in eyes and teeth of fossil primates suggest that a shift to diurnal foraging and a shift from insectivory to frugivory took place roughly 35 million years ago in the lineage leading to anthropoids. The evolutionary implication is that at this point regular foraging on fruit introduced a semireliable extrinsic source of ascorbic acid into the diet. Under these conditions, there would be no selective disadvantage of inheriting or transmitting a nonfunctional variant of the GULO gene. Selection would be masked by an acquired behavioral adaptation and by the ascorbic acid rich niche that was thereby created. The eventual complete loss of function of the GULO gene would lead to the equivalent of an evolutionary addiction to foods providing ascorbic acid (depicted in Figure 35.3B).

This example of extrinsic ascorbic acid dependency provides us with an opportunity to look at some of the secondary consequences of this degradation. The masking of selection maintaining this enzyme in turn would have unmasked selection on a variety of other traits that help guarantee the availability of this now essential nutrient. Quite possibly, the evolution of three-color vision and various tooth and digestive adaptations were also related to this evolutionary addiction, as the need for extrinsic ascorbic acid would become a new selection pressure. In other words, the behavioral flexibility that initially allowed primates to regularly forage on fruit and led to the spontaneous degradation of the ascorbic acid synthesis pathway, eventually "addicted" anthropoid primates to a behavioral niche in which fruit acquisition and digestion were critical. This addiction would have unmasked selection on many diverse traits that coincidentally supported this "addiction," including, for example, the capacity to judge the ripeness of fruit, forage on the outer limbs of trees, find the sugar-rich and slightly acidic content of fruit attractive, and metabolize the sugars and tolerate the ethanol that ripe fruits contain. All of these could be considered part of an adaptive suite for guaranteeing the presence of ascorbic acid.

This process shares a number of features in common with the evolutionary process now generally

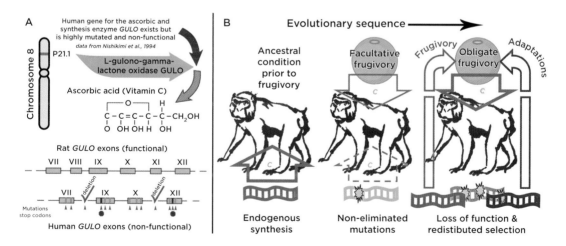

Figure 35.3 Degradation of endogenous ascorbic acid (vitamin C) production in primates due to relaxed selection caused by foraging on fruit. (A) Comparison of the GULO gene in rat and human. The rat gene produces a protein that catalyzes the final step in ascorbic acid synthesis. The human pseudogene for GULO has incorporated many deleterious mutations, including deletions of entire exons and the insertion of stop codons. (B) Schematic depiction of the stages in the evolution of primate dependence on environmental sources of ascorbic acid (e.g., via frugivory). In the third stage (far right) the GULO gene has become entirely nonfunctional and selection has shifted to any loci in the genome that produce phenotypic effects that help maintain reliable access to extrinsic ascorbic acid (e.g., digestive adaptations and 3-color vision; depicted in green and blue).

referred to as *niche construction* (Odling-Smee et al., 2003; see also West et al., 1988). One of the classic examples of niche construction is the production of beaver dams. Beaver dams produce an artificial aquatic environment. Beaver bodies currently exhibit adaptations to this aquatic niche as do a variety of beaver behavioral tendencies. So the artificial niche created by beaver behaviors has played a role in the evolution of many other beaver adaptations, in the same way that independent environmental features play a role in selectively favoring the preservation of other traits. This self-made environment introduces a sort of short circuit in the cause–effect cycle of natural selection. Beavers today are essentially unable to successfully reproduce unless they live in such a beaver-made niche.

The development of stone tool technology in our own evolutionary prehistory was a niche construction event with similarly ramifying consequences. For example, the use of stone tools in hominid ancestry appears to have mitigated the intense masticatory processing of vegetable foods that characterized the australopithecines. Within a half million years of the appearance of the first stone tools, there was a radical reduction in the large flat molars, thick enamel, robust face and jaw structure, and powerful jaw muscles of the australopithecines. As I will argue below, this initial step of niche construction was only the first of many niche construction innovations that radically altered the forces of natural selection affecting our ancestors and their cognitive traits. This artificial niche did not merely create new selection pressures, it also eliminated many others. As I will argue below, both effects are relevant to explaining the anomalous trajectory of human evolution.

To provide a mnemonic aphorism that characterizes the special evodevo logic that is implicit in all these examples, I call it the *Lazy Gene* hypothesis. The Lazy Gene hypothesis suggests that we should not assume genetic micromanagement of epigenetic processes, but rather only genetic regulation of the boundary conditions affecting processes that have the potential of arising by self-organization, self-assembly, or other extragenomic organizing processes.

This view shares some features in common with the perspective called developmental systems theory (e.g., see Oyama et al., 2001; and also Chapter 2), which argues that the inheritance of extragenomic factors is as important as genetic inheritance. One difference in emphasis, however, is that the lazy gene approach assumes that genetic information plays the primary role maintaining the conditions for inheritance, without which the various extragenomic influences would not be reliably available. In other words, there is an important sense in which genetic information is primarily responsible for inheritance even if it is not the sole or even the major source of the morphogenetic processes contributing to epigenesis. More importantly, the lazy gene approach attempts to explain how such extragenomic factors might evolve to become reliable epigenetic mechanisms in the first place, even though their ultimate origin might be extrinsic to the organism.

The most relevant (and also counterintuitive) extragenomic influences are those that arise from systemic effects, often involving what are often described as self-organizing processes, since these do not arise from specific structural or molecular effects, but rather from interaction dynamics. A classic example of a self-organized developmental process is the mathematically regular Fibonacci spirals observed in pinecones, sunflowers, celery stalks, and a myriad of other plants. This complex and highly regular pattern contributes to optimal spacing around a stalk and to scalable self-similar growth patterns over many orders of magnitude. However, its characteristic 3–5, 5–8, 8–13, 13–21, 21–33, … pattern of interlocking spirals is not explicitly coded in the genome. It is a self-organizing effect that emerges from cell–cell interactions in response to differential sensitivity to growth hormone expression. Only this hormonal response is passed from generation to generation by genetic inheritance. Indeed, many of the form-generating processes of embryogenesis involve the self-organizing consequences of recurrent cell–cell interactions and the spontaneous geometry of molecular diffusion processes. Like the duplication-masking effects at the genomic, phenotypic, and behavioral levels, such emergent organizing constraints will likewise promote degradation of redundant genomic influences and increasing dependency on and synergistic adaptation to these extrinsic factors.

The lazy gene hypothesis is an epigenetic parsimony principle. Epigenetic biases and constraints that are reliably present or that reliably emerge during development, due to adaptive flexibility or extragenomic influences, will tend to mask selection maintaining corresponding genetically inherited information. Thus the genome will tend to offload morphogenetic control, in the course of evolution, in a way that takes advantage of the emergent regularities that characterize many epigenetic processes. This does not mean, however, that we should treat genetic and epigenetic inheritance as simply parallel inheritance systems that are interchangeable, as is sometimes argued by proponents of developmental systems theory. Although gene expression depends upon epigenetic processes and epigenetic processes depend on conditions produced by genes, the genetic information is embodied in a structural artifact whereas epigenetic information is dynamical in origin and must emerge anew in each new developing organism. In this sense, the lazy gene argument recognizes that the ultimate source of genetic information is vested in self-organizing epigenetic interactions, but it also recognizes that because these effects are highly context sensitive, only an independent nonlabile nondynamical means for "remembering" these conditions from generation to generation (e.g., genetic information) is able to guarantee their reliable emergence in development. In this way, we avoid the greedy reductionism of the new synthesis gene-centered view but do not confuse the complementary roles of genetic and epigenetic inheritance.

On the one hand, this tendency to spontaneously offload morphogenetic control in evolution obviates the possibility that such emergent effects will ever be fully replaced by genetic prespecification, as Baldwin believed. On the other hand, it suggests a powerful non-Darwinian mechanism that may contribute to the evolution of complex functional synergies and to the emergence of highly distributed control of development. Because spontaneous self-organizing biases arise irrespective of natural selection, the two processes can complement one another. Natural selection captures and stabilizes the conditions for useful self-organizing processes, if they emerge, but stabilizing selection will tend to inhibit the expression of variant or alternative self-organizational tendencies. Without the selective elimination of most variants of the information embodied in the physical structure of genes, the fragile conditions conducive to self-organizing epigenetic effects would quickly be lost. But novel self-organizing effects can only emerge if these strictures periodically loosen.

Relaxed Selection and Brain Complexity: A Birdsong Example

With respect to brain evolution and development, a spontaneous tendency for genomes to offload epigenetic control to any and all reliably present organizing influences outside the genome has interesting implications. The brain, more than any other organ, is likely to be strongly coupled with extrinsic regularities in the world. Also, because of the brain's highly reentrant network architecture and activity-dependent modifiability, nervous system functions are likely to generate complex emergent higher-order regularities. Brain evolution should therefore be highly susceptible to lazy gene effects.

The effect of relaxed selection on brain organization and control of complex behavior is dramatically demonstrated by a recent series of studies comparing a wild finch, the White-Rump Munia, to a long domesticated breed of the same species, the Bengalese Finch (Okanoya, 2004). The Bengalese Finch has been bred for coloration in Japan for about 250 years, but not for singing. And yet, surprisingly, it appears that in the absence of breeding for singing, being shielded from natural and sexual selection has produced increased song complexity, greater involvement of social learning in song development, and more diverse neural control of singing behaviors, as compared to its wild cousin. Since it is generally believed that complexity of singing behavior in songbirds is a consequence of sexual selection for male display (Catchpole & Slater 1996; Darwin, 1871; Okanoya, 2002; Zahavi & Zahavi, 1997), this result appears paradoxical.

The song of the Bengalese Finch is complex and variable and exhibits what amounts to a form of song "syntax" (here understood only to refer to combinatorial reordering possibilities). The specific details of song structure, including specific song elements, and variants of song syntax are acquired by early social learning from adult singers. It learns its song shortly after hatching, as is typical of many songbirds. And like other songbird species that acquire their songs via social learning, the Bengalese Finch makes use of multiple brain areas for song acquisition and production. In contrast, its wild cousin has a simpler and much more stereotypic song, for which learning plays a relatively lesser role. This raises a troubling question: How could an increase in the complexity of both song structure and of neural systems for producing song have evolved in the absence of overt selection acting on these traits? More generally, it raises questions concerning the evolution of the wide range and phylogenetic distribution of species differences in the flexibility, the extent of social learning, and the recruitment of brain structures in singing behavior. It also may shed light on some surprising seemingly incidental effects of domestication (e.g., see Belyaev, 1979; Trut, 1999).

Whereas such an effect makes little sense for classical neo-Darwinian accounts, the lazy gene perspective developed here offers a plausible mechanism for the shift away from congenitally prespecified stereotypic song to socially acquired flexible singing behavior, in the absence of selection. I have argued that prolonged domestication masked selection that in the wild had maintained highly canalized control over song structure and production (Deacon, 2006). Relaxing these environmental pressures and undermining sexual selection effects led to spontaneous degradation of previously strong genetic constraints and opened the door to increased epigenetic variability and conditionality. This diminution of bottom-up constraints allowed a wider range of neural substrates and sensory experiences to influence singing behavior. But more importantly, I will argue that this relaxation-degradation effect and the upward shift of morphogenetic control that it produces, can under certain circumstances also lead to an increase in complexity of both brain and behavior.

The Bengalese Finch example provides a model of how this process might begin. Homologous nuclei and connections are present in both social learners of song and stereotypic singers, as well as in both males and females (though typically only males sing). The differences mostly involve the relative size of telencephalic nuclei, the level of their interconnectivity and the differential expression of molecular features (MacDougall-Shackleton & Ball, 1999; Tobari et al., 2006). So the potential substrates for complex learned song are present generally, but they serve other functions in birds that do not sing or do so stereotypically and probably did not play a role in complex vocal behavior in the common ancestor to songbirds and their other avian cousins (Jarvis, 2004).

As a consequence of having their mate choice determined by breeders on the basis of coloration patterns, and irrespective of singing, selection in this species was relaxed on all aspects of song production. In the absence of either sexual selection for the display characteristic of song, or selection with respect to species identification or predator avoidance, genetic influences constraining song production would tend to exhibit random drift. Any mutations degrading such genetically based constraints on song structure would no longer be selected against, so long as they did not otherwise impose costs on other essential systems. The result,

over time, would be a kind of focal degeneration of song-constraining genetic influences in the domesticated lineage. As with other cases of genetic drift, the expected consequence would be an increase in phenotypic variability (i.e., song variability) and a decrease in its autonomy from other related influences.

Analyzing the ethogram of the two breeds, Okanoya and colleagues observed evidence of increased song variability in the domesticated finch compared to the wild finch, but not merely an increase in variability. The songs can be analyzed into relatively discrete song elements, sometimes referred to as "notes." Transitions between characteristic notes have different probabilities characteristic of a particular song type or singer. The White-Rump Munia song is characterized by a limited and relatively invariant set of notes, as well as a very distinct distribution of transition probabilities between the different notes. In other words, most transitions are of either very high probability or very low probability (including many of near zero probability), resulting in highly predictable sequences of notes. Moreover, there are few if any loop-backs in this ethogram, which results in a very linear progression of notes from start to finish of a singing bout, and seldom any recurring note cycles. Different individuals within the species sing very similar versions of the same song. In contrast, the song ethogram of the Bengalese Finch includes both a larger repertoire of notes, many more nonzero transition probabilities between notes, and fewer very high probability transitions. This results in a far more complex ethogram, with many more transitions possible, including many possible loop-backs. Individuals thus sing a more varied song and the individual differences are also considerably greater.

The Bengalese Finch song variability is not, however, just randomly distributed. It is strongly affected by experience listening to model singers during development. Interestingly, there is also evidence of individuals who learn from two different adult singers who produce a hybrid song as an adult, borrowing from each of its models. And Bengalese Finches can also learn to sing the White-Rump Munia song, if raised hearing only that song. The reverse in not true. White-Rump Munia chicks do not appear to be influenced by what they hear, or whether they hear another Munia singing at all. Thus if cross-fostered with Bengalese Finch parents they nevertheless mature to sing the typical Munia song.

The effect of genetic drift on ethogram structure can be expected to decrease stereotypy in two respects. First, note structure should simplify and note specificity should become more variable both within and across individuals. Second, the specificity of the transition probabilities between notes should also be relaxed, causing probability differences to regress toward the mean, eventually making all transitions more equiprobable. Both effects are characteristic of the difference between Munia and Bengalese Finch song.

A recent computer simulation test of this hypothesis (Ritchie & Kirby, 2007) demonstrated that analogous relaxation of selection on "song" production of a population of algorithmic "agents" resulted in an analogous song complexification effect, as well as a serendipitous coupling between song structure and learning mechanism. These agents were initially selected so that "reproduction" of new agents from the prior generation was initially predicated on intense selection for song matching, and thus produced highly invariant songs. Increased complexity following relaxation of this restriction could be understood as merely increased variability, but the increased role of learning complicates this interpretation.

In a songbird species that does not learn its regional variant of the species' song, there are relatively few forebrain structures playing a critical role in song production. A motor nucleus located posteriorly in the forebrain called the robust nucleus of the archopallium (RA) plays the major role in production of song in songbirds (e.g., Nottebohm et al., 1976). Damage to it can severely simplify or even eliminate singing ability in most bird species. In species with highly stereotypic songs, however, damage to other forebrain nuclei generally has minimal detrimental effects on singing so long as it spares RA (except where it produces deafness prior to song development near maturity). This is not the case with species that acquire their regional song variant via social learning, and which have more variation in song style across individuals. In such species, numerous forebrain nuclei and interconnections also play supportive roles both in learning and in the production of songs. Included among these structures are auditory areas critical for "recording" the songs sung by nearby adult singers and for remembering the perceptual models against which to compare one's own singing. In addition, there are a handful of more anteriorly located forebrain neostriatal nuclei (e.g., area X, MAN, Nif) that play critical roles in learning to replicate the acquired song. Finally, a premotor structure, the caudal region of the hyperstriatum ventrale (Hvc)

plays a crucial role in both integrating these influences and contributing higher-order regulatory control over RA and thus critically important in song complexity and flexibility (see Figure 35.4).

The Bengalese Finch and White-Rump Munia fit on either end of this spectrum. Whereas Munia song is only disrupted by damage to the RA nucleus in the forebrain, Bengalese Finch song is drastically simplified by damage to Hvc, resulting in a highly stereotypic song. And song learning is significantly impaired by damage to auditory or rostral striatal regions of the forebrain.

While it is not difficult to imagine how domestication might produce increased behavioral variability, it is less obvious how the effects of drift could explain this increase in the complexity of neural control. Perhaps one reason that this seems counterintuitive is that we tend to think of increasing complexity as the addition of something. Thus the above difference could be described as adding each of these new structures to the song control system of the bird brain. However, this is misleading in two senses. First, these additional structures function in multiple contexts in every songbird brain, irrespective of the kind of song, and connections between them, some of which include RA, exist even in species where they play no role in singing. They are not specifically limited to "song circuits," but are to some extent specialized to each provide a distinct computational contribution to the learning, planning, motor coordination, perceptual memory, etc., involved in many different behaviors. Second (assuming that bird and mammal brains involve roughly analogous developmental processes) in the immature brain, there is likely to be less exclusive specificity of connectivity between these and other forebrain nuclei, which is only later reduced and/or limited in its influence. So we can also describe this effect of domestication as disinhibiting the influence of these connections and/or less effectively and less selectively culling the diversity of immature connections. Additionally, we might expect that the circuitry within RA of the domesticated finch is also less differentiated and thus less constraining of motor output. In other words, drift should allow a slight degeneration of the genetic specificity of certain features of brain development, and the result would not so much appear as loss of function, but rather degeneracy leading to reduction of constraint on factors controlling production.

In summary, reduced selection can be expected to produce progressive despecialization of the circuits that contribute tight constraints on motor

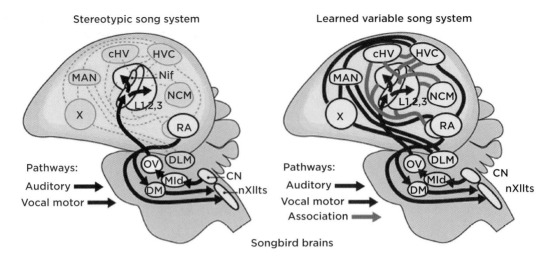

Figure 35.4 Comparison of the general organization of the songbird brain singing circuits in species/breeds with stereotypic songs that are minimally affected by social learning (left) and species/breeds with variable songs acquired via social learning (right). Red arrows indicate motor output circuits, blue arrows indicate auditory input circuits, and green arrows indicate association connections linking auditory, motor and higher-order motor learning systems. Birds with highly canalized stereotypic songs (like the Munia) have minimal forebrain involvement in song control, but birds that acquire their song socially (like the Bengalese Finch) utilize numerous forebrain nuclei and large numbers of association fiber tracts in the acquisition and production of their songs.

patterning that specify song structure. With this relaxation of inherited context independent biases, other previously inhibited or ineffectual influences, contributed by other brain systems—such as the trace of early auditory experience—could begin to play a larger role in biasing song formation. Both the weakening of constraints intrinsic to RA circuits and the possible mature persistence of significant immature projection patterns from other forebrain nuclei could thus contribute to a more distributed and thus multifaceted control of singing and song structure.

This pattern of redistributed control of function among brain systems is loosely analogous to the redistribution of the control over ascorbic maintenance that resulted from degradation of the GULO gene in primate evolution (described above), in the sense that degradation of this highly constrained mechanism opened the door to many other contributions from diverse and previously irrelevant mechanisms, such as specialized digestive and visual adaptations. However, in the case of the Bengalese Finch, there is no selection to shape up these more indirect influences. Their emergent roles in song production are merely incidental to their other functional and developmental features. Nevertheless, despite the nonfunctional and purely serendipitous changes in song control, and the fact that they are due entirely to degenerate genetic

influences and the associated despecialization of certain epigenetic processes, the result is appropriately described as an increase in complexity for the following reasons.

1. There is a considerable increase in the number of song variables able to be modified and an expansion of the range of extrinsic factors with respect to which these song features can be adjusted.

2. The resulting behavioral function is not merely more variable, it is also more conditionally responsive to contextual influences, including social influences.

3. The prior adaptive functions of the many neural systems that ultimately came to play a role in singing provided a large and previously untapped domain of functional overlap where new interrelationships contribute considerably increased structural complexity.

Of course, specificity of these prior functions and the constrained variation of song in the wild were adaptive. So the domesticated species' less precise and more flexible behaviors would likely not serve it well if released again into the same ancestral environment. In this respect, increased complexity is not necessarily an adaptive advantage, though increased flexibility might make Bengalese Finches better able to adapt to non-native environments.

Of course, singing behavior is only one of many systems that is likely to be dedifferentiated by domestication. Since domestication globally reduces selection on a large number of behavioral systems and physical capacities, it should be expected to lead to widespread patterns of dedifferentiation involving many nonessential systems, not just the genes and corresponding brain structures involved in song control. In the Bengalese Finch, these appear to extend to mate choice, nesting behavior, offspring care, and toleration of environmental disturbance, among other features (Okanoya, personal communication). Considering that the widespread genetic drift associated with long-term domestication is likely to be expressed developmentally as less differentiated adult features, it also should not surprise us that domestication tends to produce animals that appear superficially altricial in both behavioral and physiognomic characteristics (e.g., see Beylaev, 1979; Trut, 1999).

Neural Developmental Degeneracy and the Evolution of Language

The process of relaxing selection on neurobehavioral traits in domesticated birds, described above, provides a suggestive analogy for rethinking the evolution of a similarly complexified neurobehavioral trait in humans: language. It is almost universally assumed that the human language capacity evolved under the influence of intense selection favoring the evolution of supportive neural mechanisms. There are, however, serious difficulties in using the simple neo-Darwinian paradigm to explain some of the more enigmatic features of this uniquely human adaptation. First there are the many functional discontinuities with respect to other species' vocal and behavioral communication systems. Second, there is the unprecedented complexity of language and the apparent miracle of rapid language acquisition in infancy. And third, there is the extensive synergy of diverse brain systems involved in the comprehension and production of language. These curious attributes have frustrated attempts to move beyond highly generic claims about selection for "increased neural complexity" or appeals to "big bang" lucky mutations that simply posit the introduction of these unprecedented faculties. But reflecting on these challenges in the context of the "lazy gene" hypothesis provides many striking parallels. Although it seems undeniable that many aspects of the language adaptation have been honed by natural selection, there are many other aspects involving individual and cultural variability, flexibility

of form and expression, complexity of behavioral output, dependence on social learning, and highly distributed synergistic neurological organization, that are reminiscent of the relaxed selection effects described above for Bengalese Finch singing.

The most obvious place to start to explore these parallels is to ask whether there are aspects of the human language adaptation that are similar to the reorganization of song control in the Bengalese Finch. Potential examples might include the following features of language and its correlates.

First, there appears to have been significant loss, simplification, and cooption of many species typical stereotypic calls, which are characteristic of the communication of our close relatives the chimpanzees. With the exception of laughter, sobbing, and shrieks of fright, we inherit a very limited repertoire of this sort of prespecified vocalizations specialized for distinct social messages or objects in our environment. Since stereotypic calls are neither produced by prelinguistic infants nor in cases of global aphasia, it is unlikely that they are merely suppressed or superseded by language use. More likely their neural substrates have been subject to degeneration, perhaps analogous to the degeneration of song stereotypy in the Bengalese Finch.

There has also been an analogous degeneration of the vocalization transition biases that are typical of calls (e.g., as is still present in the stereotypic "ha-ha-ha" of laughter), allowing spoken language to take advantage of the ability to combine almost any oral–vocal articulations that are mechanically possible for the production of words and sentences.

There has been a corresponding decoupling of the correlations between particular vocalizations and arousal states that are also be characteristic of stereotypic calls. So except for the few preserved human calls, there is effectively a completely arbitrary link between any specific vocalization and emotional state.

What might be termed "evolutionary disinhibition" is dramatically exemplified by a related human-unique behavior: infant babbling (see also Chapter 34 for a somewhat different view). In the context of other species' vocal predispositions, infant babbling can be compared to a neurological disinhibition effect. A young child begins to babble in low arousal contexts, when stereotypic calls like crying are unlikely, and prior to its use for communication. The organization of babbled "syllables" is largely unconstrained except perhaps by mechanical limitations, though later it tends to show mimicry of the tonal characteristic of the surrounding speakers' language.

Finally, some features characteristic of other species' call mechanisms seem to be incorporated into speech, but in quite a different way. Speech prosody seems to coopt many of these call arousal correlations, subordinated to the articulation of speech phonemes. The prosody of speech appears to have borrowed many of the tonal and rhythmic features that are associated with specific emotional states in ways analogous to these features in the calls of other species. So in human speech, we communicate our emotional tone, our interest, and our attention to things we consider important using generic vocal changes that are more universal than any sound-meaning couplings in language. So not only has there been partial degeneracy of this call system but, again analogous to the new conditionality of vocalization in the Bengalese Finch example, this has enabled two independent mechanisms to work in concert.

Not only does language require vocal flexibility and decoupling of specific vocalizations from specific cognitive-emotional states, but it also requires coupling with auditory analysis and memory and with motor skill learning systems. The functional linkage of these otherwise largely autonomous neural subsystems in the evolution of the human brain is also paralleled by the effects of relaxed selection on the brain systems controlling song in the Bengalese Finch. The neuroanatomical contrast between song-learners' brains and stereotypic singers among songbirds is, in many respects,

strikingly analogous (perhaps even in the evolutionary sense) to the neuroanatomical differences in the substrates for stereotypic calls and language (see Figure 34.5).

A generation of using lesion and stimulation techniques to study call production systems in primate brains has mapped out an elaborate limbic-midbrain system, in which distinct basal and midline forebrain structures and pathways associated with specific drives and arousal states are also centers from which electrical stimulation can induce the production of stereotypic calls typically associated with those states. Cerebral cortical sites associated with call production are limited almost exclusively to the anterior midline, in perilimbic regions such as the anterior cingulate cortex (Jürgens, 1979). Motor and premotor cortex appears uninvolved (Jürgens et al., 1982). In general, these forebrain sites are few, overlapping, and highly interconnected. In contrast, language is significantly dependent on cerebral cortical systems that are widely separated between frontal motor and premotor, temporal auditory, parietal multisensory, and prefrontal executive systems, as well as with striatal and thalamic structures to which each of these cortical regions are linked (Deacon, 1997). Even the cerebellum appears to play a role in cognitive aspects of language processing. Thus language is characterized by a largely independent and quite widely distributed network of forebrain systems, which in other species do not share this kind of close synergistic contribution to a single cognitive-behavioral function.

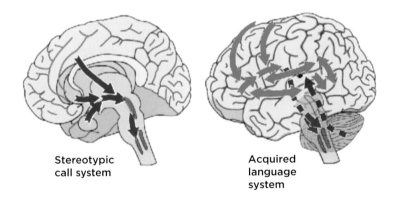

Stereotypic call system

Acquired language system

Figure 35.5 Comparison of the general organization of neural circuits controlling stereotypic species typical calls (e.g., laughing, sobbing) and language in humans. Analogous to the Munia-Bengalese finch comparison, the difference shows minimal forebrain involvement (e.g., few cortical areas are involved in stereotypic call production), but highly distributed forebrain (especially cortical) involvement in language processes. The depiction of language circuits is extremely simplified and only show major cortico-cortical pathways involved in language processing, and also does not depict the numerous cortico-subcortical connections that are also implicated in various aspects of language processing. Color coding as in Figure 35.4.

Of course, one of the most significant features of language, also paralleled by the Bengalese Finch example, is its critical dependence on social transmission. The level of this social influence of the local speech environment on human neurological function is unparalleled in any other species. Although we take this for granted, it is hard to overemphasize the extent to which the developmental neurology of language has become dependent on the social transmission of information. Some degree of genetic and epigenetic control of brain development relevant to language has likely been "offloaded" to this extrinsic source of information. Like the addiction to ascorbic acid, this has almost certainly had a secondary reorganizing effect on many other systems, which now serve to help stabilize and maintain this extrinsic epigenetic information source. It is perhaps the most extreme development of the trend in large brained species to rely on extrinsically driven activity-dependent shaping of neural circuits to complete neural circuit specification.

Unlike the Bengalese Finch example, however, the story of human brain and language evolution is not merely one of relaxed selection. Relaxed selection may have played an important role in allowing complex functional synergies to emerge, both among brain systems now contributing to language and between these brain systems and socially transmitted information. But once these capacities became available and the reproductive advantages of symbolically transmitted knowledge and social organization became reliable there would certainly have been selection favoring not only the stabilization of this unprecedented neural synergy but for optimizing its functionality (Deacon, 1997). So while we may be able to attribute many features of this unprecedented capacity to relaxation of selection and the complexity afforded by degeneracy of previously more autonomously specialized systems, we need to also consider how this may have unmasked selection on other neurological features.

Conclusions

This analysis has suggested that certain critical human language adaptations may be consequences of the evolutionary degradation of genetic and neurological substrates due to the removal of selective pressures. This appears to be the opposite of the view of most students of human mental evolution who hold that our special propensity for language can be understood as an "adaptation," honed by natural selection. What I have loosely called the lazy gene effect is merely an amplification of the

evodevo paradigm for integrating the formative influences contributed by epigenetic mechanisms with those that can be ascribed to natural selection. It can be seen as the exception that proves the rule that natural selection and epigenetic processes both contribute to the form that adaptations can take. Specifically, the reduction of natural selection is shown to release what might be described as "latent" potentials implicit in the epigenetic mechanisms that translate genetic information into phenotypic consequences. These mechanisms should be quite general, applying to many cases of the evolution of complex functional synergies at all levels of scale. The interplay between the genetically degenerate effects of relaxed selection, which can expose novel epigenetic synergies, and the sculpting effects of selection, which can preserve useful emergent consequences, provide complementary mechanisms contributing to the evolution of functional complexity. The role of relaxed selection may be particularly relevant to the evolution of nervous system complexity because of the potential for brain development to entrain many levels of morphological biases, including those imposed from environmental and social sources.

The neurological specializations for language that aid in its transmission, acquisition, and use exhibit many features that may be better understood in these non-Darwinian terms. The advantage of considering this possibility is that it refocuses attention on the multitude of processes involved in neural development that can potentially provide sources of information contributing to language organization, and the particular processes by which language competence is acquired. From this vantage point, many converging factors appear likely to have played a formative role in the emergence of this unique social-cognitive-biological phenomenon. By turning our attention away from the search for hypothetical selection pressures favoring the evolution of language, to the exploration of epigenetic mechanisms that were modified and coopted for this novel function, we can avoid many of the pitfalls of inventing evolutionary scenarios to explain the many complex idiosyncrasies of language. More importantly, it opens up a whole new domain of experimental inquiry into what was once considered terra incognita.

For linguists, the lazy gene approach to language adaptation suggests some quite counterintuitive hypotheses. Languages are vast systems of socially transmitted and maintained behavioral algorithms. In this respect, there is an enormous capacity for masking effects. To whatever extent that intrinsic semiotic constraints, neural processing limitations, and social transmission effects might contribute emergent self-organizing and selection effects which structure language, we should expect them to impede the evolution of corresponding innate language universals. This will be a difficult view for theorists who have argued that innate grammatical biases could have arisen due to the Baldwin effect (e.g., Pinker, 1994), because as we have seen the reverse effect is more likely. However, as highly canalized adaptations for social communication become increasingly degraded in the context of socially transmitted language, the increasing dependence on social transmission will "unmask" selection on any mental capacities that enhance social transmission. This will have the effect of redistributing selection to diverse genetic loci and extrinsic factors, in much the same way as happened with the loss of ascorbic acid synthesis capacity. The inevitable diversity, indirectness, and combinatorial synergies of such acquisition and transmission biases will make this a far more complex explanation of language universals than simply postulating an innate language faculty. But lacking a clear mechanism for its evolution, and now recognizing the plausibility of a mechanism that would tend to degrade such a genetic endowment even if it had been present in our ancestry, innate universal grammar cannot claim the status of being a parsimonious biological explanation. Additionally, there are many features of language that make better sense in the context of a highly distributed control of language genesis, such as its remarkable robustness despite its unprecedented complexity and flexibility, and the rarity of specific inherited language impairments.

Finally, for paleontologists and anthropologists, this analysis brings our attention to one final question about our genome and our brains in general. Are we genetically augmented apes with numerous genetic and neural improvements that make us better than our cousins? Or is it more parsimonious to recognize that many of these presumed "adaptations" are better understood as consequences of degenerative processes due to a reduction of selection pressures? Almost certainly, the unique combination of traits that support our language capacities and our social dependence are a consequence of both kinds of influences.

We are in many ways a self-domesticated species. Would it be too humbling to see ourselves as a somewhat genetically degenerate, neurologically dedifferentiated ape? Reframing humanness in biologically degenerate terms is not, as we have seen, to deny that we are in many respects more complex, both neurologically and behaviorally than other ape species. Moreover, the dedifferentiating effects of domestication may explain certain other enigmatic features of human nature, such as our cultural variability and even our fascination with art and music.

Perhaps our great leap forward required first taking a few steps back.

References

Alberch, P. (1989). The logic of monsters: Evidence for internal constraint in development and evolution. *Geobios, 19*, 21–57.

Balaban, E. (1997). Changes in multiple brain regions underlie species differences in a complex, congenital behavior. *Proceedings of National Academy of Science USA, 94*, 2001–2006.

Baldwin, J. M. (1896). A new factor in evolution. *American Naturalist, 30*, 441–451, 536–533.

Beylaev, D. K. (1979). Destabilizing selection as a factor in domestication. *Journal of Heredity, 70*, 301–308.

Butler, A. B., & Hodos, W. (1996). *Comparative vertebrate neuroanatomy*. New York: Wiley-Liss.

Carroll, S. B. (2000). Endless forms: the evolution of gene regulation and morphological diversity. *Cell, 101*, 577–580.

Catchpole, C. K., & Slater, P. J. B. (1996). *Bird song: Biological themes and variations*. Cambridge: Cambridge University Press.

Chatterjee, I. B. (1973). Evolution and the biosynthesis of ascorbic acid. *Science, 182*, 1271–1272.

Cowan, W. M., Fawcett, J. W., O'Leary, D. D. M., & Stanfield, B. B. (1984). Regressive events in neurogenesis. *Science, 255*, 1258–1265.

Darwin, C. (1871). *The descent of man and selection in relation to sex*. London: John Murray.

Deacon, T. (1990). Rethinking mammalian brain evolution. *American Zoologist, 30*, 629–705.

Deacon, T. (1997). *The symbolic species: the coevolution of language and the brain*. New York: W. W. Norton & Co.

Deacon, T. (2003). Multilevel selection in a complex adaptive system: the problem of language origins. In B. Weber & D. Depew (Eds.), *Evolution and learning: The Baldwin effect reconsidered* (pp. 81–106). Cambridge, MA: MIT Press.

Deacon, T. (2006). Evolution of language systems in the human brain. In J. Kaas (Ed.), *Evolution of Nervous Systems. Vol. 5, The Evolution of Primate Nervous Systems*. London: Elsevier Press.

Finlay, B. L., & Darlington, R. B. (1995). Linked regularities in the development and evolution of mammalian brains. *Science 268*, 1578–1584.

Finlay, B. L., Wikler, K. C., & Sengelaub, D. R. (1987). Regressive events in brain development and scenarios for vertebrate brain evolution. *Brain Behavior and Evolution, 30*, 102–117.

Frost, D. O. (1981). Orderly anomalous retinal projections to the medial geniculate, ventrobasal and lateral posterior nuclei of the hamster. *The Journal of Comparative Neurology, 203*, 227–256.

Gerhart J., & Kirschner, M. (1997). *Cells, embryos, and evolution: Toward a cellular and developmental understanding of phenotypic variation and evolutionary adaptability.* Malden: Blackwell Science.

Gilad Y., Man O., Pääbo S., & Lancet D. (2003). Human specific loss of olfactory receptor genes. *Proceedings of the National Academy of Sciences USA, 100,* 3324–3327.

Gilbert, S. F. (1997). *Developmental biology.* Sunderland: Sinauer.

Gilbert, S. F. (2000). Diachronic biology meets evo-devo: C. H. Waddington's approach to evolutionary developmental biology. *American Zoologist, 40,* 729–737.

Gilbert, S. F. (2000). Genes classical and genes developmental: The different uses of genes in evolutionary theory. In P. Buerton, R. Falk, & H.-J. Rheinberger (Eds.), *The concept of the gene in development evolution* (pp. 178–192). New York: Cambridge University Press.

Gilbert, S. F. (2003). The morphogenesis of evolutionary developmental biology. *International Journal of Developmental Biology, 47,* 467–477.

Gould, S. J. (1975). Allometry in primates, with emphasis on scaling and the evolution of the brain. In Szalay (Ed.), *Approaches to primate paleobiology.* Basel: Karger.

Holliday, M., & Hamburger, V. (1976). Reduction of naturally occurring motoneuron loss by enlargement of the periphery. *The Journal of Comparative Neurology, 170*: 311–320.

Holloway, R. (1979). Brain size, allometry, and reorganization: Toward a synthesis. In M. Hahn, C. Jensen, & B. Dudek (Eds.), *Development and evolution of brain size.* New York: Academic Press.

Isacson, O., & Deacon, T. (1996). Specific axon guidance factors persist in the adult brain as demonstrated by pig neuroblasts transplanted to the rat. *Neuroscience 75,* 827–837

Jarvis, E. (2004). Learned birdsong and the neurobiology of human language. *Proceedings of the National Academy of Sciences, 1016,* 749–777.

Jerison, H. J. (1973). *Evolution of the brain and intelligence.* New York: Academic Press.

Jürgens, U. (1979). Neural control of vocalization in non-human primates. In H. D. Steklis & M. J. Raleigh (Eds.), *Neurobiology of social communication in primates.* New York: Academic Press.

Jürgens, U., Kirzinger, A., & von Cramon, D. (1982). The effects of deep-reaching lesions in the cortical face area on phonation. A combined case report and experimental monkey study. *Cortex, 18,* 125–139.

Katz, M. J. (1982). Ontogenetic mechanisms: The middle ground of evolution. In J. T. Bonner (Ed.), *Evolution and development* (pp. 207–212). Berlin: Springer Verlag.

Katz, M. J., Lasek, R. J., & Kaiserman-Abramof, I. R. (1981). Ontophyletics of the nervous system: eyeless mutants illustrate how ontogenetic buffer mechanisms channel evolution. *Proceedings of National Academy of Sciences USA, 78,* 397–401.

Karten, H. J. (1969). The organization of the avian telencephalon and some speculations on the phylogeny of the amniote telencephalon. *Annals of New York Academy of Sciences, 167,* 164–179.

Killackey, H. P. (1990). Neocortical expansion: an attempt toward relating phylogeny and ontogeny. *Journal of Cognitive Neuroscience, 2,* 1–17.

Krubitzer, L. (1995). The organization of neocortex in mammals: are species differences really so different? *Trends in Neuroscience, 18,* 408–417.

Krubitzer. L., & Kaas, J. (2005). The evolution of the neocortex in mammals: how is phenotypic diversity generated? *Current Opinions in Neurobiology, 15,* 444–453.

Lamarck, J. B. (1809/1914). *Zoological philosophy.* London: Macmillan.

Li, W. H. (1983). Evolution of duplicate genes and pseudogenes. In M. Nei & R. Koehn (Eds.), *Evolution of genes and proteins* (pp. 14–37). Sunderland, MA: Sinauer.

Lumsden, A., & Krumlauf, R. (1996). Patterning the vertebrate neuroaxis. *Science, 274,* 1109–1114.

Lynch, M., & Conery, J. S. (2003). The origin of genome complexity. *Science, 302,* 1401–1404.

MacDougall-Shackleton, S. A., & Ball, G. F. (1999). Comparative studies of sex differences in the song-control system of songbirds. *Trends in Neuroscience, 22,* 432–436.

Mallamaci, A., & Stoykova, A. (2006). Gene networks controlling early cerebral cortex arealization. *European Journal of Neuroscience, 23,* 847–856.

Maynard Smith, J. (1987). When learning guides evolution. *Nature, 329,* 761–762.

McGinnis, W., Levine, M. S., Hafen, E., Kuroiwa, A., & Gehring, W. J. (1984). A conserved DNA sequence in homoeotic genes of the Drosophila Antennapedia and bithorax complexes. *Nature, 308,* 428–433.

Morgan, C. L. (1896). On modification and variation. *Science, 4,* 733–740.

Nishikimi, M., Fukuyama, R., Minoshima, S., Shimizu, N., & Yagi. K. (1994). Cloning and chromosomal mapping of the human nonfunctional gene for L-gulono-gamma-lactone oxidase, the enzyme for L-ascorbic acid biosynthesis missing in man. *Journal of Biological Chemistry, 269,* 13685–13688.

Nottebohm, F., Stokes, T. M., & Leonard, C. M. (1976). Central control of song in the canary, *Serinus canarius. The Journal of Comparative Neurology, 165,* 457–486.

Odling-Smee, F. J., Laland, K. N., & Feldman, M. W. (2003). *Niche construction: The neglected process in evolution.* Princeton, NJ: Princeton University Press.

Ohno, S. (1970). *Evolution by gene duplication.* Berlin: Springer.

Ohta, T. (1994). Further examples of evolution by gene duplication revealed through DNA sequence comparisons. *Genetics, 138,* 1331–1337.

Ohta, Y., & Nishikimi, M. (1999). Random nucleotide substitutions in primate nonfunctional gene for l-gulono-gamma-lactone oxidase, the missing enzyme in l-ascorbic acid biosynthesis. *Biochimica Biophysica Acta, 1472,* 408–411.

Okanoya, K. (2002). Sexual display as a syntactic vehicle: The evolution of syntax in birdsong and human language through sexual selection. In A. Wray (Ed.), *The transition to language.* Oxford: Oxford University Press.

Okanoya, K. (2004). The Bengalese Finch: A window on the behavioral neurobiology of birdsong syntax. *Annals of the New York Academy of Sciences, 1016,* 724–735.

O'Leary, D. D. M. (1989). Do cortical areas emerge from a protocortex? *Trends in Neuroscience, 12,* 400–406.

O'Leary, D. D. M. (1992). Development of connectional diversity and specificity in the mammalian brain by the pruning of collateral projections. *Current Opinions in Neurobiology, 2,* 70–77.

O'Leary, D. D. M., & Nakagawa, Y. (2002). Patterning centers, regulatory genes and extrinsic mechanisms controlling arealization of the neocortex. *Current Opinion in Neurobiology, 12,* 14–25.

Oppenheim, R. W. (1981). Neuronal cell death and some related regressive phenomena during neurogenesis: a selective historical review and progress report. In W. M. Cowan (Ed.), *Studies in developmental neurobiology: Essays in honor of Victor Hamburger* (pp. 74–133). New York: Oxford University Press.

Orgel, L. E. (1977). Gene duplication and the origin of proteins with novel functions. *Journal of Theoretical Biology, 67*, 773.

Osborn, H. F. (1896). Ontogenic and phylogenic variation. *Science, 4*, 786–789.

Oyama, S., Griffiths, P. E., & Gray, R. D. (Eds.). (2001). *Cycles of contingency: Developmental systems and evolution.* Cambridge, MA: MIT Press.

Provine, R. (2000). *Laughter: A scientific investigation.* New York: Viking.

Purves, D. (1988). *Body and brain: A trophic theory of neural connections.* Cambridge, MA: Harvard University Press.

Purves, D., & Lichtman, J. W. (1980). Elimination of synapses in the developing nervous system. *Science, 210*, 153–157.

Raff, R. A. (1996). *The shape of life: Genes, development, and the evolution of animal form.* Chicago: Chicago University Press.

Rakic, P. (1988). Specification of cerebral cortical areas. *Science, 241*, 170–176.

Ritchie, G., & Kirby, S. (2007). A possible role for selective masking in the evolution of complex, learned communication systems. In Lyon, C., Nehaniv, C., & Cangelosi, A. (Eds.), *Emergence of communication and language* (pp. 387–402). Berlin: Springer Verlag.

Rouquier, S., Taviaux, S., Trask, B., Brand-Arpon, V., van den Engh, G., Demaille, J., et al. (1998). Distribution of olfactory receptor genes in the human genome. *Nature Genetics, 18*, 243–250.

Rubenstein, J. R., Martinez, S., Shimamura, K., & Puelles, L. (1994). The embryonic vertebrate forebrain: The prosomeric model. *Science, 266*, 578–580.

Rutherford, S. L., & Lindquist, S. (1998). Hsp90 as a capacitor for morphological evolution. *Nature, 396*, 336–342.

Sacher, G. A. (1970). Allometric and factorial analysis of brain structure in insectivores and primates. In C. R. Noback & W. Montagna (Eds.), *The primate brain* (pp. 245–287). New York: Appleton-Century-Crofts.

Scott, M. P., & Weiner, A. J. (1984). Structural relationships among genes that control development: sequence homology between the Antennapedia, Ultrabithorax, and fushi tarazu loci of Drosophila. *Proceedings of the National Academy of Sciences, USA, 81*, 4115–4119.

Simpson, G. C. (1953). The Baldwin effect. *Evolution 7*: 110–117.

Stanfield, B. B., & O'Leary, D. D. M. (1985). Fetal occipital cortical neurons transplanted to the rostral cortex can extend and maintain a pyramidal tract axon. *Nature, 313*, 135–137.

Stanfield, B. B., Nahin, B. R., & O'Leary, D. D. M. (1987). A transient postmamillary component of the rat fornix during development: Implications for interspecific differences

in mature axonal projections. *Journal of Neuroscience, 7*, 3350–3361.

Stephan H. H., Frahm B., & Baron G. (1981). New and revised data on volumes of brain structures in insectivores and primates. *Folia Primatologia* (Basel), *35*, 1–29.

Striedter, G. F. (1997). The telencephalon of tetrapods in evolution. *Brain Behavioral Evolution, 49*, 179–213.

Striedter, G. F. (2005). *Principles of brain evolution.* Sunderland, MA: Sinauer.

Sur, M., Garraghty, P. E., & Roe, A. W. (1988). Experimentally induced visual projections into auditory thalamus and cortex. *Science, 242*, 1437–1441.

Tobari, Y., Okumura, T., Tani, J., & Okanoya, K. (2006). Non-singing female Bengalese Finches (*Lonchura striata var. domestica*) possess neuronal projections connecting a song learning region to a song motor region. *Ornithological Science, 5*, 47–55.

Trut, L. M. (1999). Early canid domestication: the farm-fox experiment. *American Scientist, 87*, 160–168.

Van de Peer, Y., Taylor, J. S., Braasch, I., & Meyer, A. (2001). The ghost of selection past: rates of evolution and functional divergence of anciently duplicated genes. *Journal of Molecular Evolution, 53*, 436–446.

Waddington, C. H. (1942). Canalization of development and the inheritance of acquired characters. *Nature, 150*, 563–565.

Waddington, C. H. (1953). Genetic assimilation of an acquired character. *Evolution, 7*, 118–126.

Walsh, J. B. (1995). How often do duplicated genes evolve new functions? *Genetics, 139*, 421–428.

West, M. J., King, A. P., & Arberg, A. A. (1988). The inheritance of niches: The role of ecological legacies in ontogeny. In E. M. Blass (Ed.), *Handbook of behavioral neurobiology* (Vol. 9, pp. 41–62). New York: Plenum Press.

Wilczynski, W. (1984). Central neural systems subserving a homoplasous periphery. *American Zoologist, 24*, 755–763.

Yamauchi, H. (2004). *Baldwinian accounts of language evolution.* PhD Thesis, University of Edinburgh.

Zahavi, A., & Zahavi, A. (1997). *The handicap principle.* Princeton: Princeton University Press.

Zhang, J. (2003). Evolution by gene duplication: An update. *Trends in Ecology and Evolution, 18*, 292–298.

Notes

1 Selection can be understood as a constraint or bias on the variance of a trait over time. "Relaxation" refers to reduction of that constraining influence, and will tend to allow "drift" within a wider domain of variance. Complete relaxation of selection is no constraint, or so-called "neutral" selection.

2 In most vertebrates there has been yet an additional duplication effect involving the entire linked family of Hox genes. The entire cluster appears to have undergone two duplications, and each resulting Hox gene cluster has subsequently undergone modification with a number of whole gene deletion and duplication effects distinguishing each cluster. This has produced a more cryptic segmental organization of the body plan in vertebrates in contrast to arthropods. But still the theme-and-variation logic is visible in parallels between limbs and their digits, vertebrae, ribs, teeth, and many other segmental features.

INDEX

Note: Page numbers in *italics* denote figures and tables.